Renal and Electrolyte Disorders

D1581828

Renal and Electrolyte Disorders

FIFTH EDITION

EDITED BY
ROBERT W. SCHRIER, M.D.
Professor and Chairman, Department of Medicine, University of Colorado
Health Sciences Center, Denver

Lippincott - Raven
PUBLISHERS

Philadelphia • New York

Acquisitions Editor: Vickie Thaw
Manufacturing Manager: Dennis Teston
Production Services: Colophon
Cover Designer: Patricia Read Barry
Indexer: Michael Loo
Compositor: Maryland Composition
Printer: Maple Press

Fifth Edition
Previous editions © 1976, 1980, 1986, and 1992 by Little, Brown and Company, Inc.

Printed in the United States of America
9 8 7 6 5 4 3 2

Library of Congress Cataloging-in-Publication Data

Renal and electrolyte disorders / edited by Robert W. Schrier.—5th
ed.
    p.   cm.
  Includes bibliographical references and index.
  ISBN 0-316-77454-5
  1. Kidneys—Diseases. 2. Water-electrolyte imbalances.
I. Schrier, Robert W.
  [DNLM: 1. Kidney Diseases—physiopathology. 2. Water-Electrolyte
Imbalance—physiopathology.   WJ 300 R391 1997]
RC903.R47 1997
616.6′ 1—dc21
DNLM/DLC
for Library of Congress   97-5943
                                      CIP

To Barbara
and
David, Debbie, Doug, Derek, and Denise

Contents

Contributing Authors

William T. Abraham, M.D.
Assistant Professor, Division of Cardiology, University of Colorado Health Sciences Center, Denver

Allen C. Alfrey, M.D.
Professor of Medicine, University of Colorado School of Medicine; Chief, Division of Nephrology and Hypertension, Department of Veterans Affairs Medical Center, Denver

Ahmed M. Alkhunaizi, M.D.
Division of Renal Diseases and Hypertension, Department of Medicine, University of Oregon School of Medicine, Portland

Tomas Berl, M.D.
Professor of Medicine, University of Colorado School of Medicine; Head, Division of Nephrology and Hypertension, University of Colorado Health Sciences Center, Denver

Verena A. Briner, M.D.
P.D. Doctor, Chairman of Department of Medicine, Kantonsspital, Luzern, Switzerland

Laurence Chan, M.D., Ph.D., F.R.C.P.
Associate Professor of Medicine, University of Colorado School of Medicine; Director, Transplant Nephrology, Division of Renal Diseases and Hypertension, University of Colorado Health Sciences Center, Denver

Arlene B. Chapman, M.D.
Associate Professor, Division of Renal Diseases and Hypertension, University of Colorado School of Medicine, Denver

John D. Conger, M.D.
Professor, Department of Medicine, University of Colorado School of Medicine; Chief of Staff, Denver Veterans Affairs Medical Center, Denver

Paul R. Conlin, M.D.
Assistant Professor of Medicine, Harvard Medical School; Assistant Physician, Endocrine-Hypertension Division, Department of Medicine, Brigham and Women's Hospital, Boston

Robert G. Dluhy, M.D.
Associate Professor of Medicine, Harvard Medical School; Associate Physician, Endocrine-Hypertension Division, Department of Medicine, Brigham and Women's Hospital, Boston

Charles L. Edelstein, M.D.
Instructor, Renal Medicine, Division of Renal Diseases and Hypertension, Department of
Medicine, University of Colorado School of Medicine, Denver

Richard J. Glassock, M.D.
Professor and Chair, Department of Medicine, University of Kentucky College of
Medicine; Kentucky Clinic, Lexington

William D. Kaehny, M.D.
Professor of Medicine, University of Colorado School of Medicine; Associate Chief,
Medical Service, Veterans Affairs Medical Center, Denver

George A. Kaysen, M.D.
Professor of Medicine, Division of Nephrology, University of California, Davis, School of
Medicine, Davis; Chief, Division of Nephrology, UC Davis Medical Center, Sacramento

Saulo Klahr, M.D.
Simon Professor, Department of Medicine, Washington University School of Medicine;
Physician-in-Chief, The Jewish Hospital of St. Louis, St. Louis

James P. Knochel, M.D.
Professor, Department of Internal Medicine, University of Texas Southwestern Medical
School; Chairman, Department of Internal Medicine, Presbyterian Hospital, Dallas

Rajiv Kumar, M.B.B.S.
Professor of Medicine, Biochemistry, and Molecular Biology, and Chair, Division of
Nephrology, Mayo Medical School, Rochester, Minnesota

Moshe Levi, M.D.
Associate Professor of Internal Medicine, University of Texas Southwestern Medical
Center; Chief, Nephrology Section, Dallas Veterans Administration Medical Center,
Dallas

Charles R. Nolan, M.D.
Associate Professor, Department of Medicine, University of Colorado Health Sciences
Center, Denver

Linda N. Peterson, Ph.D.
Professor, Departments of Physiology and Paediatrics, University of Ottawa, Ottawa,
Ontario, Canada

Mordecai M. Popovtzer, M.D.
Professor of Medicine, Hebrew University-Hadassah Medical School; Chief of Nephrology
and Hypertension Services and Director, The Jerusalem Osteoporosis Center, Hadassah
University Hospital, Jerusalem, Israel

Robert W. Schrier, M.D.
Professor and Chairman, Department of Medicine, University of Colorado Health
Sciences Center, Denver

Joseph I. Shapiro, M.D.
Assistant Professor of Medicine, Chief, Nephrology Division, Medical College of Ohio, Toledo

Gordon H. Williams, M.D.
Professor of Medicine, Harvard Medical School; Chief, Endocrine-Hypertension Division, Department of Medicine, Brigham and Women's Hospital, Boston

Muhammad M. Yaqoob, M.D.
Department of Renal Medicine and Transplantation, Royal London Hospital, London

Preface

The fifth edition of *Renal and Electrolyte Disorders* has been an exciting challenge to edit because of the many advances that have occurred in the various areas of renal pathophysiology over the past four years. We are in a revolutionary era of biomedical science. Since the kidney is responsible for maintaining the *milieu intérieur* in health and disease, it is very difficult for any physician to practice state-of-the-art medicine without an up-to-date knowledge of renal physiology and pathophysiology.

For over twenty years, virtually thousands of medical students, house officers, and fellows have been introduced to the intricacies of renal physiology and pathophysiology by reading and studying *Renal and Electrolyte Disorders*. This is both a remarkable tradition and a demanding responsibility to which a brilliant group of authors have responded in the fifth edition of *Renal and Electrolyte Disorders*.

The recent developments in sodium and water metabolism have been very exciting. These findings have elucidated on the mechanisms involved in body fluid volume regulation in edematous disorders—particularly cardiac failure and cirrhosis—as well as in pregnancy. The vasopressin receptor has been cloned, as have several water channels including the collecting duct water channel, which responds to vasopressin. This has delineated the defects in nephrogenic diabetes insipidus, as well as the role of nonosmotic release of vasopressin in edematous disorders. Now there are nonpeptide, orally active vasopressin antagonists that will become clinically available as "aquaretics," i.e., drugs that increase solute-free water excretion and thus treat hyponaturemic disorders such as the syndrome of inappropriate antidiuretic hormone secretion (SIADH), cirrhosis, and cardiac failure.

In addition to the role of angiotensin-converting enzyme (ACE) inhibitors, there are now inhibitors of the angiotensin II receptor that are clinically available. Gordon H. Williams and his colleagues bring several decades of knowledge and experience to the field of the renin-angiotensin-aldosterone system. The same is true of Linda N. Peterson, who has been joined by Moshe Levi in writing the chapter on potassium metabolism. Few can teach acid-base metabolism at the level of William D. Kaehny, and Joseph I. Shapiro has added substance to the arguments about the role of sodium bicarbonate in the treatment of metabolic acidosis.

Three world-renowned clinician-scientists, Mordecai M. Popovtzer, James P. Knochel, and Rajiv Kumar, provide the most up-to-date information on calcium, phosphorus, vitamin D, and parathyroid hormone activity. Charles R. Nolan, a premier clinician-educator, discusses the pivotal role of the kidney in the pathogenesis of hypertensive states, and Arlene B. Chapman updates the knowledge about renal disease and hypertension during pregnancy.

There is an explosion of knowledge regarding the mechanisms of renal vascular and epithelial injury during ischemia, which is discussed relative to the pathophysiology of acute renal failure. Allen C. Alfrey has been a pioneer in all aspects of chronic renal failure for three decades. His insights form the basis of the chapter on chronic renal failure. Saulo Klahr and his colleagues have been primarily responsible for advancing the study of the pathophysiology of obstructive nephropathy. George A. Kaysen has been a major contributor to our understanding of proteinuric states, particularly the nephrotic syndrome. Last, Richard J. Glassock writes expertly about the glomerulopathies, an area in which he is an internationally known expert.

Thus, taken together, we are very fortunate to have these distinguished authors contribute to the fifth edition of *Renal and Electrolyte Disorders*. I also thank Shirley Artese for her excellent editorial support.

R.W.S.

Renal and Electrolyte Disorders

Disorders of Water Metabolism

Tomas Berl and Robert W. Schrier

Historical and Evolutionary Aspects of Renal Concentrating and Diluting Processes

In *From Fish to Philosopher*, Homer Smith [1] suggested that the concentrating capacity of the mammalian kidney may have played an important role in the evolution of various biologic species, including *Homo sapiens*. He suggested that the earliest protovertebrates resided in a saltwater environment that had a composition similar to their own extracellular fluid (ECF). These species could therefore ingest freely from the surrounding sea without greatly disturbing the composition of their own *milieu interieur*. However, when these early vertebrates migrated into freshwater streams, the evolution of a relatively water-impermeable integument was mandatory to avoid fatal dilution from their hyposmotic, freshwater environment. Thus a vascular tuft, which we now call the glomerulus, developed, enabling the fish to filter the excess fluid from their blood.

The proximal tubule, which reabsorbed isotonic fluid, evolved in response to the need for salt preservation. However, this did not allow the excretion of hypotonic urine, which is mandatory for organisms ingesting hypotonic fluid from their freshwater environment. This need was met by the development of the distal tubule, which could dilute urine. In this portion of the nephron, salt was reabsorbed without water, since the distal tubular epithelium was relatively impermeable to water. The fish could then excrete the excess solute-free water they had obtained from their freshwater environment without concomitantly losing their body salts.

Several million years later, vertebrates began to reside on dry land. In this terrestrial environment, the problem of salt conservation persisted, but the excretion of large volumes of fluid was no longer necessary; paradoxically, conservation of fluid was of primary importance in the new arid environment. The kidneys of reptiles, birds, and mammals, however, had glomeruli, which filtered large amounts of fluid and salt, even though excretion of only minute amounts of these substances was needed to maintain daily balance. In reptiles and birds, the kidneys responded to this challenge by a decrease in the number of capillary loops in their glomerular tufts. In some fish, such as the sea horse and pipefish, which may have been the first vertebrates to return to the sea, aglomerular kidneys actually evolved. Tubular secretory systems also evolved in the nephron to allow elimination of nitrogenous wastes without the need for extremely large filtered volumes of fluid. Lastly, a relatively insoluble nitrogenous end product, uric acid, was produced and could be excreted in supersaturated solutions with a minimal amount of water loss.

In mammals, however, the high-pressure glomerular filters were maintained, but a system developed for concentrating urine, namely, the countercurrent mechanism. Mammals, along with birds, are unique among vertebrates in possessing loops of Henle and in their ability to compensate for water deficits by elaborating a urine more concentrated than blood.

Countercurrent Concentrating Mechanism

By analogy with heat exchangers, in 1942 the functional significance of the loops of Henle was proposed when Dr. Kuhn and Dr. Ryffel of the physical chemistry department at the University of Basel, Switzerland, originated the concept of the countercurrent multiplier system for urine concentration [2]. The hypothesis states that a small difference in osmotic concentration (single effect, or *einzeln Effekt*) at any point between fluid flowing in opposite directions in two parallel tubes connected in hairpin manner can be multiplied many times along the length of the tubes. The countercurrent multiplier system is illustrated in Figure 1-1 for a 200-mOsm gradient. In the kidney, such a gradient would result in a high osmolar concentration difference between the corticomedullary junction and the hairpin loop at the tip of the papilla. Since then, numerous experiments have confirmed the operation of a countercurrent multiplier in the kidney, with the thick ascending limb of Henle as the water impermeated site of active solute reabsorption [3].

Basic Determinants of the Concentrating and Diluting Process in the Kidney

We shall briefly discuss some of the factors that affect the concentrating and diluting processes in the mammalian kidney [4] before we proceed to the clinical disorders of water metabolism. Several aspects of the countercurrent mechanism are depicted in Figure 1-2. It is important to emphasize that many of these events are the same whether the final excreted urine is hypotonic or hypertonic to plasma.

Glomerular Filtration Rate and Proximal Tubular Reabsorption

The rates of glomerular filtration and proximal tubular reabsorption are important primarily in determining the rate of sodium and water delivery to the more distal portions of the nephron, where the renal concentrating and diluting mechanisms are operative. Since fluid reabsorption in the proximal tubule is isosmotic, owing to the water permeability of tubular epithelium, tubular fluid is neither concentrated nor diluted in the proximal portion of the nephron. Rather, after approximately 70

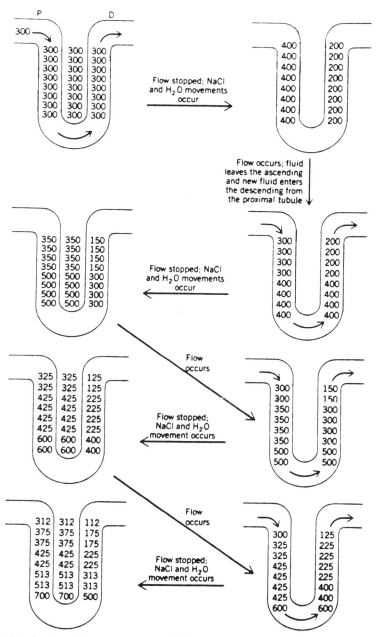

Fig. 1-1. Mechanism of countercurrent multiplication. See text for details. (From A. Vander, *Renal Physiology*. New York: McGraw-Hill, 1980. P. 84.)

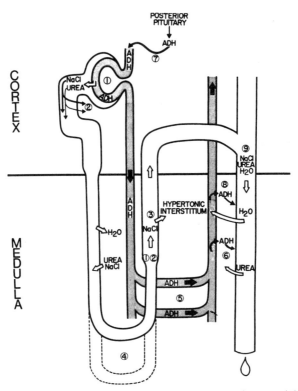

Fig. 1-2. Potential determinants of the renal concentrating mechanism. (1) Glomerular filtration rate as a determinant of fluid and solute delivery to the ascending limb of the loop of Henle. (2) Proximal tubular reabsorption as a determinant of fluid and solute delivery to the ascending limb of the loop of Henle. (3) Sodium chloride and potassium cotransport in the water-impermeable ascending limb. (4) Length and integrity of the long loops of Henle in the inner medulla and papilla. (5) Rate of medullary blood flow in the vasa recta. (6) Urea availability. (7) Presence of antidiuretic hormone (ADH). (8) Response of the cortical and medullary collecting ducts to ADH. (9) Rate of solute and water delivery as a determinant of the completeness of osmotic equilibration with the interstitium.

percent of glomerular filtrate is reabsorbed in the proximal tubules, the remaining 30 percent of fluid entering the loop of Henle is still isotonic to plasma. A decrease in glomerular filtration rate (GFR) or an increase in proximal tubular reabsorption, or both, may diminish the amount of fluid delivered to the distal nephron and thus limit the renal capacity to excrete water. Similarly, a diminished GFR and increased proximal tubular reabsorption may limit the delivery of sodium chloride to the ascending limb, where the tubular transport of these ions without water initiates the formation of the hypertonic medullary interstitium. With diminished delivery of sodium chloride to the ascending limb, the resultant lowering of medullary hypertonicity will impair maximal renal concentrating capacity by limiting the osmotic gradient for water movement from the collecting duct.

Descending and Ascending Limbs of the Loops of Henle, Distal Tubule, and Collecting Ducts

Since the urine that emerges from the proximal tubule is isosmotic, the first nephron segment actually involved in urinary concentration is the descending limb of Henle's loop. There are two types of descending limbs (Fig. 1-3). The short loops originate in superficial and midcortical glomeruli and turn in the outer medulla. The long loops originate in deep cortical and juxtamedullary glomeruli and penetrate variable

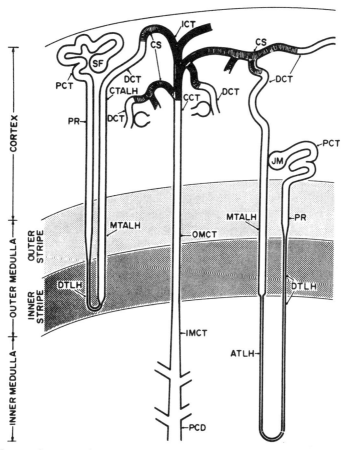

Fig. 1-3. Two nephron populations, superficial (SF) and juxtamedullary (JM), are depicted. The major nephron segments are labeled as follows: PCT = proximal convoluted tubule; PR = pars recta; DTLH = descending thin limb of Henle; ATLH = ascending thin limb of Henle; MTALH = medullary thick ascending limb of Henle; CTALH = cortical thick ascending limb of Henle; DCT = distal convoluted tubule; CS = connecting segment; CCT = cortical collecting tubule; OMCT = outer medullary collecting tubule; IMCT = inner medullary collecting tubule; PCD = papillary collecting duct. (From H. R. Jacobson, Functional segmentation of the mammalian nephron. *Am. J. Physiol.* 241:F203, 1981.)

distances into the inner medulla. Short and long descending limbs are anatomically distinct, and the long limbs in particular display considerable interspecies variability [5, 6]. It is of interest that no correlation is apparent between a species' maximal concentrating ability and the ratio of short and long loops. In fact, in rodents with highest urinary concentrations, the number of short loops is considerably greater than the number of long loops. In the human kidney, approximately 15 percent of nephrons possess long loops, and the other 85 percent of nephrons have short loops. The descending thin limb is devoid of vasopressin*-sensitive adenylate cyclase in all species [7, 8]. This nephron segment is very water permeable in most species but is also solute permeable in some species [9].

Somewhat proximal to the hairpin turn, there is a transition from the descending limb to the ascending thin limb of Henle's loop [7]. Although its functional significance is not known, vasopressin-sensitive adenylate cyclase has been demonstrated in the thin ascending limb of the rabbit and rat but remains untested in the mouse and humans [8]. As is the remainder of the ascending limb, this segment is water impermeable. Whether the movement of solute out of this segment is passive or active remains controversial [9]. Active sodium transport has not been convincingly demonstrated, and this segment's morphologic appearance with few mitochondria does not suggest active metabolic work.

The thick ascending limb of Henle's loop appears both structurally and functionally distinct from its thin counterpart [7]. The epithelium is remarkably uniform among species with tall, heavily interdigitating cells with large mitochondria. Despite interspecies morphologic homogeneity, the pattern of vasopressin-responsive adenylate cyclase has shown considerable variability. This effect of vasopressin to stimulate adenylate cyclase is strongly present in the mouse and rat, modestly present in the rabbit, and absent in humans. The observation that fluid emerges into the early distal tubule hypotonic (about 100 mOsm/kg H_2O) supports the view that active sodium chloride transport out of this water-impermeable segment provides the single effect required for the operation of the countercurrent multiplier. The primary mechanism of chloride absorption in the thick ascending limb is mediated by an electroneutral sodium, potassium, and chloride ($Na^+ : K^+ : 2Cl^-$) cotransport [10]. The possibility that vasopressin is involved in the control of sodium chloride reabsorption in this nephron has been suggested from studies in experimental animals [11, 12].

The distal convoluted tubule is the segment between the macula densa and the collecting ducts. This is a morphologically heterogeneous segment [6] with no biochemical responsiveness to vasopressin in the rabbit, mouse, and humans [8] and no water permeability in either the presence or the absence of the hormone. The collecting ducts are formed in the cortex by the confluence of several distal tubules. They descend through the cortex and outer medullary individually, but on entering the inner medulla, they successively fuse together. In humans, a terminal inner medullary collecting duct draws from as many as 7800 nephrons. The collecting tubules possess vasopressin-sensitive adenylate cyclase in all species studied [8], and

---

* Since vasopressin is the primary antidiuretic hormone (ADH) in humans, the terms *ADH* and *vasopressin* are used interchangeably in this chapter.

they are virtually impermeable to water in the absence of the hormone. The inner medulla itself consists of two functionally and morphologically distinct segments with different urea permeabilities [13].

Kokko and Rector [14] have proposed a model of urinary concentration that is in concert with (1) the anatomic features described above, (2) the permeability characteristics of the various segments of the system, and (3) in particular, limiting the active transport of solute to the thick portion of the ascending limb of Henle in the outer medulla. As depicted in Figure 1-4, the components of the mechanism are as follows:

1. The water-impermeable thick ascending limb of Henle's loop actively cotransports sodium, chloride, and potassium, thereby increasing the tonicity of the surrounding interstitium and delivering hypotonic fluid to the distal tubule. Urea is poorly reabsorbed and therefore retained in the tubule.

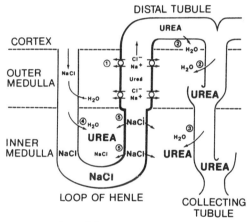

Fig. 1-4. Schematic representation of the passive urinary concentrating mechanism. Both the thin ascending limb in the inner medulla and the thick ascending limb in the outer medulla, as well as the first part of the distal tubule, are impermeable to water, as indicated by the thickened lining. In the thick ascending limb, active sodium, chloride, and potassium cotransport (1) renders the tubule fluid dilute and the outer medullary interstitium hyperosmotic. In the last part of the distal tubule and in the collecting tubule in the cortex and outer medulla, water is reabsorbed down its osmotic gradient (2), increasing the concentration of urea that remains behind. In the inner medulla, both water and urea are reabsorbed from the collecting duct (3). Some urea reenters the loop of Henle (not shown). This medullary recycling of urea, in addition to trapping of urea by countercurrent exchange in the vasa recta (not shown), causes urea to accumulate in large quantities in the medullary interstitium (indicated by UREA), where it osmotically extracts water from the descending limb (4) and thereby concentrates sodium chloride in descending-limb fluid. When the fluid rich in sodium chloride enters the sodium chloride–permeable (but water-impermeable) thin ascending limb, sodium chloride moves passively down its concentration gradient (5), rendering the tubule fluid relatively hyposmotic to the surrounding interstitium. (From R. L. Jamison and R. H. Maffly, The urinary concentrating mechanism. *N. Engl. J. Med.* 295:1059, 1976. Reprinted by permission.)

2. Under the influence of vasopressin in the distal tubule (in the rat) and in the cortical and outer medullary collecting ducts (in most species), tubular fluid equilibrates with the isotonic and hypertonic interstitium, respectively. Low urea permeability in this portion of the nephron allows its concentration to increase.

3. The inner medullary collecting duct is more permeable to urea. Therefore, in this segment of nephron, in addition to water reabsorption, urea is also reabsorbed as it diffuses passively along its concentration gradient into the interstitium, where it constitutes a significant component of the medullary interstitial tonicity.

4. The resulting increase in interstitial tonicity creates the osmotic gradient that abstracts water from a highly water-permeable and solute-impermeable descending limb of Henle's loop. This process elevates the concentration of sodium chloride in the tubular fluid. When tubular fluid arrives at the bend of the loop, its tonicity is the same as that of the surrounding interstitium. However, the sodium chloride concentration of the tubular fluid is higher and the urea concentration lower than of the interstitium.

5. Tubular fluid then enters the thin ascending limb, which is more permeable to sodium than urea. The sodium gradient provides for passive removal of sodium chloride from this segment into the interstitium.

To prevent urea removal from the inner medulla to the cortex, the ascending and descending vasa recta act as a countercurrent exchanger and "trap" urea in the inner medulla. The ascending vasa recta may also deposit urea into adjacent descending thin limbs of a short loop of Henle, thereby recycling it to the inner medullary collecting tubule. As shown in Figure 1-3, the descending limbs of short loops do not enter the inner medulla; thus the addition of urea to these loops does not interfere with the removal of water from the descending thin limb in the inner medulla, a step that is so crucial to the concentrating process.

This model of urinary concentration is very attractive [9], and many of its aspects have been experimentally supported [3]. Thus, in most species, particularly in the rabbit, the water permeability of the thin descending limb is very high [3, 15]. In contrast, the thick ascending limb has very low osmotic water permeability, high permeability to sodium, and lower permeability to urea [16]. With the low urea permeability of the thick ascending limb and cortical collecting ducts [17], urea is concentrated as it enters the inner medullary collecting duct. The initial portion of this segment has low urea permeability, while the terminal segment is highly permeable in the presence of vasopressin [18]. This allows for urea reabsorption at the terminal inner medullary collecting duct and its recycling into the anatomically adjacent thin ascending limbs [19]. Since this urea entry could rapidly dissipate the sodium gradient needed for passive sodium reabsorption, a model has been proposed in which the passive system operates only at the very tip of the loop, but the loop of Henle turns at multiple levels within the inner medulla [20].

It should be recalled that the single effect in the ascending limb of Henle serves also to dilute the urine. In the absence of ADH, and thus with water impermeability of the collecting ducts, the continued reabsorption of solute in the remainder of the distal nephron results in a maximally dilute urine (50 mOsm/kg). It thus should be apparent that impairment of sodium, chloride, and potassium cotransport in the ascending limb of the loop of Henle will limit the renal capacity both to concentrate and to dilute the urine.

Medullary Blood Flow

Medullary blood flow, whose rate can be regulated independently of whole kidney blood flow, may also affect the renal capacity both to concentrate and to dilute the urine, since the preservation of the medullary hypertonicity in the interstitium is dependent on the countercurrent exchange mechanism in the vasa recta [21]. Although medullary blood flow constitutes only 5 to 10 percent of total renal blood flow, this flow is still several times more rapid than the tubular flow. As previously noted, the vasa recta serve as a countercurrent exchanger that permits the preservation of interstitial tonicity. Blood that enters the descending vasa recta becomes increasingly concentrated as water diffuses out of and solutes diffuse into this portion of the nephron. The hairpin configuration of the vasa recta, however, does not allow the solute-rich blood to leave the medulla. In the ascending portion of the vasa recta, water diffuses into the vasa recta and solute moves out, thus maintaining interstitial hypertonicity. Even with an intact countercurrent exchange system in the vasa recta, circumstances that increase medullary blood flow may "wash out" the medullary concentration gradient and thereby diminish renal concentrating capacity. Moreover, even in the absence of ADH, the collecting duct is not completely water impermeable; therefore, a further decrease in the hypertonic medullary interstitium during an increase in medullary blood flow may decrease the ADH-independent osmotic water movement from the collecting duct and thereby increase water excretion. It is of interest that medullary blood flow increases in response to a decrease in vasopressin, presumably by diminished activation of V_1 receptors [22]. However, the role of vasopressin on the renal circulation in the process of the renal concentrating mechanism is probably limited, since V_1 antagonists do not impair urinary concentration [22].

Distal Solute Load

The rate of solute delivery to the collecting duct is a known determinant of renal concentrating capacity [23]. As shown in Figure 1-5, in spite of maximal levels of ADH, urinary osmolality in normal humans progressively diminishes as solute excretion increases. At high rates of solute excretion, urinary osmolality may reach isotonicity in humans even though supraphysiologic doses of ADH are infused [24]. With the infusion of submaximal doses of ADH in patients with pituitary diabetes insipidus, an increase in solute excretion may even be associated with hypotonic urine [23]. Hypotonic urine resistant to ADH also has been observed both in the dog [25] and in the monkey [26] during a solute diuresis and administration of large doses of vasopressin.

At least two factors may be responsible for this effect of solute excretion on renal concentrating capacity. First, a solute diuresis generally is associated with an increase in medullary blood flow, which could lower the medullary solute concentration profile. Second, the rapid rate of tubular flow through the medullary collecting duct could shorten contact time sufficiently so that complete osmotic equilibrium of fluid would not be allowed between the collecting duct and medullary interstitium,

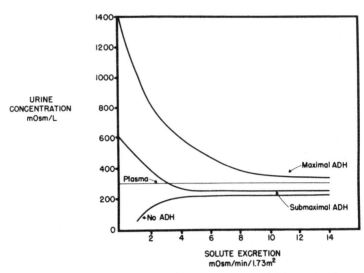

Fig. 1-5. Effect of solute excretion on renal concentration and diluting mechanisms. The submaximal response to ADH may be due to the presence of submaximal amounts of ADH or the diminished response of the collecting duct to maximal amounts of ADH. (From H. E. de Wardener and F. del Greco, Influence of solute excretion rate on production of hypotonic urine in man. *Clin. Sci.* 14:715, 1955.)

even though ADH had made the collecting duct membrane maximally permeable to water.

Antidiuretic Hormone

Arginine vasopressin (AVP), a cyclic hexapeptide (mol wt 1099) with a tail of three amino acids, is the ADH in humans (Fig. 1-6). In the final analysis, the renal concentrating and diluting processes are ultimately dependent on the presence or absence, respectively, of ADH to modulate collecting duct water permeability [27]. The presence of a basic amino acid (arginine or lysine) in the middle of the intact hormone at position 8 is crucial for antidiuresis, as is the asparagine at position 5. AVP is synthesized in the supraoptic and paraventricular magnocellular nuclei in the hypothalamus. In these nuclei, a biologically inactive macromolecule is cleaved into the smaller, biologically active AVP. Both oxytocin and AVP are encoded in

Arginine-vasopressin

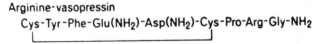

Fig. 1-6. Structure of the human antidiuretic hormone, arginine vasopressin (AVP). (Modified from R. W. Schrier and P. D. Miller, Water Metabolism in Diabetes Insipidus and the Syndrome of Inappropriate Antidiuretic Hormone Secretion. In N. A. Kurtzman and M. Martinez-Maldonado [eds.], *Pathophysiology of the Kidney*. Springfield, Ill.: Thomas, 1977. Courtesy of Charles C Thomas, Publisher.)

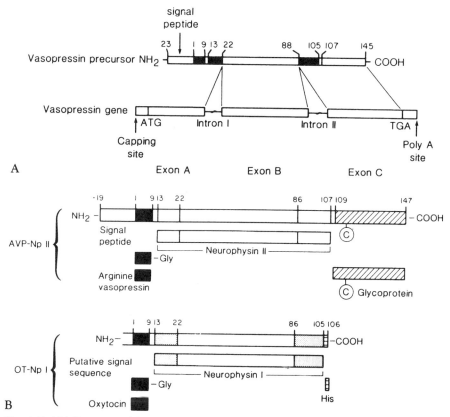

Fig. 1-7. (A) Structure of the gene that codes for the synthesis of proprevasopressin. (B) The structure of the biosynthetic peptide precursors of arginine vasopressin (prepro-vasopressin) and oxytocin (pro-oxyphysin). (From G. L. Robertson and T. Berl, Pathophysiology of Water Metabolism. In B. M. Brenner and F. C. Rector, Jr. [eds.], *The Kidney* [4th ed.]. Philadelphia: Saunders, 1991.)

human chromosome 20 in close proximity to each other [28]. The preprohormone gene is approximately 2000 base pairs in length and comprises three exons [29] (Fig. 1-7). Following a signal peptide, AVP is encoded in the first exon. Although spanning all three exons, the binding protein neurophysin is primarily encoded in exon B, and the glycoprotein in exon C. The promoter has cis-acting elements including a glucocorticoid response element, a cyclic adenosine monophosphate response element, and four AP-2 binding sites [30]. It is of interest that the Brattleboro rat, a strain with an autosomal recessive defect that causes AVP deficiency, is afflicted by a single base deletion in exon B [31]. This leads to a shift in the reading frame, with loss of the translational stop code. Although transcribed and translated in the hypothalamus, the translational product is neither transported nor processed in these mutant rats. After translation, the precursor prehormone, called propressophysin, is cleaved by removal of the signal peptide. Vasopressin, with its

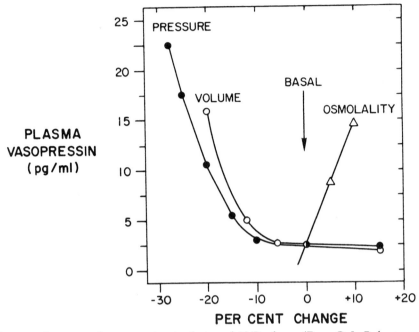

Fig. 1-8. Osmotic and nonosmotic stimulation of AVP release. (From G. L. Robertson and T. Berl, Pathophysiology of Water Metabolism. In B. M. Brenner and F. C. Rector, Jr. [eds.], *The Kidney* (4th ed.). Philadelphia: Saunders, 1991. P. 677.)

binding protein neurophysin II, and the glycoprotein are transported in neurosecretory granules down the axons and stored in nerve terminals in the pars nervosa. There is no known physiologic role of the neurophysins, but they do neutralize the negative charge of vasopressin. The release of stored peptide hormone and its neurophysin into the systemic or hypophyseal portal circulation occurs by an exocytosis. With increased plasma osmolality, electrical impulses travel along the axons and depolarize the membrane of the terminal axonal bulbs. The membrane of the secretory granules fuses with the plasma membrane of the axonal bulbs, and the peptide contents are then extruded into the adjacent capillaries.

The regulation of ADH release from the posterior pituitary is dependent primarily on two mechanisms: osmotic and nonosmotic pathways (Fig. 1-8).

The osmotic regulation of ADH is dependent on "osmoreceptor" cells in the anterior hypothalamus in proximity but separate from supraoptic nuclei [32]. These cells, most likely by altering their cell volume, recognize changes in ECF osmolality. Cell volume is decreased most readily by substances that are restricted to the ECF, such as hypertonic saline or hypertonic mannitol, and thus enhance osmotic water movement from cells; these substances are very effective in stimulating ADH release. In contrast, urea moves readily into cells and therefore does not alter cell volume; hypertonic urea does not effectively stimulate ADH release. A similar response pattern is evident when vasopressin release is studied in the hypothalamoneurohypophyseal complex in organ culture. Specifically, sodium chloride, sucrose, and manni-tol at 310 mOsm/kg H_2O cause a threefold increase in AVP release, while urea and glucose fail to stimulate vasopressin. These studies also support the view that the receptor responds to changes in osmolality rather than sodium. The effects of increased osmolality on vasopressin release are associated with measurable (two-to fivefold) increases in vasopressin precursor messenger RNA (mRNA) in the hypothalamus [34, 35] and salt-loading increases vasopressin RNA in the pituitary [36]. The osmoreceptor cells are very sensitive to changes in ECF osmolality. Fluid deprivation or an increase in the concentration of an impermeative solute sufficient to increase ECF osmolality by 1 percent stimulates ADH release, while water inges-tion causing a 1 percent decrease in ECF osmolality suppresses ADH release (Fig. 1-8). Although there are considerable genetically determined individual variations in both the threshold and sensitivity [37], a close correlation between AVP and plasma osmolality has been demonstrated in subjects with various states of hydra-tion. There is also a close correlation between AVP and urinary osmolality (Fig. 1-9).

Vasopressin release also can occur in the absence of changes in plasma osmolality [37]. While a number of such nonosmotic stimuli exist, physical pain, emotional stress, and a decrement in blood pressure or blood volume are the most prominent ones. A 7 to 10 percent decrement in either blood pressure or blood volume causes the prompt release of vasopressin (see Fig. 1-8). Since the integrity of the circulatory volume takes precedence over mechanisms that maintain tonicity, activation of these nonosmotic pathways overrides any decline in the osmotic stimulus that other-

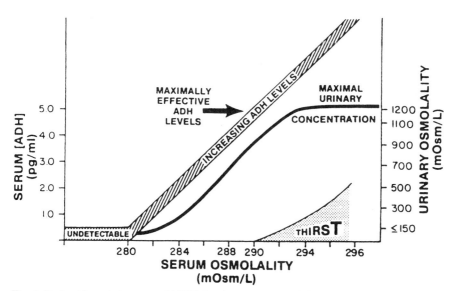

Fig. 1-9. Antidiuretic hormone (ADH) levels, urinary osmolality, and thirst as functions of serum osmolality. (From R. G. Narins and G. C. Krishna, Disorders of Water Balance. In J. H. Stein [ed.], *Internal Medicine*. Boston: Little, Brown, 1987. P. 794.)

wise would suppress the hormone's release. This process accounts for the pathogenesis of hyponatremia in various pathophysiologic states, including cirrhosis and heart failure.

There is considerable evidence for the existence of baroreceptor sensors in the low-pressure (venous) areas of the circulation, particularly in the atria. Atrial distention causes a decrease in AVP levels, a process that may be mediated in part by the secretion of atrial natriuretic peptide. Alternatively, stretch receptors in the left atrium, aorta, and carotid sensors send impulses through the vagus and glossopharyngeal nerves to the nucleus tractus solitarii of the medulla. Postsympathetic pathways transmit this information to the hypothalamus. The importance of these neural pathways is underlined by the fact that denervation of baroreceptors abolishes the release of AVP in response to many nonosmotic stimuli. Both arterial and venous receptors most likely act in concert by this final common pathway.

Since many of the pathophysiologic states associated with nonosmotic AVP release are also characterized by enhanced plasma renin activity and therefore high angiotensin II levels, it is possible that angiotensin II is a mediator of AVP release in these states. Likewise, activation of the sympathetic nervous system could be involved in the process. In this regard, the supraoptic nuclei are heavily innervated by noradrenergic neurons, and β-adrenergic stimulation causes an antidiuresis. However, even this antidiuresis requires intact baroreceptor pathways. Other pathways that could stimulate the nonosmotic secretion of AVP have been proposed. For example, the profound antidiuresis associated with vomiting and pain has been ascribed to an emetic and cerebral pain center, respectively. However, not even in these settings has a role for baroreceptor pathways been convincingly excluded. In addition to catecholamines, other biogenic amines, polypeptides, and even cytokines have been implicated as modulators of AVP release [39, 40].

Cellular Action of Vasopressin

Once released from the posterior pituitary, vasopressin exerts its biologic action on water excretion by binding to receptors in the basolateral membrane of the collecting duct [41, 42] (Fig. 1-10). The receptors to which vasopressin binds have now been cloned and fully described. The V_1 receptor is a widely distributed 394-amino-acid protein with seven transmembrane domains [43]. The 370-amino-acid V_2 receptor, which is only in the kidney and has a similar configuration, has been cloned for both rat [44] and humans [45]. Employing reverse transcription and polymerase chain reaction, both forms of the receptor have been found in various segments of the nephron [46]. While the V_1 receptor messenger is plentiful in the glomerulus, it is also detected in the collecting duct, where the V_2 message predominates. It must be noted, however, that others have not detected V_1 mRNA in the terminal inner medulla [27], and in situ hybridization studies suggest localization to the vasa recta rather than the collecting ducts themselves [47]. In vascular smooth muscle cells, the V_1 receptor is internalized and then returns to the cell membrane without requiring new protein synthesis [48]. A similar endocytosis of receptors occurs in kidney cells [49].

Binding of AVP to its V_2 receptor results in increased adenylate cyclase activity, which catalyzes the formation of cyclic adenosine 3',5'-monophosphate (cyclic

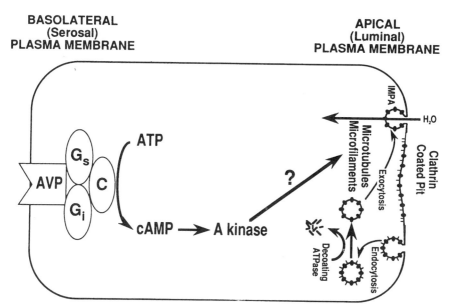

Fig. 1-10. Schematic representation of the cellular action of vasopressin. The figure depicts the proposed pathway of water channel recycling in collecting duct principal cells. Intramembranous particles that are believed to represent water channels are concentrated in clathrin-coated pits at the cell surface and are endocytosed in coated vesicles. These vesicles are rapidly decoated, and while their fluid-phase content may eventually reach multivesicular lysosomes, water channels themselves may escape degradation and be recycled back to the apical membrane. The nature of the vesicles carrying water channels to the membrane has not been elucidated in the collecting duct, nor have the sites of fusion of these vesicles at the apical membrane been described following vasopressin administration in this tissue. AVP = arginine vasopressin; G_s, G_i = stimulatory and inhibitory guanine nucleotide–binding regulatory proteins; C = catalytic unit of adenylate cyclase; ATP = adenosine triphosphate; cAMP = cyclic adenosine monophosphate; A kinase = cyclic nucleotide-dependent protein kinase; IMPA = intramembrane particle aggregates. (From I. Teitelbaum, C. R. Kleeman, and T. Berl, The Physiology of the Renal Concentrating and Diluting Mechanisms. In R. G. Narins [ed.], *Clinical Disorders of Fluid and Electrolyte Metabolism* [5th ed.]. New York: McGraw-Hill, 1994. P. 101.)

AMP) from adenosine triphosphate. The V_2 receptor is coupled to the catalytic unit of adenylate cyclase by the stimulatory guanine nucleotide–binding regulatory protein, G_s [50, 51]. This is a heterotrimeric protein whose α subunit binds and hydrolyzes guanosine triphosphate (GTP). In the absence of AVP, the α chain is bound to guanosine diphosphate (GDP) and does not stimulate the catalytic unit. Receptor occupancy catalyzes the exchange of GDP for GTP; this results in a conformational change in the α subunit that allows it to stimulate the catalytic unit to form cyclic AMP. Hydrolysis of the bound nucleotide then returns the system to the inactive state. In similar fashion, the activity of the catalytic unit is subject to modulation by G_i, a family of proteins that mediate inhibition of adenylate cyclase [50, 51].

The AVP-induced increase in adenylate cyclase activity results in heightened cyclic AMP formation, which ultimately causes the apical (luminal) cell membrane to become more permeable to water [52]. Administration of exogenous cyclic AMP or its analogues mimics the effect of ADH on the collecting tubule [53]. The cellular effect of cyclic AMP appears to relate to its ability to activate protein kinase A, which in turn phosphorylates serine and threonines. Activation of protein kinase(s) by cyclic AMP occurs in a dose-dependent fashion [54]. It is of interest that H89 and Rp-cAMPs, inhibitors of protein kinase A, block the hydro-osmotic response to vasopressin in perfused collecting ducts [55].

In response to ADH, the apical membranes form intramembranous particle aggregates [56]. Their formation coincides temporally with osmotic water flow [57]. Inhibitors of microtubule formation decrease the formation of these aggregates [58] as well as the osmotic response to vasopressin and cyclic AMP [59]. It is now believed that these intramembranous particles contain the water channel whose incorporation into the apical membrane may be facilitated by an AVP-mediated depolymerization of F-actin [60]. It has been proposed that this water channel undergoes a recyclic process in collecting duct cells in response to vasopressin [61–63]. Figure 1-10 depicts the exocytosis and endocytosis to which the channel is subjected as it is transported in clathrin-coated pits. The water channel responsible for the high water permeability of the luminal membrane in response to vasopressin has been recently cloned and designated as AQP-CD [64]. This is a 271-amino-acid single-chain polypeptide with six membrane-spanning domains found only in the kidney. Studies in microdissected tubules and immunolocalization place the protein solely to the collecting duct [64, 65]. This is thus most likely to be the vasopressin-regulated water channel in the kidney. Details of both its short- and long-term regulations are presently lacking [27].

Means of Quantitating Renal Water Excretion

The quantitation of water excretion has been facilitated by the concept that urine flow (V) is divisible into two components. One component is the urine volume needed to excrete solutes at the concentration of solutes in plasma. This isotonic component has been termed *osmolar clearance* (C_{osm}). The other component is called *free-water clearance* (C_{H_2O}) and is the theoretic volume of solute-free water that has been added to (positive C_{H_2O}) or reabsorbed from (negative C_{H_2O} or $T^c_{H_2O}$) the isotonic portion of urine (C_{osm}) to create either hypotonic or hypertonic urine, respectively. These terms are calculated as follows:

$$V = C_{osm} + C_{H_2O}$$

$$C_{H_2O} = V - C_{osm}$$

$$\text{Since, } C_{osm} = \frac{\text{urine osmolality } (U_{osm}) \times \text{urine flow } (V)}{\text{plasma osmolality } (P_{osm})}$$

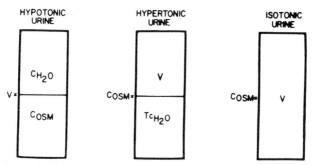

Fig. 1-11. Relationship between urine flow (V), C_{osm}, C_{H_2O}, and $T^c_{H_2O}$ in hypotonic, hypertonic, and isotonic urine.

$$C_{H_2O} = V - \frac{U_{osm} + V}{P_{osm}}$$

$$C_{H_2O} = V \left(1 - \frac{U_{osm}}{P_{osm}} \right)$$

Further inspection of these relationships will reveal the following:

1. When U_{osm} equals P_{osm} (isotonic urine), V equals C_{osm}; therefore, C_{H_2O} is zero.
2. When U_{osm} is greater than P_{osm} (hypertonic urine), C_{osm} is greater than V; therefore, C_{H_2O} will be negative (also denoted as $T^c_{H_2O}$).
3. When U_{osm} is less than P_{osm} (hypotonic urine), C_{osm} is less than V, and C_{H_2O} is positive.

This relationship is depicted further in Figure 1-11.

To summarize, C_{H_2O} represents the volume of water that must be removed from hypotonic urine, and $T^c_{H_2O}$ represents the volume of water that would have to be added to hypertonic urine to make the urine isotonic with plasma. The excretion of a hypertonic urine has the net effect of returning solute-free water to the organism and thereby dilutes body fluids. In contrast, the excretion of a hypotonic urine has the net effect of ridding the organism of solute-free water and thus concentrating body fluids. The urine osmolality alone does not give the volume of water added to or removed from the organism; the calculation of C_{H_2O} or $T^c_{H_2O}$ better allows the quantitation of water balance.

The clearance formulas utilize terms that include the total serum and urine osmolality. Urea is an important component of urine osmolality. As urea readily crosses cell membranes, it does not establish transcellular osmotic gradients and therefore does not cause water movement between body fluid compartments. Therefore, urea influences neither the serum sodium concentration nor the release of vasopressin, and its inclusion in the urine osmolality does not predict changes in serum sodium. This is better reflected if specifically electrolyte-free water clearance ($C_{H_2O}[e]$) is measured. In this formulation, the serum osmolality is replaced by serum sodium and urine osmolality by $U_{Na} + U_K$. Therefore,

$$C_{H_2O}(e) = V\left(1 - \frac{U_{Na} + U_K}{P_{Na}}\right)$$

If a patient's $U_{Na} + U_K < P_{Na}$, $C_{H_2O}(e)$ is positive, a process that will raise the concentration of sodium. Conversely, if $U_{Na} + U_K > P_{Na}$, $C_{H_2O}(e)$ is negative, a process that tends to lower the concentration of sodium in serum.

Relationship Between Daily Solute Load, Renal Concentrating Capacity, and Daily Urine Volume

A person ingesting a diet containing average amounts of sodium and protein has to dispose of approximately 600 mOsm of solute per day. The daily volume of urine in which this solute is excreted will depend on the fluid intake. The 600 mOsm can be excreted in 6 liters of urine at 100 mOsm/kg H_2O* if the daily fluid intake is generous; if water ingested is limited and renal concentrating capacity is intact, the 600-mOsm solute load can be excreted in 500 ml of urine at 1200 mOsm/kg H_2O.

This flexibility in daily urine volumes for a given solute load is limited if renal concentrating ability is impaired. For example, if the maximal renal concentrating ability is reduced to 300 mOsm/kg H_2O, the 600 mOsm obligates 2 liters of urine per day. With a more severe concentrating defect that does not allow urine to be concentrated above 60 mOsm/kg H_2O, the 600 mOsm of daily solute requires 10 liters of urine per day.

In terms of water conservation, the kidney's ability to increase urine osmolality from 60 to 300 mOsm/kg H_2O is quantitatively more important than its ability to increase urine osmolality from 300 to 1200 mOsm/kg H_2O. For example, with a daily solute load of 600 mOsm, a decrease in maximal urine osmolality from 1200 to 300 mOsm/kg H_2O increases obligatory urine flow from 0.5 to 2.0 L/day. Thus, even in the absence of the renal capacity to concentrate urine above plasma, severe polydipsia and polyuria should not be observed. However, for the same solute load, a further decrease in maximal urinary concentration from 300 to 60 mOsm/kg H_2O requires the excretion of 10 liters of urine per day. This degree of defect in water conservation obviously is associated with overt polyuria and polydipsia. In the absence of an intact thirst mechanism and a large intake of water, a severe water deficit and hypernatremia would occur.

Renal Capacity to Reabsorb Solute-Free ($T^c_{H_2O}$) Versus Capacity to Excrete Solute-Free Water (C_{H_2O})

In quantitative terms, the normal kidney's ability to reabsorb $T^c_{H_2O}$ is more limited than its ability to excrete C_{H_2O}. With maximal urine osmolality of 1200 mOsm/kg H_2O and a daily urine volume of 500 ml, $T^c_{H_2O}$ can be calculated as follows:

---

* The expression mOsm/kg H_2O is used to express osmolar concentration, and a kilogram of water can be equated to a liter of water.

$$C_{osm} = \frac{UV}{P} \text{ or } C_{osm} = \frac{1200 \text{ mOsm/kg } H_2O \times 500 \text{ ml/day}}{300 \text{ mOsm/kg } H_2O}$$

$$C_{osm} = 2000 \text{ ml/day}$$

$$T^c_{H_2O} = C_{osm} - V$$

$$T^c_{H_2O} = 2000 - 500 \text{ ml/day}$$

$$T^c_{H_2O} = 1500 \text{ ml/day}$$

Thus, only 1500 ml of solute-free water is returned to body fluids during this maximal antidiuresis. In contrast, with the same daily solute load of 600 mOsm, a minimal urine osmolality of 60 mOsm/kg H_2O, and a daily urine volume of 10 liters, the renal capacity to excrete C_{H_2O} is much greater than the capacity to return solute-free water ($T^c_{H_2O}$) to the body. More specifically,

$$C_{osm} = \frac{UV}{P} \quad \text{or} \quad \frac{60 \text{ mOsm/kg}}{300 \text{ mOsm/kg}} \times 10 = 2 \text{ L/day}$$

$$C_{H_2O} = V - C_{osm} \quad \text{or} \quad 10 \text{ L} - 2 \text{ L} = 8 \text{ L/day}$$

Thus, with comparable solute loads and relatively maximal and minimal urine osmolalities, the $T^c_{H_2O}$ of 1.5 L/day is substantially less than the C_{H_2O} of 8 L/day.

Prevention of a total body water deficit is thus largely dependent on water intake as modulated by thirst. The thirst center appears to be closely associated anatomically with the osmoreceptor in the region of the hypothalamus. Defects in thirst response may involve either organic or generalized central nervous system lesions and can lead to severe water deficit even in the presence of a normal concentrating mechanism. Of course, the water deficit will occur more promptly if renal concentrating ability is also impaired.

Clinical Disorders of Urinary Concentration Causing Hypernatremic States

The renal concentrating mechanism represents the first defense against water depletion and hyperosmolality. A perturbation in any component of the concentrating mechanism culminates in an inability to maximally concentrate urine. When renal concentration is impaired, thirst becomes a very effective mechanism for preventing further increases in serum sodium [66]. The threshold for thirst appears to be approximately 10 mOsm/kg H_2O above that of vasopressin release (see Fig. 1-9). Thirst is in fact so effective that even patients with complete diabetes insipidus avoid hypernatremia by fluid intake in excess of 10 L/day. Hypernatremia supervenes therefore only when hypotonic fluid losses occur in combination with a disturbance in water intake [67]. This is most commonly seen in the aged with an alteration in level of consciousness, in the very young with inadequate access to water, or in a rare subject with a primary disturbance in thirst.

As shown in Figure 1-12, hypernatremia can develop with either low, normal, or, more rarely, high total body sodium [68].

Hypernatremia in Patients with Low Total Body Sodium

Patients who sustain losses of both sodium and water but with a relatively greater loss of water are classified as having hypernatremia with low total body sodium. Such patients exhibit the signs of hypovolemia such as orthostatic hypotension, tachycardia, flat neck veins, poor skin turgor, and dry mucous membranes. The causes underlying the hypovolemic state are similar to those that cause hypovolemic hyponatremia. The effect on serum sodium is determined by the failure to ingest water (hypernatremia) or excessive free water intake (hyponatremia). Extrarenal loss of hypotonic fluid can occur either through the skin due to profuse sweating in a hot or humid environment or, more frequently, from the gastrointestinal tract in the form of diarrhea. Although primarily recognized in children, lactulose-induced diarrhea leading to hypernatremia appears to be common. Since the renal water- and sodium-conserving mechanisms operate normally in these patients, urine osmolality is high (usually >800 mOsm/kg H_2O) and urinary sodium concentration is low (<10 mEq/L). Hypotonic losses can also occur by the renal route during a loop diuretic–induced hypotonic diuresis or an osmotic diuresis with either mannitol, glucose, glycerol, or, more rarely, urea. Elderly patients with partial urinary tract obstruction can excrete large volumes of hypotonic urine. The urine in these cases is hypotonic or isotonic, and the urinary sodium concentration is greater than 20 mEq/L. It must be emphasized, however, that since glucose and mannitol enhance osmotic water movement from the intracellular fluid to the ECF compartment, some of these patients may have a normal or even low serum sodium concentration in spite of serum hypertonicity.

Hypernatremia in Patients with Normal Total Body Sodium

Loss of water without sodium does not lead to overt volume contraction unless the water losses are massive. Patients with hypernatremia secondary to water loss therefore appear to be euvolemic with a normal total body sodium. The extrarenal sources of such water losses are the skin and the respiratory tract. A high environmental temperature as well as a febrile or hypermetabolic state can cause considerable water losses. If such hypotonic losses are not accompanied by appropriate water intake, hypernatremia supervenes. Urine osmolality is very high, reflecting an intact osmo-receptor-vasopressin-renal response. Urinary sodium concentration will vary according to the patient's sodium intake.

More frequently the losses of water are of renal origin, as in diabetes insipidus. Diabetes insipidus is a polyuric disorder characterized by high rates of electrolyte-free

21

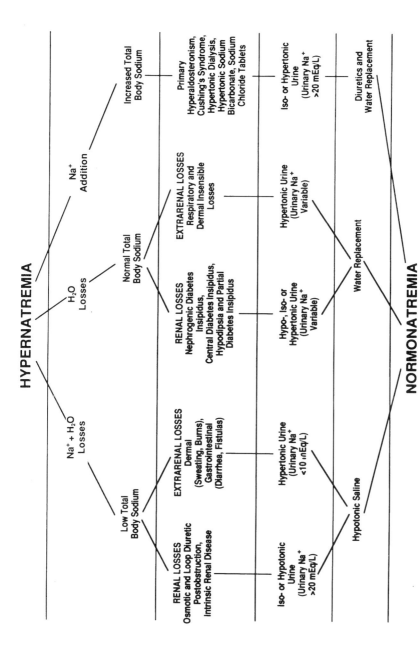

Fig. 1-12. Diagnostic and therapeutic approach to the hypernatremic patient. (Reprinted from T. Berl, R. J. Anderson, K. M. McDonald, et al., Clinical disorders of water metabolism. *Kidney Int.* 10:117, 1976.)

water excretion. When these losses are not appropriately replaced, hypernatremia supervenes. Depending on whether the water losses are due to a failure to secrete vasopressin or to a renal resistance to the hormone, the disease is designated as being central or nephrogenic, respectively.

Central Diabetes Insipidus

Failure to normally synthesize or secrete vasopressin limits maximal urinary concentration and, depending on the severity of the disease, causes varying degrees of polyuria and polydipsia. The causes of central diabetes insipidus are listed in Table 1-1. The disease is very rarely inherited. Families with an autosomal dominant inheritance pattern have been described [69]. These patients display a marked deficiency of neurosecretory cells, particularly in the supraoptic nucleus. Molecular analysis of these patients has most often revealed a single base substitution in either exon A or exon B of the gene that codes for proprevasopressin [70] (see Fig. 1-7). This is unlike the animal model of congenital central diabetes insipidus in which a base deletion causes a frame shift, producing an abnormal protein. There is also a rare inherited autosomal recessive form of central diabetes insipidus that occurs

Table 1-1. Causes of central diabetes insipidus

Hereditary
  Autosomal dominant
  Autosomal recessive (Wolfram syndrome)
Acquired
  Head trauma, skull fracture, and orbital trauma
  Posthypophysectomy
  Suprasellar and intrasellar tumors
    Primary (suprasellar cyst, craniopharyngioma, pinealoma, meningioma, and glioma)
    Metastatic (breast or lung cancer, leukemia, and lymphomas)
  Granulomas
    Sarcoid
    Wegener's granulomatosis
    Tuberculosis
    Syphilis
  Histiocytosis
    Eosinophilic granuloma
    Hand-Schüller-Christian disease
  Infections
    Encephalitis
    Meningitis
    Guillain-Barré syndrome
  Vascular
    Cerebral aneurysm
    Cerebral thrombosis or hemorrhage
    Sickle cell disease
    Postpartum necrosis (Sheehan's syndrome)
    Pregnancy (transient)

Source: M. Levi and T. Berl, Water Metabolism. In H. C. Gonick (ed.), *Current Nephrology*. Vol. 5, p. 23. Copyright © 1982 by Year Book Medical Publishers, Inc., Chicago.

in association with diabetes mellitus, optic atrophy, and deafness (Wolfram syndrome) [69]. Of acquired causes, in approximately half of the patients, the loss of vasopressin secretory capacity is idiopathic. Histologically, this form of diabetes insipidus is similar to the previously described inherited form and may well have an autoimmune etiology [71]. Head trauma, hypophysectomy, and neoplasms, either primary or metastatic (mainly from lung and breast tumors), constitute most of the other causes [72, 73]. Other etiologic factors include encephalitis, sarcoidosis, eosinophilic granuloma, and histiocytosis [74, 75]. Finally, central diabetes insipidus has recently been described following development of cerebral edema in 11 postoperative hyponatremic women [76].

Clinical Features. Polyuria and polydipsia are the hallmarks of central diabetes insipidus and must be considered in the differential diagnosis of any patient who presents with such symptoms. As illustrated in Figure 1-11, polyuria can occur also from a solute diuresis, in which case C_{osm} is increased and the urine osmolality is greater than 300 mOsm/kg. When polyuria is due to an increase in C_{H_2O} and urine osmolality is less than 150 mOsm/kg, a diagnosis of diabetes insipidus should be considered. Urine flow can range between 3 and 15 L/day, depending on the severity of the disease. The disorder frequently has an abrupt onset and occurs with equal frequency in both sexes. Although the time of onset is extremely variable, it is rare in infancy and is most frequent in the 10- to 20-year age group. Patients with central diabetes insipidus often have a predilection for cold water. Since there is little diurnal variation in the polyuria, nocturia is frequently marked. In untreated patients, however, bladder capacity may be increased so that nocturia may not be a prominent symptom. In general, however, nocturia is frequent, and sleep deprivation commonly leads to fatigue and irritability [77]. If the thirst mechanism is intact and water is available, patients with central diabetes insipidus do not develop hypernatremia and thus have no symptoms except for the inconvenience associated with the marked polyuria and polydipsia. With concomitant hypodipsia, no access to water, or an illness that precludes adequate water intake, however, severe and even life-threatening hypernatremia can supervene.

Diagnosis. The development of severe polyuria and polydipsia (>6–8 L/day) in an adult patient who does not have diabetes mellitus (the most common cause of a solute diuresis) indicates the possibility of either (1) a failure of vasopressin release, that is, central diabetes insipidus; or (2) excessive water intake, that is, compulsive water-drinking (perhaps better termed dipsogenic diabetes insipidus). Profound polyuria in childhood is more likely to be congenital nephrogenic diabetes insipidus, a disorder that will be discussed later.

The differential diagnosis between central diabetes insipidus and compulsive water-drinking may be very difficult [78]. Plasma vasopressin levels are diminished in both circumstances. In central diabetes insipidus, this is due to impaired synthesis or secretion of vasopressin. Thus the patient has polydipsia because, in the absence of ADH, renal water conservation is impaired. In contrast, the compulsive water-drinker ingests large amounts of fluids, which functionally suppress endogenous ADH release, and thus the large water intake is excreted. In other words, the patient with central diabetes insipidus has polydipsia because of polyuria, while the compulsive water-drinker has polyuria because of polydipsia. With the use of the computed tomography scan, abnormalities in the hypothalamopituitary region can be seen in a majority of patients with central diabetes insipidus [79]. Magnetic resonance may further improve the sensitivity. Normally on T1-weighted images the posterior pituitary produces a bright signal that is indistinguishable from fatty tissue, but this signal is lost in patients with central diabetes insipidus [80, 81].

The patient's history can be helpful in making the differential diagnosis. Whereas with central diabetes insipidus the patient has an abrupt onset of polyuria and polydipsia, the patient who is a compulsive water-drinker has a more vague history of the onset of polydipsia and polyuria. The compulsive or psychogenic water-drinker also may have a history of considerable variation in water intake and urine output on an hour-to-hour or day-to-day basis, while the patient with central diabetes insipidus has a very consistent need for water intake. Large variations in water intake, in the patient whose intakes and outputs are measured, are therefore a clue to the diagnosis of compulsive water-drinking. Nocturia is more severe and frequent in subjects with central diabetes insipidus. Finally, the previously noted preference for ice water usually is not described by subjects with compulsive water-drinking. Compulsive water-drinkers also may have a history of psychiatric disorders and not infrequently are women during their menopause. Since the psychogenic water-drinker is generally in modest positive fluid balance and the patient with central diabetes insipidus is generally in modest negative fluid balance, a plasma osmolality below 270 mOsm/kg H_2O suggests compulsive water-drinking, while a plasma osmolality above 295 mOsm/kg H_2O suggests central diabetes insipidus. While the differentiation between central and dipsogenic diabetes insipidus in their classic forms may thus pose no difficulties, the correct diagnosis is frequently not easy to make, particularly when the defect in vasopressin release is partial.

A fluid deprivation test may provide the most reliable information regarding the assessment of these polyuric disorders [82] (Table 1-2). Fluid deprivation must be instituted with careful monitoring of body weight and vital signs, since the patient with central diabetes insipidus may rapidly develop a severe negative fluid balance. During the fluid deprivation, the patient should not be permitted to lose more than 3 to 5 percent of body weight. Normal subjects require 16 to 18 hours to achieve a mean maximum urine osmolality of approximately 1000 to 1200 mOsm/kg H_2O. After this period of fluid deprivation, the injection of 5 units of aqueous vasopressin subcutaneously causes no further increase in their urine osmolality. This suggests that the dehydration test has maximally stimulated endogenous vasopressin release. One might suspect, therefore, that fluid deprivation readily discriminates between those with a normal neurohypophyseal system, such as the compulsive water-drinker, and the patient with central diabetes insipidus. Observations of normal men who have drunk large daily volumes of water have, however, demonstrated a blunted response to vasopressin [83]. A decrease in medullary tonicity occurs, perhaps as a result of an increase in medullary blood flow, and this is associated with the diminution in renal concentrating capacity. For this reason, patients with compulsive water-drinking may demonstrate submaximal concentrating ability after fluid deprivation, but their urine osmolality still exceeds 500 mOsm/kg. Since with

Table 1-2. Water-deprivation test*

	Urinary osmolality with water deprivation (mOsm/kg H$_2$O)	Plasma AVP after dehydration	Increase in urinary osmolality with exogenous AVP
Normal	>800	>2 pg/ml	Little or no increase
Complete central diabetes insipidus	<300	Undetectable	Substantially increased
Partial central diabetes insipidus	300–800	<1.5 pg/ml	Increase of greater than 10% of urinary osmolality after water deprivation
Nephrogenic diabetes insipidus	<300–500	>5 pg/ml	Little or no increase
Primary polydipsia	>500	<5 pg/ml	Little or no increase

* Water intake is restricted until the patient loses 3 to 5 percent of his or her body weight or until three consecutive hourly determinations of urinary osmolality are within 10 percent of each other. (Caution must be exercised to ensure that the patient does not become excessively dehydrated.) Aqueous AVP (5 U SQ) is given, and urinary osmolality is measured after 60 minutes. The expected responses are given above.
Source: D. Lanese and I. Teitelbaum, Hypernatremia. In H. R. Jacobson, G. E. Striker, and S. Klahr (eds.), *The Principles and Practice of Nephrology* (2nd ed.). St. Louis: Mosby, 1995. P. 895.

fluid deprivation endogenous vasopressin secretion is maximal, there is no further increase with exogenous vasopressin. This serves to differentiate such patients from those with neurogenic diabetes insipidus, whose urine osmolality substantially increases (>10%) following the administration of vasopressin [82]. Of particular importance is the recognition of patients who have only a partial defect in ADH secretion. Urine osmolalities in these patients and in compulsive water-drinkers may be similar after fluid deprivation, but only the patient with partial diabetes insipidus will respond further to exogenous vasopressin. Miller and associates [82] have argued that if exogenous vasopressin increases urine osmolality by more than 10 percent after fluid deprivation, a defect in ADH release is probably present. Only patients with complete diabetes insipidus may demonstrate overt clinical symptoms of polyuria and polydipsia, while patients with partial central diabetes insipidus may remain asymptomatic.

Although the described water deprivation test is useful in the differential diagnosis of polyuric disorders, it is time-consuming and requires considerable patient cooperation. Occasionally the diagnosis of central diabetes insipidus needs to be made more promptly or in acutely ill subjects. An examination of the relationship between plasma osmolality (excluding glucose and urea) and urine osmolality can be helpful. The finding of a low urine osmolality as plasma tonicity rises during a brief period of water withdrawal suggests the diagnosis of central diabetes insipidus [84].

Measurements of circulating AVP can serve as a valuable adjunct to the water deprivation test. A correlation between the test with directly measured radioimmunoassayable levels of the hormone has been undertaken [86]. In all patients with complete central diabetes insipidus, vasopressin measurements confirmed the diagnosis reached by the dehydration test. However, in 2 of 6 patients thought to have partial diabetes insipidus by the criteria of the test, vasopressin levels were more compatible with nephrogenic diabetes insipidus and primary polydipsia. Furthermore, 3 of 10 patients classified as having primary polydipsia by the dehydration test had evidence for partial diabetes insipidus [85]. An alternative and perhaps more definite diagnostic approach is provided by the measurement of plasma vasopressin following fluid deprivation [86] (see Fig. 1-13). It would appear, therefore, that incorporation of vasopressin measurements by a sensitive radioimmunoassay may complement and refine the accuracy of previously available tests in the differential diagnosis of polyuric syndromes. More recently, the measurement of AQP-CD antibody to the vasopressin-sensitive water channel in urine has been described as a

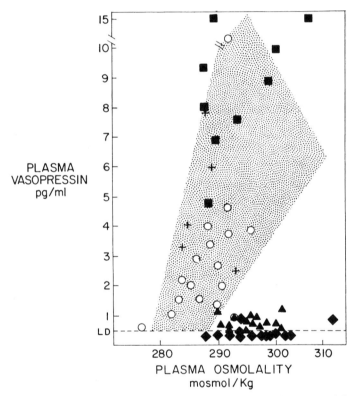

Fig. 1-13. The relationship of plasma vasopressin to concurrent plasma osmolality in patients with polyuria of diverse causes. All measurements were made at the end of a standard dehydration test. The shaded area represents the range of normal. In patients with severe (*closed diamonds*) or partial (*closed triangles*) neurogenic diabetes insipidus, plasma vasopressin was almost always subnormal relative to plasma osmolality. In contrast, the values from patients with dipsogenic (*open circles*) or nephrogenic (*closed squares*) diabetes insipidus were consistently within or above the normal range. (From G. L. Robertson, Diagnosis of Diabetes Insipidus. In A. P. Czernichow and A. Robinson [eds.], *Diabetes Insipidus in Man, Frontiers of Hormone Research.* Basel: S. Karger, 1985.)

Table 1-3. Therapeutic regimens for the treatment of diabetes insipidus

	Drug	Dose
Complete central diabetes insipidus	DDAVP	10–20 μg intranasally q12–24h
Partial central diabetes insipidus	Vasopressin tannate	2–5 U IM q24–48h
	Aqueous vasopressin	5–10 U SQ q4–6h
	Chlorpropamide	250–500 mg daily
	Clofibrate	500 mg tid–qid
	Carbamazepine	400–600 mg daily
Nephrogenic diabetes insipidus	Thiazide diuretics	Conventional doses
	Nonsteroidal anti-inflammatory drugs	Conventional doses

Source: Modified from D. Lanese and I. Teitelbaum, Hypernatremia. In H. R. Jacobson, G. E. Striker, and S. Klahr (eds.), *The Principles and Practice of Nephrology* (2nd ed.) St. Louis: Mosby, 1995. P. 897.

tool to differentiate polyuric disorders. Vasopressin increases the water channel excretion in urinary cells when the renal tubule responds to the hormone, as in central disorders [87]. The clinical utility of this approach is limited at this time.

Treatment. If the thirst mechanism is intact and water available, patients with central diabetes insipidus do not develop hypernatremia and thus have no symptoms except for the inconvenience associated with marked polyuria and polydipsia. Hormonal replacement and pharmacologic agents both are available for the treatment of central diabetes insipidus (Table 1-3). In acute settings, such as after hypophysectomy, the aqueous vasopressin (Pitressin) preparation is preferable. Its short duration of action allows for more careful monitoring and decreases the likelihood of complications such as water intoxication. In chronic settings, vasopressin tannate in oil (Pitressin Tannate) is potent and effective for 24 to 72 hours. It requires a deep subcutaneous or intramuscular injection by a fairly large-gauge needle because of the viscosity of the oil vehicle. This material can cause sterile abscesses in some subjects and on occasion be associated with resistance due to development of antibodies [88]. Care must be taken to allow return of polyuria and polydipsia between injections to avoid cumulative water retention and severe hyponatremia.

A modification of the natural vasopressin molecule to form desmopressin acetate (DDAVP) has resulted in a compound with prolonged antidiuretic activity (6–24 hours) and virtual elimination of vasopressor activity (antidiuretic-to-pressor ratio of approximately 2000:1) as compared with the natural hormone AVP (duration of action of 2 to 4 hours and antidiuretic-to-pressor ratio of 1:1) [89–91]. Substitution of D-arginine for L-arginine at position 8 resulted in a peptide DAVP with diminished vasopressor activity, and deamination of the hemicysteine at position 1 gave rise to a second peptide, with enhanced antidiuretic-to-pressor activity and prolonged duration of action (Fig. 1-14). DDAVP is administered intranasally in a dosage ranging from 10 to 20 μg every 8 to 12 hours. There are considerable individual variations in the required dosage, but most patients require twice daily administration for good

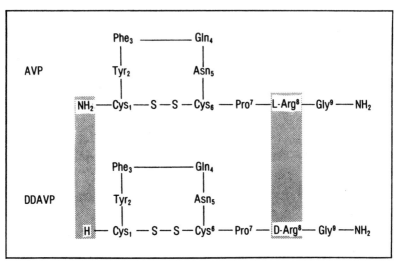

Fig. 1-14. Changes in arginine vasopressin molecule (AVP) to form desmopressin acetate (DDAVP). Amino group on hemicysteine is replaced with proton, and L-arginine is replaced by D-arginine. (From F. Ziai, R. Walles, and I. M. Rosenthal, Treatment of central diabetes insipidus in adults and children with desmopressin. *Arch. Intern. Med.* 138:1382, 1978. Copyright 1978, American Medical Association.)

control [92]. DDAVP can be administered intravenously (1–2 μg) and is also active orally at large doses (between 100 and 400 μg) [93, 94].

Large doses of DDAVP may cause transient headaches, nausea, and a slight increase in blood pressure; these symptoms disappear if the dosage is reduced. Nasal congestion, mild abdominal cramps, and vulval pain have occurred rarely.

Though intranasal DDAVP is now the treatment of choice for central diabetes insipidus, it is well to remember that alternatives to hormone replacement may be helpful at times. Since with a very dilute urine of fixed osmolality the urine volume is determined by the solute load requiring excretion, a reduction of salt and protein in the diet will reduce the major urinary solutes and thus the volume of urine necessary to accommodate their excretion. Also, a number of pharmacologic agents with antidiuretic properties are also used [95]. Chlorpropamide (Diabinese) is the most commonly employed [96]. Its antidiuretic effects are manifested only if some vasopressin is present and is therefore useful only in partial diabetes insipidus. In Brattleboro rats with diabetes insipidus, chlorpropamide augmented the antidiuretic responses to DDAVP [97]. A trial of 250 mg every day or twice a day may be offered to patients with partial central diabetes insipidus and at least 7 days allowed for an effect to occur. The anticonvulsant carbamazepine (Tegretol) [98] has also caused antidiuresis in subjects with diabetes insipidus. A combination of chlorpropamide and carbamazepine has been found to provide an effect that could be synergistic [90]. Clofibrate also has been used to treat partial central diabetes insipidus. At present, however, none of these approaches can be recommended over intranasal DDAVP.

Congenital Nephrogenic Diabetes Insipidus

Congenital nephrogenic diabetes insipidus is a rare hereditary disorder in which the renal tubule is insensitive to vasopressin [99]. The disease manifests itself in the complete clinical form only in males and in a subclinical form in females, suggesting a sex-linked dominant inheritance with variable penetrance in the female. The gene responsible for the defect has, in fact, been mapped to region 28 on the long arm of the X chromosome (Xq28) [100, 101].

Since the insertion of the normal human Xq28 chromosome region into rodent cell lines devoid of V_2 receptors results in the expression of functional receptors, the suggestion that a defect in the gene encoding the V_2 receptor is responsible for hereditary nephrogenic diabetes insipidus seemed most attractive. Also, the failure to increase cyclic AMP in response to DDAVP but not in response to norepinephrine pointed to a receptor defect [102]. In fact, this has proved to be the case. Since the first description of the molecular identification of the gene responsible for the disease [103], a number of mutations, probably more than 20, have been described in affected families [104–106]. It is now clear that the defect observed in an experimental mouse model with vasopressin-resistant concentrating defect is distinct from that in the human disease, as the disorder in mice appears to reside in enhanced phosphodiesterase activity in the rolipram-sensitive isoenzyme [107, 108]. It is also of interest that there appears to be an even rarer variant of congenital nephrogenic diabetes insipidus, inherited as an autosomal recessive. Unlike the X-linked form in which there is also a failure of the endothelium to release coagulation and fibrinolytic products in response to DDAVP [109], this form is limited to the kidney [110]. This disease has recently been found to be due to a mutation in the gene encoding the vasopressin-sensitive water channel [111].

Clinical Manifestations. Although the disease is most probably inborn, the diagnosis of congenital nephrogenic diabetes insipidus is usually not made until the infant presents with a hyposmolar urine in the face of severe dehydration, hypernatremia, vomiting, and fever. Unlike some of the females, who have partial responsiveness to vasopressin, the male with the full-blown complete form of this disorder will not elaborate a hypertonic urine even in the face of severe dehydration. The impaired growth and occasional mental retardation that occur in these cases are most likely due to repeated episodes of dehydration and hypernatremia rather than being integral components of the disease. Hydronephrosis is also common in these patients, perhaps because of voluntary retention of large volumes of urine, with subsequent vesicoureteral reflux [112].

Treatment. Neither vasopressin nor other pharmacologic agents that potentiate its action or stimulate its release, such as chlorpropamide [95], are effective in concentrating the urine of patients with nephrogenic diabetes insipidus. An intact thirst mechanism is therefore indispensable for the maintenance of good hydration in children with this disorder, as is careful monitoring of fluid balance. Since the excretion of solute requires further water losses, children with this disorder who need rehydration should receive hypotonic (2.5%) rather than isotonic (5%) glucose solutions. Glucosuria may occur with the latter solution and thus aggravate fluid losses [113].

Limitation of oral solute intake (low-sodium diet) may also lead to a decrease in urine flow in patients with nephrogenic diabetes insipidus. Thiazide diuretics, which inhibit sodium reabsorption in the cortical diluting segment of the nephron, have met with some success in the management of these patients [113]. The ability of thiazides to diminish sodium reabsorption in this water-impermeable portion of the nephron would by itself decrease C_{H_2O} but not urine flow. It seems most likely that the decrease in urine flow is secondary to the sodium loss and ECF volume contraction. ECF volume depletion in turn decreases GFR and increases proximal tubular sodium and water reabsorption. These secondary effects of the diuretic agent then decrease urine flow. The ECF volume contraction can be maintained with a low sodium intake after discontinuance of the diuretic, so that the therapy still remains effective. The addition of amiloride to hydrochlorothiazide may provide added benefit [114]. Nonsteroidal anti-inflammatory agents have been found to be effective [115], and in this regard, tolmetin appears to be particularly well tolerated in children [116]. It should be noted that none of these modalities results in the elaboration of a hypertonic urine. Even an increase in urine osmolality from 50 to 200 mOsm/kg H_2O is very important, however, because it significantly reduces obligatory urine loss from 10 to 12 L/day to a tolerable 3 to 4 L/day. Such a change in urine flow also minimizes the dilatation of the urinary tract.

Acquired Nephrogenic Diabetes Insipidus

The acquired form of nephrogenic diabetes insipidus is much more common than the congenital form of the disease, but it is rarely severe. In fact, while maximal concentrating ability is impaired in this disorder, the ability to elaborate a hypertonic urine is usually preserved. Nocturia, polyuria, and polydipsia may occur in this acquired form of nephrogenic diabetes insipidus, but the urine volumes are generally less (<3–4 L/day) than those observed with complete central diabetes insipidus, psychogenic water-drinking, or congenital nephrogenic central diabetes insipidus. The more common causes of acquired nephrogenic diabetes insipidus are listed in Table 1-4.

Chronic Renal Failure. A defect in renal concentrating capacity is a consistent accompaniment of most forms of advanced renal failure. Thus, chronic renal failure constitutes a form of acquired nephrogenic diabetes insipidus [117]. Advanced renal insufficiency of any cause can cause a vasopressin resistance associated with hypotonic urine [118].

In some forms of kidney disease, listed in Table 1-4, vasopressin unresponsiveness can occur at a stage when GFR is not markedly diminished [119]. The occurrence of a profound diuresis in association with a concentrating defect in glomerular diseases of the kidney is rare, and in general, a close correlation exists between GFR and maximal urine osmolality.

The causes of the defect in renal concentrating capacity associated with chronic renal failure are probably multiple [118, 119]. These include (1) a disruption of inner medullary structures or local alterations in medullary blood flow as is seen in

Table 1-4. Causes of acquired nephrogenic diabetes insipidus

Chronic renal disease
   Polycystic disease
   Medullary cystic disease
   Ureteral obstruction
   Amyloidosis
   Advanced renal failure of any etiology
Electrolyte disorders
   Hypokalemia
   Hypercalcemia
Drugs
   Alcohol
   Lithium
   Demeclocycline
   Glyburide
   Amphotericin
   Foscarnet
Sickle cell disease
Dietary abnormalities
   Excessive water intake
   Decreased sodium chloride intake
   Decreased protein intake
Miscellaneous
   Gestational diabetes insipidus

tubulointerstitial diseases, sickle cell disease, and analgesic nephropathy, (2) an impairment in sodium chloride transport out of the thick ascending limb of Henle's loop, a process that limits maximal interstitial tonicity, and (3) an increase in solute excretion in the remaining few functioning nephrons, an adaptive response to the need to excrete the same solute load as the normal kidney. Solute diuresis in normal humans may cause isotonic urine in the presence of maximal amounts of vasopressin [24]. However, none of these pathogenic mechanisms alone can explain the observation that vasopressin-resistant hypotonic urine may be found in patients with advanced renal failure [118]. If the assumption is made that even in the absence of a countercurrent system the tonicity of the renal medulla is never less than that of plasma, a failure of complete osmotic equilibration between the collecting duct and medullary interstitium must occur to explain vasopressin-resistant hypotonic urine. One possibility is that the response to ADH of the collecting duct membranes in the damaged kidney is submaximal. In fact, studies in the isolated collecting duct of uremic rabbits have demonstrated impaired water permeability and abnormal adenylate cyclase responsiveness to vasopressin [120]. A recent study suggests that the vasopressin resistance in chronic renal failure may be due to a selective down-regulation of the V_2 receptor, since membranes from the inner medulla of rats with renal failure have markedly diminished V_2 receptor mRNA [121].

Recognition of the renal concentration defect is foremost in the therapeutic approach. If the maximal renal concentrating capacity of a patient with chronic renal failure is 300 mOsm/kg H_2O and the daily solute load is 600 mOsm, a urine volume of 2 L/day is necessary to excrete the solute load. The patient's fluid intake, including 500 ml for insensible losses, must therefore be at least 2500 ml/day. Thus, if the patient is ill and cannot ingest fluids for several days, severe volume depletion can occur because of the failure of the kidney to concentrate the urine. Recognition of the subclinical concentrating defect, which can emerge as an important clinical problem during an acute illness, is therefore pivotal in the long-term management of patients with chronic renal failure.

Electrolyte Abnormalities. Hypokalemia has long been known to cause polyuria as a consequence of a vasopressin-resistant renal concentrating defect [122]. Initially the polyuria is due to a primary effect of potassium depletion to stimulate water intake [123]. A renal concentrating defect that is independent of the high rate of water turnover eventually supervenes. The defect is in part due to a decrement in interstitial tonicity, which most likely relates to a decrease in sodium chloride reabsorption in the thick ascending limb [124]. The elaboration of hypotonic urine suggests a defect in the collecting duct's response to vasopressin, independent of the decreased medullary tonicity. A direct effect of hypokalemia on the collecting tubule is supported by studies in the toad bladder that show a decrease in cyclic AMP and vasopressin-stimulated water flow when potassium is removed from the bathing solution [125]. These findings suggest both a pre–cyclic AMP and post–cyclic AMP defect. The hypokalemia-induced resistance to vasopressin is associated with decreased cyclic AMP accumulation, apparently due to decreased adenylate cyclase activity [126]. A decrement in the vasopressin-sensitive water channel (aquaporin 2) has been described in hypokalemic rats [126a]. Hypokalemia from any cause, such as diarrhea, chronic diuretic use, or primary aldosteronism, may be associated with a urinary concentrating defect. The defect is generally reversible but requires a longer time (1–3 months) than would be expected from a purely functional defect [127].

Hypercalcemia is another well-recognized cause of impaired urinary concentrating ability [122]. While due in part to mild polydipsia [128], the defect is primarily intrarenal. A decrement in medullary interstitial tonicity is clearly present with hypercalcemia [128], which may be related to diminished solute reabsorption in the thick ascending limb [129]. This defect is associated with a decrement in AVP-stimulated adenylate cyclase in this nephron segment [130]. The concentrating defect is, however, multifactorial, as the elaboration of a hypotonic urine implies an intrinsic defect in the collecting tubule. In this regard, studies in isolated toad bladders [131] as well as papillary collecting ducts reveal a decreased response to vasopressin in hypercalcemia. A similar inhibition of cyclic AMP accumulation and hydro-osmotic response to AVP is seen with maneuvers that increase cell calcium [132, 133]. The cause of the hypercalcemia does not appear to be important in the occurrence of the concentrating defect, since it has been observed with hypercalcemia of various etiologies.

Pharmacologic Agents. Various pharmacologic agents have been found to impair the renal capacity to concentrate urine [134] (see Table 1-4). Ethanol and phenytoin

(Dilantin) [135] seem to exert their action by a central effect on vasopressin release. Some hypoglycemic agents cause a diuresis by a mechanism probably unrelated to suppression of vasopressin release [136]. The renal toxicity of amphotericin can manifest in the form of a concentrating defect [137]. Foscarnet, an agent increasingly employed in the treatment of cytomegalovirus infection in patients with acquired immune deficiency syndrome (AIDS), has been described to cause a nephrogenic diabetes insipidus [138].

The drugs most commonly associated with nephrogenic diabetes insipidus are demeclocycline and lithium. Since it was first recognized as a cause of nephrogenic diabetes insipidus [139], demeclocycline has become the drug of choice for the treatment of the syndrome of inappropriate ADH secretion (SIADH). It has yet to be determined if demeclocycline reduces AVP secretion. It is clear, however, that demeclocycline induces dose-dependent decreases in human renal medullary adenylate cyclase activity [52]. Since the drug decreases not only vasopressin but also cyclic AMP–stimulated water flow, a post–cyclic AMP defect may be operant [139]. In fact, demeclocycline has been shown to decrease protein kinase activity; phosphodiesterase activity is mildly diminished as well [52]. The precise biochemical mechanism of demeclocycline, however, has eluded elucidation.

By virtue of its widespread use in the treatment of affective disorders, lithium has emerged as perhaps the most common cause of nephrogenic diabetes insipidus, effecting as many as 50 percent of patients on the drug [140, 141]. There is no evidence that lithium impairs vasopressin release [142, 143]. In terms of the mechanism of its renal action, lithium does not interfere with accumulation of medullary solutes [144]. Thus, an intrinsic tubular defect is postulated. In this regard, lithium decreases vasopressin-stimulated water transport in the perfused cortical collecting duct [145]. An inhibition in adenylate cyclase or in cyclic AMP generation is observed in human tissue [146] and cultured cells [147, 148] exposed to the cation as well as animals chronically treated with lithium [149]. More recently a down-regulation of the vasopressin-regulated water channel (aquaporin) has been described in lithium-treated rats [150]. It is of interest that the urinary aquaporin levels remained low after removal of lithium, in line with the slow recovery of concentrating ability seen in humans [140].

Sickle Cell Anemia. A renal concentrating defect is a common accompaniment of sickle cell anemia and sickle cell trait. Sickling of red blood cells in the hypertonic medullary interstitium with occlusion of the vasa recta appears to cause inner medullary and papillary damage. Microradioangiographic studies have failed to demonstrate vasa recta blood flow in patients with sickle cell disease [151]. The resultant medullary ischemia may impair sodium chloride transport in the ascending limb and thus diminish medullary tonicity. Transfusions of normal blood have been shown to restore renal concentrating capacity in children, thus indicating that the sickled red blood cells have a role in the defect. With more prolonged disease, medullary infarcts occur, and the concentrating defect is no longer reversible with transfusions. The diminished maximal urine osmolality also occurs in sickle cell anemia in association with papillary edema [152], thus providing a situation analogous to experimental papillectomy.

Dietary Abnormalities. As noted in the discussion of primary polydipsia, excessive water intake culminates in an impairment of maximal urinary concentration. While this is most likely due to a decrease in medullary interstitial tonicity, an alteration in the cellular action of vasopressin has not been assessed. A marked restriction in sodium chloride intake also impairs the urinary concentrating mechanism [153]. A similar defect is encountered in states of severe protein restriction [154]. Since urea and sodium chloride account for virtually all interstitial tonicity, their decreased availability may account in large part for the observed defect. A defect in water reabsorption related to decrement in aquaporin expression has been invoked [154a].

Gestational Diabetes Insipidus. A form of diabetes insipidus has been described in pregnancy that is vasopressin unresponsive [155, 156]. This resistance is not due to renal unresponsiveness to the hormone but rather to an increase in circulating vasopressinase, leading to excessive catabolism [157]. Since DDAVP is not affected by the enzyme, this agent can reduce urine flow and can serve as a diagnostic tool of this entity.

Hypodipsic Essential Hypernatremia

The term *hypodipsic essential hypernatremia* has been used to describe the condition in a group of euvolemic hypernatremic patients who have the capacity to release vasopressin and have a normal renal response to the hormone. Most [158, 159], but not all [160], of these patients have cerebral lesions in the vicinity of the hypothalamus. A partial list of causes of the hypodipsia-hypernatremia syndrome is shown in Table 1-5. These patients are characterized by (1) persistent hypernatremia not explained by any apparent extracellular volume loss, (2) absence or attenuation of thirst, (3) partial diabetes insipidus, and (4) a normal renal response to AVP [158–161]. It has been proposed that these patients have a "resetting" of the osmoreceptor, since these patients tend to concentrate and dilute urine at inappropriately high levels of plasma osmolality. However, using the regression analysis of plasma AVP level versus plasma osmolality, it has been shown that in some of these patients the tendency to concentrate and dilute urine at inappropriately high levels of plasma osmolality is due solely to a marked reduction in sensitivity or gain of the osmoregulatory mechanism [162]. In other patients, however, plasma AVP levels fluctuate in a random manner, bearing no apparent relationship to changes in plasma osmolality. Such patients frequently display large swings in serum sodium concentration. It appears that most patients with essential hypernatremia fit one of these two patterns [162, 163] (Fig. 1-15). Both of these groups of patients consistently respond normally to nonosmolar AVP release. These observations suggest that (1) the osmoreceptor must be anatomically as well as functionally separate from the neurosecretory neurons, since a hypothalamic lesion could impair the osmoreceptor but not nonosmotic pathways for AVP release, and (2) the osmoreceptor neurons that regulate vasopressin secretion are not totally synonymous with those that regulate thirst, but they appear to be anatomically close if not overlapping. In the elderly, hypodipsia appears to occur without overt hypothalamic lesions and can culminate in severe hypernatremia [164]. A decre-

Table 1-5. Causes of the hypodipsia-hypernatremia syndrome

Ectopic pinealoma
Dysgerminoma/germinoma
Craniopharyngioma
Teratoma
Meningioma
Metastatic bronchial carcinoma
Eosinophilic granuloma
Schüller-Christian disease
Granulomatous tumor
Hypothalamic neuronal degeneration
Subarachnoid hemorrhage
Posttraumatic carotid cavernous fistula
Microcephaly
Occult hydrocephalus
Head trauma
Aneurysectomy (anterior communicating artery)
Sarcoidosis

Source: M. Levi and T. Berl, Water Metabolism. In H. C. Gonick (ed.), *Current Nephrology.* Vol. 5, p. 37. Copyright © 1982 by Year Book Medical Publishers, Inc., Chicago.

ment in angiotensin II–mediated thirst in the elderly has been suggested [165] as the cause for a well-documented decrement in an osmotically regulated thirst sensitivity [166].

Hypernatremia in Patients with Increased Total Body Sodium

Hypernatremia with increased total body sodium is the least common type of hypernatremia and is usually due to exogenous administration of hypertonic sodium–containing solutes [167] (Table 1-6). Hypernatremia supervenes during resuscitative efforts with hypertonic sodium bicarbonate, inadvertent intravascular infusion of hypertonic saline in therapeutic abortions, inadvertent dialysis against a high sodium concentration dialysate, seawater drowning, and even after ingestion of large quantities of sodium chloride tablets. Patients with primary hyperaldosteronism and Cushing's syndrome have slight, clinically unimportant elevations in serum sodium concentration. As expected, patients with hypernatremia and high total body sodium excrete generous quantities of the cation in the urine.

Signs and Symptoms of Hypernatremia

Hypernatremia always reflects a hyperosmolar state. The most prominent manifestations of hyperosmolar disorders are of a neurologic nature [168]. These follow move-

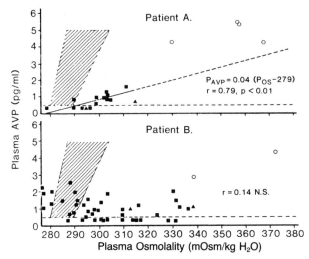

Fig. 1-15. Plasma vasopressin as a function of "effective" plasma osmolality in two patients with adipsic hypernatremia. Effective plasma osmolality was determined by subtracting the contribution of excess urea and glucose, solutes that normally do not stimulate vasopressin release. Open circles represent values obtained on admission; closed squares, values obtained during forced hydration; closed triangles, values obtained after 1–2 weeks of ad libitum water intake; and shaded areas indicate the range of normal values. (From G. L. Robertson, The Physiopathology of ADH Secretion. In G. Tolis et al. [eds.], *Clinical Neuroendocrinology: A Pathophysiological Approach.* New York: Raven, 1979. P. 247.)

ment of water out of cells, resulting in a cellular dehydration, particularly in the brain [169]. The signs and symptoms of hypernatremia are listed in Table 1-7. Restlessness, irritability, depression of sensorium, lethargy, muscular twitching, hyperreflexia, and spasticity may occur and culminate in coma, seizures, and death. The morbidity and mortality of hypernatremia, particularly in the acute forms, are very high [168]. In children, the mortality of acute hypernatremia ranges between 10 and 70 percent, with a mean of approximately 45 percent. Unfortunately, even in survivors neurologic sequelae are common, affecting as many as two-thirds of the children [170]. Mortality in chronic hypernatremia is approximately 10 percent. In adults, acute elevation of serum sodium above 160 mEq/L is associated with a 75 percent mortality, while the mortality in chronic cases is approximately 60 percent. It must be pointed out, however, that in the adult, hypernatremia frequently occurs in the setting of serious underlying diseases, which may be the primary cause of the high mortality. The sequelae of hypernatremia in adults have not been studied systematically.

The signs and symptoms of hypernatremia are most likely related to a variety of anatomic derangements. The loss of volume and shrinkage of brain cells associated with the hyperosmolar states cause tearing of cerebral vessels [171]. In addition to these gross anatomic changes, the brain sustains alterations in the composition of water and solutes that may be of great importance in the pathophysiology of the

Table 1-6. Therapeutic hypertonic solutions

Solute	Molecular weight	Concentration (mg/dl)	Osmolality (mOsm/kg H_2O)	Typical container size (ml)	Use
Sodium chloride	58.5	3 5 20	1026 1711 6845	500 500 250	Emergency treatment of hypotonic states; intra-amniotic instillation for therapeutic abortion
Sodium bicarbonate	84.0	5 7.5	1190 1786	500 50	Treatment of metabolic acidosis, hyperkalemia, cardiopulmonary arrest

Source: Modified from G. Morrison and I. Singer, Hyperosmolal States. In R. G. Narins (ed.), *Clinical Disorders of Fluid and Electrolyte Metabolism*. New York: McGraw-Hill, 1994. Part 1, p. 646.

Table 1-7. Signs and symptoms of hypernatremia

Depression of sensorium
Irritability
Seizures (unusual in adults)
Focal neurologic deficits
Muscle spasticity (unusual in adults)
Signs of volume depletion (variable)
Fever
Nausea or vomiting
Labored respiration
Intense thirst

Source: D. Lanese and I. Teitelbaum, Hypernatremia. In H. R. Jacobson, G. E. Striker, and S. Klahr (eds.), *The Principles and Practice of Nephrology* (2nd ed.). St. Louis: Mosby, 1995. P. 896.

symptoms of hypernatremia [172]. These are responses designed to regulate volume and restore cell size. Thus, the water losses are not as severe as would be predicted. In the early phase, the entry of sodium and chloride into brain cells greatly mitigates the loss of water that would otherwise occur from ideal osmotic behavior [173, 174]. After 7 days of hypernatremia, brain water has returned to control levels as brain osmolality remains elevated. At this time, idiogenic osmoles account for as much as 60 percent of the increase in intracellular osmolality. It now seems possible that some of these idiogenic osmoles are due to an increase in intracellular amino acids [175], particularly taurine [176]. In addition, accumulation of osmolytes such as urea, glutamine, glycerolphosphorylcholine, and *myo*-inositol has been documented in hypernatremic rats [177].

Therapy of Hypernatremia

The primary goal in the treatment of hypernatremia is the restoration of serum tonicity. The specific approach depends on the patient's ECF volume (see Fig. 1–12). The following principles are useful:

1. When the patient has low total body sodium, as evidenced by circulatory manifestations (e.g., orthostatic hypotension), isotonic sodium chloride should be given until systemic hemodynamics are stabilized. Thereafter, the hypernatremia can be treated with 0.45% sodium chloride or 5% dextrose.
2. When the patient is hypervolemic and hypernatremic, the removal of excess sodium is the goal, which can be achieved either by administration of diuretics along with 5% dextrose or, if renal function is impaired, by dialysis.
3. The euvolemic hypernatremic patient who has sustained pure water losses requires water replacement as a 5% dextrose infusion. The water deficit in this setting can be calculated on the basis of the serum sodium concentration and on the assumption that 60 percent of the body's weight is water. Example:

$$\text{Weight} = 75 \text{ kg} \times 0.6 = 45 \text{ L total body water}$$

Serum sodium = 154 mEq/L

The water needed to lower the serum sodium concentration to 140 mEq/L can be calculated as follows:

$$154/140 \times 45 \text{ L} = 49.5 \text{ L}$$
$$49.5 - 45.0 = 4.5 \text{ L}$$

This represents the water deficit and is the net positive water balance necessary to correct the hypernatremia. The water deficit can be expressed in a single equation as follows:

$$\text{Water deficit} = 0.6 \times \text{body weight (kg)} \times (P_{Na}/140 - 1)$$

Thus, $0.6 \times 45 \times (154/140 - 1)$

$45 \times (1.1 - 1)$

$45 \times 0.1 = 4.5 \text{ L}$

The rapidity with which the correction should be made has been a matter of some controversy, primarily as concerns the pediatric population [178]. Most authors feel that it should be achieved in more than 48 hours and at a rate not greater than 2 mOsm/hr. Hypernatremic animals treated rapidly with intravenous solution have a higher incidence of seizures [179]. It is likely that the described cerebral adjustments to hypernatremia, whereby brain water content is corrected and new solutes are generated, contribute to this phenomenon. As extracellular osmolality is rapidly decreased, an osmotic gradient may develop between brain and plasma. This would result in net movement of water into the brain, causing cerebral edema. A slower rate of correction probably can prevent this sequence of events by allowing idiogenic osmoles time to be dissipated.

In patients with essential hypernatremia and the elderly with hypodipsia, 1 to 2 liters of water per day may need to be administered as a prescription. Chlorpropamide itself augments thirst, and its use in conjunction with desmopressin in patients with adipsia has been proposed [180].

Clinical Disorders of Renal Diluting Capacity: Hyponatremic States

While the disorders of renal concentrating capacity described in this chapter may be associated with water depletion and hypernatremia, disorders of renal diluting capacity most frequently present with hyponatremia. Sodium and its accompanying anions account for nearly all the osmotic activity of plasma [181].

Calculated serum osmolality

$$= [2Na^+ + \text{blood urea nitrogen (mg/dl)}/2.8 + \text{glucose (mg/dl)}/18]$$

Thus, while an increase in serum sodium always reflects hyperosmolality, hyponatremia usually is associated with hypo-osmolality. The most common setting in which the serum sodium does not reflect serum osmolality occurs when there is an additional osmolyte such as ethanol, methanol, or ethylene glycol in the extracellular fluid. An osmolar gap is said to be present when the above calculated serum osmolality is more than 10 mOsm lower than the one directly measured by the osmometer [181–183]. It must also be noted that the nature of the solute determines whether there is an increase merely in measured osmolality, whether effective osmolality is also increased, and whether it alters the serum sodium concentration (Table 1-8). Solutes that are permeative across cell membranes such as urea, methanol,

Table 1-8. Relationship between serum tonicity and sodium concentration in the presence of other substances

	Serum tonicity	Serum sodium
Glucose, mannitol, maltose, glycine (translocational hyponatremia)	↑ or ↔	↓
Azotemia (high BUN), ethanol, methanol, ethylene glycol	↑	↔
Pseudohyponatremia (high lipids and protein)	↔	↓

Source: G. L. Robertson and T. Berl, Pathophysiology of Water Metabolism. In B. M. Brenner and F. C. Rector, Jr. (eds.), *The Kidney* (4th ed.). Philadelphia: Saunders, 1991. P. 677.

ethanol, and ethylene glycol do not cause water movement and thus cause hypertonicity without causing cellular dehydration. As such there is no alteration in serum sodium. A high blood urea nitrogen (BUN) and ethanol intoxication are the most common settings in which this occurs. In contrast, glucose, in the insulinopenic state, is not permeative and as such establishes an effective gradient for water to leave the cell and move into the ECF compartment. This process lowers the serum sodium concentration, and hyponatremia can coexist with a normal or even elevated tonicity. Conceptually, this can be viewed as "translocational" hyponatremia, as an alteration in the plasma sodium level does not reflect a change in total body water but rather reflects water movement from the intracellular to the extracellular space. Hyperglycemia accounts for 15 percent of hyponatremia in hospitalized patients. This effect of hyperglycemia must be considered in the interpretation of the serum sodium, and an appropriate correction must be made. The decrease in plasma sodium is approximately 1.6 mEq/L for every 100 mg/dl increase in plasma glucose. As the glucose is lowered, the sodium concentration returns to normal without specific intervention. Similar decrements in serum sodium concentration following the infusion of other osmotically active substances, such as mannitol, maltose, or the absorption of glycine during transurethral prostate resection or hysterectomies, are not infrequent causes of translocational hyponatremia [184].

Pseudohyponatremia occurs when the solid phase of plasma (normally 6–8%) is markedly increased by large increments in serum lipids or protein, as the flame photometer measures sodium concentration of the entire plasma and not just the liquid phase. A rise in plasma lipids of 4.6 g/L will lead to a decrease in sodium concentration of approximately 1 mEq/L. Plasma protein concentrations of greater than 10 g/dl will have a similar effect. The use of a direct ion selective electrode, measuring only the sodium concentration of the liquid phase, eliminates this problem [185].

Hyponatremia is among the most common electrolyte disorders seen in clinical practice [186]. Hyponatremia may be associated with decreased, increased, or near normal amounts of total body sodium [186]. This section will attempt to discuss and categorize the disorders of renal diluting capacity and associated hyponatremia in relationship to total body sodium and ECF volume status. In each instance, the pathogenetic mechanisms that may be involved will be considered.

Disorders of diluting capacity are due to (1) the continued secretion of ADH in spite of the presence of serum hypo-osmolality, which by itself would suppress vasopressin secretion, or (2) intrarenal factors, such as a decrease in GFR or an increase in proximal tubular fluid and sodium reabsorption, or both, which diminish the delivery of fluid to the distal diluting segments of the nephron. A defect in sodium chloride transport out of the water-impermeable portions of the nephron, including the cortical and medullary ascending limb of the loop of Henle, is another intrarenal factor that will impair the nephron's capacity to dilute tubular fluid and urine.

Figure 1-16 summarizes the diagnostic and therapeutic approach to hyponatremia discussed in this chapter. After the patient's hyponatremia is shown to reflect a truly hypotonic state, a thorough history and physical examination to assess the volume status of the patient with hyponatremia are essential. Once the patient is placed in one of the three categories (edematous states, hypovolemic states, or

41

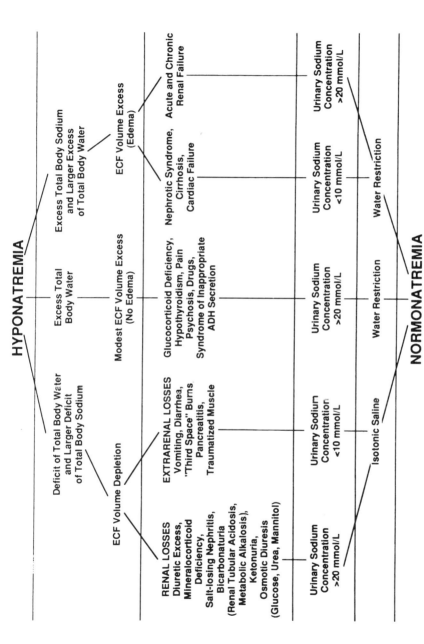

Fig. 1-16. Diagnostic and therapeutic approach to the hyponatremic patient. (From T. Berl, R. J. Anderson, K. M. McDonald, and R. W. Schrier. Clinical disorders of water metabolism. *Kidney Int.* 10:117, 1976.)

neither), the diagnostic possibilities are narrowed to a great extent. Examination of the urinary sodium concentration provides supportive evidence for the diagnosis. This diagnostic approach to hyponatremia also makes the appropriate therapy easy to define [187].

Hyponatremia Associated with Low Total Body Sodium

In addition to hypothalamic osmoreceptors, another "physiologic" control of ADH release is the person's volume status (see Fig. 1-8). As already discussed, when the osmoreceptor and volume receptors for control of ADH receive opposing stimuli, the effect of the volume receptors on ADH release generally predominates. Thus, in the presence of hypovolemia, ADH release is stimulated and water is retained, even at the expense of the occurrence of hypo-osmolality. The glossopharyngeal afferent pathways from the aortic arch and carotid sinus are the main pathways whereby changes in arterial pressure are associated with alterations in ADH [188]. Receptors in the left atrium that are also present may modulate vagal afferent tone and ADH release [189]. In the presence of volume depletion, a fall in pressure at the level of both the arterial baroreceptors and the left atrium may inhibit afferent neural tone, an effect known to stimulate ADH release [189]. Thus, the baroreceptor-stimulated secretion of vasopressin, coupled with high water intake (either oral or parenteral), culminates in hyponatremia.

Gastrointestinal and Third Space Losses

The presence of hypovolemia, as judged by weight loss, orthostatic hypotension and tachycardia, and decreased central venous pressure, in association with hyponatremia, raises the question as to the source of the fluid and electrolyte losses. There are primarily two main sources for such losses, the kidney and the gastrointestinal tract. In the presence of gastrointestinal losses (through either vomiting or diarrhea), the kidney responds by conserving sodium chloride. A similar pattern is observed with sequestration of fluids into third spaces, as the peritoneal cavity in peritonitis and pancreatitis or the bowel lumen with ileus and burns. In these entities, if renal function is normal, the urinary sodium concentration should be less than 10 mEq/L and usually is as low as 1 to 3 mEq/L. The urine osmolality should also be in the hyperosmolar range. An exception is with vomiting and metabolic alkalosis in which bicarbonaturia is present. The urinary bicarbonate anion obligates cations and therefore may be associated with a urinary sodium concentration greater than 20 mEq/L. The urinary chloride concentration, however, will be less than 10 mEq/L. Ketonuria with starvation or diabetes also can obligate renal sodium loss despite the presence of hypovolemia. Also, if renal function is severely impaired, examination of the urinary sodium chloride concentration and osmolality may be misleading. In this setting, the damaged kidney may not possess the capacity for maximal conservation of sodium chloride or concentration of urine [190].

Diuretics

The kidney may sometimes be the source of the fluid and electrolyte losses. Excessive use of diuretics is one of the most common situations in which hyponatremia is associated with hypovolemia [191]. Advanced age in underweight women appears to be an important risk factor [191, 192]. Hyponatremia occurs almost exclusively with thiazide rather than loop diuretics, presumably because the former do not affect urinary concentrate but the latter do. Hyponatremia supervenes within 14 days of initiating diuretic therapy [193, 194]. Diuretics cause hyponatremia by at least three mechanisms: (1) volume depletion, which will result in impaired water excretion by both an enhanced antidiuretic hormone release and decreased fluid delivery to the diluting segment, (2) a direct effect of diuretics on the diluting segment, and (3) potassium depletion. The mechanism whereby potassium depletion itself leads to hyponatremia is not entirely understood. It appears, however, that it can occur independently of the sodium depletion that frequently accompanies diuretic use [195]. An effect of hypokalemia to increase water intake [122] could aggravate any of the aforementioned mechanisms. It must be noted that the concomitant administration of potassium-sparing diuretics does not prevent the development of hyponatremia [191]. Although the diagnosis of diuretic-induced hyponatremia is frequently obvious, surreptitious diuretic abuse is being increasingly recognized and should be considered in patients whose other electrolyte abnormalities and high urinary chloride excretion suggest this possibility.

Salt-Losing Nephritis

Salt-losing nephritis is another condition with which hyponatremia and hypovolemia may be associated. In most circumstances, salt-losing nephritis is associated with advanced chronic renal failure (GFR < 10 ml/min). With certain diseases, such as medullary cystic disease, polycystic disease, analgesic nephropathy, obstructive nephropathy, and chronic pyelonephritis, however, salt-losing nephritis may occur with less severe renal impairment. The term *salt-losing nephritis* has been used to describe a wide variety of conditions, and thus the following classifications may be helpful.

In most patients with chronic renal failure and a GFR of less than 10 to 15 ml/min, the rapidity of the renal response to a low sodium intake is blunted, and the minimal urinary sodium concentration achieved is often higher than expected with normal renal function [190]. In normal subjects placed on a low-sodium diet, urinary sodium concentration decreases to a level of 1 to 3 mEq/L within 3 to 5 days. In contrast, patients with advanced chronic renal failure may need 7 to 21 days to achieve a minimal urinary sodium concentration, and this minimal level may be greater than 10 to 15 mEq/L [190]. These patients may then be classified as mild renal salt-wasters, and they constitute the most common category of subjects with advanced renal failure. With water balance maintained constant, the negative sodium balance in these patients is not of a degree sufficient to cause severe hyponatremia. Other patients with advanced renal failure exhibit an even greater degree of impairment in sodium conservation and, when they are placed on a low-sodium diet, develop progressive hyponatremia [190]. As in the milder cases, these patients are capable of maintaining sodium balance when on a normal sodium intake and exhibit hyponatremia only with dietary sodium restriction or extrarenal sodium losses. They may thus be classified as moderate renal salt-wasters. Finally, there are a few reports in the literature of patients who must receive large supplemental intakes of sodium to avoid volume depletion and hyponatremia [196]. When these cases were first described, the presence of renal salt-wasting, increased skin pigmentation, hypotension, and hyponatremia suggested the diagnosis of Addison's disease [196]. These rare patients may be classified as severe renal salt-wasters.

Certain patients with renal tubular acidosis, particularly that of the proximal or type II variety, may exhibit renal sodium and potassium wastage despite only modest decreases in GFR [197]. These patients have prominent bicarbonaturia because of a defect in the proximal tubule affecting the reclamation of bicarbonate (see Chap. 3). As already mentioned, bicarbonate is a relatively impermeative anion that obligates the renal excretion of cations, including primarily sodium and potassium. In this setting of renal tubular acidosis, the bicarbonaturia obligates the excretion of sodium, so that a minimal urinary sodium concentration is not achieved despite the presence of hypovolemia.

Mineralocorticoid Deficiency

A finding of hyponatremia and ECF volume depletion also suggests the possibility of primary adrenal insufficiency, particularly in the presence of a urinary sodium concentration higher than minimal, that is, greater than 20 mEq/L. Because of the mineralocorticoid deficiency, a diminished urinary excretion of potassium and hyperkalemia is an indication that primary adrenal insufficiency is the cause of the hyponatremia. It is worthy of mention that when hypopituitarism is associated with hyponatremia, urinary sodium concentration may become minimal, since mineralocorticoid function is intact.

The mechanisms whereby adrenal insufficiency impairs renal water excretion have been the subject of considerable debate [198]. Results of recent studies in adrenalectomized dogs suggest that mineralocorticoid deficiency and an associated negative sodium balance are at least partially responsible for impaired water excretion and hyponatremia. Continued ADH secretion mediates this effect of sodium depletion on renal water excretion [198]. ECF volume depletion with increased ADH and diminished renal hemodynamics mediate the effect of mineralocorticoid deficiency to cause hyponatremia, while glucocorticoid deficiency causes ADH-mediated hyponatremia independent of volume depletion (see Hyponatremia with Normal Total Body Sodium).

Osmotic Diuresis

An osmotic diuresis also can lead to urinary losses of sodium and water, volume depletion, and hyponatremia in the face of either oral or parenteral water intake. The uncontrolled diabetic patient with glucosuria, the patient with a urea diuresis after relief of urinary tract obstruction, and the patient undergoing a mannitol diuresis [199] are examples of such causes of hyponatremia. The urinary sodium concentration is generally greater than 20 mEq/L because the osmotic diuresis obligates cation excretion in spite of concomitant volume depletion. In patients with diabetes, the sodium wasting caused by the glycosuria can be accentuated by ketonuria as β-hydroxybutyrate and acetoacetate, which also obligate urinary electrolyte losses. Ketonuria may also contribute to the renal sodium wasting and hyponatremia seen in starvation and alcoholic ketoacidosis [200].

Hyponatremia Associated with Increased Total Body Sodium

Hyponatremia is perhaps most frequently observed in the edematous disorders. In this setting, both total body sodium and total body water are increased, but total body water is increased to a greater extent. Since diuretics are used frequently in edematous disorders, hyponatremia presents a diagnostic dilemma as to whether the impairment in water excretion is due to the diuretic therapy or to the primary disease. This is because the edematous disorders, including cirrhosis, cardiac failure, and nephrotic syndrome, may impair renal water excretion and be associated with hyponatremia in the absence of diuretic use.

Congestive Heart Failure

The common association between congestive heart failure and sodium and water retention is well established [201–205]. The hyponatremia may be mediated by either a decreased delivery of tubular fluid to the distal nephron or an increased release of vasopressin, or both.

In an experimental model of low cardiac output, both AVP and diminished delivery to the diluting segment were found to be important in mediating the abnormality in water excretion [206]. It thus appears that the decrement in "effective arterial blood volume" [205, 207] with the decrease in arterial filling being sensed by aortic and carotid sinus baroreceptors causes stimulation of vasopressin release. This stimulation must supersede the inhibition in ADH release that accompanies at least acute distention of the left atrium [208]. In fact, there is evidence that chronic distention of the atria blunts the sensitivity of the atrial receptors [207], and therefore the effects of the high-pressure baroreceptors may act in an uninhibited manner to stimulate vasopressin release. Experiments using an AVP antagonist in a model of low cardiac output also point to an important role for the hormone in abnormal urinary dilution [209].

A number of studies have demonstrated elevated AVP levels in patients with heart failure [210–212]. Likewise, the mRNA message for AVP preprohormone is elevated in the hypothalamus of animals with chronic heart failure [213]. It is most likely that nonosmotic pathways, whose activation is suggested by the increase in sympathetic activity seen in congestive heart failure [214, 215], are the mediator of the hormone's release. Thus, an improvement of cardiac function with afterload reduction decreased AVP levels and improved water excretion in such patients [216]. The normalization of the serum sodium concentration in hyponatremic patients with heart failure receiving captopril either with [217] or without [218] diuretics is most likely explained by these mechanisms. A decrease in AVP levels also accompanied improvement of cardiac function by hemofiltration. The effect of the recently described orally active V_2 antagonist OPC-31260 [219] in these patients is highly awaited.

Hepatic Failure

Patients with advanced cirrhosis and ascites frequently present with hyponatremia as a consequence of their inability to excrete a water load [201, 204, 205, 220–222]. Since plasma volume expansion precedes ascites formation, the classic underfilling theory whereby ascites formation causes plasma volume depletion with resultant renal sodium retention has been discarded. Moreover, the overflow theory of sodium retention in cirrhosis is unlikely since in cirrhosis the activation of the neural humoral axis of norepinephrine, renin-angiotensin-aldosterone, and the nonosmotic stimulation of vasopressin does not suggest expansion of the intravascular space. The peripheral arterial vasodilation theory of sodium and water retention in cirrhosis therefore has been proposed [220–223]. In this theory, which has been accepted by many major experts in the field, splanchnic arterial vasodilation occurs very early in cirrhosis and leads to arterial underfilling, with activation of the above neurohumoral axis, leading to sodium and water retention (see Chap. 2).

As with cardiac failure, the relative role of intrarenal and extrarenal factors in the impaired water excretion has been a matter of controversy [201]. Experimental models of deranged liver function have demonstrated a predominant role for AVP secretion in the pathogenesis of the disorder. Also an increment in mRNA in the hypothalamus of cirrhotic rats has been reported [224]. In some of these studies, however, a small vasopressin-independent intrarenal mechanism has also contributed to the defective water excretion [201].

While patients with cirrhosis who have no edema or ascites excrete a water load normally [225], those with ascites usually do not. Two studies have demonstrated elevated AVP levels in such patients [226, 227]. Patients who had a defect in water excretion had higher levels of vasopressin as well as higher plasma renin activity, plasma aldosterone, and norepinephrine. Likewise, their serum albumin concentration was lower, as was their urinary excretion of sodium, all suggesting a decrease in effective arterial blood volume. Sympathetic tone is high in cirrhosis [228]. In fact, the plasma concentration of norepinephrine, a good index of baroreceptor sympathetic activity in humans, appears to correlate well with the levels of AVP and the excretion of water [229]. These studies therefore offer strong support for the view that effective arterial blood volume is contracted rather than expanded in decompensated cirrhosis [230]. This view is further strengthened by the improved water excretion that accompanies head-out water immersion, a maneuver that translocates peripheral fluid to the central blood volume [201]. In fact, the combination of head-out water immersion and maintenance of peripheral vascular resistance with an infusion of norepinephrine normalizes water excretion in decompensated cirrhotic patients [231].

Nephrotic Syndrome

The incidence of hyponatremia in the nephrotic syndrome is lower than in either congestive heart failure or cirrhosis [201]. An elevated level of plasma vasopressin has also been shown to occur in patients with nephrotic syndrome [232]. In view of the alterations in Starling forces that accompany hypoalbuminemia and that allow transudation of salt and water across capillary membranes into the interstitial space, patients with the nephrotic syndrome have been considered to have intravascular volume contraction. The possibility that such volume contraction stimulates vasopressin release was suggested by studies in which neck-out water immersion increased water excretion in nephrotic subjects [233]. However, this mechanism may not be applicable to all patients with the disorder. Some patients with the nephrotic syndrome have been shown to have increased plasma volumes with suppressed plasma renin activity and aldosterone levels [234, 235]. It appears likely that the underfilling mechanism is operant in patients with normal GFR, while those nephrotic patients with decreased renal function may retain sodium and water and become hypervolemic. The incidence of hyponatremia and its pathogenesis in these patients remain unexplored. However, a correlation between the decrement in blood volume and increased plasma vasopressin concentrations has been reported in adult nephrotic patients of different causes but with normal GFR [232]. Also, in nephrotic rats, AVP mRNA is elevated in the hypothalamus [236].

Advanced Chronic Renal Failure

The combination of hyponatremia and edema also may occur in patients with advanced renal failure whether due to acute or chronic renal failure [117, 237]. Unlike subjects with edematous disorders, these patients do not have a minimal urinary sodium concentration because of the accompanying tubular dysfunction. The chronically diseased kidney may also exhibit a profound increase in fractional sodium excretion in an effort to maintain sodium balance despite its reduced number of functioning nephrons [120]. Generally edema develops because larger intakes of sodium are ingested than can be excreted by the diseased kidneys, which are filtering only a fraction of the amount of sodium filtered by normal kidneys. For example, at a GFR of 100 ml/min (144 L/day) and a plasma sodium concentration of 140 mEq/L, the daily filtered load of sodium (GFR $\times$ plasma sodium concentration) is 20,160 mEq. With a reduction in GFR to 5 ml/min, the daily amount of sodium filtered is only 1008 mEq. Obviously the fractional excretion of sodium necessary to maintain sodium balance is much greater in the latter circumstance.

The narrow range of water-handling by the diseased kidney is probably also due in large part to the smaller volumes of fluid that are filtered daily by the diseased kidney. At a GFR of 5 ml/min, only 7.2 liters of filtrate is formed daily, and perhaps 30 percent, or 2.2 liters, of this filtered fluid will reach the diluting segment of the nephron. Thus, even with total suppression of ADH and water impermeability of the collecting duct, a maximum of 2.2 liters of solute-free water could be excreted daily. If the daily water intake exceeds this volume, plus insensible losses, a positive water balance and hyponatremia will occur. Thus, in advanced chronic renal failure, the volume of fluid filtered and delivered to the diluting segment is of paramount importance to the renal capacity to excrete water. While most patients with advanced renal failure (GFR $<$ 10 ml/min) have little capacity to concentrate urine, some capacity to dilute urine may be preserved [190]. As should be apparent from the foregoing discussion, however, the capacity to maintain water balance is dependent not only on the ability to dilute urine but also on the quantitative capacity of the kidney to excrete C_{H_2O}. With acute renal failure, the near absence of GFR provides a sufficient explanation for the virtual absence of the kidney to respond to a water load.

Hyponatremia with Normal Total Body Sodium

Figure 1-16 lists the causes of euvolemic hyponatremia.

Glucocorticoid Deficiency

Glucocorticoid deficiency is important in the impaired water excretion of primary and secondary adrenal insufficiency [77]. An elevation of AVP levels accompanies the water excretory defect of anterior pituitary insufficiency [238], and particularly adrenocorticotropic hormone deficiency [239], which is corrected by physiologic doses of glucocorticoids [240]. A sensitive radioimmunoassay technique has demonstrated inappropriately elevated levels of ADH in association with pure glucocorticoid hormone deficiency in the absence of ECF volume depletion [241]. It seems clear, however, that ADH-independent factors also are involved in impaired water excretion with glucocorticoid deficiency. Whereas the ADH-dependent component may be observed in adrenalectomized, mineralocorticoid-replaced rats deprived of glucocorticoid hormone for 24 hours, an ADH-independent impairment in water excretion occurs after 2 weeks of glucocorticoid deficiency in ADH-deficient Brattleboro rats. The ADH-independent effect is associated with impaired renal hemodynamics and decreased distal fluid delivery to the diluting segment of the nephron [242]. An inhibitor of the hydro-osmotic effect of vasopressin has demonstrated similar vasopressin-dependent and independent mechanisms [243].

Hypothyroidism

Hyponatremia may develop in some patients with hypothyroidism, even in the absence of cardiac failure. Several mechanisms have been proposed to explain this impaired diluting capacity with hypothyroidism [77]. Studies in hypothyroid humans [244] and hypothyroid rats [245] have demonstrated elevated radioimmunoassayable titers of vasopressin, thus implicating ADH in the impaired water excretion associated with thyroid hormone deficiency. On the other hand, studies of osmoregulation in hypothyroid patients have found that both the threshold [246] and the sensitivity of the vasopressin response are intact [247]. Such an observation incriminates an intrarenal hemodynamic disturbance as suggested by studies in hypothyroid vasopressin-deficient Brattleboro rats [248]. Although increased tubular sensitivity to AVP in hypothyroidism has been proposed, an actual resistance has been described. This resistance appears to be mediated by a defective generation in AVP-stimulated cyclic AMP generation in the thick ascending limb of hypothyroid rats [249]. Thus, other factors must override this AVP resistance and lead to hyponatremia in hypothyroidism. Taken together, the available studies suggest that both an intrarenal mechanism (e.g., decreased GFR) and a persistent AVP release may be operant in the hyponatremia associated with severe hypothyroidism, for example, myxedema.

Psychosis

Acutely psychotic patients, particularly those with schizophrenia, are at risk of developing hyponatremia [250]. This risk is enhanced by the propensity of these patients to increase their water intake. The incidence of hyponatremia in this population is unknown. The elucidation of the mechanism has been confounded, since the possible contribution of pharmacologic agents, such as thiazide and carbamazepine, are frequently implicated [251]. However, reports of psychotic patients with water intoxication who are not taking medications also exist. The mechanism of the hyponatremia associated with psychosis thus appears to be multifactorial [252]. Thirst perception is increased, there is a mild defect in osmoregulation that causes AVP to be secreted at lower osmolality, and the renal response to AVP may be enhanced. While each derangement alone would be insufficient to cause overt hyponatremia, their combination very well may [253].

Postoperative Hyponatremia

It is being increasingly recognized that the incidence of hospital-acquired, and particularly postoperative, hyponatremia [254, 255] is high. Most of the patients are euvolemic and have measurable AVP levels [255, 256]. In most of the patients, the hyponatremia is asymptomatic; but, as will be discussed, there is a subgroup of postoperative women with cerebral edema who have seizures and hypoxia with catastrophic neurologic events [257].

Pharmacologic Agents

Drugs associated with water retention are listed in Table 1-9. Some cause water retention by releasing vasopressin, others by potentiating ADH action. One of

Table 1-9. Drugs associated with hyponatremia

Antidiuretic hormone analogues
   Deamino-D-arginine vasopressin
   Oxytocin
Drugs that enhance antidiuretic hormone release
   Chlorpropamide
   Clofibrate
   Carbamazepine-oxycarbazepine
   Vincristine
   Nicotine
   Narcotics
   Antipsychotic/antidepressants*
   Ifosfamide
Drugs that potentiate renal action of antidiuretic hormone
   Chlorpropamide
   Cyclophosphamide
   Non-steroidal anti-inflammatory drugs
   Acetaminophen
Drugs that cause hyponatremia by unknown mechanisms
   Haloperidol
   Fluphenazine
   Amitriptyline
   Thioridazine
   Fluoxetine

* Antidiuretic hormone release may be secondary to underlying pyschosis.
Source: J. H. Veis, and T. Berl, Hyponatremia. In H. R. Jacobson, G. E. Striker, and S. Klahr (eds.), *The Principles and Practice of Nephrology* (2nd ed.) St. Louis: Mosby, 1995. P. 890.

the drugs that is frequently associated with hyponatremia is chlorpropamide. The incidence of mild hyponatremia in patients on this drug may be as high as 7 percent, but severe hyponatremia (<130 mEq/L) occurs in only 2 percent [258]. The drug increases urinary concentration in patients with central, but not nephrogenic, diabetes insipidus [259] by enhancing the renal effect of the hormone, perhaps by up-regulating the vasopressin receptor [260]. Alternatively, studies in chlorpropamide-treated animals have suggested an effect of the drug to enhance solute reabsorption in the medullary ascending limb, thereby increasing interstitial tonicity and the osmotic driving force for water reabsorption rather than a cyclic AMP–mediated alteration in collecting duct water permeability [261]. The anticonvulsant carbamazepine [262] as well as oxycarbazepine [263] also has antidiuretic properties. Both central and renal mechanisms have been proposed [95]. An increasing number of antipsychotic agents have been associated with hyponatremia, and they are frequently implicated in an explanation for the water intoxication in psychotic patients. The role of the drugs in the etiology of the impaired water excretion in patients receiving the agents has not been dissociated, in most cases, from the role of the underlying psychiatric disorder for which the patient is receiving the drug. Therefore, while the clinical association between antipsychotic drugs and hyponatremia is frequently encountered, the pharmacologic agents themselves may not be the primary factors responsible for the water retention. Furthermore, the mechanism whereby they cause hyponatremia is not known.

Several drugs used in cancer treatment also caused an antidiuresis. The effect of vincristine on ADH release may be mediated by the neurotoxicity of the drug. The antidiuresis caused by cyclophosphamide seems to be temporally related to the excretion of a metabolite, though nausea-mediated ADH release may also be involved. It is important to be aware of potential acute hyponatremia in cyclophosphamide-treated patients who are vigorously hydrated to avert urologic complications. The cyclophosphamide analogue ifosfamide can also cause hyponatremia [265].

Syndrome of Inappropriate Antidiuretic Hormone Secretion

Pathophysiology. The chronic administration of AVP when accompanied with intake of water culminates in the development of hyponatremia (Fig. 1-17). It is of interest that, as depicted in Figure 1-17, the continued administration of AVP is accompanied by a decline in the hydro-osmotic effect of the hormone as urine osmolality falls and serum sodium stabilizes, a phenomenon denoted as vasopressin escape [269]. A down-regulation of receptors [270], possibly by activation of an inhibitory G protein, has been suggested [271]. In addition to a renal mechanism, however, a decrease in hypothalamic vasopressin in RNA has also been described in chronic hyponatremia [272].

Clinical Settings. The diagnosis of SIADH is made primarily by excluding other causes of hyponatremia [186]. A diagnosis of SIADH should be considered in the absence of hypovolemia, edematous disorders, endocrine dysfunction (including primary and secondary adrenal insufficiency and hypothyroidism), renal failure, and drugs, all of which may impair water excretion. In Table 1-10 are listed various diseases in which SIADH may occur. These associated diseases generally fall into three categories: malignancies, pulmonary disorders, and central nervous system

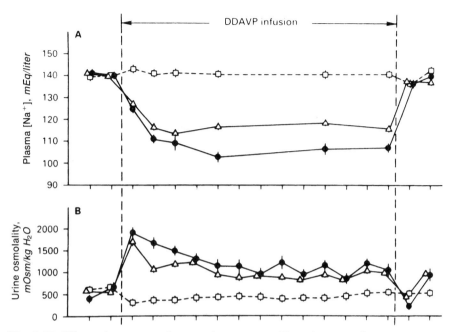

Fig. 1-17. Effects of pitressin and water administration. Note that urine flow increases, urine osmolality decreases, and serum sodium stabilizes. DDAVP = desmopressin acetate. (From J. G. Verbalis and M. Drutarosky, Adaptation to chronic hypo-osmolality in rats. *Kidney Int.* 34:351, 1988.)

disorders. In addition, an increasing number of patients with AIDS are being reported to have hyponatremia [273]. In patients with SIADH, the urine is concentrated despite the presence of hyponatremia. The urinary sodium concentration generally is greater than 20 mEq/L, but if the patients are placed on a low-sodium diet or become volume depleted, the urinary sodium concentration may decrease to less than 1 mEq/L [274].

It has now become apparent that most patients with SIADH have a defect in the osmoregulation of vasopressin. Robertson [162] has reported plasma vasopressin measurements in 106 patients who fulfilled the clinical criteria for the diagnosis of SIADH before the correction of their hyponatremia. In the vast majority, plasma vasopressin concentration was inadequately suppressed relative to the hypotonicity present. Interestingly, in most patients, plasma vasopressin was between 1 and 10 pg/ml, the same range as in normally hydrated, healthy adults, which indicates that inappropriate secretion often can be demonstrated only by measuring vasopressin under hypotonic conditions. Even with this approach, however, abnormalities in plasma vasopressin were not apparent in almost 10 percent of the patients with clinical evidence of SIADH. In an effort to define better the nature of the osmoregulatory defect in these patients, Robertson obtained additional measurements of plasma vasopressin during the infusion of hypertonic saline. When this method of

Table 1-10. Disorders associated with the syndrome of inappropriate antidiuretic hormone secretion

Carcinomas	Pulmonary disorders	Central nervous system disorders
Bronchogenic carcinoma	Viral pneumonia	Encephalitis (viral or bacterial)
Carcinoma of the duodenum	Bacterial pneumonia	Meningitis (viral, bacterial, tuberculous, and fungal)
	Pulmonary abscess	
Carcinoma of the pancreas	Tuberculosis	Carcinoma of the ureter
	Aspergillosis	Head trauma
Thymoma	Positive pressure breathing	Brain abscess
Cardinoma of the stomach		Brain tumors
	Asthma	Guillain-Barré syndrome
Lymphoma	Pneumothorax	Acute intermittent porphyria
Ewing's sarcoma	Mesothelioma	Subarachnoid hemorrhage or subdural hematoma
Carcinoma of the bladder	Cystic fibrosis	
		Cerebellar and cerebral atrophy
Prostatic carcinoma		Cavernous sinus thrombosis
Oropharyngeal tumor		Neonatal hypoxia
		Hydrocephalus
		Shy-Drager syndrome
		Rocky Mountain spotted fever
		Delirium tremens
		Cerebrovascular accident (cerebral thrombosis or hemorrhage)
		Acute psychosis
		Peripheral neuropathy
		Multiple sclerosis

Source: M. Levi and T. Berl, Water Metabolism. In H. C. Gonick (ed.), *Current Nephrology.* Vol. 5, p. 45. Copyright © 1982 by Year Book Medical Publishers, Inc., Chicago.

analysis was applied to 25 patients with SIADH, four different types of osmoregulatory defects were identified.

As seen in Figure 1-18, in type I, the infusion of hypertonic saline was associated with large and erratic fluctuations in plasma vasopressin, which bore no relationship to the rise in plasma osmolality. This pattern was found in 6 of 25 patients studied, who had acute respiratory failure, bronchogenic carcinoma, pulmonary tuberculosis, schizophrenia, and rheumatoid arthritis. This pattern indicates that the secretion of vasopressin either had been totally divorced from osmoreceptor control or was responding to some periodic nonosmotic stimulus. A completely different type of osmoregulatory defect is exemplified by type II response, as seen in Figure 1-18. The infusion of hypertonic saline resulted in a prompt and progressive rise in plasma osmolality. Regression analysis showed the precision and sensitivity of this response to be essentially the same as in healthy subjects but the intercept or threshold value at 253 mOsm/kg to be well below the normal range. This pattern, which reflects the "resetting of the osmoreceptor," was found in 9 of the 25 patients who had the

Physiopathology of ADH Secretion

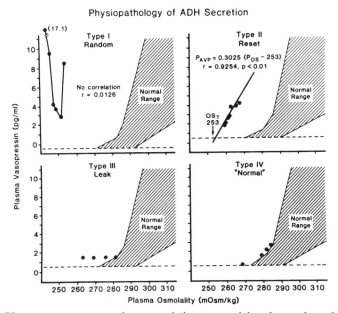

Fig. 1-18. Plasma vasopressin as a function of plasma osmolality during the infusion of hypertonic saline in four groups of patients with clinical syndrome of inappropriate antidiuretic hormone secretion (SIADH). Shaded area is range of normal values. (From G. L. Robertson, The Physiopathology of ADH Secretion. In G. Tolis et al. [eds.], *Clinical Neuroendocrinology: A Pathophysiological Approach.* New York: Raven, 1979. P. 247.)

diagnosis of bronchogenic carcinoma, cerebrovascular disease, tuberculous meningitis, acute respiratory disease, and carcinoma of the pharynx. Another patient with hyponatremia and acute idiopathic polyneuritis had an identical pattern to a hypertonic saline infusion and was determined to have resetting of the osmoreceptor. This and other patients with a reset osmostat have been able to dilute their urine maximally and sustain a urine flow sufficient to prevent a further increase in body water. Thus, an abnormality in AVP regulation can exist in spite of the ability to dilute the urine maximally and excrete a water load, a situation reminiscent of the hypotonicity seen in pregnancy.

As seen in Figure 1-18, in the type III response, plasma vasopressin was elevated initially but did not change during the infusion of hypertonic saline until plasma osmolality reached the normal range. At that point, plasma AVP began to rise appropriately, indicating a normally functioning osmoreceptor mechanism. This response was found in 8 of the 25 patients with the diagnosis of central nervous system disease, bronchogenic carcinoma, carcinoma of the pharynx, pulmonary tuberculosis, and schizophrenia. Its pathogenesis is unknown, but it was speculated that this variety of SIADH may be due to a constant, nonsuppressible leak of AVP despite otherwise normal osmoregulatory function. Unlike type II, or the resetting type of defect, it results in impaired urinary dilution and water excretion.

As seen in Figure 1-18, in the type IV response, the osmoregulation of vasopressin appeared to be completely normal despite the marked inability to excrete a water load. The plasma AVP was appropriately suppressed under hypotonic conditions and did not rise until plasma osmolality reached the normal threshold level. When this procedure was reversed by water loading, plasma osmolality and plasma AVP again fell normally, but urinary dilution did not occur and the water load was not excreted. This defect was present in 2 out of 25 patients with the diagnosis of bronchogenic carcinoma and diabetes mellitus. This finding may indicate that in these patients the antidiuretic defect was due to some abnormality other than inappropriate secretion of AVP and could be due to either increased renal tubular sensitivity to AVP or the existence of an antidiuretic substance other than AVP. Alteratively, the possibility that the assay was not sufficiently sensitive to detect significant levels of AVP must also be considered.

Signs and Symptoms of Hyponatremia

The most common signs and symptoms of hyponatremia are listed in Table 1-11. Most patients with hyponatremia are asymptomatic. Although gastrointestinal complaints occur early, the majority of the manifestations of hyponatremia are of a neuropsychiatric nature and include lethargy, psychosis, seizures, and coma. Elderly and young children with hyponatremia are most likely to become symptomatic. It has also become apparent that neurologic complications occur more frequently in menstruating women. In a case-control study, despite approximately equal incidence of postoperative hyponatremia in males and females, 97 percent of those with permanent brain damage were women and 75 percent of them were menstruant [275]. The severity of symptoms is also dependent on the rate at which serum sodium concentration is lowered. There is considerable disagreement as to the mortality of acute hyponatremia. This has been reported to be as high as 50 percent and as low as 3 percent [276]. There is general agreement that the mortality of chronic hyponatremia in hospitalized patients is between 10 and 27 percent [237, 254, 277].

Table 1-11. Symptoms and signs that may be associated with hyponatremia

Symptoms	Signs
Lethargy, apathy	Abnormal sensorium
Disorientation	Depressed deep tendon reflexes
Muscle cramps	Cheyne-Stokes respiration
Anorexia, nausea	Hypothermia
Agitation	Pathologic reflexes
	Pseudobulbar palsy
	Seizures

Source: T. Berl, R. J. Anderson, K. M. McDonald, and R. W. Schrier, Clinical disorders of water metabolism. *Kidney Int.* 10: 117, 1976.

Furthermore, the deaths are generally due to the underlying disorder rather than the hyponatremia per se. While no predictable correlation exists between changes in sensorium and the degree of hyponatremia [278], most patients who have seizures and coma have plasma sodium concentrations of less than 120 mEq/L. The signs and symptoms are most likely related to the cellular swelling and cerebral edema that are associated with hyponatremia [169]. In fact, such cerebral edema with occasional herniation has been noted in postmortem examination of both humans [257] and experimental animals [278]. It is of note, however, that in the animal studies the increase in brain water was less marked than would be predicted from the decrease in tonicity if the brain were to operate as a passive osmometer. The volume regulatory responses that protect against cerebral edema have been extensively studied and reviewed [268, 279]. Studies in rats demonstrate a prompt loss of both electrolyte and organic osmolytes after the onset of hyponatremia [280]. While some of the osmolyte losses occur within 24 hours [281], the loss of such solutes becomes more marked in subsequent days (Fig. 1-19) and account for almost complete restoration of cerebral water. The electrolytes and other osmolytes lost in the adaptation to hyponatremia are shown in Figure 1-20. The rate at which the brain restores the lost electrolytes and osmolytes when hyponatremia is corrected is of great pathophysiologic importance. Sodium and chloride recover quickly and even overshoot [280, 282]. However, the reaccumulation of osmolytes is considerably delayed (Fig. 1-19). This process is likely to account for the more marked cerebral dehydration that accompanies the correction in previously adapted animals.

Therapy of Hyponatremia

The treatment of hyponatremia has been the subject of considerable interest and controversy [276, 283]. The strategy is dictated by both the underlying cause of the disorder and the clinical severity. Unfortunately, the identification of the underlying pathology is not immediately evident. Management should be based on whether the patient is or is not symptomatic and whether the disorder is acute or chronic [184].

Symptomatic Hyponatremia

Acute. The neurologic symptoms of acute hyponatremia are most commonly seen in premenopausal females in the postoperative state [257, 275], in elderly persons on thiazide diuretics [192], and in patients with psychogenic polydipsia [285]. It is generally agreed that these patients should be treated promptly. In this setting, the risks of cerebral edema and seizures outweigh any risk of rapid correction. The mortality rate in these patients is considerable, and those that survive frequently do so with neurologic residual [257]. The female preponderance of the syndrome is not fully understood. The volume adaptive response whereby the brain decreases its volume in acute hyponatremia may be inhibited by female hormones [286]. A contribution of hypoxia may also be important, since in experimental animals when hypoxia is combined with hyponatremia the volume adaptive response is abrogated, resulting in brain edema and increased mortality [287]. Since the neurologic compli-

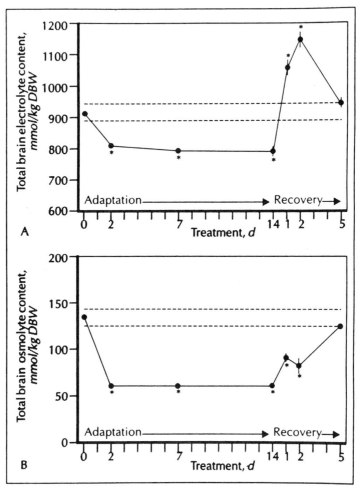

Fig. 1-19. Comparison of changes in brain electrolyte (A) and organic osmolyte (B) contents during adaptation to hyponatremia and after rapid correction of hyponatremia in rats. Both electrolytes and organic osmolytes are lost quickly following the induction of hyponatremia beginning on day 0. Brain content of both solutes remains depressed during maintenance of hyponatremia from days 2 through 14. After rapid correction of the hyponatremia on day 14, electrolytes reaccumulate rapidly and overshoot normal brain contents on the first 2 days after correction before returning to normal levels by the fifth day after correction. In contrast, brain organic osmolytes recover much more slowly and do not return to normal brain contents until the fifth day after correction. The dotted lines indicate ±SEM from the mean values of normonatremic rats on day 0. Asterisks denote $p < 0.01$ compared with brain contents of normonatremic rats. DBW = dry brain weight. (Adapted from J. G. Verbalis and S. R. Gullans, Hyponatremia causes large sustained reductions in brain content of multiple organic osmolytes in rats. *Brain Res.* 567:274–282, 1991; and J. G. Verbalis and S. R. Gullans, Rapid correction of hyponatremia produces differential effects on brain osmolyte and electrolyte reaccumulation in rats. *Brain Res.* 606:19–27, 1993.)

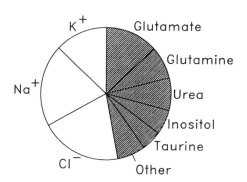

Fig. 1-20. Relative decreases in individual osmolytes during adaptation to chronic hyponatremia. The category "other" represents glycerolphosphorylcholine, urea, and several other amino acids. (From S. R. Gullans and J. G. Verbalis, Control of brain volume during hyperosmolar and hypoosmolar conditions. *Annu. Rev. Med.* 44:289–301, 1993. Reproduced, with permission, from the *Annual Review of Medicine,* Volume 44, © 1993, by Annual Reviews Inc.)

cations associated with acute symptomatic hyponatremia are devastating, these patients require prompt treatment [288] with hypertonic saline [289, 290], preferably in combination with furosemide, to prevent both sodium overload and to enhance water excretion [291]. This approach should be continued until seizures subside.

Chronic. Patients in whom the adaptive process to hyponatremia has occurred (>48 hours), when treated, are at risk of developing a demyelinating syndrome. In this setting, the rapid increase in serum tonicity leads to a greater degree of cerebral water loss than a previously normonatremic brain [276] and makes the development of a demyelinating process more likely [292]. Some believe that the correction rate in this setting is critical. Others maintain that the absolute change is more critical. Specifically, patients with an absolute change in serum sodium of more than 25 mmol/L over a 48-hour period are particularly at risk for neurologic consequences. It would appear prudent, therefore, to approach a symptomatic patient whose duration of hyponatremia is unknown, but most likely chronic, by increasing the serum sodium by approximately 10 percent over 24 hours (since brain water is rarely increased by more). Thus, serum sodium would be increased by less than 20 mmol/L/24 hr. At no time should the correction rate be allowed to exceed 1 mmol/L/hr. Once symptoms subside, water restriction can be instituted.

Although small demyelinating lesions produce minimal symptoms, patients with more extensive diseases have flaccid quadriplegia, dysphagia, and dysarthria. The factors that predispose to this neurologic complication have not been fully delineated. In the view of some, the rate of correction is critical [293]. Other data suggest that the process is independent of rate of correction and is due to the absolute change in serum sodium over a given time period [294]. This concept is also supported by experimental data [295, 296]. These two variables are not entirely independent. Therefore attention to both correction rate and magnitude is indicated. In this regard, in experimental animals [297], correction at an excessive rate (>2 mmol/L/hr) or magnitude (>20 mmol/L/24 hr) was associated with the development of cerebral lesions (Fig. 1-21). Others would propose more conservative correction rates of approximately 0.4 mmol/L/hr and 12 mmol/L in any 24-hour period [298].

In summary, rapid correction is most indicated for patients with acute (<48

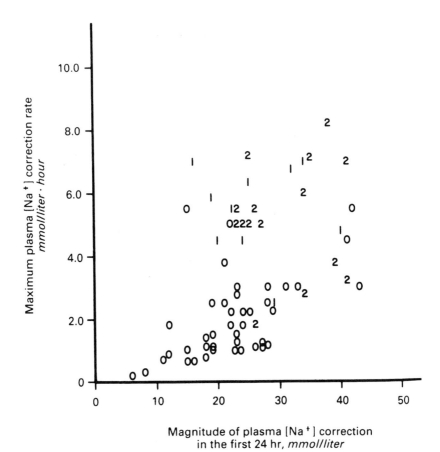

Fig. 1-21. Incidence of demyelinative lesions in individual rats as a function of both the maximal rate of correction of hyponatremia and the magnitude of the increase in plasma sodium concentration over the first 24 hours of the correction. Each rat in one of the three correction groups (water restriction, water diuresis, and hypertonic saline) is plotted as a function of the maximal rate of increase in plasma sodium achieved over any 4-hour period during the correction (abscissa) and the total magnitude of the increase in plasma sodium achieved during the first 24 hours of the correction (ordinate). Rats are depicted by their neuropathology score (0 = no demyelinative lesions; 1 = focal demyelinative lesions; 2 = diffuse demyelinative lesions). (From J. G. Verbalis, A. J. Martinez, and M. D. Drutarosky, Neurological and neuropathological sequelae of correction of chronic hyponatremia. Used with permission from *Kidney International* 39:1274, 1991.)

hours) and symptomatic hyponatremia. This should probably aim to raise serum sodium concentrations by approximately 1 to 2 mmol/L/hr until seizures subside. An absolute change of greater than 20 mEq/L over 24 hours should be avoided. This correction can be achieved by the administration of hypertonic saline. As long as the electrolyte concentration (sodium plus potassium) of the fluid administered is higher than that of urine electrolytes (sodium plus potassium), the level of plasma sodium will increase. This is so because, as noted previously, electrolyte free water is excreted whenever urinary sodium plus potassium exceeds serum sodium. For example: A 70-kg man has a serum sodium of 110 mEq/L. Assuming that 60 percent of body weight is water:

Total body water (TBW) $= 70 \times 0.6 = 42$ L

Since serum sodium concentration $= \dfrac{\text{total body cation (Na + K) content}}{\text{TBW}}$

In this patient, total body cation content $= 42$ L $\times$ 110 mEq/L $= 4620$ mEq.

Over the next 2 hours, this patient receives 200 ml of 3% NaCl and excretes 1000 ml of urine. The urinary sodium is 70 mEq/L, and the urinary potassium is 30 mEq/L. In this case, there is no net cation gain or loss, as 100 mEq of sodium was given (the sodium content of 200 ml of 3% NaCl) and 100 mEq of cation was excreted. However, total body water has decreased by 800 ml (1000 ml excreted $-$ 200 ml given with the hypertonic saline). Thus, the 4620 mEq of body cation is now in 41.2 liters, which would increase serum sodium to 112 mEq/L (4620/41.2). The rate at which serum sodium will rise will therefore depend not only on the volume of hypertonic saline administered but also on the volume and cation content of urine excreted. Since sodium and potassium balance is maintained, cation excretion is dependent on the amount infused, but the urine volume is in large measure determined by the kidney's ability to generate solute-free water. The concomitant administration of loop diuretics will increase solute-free water excretion and therefore the rate of correction if needed.

The excess water that needs to be excreted to achieve an increment in sodium can likewise be calculated. Assuming that a patient weighs 70 kg when his serum sodium is 115 mEq/L, the excess water that needs to be excreted to correct the hyponatremia to 130 mEq/L can be estimated as follows:

Total body water (TBW) $=$ body weight (kg) $\times$ 60%

In this case, TBW $= 70 \times 0.6 = 42$ L

Excess water $=$ TBW $-$ (actual plasma Na/desired plasma Na) $\times$ TBW

Excess water $= 42 - (115/130 \times 42) = 42 - 37.2 = 4.8$ L

During therapy, serum and urine electrolytes should be frequently obtained to avoid overcorrection. Once symptoms have decreased and a small degree of correction achieved, further therapy can proceed more slowly with either decreased rates of saline or with fluid restriction alone.

Asymptomatic. Patients with asymptomatic hyponatremia invariably have a chronic component to their disease. Such patients should be managed solely by water restriction even when the serum sodium is very low. The degree of the restriction depends on the severity of the diluting impairment. Over a long time, water restriction is difficult to enforce, and therefore agents that antagonize the renal action of AVP have been employed [299]. It appears that demeclocycline is more effective and safer than lithium in the treatment of SIADH [300]. In hyponatremic subjects with cirrhosis, however, demeclocycline causes nephrotoxicity and thus should be avoided [301].

As the level of urinary concentration is more or less fixed in the SIADH secretion, urine flow can be increased by increasing solute excretion. A dosage of 30 to 60 g of urea per day can successfully treat the syndrome [302]. A similar benefit occurs with the use of furosemide (40 mg/day) with a high salt intake (200 mEq/day). The development of orally active, nonpeptide antagonists of the hydro-osmotic effect of AVP provides an exciting potential therapeutic tool in the management of patients with water excess [303]. These agents antagonize both endogenous and exogenous AVP, causing a water diuresis in the absence of any alterations in filtration rate or solute excretion [304]. These antagonists appear to block the action of AVP to stimulate adenylate cyclase in cortical, medullary, and papillary collecting ducts; to interfere with binding of radioactive vasopressin to papillary membranes; and to block AVP-mediated water flow in isolated rabbit collecting ducts [305]. The development and use of oral antagonist of the V_2 receptor [219, 306] is extremely exciting, particularly since it has been found to be effective in a rat model of SIADH [307]. Its effectiveness in other pathologic states as well as in forthcoming human trials will be of great interest.

References

1. Smith HW: *From Fish to Philosopher: The Story of Our Internal Environment.* Boston, Little, Brown, 1953.
2. Kuhn W, Ryffel K: Herstellung konzentrierter Losungen aus verdunnten durch blosse Membranwirkung: Ein Modellversuch zur Funktion der Niere. *Z Physiol Chem* 276:145, 1942.
3. Sands JM, Kokko JP: Countercurrent system. *Kidney Int* 38:695, 1990.
4. Pitts RF: *Physiology of the Kidney and Body Fluids* (3rd ed). Chicago, Year Book, 1974.
5. Jamison RL, Kriz W: *Urinary Concentrating Mechanism: Structure and Function.* New York, Oxford University Press, 1982, p 133.
6. Kriz W: Structural organization of the renal medullary counterflow system. *Fed Proc* 42:2379, 1983.
7. Jacobson RH: Functional segmentation of the mammalian nephron. *Am J Physiol* 241:F203, 1981.
8. Morel F: Sites of hormone action in the mammalian nephron. *Am J Physiol* 240:F159, 1981.
9. Andreoli TE, Berliner RW, Kokko JH, et al: Questions and replies: Renal mechanisms of urinary concentrating and diluting processes. *Am J Physiol* 235:F1, 1978.
10. Molony DA, Reeves BW, Andreoli TE: $Na:K:2Cl^-$ cotransport and the thick ascending limb. *Kidney Int* 36:418, 1989.
11. Culpepper RM, Andreoli TE: Interactions among prostaglandin E_2, antidiuretic hormone, and cyclic adenosine monophosphate in modulating Cl-absorption in single mouse medullary thick ascending limbs of Henle. *J Clin Invest* 71:1588, 1983.
12. Schlatter E, Greger R: cAMP increases the basolateral Cl^- conductance in the isolated perfused medullary thick ascending limb of Henle's loop of the mouse. *Pflugers Arch* 405:367, 1985.
13. Clapp WH, Madsen KM, Verlander JW, Tisher CC: Morphologic heterogeneity along the inner medullary collecting duct. *Lab Invest* 60:219, 1989.
14. Kokko JP, Rector FC Jr: Countercurrent multiplication system without active transport in inner medulla. *Kidney Int* 2:214, 1972.

15. Imai M, Tanguchi J, Yoshitomi K: Transition of permeability properties along the descending limb of long-loop nephron. *Am J Physiol* 254:F323, 1988.

16. Kondo Y, Imai M: Effect of glutaraldehyde on renal tubular function: II. Selective inhibitor of Cl^- transport in the hamster thin ascending limb of Henle's loop. *Pflugers Arch* 408:484, 1987.

17. Knepper MA: Urea transport in isolated thick ascending limb and collecting ducts from rats. *Am J Physiol* 245:F634, 1983.

18. Sands JM, Knepper MA: Urea permeability of mammalian inner medullary collecting duct system and papillary surface epithelium. *J Clin Invest* 79:138, 1987.

19. Lemley KV, Kriz W: Cycles and separations: The histotopography of the urinary concentrating process. *Kidney Int* 31:538–548, 1987.

20. Layton HE: Urea transport is a distributed model of the urinary concentrating mechanism. *Am J Physiol* 258:F1110, 1990.

21. Chou SY, Porush J, Fanbert P: Renal medullary circulation: Hormonal control. *Kidney Int* 37:1, 1990.

22. Zimmerhackle B, Robertson CR, Jamison RL: Effect of arginine vasopressin on renal medullary blood flow: A video-microscopic study in the rat. *J Clin Invest* 76:770, 1985.

23. de Wardener HE, del Greco F: Influence of solute excretion rate on production of hypotonic urine in man. *Clin Sci* 14:715, 1955.

24. Zak GA, Brun C, Smith HW: The mechanism of formation of osmotically concentrated urine during the antidiuretic state. *J Clin Invest* 33:1064, 1954.

25. Orloff J, Wagner HN Jr, Davidson DG: The effect of variations in solute excretion and vasopressin dosage on the excretion of water in the dog. *J Clin Invest* 37:458, 1958.

26. Tisher CC, Schrier RW, McNeil JS: Nature of the urine concentrating mechanism in the macaque monkey. *Am J Physiol* 223:1128, 1972.

27. Knepper MA, Nielsen S, Chan C, et al: Mechanism of vasopressin action in the renal collecting duct. *Semin Nephrol* 14:302, 1994.

28. Schmale H, Fehr S, Richter D: Vasopressin biosynthesis—from gene to peptide hormone. *Kidney Int* 32(Suppl. 21):S8, 1987.

29. Riddell DC, Mallonee R, Phillips L: Chromosome assignment of human sequence encoding arginine vasopressin, neurophysin II and growth hormone releasing factor. *Somat Cell Mol Genet* 11:189, 1987.

30. Richter D, Mohr E, Schmale H: Molecular Aspects of the Vasopressin Gene Family. In Jard S, Jamison R (eds): *Vasopressin*. London, John Libbey Eurotext, 1991, p 3–11.

31. Schmale H, Richter D: Single base deletion in the vasopressin gene is the cause of diabetes insipidus in Brattleboro rats. *Nature* 309:705, 1984.

32. Thrasher TN, Keil LC: Regulation of drinking and vasopressin secretion: Role of organum vasculosum laminae terminalis. *Am J Physiol* 253:R108, 1987.

33. Ishikawa S, Saito T, Yoshida S: The effect of osmotic pressure and angiotensin II on arginine vasopressin release from guinea pig hypothalamoneurohypophyseal complex in organ culture. *Endocrinology* 106:1591, 1980.

34. Majzoub JA, Rich A, Vanborn J, et al: Vasopressin and oxytocin mRNA regulation in the rat assessed by hybridization with synthetic oligonucleotide. *J Biol Chem* 258:14061, 1983.

35. Uhl GR, Zingg HH, Habener J: Vasopressin mRNA in situ hybridization: Localization and regulation studied with oligonucleotide cDNA probes in normal and Brattleboro rat hypothalamus. *Proc Natl Acad Sci USA* 82:5555, 1985.

36. Murphy D, Levy A, Lightman S, Conti D: Vasopressin RNA in the neural lobe of the pituitary: Dramatic accumulation in response to salt loading. *Proc Natl Acad Sci USA* 86:9002, 1989.

37. Zerbe RL: Genetic Factors in Normal and Abnormal Regulation of Vasopressin Secretion. In Schrier RW (ed): *Water Balance and Antidiuretic Hormone*. New York, Raven, 1985, p 213.

38. Dunn FL, Brennan TJ, Nelson AE, et al: The role of blood osmolality and volume in regulating vasopressin secretion in the rat. *J Clin Invest* 52:3212, 1973.

39. Sklar AH, Schrier RW: Central nervous system mediators of vasopressin release. *Physiol Rev* 63:1243, 1983.

40. Yamashita H, Inenaga K, Yamamoto S, et al: Chemical Control of Vasopressin Neurons. In Gross P, Richter D, Robertson GL (eds), *Vasopressin*. London, John Libbey Eurotext, 1993, p 199–203.
41. Dousa TP, Valtin H: Action of antidiuretic hormone in mice with inherited vasopressin-resistant urinary concentration defects. *J Clin Invest* 54:753, 1974.
42. Verkman AS: Mechanisms and regulation of water permeability in renal epithelia. *Am J Physiol* 257:C837–C850, 1989.
43. Morel A, O'Carroll AM, Brownstein M, et al: Molecular cloning and expression of a rat V1a arginine vasopressin receptor. *Nature* 356:523–526, 1992.
44. Lolait SS, O'Carroll AM, McBride O, et al: Cloning and characterization of a vasopressin V2 receptor and possible link to nephrogenic diabetes insipidus. *Nature* 357:336–339, 1992.
45. Birnbaumer M, Seibold A, Gilbert S: Molecular cloning of the receptor for human antidiuretic hormone. *Nature* 357:333–335, 1992.
46. Terada Y, Tomita K, Nonoguchi H, et al: Different localization and regulation of two types of vasopressin receptor messenger RNA in microdissected rat nephron segments using reverse transcription polymerase chain reaction. *J Clin Invest* 92:2339–2345, 1993.
47. Ostronesta NL, Young WS, Knepper MA, et al: Expression of vasopressin V1a and V2 receptor messenger ribonucleic acid in the liver and kidney of embryonic developing and adult rats. *Endocrinology* 33:1849–1859, 1993.
48. Briner VA, Williams B, Tsai P, et al: Demonstration of processing and recycling of biologically active V1 vasopressin receptor in vascular smooth muscle. *Proc Natl Acad Sci USA* 89: 2854–2858, 1992.
49. Carmichael MC, Lutz W, Kumar R: Endocytosis of the Vasopressin Receptor. In Gross P, Richter D, Robertson GL (eds): *Vasopressin*. London, John Libbey Eurotext, 1993, pp 79–92.
50. Johnson GL, Dhanasekaran N: The G protein family and their interaction with receptors. *Endocrinol Rev* 10:317, 1989.
51. Miller TR: Transmembrane signalling through G protein. *Kidney Int* 39:421, 1991.
52. Dousa TP, Valtin H: Cellular actions of vasopressin in the mammalian kidney. *Kidney Int* 10:46, 1976.
53. Grantham JJ, Burg MB: Effect of vasopressin and cyclic AMP on permeability of isolated collecting tubules. *Am J Physiol* 211:255–259, 1966.
54. Dousa TP, Barnes LD: Regulation of protein kinase by vasopressin in renal medulla in situ. *Am J Physiol* 232:F50, 1977.
55. Snyder HM, Noland TD, Breyer MP: cAMP dependent protein kinase mediates hydroosmotic effect of vasopressin in collecting duct. *Am J Physiol* 263:C147–C153, 1992.
56. Kachadorian WA, Wade JB, Discala V: Vasopressin-induced structural change in toad bladder luminal membrane. *Science* 190:67, 1975.
57. Kachadorian WA, Levine SD, Wade JB, et al: Relationship of aggregated intramembranous particles to water permeability in vasopressin-treated toad urinary bladders. *J Clin Invest* 59: 576, 1977.
58. Kachadorian WA, Ellis JS, Miller J: Possible roles for microtubules and microfilaments in ADH action on toad urinary bladder. *Am J Physiol* 236:F14, 1979.
59. Taylor A: Role of Microtubules and Microfilaments in the Action of Vasopressin. In Andreoli TE, Grantham JJ, Rector FC Jr (eds): *Disturbances in Body Fluid Osmolality*. Bethesda, Md, American Physiological Society, 1977, p 97.
60. Simon H, Gao Y, Franki N, et al: Vasopressin depolymerizes apical factor in rat inner medullary collecting duct. *Am J Physiol* 265:C757–C762, 1993.
61. Ausiello D: Cellular biology of the water channel. *Kidney Int* 30:497, 1989.
62. Brown D: Membrane recycling and epithelial cell function. *Am J Physiol* 250:F1, 1989.
63. Verkman AS: Mechanism and regulation of water permeability in renal epithelia. *Am J Physiol* 257:C837, 1989.
64. Fushimi K, Uchida S, Husa Y, et al: Cloning and expression of apical membrane water channel of rat kidney collecting tubule. *Nature* 361:549–552, 1993.
65. Nielsen S, DiGiovanni SR, Christensen E: Cellular and subcellular immunolocalization of vasopressin regulated water channel in rat kidney. *Proc Natl Acad Sci USA* 90:11663–11667, 1993.

66. Anderson B: Regulation of water intake. *Physiol Rev* 58:582, 1978.
67. Perez GO, Oster JR, Robertson GL: Severe hypernatremia with impaired thirst. *Am J Nephrol* 9:421, 1989.
68. Berl T, Anderson RJ, McDonald KM, et al: Clinical disorders of water metabolism. *Kidney Int* 10:117, 1976.
69. Robertson GL, McLeod JF, Zerbe RL, et al: Vasopressin Function in Heritable Forms of Diabetes Insipidus. In Gross P, Richter D, Robertson GL (eds): *Vasopressin*. London, John Libbey Eurotext, 1993, pp 493–502.
70. McLeod JF, Koracs L, Gaskill M, et al: Familial neurohypophyseal diabetes insipidus associated with a single peptide mutation. *J Clin Endocrinol Metab* 77:599A–599G, 1993.
71. Scherbaum WA, Boltazzo GL: Antibodies to vasopressin cells in idiopathic diabetes insipidus: Evidence for an autoimmune variant. *Lancet* 1:897, 1984.
72. Yap HY, Tashima CK, Blumenschein GR: Diabetes insipidus and breast cancer. *Arch Intern Med* 139:1009, 1979.
73. Coggins CH, Leaf A: Diabetes insipidus. *Am J Med* 42:807, 1967.
74. Dunger DB, Broadbent V, Yeoman V, et al: The frequency and natural history of diabetes insipidus in children with Langerhans cell histiocytosis. *N Engl J Med* 321:1157, 1989.
75. Winnacker J, Becker K, Katz S: Endocrine aspects of sarcoidosis. *N Engl J Med* 278:483, 1968.
76. Fraser CL, Arieff AI: Fatal central diabetes mellitus and insipidus resulting from untreated hyponatremia: A new syndrome. *Ann Intern Med* 112:113, 1990.
77. Weiss NM, Robertson GL: Water metabolism in endocrine disorders. *Semin Nephrol* 4:303, 1984.
78. Moses AM, Streeten DHP: Differentiation of polyuric states by measurement of responses to changes in plasma osmolality induced by hypertonic saline infusions. *Am J Med* 42:368, 1967.
79. Manelfe C, Louvet S: Computed tomography in diabetes insipidus. *J Comput Assist Tomogr* 3:309, 1979.
80. Fujisawa I, Nishimura K, Asato R, et al: Posterior lobe of the pituitary in diabetes insipidus MR findings. *J Comput Assist Tomogr* 11:22, 1987.
81. Halim P, Sigal R, Doyan D, et al: Post-traumatic diabetes insipidus: MR demonstration of pituitary stalk rupture. *J Comput Assist Tomogr* 12:135, 1988.
82. Miller M, Dalakos T, Moses AM, et al: Recognition of partial defects in antidiuretic hormone secretion. *Ann Intern Med* 73:721, 1970.
83. de Wardener HE, Herxheimer A: The effect of a high water intake on the kidney's ability to concentrate the urine in man. *J Physiol* (Lond) 139:42, 1957.
84. Richman RA, Post EM, Notman DD: Simplifying the diagnosis of diabetes insipidus in children. *Am J Dis Child* 135:839, 1981.
85. Zerbe RL, Robertson GL: A comparison on plasma vasopressin measurements with a standard indirect test in the differential diagnosis of polyuria. *N Engl J Med* 304:1529, 1981.
86. Milles J, Spruce B, Baylis PH: A comparison of diagnostic methods to differentiate diabetes insipidus from primary polyuria: A review of 21 patients. *Acta Endocrinol* 104:410, 1983.
87. Kanno K, Sasaki S, Hirata Y, et al: Urinary excretion of aquaporin-2 in patients with diabetes insipidus. *N Engl J Med* 332:1540–1545, 1995.
88. Vokes T, Gaskell MB, Robertson GL: Antibodies to vasopressin in patients with diabetes insipidus. *Ann Intern Med* 108:190, 1988.
89. Harris AS: Clinical experience with desmopressin: Efficacy and safety in central diabetes insipidus and other conditions. *J Pediatr* 114:711, 1984.
90. Seck JR, Dinger DB: Diabetes insipidus: Current treatment recommendation. *Drugs* 44:216–224, 1992.
91. Robertson GL, Harris A: Clinical use of vasopressin analogues. *Hosp Prac* 24:114, 1989.
92. Rado JP, Maros J, Borbely L: Individual differences in antidiuretic response induced by dDAVP in diabetes insipidus. *Horm Metab Res* 8:155, 1976.
93. Cunnah D, Ross G, Besser GM: Management of cranial diabetes insipidus with oral desmopressin (dDAVP). *Clin Endocrinol* 24:253, 1986.
94. Fjellestad-Paulesen A, Tubiana-Ruf N, Harris A, et al: Central diabetes insipidus in children: Antidiuretic effect and pharmacokinetics of intranasal and peroral L-deamino D-arginine vasopressin. *Acta Endocrinol* 115:307, 1987.

95. Gardenswartz MH, Berl T: Drug induced changes in water excretion. *Kidney* 15:19, 1981.
96. Froyshov I, Haugen HN: Chlorpropamide treatment in diabetes insipidus. *Acta Med Scand* 183:397, 1968.
97. Moses AM, Coulson R: Augmentation by chlorpropamide of L-deamino-8-D-arginine vasopressin–induced antidiuresis and stimulation of renal medullary adenylate cyclase and accumulation of adenosine 3′,5′-monophosphate. *Endocrinology* 106:367, 1980.
98. Wales JK: Treatment of diabetes insipidus with carbamazepine. *Lancet* 2:948, 1975.
99. Bichet DG: Hereditary nephrogenic diabetes insipidus. *Adv Nephrol Necker Hosp* 20:175–189, 1991.
100. Kambouris M, Dlouhy SR, Trofatter JA, et al: Localization of the gene for x-linked nephrogenic diabetes insipidus to Xq28. *Am J Med Genet* 29:239, 1988.
101. Knoers N, Heyden VD, Van Oost BA: Nephrogenic diabetes insipidus: Close linkage with markers from the distal long area of the human X-chromosome. *Hum Genet* 80:31, 1988.
102. Bichet D, Razi M, Arthur MF: Epinephrine and dDAVP administration in patients with congenital nephrogenic diabetes insipidus. *Kidney Int* 36:859, 1989.
103. Rosenthal W, Seibold A, Antaramian A, et al: Molecular identification of the gene responsible for congenital nephrogenic diabetes insipidus. *Nature* 359:233–234, 1992.
104. Holtzman E, Harris W, Kolakowski L, et al: A molecular defect in the vasopressin V2 receptor gene causing nephrogenic diabetes insipidus. *N Engl J Med* 328:1534–1537, 1993.
105. Meredino JJ, Spiegel AM, Crawford JD: A mutation in the vasopressin V2 receptor gene in a kindred with X-linked nephrogenic diabetes insipidus. *N Engl J Med* 328:1538–1541, 1993.
106. Bichet D, Birnbaumer M, Lonegren M, et al: Nature and recurrence of AVPR2 mutation in X-linked nephrogenic diabetes insipidus. *Am J Hum Genet* 55:278–286, 1994.
107. Gapstur S, Homma R, Coffey A, et al: Abnormal cAMP catabolism in collecting tubules of mice with hereditary nephrogenic diabetes insipidus (NDI mice). *Kidney Int* 33:264, 1988.
108. Homma S, Gapstur S, Dousa T: Catabolism of cAMP and cGMP in collecting tubule of normal mice and mice with hereditary nephrogenic diabetes insipidus (NDI). *Kidney Int* 33: 267, 1988.
109. Bichet D, Razi M, Lonergan M: Hemodynamic and coagulation responses to L-desamino 8-D-arginine vasopressin in patients with congenital nephrogenic diabetes insipidus. *N Engl J Med* 318:881, 1988.
110. Knoers N, Monnens LA: A variant of nephrogenic diabetes insipidus: V2 receptor abnormality restricted to the kidney. *Eur J Pediatr* 150:370, 1991.
111. Deen P, Verdijk M, Knoers N: Requirement of human renal water channel, Aquaporin 2, for vasopressin dependent concentration of urine. *Science* 264:92–95, 1994.
112. Carter RD, Goodman AD: Nephrogenic diabetes insipidus accompanied by massive dilation of the kidneys, ureters and bladder. *J Urol* 89:366, 1963.
113. Orloff J, Burn MB: Vasopressin-Resistant Diabetes Insipidus. In Stanbury J, Wyngaarden JB, Frederickson NS (eds): *The Metabolic Basis of Inherited Disease* (3rd ed). New York, McGraw-Hill, 1972, p 1567.
114. Alon U, Chan JCM: Hydrochlorothiazide-amiloride in the treatment of congenital nephrogenic diabetes insipidus. *Am J Nephrol* 5:9, 1985.
115. Libber S, Harrison H, Spector D: Treatment of nephrogenic diabetes insipidus with prostaglandin synthesis inhibitors. *J Pediatr* 108:305, 1981.
116. Chevalier RL, Rogol AD: Tolmetin sodium in the management of nephrogenic diabetes insipidus. *J Pediatr* 101:787, 1982.
117. Fine LG, Salehmoghaddam S: Water homestasis in acute and chronic renal failure. *Semin Nephrol* 4:289, 1984.
118. Tannen RL, Regal EM, Dunn MJ, et al: Vasopressin-resistant hyposthenuria in advanced chronic renal disease. *N Engl J Med* 280:1135, 1969.
119. Gabow PA, Kaehny WD, Johnson AM, et al: The clinical utility of renal concentrating capacity in polycystic kidney disease. *Kidney Int* 35:675, 1989.
120. Fine LG, Schlondorf D, Trizna W, et al: Functional profile of isolated uremic nephron: Impaired water permeability and adenylate cyclase responsiveness of the cortical collecting duct to vasopressin. *J Clin Invest* 61:1519, 1978.

121. Teitelbaum I, McGuinness S: Vasopressin resistance in chronic renal failure: Evidence for the role of decreased V2 receptor m-RNA. *J Clin Invest* 96:378, 1995.
122. Teitelbaum I, Berl T: Water metabolism in patients with electrolyte disorders (editorial). *Semin Nephrol* 4:354, 1984.
123. Berl T, Linas S, Aisenbrey G, et al: On the mechanism of polyuria in potassium depletion: The role of polydipsia. *J Clin Invest* 60:620, 1977.
124. Gutsche HU, Peterson LW, Levine DZ: In vivo evidence of impaired solute transport by the thick ascending limb in potassium-depleted rats. *J Clin Invest* 73:908, 1984.
125. Finn AL, Handler JS, Orloff J: Relation between toad bladder potassium content and permeability response to vasopressin. *Am J Physiol* 210:1279, 1966.
126. Kim JK, Summer SN, Berl T: Studies on the cyclic AMP system in the papillary collecting duct of the potassium depleted rat. *Kidney Int* 26:384, 1984.
126a. Marples D, Frokiaer J, Dorup M, et al: Hypokalemia induced down regulation of aquaporin 2-water channel expression in rat kidney medulla and cortex. *J Clin Invest* 97:1960, 1996.
127. Relman AS, Schwartz WB: The kidney in potassium depletion. *Am J Med* 24:764, 1958.
128. Levi M, Peterson L, Berl T: Mechanism of concentrating defect in hypercalcemia: Role of polydipsia and prostaglandins. *Kidney Int* 23:489, 1983.
129. Peterson LN: Vitamin D–induced chronic hypercalcemia inhibits thick ascending limb NaCl reabsorption in vivo. *Am J Physiol* 259:F122, 1990.
130. Berl T: The cAMP system in vasopressin sensitive nephron segments of the vitamin D treated rat. *Kidney Int* 31:1065, 1987.
131. Omachi RS, Robbie DE, Handler JS, Orloff J: Effects of ADH and other agents on cyclic AMP accumulation in toad bladder epithelium. *Am J Physiol* 226:1152, 1974.
132. Ando Y, Jacobson H, Breyer M: Phorbol ester and A23187 have additive but mechanistically separate effects on vasopressin action in rabbit collecting tubule. *J Clin Invest* 81:1578, 1988.
133. Teitelbaum I, Berl T: Effects of calcium on vasopressin-mediated cAMP formation in cultured rat inner medullary collecting tubule cells. *J Clin Invest* 77:1574, 1986.
134. Singer I, Forrest JV: Drug-induced states of nephrogenic diabetes insipidus. *Kidney Int* 10:82, 1976.
135. Kleeman CR, Rubini ME, Lamdin E, et al: Studies in alcohol diuresis: II. The evaluation of ethyl alcohol as an inhibitor of the neurohypophysis. *J Clin Invest* 34:448, 1955.
136. Moses AM, Van Gemert M, Miller M: Evidence that glyburide-induced diuresis is not mediated by inhibition of ADH. *Horm Res* 5:359, 1974.
137. Douglas JB, Healy JK: Nephrotoxic effects of amphotericin B, including renal tubular acidosis. *Am J Med* 46:154, 1969.
138. Farese R, Schambelan M, Hollander H, et al: Nephrogenic diabetes insipidus associated with foscarnet treatment of cytomegalovirus retinitis. *Ann Intern Med* 112:955–956, 1990.
139. Singer I, Rotenberg D: Demeclocycline-induced nephrogenic diabetes insipidus. *Ann Intern Med* 79:679, 1973.
140. Baton R, Gaviria M, Battle D: Prevalence, pathogenesis and treatment of renal dysfunction associated with chronic lithium therapy. *Am J Kidney Dis* 10:329–345, 1987.
141. Walker RG: Lithium nephrotoxicity. *Kidney Int* 42:593–598, 1993.
142. Baylis PH, Heath DA: Water disturbances in patients treated with oral lithium carbonate. *Ann Intern Med* 88:607, 1978.
143. Forrest JN Jr, Cohen AD, Torretti J, et al: On the mechanism of lithium-induced diabetes insipidus in man and the rat. *J Clin Invest* 53:1115, 1974.
144. Christensen S: Acute and chronic effects of vasopressin in rats with lithium-polyuria. *Acta Pharmacol Toxicol* (Copenh) 38:241, 1976.
145. Cogan E, Abramow M: Inhibition by lithium of the hydroosmotic action of vasopressin in the isolated perfused collecting duct of the rabbit. *J Clin Invest* 77:1507, 1986.
146. Dousa TP: Interaction of lithium with vasopressin-sensitive cyclic AMP system of human renal medulla. *Endocrinology* 95:1359, 1974.
147. Anger MS, Shanley P, Mansour J, et al: Effects of lithium on cAMP generation in cultured rat inner medullary collecting tubule cells. *Kidney Int* 37:1211, 1990.
148. Goldberg H, Clayman S, Skorecki R: Mechanisms of lithium inhibition of vasopressin-sensitive adenylate cyclase in cultured epithelial cells. *Am J Physiol* 255:F995, 1988.

149. Christensen S, Kussano A, Yusufi N, et al: Pathogenesis of nephrogenic diabetes insipidus due to chronic administration of lithium salts. *J Clin Invest* 75:1869–1879, 1985.

150. Marples D, Christensen S, Christensen E, et al: Lithium induced downregulation of Aquaporin-2 water channel expression in rat kidney medulla. *J Clin Invest* 95:1838–1845, 1995.

151. Statius Van Eps LW, Pinedo-Veels C, De Vries GH, et al: Nature of concentrating defect in sickle-cell nephropathy: Microradioangiographic studies. *Lancet* 1:450, 1970.

152. Buckalew VM Jr, Someren A: Renal manifestations of sickle cell disease. *Arch Intern Med* 133:660, 1974.

153. Goldsmith C, Beasly HK, Whalley PJ, et al: Effect of salt deprivation on urinary concentrating mechanism in dog. *J Clin Invest* 40:2043, 1961.

154. Epstein FH, Kleeman CR, Pursel S, et al: The effect of feeding protein and urea on renal concentrating process. *J Clin Invest* 36:635, 1957.

154a. Sands J, Naruse M, Jacobs J, et al: Changes in aquaporin 2 protein contribute to the urinary concentrating defect in rat fed a low-protein diet. *J Clin Invest* 97:2807, 1996.

155. Barron WM, Cohen LH, Ulland LA, et al: Transient vasopressin resistant diabetes insipidus in pregnancy. *N Engl J Med* 310:442, 1984.

156. Ford SM Jr: Transient vasopressin resistant diabetes insipidus of pregnancy. *Obstet Gynecol* 68:288, 1986.

157. Durr JA, Hoggard JG, Hunt JM, Schrier RW: Diabetes insipidus in pregnancy associated with abnormally high vasopressinase activity. *N Engl J Med* 316:1070, 1987.

158. De Rubertis F, Michelis M, Beck N, et al: "Essential" hypernatremia due to ineffective osmotic and intact volume regulation of vasopressin secretion. *J Clin Invest* 50:97, 1975.

159. Sridhar CB, Calvert GD, Ibbertson HK: Syndrome of hypernatremia, hypodipsia and partial diabetes insipidus: A new interpretation. *J Clin Endocrinol Metab* 38:890, 1974.

160. Alford FP, Scoggins BA, Wharton C: Symptomatic normovolemic essential hypernatremia. *Am J Med* 54:359, 1973.

161. Halter J, Goldberg A, Robertson G, et al: Selective osmoreceptor dysfunction in the syndrome of chronic hypernatremia. *J Clin Endocrinol Metab* 44:609, 1977.

162. Robertson GL: The Physiopathology of ADH Secretion. In Tolis G, Labrie F, Martin J, Naftolin F (eds): *Clinical Neuroendocrinology: A Pathophysiological Approach*. New York, Raven, 1979, p 247.

163. Brezis M, Weiler-Rowell D: Hypernatremia, hypodipsia and partial diabetes insipidus: A model for defective osmoregulation. *Am J Med Sci* 279:37, 1980.

164. Miller PD, Krebs RA, Neal BJ, et al: Hypodipsia in geriatric patients. *Am J Med* 73:354, 1983.

165. Yamamoto T, Horada H, Fukuyama J: Impaired arginine vasopressin secretion associated with hypoangiotensinemia in hypernatremic dehydrated elderly patients. *JAMA* 259:1039, 1988.

166. Phillips PA, Rolls BJ, Ledingtrom JG: Reduced thirst after water deprivation in healthy elderly men. *N Engl J Med* 311:753, 1984.

167. Feig PU, McCurdy DK: The hypertonic state. *N Engl J Med* 297:1444, 1977.

168. Arieff AI, Guisado R: Effects on the central nervous system of hypernatremic and hyponatremic states. *Kidney Int* 10:104, 1976.

169. Pollack AS, Arieff AI: Abnormalities of cell volume regulation and their functional consequences. *Am J Physiol* 239:F195, 1980.

170. Macaulay D, Watson M: Hypernatremia as a cause of brain damage. *Arch Dis Child* 42:485, 1967.

171. Fineberg L, Luttrell C, Redd H: Pathogenesis of lesion in the nervous system in hypernatremic states: Experimental studies of gross anatomic changes and alterations of chemical composition of tissues. *Pediatrics* 23:46, 1959.

172. Arieff AI, Guisado R, Lazarowitz VC: The Pathophysiology of Hyperosmolar States. In Andreoli TE, Grantham JJ, Rector FC Jr (eds): *Disturbances in Body Fluid Osmolality*, for the American Physiological Society. Baltimore, Williams & Wilkins, 1977, p 227.

173. Cserr H, DePasquale M, Patlak CS: Regulation of brain water and electrolytes during acute hyperosmolality in rats. *Am J Physiol* 253:F522, 1987.

174. Cserr H, DePasquale M, Patlak CS: Volume regulatory influx of electrolytes from plasma to brain during acute hyperosmolality. *Am J Physiol* 253:F530, 1987.

175. Fishman RA, Chan PH: Changes in ammonia and amino acid metabolism induced by hyperosmolality in vivo and in vitro. *Trans Am Neurol Assoc* 101:1, 1976.

176. Thurston JH, Hanhart RE, Dirgo JA: Taurine: A role in osmotic regulation of mammalian brain and possible clinical significance. *Life Sci* 26:1561, 1980.

177. Lien Y-H, Shapiro JI, Chan L: Effects of hypernatremia on organic brain osmoles. *J Clin Invest* 85:1427, 1990.

178. Fineberg L: Hypernatremic dehydration in infants. *N Engl J Med* 289:196, 1973.

179. Hogan GR, Dodge PR, Gill SR, et al: The incidence of seizures after rehydration of hypernatremic rabbits with intravenous or ad-lib oral fluids. *Pediatr Res* 18:340, 1984.

180. Redmond GP, Rother D, Halim JF: Combined desmopressin (dDAVP) and chlorpropamide therapy for diabetes insipidus with absent thirst. *Cleve Clin Q* 50:351, 1983.

181. Gennari FJ: Serum osmolality: Uses and limitation. *N Engl J Med* 310:102, 1984.

182. Smithline N, Gordior K: Gaps—anion and osmolal. *JAMA* 236:1594, 1976.

183. Gabow PA: Ethylene glycol intoxication. *Am J Kidney Dis* 11:277, 1988.

184. Veis JH, Berl T: Hyponatremia. In Jacobson HR, Striker GE, Klahr S (eds): *Principles and Practice of Nephrology*. St. Louis, Mosby, 1995, pp 888–893.

185. Vaswani SK, Sprague R: Pseudohyponatremia in multiple myeloma. *South Med J* 86:251, 1993.

186. Berl T, Schrier RW: Water Metabolism and the Hypo-osmolar Syndromes. In Brenner BM, Stein JH (eds): *Sodium and Water Homeostasis*, Contemporary Issues in Nephrology, vol 1. New York, Churchill Livingstone, 1978, p 1.

187. Meyer-Lehnert H, Schrier RW: Hyponatremia: Diagnosis and Treatment. In Seldin DW, Giebisch G (eds): *The Regulation of Sodium and Chloride Balance*. New York, Raven, 1990, p 443.

188. Berl T, Cadnapaphornchai P, Harbottle JA, et al: Mechanism of suppression of vasopressin during alpha adrenergic stimulation with norepinephrine. *J Clin Invest* 53:219, 1974.

189. Schrier RW: Body fluid volume regulation in health and disease: A unifying hypothesis. *Ann Intern Med* 113:155, 1990.

190. Schrier RW, Regal EM: Influence of aldosterone on sodium, water and potassium metabolism in chronic renal disease. *Kidney Int* 1:156, 1972.

191. Abramow M, Cogan E: Clinical aspects of pathophysiology of diuretic-induced hyponatremia. *Adv Nephrol* 13:1, 1984.

192. Ashouri OS: Severe diuretic-induced hyponatremia in the elderly. *Arch Intern Med* 146:1355, 1986.

193. Sonnenblick M, Friedlander Y, Rosin AJ: Diuretic induced severe hyponatremia: Review and analysis of 129 reported patients. *Chest* 103:601–606, 1993.

194. Rose BD: A physiologic approach to solute and water balance in hyponatremia. *Kidney Int* 17:1, 1984.

195. Fichman MP, Vorherr H, Kleeman CR, et al: Diuretic-induced hyponatremia. *Ann Intern Med* 75:853, 1971.

196. Thorn GW, Koepf GF, Clinton M Jr: Renal failure simulating adrenocortical insufficiency. *N Engl J Med* 231:76, 1944.

197. Sebastian A, McSherry E, Morris RC Jr: On the mechanism of renal potassium wasting in renal tubular acidosis associated with the Fanconi syndrome (type 2 RTA). *J Clin Invest* 50: 231, 1971.

198. Schrier RW, Linas SL: Mechanisms of the defect in water excretion in adrenal insufficiency. *Miner Electrolyte Metab* 4:1, 1980.

199. Gennari FJ, Kassirer JP: Osmotic diuresis. *N Engl J Med* 291:714, 1974.

200. DeFronzo RA: The effect of insulin on renal sodium metabolism: A review with clinical implications. *Diabetologia* 21:165, 1981.

201. Bichet DG, Schrier RW: Water metabolism in edematous disorders (editorial). *Semin Nephrol* 4:325, 1984.

202. Dzau VJ, Colucci WS, Williams GH, et al: Sustained effectiveness of converting enzyme inhibition in patients with severe congestive heart failure. *N Engl J Med* 302:1373, 1980.

203. Dzau VJ, Packer M, Lilly L, et al: Prostaglandins in severe congestive heart failure: Relation to activation of the renin-angiotensin system and hyponatremia. *N Engl J Med* 310:347, 1984.

204. Schrier RW: Pathogenesis of sodium and water retention in high and low cardiac output cirrhosis, nephrotic syndrome, and pregnancy (Parts 1 and 2). *N Engl J Med* 319:1065, 319: 1127, 1988.
205. Schrier RW, Niederberger M: Paradoxes of body fluid volume regulation in health and disease: A unifying hypothesis. *West J Med* 161:393–408, 1994.
206. Anderson RJ, Harbottle J, McDonald KM, et al: Mechanism of effect of thoracic inferior vena cava constriction on renal water excretion. *J Clin Invest* 54:1473, 1974.
207. Berns AS, Schrier RW: The Kidney in Heart Failure. In Suki WN, Eknoyan G (eds): *The Kidney in Systemic Disease* (2nd ed). New York, Wiley, 1981, p 569.
208. de Torrente A, Robertson GL, McDonald KM, et al: Mechanism of diuretic response to increased left atrial pressure in the anesthetized dog. *Kidney Int* 8:355, 1975.
209. Ishikawa S, Saito T, Okada K, et al: Effect of a vasopressin antagonist on water excretion in vena cava constriction. *Kidney Int* 30:49, 1986.
210. Goldsmith SR, Francis GS, Cowley AW, et al: Increased plasma arginine vasopressin levels in patients with congestive heart failure. *J Am Coll Cardiol* 1:1385, 1983.
211. Riegger GAJ, Liebau G, Kochsie K: Antidiuretic hormone in congestive heart failure. *Am J Med* 72:49, 1982.
212. Szatalowicz VL, Arnold PE, Chaimovitz C, et al: Radioimmunoassay of plasma arginine vaso-pressin in hyponatremic patients with congestive heart failure. *N Engl J Med* 305:263, 1981.
213. Kim JK, Michel JB, Soubrier F, Schrier RW: Arginine vasopressin gene expression in chronic cardiac failure in rats. *Kidney Int* 38:818, 1990.
214. Levine TB, Francis GS, Goldsmith SR, et al: Activity of the sympathetic nervous system and renin-angiotensin system assessed by plasma hormone levels and their relation to hemody-namic abnormalities in congestive heart failure. *Am J Cardiol* 49:1659, 1982.
215. Ferguson DW, Berg WJ, Sanders JS: Clinical and hemodynamic correlates of sympathetic nerve activity in normal humans and patients with heart failure: Evidence from direct micro-neurographic recordings. *J Am Coll Cardiol* 16:1125, 1990.
216. Bichet D, Kortos G, MeHauer B, et al: Modulation of plasma and platelet vasopressin by cardiac function in patients with heart failure. *Kidney Int* 29:1188, 1986.
217. Dzau VJ, Hollenberg NK: Renal response to captopril in severe heart failure: Role of furose-mide in natriuresis and reversal of hyponatremia. *Ann Intern Med* 100:777, 1984.
218. Packer M, Medina M, Yusha K: Correction of dilutional hyponatremia in severe chronic heart failure by converting enzyme inhibition. *Ann Intern Med* 100:782, 1984.
219. Ohnishi A, Orita Y, Okahara R, et al: Potent aquaretic agent: A novel nonpeptide selective vasopressin 2 antagonist (OPC-31260) in men. *J Clin Invest* 92:2653, 1993.
220. Schrier RW, Arroyo V, Bernardi M, et al: Peripheral arterial vasodilation hypothesis: A proposal for the initiation of renal sodium and water retention in cirrhosis. *Hepatology* 8: 1151–1157, 1988.
221. Schrier RW: A unifying hypothesis of body fluid volume regulation. *J R Coll Physicians Lond* 26:295–306, 1992.
222. Schrier RW: An odyssey into the milieu intirieur: Pondering the enigmas (editorial). *J Am Soc Nephrol* 2:1549–1559, 1992.
223. Schrier RW, Niederberger M, Weigert A, Gines P: Peripheral Arterial Vasodilation: Determi-nant of Functional Spectrum of Cirrhosis. In Blendis LM (ed): *Seminars in Liver Disease*. New York, Thieme, 1994, vol 22, pp 14–22.
224. Kim J, Summer S, Howard R, Schrier RW: Vasopressin gene expression in rats with experi-mental cirrhosis. *Hepatology* 17:143, 1993.
225. Madsen M, Pedersen EB, Danielson H: Impaired renal water excretion in early hepatic cirrho-sis. *Scand J Gastroenterol* 21:749, 1986.
226. Bichet DG, Groves B, Schrier RW: Mechanisms of improvement of water and sodium excre-tion by enhancement of central hemodynamics in decompensated cirrhotic patients. *Kidney Int* 24:788, 1983.
227. Bichet DG, Szatalowicz V, Chaimovitz C, et al: Role of vasopressin in abnormal water excre-tion in cirrhotic patients. *Ann Intern Med* 96:413, 1982.
228. Floras J, Legaut L, Morali GA: Increased sympathetic outflow in cirrhosis and ascites: Direct evidence from intraneural recordings. *Ann Intern Med* 114:373, 1991.

229. Bichet DG, Van Putten VJ, Schrier RW: Potential role of increased sympathetic activity in impaired sodium and water excretion in cirrhosis. *N Engl J Med* 307:1552, 1982.
230. Epstein FM: Underfilling versus outflow in hepatic ascites (editorial). *N Engl J Med* 307: 1577, 1983.
231. Shapiro MD, Nicholls KM, Groves BM, et al: Interrelationship between cardiac output and vascular resistance as determinants of effective arterial blood volume in cirrhotic patients. *Kidney Int* 18:206, 1985.
232. Usberti M, Federico S, Cianciaruso B, et al: Role of plasma vasopressin in the impairment of water excretion in nephrotic syndrome. *Kidney Int* 25:422, 1984.
233. Krishna GG, Danovitch GM: Effects of water immersion on renal function in the nephrotic syndrome. *Kidney Int* 21:395, 1982.
234. Dorhout Mees EJ, Geers H, Koomans HA: Blood volume and sodium retention in the nephrotic syndrome: A controversial pathophysiological concept. *Nephron* 36:201, 1986.
235. Meltzer JI, Keim HJ, Laragh JH, et al: Nephrotic syndrome: Vasoconstriction and hypervolemic types indicated by renin-sodium profiling. *Ann Intern Med* 91:688, 1979.
236. Kim JK, Pyo H, Schrier RW: Vasopressin Gene Expression in Disease States. In Gross P, Richter D, Robertson GL (eds): *Vasopressin*. London, John Libbey Eurotext, 1993, p 455.
237. Gross PA, Pehrisch H, Rascher W, et al: Pathogenesis of clinical hyponatremia: Observation of vasopressin and fluid intake in 100 hyponatremic medical patients. *Eur J Clin Invest* 17: 123, 1987.
238. Oelkers W: Hyponatremia and inappropriate secretion of vasopressin in patients with hypopituitarism. *N Engl J Med* 321:492, 1989.
239. Ishikawa S, Fujisawa G, Tsuboi Y, et al: Role of antidiuretic hormone in hyponatremia in patients with isolated adrenocorticotropic hormone deficiency. *Endocrinol Jpn* 38:325, 1991.
240. Agus ZS, Goldberg M: Role of antidiuretic hormone in the abnormal water diuresis of anterior hypopituitarism in man. *J Clin Invest* 50:1478, 1971.
241. Boykin J, de Torrente A, Erickson A, et al: Role of plasma vasopressin in impaired water excretion of glucocorticoid deficiency. *J Clin Invest* 62:738, 1978.
242. Linas SL, Berl T, Robertson G, et al: Evidence for vasopressin dependent and independent mechanisms in the impaired water excretion of glucocorticoid deficiency. *Kidney Int* 18:58, 1980.
243. Ishikawa S, Schrier RW: Effect of arginine vasopressin antagonist on renal water excretion in glucocorticoid and mineralocorticoid deficient rats. *Kidney Int* 22:587, 1982.
244. Skowsky WR, Kikuchi TH: The role of vasopressin in the impaired water excretion of myxedema. *Am J Med* 64:613, 1978.
245. Seif S, Robinson A, Zenser T, et al: Neurohypophyseal peptides in hypothyroid rats: Plasma levels and kidney response. *Metabolism* 28:137, 1979.
246. Hochberg Z, Benderly A: Normal osmotic threshold for vasopressin release in the hyponatremia of hypothyroidism. *Horm Res* 18:128, 1983.
247. Iwasaki Y, Oiso Y, Yamauch K: Osmoregulation of plasma vasopressin in myxedema. *J Clin Endocrinol Metab* 70:534, 1990.
248. Emmanouel DS, Lindheimer MD, Katz AI: Mechanism of impaired water excretion in hypothyroid rats. *J Clin Invest* 54:926, 1974.
249. Kim JK, Summer SN, Schrier RW: Cellular action of arginine vasopressin in the isolated renal tubules of hypothyroid rats. *Am J Physiol* 253:F104, 1987.
250. Riggs AT, Dysken MW, Kim SW, Opsahl JA: A review of disorders of water homeostasis in psychiatric patients. *Psychosomatics* 32:133, 1991.
251. Emseley RA, Van der Meer H, Aalbers C, et al: Inappropriate antidiuretic state in long-term psychiatric patients. *S Afr Med J* 77:307, 1990.
252. Goldman M, Luchins DJ, Robertson GL: Mechanism of altered water metabolism in psychotic patients with polydipsia and hyponatremia. *N Engl J Med* 318:397, 1988.
253. Berl T: Psychosis and water balance. *N Engl J Med* 318:441, 1988.
254. Anderson RJ: Hospital associated hyponatremia. *Kidney Int* 29:1237, 1986.
255. Chung H-M, Kluge R, Schrier RW, et al: Post-operative hyponatremia. *Arch Intern Med* 140: 333, 1986.

256. Anderson RJ, Chung H-M, Kluge R, et al: Hyponatremia: A prospective analysis and the pathogenetic role of vasopressin. *Ann Intern Med* 102:164, 1985.
257. Arieff AI: Permanent neurological disability from hyponatremia in healthy women undergoing elective surgery. *N Engl J Med* 314:1529, 1986.
258. Hirokawa CA, Gray DR: Chlorpropamide-induced hyponatremia in the veteran population. *Ann Pharmacotherapy* 10:1243, 1992.
259. Miller M, Moses AM: Drug-induced states of impaired water excretion in mammalian kidney. *Kidney Int* 10:38, 1976.
260. Haenelt M, Hensen J, Distler A, Gross P: Upregulation by Chlorpropamide of Rat Renal Papillary Vasopressin Receptor. In Gross P, Richter D, Robertson GL (eds): *Vasopressin*. London, John Libbey Eurotext, 1993, p 588.
261. Kusano B, Brain-Wemess JL, Vich DJ, et al: Chlorpropamide action on renal concentrating mechanism in rats with hypothalamic diabetes insipidus. *J Clin Invest* 72:1298, 1983.
262. Cooney JA: Carbamazepine and SIADH. *Am J Psychiatry* 147:1101, 1990.
263. Steinhoff BJ, Stoll KD, Stodieck SR, Paulus W: Hyponatremic coma under oxcarbazepine therapy. *Epilepsy Res* 11:67–70, 1992.
264. Harlow PJ, DeClerch YA, Share NA, et al: A fatal case of inappropriate ADH secretion induced by cyclophosphamide therapy. *Cancer* 44:896, 1979.
265. Culine S, Ghosn M, Droz J: Inappropriate antidiuretic hormone secretion induced by ifosfamide. *Eur J Cancer* 26:922, 1990.
266. Verbalis JG: Pathogenesis of hyponatremia in an experimental model of inappropriate antidiuresis. *Am J Physiol* 36:R1617–R1625, 1994.
267. Kovacs L, Robertson GL: Disorders of water balance: Hyponatremia and hypernatremia. *Baillieres Clin Endocrinol Metab* 6:107–127, 1992.
268. Verbalis JG: Hyponatremia: Epidemiology, pathophysiology and therapy. *Curr Opin Nephrol Hypertension* 2:636, 1993.
269. Verbalis J, Drutarosky M: Adaptation to chronic hypoosmolality in rats. *Kidney Int* 34:351, 1988.
270. Eggena P, Ma CL: Downregulation of vasopressin receptors in toad bladder. *Am J Physiol* 250:C453, 1986.
271. Wilson PD, Dixon BS, Dillingham MA, et al: Pertussis toxin prevents homologous desensitization of adenylate cyclase in cultured renal epithelial cells. *J Biol Chem* 261:1509, 1986.
272. Robinson AJ, Roberts MM, Evron WA, et al: Hyponatremia in rats induced down-regulation of vasopressin synthesis. *J Clin Invest* 86:1023, 1990.
273. Tang WW, Kaptein E, Feinstein E: Hyponatremia in hospitalized patients with the acquired immune deficiency syndrome (AIDS) and AIDS related complex. *Am J Med* 94:169–174, 1993.
274. Nolph KD, Schrier RW: Sodium, potassium and water metabolism in the syndrome of inappropriate antidiuretic hormone secretion. *Am J Med* 49:534, 1970.
275. Ayus JC, Wheeler J, Arieff AI: Postoperative hyponatremic encephalopathy in menstruant women. *Ann Intern Med* 117:891–897, 1992.
276. Berl T: Treating hyponatremia: Damned if we do and damned if we don't (Nephrology Forum). *Kidney Int* 37:1006, 1990.
277. Tierney WM, Martin DK, Greenlee MC, et al: The prognosis of hyponatremia at hospital admission. *J Gen Intern Med* 1:380, 1986.
278. Arieff AI, Llach F, Massry SG: Neurological manifestations and morbidity of hyponatremia: Correlation with brain water and electrolytes. *Medicine* (Baltimore) 55:121, 1976.
279. Gullans SR, Verbalis JG: Control of brain volume during hyperosmolar and hypoosmolar conditions. *Annu Rev Med* 44:289–301, 1993.
280. Lien YH, Shapiro UI, Chan L: Study of brain electrolytes and organic osmolyte during correction of chronic hyponatremia: Implication for the pathogenesis of central pontine myelinolysis. *J Clin Invest* 88:303–309, 1991.
281. Sterns RH, Baer J, Ebersol S, et al: Organic osmolytes in acute hyponatremia. *Am J Physiol* 264:F833, 1993.
282. Verbalis JG, Gullans SR: Rapid correction of hyponatremia produces differential effects on brain osmolyte and electrolyte reaccumulation in rats. *Brain Res* 606:19–27, 1993.

283. Cluitmans FH, Meinders AE: Management of severe hyponatremia: Rapid or slow correction? *Am J Med* 88:161, 1990.
284. Sterns RH: The treatment of hyponatremia. *Am J Med* 88:557, 1990.
285. Cheung J, Zikos D, Spokicki H, et al: Long term neurologic outcome in psychogenic water drinkers with severe symptomatic hyponatremia: The effect of rapid correction. *Am J Med* 88:561, 1990.
286. Fraser CL, Sarnacki P: Na-K-ATPase pump function in male rat brain synaptosomes is different from that of females. *Am J Physiol* 257:E284, 1989.
287. Vexler Z, Ayus C, Roberts T, et al: Hypoxic and ischemic hypoxia exacerbates injury associated with metabolic encephalopathy in laboratory animals. *J Clin Invest* 93:256, 1994.
288. Ayus JC, Arieff AI: Pathogenesis and prevention of hyponatremic encephalopathy. *Endocrinol Metab Clin North Am* 22:425, 1993.
289. Ayus IC, Olivero JJ, Fromer JP: Rapid correction of severe hyponatremia with intravenous hypertonic saline solution. *Am J Med* 72:43, 1982.
290. Worthley LG, Thomas PD: Treatment of hyponatremic seizures with intravenous 29.2% saline. *Br Med J* 292:168, 1986.
291. Hantman D, Rossier B, Zohlman R, et al: Rapid correction of hyponatremia in the syndrome of inappropriate secretion of antidiuretic hormone: An alternative treatment to hypertonic saline. *Ann Intern Med* 78:870, 1973.
292. Sterns RH, Riggs JE, Schochet SS Jr: Osmotic demyelination syndrome following correction of hyponatremia. *N Engl J Med* 314:1535, 1986.
293. Sterns RH: Severe symptomatic hyponatremia: Treatment and outcome. A study of 64 cases. *Ann Intern Med* 107:656, 1987.
294. Ayus JC, Krothapalli RK, Arieff AI: Treatment of symptomatic hyponatremia and its relation to brain damage. *N Engl J Med* 317:1190, 1987.
295. Soupart A, Penninckx R, Stenuit R, et al: Treatment of chronic hyponatremia in rats by intravenous saline: Comparison of rate versus magnitude of correction. *Kidney Int* 41:1662–1667, 1992.
296. Ayus IC, Krothapalli RK, Armstrong DL, et al: Symptomatic hyponatremia in rats: Effect of treatment on mortality and brain lesions. *Am J Physiol* 257:18, 1989.
297. Verbalis JG, Martinez AJ: Neurological and neuropathological sequelae of correction of chronic hyponatremia. *Kidney Int* 39:1274–1282, 1991.
298. Stern RH: Severe hyponatremia: The case for conservative management. *Crit Care Med* 20:534–539, 1992.
299. de Troyer A, Demanet JC: Correction of antidiuresis by demeclocycline. *N Engl J Med* 293:915, 1975.
300. Schrier RW: New treatments for hyponatremia. *N Engl J Med* 298:214, 1978.
301. Miller PD, Linas SL, Schrier RW: Correlation between plasma demeclocycline levels and nephrotoxic effect in hyponatremic cirrhotic individuals. *JAMA* 243:2513, 1980.
302. Decaux G, Prospert F, Pennickx R, et al: 5 year treatment of the chronic syndrome of inappropriate secretion of ADH with oral urea. *Nephron* 63:468–470, 1993.
303. Schrier RW: Update on treatment of hyponatremia disorders (editorial). *N Engl J Med* 312:1121, 1985.
304. Ishikawa S, Kim JK, Schrier RW: Further in vivo evidence for antagonist to antidiuretic action of arginine vasopressin. *Am J Physiol* 245:R713, 1983.
305. Kim JK, Dillingham MD, Summer SN, et al: Effects of vasopressin antagonist on vasopressin binding, adenylate cyclase activation and water flux. *J Clin Invest* 76:1530, 1985.
306. Yamamura Y, Ogawa H, Kondo K, et al: Development and Pharmacology of Non-peptide V_1 and V_2 Vasopressin Receptor Antagonists. In Gross P, Richter D, Robertson GL (eds): *Vasopressin.* London, John Libbey Eurotex, 1993, p 507.
307. Fujisawa G, Ishikawa S, Okada K, Saito T: Therapeutic efficacy of non-peptide ADH antagonist OPC-31260 in SIADH rats. *Kidney Int* 44:19, 1993.

2

Renal Sodium Excretion, Edematous Disorders, and Diuretic Use

William T. Abraham and Robert W. Schrier

An understanding of body fluid volume regulation, as modulated by renal sodium and water excretion, is critical for the practice of clinical medicine. Since the sodium ion is the primary determinant of extracellular fluid (ECF) volume, knowledge of the intrarenal and extrarenal factors affecting renal sodium excretion is important to comprehend the mechanism of body fluid volume regulation in health and disease. In this regard, the edematous disorders—cardiac failure, liver disease, and the nephrotic syndrome—present a particular challenge to our understanding of body fluid volume regulation. In normal humans, if the ECF volume is expanded by the administration of isotonic saline, the kidney will excrete the excess amount of sodium and water in the urine, thus returning the ECF volume to normal. However, in these edematous states, avid renal sodium and water retention persist despite expansion of ECF volume and the presence of total-body sodium and water excess. In circumstances where advanced kidney disease is present and renal function and excretory capacity are diminished, such as in acute or chronic intrinsic renal failure, it is obvious why the decreased glomerular filtration rate (GFR) may be associated with retention of sodium and water to the point of pulmonary and/or peripheral edema. However, in patients with heart failure or liver disease and in some patients with the nephrotic syndrome, it is clear that the integrity of the kidney as the ultimate effector organ of body fluid volume regulation is intact. Thus, in these edematous disorders, the kidney must be responding to extrarenal signals from the afferent limb of a volume regulatory system. The study of these edematous disorders has led to our proposal of a unifying hypothesis of body fluid volume regulation that applies to both health and disease [1–6]. The purpose of this chapter is to review the afferent and efferent mechanisms that determine renal sodium and water handling, particularly in the context of the edematous disorders, and to discuss the treatment of edema with diuretic agents.

Sodium Ion as Determinant of Extracellular Fluid Volume

Sodium ions reside primarily in the ECF compartment, to which they are extruded from cells by active transport mechanisms [7]. These transport processes result in an intracellular sodium concentration of 10 mEq/L and an ECF sodium concentration of 145 mEq/L. The sodium ion and its major anions, chloride and bicarbonate, constitute more than 90 percent of the total solute in the ECF space. Thus, total body sodium and its accompanying anions are the osmotically active solutes that are the major determinants of ECF volume. In turn, the regulation of sodium balance is determined by the relationship between sodium intake, extrarenal sodium loss, and renal sodium excretion. Practically, renal sodium excretion may be considered to be the primary determinant of sodium balance, since the kidney is able to excrete virtually sodium-free urine as well as rapidly excrete large sodium loads in response to diminished or increased sodium intakes, respectively.

A positive sodium balance is associated with increased amounts of sodium, located predominantly in the ECF compartment. Since cellular membranes are freely permeable to water, the osmotic gradient created by the addition of ECF sodium will cause water to move from cells into the ECF compartment, thus expanding ECF volume. In addition, an increase in ECF osmolality stimulates the hypothalamic thirst center and leads to increased fluid intake [8] and also releases arginine vasopressin (AVP) from the posterior pituitary, which, by increasing the water permeability of collecting duct epithelium, decreases renal water excretion [9]. These latter two effects of an increased ECF osmolality results in a positive water balance, and the combined influence of positive sodium and water balances leads to further expansion of ECF volume. If this expansion of ECF is of sufficient magnitude, an alteration of the Starling forces that govern the transfer of fluid from the vascular compartment to the surrounding interstitial spaces occurs, and edema results [10]. Conversely, a negative sodium balance results in a depletion of ECF volume. A decrease in ECF volume may result in a parallel decline in plasma volume. Maintenance of ECF volume and plasma volume is necessary for adequacy of circulation and survival of the organism. Thus, in situations of ECF volume depletion, renal sodium and water retention is clearly appropriate. However, in edematous disorders, continued renal sodium and water retention despite total-body sodium and water excess defines a paradoxical clinical situation.

It is worth mentioning that the osmolality of ECF is regulated by the AVP-thirst-renal axis (as discussed in depth in Chap. 1). The osmolality of the ECF, however, is not a reliable index of ECF volume. ECF volume and its determinant total-body sodium are best assessed by physical examination and determination of urinary sodium concentration. For example, a finding of generalized edema suggests an expanded ECF volume and increased total-body sodium. Conversely, orthostatic tachycardia and/or hypotension, flat neck veins, and decreased skin turgor suggest depletion of ECF volume and decreased total-body sodium. In fact, alterations in the osmolality of the ECF can occur in association with normal, increased, or decreased ECF volume (see Chap. 1).

In summary, the control of ECF volume is dependent on the regulation of sodium balance. The kidneys play the pivotal role in the regulation of sodium balance and therefore of ECF volume homeostasis. In certain edema-forming states associated with normal filtration rates of sodium, the kidney retains sodium and water despite expansion of the ECF volume and total-body sodium and water. A knowledge of the afferent ("sensor") and efferent ("effector") mechanisms of sodium and water retention associated with the edematous disorders forms the basis for our understanding of body fluid volume regulation.

Afferent Mechanisms Involved in Body Fluid Volume Regulation

The Concept of "Effective Blood Volume" or the Compartment Sensed

If the afferent receptors of body fluid volume regulation sense primarily total blood volume, then the kidneys of edematous patients should increase their excretion of sodium and water as their total blood volume increases. However, as mentioned, in patients with advanced cardiac failure, liver disease, or the nephrotic syndrome, this does not occur. Thus, there must be some body fluid compartment that is still "underfilled"—even in the presence of expansion of total ECF and blood volumes—and comprises the afferent limb of renal sodium and water retention in patients with edematous disorders. In 1948, Peters coined the term "effective blood volume" as a reference to such an underfilled body fluid compartment [11]. Accordingly, extrarenal signals must be initiated by this decrease in effective blood volume, which enhances tubular sodium and water reabsorption by the otherwise normal kidney. In this regard, it is clear that renal sodium and water retention can occur in patients with cardiac failure or cirrhosis and in some patients with the nephrotic syndrome prior to any diminution in GFR.

Borst and deVries [12] first suggested cardiac output as the primary modulator of renal sodium and water excretion. In this context, the level of cardiac output would constitute effective blood volume and thus serve as the primary stimulus for renal sodium and water retention in patients with edematous disorders. While this concept is appealing, substantial renal sodium and water retention may occur in the presence of an increase in cardiac output. For example, a significant elevation in cardiac output may occur in the presence of avid renal sodium and water retention and expansion of ECF volume in association with cirrhosis, pregnancy, arteriovenous (AV) fistulae, and other causes of high-output cardiac failure such as thyrotoxicosis and beriberi. Thus, there must exist some other or additional determinant(s) of effective blood volume.

Primacy of the Arterial Circulation in Volume Regulation

The unifying hypothesis of body fluid volume regulation in health and disease states that the fullness of the arterial vascular compartment or the so-called effective *arterial* blood volume (EABV) is the primary determinant of renal sodium and water excretion [1–6]. In a 70-kg man, total-body water approximates 42 L of which only

Table 2-1. Body fluid distribution

Compartment	Amount	Volume in 70-kg man
Total body fluid	60% of body weight	42 L
Intracellular fluid	40% of body weight	28 L
Extracellular fluid (ECF)	20% of body weight	14 L
Interstitial fluid	Two-thirds of ECF	9.4 L
Plasma fluid	One-third of ECF	4.6 L
Venous fluid	85% of plasma fluid	3.9 L
Arterial fluid	15% of plasma fluid	0.7 L

0.7 L (1.7% of total-body water) resides in the arterial circulation (Table 2-1). From a teleologic viewpoint, it is attractive to propose that the primacy for regulation of renal sodium and water excretion, and thus body fluid volume homeostasis, is modulated by the smallest body fluid compartment—thus endowing the system with exquisite sensitivity to relatively small changes in body fluid volume—and resides in that fluid compartment that is responsible for the arterial perfusion of the body's vital organs and tissues. Thus total ECF, interstitial fluid, or intravascular volumes are not primary determinants of renal sodium and water excretion, and the venous component of intravascular volume is likewise excluded as the primary determinant of sodium and water excretion, since all of these body fluid compartments may be expanded while the renal sodium and water retention persists in edematous patients. It is acknowledged, however, that there are experimental and clinical circumstances in which selective rises in right and left or left atrial pressure stimulate the release of atrial natriuretic peptide (ANP) [13] or suppression of AVP [14], respectively, which may enhance sodium and water excretion. These events must, however, be subservient to more potent determinants of body fluid volume regulation, since the patient with advanced left or right ventricular dysfunction or both exhibits avid sodium and water retention despite markedly elevated atrial and ventricular pressures.

Cardiac Output and Peripheral Arterial Resistance as the Determinants of the Fullness of the Arterial Circulation and Renal Sodium and Water Excretion

The EABV is a measure of the adequacy of arterial blood volume to "fill" the capacity of the arterial circulation. Normal EABV exists when the ratio of cardiac output to peripheral vascular resistance maintains venous return and cardiac output at normal levels. Thus, diminished EABV may be initiated by either a decrease in cardiac output or a fall in peripheral arterial resistance (i.e., an increase in the holding capacity of the arterial vascular tree). Decreased EABV results in unloading of high-pressure baroreceptors with subsequent activation of the three major neurohormonal vasoconstrictor systems—namely the sympathetic nervous system, the

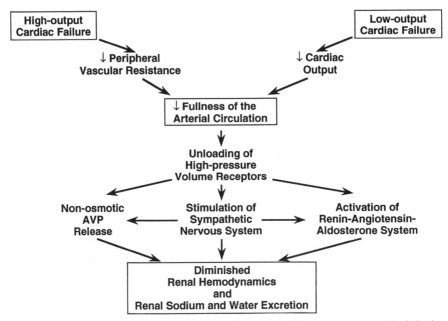

Fig. 2-1. Mechanism for the initiation of renal sodium and water retention in both high-output and low-output heart failure. AVP = arginine vasopressin.

renin-angiotensin-aldosterone system, and the nonosmotic release of AVP—which diminish renal hemodynamics and promote renal sodium and water retention. This hypothesis accounts for the initiation of sodium and water retention in low- and high-output cardiac failure, liver disease, and other states of arterial underfilling (Figs. 2-1 and 2-2).

Afferent Volume Receptors

As mentioned previously, the afferent volume receptors for such a volume regulatory system must reside in the arterial vascular tree, such as the high-pressure baroreceptors in the carotid sinus, aortic arch, left ventricle, and juxtaglomerular apparatus. While the low-pressure volume receptors of the thorax (cardiac atria, right ventricle, and pulmonary vessels) must be of some importance to the volume regulatory system, there is considerable evidence that arterial receptors predominate over low-pressure receptors in volume control in mammals [15–23].

High-Pressure Volume Receptors

In humans, the presence of volume-sensitive receptors in the arterial circulation was first suggested by Epstein et al. [24] based on observations made in patients with traumatic AV fistulae. Closure of traumatic AV fistulae is associated with an immediate increase in renal sodium excretion independent of concomitant changes in either GFR or renal blood flow (RBF) [24]. Closure of AV fistulae is associated

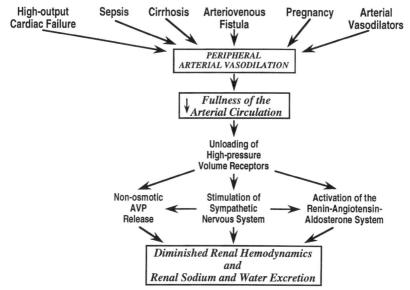

Fig. 2-2. Mechanism for the initiation of renal sodium and water retention in cirrhosis and in other states of arterial underfilling due to peripheral arterial vasodilation. AVP = arginine vasopressin.

with a decreased rate of emptying of the arterial blood into the venous circulation, as demonstrated by closure-induced increases in diastolic arterial pressure and decreases in cardiac output [24]. Further evidence implicating the relative "fullness" of the arterial vascular tree as a sensor in modulating renal sodium excretion can be found in denervation experiments. In these studies, surgical or pharmacologic interruption of sympathetic efferent neural pathways emanating from high-pressure areas inhibited the natriuretic response to volume expansion [25–29]. Moreover, reduction of pressure or stretch at the carotid sinus, similar to that produced by decreased cardiac output or arterial hypotension, has been shown to activate the sympathetic nervous system and to promote renal sodium and water retention [30, 31]. High-pressure baroreceptors also appear to be important factors in regulating nonosmotic release of AVP and thus renal water excretion [32, 33]. One of the best-defined high-pressure receptors that is known to act in an appropriate manner to maintain constancy of the effective circulating arterial volume is the renal afferent arteriolar baroreceptor or juxtaglomerular apparatus. This baroreceptor is an important factor in the control of renal renin secretion and thus angiotensin II formation and aldosterone synthesis and release [30]. The vasoconstrictor and sodium-retaining effects of angiotensin II and the sodium-retaining effect of aldosterone then act to restore the effective circulating arterial volume.

Low-Pressure Volume Receptors

Low-pressure sensors may also have an important role to play in body fluid volume regulation because the more compliant venous side of the circulation contains up to 85 percent of the total blood volume at any given time (see Table 2-1). In fact, a variety of maneuvers that decrease thoracic venous return, such as prolonged standing [34], lower-extremity tourniquets [35, 36], and positive pressure breathing [37], are associated with diminished renal sodium excretion. Conversely, maneuvers that augment venous filling, such as recumbency [38] and negative pressure breathing [39], are associated with increased renal sodium excretion. Moreover, a direct correlation between renal sodium excretion and left atrial pressure has been demonstrated in the dog, suggesting a role for an atrial receptor as one type of intrathoracic sensor [40, 41]. Immersion in water to the neck or so-called head-out water immersion results in a pressure gradient from 80 mm Hg at the foot to 0 mm Hg at water level. This maneuver increases venous return to the heart. In response to head-out water immersion, a profound increase in renal excretion of salt and water occurs independent of major changes in either GFR or renal hemodynamics [42]. As first suggested by Gauer and Henry and associates [39, 43], physiologically significant left atrial receptors have been shown to contribute to ECF volume regulation by exerting nonosmotic control over AVP secretion and thus over renal water excretion [14, 35, 40, 43]. In addition, the atria have been demonstrated to be the site for synthesis, storage, and release of vasoactive and natriuretic humoral agents [13, 44, 45].

Thus, increased filling of the thoracic vascular and cardiac atria would be expected to signal the kidney to increase urinary sodium excretion in order to return the blood volume to normal. However, in the setting of chronic heart failure, renal sodium and water retention occur despite loading of the low-pressure baroreceptors. Thus, in chronic heart failure, diminished cardiac output and decreased EABV must exert the predominant effect via unloading of high-pressure arterial baroreceptors. Chronic studies in animals employing either experimental tricuspid insufficiency [46] or right atrial distention with an inflatable balloon [47] support this hypothesis. In these animal models, the increase in right atrial pressure was associated with avid renal sodium retention rather than the expected natriuresis. However, a concomitant fall in cardiac output could explain the sodium retention. Alternatively, alterations in cardiopulmonary baroreceptor function may occur in chronic but not in acute heart failure.

Zucker et al. [48] have demonstrated that the inhibition of renal sympathetic nerve activity that is seen during acute left atrial distention is lost during chronic heart failure in the dog. Moreover, a decrease in cardiac preload fails to produce the expected parasympathetic withdrawal and sympathetic activation in humans with heart failure [49–51]. Nishian and colleagues [51] have recently described paradoxical forearm vasodilation and hemodynamic improvement during lower-body negative pressure in patients with severe chronic heart failure. This paradoxical response to acute unloading of low-pressure baroreceptors was associated with static, rather than the expected increased, plasma norepinephrine levels [51], further demonstrating this altered response to low-pressure baroreceptor unloading in heart failure. These observations confirm those made in heart failure patients during other forms of orthostatic stress [49, 50]. These findings are also consistent with the observation of a strong positive correlation between left atrial pressure and coronary sinus norepinephrine, a marker of cardiac adrenergic activity, in patients with chronic heart failure [52]. Taken together, these findings suggest that the normal inhibitory control of sympathetic activation accompanying increased atrial pressures is lost in heart failure patients and may somehow be converted to a stimulatory signal.

Finally, cardiac, pulmonary, and hepatic chemoreceptors have also been implicated as physiologically important modulators of renal sodium and water excretion [53–56]. However, the exact role of such chemically responsive receptors in body fluid volume regulation remains to be defined.

In summary, the afferent or sensor mechanisms for sodium and water excretion may be preferentially located on the arterial side of the circulation where diminished fullness of the arterial vascular tree due to decreased cardiac output or to peripheral arterial vasodilation results in unloading of high-pressure receptors and subsequent renal sodium and water retention. Reflexes from low-pressure volume receptors may also be altered so as to influence renal sodium and water handling. In any event, changes in systemic and renal hemodynamics and activation of various neurohormonal systems largely comprise the efferent limb of the volume regulatory system.

Efferent Mechanisms Involved in Body Fluid Volume Regulation

The Neurohormonal Response to Arterial Underfilling

Arterial underfilling secondary to a diminished cardiac output or peripheral arterial vasodilation elicits a number of compensatory neurohormonal responses that act to maintain the integrity of the arterial circulation by promoting peripheral vasoconstriction as well as expansion of the ECF volume through renal sodium and water retention. As mentioned previously, the three major neurohormonal vasoconstrictor systems activated in response to a diminished EABV are the sympathetic nervous system, the renin-angiotensin-aldosterone system, and the nonosmotic release of AVP. Baroreceptor activation of the sympathetic nervous system appears to be the primary integrator of the hormonal vasoconstrictor systems involved in the volume control system, since the nonosmotic release of AVP involves sympathetic stimulation of the supraoptic and paraventricular nuclei in the hypothalamus [57] and activation of the renin-angiotensin-aldosterone system involves renal β-adrenergic stimulation [58]. Thus, in low-output cardiac failure, diminished integrity of the arterial circulation as determined by decreased cardiac output causes unloading of arterial baroreceptors in the carotid sinus and aortic arch. Peripheral vasodilation produces unloading of these arterial baroreceptors in the setting of high-output cardiac failure, cirrhosis, and other states of arterial underfilling. This baroreceptor inactivation results in diminution of the tonic inhibitory effect of afferent vagal and glossopharyngeal pathways to the central nervous system and initiates an increase in sympathetic efferent adrenergic tone with subsequent activation of the other two major vasoconstrictor hormonal systems. Various counterregulatory, vasodilatory hormones may also be activated in heart failure, including natriuretic peptides and vasodilating renal prostaglandins. Activation of these various neurohormonal vaso-constrictor and vasodilator systems substantially determines renal sodium and water handling in the edematous disorders and comprises a major part of the efferent limb of body fluid volume regulation. The pathogenesis of sodium and water retention associated with cardiac failure, liver disease, and the nephrotic syndrome will now be reviewed in the context of the unifying hypothesis of body fluid volume regulation.

Pathogenesis of Sodium and Water Retention in Cardiac Failure

Sodium and water retention and resultant edema formation are cardinal features of chronic cardiac failure. In fact, the inability to excrete a sodium load has been used as an index of the presence of heart failure [59], and a defect in water excretion is routinely encountered in such patients [60]. Two theories have been proposed to explain the renal response to cardiac failure. The "backward" theory of heart failure, proposed in 1832, suggests that increased venous hydrostatic pressure due to in-creased ventricular filling pressures causes edema by promoting transudation of fluid from the intravascular to the interstitial compartment, thus resulting in edema formation [61]. The reduced intravascular volume then signals the kidneys to retain sodium and water, further exacerbating the venous hypertension and formation of edema. The alternative "forward" theory of cardiac failure suggests that a primary decrease in cardiac output activates afferent and efferent pathways and results in renal sodium retention [62]. As pointed out by Smith [36], these theories are not mutually exclusive, and both are operant in the pathophysiology of heart failure, since, as noted previously, both central venous hypertension and arterial underfilling are implicated in the afferent limb of body fluid volume regulation. In the case of low-output heart failure, decreased cardiac output is the cause of the arterial underfilling, while in the circumstance of high-output cardiac failure, peripheral arterial vasodilation initiates the afferent limb of sodium and water retention (see Fig. 2-1).

Renal Hemodynamics in Cardiac Failure

Glomerular Filtration Rate. Many early investigators believed that the cause of sodium retention in heart failure was a decrease in GFR. However, recent studies have failed to confirm such a correlation [63–65]. In fact, GFR is often normal in heart failure and can even be elevated in states of high-output cardiac failure [66]. It is acknowledged, however, that the contribution of GFR to sodium balance is difficult to evaluate because very minute changes in GFR can be difficult to detect and may account for important changes in sodium excretion [67]. Nevertheless, although GFR may be diminished in patients with advanced heart failure, an in-crease in tubular sodium reabsorption is no doubt an important cause of sodium and water retention in cardiac failure.

Renal Blood Flow. Heart failure is commonly associated with an increase in renal vascular resistance and a decrease in RBF. In general, RBF decreases in proportion to the decrease in cardiac output. Some investigators have also shown a redistribution of RBF from outer cortical nephrons to juxtamedullary nephrons in experimental heart failure [46, 68–70]. It was proposed that deeper nephrons with longer loops of Henle reabsorb sodium more avidly. Thus, the redistribution of blood flow to these nephrons with heart failure results in renal sodium retention. However, other investigators have not been able to demonstrate such a redistribution of blood flow in other models of cardiac failure [71]. At the present time, the role of redistribution of RBF in the sodium retention of cardiac failure remains uncertain.

Filtration Fraction. Since RBF falls as cardiac output decreases and GFR is usually preserved, filtration fraction is often increased in heart failure. An increase in filtration fraction results in increased protein concentration and oncotic pressure in the efferent arterioles and peritubular capillaries that surround the proximal tubules [72]. Such an increase in peritubular oncotic pressure has been proposed to increase sodium and water reabsorption in the proximal tubule [73, 74]. These changes in renal hemodynamics and filtration fraction, which favor proximal tubular sodium reabsorption, are primarily a consequence of constriction of the efferent arterioles within the kidney (Fig. 2-3). These renal hemodynamic changes are mediated mainly by activation of neurohormonal vasoconstrictor systems, as both activation of renal nerves and increased circulating norepinephrine and angiotensin II have been implicated in efferent arteriolar vasoconstriction [75, 76]. In addition, decreased activity of such substances as vasodilating renal prostaglandins may also play a role in the renal vasoconstriction [77, 78].

Of note, micropuncture studies in dogs with vena caval constriction and AV

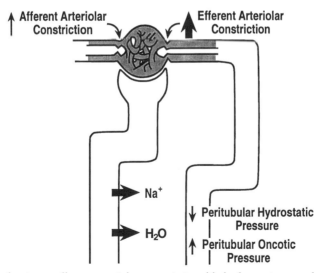

Fig. 2-3. Predominant efferent arteriolar constriction, likely due to increased renal sympathetic activity and angiotensin II, alters net postglomerular Starling forces in a direction to favor enhanced proximal tubular sodium reabsorption in states of arterial underfilling.

fistulae have demonstrated the importance of distal nephron sites of increased sodium reabsorption [79, 80]. Increased filtration fraction primarily affects proximal tubular sodium reabsorption. Thus, while clearance and micropuncture studies in animals with heart failure have demonstrated increased sodium reabsorption in the proximal tubule [81], distal sodium reabsorption also seems to be involved. Furthermore, changes in filtration fraction have been observed in heart failure long before changes in sodium balance occur, thus questioning the dominance of peritubular factors and proximal reabsorption in the sodium retention of cardiac failure [64, 82].

The Sympathetic Nervous System in Cardiac Failure

The sympathetic nervous system is unquestionably activated in patients with heart failure. Various studies have demonstrated elevated peripheral venous plasma norepinephrine concentrations in heart failure patients [83–86]. Using tritiated norepinephrine in patients with advanced heart failure, Davis and co-workers [84] and Hasking et al. [85] have shown that both increased norepinephrine secretion and decreased norepinephrine clearance contribute to the high venous plasma norepinephrine concentrations seen in these patients, suggesting that increased sympathetic activity is at least partially responsible for the elevated circulating plasma norepinephrine. Recently, we have demonstrated that the initial rise in plasma norepinephrine in heart failure is solely due to increased norepinephrine secretion, providing evidence of increased sympathetic nervous system activity early in the course of cardiac failure [86]. Moreover, plasma norepinephrine is increased in patients with asymptomatic left ventricular dysfunction (i.e., prior to the onset of overt heart failure) [87]. Finally, studies employing peroneal nerve microneurography to directly assess sympathetic nerve activity to muscle have confirmed the presence of increased sympathetic activity in heart failure patients [88]. Significantly, the degree of activation of the sympathetic nervous system—as assessed by the peripheral venous plasma norepinephrine concentration—has been correlated with poor prognosis in heart failure [89].

Activation of Renal Nerves. Renal nerves are also activated in human heart failure [85]. By promoting renal vasoconstriction, stimulation of the renin-angiotensin-aldosterone system, and direct effects on the proximal convoluted tubule, enhanced renal sympathetic activity may contribute to the avid sodium and water retention of heart failure. Indeed, intrarenal adrenergic blockade has been shown to cause a natriuresis in experimental animals and humans with heart failure [90, 91]. In addition, in the rat, renal nerve stimulation has been demonstrated to produce approximately a 25 percent reduction in sodium excretion and urine volume [92]. The diminished renal sodium excretion that accompanies renal nerve stimulation may be mediated by at least two mechanisms. As mentioned previously, studies performed in rats have demonstrated that norepinephrine-induced efferent arteriolar constriction alters peritubular hemodynamic forces in favor of increased tubular sodium reabsorption [75]. In addition, renal nerves have been shown to exert a direct influence on sodium reabsorption in the proximal convoluted tubule [92, 93].

Bello-Reuss et al. [92] demonstrated this direct effect of renal nerve activation to enhance proximal tubular sodium reabsorption in whole-kidney and individual nephron studies in the rat. In these animals, renal nerve stimulation produced an increase in the tubular fluid–to–plasma inulin concentration ratio in the late proximal tubule, an outcome of increased fractional sodium and water reabsorption in this segment of the nephron [92]. Hence, increased renal nerve activity may promote sodium retention by a mechanism independent of changes in renal hemodynamics. On the other hand, sodium retention persists in dogs with denervated transplanted kidneys and chronic vena caval constriction [76]. Moreover, renal denervation does not prevent ascites in the dog with chronic vena caval constriction [94]. Thus, renal nerves probably contribute but do not fully account for the avid sodium retention of heart failure.

The role of renal nerves in renal sodium-retaining, edema-forming states has recently been reassessed in conscious chronically instrumented rats with heart failure secondary to myocardial infarction [91]. Renal sodium and water excretion of an acutely administered oral or intravenous isotonic saline load was significantly less than in control rats. Bilateral renal denervation of the experimental heart failure rats restored their renal excretory response to that of the control rats. In addition, in response to the acute administration of a standard intravenous isotonic saline load, the decrease in efferent renal sympathetic activity was significantly less, as compared with that of control rats. These results support an increased basal efferent renal sympathetic nerve activity in heart failure, which fails to suppress normally in response to the isotonic saline load.

Finally, recent experience with the partial β_1-adrenergic receptor agonist xamoterol in heart failure suggests a role for renal nerves in modulating proximal tubular sodium reabsorption [95]. Botker et al. [95] examined the acute renal effects of xamoterol in 12 patients with mild to moderate heart failure. Each patient was given xamoterol (0.2 mg/kg) or placebo in random order separated by 2 weeks of clinically stable drug washout. Renal clearance and excretion measurements were made in the supine position at 30- to 60-minute intervals before, during, and up to 6 hours after infusion. Lithium clearance was used as a measure of proximal tubular sodium handling [96]. Blood pressure, heart rate, renal plasma flow, GFR, and urine flow rate remained unchanged, while xamoterol significantly decreased renal sodium excretion by 30 percent. This acute decrease in sodium excretion with xamoterol was associated with an increase in proximal tubular sodium reabsorption, as indicated by decreased lithium clearance. Of note, plasma concentrations of angiotensin II and aldosterone were unaffected by xamoterol. These observations suggest a direct effect of acute xamoterol to enhance proximal tubular sodium reabsorption in heart failure. In patients with heart failure, the endogenous adrenergic receptor agonist and neurotransmitter norepinephrine may thus exert a similar effect on the proximal renal tubule.

The Renin-Angiotensin-Aldosterone System in Cardiac Failure

The renin-angiotensin-aldosterone system is also activated in heart failure, as assessed by plasma renin activity (PRA) [97]. Renin acts on angiotensinogen to produce angiotensin I, which is then converted by angiotensin-converting enzyme (ACE) to angiotensin II. In heart failure, the resultant increased plasma concentration of angiotensin II exerts important circulatory effects, including peripheral arterial and venous vascular constriction, renal vasoconstriction, and cardiac inotropism. Angiotensin II also acts to promote the secretion of the sodium-retaining hormone aldosterone by the adrenal cortex and in positive-feedback stimulation of the sympathetic nervous system. In the kidney, activation of this hormonal system may promote sodium retention via several mechanisms, as will be discussed. Moreover, like adrenergic activation, stimulation of the renin-angiotensin-aldosterone system is associated with an unfavorable prognosis in heart failure [98].

Renal Effects of Increased Angiotensin II and Aldosterone. Angiotensin II may contribute to the sodium and water retention of heart failure through direct and indirect effects on proximal tubular sodium reabsorption and, as mentioned, by stimulating the release of aldosterone from the adrenal gland. Angiotensin II causes renal efferent arteriolar constriction, resulting in decreased renal blood flow and an increased filtration fraction. As with renal nerve stimulation, this results in increased peritubular capillary oncotic pressure and reduced peritubular capillary hydrostatic pressure, which favors the reabsorption of sodium and water in the proximal tubule [76]. Moreover, angiotensin II has been shown to enhance sodium reabsorption in the proximal tubule [99]. In a study of the rat proximal tubule, Liu and Cogan [99] demonstrated increased tubular sodium chloride reabsorption during the infusion of angiotensin II, while the angiotensin II receptor antagonist saralasin decreased proximal tubular sodium chloride reabsorption. Finally, in a recent report from Abassi and associates [100], the administration of the angiotensin II receptor antagonist losartan to decompensated sodium-retaining rats with heart failure secondary to AV fistulae produced a marked natriuresis. While proximal tubular sodium handling was not examined in this investigation, the observation that losartan restored renal responsiveness to ANP is consistent with a losartan-induced increase in the delivery of sodium to the distal tubular site of ANP action. The role of distal tubular sodium delivery in the renal sodium retention of heart failure is discussed below.

To define more precisely the role of the renin-angiotensin-aldosterone axis in cardiac failure, Watkins and co-workers [101] studied a conscious dog model of heart failure. Using either partial constriction of the pulmonary artery or thoracic inferior vena cava, these workers acutely produced a low cardiac output state characterized by reduced blood pressure, increased PRA and aldosterone concentrations, and renal sodium retention. As plasma volume and body weight increased over several days, the aforementioned variables all returned toward control levels. During the initial hyperreninemic period, a single injection of an ACE inhibitor significantly lowered blood pressure. Also, chronic administration of the converting enzyme inhibitor prevented a rise in aldosterone and prevented 30 percent of the sodium retention and subsequent volume expansion. These studies lend support to the hypothesis that aldosterone is an important factor in the pathogenesis of cardiac edema and suggest that angiotensin II plays an important physiologic role in heart failure by supporting blood pressure due to its vasoconstrictor effect and maintaining blood volume secondary to the sodium-retaining effects of angiotensin II and aldosterone. It likewise becomes clear that, depending on the status of cardiac decompensation and plasma volume, the patient with heart failure may have a high or normal PRA and aldosterone level. This may explain some of the controversy that currently exists regarding the levels of these hormones in patients with heart failure.

A role for renin-angiotensin-aldosterone system activation in the sodium retention of human heart failure is supported by the finding that urinary sodium excretion inversely correlates with PRA and urinary aldosterone excretion in heart failure patients [102]. However, the administration of an ACE inhibitor during heart failure does not consistently increase urinary sodium excretion in spite of a consistent fall in plasma aldosterone concentration [103]. The simultaneous fall in blood pressure due to decreased circulating concentrations of angiotensin II, however, may activate hemodynamic and neurohormonal mechanisms that could obscure the natriuretic response to lowered angiotensin II and aldosterone concentrations. Support for this hypothesis comes from a recent study performed by Hensen and associates [104]. We examined the effect of the specific aldosterone antagonist spironolactone on urinary sodium excretion in patients with mild to moderate heart failure who were withdrawn from all medications prior to study. Sodium was retained in all patients throughout the period prior to aldosterone antagonism. During therapy with spironolactone, all heart failure patients exhibited a significant increase in urinary sodium excretion and reversal of the positive sodium balance (Fig. 2-4). Moreover, the urinary sodium-to-potassium concentration ratio significantly increased during spironolactone administration, consistent with a decrease in aldosterone action in the distal nephron. Of note, PRA and norepinephrine increased and ANP decreased during the administration of spironolactone. Thus, this investigation demonstrates reversal of the sodium retention of heart failure with the administration of an aldosterone antagonist, despite further activation of various antinatriuretic influences including stimulation of the renin-angiotensin and sympathetic nervous systems, and supports a role for aldosterone in the renal sodium retention. Ongoing multicenter trials of spironolactone in patients with heart failure should clarify further the role of aldosterone antagonism in the treatment of cardiac failure.

The Nonosmotic Release of Arginine Vasopressin in Cardiac Failure

Plasma AVP is often elevated in patients with congestive heart failure and correlates in general with the clinical and hemodynamic severity of disease and with the serum sodium level [105–109]. Using a sensitive radioimmunoassay for AVP, Szatalowicz and associates [105] showed that, in 30 of 37 patients with cardiac failure and hyponatremia, plasma AVP was detectable. Because all of these patients had sufficient hyponatremia and hypo-osmolality to suppress the osmotic release of AVP, it was concluded that the nonosmotic AVP release in these patients was the result of baroreceptor stimulation secondary to diminished cardiac output. Riegger and colleagues [106] have also reported that several patients with heart failure had inappropriately high AVP levels. When two of these patients were treated with hemofiltration to remove excess body fluid, cardiac output increased and AVP levels normalized [106]. Taken together, these observations demonstrate enhanced AVP release in cardiac failure and support the notion that nonosmotic mechanisms, such as a decrease in EABV, are responsible.

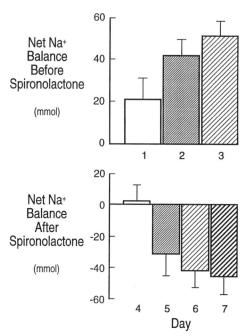

Fig. 2-4. Reversal of sodium retention with aldosterone antagonism in patients with heart failure. Net positive cumulative sodium balance, by day, for the period before spironolactone (*upper panel*) and net negative cumulative sodium balance after the initiation of spironolactone, 400 mg/day (*lower panel*), are shown. (From J. Hensen, W. T. Abraham, J. A. Durr, and R. W. Schrier, Aldosterone in congestive heart failure: Analysis of determinants and role in sodium retention. *Am. J. Nephrol.* 11:441, 1991. Reprinted by permission of S. Karger AG [Basel].)

Renal Effects of Arginine Vasopressin. AVP, via stimulation of its renal or V_2 receptor subtype, enhances water reabsorption in the distal nephron, including cortical and medullary collecting ducts. Several lines of evidence implicate nonosmotic AVP release in the abnormal water retention of heart failure. First, in animal models of heart failure, the absence of a pituitary source of AVP is associated with normal or near normal water excretion [21, 110]. This observation was first made by Anderson and colleagues [21] in the dog during acute thoracic vena caval constriction. In these animals, acute removal of the pituitary source of AVP by surgical hypophysectomy virtually abolished the defect in water excretion. Abnormal water excretion also occurs in the rat with an aortocaval fistula [110]. The impairment in water excretion seen in this high-output model of cardiac failure is presumably the result of AVP release, since the defect is not demonstrable in rats with central diabetes insipidus [110].

The second line of evidence supporting a role for AVP in the water retention of heart failure comes from studies using selective peptide and nonpeptide antagonists of the V_2 receptor of AVP in several animal models of cardiac failure [111–114]. Ishikawa et al. [111] have assessed the antidiuretic effect of plasma AVP in a low-output model of cardiac failure secondary to vena caval constriction in the rat. In these animals, plasma AVP concentrations were increased, and an antagonist of the antidiuretic effect of AVP reversed the defect in water excretion. Yared et al. [112] have also shown a reversal of water retention using an antagonist to the antidiuretic effect of AVP in another model of heart failure, the rat coronary artery ligation model. Recently, an orally active nonpeptide V_2 receptor AVP antagonist, OPC-31260, has been described [115]. The intravenous administration of OPC-31260 during a dose-ranging study in normal human subjects has been shown to increase urine output to a similar extent as 20 mg of furosemide given intravenously [116]. In these healthy volunteers, urine osmolality was significantly lower after administration of the V_2 receptor antagonist, thus indicating an increase in solute-free water clearance. Moreover, this agent has been shown to reverse the impairment in renal water excretion in rats with experimental heart failure due to myocardial infarction [113] and in dogs with pacing-induced heart failure [114], further supporting a role for AVP in the renal water retention of heart failure. This effect of the nonosmotic release of AVP to cause water retention in cardiac failure recently has been associated with increased transcription of messenger RNA (mRNA) for the AVP preprohormone in the rat hypothalamus [117].

Finally, in a study by Bichet et al. [107], the effect of the ACE inhibitor captopril and the α_1-adrenergic blocker prazosin to reverse the abnormality in water retention in patients with class III and IV heart failure was examined. The afterload reduction and increased cardiac output with either agent were associated with improved water excretion and suppression of AVP in response to an acute water load. A role of angiotensin II in modulating the effect of AVP in heart failure seems unlikely, since captopril and prazosin had different effects on the renin-angiotensin system; yet their effects to improve water excretion as plasma AVP was suppressed were comparable. In this regard, it is important to note that in this study by Bichet and co-workers [107], the average decrease in mean arterial pressure was 5 mm Hg, a decrement that is less than the 7 to 10 percent necessary to activate the nonosmotic release of AVP [118]. Thus, these results are compatible with the suggestion that a decrease in stroke volume and cardiac output, rather than a fall in mean arterial pressure, is the primary stimulus for the nonosmotic release of AVP in low-output cardiac failure. The association of improved cardiac output and water excretion during afterload reduction is compatible with an influence of high-pressure baroreceptors sensing pulse pressure in modulating AVP release.

In addition to persistent AVP secretion, altered renal hemodynamics may contribute to water retention in heart failure. Decreased RBF and increased filtration fraction would be expected to increase proximal reabsorption of sodium and water, thereby diminishing fluid delivery to distal diluting segments [81, 119]. Increasing distal fluid delivery by administration of mannitol or furosemide improves the diluting ability of patients with heart failure [119–121]. Mannitol, however, also expands intravascular volume and could suppress nonosmotic release of AVP, and furosemide may impair the renal response to AVP, since furosemide improves solute-free water excretion in patients also receiving infusions of AVP [120]. Therefore, these studies do not exclude the possibility that AVP secretion is primarily responsible for the inability of patients with cardiac failure to dilute their urine.

In summary, activation of the sympathetic nervous system, the renin-angiotensin-aldosterone system, and the nonosmotic release of AVP—by exerting direct (tubular) and indirect (hemodynamic) effects on the kidneys—are implicated in the renal sodium and water retention of heart failure. These neuroendocrine mechanisms appear to be activated in response to arterial underfilling and suppressed by maneuvers that restore the EABV to or toward normal. In addition, the effects of these neurohormonal vasoconstrictor systems may be counterbalanced by endogenous vasodilatory and natriuretic hormones.

Natriuretic Peptides in Cardiac Failure

The natriuretic peptides, including ANP and brain natriuretic peptide (BNP), circulate at increased concentrations in patients with heart failure [122–124]. These peptide hormones possess natriuretic, vasorelaxant, and renin-, aldosterone-, and possibly AVP- and sympatho-inhibiting properties [44, 45, 125–128]. Both ANP and BNP appear to be released primarily from the heart in response to increased atrial or ventricular end-diastolic or transmural pressures [13, 129]. In a recent study of ANP kinetics in patients with cardiac failure, we demonstrated that increased ANP production rather than decreased metabolic clearance was the major factor contributing to the elevated plasma ANP concentrations in these patients [130]. This finding is consistent with the observed increase in expression of both ANP and BNP mRNA in the cardiac ventricles of humans and animals with heart failure [131, 132]. In a coronary ligation model of heart failure in the rat, the infusion of a monoclonal antibody shown to specifically block endogenous ANP in vivo caused a significant rise in right atrial pressure, left ventricular end-diastolic pressure, and peripheral vascular resistance [133]. Thus, natriuretic peptides appear to attenuate to some degree the arterial and venous vasoconstriction of heart failure.

Renal Effects of the Natriuretic Peptides. In normal humans, ANP and BNP increase GFR and urinary sodium excretion with no change or only a slight fall in renal blood flow [129, 134]. These changes in renal hemodynamics are likely mediated by afferent arteriolar vasodilation with constriction of the efferent arterioles. However, in addition to increasing GFR and filtered sodium load as a mechanism of their natriuretic effect, ANP and BNP are specific inhibitors of sodium reabsorption in the collecting tubule [135–137]. An important role for endogenous ANP in the renal sodium balance of heart failure has been demonstrated by Lee and associates [138]. Similar decreases in cardiac output were induced in two groups of dogs by constriction of the thoracic inferior vena cava (TIVC) or by acute rapid ventricular pacing. In the TIVC constriction group, sodium retention paralleled the activation of the renin-angiotensin-aldosterone system. Atrial pressures and plasma ANP were not increased in this group of dogs. In comparison, the ventricular pacing group did not experience sodium retention or activation of the renin-angiotensin-aldosterone system. This group had similar reductions in cardiac output and arterial pressure as did the TIVC constriction group but, unlike the TIVC constriction group, had increased atrial pressures and circulating endogenous ANP levels. In a third group, exogenous ANP was administered to TIVC constriction dogs to increase plasma ANP levels to those observed in the pacing model. The ANP infusion prevented the sodium retention and the activation of the renin-angiotensin-aldosterone system.

Unfortunately, the administration of synthetic ANP to patients with low-output heart failure results in a much smaller increase in renal sodium excretion and less significant changes in renal hemodynamics compared to normal subjects [129]. Like ANP, the natriuretic effect of BNP is blunted in rats with high-output heart failure produced by AV fistulae [139]. Since ANP and BNP appear to share the same receptor sites [140], it is possible that the natriuretic effect of BNP is also blunted in sodium-retaining patients with heart failure. Support for this hypothesis may be found in a recent report from our laboratory [141]. In 10 patients with advanced decompensated NYHA class III heart failure due to either ischemic or idiopathic dilated cardiomyopathy (left ventricular ejection fraction 16 $\pm$ 2 percent, cardiac index 1.8 $\pm$ 0.2 L/min/m^2, pulmonary capillary wedge pressure 27 $\pm$ 3 mm Hg), the administration BNP at either 0.025 or 0.05 μg/kg/min for 4 hours produced a natriuresis in only 4 patients. The effect of BNP on GFR and renal blood flow was inconsistent in these patients and did not predict the natriuretic response. While the renal effects of BNP were blunted in some of these heart failure patients, BNP did produce a significant 50 percent decrease in pulmonary capillary wedge pressure, significantly lowered peripheral vascular resistance, and increased plasma cyclic guanosine monophosphate (cyclic GMP) concentration in these patients, supporting the biologic responsiveness of vascular BNP receptors in heart failure.

Recently, Elsner and associates [142] have suggested that renal responsiveness to a slightly extended form of ANP, urodilatin or ANP$_{95-126}$, is preserved in heart failure. In normal humans, this natriuretic peptide of renal origin produces hemodynamic and renal effects that are similar to ANP [143]. While the six heart failure patients studied by Elsner et al. [142] demonstrated a modest natriuresis during urodilatin infusion, it should be noted that patient selection and methodologic considerations confound the interpretation of their findings. Thus, we await further studies of urodilatin in heart failure to determine its efficacy.

The mechanism of the relative renal resistance to natriuretic peptides in heart failure remains controversial. Possible mechanisms include (1) down-regulation of renal ANP receptors, (2) secretion of inactive immunoreactive ANP, (3) enhanced renal neutral endopeptidase activity limiting the delivery of ANP to receptor sites, (4) hyperaldosteronism by an increased sodium reabsorption in the distal renal tubule, and (5) diminished delivery of sodium to the distal renal tubule site of ANP action. In sodium-retaining patients with heart failure, we have reported a strong positive correlation between plasma ANP and urinary cyclic GMP (the second messenger for the natriuretic effect of ANP, BNP, and urodilatin in vivo [144]. This observation supports the active biologic responsiveness of renal ANP receptors in heart failure and thus suggests that diminished distal tubular sodium delivery may be involved in the natriuretic peptide resistance observed in patients with cardiac failure. Further support for this hypothesis is found in our experience with cirrhosis, another edematous disorder associated with renal ANP resistance, where maneuvers that increase distal tubular sodium delivery have been shown to reverse the ANP resistance [145]. Moreover, in heart failure, the administration of an angiotensin II receptor antagonist or furosemide, which is expected to increase distal

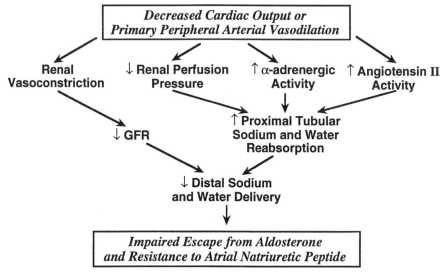

Fig. 2-5. Proposed mechanism of natriuretic peptide resistance and impaired aldosterone escape in states of arterial underfilling. GFR = glomerular filtration rate. (From R. W. Schrier and O. S. Better, Pathogenesis of ascites formation: Mechanism of impaired aldosterone escape in cirrhosis. *Eur. J. Gastroenterol. Hepatol.* 3:721, 1991.)

tubular sodium delivery, also improves the renal response to ANP [100, 146]. Finally, studies in rats with experimental heart failure have demonstrated that renal denervation reverses the ANP resistance [147], an effect likely mediated by increased distal tubular sodium delivery. Figure 2-5 shows the proposed role of diminished distal tubular sodium delivery in natriuretic peptide resistance and impaired aldosterone escape in states of arterial underfilling.

Renal Prostaglandins in Cardiac Failure

In normal subjects and in intact animals, renal prostaglandins do not regulate renal sodium excretion or renal hemodynamics to any significant degree [148, 149]. In patients with heart failure, prostaglandin activity is increased and has been shown to correlate with the severity of disease as assessed by the degree of hyponatremia [150]. Moreover, it has been well documented that the administration of a cyclooxygenase inhibitor in heart failure patients may result in acute reversible renal failure, an effect proposed to be due in part to inhibition of renal prostaglandins [151]. A recent investigation in patients with moderate heart failure and a normal sodium intake demonstrated that the administration of acetylsalicylic acid in doses that decrease the synthesis of renal prostaglandin E_2 results in a significant reduction in urinary sodium excretion [152]. These observations suggest a possible role for vasodilating prostaglandins in heart failure; however, their exact role in renal sodium handling in this edematous disorder remains to be elucidated.

	COMPENSATED CIRRHOSIS (NO ASCITES)	DECOMPENSATED CIRRHOSIS (ASCITES)	HEPATORENAL SYNDROME
Peripheral Arterial Vasodilation	↑	↑↑	↑↑↑
Plasma Hormones (AVP, Renin, Aldosterone, NE)	Normal	↑	↑↑
Plasma Volume	↑	↑↑	↑↑↑

Fig. 2-6. The range of pathophysiology from compensated to decompensated cirrhosis to the hepatorenal syndrome. According to the peripheral arterial vasodilation hypothesis, progressive arterial vasodilation is associated with progressive stimulation of neurohormonal vasoconstrictor systems, despite expansion of plasma volume. AVP = arginine vasopressin; NE = norepinephrine.

Pathogenesis of Sodium and Water Retention in Cirrhosis

Like cardiac failure, two theories have attempted to explain the pathogenesis of sodium and water retention in cirrhosis [153, 154]. The classic "underfill hypothesis" suggested that ascites formation secondary to portal hypertension decreased plasma volume and then secondarily caused renal sodium and water retention [154]. However, results of animal studies have shown that sodium and water retention precede ascites formation in cirrhotic animals, thus contradicting the hypothesis [153]. Moreover, plasma volume is decreased, not expanded, in cirrhosis. Alternatively, primary renal sodium and water retention, secondary to a hepatorenal reflex, was proposed to lead to plasma volume expansion of both the venous and arterial compartments and cause overflow ascites [153]. This "overfill hypothesis" of ascites formation in cirrhotic patients, however, did not explain the progressive stimulation of the neurohumoral profile that is observed in cirrhotic patients and is characteristic of arterial underfilling. Against this background, we have suggested a primary role for peripheral arterial vasodilation for the initiation of renal sodium and water retention in cirrhosis [1–6, 155, 156] (see Fig. 2-2). This theory encompasses the entire range from compensated to decompensated cirrhosis to the hepatorenal syndrome and explains the progressive increases in both plasma volume and neurohormonal activation that occur as cirrhosis worsens (Fig. 2-6).

Peripheral Arterial Vasodilation Hypothesis

According to this hypothesis, splanchnic arterial vasodilation occurs early in cirrhosis, and the resultant arterial underfilling stimulates sodium and water retention with plasma volume expansion prior to ascites formation. The normal plasma hormone concentrations in these compensated cirrhotic patients are relatively increased for the degree of sodium and water retention and plasma volume expansion. The mediators of the early splanchnic vasodilation in cirrhosis may include the opening of existing shunts, activation of vasodilating hormones, and ultimately the development of collaterals. As cirrhosis progresses, vasodilation may occur at other sites including the skin, muscle, and lung. However, while the presence of splanchnic arterial vasodilation is well documented in experimental and human cirrhosis, the development of arterial vasodilation involving other vascular territories is less certain.

Increased synthesis and release of the potent vasodilator nitric oxide, perhaps due to increased circulating levels of endotoxin in cirrhosis, have been proposed to account for the arterial vasodilation and hyperdynamic circulation seen in cirrhotic patients [157–161]. While nitric oxide activity is difficult to assess in vivo, indirect evidence supports this hypothesis. For example, urinary cyclic GMP, the second messenger of nitric oxide as well as the natriuretic peptides [162], is increased in patients with cirrhosis prior to the development of ascites and in some patients prior to an increase in circulating ANP concentrations [161]. In addition, our laboratory recently has demonstrated markedly increased cyclic GMP concentrations in aortic tissue from rats with experimental cirrhosis [159]. In these animals, aortic cyclic GMP concentrations correlated inversely with arterial pressure ($r = -0.54$, $p < 0.0001$). Significantly, the chronic administration of the nitric oxide synthesis inhibitor N^G-nitro-L-arginine-methyl-ester (L-NAME, 10 mg/kg/day for 7 days) induced a marked reduction in aortic cyclic GMP concentration and an increase in arterial blood pressure in cirrhotic rats to similar levels obtained in L-NAME–treated control animals, indicating that the high aortic cyclic GMP content and decreased arterial blood pressure in cirrhotic rats were due to an increased nitric oxide synthesis [159]. We also have shown that normalization of vascular nitric oxide production by chronic nitric oxide synthesis inhibition corrects the systemic hemodynamic abnormalities in cirrhotic rats with ascites [160]. Specifically, L-NAME, 0.5 mg/kg/day for 10 days in drinking water, normalized mean arterial pressure, cardiac output, and systemic vascular resistance in these cirrhotic animals. Moreover, Guarner et al. [158] have recently demonstrated elevated serum nitrite and nitrate levels—a crude index of in vivo nitric oxide generation—in 51 cirrhotic patients. Of note, in these patients, the elevated serum nitrite and nitrate levels significantly correlated with plasma endotoxin levels and decreased in response to a reduction in plasma endotoxin concentration following the administration of colistin [158]. In addition, an enhanced sensitivity to mediators of endothelium-dependent vasodilation has recently been demonstrated in human cirrhosis [163]. Taken together, these observations are compatible with the presence of nitric oxide–induced arterial vasodilation in cirrhosis.

Endogenous opioids may also contribute to the peripheral vasodilation and to the renal sodium and water retention of cirrhosis as the administration of opioid antagonists (e.g., naloxone or naltrexone) increases sodium and water excretion after water loading in humans [164] and animals [165] with cirrhosis and ascites. Other factors that have been proposed to mediate the splanchnic vasodilation in cirrhosis include vasodilating prostaglandins, glucagon, calcitonin gene–related peptide, platelet activating factor, substance P, and vasoactive intestinal peptide; however, definitive proof is lacking for all of them. In this regard, the recent observation of improved sodium and water excretion following administration of vasoactive intestinal peptide antiserum to rats with carbon tetrachloride–induced cirrhosis supports a possible role for this peptide hormone in the salt and water retention of cirrhosis [166].

As with cardiac failure, pretreatment hyponatremia and high plasma concentrations of renin, norepinephrine, and aldosterone portend a poor prognosis in the cirrhotic patient. The highest plasma concentrations of these hormones and the lowest blood pressures occur as the decompensated cirrhotic patient with ascites progresses toward the hepatorenal syndrome (see Fig. 2-6).

Nephron Sites of Sodium Retention in Cirrhosis

There is indirect evidence for both enhanced proximal and distal tubular reabsorption in human cirrhotic subjects. The following findings support enhanced proximal tubular reabsorption in hepatic cirrhosis: (1) maneuvers that expand plasma volume and increase distal nephron delivery of fluid (i.e., neck immersion and infusion of saline or mannitol) result in increased renal sodium excretion and solute-free water formation independent of changes in GFR [167, 168]; (2) in some water-loaded cirrhotics with ascites and minimal urine osmolalities, urine flow rates (an index of distal delivery of tubular fluid under these circumstances) are lower than in normal subjects [169, 170]; and (3) enhanced proximal reabsorption of tubular fluid has been found in micropuncture and clearance studies of dogs and rats with chronic bile duct ligation as well as rats with cirrhosis secondary to carbon tetrachloride exposure [171–173].

Evidence for enhanced distal nephron sodium reabsorption is based on the following observations: (1) water-loaded patients with sodium retention and cirrhosis with minimal urine osmolalities often have urine flow rates comparable to normal controls [174]; (2) water-loaded cirrhotics with minimal urine osmolalities have increased calculated distal fractional sodium reabsorption after receiving hypotonic saline infusions [174]; (3) acetazolamide, a diuretic acting at the proximal tubule, produces a significant natriuresis in cirrhotic subjects only when there is concomitant distal nephron blockade of sodium reabsorption with ethacrynic acid [175]; and (4) micropuncture studies in the dimethylnitrosamine and bile duct ligation models of cirrhosis demonstrate enhanced distal nephron sodium reabsorption [176, 177]. In summary, clinical and experimental studies suggest that both proximal and distal nephron sites participate in enhanced renal tubular sodium reabsorption in cirrhosis. As in cardiac failure, neurohormonal activation appears to play a major role in the sodium (and water) retention of cirrhosis.

The mechanisms responsible for enhanced sodium and water reabsorption in cirrhosis are no doubt multifactorial. A decrease in GFR is not observed in many sodium-retaining cirrhotic patients, suggesting that sodium retention can occur independently of a decrease in GFR. An increase in renal vascular resistance and in filtration fraction is often seen in decompensated cirrhosis. Thus, peritubular physical forces (decreased hydrostatic pressure and increased oncotic pressure [see Fig. 2-3]) may act to enhance proximal tubular sodium reabsorption in cirrhosis.

The Sympathetic Nervous System in Cirrhosis

Recently, elevated plasma levels of norepinephrine have been observed in cirrhotic patients with ascites. Plasma norepinephrine levels correlate positively with plasma AVP concentrations and with PRA and negatively with urinary sodium excretion [167]. Moreover, we have demonstrated elevated norepinephrine spillover rates in cirrhotic patients compared to normal controls (1.5 ± 0.25 versus 0.26 ± 0.08 μg/min/m^2, $p < 0.001$), while norepinephrine clearance rates were comparable between the two groups (3.13 ± 0.5 versus 2.6 ± 0.3 L/min, $p =$ NS) [178]. Floras et al. [179], using the technique of peroneal nerve microneurography to directly measure sympathetic nerve activity to muscle, have also demonstrated adrenergic activation in cirrhotic patients. Finally, Ring-Larsen and co-workers [180] have demonstrated normal hepatic norepinephrine clearances and increased renal norepinephrine release in cirrhotic patients. Taken together, these findings are compatible with the presence of systemic and renal adrenergic activation in cirrhosis.

These findings suggest that increased activity of the sympathetic nervous system and renal nerves could also result in enhanced renal sodium reabsorption in cirrhosis. As previously mentioned, renal adrenergic stimulation has been shown to increase proximal tubular sodium reabsorption. In addition, we have shown a negative correlation between plasma norepinephrine and urinary sodium excretion ($r = -0.76$, $p < 0.001$) in cirrhotic patients [181]. Ring-Larsen et al. [182] have demonstrated an inverse correlation between plasma norepinephrine and renal blood flow. Moreover, in the report from Floras et al. [179], muscle sympathetic nerve activity was inversely correlated with urinary sodium excretion.

Role of Aldosterone in Cirrhosis

There have been reports of natriuresis occurring after either removal of the source of aldosterone by adrenalectomy [183] or administration of spironolactone [184], a competitive inhibitor of aldosterone. However, inhibition of aldosterone synthesis with aminoglutethimide [185] or adrenalectomy [183] did not entirely restore renal sodium excretion to normal in other cirrhotic patients. Moreover, water immersion of patients with cirrhosis results in natriuresis even in the presence of pharmacologic doses of mineralocorticoids [186]. Furthermore, in one study of cirrhotics given excess sodium intake, 3 of 11 patients had suppressed levels of PRA and aldosterone, yet gained approximately 1 kg of weight per day [187]. These patients retained as much sodium as the 6 patients who had persistently elevated plasma aldosterone levels [187]. On the other hand, the near-uniform response to spironolactone in cirrhotic patients suggests that the increased levels of aldosterone contribute to the increased distal sodium reabsorption.

The Nonosmotic Release of Vasopressin in Cirrhosis

Hyponatremia with impaired ability to excrete a water load occurs in a substantial number of patients with cirrhosis of the liver, thereby demonstrating an impairment in urinary dilution in these patients [188–190]. Decompensated cirrhotic patients with ascites and/or edema have an abnormal response to water administration, while cirrhotic patients without ascites or edema usually excrete water normally [190, 191]. There are two potential mechanisms for this inability to excrete solute-free water in decompensated cirrhotic patients with ascites: (1) a derangement in renal hemodynamics with decreased fluid delivery to the distal nephron and (2) an extra-renal mechanism involving nonosmotic AVP release. Maneuvers that improve distal fluid delivery such as infusion of mannitol, saline [168, 192], saline plus albumin, and ascitic fluid [193], as well as head-out water immersion [167], improve urinary dilution and water excretion in cirrhosis. These maneuvers also increase central blood volume and could improve water excretion by suppressing baroreceptor-mediated AVP release. In this regard, administration of either alcohol to suppress AVP release [194] or demeclocycline to antagonize vasopressin action [195, 196] improves water excretion in cirrhosis, thus also suggesting a role for AVP. In addition, we have studied four experimental models of altered liver function in our laboratory: (1) TIVC constriction in the dog as a model of hepatic congestion [32]; (2) acute portal vein constriction in the dog as a model of portal venous hypertension [21]; (3) chronic bile duct ligation in the rat as a model of obstructive jaundice [197]; and (4) carbon tetrachloride–induced liver disease in the rat as a model of chronic cirrhosis [177, 198]. In each of these experimental models, a predominant role of AVP in the impairment of water excretion was demonstrated. However, in each case, there was also evidence that diminished fluid delivery to the distal diluting segment also contributed to the abnormal water excretion.

Studies of patients with cirrhosis also implicate the nonosmotic release of AVP as a major factor responsible for water retention in cirrhosis. Bichet and colleagues [199] studied 26 cirrhotic patients who received a standard water load (20 ml/kg). On the basis of their ability to excrete this water load, patients could be separated into two groups: those able to excrete more than 80 percent of the water load in 5 hours ("excretors") and those unable to excrete a water load normally ("nonexcretors"). Nonexcretors had lower serum sodium concentrations and higher plasma AVP levels after the water load. These nonexcretors were also found to have higher pulse rates, lower plasma albumin concentrations, higher PRA and aldosterone concentrations, and higher plasma norepinephrine levels than normonatremic cirrhotic patients with normal water excretion [199]. A greater decrease in EABV in the nonexcretors is suggested by these studies and may provide the nonosmotic stimulus for AVP release in hyponatremic cirrhotic patients. In subsequent experiments, enhancement of central blood volume by water immersion to the neck suppressed AVP release and improved, but did not normalize, water excretion [167]. However, a comparable suppression of AVP with head-out water immersion and norepinephrine infusion normalized water excretion in decompensated cirrhotic patients [200]. The increment in water excretion with this combined maneuver, which increases renal perfusion pressure, must have been due to an increase in distal fluid delivery.

Recent studies performed in rats made cirrhotic after exposure to carbon tetrachloride and phenobarbital confirmed that AVP hypersecretion is the predominant mechanism of the impairment of water excretion, since the administration of a specific antagonist of the hydro-osmotic effect of AVP normalized water excretion in 9 of the 10 rats studied [201]. Moreover, using the orally active nonpeptide V_2 receptor AVP antagonist OPC-31260, Tsuboi et al. [202] normalized the defect in solute-free water excretion in this animal model of cirrhosis. Additional experimental data supporting a primary role for AVP in the impaired water excretion in cirrhosis come from Fujita et al. [203]. These investigators examined the effect of experimental cirrhosis on expression of the mRNA for the AVP-dependent collecting duct water channel, aquaporin-2, in the rat. Binding of AVP to the V_2 receptor initiates a chain of intracellular signaling events that ultimately leads to the transient insertion of aquaporin-2 water channels into the apical membrane of collecting duct cells, thus rendering these cells permeable to water. Thus, a marker for the induction of these collecting duct water channels, such as expression of the aquaporin-2 mRNA, may serve as a biologic assay of AVP action on collecting duct cells. In the cirrhotic rats studied by Fujita et al. [203], aquaporin-2 mRNA was markedly increased as compared to control animals. Moreover, an oral water load (30 ml/kg) did not reduce aquaporin-2 mRNA expression, but the blockade of AVP action by the V_2 receptor AVP antagonist OPC-31260 significantly diminished its expression in the cirrhotic animals. Thus, both experimental and clinical evidence suggests that AVP is a major cause of the abnormality of water excretion observed in cirrhosis.

Natriuretic Peptides in Cirrhosis

As with other edematous states associated with diminished EABV, the neurohumoral responses to the peripheral arterial vasodilation of cirrhosis are associated with factors that diminish distal sodium delivery. The impaired aldosterone escape [204] and resistance to ANP [205] that occur in cirrhosis are therefore most likely mediated by diminished distal sodium delivery. As with experimental cardiac failure, renal denervation has been shown to reverse the resistance to ANP in experimental cirrhosis [206] (Fig. 2-7). This finding supports a role of diminished distal sodium delivery in the ANP resistance. Moreover, Skorecki et al. [205] have demonstrated a normal increase in urinary cyclic GMP but no natriuresis in some cirrhotic patients infused with ANP, thus demonstrating the biologic responsiveness of renal ANP receptors in these patients. A recent report from Morali et al. [207] also supports the diminished distal tubular sodium delivery hypothesis of ANP resistance. In addition, we have recently demonstrated reversal of renal ANP resistance by increasing distal tubular sodium delivery in patients with decompensated cirrhosis [145].

Renal Prostaglandins in Cirrhosis

Zambraski and Dunn [208] have shown that prostaglandins with vasodilator properties are necessary to maintain renal blood flow and GFR in dogs with cirrhosis secondary to bile duct ligation. Similar conclusions about the importance of prostaglandins have been obtained in cirrhotic humans. Inhibition of prostaglandin synthesis in decompensated cirrhotic patients decreases renal blood flow, GFR, sodium excretion, and free water excretion and impairs the natriuretic response to diuretic agents [209, 210]. Infusion of prostaglandin has been shown to reverse these diminutions in renal blood flow and GFR observed after prostaglandin inhibition [210]. Inhibition of prostaglandin synthesis may also cause a syndrome that mimics the hepatorenal syndrome [209]. Moreover, vasodilating renal prostaglandins may play an important counterregulatory role in early or well-compensated cirrhosis [211].

In summary, numerous afferent and efferent mechanisms are involved in the abnormal sodium and water excretion seen in patients with liver disease. These

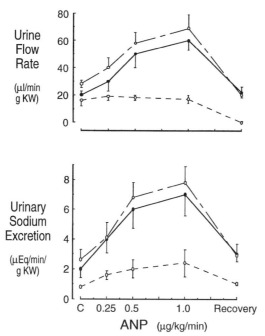

Fig. 2-7. Renal denervation reverses the renal resistance to atrial natriuretic peptide (ANP) in a rat model of cirrhosis. Solid line = control animals; dashed line = cirrhotic animals; broken line = cirrhotic plus renal denervation animals. (From J. P. Koepke et al., Renal nerves mediate blunted natriuresis to atrial natriuretic peptide in cirrhotic rats. *Am. J. Physiol.* 252:R1019 1987.)

mechanisms appear to be initiated by a diminution in EABV caused by peripheral arterial vasodilation. The sympathetic nervous system, renin-angiotensin-aldosterone axis, and the nonosmotic release of AVP are the major effector components of this increased sodium and water reabsorption, which may also be modulated by the release of natriuretic peptides and renal prostaglandins.

Pathogenesis of Sodium and Water Retention in the Nephrotic Syndrome

The two views of the pathogenesis of edema formation in the nephrotic syndrome are illustrated in Figure 2-8. According to the "underfill" theory, urinary loss of albumin occurs as a consequence of an increase in glomerular capillary permeability and results in hypoalbuminemia. This decline in serum albumin lowers intravascular colloid oncotic pressure, thereby increasing transudation of plasma from the intravascular to the interstitial space. It is this decrease in plasma volume that diminishes EABV and serves as the stimulus for renal sodium and water retention. Ultimately, the decrease in intravascular colloid oncotic pressure and the increase in interstitial hydrostatic pressure secondary to edema formation come into balance, and the

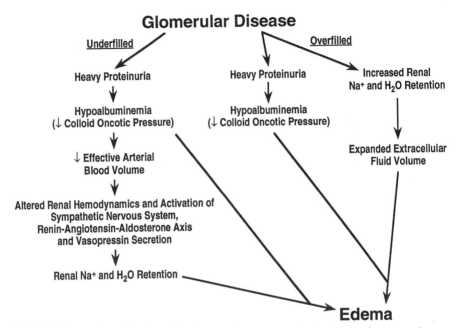

Fig. 2-8. Proposed mechanisms of sodium and water retention in the nephrotic syndrome.

edematous state stabilizes. Thus, the diminution in plasma volume is the critical afferent stimulus in inducing renal sodium and water retention and should be observed in the initiating phase of formation. Several lines of evidence support this traditional underfill theory of edema formation in the nephrotic syndrome: (1) plasma volume may be modestly decreased in some nephrotic patients in the absence of diuretic therapy [187, 212–215]; (2) systemic arterial hypotension and diminished cardiac output, correctable by plasma volume expansion, have been observed in some patients with nephrotic syndrome [215, 216]; (3) some nephrotic patients have humoral markers of arterial underfilling such as elevated plasma levels of PRA, aldosterone, and catecholamines [213, 217–223]; and (4) head-out water immersion and intravascular infusion of albumin, maneuvers that increase plasma volume, may result in substantial increases in GFR and in fractional excretion of sodium chloride and water in these patients [221, 224, 225].

Usberti and co-workers [226] recently have described two groups of nephrotic syndrome patients distinguished on the basis of their plasma albumin concentrations. Patients in group 1 had a plasma albumin concentration of less than 1.7 g/dl associated with low blood volumes and plasma ANP levels, elevated plasma angiotensin II concentrations, and increased proximal tubular reabsorption of sodium (determined by lithium clearance). In contrast, group 2 patients with a plasma albumin concentration greater than 1.7 g/dl deciliter exhibited normal blood volumes and plasma hormone concentrations. In all patients, blood volume was positively correlated with the plasma albumin concentration, and PRA was inversely correlated with both blood volume and plasma albumin. Of note, GFR was not different between group 1 and group 2 patients (100 ± 25 versus 101 ± 22 ml/min, $p = NS$), while urinary sodium excretion was substantially lower in group 1 patients (4.88 ± 5.53 versus 29.9 ± 9.3 mEq/4 hr, $p < 0.001$). Moreover, the acute expansion of blood volume in group 1 patients normalized PRA, plasma angiotensin II and aldosterone concentrations, fractional sodium excretion, and lithium clearance, while increasing circulating ANP concentrations. Taken together, all of these observations [187, 212–226] support the traditional underfill view of the pathogenesis of edema formation in the nephrotic syndrome.

To further explore the state of arterial filling in patients with the nephrotic syndrome, we recently evaluated sympathetic nervous system activity in six edematous patients with the nephrotic syndrome of various parenchymal etiologies and in six normal control subjects [223]. As previously mentioned, increased adrenergic activity is seen in states of arterial underfilling and may be the earliest sign of a decreased EABV. Sympathetic nervous system activity was assessed by determining plasma norepinephrine secretion and clearance rates using a whole-body steady-state radionuclide tracer method. Patients were withdrawn from all medications 7 days prior to study. Mean creatinine clearances and serum creatinine concentrations were normal in both the nephrotic syndrome patients and controls. However, the nephrotic syndrome patients exhibited significant hypoalbuminemia (2.0 ± 0.4 versus 3.8 ± 0.1 g/dl, $p < 0.01$). The supine plasma norepinephrine level was elevated in the patients with the nephrotic syndrome as compared to controls. More significantly, the secretion rate of norepinephrine was markedly increased in nephrotic patients (0.30 ± 0.07 versus 0.13 ± 0.02 μg/m^2/min, $p < 0.05$), whereas the clearance rate of norepinephrine was similar in the two groups (2.60 ± 0.29 versus 2.26 ± 0.27 L/min, $p = NS$) (Fig. 2-9). Plasma renin activity and plasma aldosterone, AVP, and ANP concentrations were not different in nephrotic syndrome patients compared to controls. These observations indicate that the sympathetic nervous system is activated in patients with the nephrotic syndrome prior to a significant fall in GFR or a marked activation of either the renin-angiotensin-aldosterone system or the nonosmotic release of AVP. Moreover, these data also support the presence of arterial underfilling in the nephrotic syndrome.

More recently, however, a number of investigators have challenged this traditional underfill model based on the following observations: (1) several studies of plasma and/or blood volume in edematous nephrotic patients have reported either normal or elevated values [214, 218, 220, 221, 227]; (2) hypertension and low PRA, two indices suggesting volume expansion, have been frequently reported in some patients with nephrotic syndrome [228]; (3) hypoalbuminemia in animal studies as well as in patients with analbuminemia does not necessarily lead to edema formation [229]; and (4) a low filtration fraction is often observed in patients with the nephrotic syndrome [212], in contrast to the expected relatively well-maintained GFR and increased filtration fraction usually associated with states of arterial underfilling. Thus, the "overfill" hypothesis has been proposed to account for nephrotic edema formation in some patients. According to this view, the renal retention of sodium and water occurs as a primary intrarenal phenomenon independent of systemic factors. Renal sodium and water retention produce an expanded plasma volume, and the overfilled plasma volume then leaks into the interstitium and induces edema

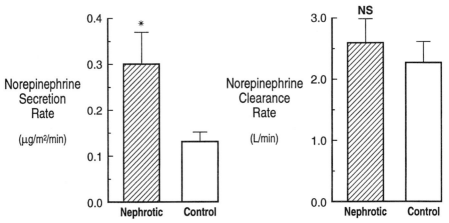

Fig. 2-9. Plasma norepinephrine secretion and clearance rates in patients with the nephrotic syndrome and normal glomerular filtration rates and in normal control subjects. The findings of increased norepinephrine secretion and normal norepinephrine clearance in the nephrotic syndrome patients are consistent with early activation of the sympathetic nervous system in the nephrotic syndrome. (From S. N. Rahman, W. T. Abraham, V. J. Van Putten et al., Increased norepinephrine secretion in patients with the nephrotic syndrome and normal glomerular filtration rates: Evidence for primary sympathetic activation. *Am. J. Nephrol.* 13:266, 1993. Reprinted by permission of S. Karger AG [Basel].)

formation. The hypoalbuminemia and decreased plasma oncotic pressure serve to enhance the formation of edema.

A possible explanation for the variable volume and humoral results obtained in patients with the nephrotic syndrome is that the afferent stimulus may not be attributed to a single mechanism. Specifically, patients with the nephrotic syndrome are heterogeneous with regard to type of renal lesion, GFR, presence of underlying systemic disease, degree of hypoalbuminemia, and diuretic usage. Experimental data supporting this possibility were published more than 20 years ago [230]. In rat studies, aminonucleoside-induced nephrosis was characterized by a decreased plasma volume, as well as a well-maintained GFR, and edema could be prevented by adrenalectomy. In contrast, nephrotic syndrome induced by nephrotoxic serum was characterized by increased plasma volume and a very low GFR, and edema occurred independently of the adrenal glands. In this regard, the studies of Meltzer et al. [228] are also of note. In 1979, these investigators characterized a group of patients with the nephrotic syndrome associated with volume depletion and stimulation of the renin-angiotensin-aldosterone system and described a second group with low or normal PRA and aldosterone concentrations and hypervolemia. The "hypovolemic" group was characterized by minimal change disease and well-preserved GFRs. These patients fit nicely into the traditional underfill schema depicted in the left panel of Figure 2-8. The "hypovolemic" patients were characterized by having chronic glomerulopathy and reduced GFR (mean, 53 ml/min) in addition to suppressed plasma concentrations of renin and aldosterone, findings consistent with intrarenal mechanisms contributing to the renal sodium and water retention and thus the overfill theory.

Nephron Sites of Sodium Retention in the Nephrotic Syndrome

The nephron site of enhanced renal sodium retention in the nephrotic syndrome has been studied predominantly in animal models of glomerulonephritis. Bernard and collaborators [231] used micropuncture and clearance methodology to study the nephron site of increased sodium reabsorption in saline-loaded rats with autologous immune complex nephritis. These rats developed heavy proteinuria, hypoalbuminemia, and hypercholesterolemia. Etiopathologic examination of kidneys from these animals revealed slight thickening of basement membranes, uniform finely granular deposits of IgG and complement distributed along the basement membranes of all glomeruli, and electron-dense subepithelial deposits. These findings are similar to those observed in human idiopathic membranous nephropathy. Arterial blood pressure, hematocrit, GFR, and renal plasma flow were comparable in control and experimental animals. Proximal tubular sodium reabsorption was actually decreased in nephrotic rats (35% versus 44%, $p < 0.05$). Absolute sodium reabsorption along the loop of Henle and in the distal convoluted tubule was comparable in nephrotic and control animals. Despite comparable sodium delivery to sites beyond the late distal convoluted tubule, the fractional excretion of sodium was significantly lower in nephrotic (2.2%) than in control (4.0%) animals. From these results, the authors conclude that nephron sites beyond the late distal convoluted tubule are responsible for the enhanced sodium reabsorption seen in this model. Alternatively, it remains possible that enhanced sodium reabsorption by deep nephrons not accessible to micropuncture could also contribute to the diminished sodium excretion.

Different results were reported by Kuroda and co-workers [232] utilizing a rat nephrotoxic serum model of nephrotic syndrome. In these studies, proteinuria, hypoalbuminemia, and hypercholesterolemia also occurred. Histologic examination of the kidneys revealed mild glomerular hypercellularity, widely dilated proximal tubules, diffuse uniform glomerular linear immunofluorescence, and electron-dense subepithelial deposits. In contrast to the study by Bernard and associates [231], these animals were actively retaining sodium. In micropuncture studies, single-nephron GFR was decreased, and the percentage of filtered water reabsorbed prior to late proximal and distal tubular convolutions was increased in the nephrotic rats. In addition, high proximal intratubular pressures were measured.

Two clearance studies have been undertaken in nephrotic patients in an attempt to clarify the nephron site of enhanced sodium reabsorption [233, 234]. Both of these studies were undertaken in patients with a wide variety of primary renal diseases and GFRs. Usberti and associates [234] measured tubular reabsorption of glucose in 21 patients with glomerulonephritis. Tubular glucose reabsorption was used as a marker for proximal tubular sodium reabsorption. The threshold for glucose reabsorption was reduced in 10 nephrotic patients, suggesting diminished proximal tubular reabsorption. In studies undertaken in 5 nephrotic patients, a similar conclusion was reached by Grausz and colleagues [233]. In these clearance studies, blockade of some of the distal tubular nephron sites of sodium reabsorption with ethacrynic acid and chlorothiazide was used to assess proximal sodium reabsorption. With this approach, proximal sodium reabsorption was found to be lower in nephrotic patients than in normal and cirrhotic patients. However, the more recent study of Usberti et al. [226] demonstrated increased proximal tubular sodium reabsorption—using the more precise technique of lithium clearance—in nephrotic syndrome patients with low albumin concentrations and blood volumes and elevated PRA.

In summary, it appears from experimental and clinical studies that distal nephron sites are involved in the avid sodium retention of the nephrotic syndrome. However, it is likely that increased proximal tubular sodium reabsorption may also be operative in selected cases, depending on the nature of the underlying renal disease and the phase of sodium retention.

Mechanisms of Enhanced Tubular Sodium Reabsorption

Several studies have been undertaken to identify the mechanism underlying the enhanced renal tubular sodium reabsorption in the nephrotic syndrome. Although a reduced GFR is frequently observed in nephrotic patients, many nephrotic patients with a normal GFR avidly retain sodium. Thus, factors in addition to a reduced filtered load of sodium are important in most patients. Based on both experimental and clinical studies, however, nephrotic patients with the lowest GFR often demonstrate the greatest degree of sodium retention [228, 230].

Peritubular capillary physical forces (oncotic and hydrostatic pressures) are believed to exert a modulating influence on renal sodium and water reabsorption. This influence is most likely exerted at the level of the proximal convoluted tubule. However, the low filtration fraction, high renal plasma flow, and normal renal vascular resistance frequently observed in nephrotic patients would suggest that factors other than peritubular capillary physical forces are responsible for enhanced tubular sodium reabsorption.

The Renin-Angiotensin-Aldosterone System in the Nephrotic Syndrome. A
potential role for the renin-angiotensin-aldosterone system in the pathogenesis of nephrotic sodium retention has been studied in detail. Two early experimental studies strongly supported a role for aldosterone in nephrotic edema [230, 235]. In rats made nephrotic with aminonucleoside, Tobian et al. [235] found an increase in juxtaglomerular cell granularity during sodium retention. Moreover, Kalant and collaborators [230] found that adrenalectomy prevented the sodium retention of aminonucleoside nephrosis. However, marked saline loading of these adrenalectomized nephrotic animals did result in edema formation [230]. A recent study has suggested that sodium retention in rat aminonucleoside nephrosis can occur independently of circulating humoral substances [236]. In these studies, aminonucleoside was administered into one renal artery. Proteinuria, a reduced GFR, and sodium retention were observed only in the kidney that received aminonucleoside. Together, these experimental observations suggest a pathogenetic role for aldosterone as well as aldosterone-independent factors in experimental nephrotic edema.

Several studies have measured components of the renin-angiotensin-aldosterone system in nephrotic humans [213, 219, 221, 223, 228, 237]. These studies have been carried out in heterogeneous patient populations at a variety of stages during the patients' illness. A wide range of values varying from very high to very low have been observed. In general, PRA values tend to be highest in patients demonstrating characteristics of underfilling and lowest in overfilled patients.

Brown and collaborators [213] have undertaken clinical studies to examine the physiologic significance of activation of the renin-angiotensin-aldosterone system in sodium-retaining nephrotic patients. Eight of 16 patients had high PRA. Administration of the ACE inhibitor captopril to these 8 patients did not induce a diuresis despite a significant reduction in plasma aldosterone to normal values. Mean arterial pressure, however, fell in these patients during converting enzyme inhibition. These results suggest that even in nephrotic patients with high plasma aldosterone, additional factors are responsible for the avid renal sodium retention. Aldosterone antagonism studies would be even more definitive, however, since no fall in blood pressure secondary to diminished angiotensin II would occur. In this regard, we have recently demonstrated reversal of the positive sodium balance in patients with the nephrotic syndrome treated with the aldosterone antagonist spironolactone [238].

Natriuretic Peptides in the Nephrotic Syndrome. Plasma ANP and BNP concentrations are elevated in animals and humans with the nephrotic syndrome [239, 241]; however, the hemodynamic and renal responses to exogenous ANP or BNP are blunted in experimental nephrosis [240] and in patients with the nephrotic syndrome [239]. Recently, Perico and Remuzzi [241] have proposed tubular insensitivity to ANP as an initiating factor in the formation of edema in the nephrotic syndrome. According to their hypothesis, renal unresponsiveness to ANP results in distal tubular sodium and water retention with subsequent edema formation. This renal ANP resistance must be due to some postreceptor mechanism, since urinary cyclic GMP responds appropriately to ANP infusion in nephrotic animals [242]. Alternatively, this blunted natriuretic response to ANP and BNP may be a secondary phenomenon due to neurohormonal vasoconstrictor activation. Our aforementioned observations of sympathetic activation and normal plasma ANP concentrations in edematous patients with the nephrotic syndrome support this latter hypothesis [223]. Moreover, Koepke and DiBona [147] have shown that renal denervation reversed the blunted diuretic and natriuretic responses to ANP in a rat model of the nephrotic syndrome. The exact role of the natriuretic peptides in the pathogenesis of the renal sodium and water retention observed in the nephrotic syndrome is therefore in need of further study.

Other humoral factors such as kinins and prostaglandins may modulate renal sodium reabsorption in nephrotic patients. For example, inhibitors of prostaglandin synthesis have been reported to reduce GFR in patients with the nephrotic syndrome and may precipitate renal insufficiency [243]. Thus, prostaglandins may attenuate factors in nephrotic syndrome that decrease GFR and cause sodium retention.

Renal Water Retention in the Nephrotic Syndrome

In contrast with the two previously described clinical edematous disorders, heart failure and cirrhosis, the nephrotic syndrome is less frequently associated with hyponatremia. In fact, serum sodium concentration is usually normal unless it is influenced by vigorous diuretic measures or during an acute water load [244, 245]. Furthermore, in nephrotic patients, high serum lipid levels may cause pseudohyponatremia unless serum sodium concentration is measured by direct ion-specific electrode. Nevertheless, abnormal water excretion was clearly demonstrated by Gur and associates [246] in six nephrotic children, since their solute-free water clearance during water loading was negative as compared to a positive value after remission of their disease. Since head-out water immersion induced an increase in free water clearance in patients with the nephrotic syndrome [221, 224], this improvement may be secondary to the suppression of the nonosmotic release of AVP. Alternatively, water immersion might improve intrarenal hemodynamics, increase the amount of fluid delivered to the distal nephron, and thereby improve water excretion. Plasma AVP concentrations have been found to be elevated in nephrotic subjects [245, 247–249] and correlated best with blood volume [249]. Water immersion and hyperosmotic albumin infusion reduced plasma levels of AVP and induced a water diuresis [247–249]. Studies by Shapiro and colleagues [250] have shown a close correlation between decrements in GFR and water excretion during a water load in nephrotic syndrome. Analysis of these studies therefore indicates that the impaired water excretion in nephrotic patients may be related both to intrarenal factors involving a fall in GFR and diminished distal fluid delivery and to extrarenal factors that primarily involve the nonosmotic release of AVP.

In summary, it appears that the effector mechanisms for sodium and water retention in the nephrotic syndrome may involve a fall in GFR, alterations in peritubular physical factors, and activation of the sympathetic nervous system, the renin-angiotensin-aldosterone system, and the nonosmotic release of AVP. Other still undefined factors may, however, also be involved in the enhanced renal tubular sodium and water reabsorption observed in nephrotic patients; some results suggest that a diminution in ANP sensitivity in the nephrotic syndrome may also be involved in the sodium retention.

Treatment of Edematous Disorders

Given the preceding background discussion of the pathophysiology of sodium and water retention in the edematous disorders, the approach to the treatment of cardiac failure, liver disease, and the nephrotic syndrome will now be considered. The general principles for such therapy are described in Table 2-2.

Evaluation of the Adequacy of Treatment of the Primary Disease Responsible for Edema

In cardiac failure, cirrhosis, and the nephrotic syndrome, the primary initiator of sodium and water retention is the decrease in EABV caused by these diseases. Initial therapeutic attempts should therefore be directed toward treatment of the primary disease. In low-output cardiac failure, the restoration of cardiac output to normal levels would abolish the decrease in EABV and thus the initiating event for renal sodium retention. Thus, the use of positive inotropic agents (e.g., digoxin) and afterload reducing agents (e.g., ACE inhibitors, arterial vasodilators) to improve

Table 2-2. General principles in the treatment of edematous disorders

Evaluation of the adequacy of treatment of the primary disease responsible for edema
Evaluation of level of salt and water intake
Mobilization of edema; bed rest and supportive stockings
Evaluation of indications for use of diuretics
  Impaired respiratory function
    Incipient or overt pulmonary edema
    Elevated diaphragms with ascites, associated with incipient or overt atelectasis
  Impaired cardiovascular function secondary to fluid overload
  Excess fluid limiting physical activity and causing discomfort
  To avoid further sodium retention and yet allow the ingestion of palatable (sodium-containing) diet
  Cosmetic effect: marginal indication

cardiac output should be aggressively pursued in heart failure patients. This approach may alleviate the need for inhibiting tubular reabsorption with diuretics, a maneuver that could further decrease cardiac output and EABV. In this regard, it should be noted that the recently published clinical practice guidelines for the treatment of heart failure from the Agency for Health Care Policy and Research recommend ACE inhibition as first-line therapy in nonedematous patients with heart failure [251]. In the nephrotic syndrome, particularly of the nil disease or lipoid nephrosis variety, administration of corticosteroids may diminish or eliminate the proteinuria and thereby correct the hypoalbuminemia [218]. In addition, treatment with ACE inhibitors [252, 253] or an angiotensin II receptor antagonist [254] has been shown to reduce the urinary protein loss associated with human nephrotic syndrome. In contrast, the administration of albumin solutions is of very little lasting value in the nephrotic syndrome, since the concomitant increase in blood volume is associated with increased clearance of albumin, and thus only a transient increase in plasma albumin concentration occurs. In extreme states of hypoalbuminemia, however, an infusion of albumin may be a lifesaving treatment for a hypotensive episode. Albumin solutions also may be of value for patients with cirrhosis, hypoalbuminemia, and edema, particularly when there is evidence of intravascular volume depletion, such as diminished central venous pressure and a fall in orthostatic blood pressure. The administered albumin is excreted less readily in cirrhotic patients because they have no defect in glomerular capillary permeability and also frequently have lower levels of GFR. A potential complication of such albumin infusions, however, is the resulting increase in portal hypertension with increased bleeding from esophageal varices and the precipitation of hepatic encephalopathy because of the protein load. In some patients with acute alcoholic hepatitis accompanying cirrhosis, corticosteroid therapy may improve liver function.

Evaluation of the Level of Sodium and Water Intake

The level of sodium and water intake of edematous patients should be evaluated. However, it should be realized that while sodium restriction alone is effective in preventing further accumulation of edema, it does not induce a negative sodium balance. Patients who are edematous are already maximally retaining sodium (<10 mEq excretion/day). Thus, at best, "sodium-free" diets that contain 10 to 20 mEq of sodium merely prevent a further increase in positive sodium balance. The diuresis that may be observed in cardiac and cirrhotic patients who are hospitalized and placed on low-sodium diets is no doubt related to the salutary consequences of bed rest on cardiac output in the former and improvement in the primary liver disease in the latter, rather than to sodium restriction per se.

The level of fluid intake also must be assessed, since most patients with edematous disorders have a defect in renal water excretion as well as in sodium excretion (see Chap. 1 and the prior discussion). If the patient is hyponatremic, the daily fluid intake should be adjusted to equal insensible losses (500–700 ml/day) plus daily urinary losses. However, severe fluid restriction is often difficult to accomplish in these patients, since increased angiotensin II and AVP concentrations may stimulate central nervous system thirst centers.

Mobilization of Edema

Bed rest alone may lead to a diuresis, particularly in patients with cardiac failure. Furthermore, patients who are resistant to diuretic agents administered on an outpatient basis may become responsive to the same or smaller doses of diuretic agents with hospitalization and bed rest. The use of professionally fitted supportive stockings may also be of value in the mobilization of edema fluid. The mechanism of the supine position or supportive stockings, or both, in mobilizing edema fluid is probably related to the diminished peripheral venous pooling and thus to an increase in EABV and renal perfusion. Finally, since upright posture in the normal person is associated with activation of the sympathetic nervous system and renin-angiotensin-aldosterone axis, the supine position may ameliorate to some extent overactivity of these neurohormonal vasoconstrictor mechanisms.

Evaluation of Indications for Use of Diuretics

If edema persists despite adequate treatment of the primary disease, diuretics should be used only for definite indications (see Table 2-2). The presence of edema alone is not an absolute indication for diuretic treatment, and any cosmetic value must be weighted against the potential deleterious effect of the drug. In general, the use of diuretic agents should be limited primarily to those situations in which impairment of respiratory or cardiac function, or both, or physical discomfort is secondary to fluid accumulation. An exception to this rule is the patient who will not restrict sodium intake; diuretics given to such patients may prevent edema accumulation despite dietary salt indiscretion. When patients find a low-salt diet unpalatable, diuretics also can be used to allow them to eat sodium in their diet.

Once the decision is made to use diuretic agents to treat an edematous disorder, there are two cardinal rules to follow in estimating the optimal rate of diuresis. In general, the daily diuresis should approximate the rate of accumulation of the edema fluid. Thus, acute pulmonary edema necessitates induction of a rapid diuresis, while

Table 2-3. Classification of diuretics by nephron site of action

Filtration diuretics
Aminophylline
Glucocorticoids
Proximal tubular diuretics
Mannitol
Acetazolamide
Loop of Henle diuretics
Ethacrynic acid
Furosemide
Bumetanide
Torsemide
Distal tubular diuretics
Potassium-losing
Thiazides
Chlorthalidone
Metolazone
Potassium-retaining
Triamterene
Spironolactone
Amiloride
Collecting duct diuretics
Lithium
Demeclocycline
Vasopressin antagonists (investigational)

chronic heart failure is best treated with a more gradual diuresis. In either case, the rate of diuresis should be such that the rate of movement of interstitial fluid into the vascular compartment will not be exceeded to any large extent. If renal excretion does exceed the rate of mobilization of interstitial fluid, intravascular volume depletion and hypotension can result, even though ECF volume is still expanded. Careful clinical monitoring of intravascular volume is therefore extremely important, particularly during the induction of an acute diuresis. Intermittent diuretic therapy, such as alternate-day therapy, may also be of value in avoiding intravascular volume depletion.

Diuretic Therapy

The judicious use of diuretic agents necessitates a knowledge of their site of action, potency, and side effects. Table 2-3 lists the primary sites of action of the available diuretic agents, but it should be emphasized that several of these diuretics also have secondary sites of action.

Site of Action of Diuretics

Filtration Diuretics. The so-called filtration diuretics are primarily aminophylline and glucocorticoids. In addition, plasma volume expansion or an increase in cardiac output secondary to use of cardiac glycosides or inotropic agents such as dopamine, dobutamine, or the phosphodiesterase inhibitors (e.g., amrinone, milrinone) may enhance GFR. Infusions of metaraminol and angiotensin II also have been shown to increase filtration rates in patients with cirrhosis, although in normal subjects these vasoconstrictor agents decrease filtration rates [170].

Proximal Tubular Diuretics. Diuretics that act primarily to decrease proximal tubular sodium reabsorption include osmotic diuretics (e.g., mannitol), carbonic anhydrase inhibitors (acetazolamide), and although their effects are less well established, probably organomercurials. Except for organomercurials, which also have a distal tubular action, the filtration and proximal tubular diuretics are not very effective when administered alone. Although the largest portion of glomerular filtrate is reabsorbed isosmotically in the proximal tubule (50–70%), the distal nephron (particularly the ascending limb of the loop of Henle) has the capacity to increase its rate of sodium reabsorption significantly [255]. Thus, an increase in glomerular filtration or depression of proximal tubular reabsorption alone may not be associated with a significant diuresis, since the increased distal sodium and fluid delivery may be reabsorbed at more distal nephron sites. The filtration and proximal tubular diuretics therefore are best used in conjunction with a diuretic that acts on the distal nephron, particularly when the patient has shown resistance to distally acting diuretics.

Loop of Henle Diuretics. The loop diuretics—ethacrynic acid, furosemide, bumetanide, and torsemide—are the most potent diuretic agents available. The inhibition by these agents of active sodium chloride transport in the medullary ascending limb of the loop of Henle exceeds the rate-limited sodium chloride reabsorption in the more distal nephron, and a maximal diuretic effect equivalent to 20 to 25 percent of the filtered load of sodium may be achieved.

Since the reabsorption of tubular sodium chloride without water in the ascending limb is a primary mechanism of urinary dilution, the loop diuretics limit maximal renal diluting capacity. It has been shown, however, that the administration of the loop diuretic furosemide may actually increase solute-free water excretion in edematous patients, who already have impaired diluting capacity [120]. Since this diuretic-induced water diuresis is unaffected by exogenous AVP administration, it has been proposed that the rapid rate of distal fluid delivery limits the osmotic equilibration between the collecting duct and interstitium. Alternatively, the diuretic may interfere with the action of AVP on the collecting duct, particularly since at comparable solute excretion rates thiazides increase and furosemide decreases urine osmolality in the presence of exogenous AVP [121]. Sodium chloride reabsorption in the ascending limb is also the major factor in the countercurrent concentrating effect that generates the hypertonicity in the medullary interstitium. Thus, loop diuretics also impair the renal capacity to concentrate the urine and conserve water. Finally, in contrast to other diuretics that may cause renal vasoconstriction, such as the thiazides and organomercurials, the loop diuretics cause renal vasodilatation, an effect that may partially contribute to their diuretic effect [256].

Distal Tubular Diuretics. The distal tubular diuretics can be classified into two groups: the potassium-losing and the potassium-retaining diuretics. The thiazide diuretics, chlorthalidone and metolazone, although chemically different, have similar diuretic effects. These distal tubular diuretics inhibit only urinary diluting capacity and not concentrating capacity, since they decrease sodium reabsorption in the cortical, but not the medullary, portion of the ascending limb and the distal convoluted tubule. As with the loop diuretics, the use of distal tubular diuretics, which also act proximal to the distal site of potassium secretion, is associated not only with a natriuresis but also with an increase in urinary potassium excretion. As will be discussed in Chapter 5, this effect of increased sodium delivery on potassium excretion has been shown not to be a stoichiometrically linked exchange of sodium for potassium. Rather, an increase in distal sodium delivery may alter potassium excretion by modulating potassium reabsorption in the collecting duct [257]. The potassium-losing tendency of mercurial diuretics is blunted by their ability to block potassium secretion selectively [258].

The clinically available potassium-conserving diuretics include triamterene, amiloride, and the aldosterone antagonist spironolactone. While the action of spironolactone is dependent on the presence of the adrenal cortex and circulating aldosterone, the ability of triamterene and amiloride to block potassium secretion is independent of adrenal function. The effect of amiloride appears to be due to inhibition of sodium entry into the cell from luminal fluid. Frequently, these diuretics are not potent enough alone, but they may be used to avoid the potassium-losing effects of diuretics that act at more proximal nephron sites, such as the thiazide and loop diuretics.

Collecting Duct Diuretics. In contrast to all the diuretics just mentioned, two diuretics act at the level of the collecting duct and induce a water diuresis rather than a natriuresis. These agents, demeclocycline and lithium, impair the ability of AVP to increase the water permeability of the renal collecting duct epithelium, thereby antagonizing the hydro-osmotic effect of AVP [259]. Because they induce a water diuresis, these agents should be given only to hyponatremic, edematous patients. Both agents are capable of inducing significant adverse effects. However, one study demonstrated superior effect with less toxicity when demeclocycline was compared with lithium in the treatment of the syndrome of inappropriate AVP secretion [260]. However, demeclocycline has been shown to be nephrotoxic in hyponatremic cirrhotic patients and thus should be avoided in the presence of liver disease [189], including heart failure with hepatic hypoperfusion and congestion. V_2 receptor AVP antagonists, which directly antagonize the renal effects of AVP, are currently entering phase II human investigation in the United States.

Potency of Diuretics

In optimal doses, all the thiazide-like drugs have reasonably comparable effects with the exception of metolazone, which is more potent than the others. The other thiazide diuretics differ from each other primarily in duration of action. Thiazide diuretics are probably the agent of choice when an oral agent of moderate potency is desired.

In optimal doses, the loop diuretics (ethacrynic acid, furosemide, bumetanide, and torsemide) are some six to eight times more potent than the thiazide diuretics. This greater potency is expected, since several times more sodium chloride is reabsorbed in the loop of Henle than in the distal convoluted tubule. Because of their potency, the loop but not the thiazide diuretics are effective in patients with advanced renal failure (GFR $<$ 25 ml/min). Metolazone also has been shown to be effective in patients with a GFR of less than 25 ml/min. The thiazide and loop diuretics both can be administered intravenously as well as orally. In contrast, mercurial diuretics are not administered orally because they may cause gastrointestinal irritation, and they are not given intravenously because they may instigate fatal reactions thought to be secondary to ventricular fibrillation. Intramuscular injection is therefore the primary route of administration for the organomercurial diuretics. In optimal doses, the potency of the mercurial diuretics is some three to four times that of the thiazide diuretics, but these agents are less potent than the loop diuretics. Because mercurial diuretics must be administered parenterally and because the more potent loop diuretics are available, the present need for mercurial diuretics is very limited. Except for the carbonic anhydrase inhibitors, the cytobiochemical mechanism of action of most diuretics remains to be defined.

Hemodynamic Effects of Diuretics

The hemodynamic actions of diuretics have been examined in normal humans, anephric subjects, patients with heart failure, and experimental animals. In 1973, Dikshit et al. [261] reported the effects of intravenous furosemide (0.5–1.0 mg/kg) in 20 patients with left heart failure complicating acute myocardial infarction. These patients exhibited a marked decrease in left ventricular filling pressure, from 20.4 to 14.8 mm Hg, occurring between 5 and 15 minutes after furosemide administration. This effect anteceded the diuretic and natriuretic effect of the drug and was associated with a 52 percent increase in mean calf venous capacitance, thus demonstrating the venodilating effect of furosemide. This early venodilating effect of furosemide has been confirmed by other workers and has also been observed in normal subjects and experimental animals. The clinical importance of this early increase in venous capacitance and diminished left ventricular filling pressure resides in the resultant early beneficial effects of furosemide on acute pulmonary edema and explains the improved clinical symptoms of pulmonary congestion that may occur with furosemide prior to the onset of the drug's diuretic response. The acute venodilation associated with furosemide administration in these patients may be mediated by vasodilating prostaglandins, since the administration of the prostaglandin synthetase inhibitor indomethacin has been shown to abolish the increase in venous capacitance initiated by furosemide in normal volunteers and anephric subjects consuming a low-sodium diet [262].

In contrast to the early venodilation observed in patients with acute left ventricular failure, intravenous furosemide has been shown to induce an acute vasoconstrictor response in patients with decompensated chronic class III and IV heart failure [263]. In these patients with advanced heart failure, intravenous furosemide (1.3 mg/kg body weight) caused a significant increase in mean arterial pressure and systemic vascular resistance, associated with a fall in stroke volume index and a rise in left ventricular filling pressure, 20 minutes after furosemide administration. This acute increase in cardiac afterload was associated with, and presumably due to, the accompanying rapid rise in circulating concentrations of three vasoconstrictor hormones, namely plasma norepinephrine, angiotensin II, and AVP. Thus, it is clear that the acute vascular effects that occur with intravenous furosemide are determined, at least in part, by whether the patient has acute [261] versus chronic heart failure [263]. With chronic treatment, however, diuretic therapy results in favorable effects on both cardiac preload and afterload, which result in an improvement in left ventricular function.

Neurohormonal Effects of Diuretics

As mentioned previously, the acute intravenous administration of furosemide is associated with activation of the sympathetic nervous system, the renin-angiotensin-aldosterone system, and the nonosmotic release of AVP in patients with acute heart failure. Likewise, chronic oral diuretic therapy (furosemide, 80–240 mg/day for 8 days) has been shown to increase plasma renin, angiotensin II, and aldosterone concentrations in chronic heart failure patients [264]. Moreover, Bayliss et al. [265] have demonstrated a similar activation of the renin-angiotensin-aldosterone system during the chronic administration of oral furosemide, 40 mg/day, plus amiloride, 5 mg/day, for 30 days to patients presenting with decompensated heart failure manifest by pulmonary and/or peripheral edema.

In addition to the effect of diuretics to increase renal renin release, the diminished concentrations of natriuretic peptides that occur in association with chronic diuretic administration may also explain the further activation of the renin-angiotensin-aldosterone system, since natriuretic peptides are known to suppress plasma renin and aldosterone synthesis and release. Support for this hypothesis may be found in studies performed in animal models of heart failure [138, 266]. Fett and associates [266] have studied the endocrine and renal effects of intravenous furosemide (1.7 mg/kg) in an animal model of acute low-output heart failure due to rapid right ventricular pacing at 250 beats/min for 3 hours. In this model, 2 hours after furosemide, there was a fall in plasma ANP, renal blood flow, and GFR as the renin-angiotensin-aldosterone system was activated. The authors then examined the effects of an exogenous infusion of ANP, sufficient to prevent the furosemide-induced fall in the elevated endogenous plasma ANP, in the same experimental model. Maintenance of plasma ANP concentrations was associated with an enhanced natriuretic response to furosemide at 1 hour (182 versus 440 μEq/min, $p < 0.05$) and at 2 hours (72 versus 180 μEq/min, $p < 0.05$), associated with suppression of plasma aldosterone and maintenance of GFR.

Intermittent Versus Continuous Intravenous Diuretic Therapy for Decompensated Edematous States

Kaojarern et al. [267] have suggested the time course of delivery of such diuretics as furosemide into the urine as an independent predictor of overall response. This observation led to the concept of a "maximally efficient excretion rate" for furosemide [267]. In this regard, it is possible that a continuous infusion of furosemide or similar diuretic at a dose that constantly maintains the most efficient urinary diuretic

Table 2-4. Complications of diuretic therapy

Metabolic complications
  Volume depletion and azotemia
  Hypokalemia and hyperkalemia
  Hyponatremia
  Acidosis and alkalosis
  Carbohydrate intolerance
  Hypomagnesemia
  Hypocalcemia and hypercalcemia
  Hyperuricemia
Hypersensitivity
  Rash
  Interstitial nephritis
  Pancreatitis
  Hematologic disorders
Miscellaneous
  Deafness
  Gastrointestinal symptoms

excretion rate may be superior to intermittent intravenous diuretic administration. Studies in heart failure patients support this hypothesis [268]. Lahav et al. [268] recently performed a prospective, randomized, crossover trial comparing intermittent intravenous furosemide administration (30–40 mg every 8 hours for 48 hours) with a continuous furosemide infusion following a single loading dose (2.5–3.3 mg/hr for 48 hours after 30–40 mg loading dose) in nine patients with advanced heart failure refractory to conventional oral therapy. Total doses of furosemide administered were equivalent in the two groups. The continuous infusion of furosemide produced greater diuresis and natriuresis compared to intermittent furosemide administration in all patients. Similar results have been obtained with furosemide or bumetanide in normal volunteers and in patients with advanced renal dysfunction [269]. These results suggest that the continuous infusion of a loop diuretic may be the preferred method for intravenous diuretic therapy in patients with decompensated disease or "diuretic resistance" (see later discussion).

Side Effects and Complications of Diuretic Therapy

The most common complications of diuretic therapy are volume depletion and potassium depletion (Table 2-4). The thiazide and loop diuretics are most commonly associated with these complications. Volume depletion can be profound and may be associated with symptoms of cerebral or coronary insufficiency, particularly in the elderly. Diminished renal perfusion also may occur, as evidenced by a rise in blood urea nitrogen and serum creatinine concentrations.

A high-potassium diet (e.g., oranges, apricots, and bananas) is frequently sufficient to avoid diuretic-induced hypokalemia. However, potassium chloride supplements or potassium-retaining diuretics may be necessary to avoid this complication in many patients treated with moderate to high doses of loop and/or thiazide-type diuretics and metolazone. It is important to note that potassium supplements and potassium-retaining diuretics should only be administered simultaneously under very close supervision due to the potential danger of fatal hyperkalemia. This is also true for the combination of potassium supplements or potassium-retaining diuretics and ACE inhibitors or angiotensin II receptor antagonists, which inhibit aldosterone and thus promote potassium retention. Spironolactone has been shown to induce or worsen renal tubular acidosis in some cirrhotic patients [270]. For patients receiving cardiac glycosides, even more careful monitoring of serum potassium concentrations is necessary during diuretic therapy, since both hypo- and hyperkalemia are known to stimulate or exacerbate arrhythmias associated with digoxin excess.

Hyponatremia may result from the impaired water excretion associated with the primary edematous disorder, from the ability of the diuretic to impair urinary diluting capacity, or from a combination thereof (see Chap. 1). In either case, if diuretic therapy is indicated, any symptomatic hyponatremia associated with edematous states is better treated by water restriction than by cessation of diuretic therapy. Metabolic acidosis is a complication of the use of carbonic anhydrase inhibition, since these agents block hydrogen ion secretion. The use of thiazide and loop diuretics may be associated with metabolic alkalosis. This is predominantly due to the excretion of sodium, chloride, and potassium without bicarbonate, which leads to a rise in serum bicarbonate concentration.

The complication of carbohydrate intolerance has been observed with both the thiazide and the loop diuretics and may be related at least in part to potassium depletion. Hypokalemia is known to blunt the insulin response to a carbohydrate load, and this mechanism accounts at least in part for the carbohydrate intolerance. Patients most affected by this complication are probably those with diabetes mellitus or those predisposed to it.

Hyperuricemia may occur with most diuretics but has been most widely reported with thiazide or furosemide therapy. The primary cause of the hyperuricemia is a reduced urine clearance, which has been attributed to the enhanced tubular sodium reabsorption associated with volume depletion, since urate reabsorption in the proximal tubule parallels the rate of tubular sodium reabsorption.

Hypercalcemia also has been described in conjunction with thiazides given to normal subjects, hyperparathyroid subjects, and hypoparathyroid subjects treated with vitamin D [271]. The negative sodium balance and positive calcium balance associated with thiazide treatment seem at least partially responsible for the hypercalcemic effect. An interrelationship between parathyroid hormone and thiazide diuretics also has been demonstrated. Because of their hypocalciuric effect, thiazide diuretics may be used in the treatment of the idiopathic hypercalciuria that afflicts some patients with renal calculi. In contrast, furosemide increases calcium excretion and therefore has been used in conjunction with saline infusions to treat hypercalcemia. Because of this hypocalcemic effect, furosemide may induce symptoms of tetany in patients with borderline hypoparathyroidism [272].

Direct nephrotoxicity due to diuretic agents is primarily restricted to the mercurial diuretics. Hypersensitivity reactions causing an interstitial nephritis may also occur in association with thiazides or furosemide. Acute renal failure may occur when a nonsteroidal anti-inflammatory agent and triamterene are administered simultaneously [273]. Skin rashes and hematologic disorders are other manifestations of hypersensitivity reactions that have been observed with diuretic therapy. A Schönlein-Henoch type of purpuric lesion of the lower extremities has been seen during treatment with ethacrynic acid [274]. In the presence of any signs of hypersensitivity reactions similar to serum sickness, the diuretic agent should be discontinued. Acute pancreatitis also has been observed in association with thiazide administration. Deafness, which is generally reversible on cessation of the diuretic administration, has been reported both with ethacrynic acid and with furosemide; in occasional cases, however, diuretic-induced deafness has been irreversible. This has generally occurred in patients with renal disease receiving acute bolus administration. Gastrointestinal disturbances may occur with any of the diuretic agents.

Causes of Diuretic Resistance

Resistance to diuretic therapy is most often due to incomplete treatment of the primary disorder, continuation of a high sodium intake, or patient noncompliance. Inadequate diuretic dose or dosing regimen and route of administration may also be implicated in some cases. For example, given the 6- to 7-hour duration of action of oral furosemide, once-daily administration of this agent may be inadequate for many patients. As noted previously, in decompensated patients, continuous intravenous diuretic therapy may be superior to intermittent dosing regimens. Once these factors have been excluded, volume depletion is the most common cause. Since the most frequently used diuretics act at sites in the loop of Henle or distal convoluted tubule, their action is dependent on adequate delivery of sodium to these sites. Thus, diuretic-induced volume depletion with attendant decreases in GFR and increases in proximal tubular sodium reabsorption impairs the response to diuretics acting in the distal nephron. Since most diuretic agents exert their diuretic effect from the luminal side of tubular cells (as opposed to the contraluminal or peritubular capillary side), the delivery of the diuretic agent to its site of action in the nephron may also be diminished during volume depletion. In this regard, it should be noted that triamterene may block the tubular secretion of furosemide, and this combination of diuretics should be avoided.

Diuretic-induced further activation of the sympathetic nervous and renin-angiotensin systems with a concomitant decrease in circulating plasma ANP may also contribute to the development of diuretic resistance, since increased renal nerve activity and angiotensin II may enhance proximal tubular sodium reabsorption, thereby obscuring the beneficial effect of a diuretic that acts in the distal nephron. This hypothesis provides the rationale for combination therapy with a diuretic and a neurohormonal antagonist, such as an ACE inhibitor, in edematous states.

Volume depletion and diuretic-induced renin release also increase aldosterone secretion. The distal tubular effect of aldosterone may blunt the natriuretic and enhance the kaliuretic response to diuretics. Avoidance of diuretic-induced volume depletion can best be obtained by initiating diuretic therapy with one of the diuretic agents of lower potency. Subsequently, the dose may be carefully titrated upward or more potent diuretics added while patient weight and orthostatic pulse and blood pressure changes are being monitored. The intermittent use of diuretics may help to avoid intravascular volume depletion. Finally, aldosterone antagonists in combination with more proximally acting diuretics may help to promote a diuresis in patients with "resistance" who do not appear to be profoundly volume depleted.

The loop diuretics and thiazides are effective in the presence of acid-base disturbances, but disorders of acid-base metabolism may impair the effect of other diuretics. For example, the intracellular dissociation of the mercuric ions from their complexes in the renal tubular cells is increased during acidosis. Thus, the effect of the organomercurial diuretics may be enhanced by the simultaneous administration of ammonium chloride or blunted by the development of metabolic alkalosis. In contrast, the diuretic effect of carbonic anhydrase inhibitors is blunted by the presence of respiratory or metabolic acidosis, possibly because of the excess of intracellular hydrogen ions even in the presence of carbonic anhydrase inhibition. Finally, the nonsteroidal anti-inflammatory agents appear capable of attenuating the action of several diuretic agents [273].

Use of Diuretics in Specific Edematous States

Cardiac Failure

In heart failure, it is the heart and not the kidney that fails. The response of the kidney can be viewed as a normal compensatory attempt to restore EABV. However, the increased renal sodium and water retention with heart failure results in increased venous return, further stretching of the diseased myocardium, pulmonary congestion, and ultimately capillary filtration of fluid (peripheral and pulmonary edema). An effective form of therapy in chronic heart failure is to increase the contractile force of the heart directly with digitalis or other inotropic agents. This direct increase in contractility results in a greater cardiac output at any level of left ventricular filling pressure.

In addition to the effect of agents directly influencing the contractile state of the myocardium, it is important to note that the myocardial contractile state is also related to preload (venous return to the heart) and afterload (impedance to left ventricular outflow). Diuretic therapy, by reducing venous return, diminishes preload. This reduction in preload can reduce left ventricular filling pressure and thus alleviate some of the congestive symptoms of heart failure. Afterload reduction by systemic vasodilator therapy (parenteral nitroprusside or oral hydralazine, ACE inhibitors, or prazosin) also potentially results in improved ventricular function. The combined reduction in both preload and afterload induced by diuretics and vasodilators also results in a favorable effect on cardiac performance.

In actuality, diuretics alone improve both congestive symptoms and exercise tolerance of patients with chronic heart failure [275]. These favorable effects may occur at the expense of a reduced cardiac output, however [275]. Thus, diuretics should be used cautiously in patients with chronic heart failure. In mild heart failure without substantial edema, ACE inhibitors alone are often effective in relieving symptoms.

In more severe degrees of heart failure, however, this form of therapy may be inadequate, and diuretics and digoxin may be needed. Again, when treating the patient with heart failure, it is important to be aware of diuretic-induced decreases in serum potassium that predispose to digitalis toxicity and cardiac arrhythmias.

Specific recommendations for the use of diuretics in heart failure are as follows:

1. Start with a loop or thiazide-type diuretic, depending on the severity of the heart failure. For severe heart failure with substantial volume overload (i.e., overt pulmonary and/or peripheral edema), use a loop diuretic, given the greater potency of this class of agents. Thiazides are usually adequate in patients with mild heart failure.
2. If a loop diuretic given twice daily in doses equivalent to furosemide, 240 mg/day, is inadequate for diuresis, add a thiazide diuretic or metolazone. This combination generally results in a synergistic effect on salt and water excretion. Note: This combination also results in a synergistic effect on renal potassium excretion, so anticipate an increase in the requirement for supplemental potassium.
3. In order to spare potassium or to enhance diuresis, a potassium-retaining diuretic may be added. However, as mentioned previously, do not combine triamterene with furosemide, since triamterene blocks the tubular secretion of furosemide, thus inhibiting furosemide effect.
4. Goal of therapy: resolution of signs and symptoms caused by pulmonary and/or peripheral edema.

Cirrhosis

Several studies suggest that diuretic therapy is associated with substantial risk of adverse effects for the cirrhotic patient [276]. The most feared complication is the induction of azotemia. This often is due to overzealous use of diuretics. Shear and associates [277] have demonstrated that the maximum rate of absorption of ascites from the peritoneum is 900 ml/day and is usually much less. A more rapid rate of diuresis (i.e., >1 L/day of negative fluid balance) occurs only at the expense of more easily mobilized peripheral edema fluid or plasma volume. Hence a profound diuresis may be associated with deterioration in renal function. Fortunately, such diuretic-induced azotemia is usually reversible. Diuretics, however, have been shown to precipitate hepatorenal syndrome.

Alterations in serum potassium concentration are often encountered during diuretic treatment of the cirrhotic patient with ascites. Since secondary hyperaldosteronism and total-body potassium depletion are frequently associated with cirrhosis [185], any diuretic that acts proximally to the distal potassium secretory site may cause profound hypokalemia unless it is accompanied by a potassium sparing diuretic. Because of the frequently observed temporal relationship between diuretic therapy and induction of hepatic encephalopathy, Gabuzda and Hall [278] have postulated that the enhanced renal ammonia production of hypokalemia may be related to the encephalopathy.

In view of these potential hazards in the use of diuretics for the cirrhotic patient, the following general principles are recommended in the treatment of ascites:

1. Daily body weight and careful clinical and biochemical monitoring is mandatory.
2. Ascertaining that liver and renal functions are stable before instituting diuretic therapy.
3. Mobilizing ascites and edema with an initial period of bed rest and restricting dietary sodium before instituting diuretic therapy, since conservative therapy alone may result in a diuresis in 5 to 15 percent of cirrhotic patients.
4. Aiming for a daily weight loss of 1 to 2 pounds in patients with ascites with peripheral edema and 0.5 to 1 pound in patients with ascites but without peripheral edema.
5. Maintaining the end point of therapy as maximum patient comfort with a minimum of drug-induced complications. Occasionally, this may require slight liberalization of sodium intake at the expense of increased usage of diuretics and maintenance of some residual ascites in selected patients.

The suggested regimen for diuretic therapy of ascites is as follows:

1. Restrict sodium (10–40 mEq/day).
2. If there is no diuresis in 3 to 4 days, add spironolactone initially (100 mg/day with increases every 3–5 days until natriuresis occurs as assessed by urinary sodium concentration). This approach results in a diuresis in 40 to 60 percent of patients.
3. If there is no diuresis with 400 mg of spironolactone per day, add hydrochlorothiazide (50–200 mg/day) or furosemide (20–80 mg/day).
4. If no diuresis is observed on this regimen after reassessment of dietary intake and hepatic and renal function show no deterioration, increasing doses of furosemide may be used.

It is of note that using a similar protocol, Gregory and associates [279] have documented that diuretic therapy can safely and efficaciously be given to the cirrhotic patient. Recently, numerous investigators have shown that repeated large-volume paracentesis (4–6 L/day) is a fast, effective, and safe therapy for ascites in patients with cirrhosis [280–284]. The subsequent administration of diuretics avoids reaccumulation of ascites in the patients responding to these drugs. Of interest, contrary to the traditional concept of the potential danger of rapid and large paracentesis, the mobilization of ascites by paracentesis associated with intravenous albumin (6 g/L of ascites removed) did not alter renal function or systemic hemodynamics, the latter being estimated either directly (by measuring plasma volume, cardiac output, or peripheral resistance) or indirectly (by measuring PRA, plasma norepinephrine, and plasma AVP concentration) [284].

Nephrotic Syndrome

The general approach to the therapy of nephrotic edema is listed in Table 2-5. As pointed out earlier, nephrotic patients may be particularly susceptible to diuretic agents that act in the distal nephron. Distal-acting diuretics of the potassium sparing variety also prove to be helpful in the management of the hypokalemia that may occur.

Table 2-5. Therapy of nephrotic edema

Treatment of primary disorder
Conservative methods of therapy
    Dietary (protein supplementation, salt restriction, water restriction)
    Physical (recumbency, lower-extremity elevation)
Diuretic therapy
    Pharmacologic agents
    Albumin infusions
    Water immersion
    Miscellaneous (converting enzyme inhibition, increase protein intake)

Acknowledgment. Studies reported in this chapter were supported, in part, by United States Public Health Services Research Grant M01-RR00051 from the General Clinical Research Centers Program of the Division of Research Resources, National Institutes of Health.

References

1. Schrier RW: Pathogenesis of sodium and water retention in high-output and low-output cardiac failure, nephrotic syndrome, cirrhosis, and pregnancy. *N Engl J Med* 319:1065, 1988.
2. Schrier RW: Body fluid volume regulation in health and disease: A unifying hypothesis. *Ann Intern Med* 113:155, 1990.
3. Schrier RW: A unifying hypothesis of body fluid volume regulation: The Lilly Lecture 1992. *J R Coll Physicians Lond* 26:295, 1992.
4. Schrier RW: An odyssey into the milieu interieur: Pondering the enigmas. *J Am Soc Nephrol* 2:1549, 1992.
5. Abraham WT, Schrier RW: Edematous disorders: Pathophysiology of renal sodium and water retention and treatment with diuretics. *Curr Opin Nephrol Hypertens* 2:798, 1993.
6. Abraham WT, Schrier RW: Body Fluid Regulation in Health and Disease. In Schrier RW, Abboud FM, Baxter JD, Fauci AS (eds): *Advances in Internal Medicine.* Chicago, Mosby Year Book, 1994, vol 39, pp 23–47.
7. Welt LG: *Clinical Disorders of Hydration and Acid-Base Balance* (2nd ed). Boston, Little, Brown, 1959, p 15.
8. Wolfe AV: Osmometric analysis of thirst in man and dog. *Am J Physiol* 161:75, 1950.
9. Verney EB: Croonian lecture: The anti-diuretic hormone and the factors which determine its release. *Proc R Soc Lond [Biol.]* 135:25, 1947.
10. Starling EH: On the absorption of fluid from the connective tissue spaces. *J Physiol* (Lond) 19:312, 1896.
11. Peters JP: The role of sodium in the production of edema. *N Engl J Med* 239:353, 1948.
12. Borst JGG, deVries LA: Three types of "natural" diuresis. *Lancet* 2:1, 1950.
13. Sato F, Kamoi K, Wakiya Y, et al: Relationship between plasma atrial natriuretic peptide levels and atrial pressure in man. *J Endocrinol Metab* 63:823, 1986.
14. de Torrente A, Robertson GL, McDonald KM, et al: Mechanism of diuretic response to increased left atrial pressure in the anesthetized dog. *Kidney Int* 8:355, 1975.
15. Goetz KL, Bond GC, Bloxham DD: Atrial receptors and renal function. *Physiol Rev* 55:157, 1975.
16. Zucker IH, Earle AM, Gilmore JP: The mechanism of adaptation of left atrial stretch receptors in dogs with chronic congestive heart failure. *J Clin Invest* 60:323, 1977.
17. Schrier RW, Lieberman RA, Ufferman RC: Mechanism of antidiuretic effect of beta adrenergic stimulation. *J Clin Invest* 51:97, 1972.

18. Schrier RW, Berl T: Mechanism of effect of alpha-adrenergic stimulation with norepinephrine on renal water excretion. *J Clin Invest* 52:502, 1973.
19. Berl T, Cadnapaphornchai P, Harbottle JA, et al: Mechanism of suppression of vasopressin during alpha-adrenergic stimulation with norepinephrine. *J Clin Invest* 53:219, 1974.
20. Berl T, Cadnapaphornchai P, Harbottle JA, et al: Mechanism of stimulation of vasopressin release during beta adrenergic stimulation with isoproterenol. *J Clin Invest* 53:857, 1974.
21. Anderson RJ, Cadnapaphornchai P, Harbottle JA, et al: Mechanism of effect of thoracic inferior vena cava constriction on renal water excretion. *J Clin Invest* 54:1473, 1974.
22. Anderson RJ, Pluss RG, Berns AS, et al: Mechanism of effect of hypoxia on renal water excretion. *J Clin Invest* 62:769, 1978.
23. Schrier RW, Berl T: Mechanism of antidiuretic effect of interruption of parasympathetic pathways. *J Clin Invest* 51:2613, 1972.
24. Epstein FH, Post RS, McDowell M: Effects of an arteriovenous fistula on renal hemodynamics and electrolyte excretion. *J Clin Invest* 32:233, 1953.
25. Gilmore JP: Contribution of baroreceptors to the control of renal function. *Circ Res* 14:301, 1964.
26. Gilmore JP, Daggett WM: Response of chronic cardiac denervated dog to acute volume expansion. *Am J Physiol* 210:509, 1966.
27. Pearce JW, Sonnenberg H: Effects of spinal section and renal denervation on the renal response to blood volume expansion. *Can J Physiol Pharmacol* 43:211, 1965.
28. Schrier RW, Humphreys MH: Factors involved in the antinatriuretic effects of acute constriction of the thoracic and abdominal inferior vena cava. *Circ Res* 29:479, 1971.
29. Schrier RW, Humphreys MH, Ufferman RC: Role of cardiac output and autonomic nervous system in the antinatriuretic response to acute constricting of the thoracic superior vena cava. *Circ Res* 29:490, 1971.
30. Davis JO: The control of renin release. *Am J Med* 55:333, 1973.
31. Guyton A, Scanlon CJ, Armstrong GG: Effects of pressoreceptor reflex and Cushing's reflex on urinary output. *Fed Proc* 11:61, 1952.
32. Anderson RJ, Cronin RE, McDonald KM, et al: Mechanism of portal hypertension induces alterations in renal hemodynamics, renal water excretion and renin secretion. *J Clin Invest* 58:964, 1976.
33. Schrier RW, Berl T, Anderson RJ, et al: Nonosmolar Control of Renal Water Excretion. In Andreoli T, Grantham J, and Rector F (eds): *Disturbances in Body Fluid Osmolality*. Bethesda, Md, American Physiological Society, 1977, p 149.
34. Epstein FH, Goodyer AVN, Lawrason FD, et al: Studies of the antidiuresis of quiet standing: The importance of changes in plasma volume and glomerular filtration rate. *J Clin Invest* 30: 63, 1951.
35. Gauer OH, Henry JP: Circulating basis of fluid volume control. *Physiol Rev* 43:423, 1963.
36. Smith HW: Salt and water volume receptors: An exercise in physiologic apologetics. *Am J Med* 23:623, 1957.
37. Murdaugh HV Jr, Sieker HO, Manfredi F: Effect of altered intrathoracic pressure on renal hemodynamics, electrolyte excretion and water clearance. *J Clin Invest* 38:834, 1959.
38. Hulet WH, Smith HH: Postural natriuresis and urine osmotic concentration in hydropenic subjects. *Am J Med* 30:8, 1961.
39. Gauer OH, Henry JP, Sieker HO, et al: The effect of negative pressure breathing on urine flow. *J Clin Invest* 33:287, 1954.
40. Gillespie DJ, Sandberg RL, Koike TI: Dual effect of left atrial receptors on excretion of sodium and water in the dog. *Am J Physiol* 225:706, 1973.
41. Reinhardt HW, Kacmarczyk G, Eisele R, et al: Left atrial pressure and sodium balance in conscious dogs on a low sodium intake. *Pflugers Arch* 370:59, 1977.
42. Epstein M, Duncan DC, Fishman LM: Characterization of the natriuresis caused in normal man by immersion in water. *Clin Sci* 43:275, 1972.
43. Henry JP, Gauer OH, Reeves JL: Evidence of the atrial location of receptors influencing urine flow. *Circ Res* 4:85, 1956.
44. Currie MG, Geller DM, Cole BC, et al: Bioactive cardiac substances: Potent vasorelaxant activity in mammalian atria. *Science* 221:71, 1983.

45. Atlas SA, Kleinert HD, Camargo MJ, et al: Purification, sequencing, and synthesis of natriuretic and vasoactive rat atrial peptide. *Nature* 309:717, 1984.
46. Barger AC, Yates FE, Rudolph AM: Renal hemodynamics and sodium excretion in dogs with graded valvular damage, and in congestive failure. *Am J Physiol* 200:601, 1961.
47. Stitzer SO, Malvin RL: Right atrium and renal sodium excretion. *Am J Physiol* 228:184, 1975.
48. Zucker IH, Gorman AJ, Cornish KG, et al: Impaired atrial receptor modulation of renal nerve activity in dogs with chronic volume overload. *Cardiovasc Res* 19:411, 1985.
49. Ferguson DW, Abboud FM, Mark AL: Selective impairment of baroreceptor-mediated vasoconstrictor responses in patients with ventricular dysfunction. *Circulation* 69:451, 1984.
50. Mohanty PK, Arrowood JA, Ellenbogen KA, et al: Neurohormonal and hemodynamic effects of lower body negative pressure in patients with congestive heart failure. *Am Heart J* 118:78, 1989.
51. Nishian K, Kawashima S, Iwasaki T: Paradoxical forearm vasodilation and hemodynamic improvement during cardiopulmonary baroreceptor unloading in patients with congestive heart failure. *Clin Sci* 84:271, 1993.
52. Sandoval AB, Gilbert EM, Larrabee P, et al: Hemodynamic correlates of increased cardiac adrenergic drive in the intact failing human heart. *J Am Coll Cardiol* 13:245A, 1989.
53. Panzenbeck MJ, Tan W, Hajdu MA, et al: PGE_2 and arachidonate inhibit the baroreflex in concious dogs via cardiac receptors. *Am J Physiol* 256:H999, 1989.
54. Zucker IH, Panzenbeck MJ, Barker S, et al: PGI_2 attenuates the baroreflex control of renal nerve activity by an afferent vagal mechanism. *Am J Physiol* 254:R424, 1988.
55. Daly JJ, Roe JW, Horrocks P: A comparison of sodium excretion following the infusion of saline into systemic and portal veins in the dog: Evidence for hepatic role in the control of sodium excretion. *Clin Sci* 33:481, 1967.
56. Passo SS, Thornborough JR, Rothballer AB: Hepatic receptors in control of sodium excretion in anesthetized cats. *Am J Physiol* 224:373, 1975.
57. Sklar AH, Schrier RW: Central nervous system mediators of vasopressin release. *Physiol Rev* 63:1243, 1983.
58. Berl T, Henrich WL, Erickson AL, et al: Prostaglandins in the beta adrenergic and baroreceptor-mediated secretion on renin. *Am J Physiol* 235:F472, 1979.
59. Braunwald E, Plauth WH, Morrow AG: A method for detection and quantification of impaired sodium excretion. *Circulation* 32:223, 1965.
60. Takasu T, Lasker N, Shalhoub RJ: Mechanism of hyponatremia in chronic congestive heart failure. *Ann Intern Med* 55:368, 1961.
61. Hope JA: *Treatise on the Diseases of the Heart and Blood Vessels.* London, William Kidd, 1832.
62. Warren JV, Stead EA: Fluid dynamics in chronic congestive heart failure: An interpretation of the mechanisms producing edema, increased plasma volume and elevated venous pressure in certain patients with prolonged congestive heart failure. *Arch Intern Med* 73:138, 1944.
63. Briggs AP, Fowell DM, Hamilton WF, et al: Renal circulatory factors in the edema formation of congestive heart failure. *J Clin Invest* 27:810, 1948.
64. Davis JO: Physiology of Congestive Heart Failure. In Hamilton WF (ed): *Handbook of Physiology: Circulation.* Washington, DC, American Physiological Society, 1956, vol III, chap 59.
65. Sinclair-Smith B, Kattus AA, Kenest J, et al: The renal mechanism of electrolyte excretion and the metabolic balances of electrolytes and nitrogen in congestive cardiac failure: The effect of exercise, rest and aminophylline. *Bull Johns Hopkins Hosp* 84:369, 1949.
66. Decaux G, et al: High uric acid and urea clearance in cirrhosis secondary to increased "effective vascular volume." *Am J Med* 73:328, 1982.
67. Wesson LG Jr: Glomerular and tubular factors in the renal excretion of sodium chloride. *Medicine* (Baltimore) 36:281, 1957.
68. Barger AC, Liebowitz MR, Muldowney FP: The pathogenesis of sodium retention in congestive heart failure. *Metabolism* 5:480, 1956.
69. Barger AC, Liebowitz MR, Muldowney FP: The role of the kidney in the homeostatic adjustments of congestive heart failure. *J Chronic Dis* 9:571, 1959.
70. Kilcoyne MM, Schmidt DH, Cannon PJ: Intrarenal blood flow in congestive heart failure. *Circulation* 47:786, 1973.

71. Bourdeaux R, Mandin H: Cardiac edema in dogs: II. Distribution of glomerular filtration rate and renal blood flow. *Kidney Int* 10:578, 1976.

72. Humes HD, Gottlieb MN, Brenner BM: The Kidney in Congestive Heart Failure. In Brenner BM, Stein JH (eds): *Sodium and Water Homeostasis.* New York, Churchill Livingstone, 1978, p 51.

73. Heller BL, Jacobonson WE: Renal hemodynamics in heart disease. *Am Heart J* 39:188, 1950.

74. Vander AJ, Malvin RL, Wilde RS, et al: Reexamination of salt and water retention in congestive heart failure. *Am J Med* 25:497, 1958.

75. Meyers BD, Deen WM, Brenner BM: Effects of norepinephrine and angiotensin II on the determinants of glomerular ultrafiltration and proximal tubule fluid reabsorption in the rat. *Circ Res* 37:101, 1975.

76. Ichikawa I, Pfeffer JM, Pfeffer MA, et al: Role of angiotensin II in the altered renal function in congestive heart failure. *Circ Res* 55:669, 1984.

77. Henrich WL, Berl T, MacDonald KM, et al: Angiotensin, renal nerves and prostaglandins in renal hemodynamics during hemorrhage. *Am J Physiol* 235:F46, 1978.

78. Henriksen JH, Christensen JJ, Ring-Larsen H: Noradrenaline and adrenaline concentrations in various vascular beds in patients with cirrhosis: Relation to hemodynamics. *Clin Physiol* 1:293, 1981.

79. Auld RB, Alexander EA, Levinsky NG: Proximal tubular function in dogs with thoracic caval constriction. *J Clin Invest* 50:2150, 1971.

80. Schneider EG, Dresser TP, Lynch RF, et al: Sodium reabsorption by proximal tubule of dogs with experimental heart failure. *Am J Physiol* 220:952, 1971.

81. Bennett WM, Bagby GC, Antonovic JN, et al: Influence of volume expansion on proximal tubular sodium reabsorption in congestive heart failure. *Am Heart J* 85:55, 1973.

82. Werko L, Varnauska E, Eliasch N, et al: Studies on the renal circulation and renal function in mitral valvular disease. *Circulation* 9:687, 1954.

83. Thomas JA, Marks BH: Plasma norepinephrine in congestive heart failure. *Am J Cardiol* 41: 233, 1978.

84. Davis D, Baily R, Zelis R: Abnormalities in systemic norepinephrine kinetics in human congestive heart failure. *Am J Physiol* 254:E760, 1988.

85. Hasking GJ, Esler MD, Jennings GL, et al: Norepinephrine spillover to plasma in patients with congestive heart failure: Evidence of increased overall and cardiorenal sympathetic nervous activity. *Circulation* 73:615, 1986.

86. Abraham WT, Hensen J, Schrier RW: Elevated plasma noradrenaline concentrations in patients with low-output cardiac failure: Dependence on increased noradrenaline secretion rates. *Clin Sci* 79:429, 1990.

87. Francis GS, Benedict C, Johnstone EE, et al: Comparison of neuroendocrine activation in patients with left ventricular dysfunction with and without congestive heart failure: A substudy of the studies of left ventricular dysfunction (SOLVD). *Circulation* 82:1724, 1990.

88. Leimbach WN, Wallin BG, Victor RG, et al: Direct evidence from intraneural recordings for increased sympathetic outflow in patients with heart failure. *Circulation* 73:913, 1986.

89. Cohn JN, Levine BT, Olivari MT, et al: Plasma norepinephrine as a guide to prognosis in patients with chronic congestive heart failure. *N Engl J Med* 311:819, 1984.

90. Gill JR Jr, Mason DT, Bartter FC: Adrenergic nervous system in sodium metabolism: Effects of guanethidine and sodium-retaining steroids in normal man. *J Clin Invest* 43:177, 1964.

91. DiBona GF, Herman PJ, Sawin LL: Neural control of renal function in edema forming states. *Am J Physiol* 254:R1017, 1988.

92. Bello-Reuss E, Trevino DL, Gottschalk CW: Effect of renal sympathetic nerve stimulation on proximal water and sodium reabsorption. *J Clin Invest* 57:1104, 1976.

93. DiBona GF: Neurogenic regulation of renal tubular sodium reabsorption. *Am J Physiol* 233: F73, 1977.

94. Lifschitz MD, Schrier RW: Alterations in cardiac output with chronic constriction of thoracic inferior vena cava. *Am J Physiol* 225:1364, 1973.

95. Botker HE, Jensen HK, Krussel LR, et al: Renal effects of xamoterol in patients with moderate heart failure. *Cardiovasc Drugs Ther* 7:111, 1993.

96. Thomsen K: Lithium clearance: A new method for determining proximal and distal tubular reabsorption of sodium and water. *Nephron* 37:217, 1984.
97. Francis GS, Goldsmith SR, Levine TB, et al: The neurohumoral axis in congestive heart failure. *Ann Intern Med* 101:370, 1984.
98. Lee WH, Packer M: Prognostic importance of serum sodium concentration and its modification by converting-enzyme inhibition in patients with severe chronic heart failure. *Circulation* 73:257, 1986.
99. Liu FY, Cogan MG: Angiotensin II: A potent regulator of acidification in the rat early proximal convoluted tubule. *J Clin Invest* 80:272, 1987.
100. Abassi ZA, Kelly G, Golomb E, et al: Losartan improves the natriuretic response to ANF in rats with high-output heart failure. *J Pharmacol Exp Ther* 268:224, 1994.
101. Watkins L, Burton JA, Haber E, et al: The renin-angiotensin system in congestive failure in conscious dogs. *J Clin Invest* 57:1606, 1977.
102. Cody RJ, Covit AB, Schaer GL, et al: Sodium and water balance in chronic congestive heart failure. *J Clin Invest* 77:1441, 1986.
103. Pierpont GL, Francis GS, Cohn JN: Effect of captopril on renal function in patients with congestive heart failure. *Br Heart J* 46:522, 1981.
104. Hensen J, Abraham WT, Durr JA, Schrier RW: Aldosterone in congestive heart failure: Analysis of determinants and role in sodium retention. *Am J Nephrol* 11:441, 1991.
105. Szatalowicz VL, Arnold PA, Chaimovitz C, et al: Radioimmunoassay of plasma arginine vasopressin in hyponatremic patients with congestive heart failure. *N Engl J Med* 305:263, 1981.
106. Riegger GA, Niebau G, Kochsiek K: Antidiuretic hormone in congestive heart failure. *Am J Med* 72:49, 1982.
107. Bichet D, Kortas CK, Mattauer B, et al: Modulation of plasma and "platelet fraction" vasopressin by cardiac function in patients with severe congestive heart failure. *Kidney Int* 29:1188, 1986.
108. Pruszczynski W, Vahanian A, Ardailou R, et al: Role of antidiuretic hormone in impaired water excretion of patients with congestive heart failure. *J Clin Endocrinol Metab* 58:599, 1984.
109. Goldsmith SR, Francis GS, Cowley AW Jr: Arginine vasopressin and the renal response to water loading in congestive heart failure. *Am J Cardiol* 58:295, 1986.
110. Handelman W, Lum G, Schrier RW: Impaired water excretion in high output cardiac failure in the rat. *Clin Res* 27:173A, 1979.
111. Ishikawa S, Saito T, Okada T, et al: Effect of vasopressin antagonist on water excretion in inferior vena cava constriction. *Kidney Int* 30:49, 1986.
112. Yared A, Kon V, Brenner BM, et al: Role for vasopressin in rats with congestive heart failure. *Kidney Int* 27:337, 1985.
113. Fujita H, Yoshiyama M, Yamagishi H, et al: The effect of vasopressin V1 and V2 receptor antagonists on heart failure after myocardial infarction. *J Am Coll Cardiol* 25:234A, 1995.
114. Naitoh M, Suzuki H, Murakami M, et al: Effects of oral AVP receptor antagonists OPC-21268 and OPC-31260 on congestive heart failure in conscious dogs. *Am J Physiol* 267:H2245, 1994.
115. Yamamura Y, Ogawa H, Yamashita H, et al: Characterization of a novel aquaretic agent, OPC-31260, as an orally effective, nonpeptide vasopressin V_2 receptor antagonist. *Br J Pharmacol* 105:787, 1992.
116. Ohnishi A, Orita Y, Okahara R, et al: Potent aquaretic agent: A novel nonpeptide selective vasopressin 2 antagonist (OPC-31260) in men. *J Clin Invest* 92:2653, 1993.
117. Kim JK, Michel J-B, Soubrier F, et al: Arginine vasopressin gene expression in congestive heart failure. *Kidney Int* 33:270, 1988.
118. Dunn FL, Brennan TJ, Nelson AE, et al: The role of blood osmolality and volume in regulating vasopressin secretion in the rat. *J Clin Invest* 52:3212, 1973.
119. Bell NH, Schedl HP, Bartter FC: An explanation for abnormal water retention and hypoosmolality in congestive heart failure. *Am J Med* 36:351, 1964.
120. Schrier RW, Lehman D, Zacherle B, et al: Effect of furosemide on free water excretion in edematous patients with hyponatremia. *Kidney Int* 3:30, 1973.

121. Szatalowicz VL, Miller PD, Lacher J, et al: Comparative effects of diuretics on renal water excretion in hyponatremic edematous disorders. *Clin Sci* 62:235, 1982.
122. Nakaoka H, Imataka K, Amano M, et al: Plasma levels of atrial natriuretic factor in patients with congestive heart failure. *N Engl J Med* 313:892, 1985.
123. Raine AEG, Erne P, Bürgisser E, et al: Atrial natriuretic peptide and atrial pressure in patients with congestive heart failure. *N Engl J Med* 315:533, 1986.
124. Mukoyama M, Nakao K, Saito Y, et al: Increased human brain natriuretic peptide in congestive heart failure. *N Engl J Med* 323:757, 1990.
125. Molina CR, Fowler MB, McCrory S, et al: Hemodynamic, renal, and endocrine effects of atrial natriuretic peptide in severe heart failure. *J Am Coll Cardiol* 12:175, 1988.
126. Atarashi K, Mulrow PJ, Franco-Saenz R, et al: Inhibition of aldosterone production by an atrial extract. *Science* 224:992, 1984.
127. Samson WK: Atrial natriuretic factor inhibits dehydration and hemorrhage-induced vasopressin release. *Neuroendocrinology* 40:277, 1985.
128. Floras JS: Sympathoinhibitory effects of atrial natriuretic factor in normal humans. *Circulation* 81:1860, 1990.
129. Cody RJ, Atlas SA, Laragh JH, et al: Atrial natriuretic factor in normal subjects and heart failure patients: Plasma levels and renal, hormonal, and hemodynamic responses to peptide infusion. *J Clin Invest* 78:1362, 1986.
130. Hensen J, Abraham WT, Lesnefsky EJ, et al: Atrial natriuretic factor kinetic studies in patients with congestive heart failure. *Kidney Int* 42:1333, 1992.
131. Saito Y, Nakao K, Arai H, et al: Atrial natriuretic polypeptide (ANP) in human ventricle: Increased gene expression of ANP in dilated cardiomyopathy. *Biochem Biophys Res Comm* 148:211, 1987.
132. Hosoda K, Nakao K, Mukoyama M, et al: Expression of brain natriuretic peptide gene in human heart: Production in the ventricle. *Hypertension* 17:1152, 1991.
133. Drexler H, Hirth C, Stasch H-P, et al: Vasodilatory action of endogenous atrial natriuretic factor in a rat model of chronic heart failure as determined by monoclonal ANF antibody. *Circ Res* 66:1371, 1990.
134. Biollaz J, Nussberger J, Porchet M, et al: Four-hour infusion of synthetic atrial natriuretic peptide in normal volunteers. *Hypertension* 8:II96, 1986.
135. Koseki C, Hayashi Y, Torikai S, et al: Localization of binding sites for alpha-rat atrial natriuretic polypeptide in rat kidney. *Am J Physiol* 250:F210, 1986.
136. Healy DP, Fanestil DD: Localization of atrial natriuretic peptide binding sites within the rat kidney. *Am J Physiol* 250:F573, 1986.
137. Kim JK, Summer SN, Dürr J, et al: Enzymatic and binding effects of atrial natriuretic factor in glomeruli and nephrons. *Kidney Int* 35:799, 1989.
138. Lee ME, Miller WL, Edwards BS, et al: Role of endogenous atrial natriuretic factor in acute congestive heart failure. *J Clin Invest* 84:1962, 1989.
139. Hoffman A, Grossman E, Keiser HR: Increased plasma levels and blunted effects of brain natriuretic peptide in rats with congestive heart failure. *Am J Hypertens* 4:597, 1991.
140. Gelfand RA, Frank HJL, Levin E, et al: Brain and atrial natriuretic peptides bind to common receptors in brain capillary endothelial cells. *Am J Physiol* 261:E183, 1991.
141. Abraham WT, Lowes BD, Ferguson DA, et al: Systemic hemodynamic and renal excretory effects of a continuous 4-hour infusion of human brain natriuretic peptide in patients with heart failure. *J Am Coll Cardiol* 25:236A, 1995.
142. Elsner D, Muders F, Müntze A, et al: Efficacy of prolonged infusion of urodilatin [ANP-(95-126)] in patients with congestive heart failure. *Am Heart J* 129:766, 1995.
143. Saxenhofer H, Raselli A, Weidmann P, et al: Urodilatin, a natriuretic factor from kidneys can modify renal and cardiovascular function in men. *Am J Physiol* 259:F832, 1990.
144. Abraham WT, Hensen J, Kim JD, et al: Atrial natriuretic peptide and urinary cyclic guanosine monophosphate in patients with congestive heart failure. *J Am Soc Nephrol* 2:697, 1992.
145. Abraham WT, Lauwaars ME, Kim JK, et al: Reversal of atrial natriuretic peptide resistance by increasing distal tubular sodium delivery in patients with decompensated cirrhosis. *Hepatology* 22:737, 1995.

146. Connelly TP, Francis GS, Williams KJ, et al: Interaction of intravenous atrial natriuretic factor with furosemide in patients with heart failure. *Am Heart J* 127:392, 1994.
147. Koepke JP, DiBona GF: Blunted natriuresis to atrial natriuretic peptide in chronic sodium-retaining disorders. *Am J Physiol* 252:F865, 1987.
148. Swain JA, Heyndrickx GR, Boettcher DH, et al: Prostaglandin control of renal circulation in the unanesthetized dog and baboon. *Am J Physiol* 229:826, 1975.
149. Walker RM, Brown RS, Stoff JS: Role of renal prostaglandins during antidiuresis and water diuresis in man. *Kidney Int* 21:365, 1981.
150. Dzau VJ, Packer M, Lilly LS, et al: Prostaglandins in severe congestive heart failure: Relation to activation of the renin-angiotensin system and hyponatremia. *N Engl J Med* 310:347, 1984.
151. Walshe JJ, Venuto RC: Acute oliguric renal failure induced by indomethacin: Possible mechanism. *Ann Intern Med* 91:47, 1979.
152. Riegger GA, Kahles HW, Elsner D, et al: Effects of acetylsalicylic acid on renal function in patients with chronic heart failure. *Am J Med* 90:571, 1991.
153. Lieberman FL, Denison EK, Reynolds TB: The relationship of plasma volume, portal hypertension, ascites, and renal sodium retention in cirrhosis: The overflow theory of ascites formation. *Ann NY Acad Sci* 170:202, 1970.
154. Papper S. The role of the kidney in Laennec's cirrhosis of the liver. *Medicine* 37:299, 1958.
155. Schrier RW, Arroyo V, Bernardi M, et al: Peripheral arterial vasodilation hypothesis: A proposal for the initiation of renal sodium and water retention in cirrhosis. *Hepatology* 8:1151, 1988.
156. Rahman SN, Abraham WT, Schrier RW: Peripheral arterial vasodilation hypothesis in cirrhosis. *Gastroenterology Int* 5:192, 1992.
157. Vallance P, Moncada S: Hyperdynamic circulation in cirrhosis: A role for nitric oxide? *Lancet* 337:776, 1991.
158. Guarner C, Soriano G, Tomas A, et al: Increased serum nitrite and nitrate levels in patients with cirrhosis: Relationship to endotoxemia. *Hepatology* 18:1139, 1993.
159. Niederberger M, Ginès P, Tsai P, et al: Increased aortic cyclic guanosine monophosphate concentration in experimental cirrhosis in rats: Evidence for a role of nitric oxide in the pathogenesis of arterial vasodilation in cirrhosis. *Hepatology* 250:1625, 1995.
160. Niederberger M, Pierre-Yves M, Ginès P, et al: Normalization of nitric oxide production corrects arterial vasodilation and hyperdynamic circulation in cirrhotic rats. *Gastroenterology* 109:1624, 1995.
161. Miyase S, Fujiyama S, Chikazawa H, et al: Atrial natriuretic peptide in liver cirrhosis with mild ascites. *Gastroenterol Jpn* 25:356, 1990.
162. Burton GA, MacNeil S, de Jonge A, et al: Cyclic GMP release and vasodilation induced by EDRF and atrial natriuretic factor in the isolated perfused kidney of the rat. *Br J Pharmacol* 99:364, 1990.
163. Albillos A, Rossi I, Cacho G, et al: Enhanced endothelium-derived vasodilation in patients with cirrhosis. *Am J Physiol* 268:G459, 1995.
164. Leehey DJ, Gollapudi P, Deakin A, et al: Naloxone increases water and electrolyte excretion after water loading in patients with cirrhosis and ascites. *J Lab Clin Med* 118:484, 1991.
165. Kapusta DK, Cuntapay M: Endogenous opioid peptides in the regulation of renal function in cirrhosis with ascites. *Proceedings of the XIIIth International Congress of Nephrology*, Madrid, Spain, 1995, p 169.
166. Lonergran MA, Aglibut S, Field MI: Effect of an antiserum to vasoactive intestinal peptide (VIP) in two rat models of cirrhosis. *Proceedings of the XIIIth International Congress of Nephrology*, Madrid, Spain, 1995, p 169.
167. Bichet DG, Groves RM, Schrier RW: Mechanisms of improvement of water and sodium excretion by enhancement of central hemodynamics in decompensated cirrhotic patients. *Kidney Int* 24:788, 1983.
168. Schedl HP, Bartter FC: An explanation for and experimental correction of the abnormal water diuresis in cirrhosis. *J Clin Invest* 46:1297, 1967.
169. Klinger EL, Vaamonde CA, Vaamonde LS, et al: Renal function changes in cirrhosis of the liver. *Arch Intern Med* 125:1010, 1970.

170. Laragh JH, Cannon PJ, Bentzel CJ, et al: Angiotensin II, norepinephrine and renal transport of electrolytes and water in normal man and in cirrhosis with ascites. *J Clin Invest* 42:1179, 1963.

171. Bank N, Aynedijian HS: A micropuncture study of renal salt and water retention in chronic bile duct obstruction. *J Clin Invest* 55:994, 1975.

172. Better OS, Aisenbrey GA, Anderson RJ, et al: Role of antidiuretic hormone in impaired urinary dilution associated with chronic bile duct ligation. *Clin Sci* 58:493, 1980.

173. Lieberman FL, Reynolds TB: Renal failure with cirrhosis: Observations on the role of diuretics. *Ann Intern Med* 64:1221, 1966.

174. Chaimovitz C, Szylman P, Alroy G, et al: Mechanism of increased renal tubular sodium reabsorption in cirrhosis. *Am J Med* 52:198, 1972.

175. Schubert J, Puschett J, Goldberg M: The renal mechanisms of sodium reabsorption in cirrhosis (abstract). *Am Soc Nephrol* 3:58A, 1969.

176. Levy M: Sodium retention and ascites formation in dogs with experimental portal cirrhosis. *Am J Physiol* 233:F575, 1977.

177. Lopez-Novoa JM, Rengel MA, Rodicio JL, et al: A micropuncture study of salt and water retention in chronic experimental cirrhosis. *Am J Physiol* 232:F315, 1977.

178. Nicholls KM, Shapiro MD, Van Putten VJ, et al: Elevated plasma norepinephrine concentrations in decompensated cirrhosis. *Circ Res* 56:457, 1985.

179. Floras JS, Legault L, Morali GA, et al: Increased sympathetic outflow in cirrhosis and ascites: Direct evidence from intraneural recordings. *Ann Intern Med* 114:373, 1991.

180. Ring-Larsen H, Hesse B, Henriksen JH, et al: Sympathetic nervous activity and renal and systemic hemodynamics in cirrhosis: Plasma norepinephrine concentration, hepatic extraction and renal release. *Hepatology* 2:304, 1982.

181. Bichet DG, VanPutten VJ, Schrier RW: Potential role of increased sympathetic activity in impaired sodium and water excretion in cirrhosis. *N Engl J Med* 307:1552, 1982.

182. Ring-Larsen H, Henriksen JG, Christensen NJ: Increased sympathetic activity in cirrhosis. *N Engl J Med* 308:1029, 1983.

183. Giuseffi J, Werk EE Jr, Larson PU, et al: Effect of bilateral adrenalectomy in a patient with massive ascites and postnecrotic cirrhosis. *N Engl J Med* 257:796, 1957.

184. Eggert RC: Spironolactone diuresis in patients with cirrhosis and ascites. *Br Med J* 4:401, 1970.

185. Rosoff L, Zia P, Reynolds T, et al: Studies of renin and aldosterone in cirrhotic patients with ascites. *Gastroenterology* 69:698, 1975.

186. Epstein M, Pins DS, Schneider N, et al: Determinants of deranged sodium and water hemostasis in decompensated cirrhosis. *J Lab Clin Med* 87:822, 1976.

187. Chonko AM, Bay WH, Stein HH, et al: The role of renin and aldosterone in the salt retention of edema. *Am J Med* 63:881, 1977.

188. Arroyo V, Rodes J, Guiterrez-Lizarrage MA, et al: Prognostic value of spontaneous hyponatremia in cirrhosis with ascites. *Dig Dis* 21:249, 1976.

189. Ralli EP, Leslie SH, Stuek GH, et al: Studies of the serum and urine constituents in patients with cirrhosis of the liver during water tolerance tests. *Am J Med* 11:157, 1951.

190. Birchard WH, Prout TE, Williams TF, et al: Diuretic responses to oral and intravenous waterloads in patients with hepatic cirrhosis. *J Lab Clin Med* 48:26, 1956.

191. Rector FC: Sodium, bicarbonate and chloride absorption by the proximal tubule. *Am J Physiol* 13:F461, 1983.

192. Vlachecevic ZR, Adham NF, Zick H, et al: Renal effects of acute expansion of plasma volume in cirrhosis. *N Engl J Med* 272:387, 1965.

193. Yamahiro HS, Reynolds TB: Effects of ascitic fluid infusion on sodium excretion blood volume and creatinine clearance in cirrhosis. *Gastroenterology* 40:497, 1961.

194. Strauss MP, Birehard WH, Sazon L: Correction of impaired water excretion in cirrhosis of the liver by alcohol ingestion or expansion of extracellular fluid volume: The role of antidiuretic hormone. *Trans Assoc Am Physicians* 39:222, 1956.

195. de Troyer A, Pillay W, Broeckaert I, et al: Demeclocycline treatment of water retention in cirrhosis. *Ann Intern Med* 85:336, 1976.

196. Miller PD, Linas SL, Schrier RW: Plasma demeclocycline levels and nephrotoxicity correlation in hyponatremic cirrhotic patients. *JAMA* 243:2513, 1980.

197. Better OS, Massry SG: Effect of chronic bile duct obstruction on renal handling of salt and water. *J Clin Invest* 51:402, 1972.

198. Lopez-Novoa JM, Rengel MA, Hernando L. Dynamics of ascites formation in rats with experimental cirrhosis. *Am J Physiol* 238:F353, 1980.

199. Bichet D, Szatalowicz VL, Chaimovitz C, et al: Role of vasopressin in abnormal water excretion in cirrhotic patients. *Ann Intern Med* 96:413, 1982.

200. Shapiro MD, Nicholls KM, Groves BM, et al: Interrelationship between cardiac output and vascular resistance as determinants of effective arterial blood volume in cirrhotic patients. *Kidney Int* 28:206, 1985.

201. Claria J, Jimenez W, Arroyo V, et al: Blockade of the hydroosmotic effect of vasopressin normalizes water excretion in cirrhotic rats. *Gastroenterology* 97:1294, 1989.

202. Tsuboi Y, Ishikawa SE, Fujisawa G, et al: Therapeutic efficacy of the nonpeptide AVP antagonist OPC-31260 in cirrhotic rats. *Kidney Int* 46:237, 1994.

203. Fujita N, Ishikawa S, Sasaki S, et al: Role of water channel AQP-CD in water retention in SIADH and cirrhotic rats. *Am J Physiol* 269:F926, 1995.

204. Schrier RW, Better OS: Pathogenesis of ascites formation: Mechanism of impaired aldosterone escape in cirrhosis. *Eur J Gastroenterol Hepatol* 3:721, 1991.

205. Skorecki KL, Leung WM, Campbell P, et al: Role of atrial natriuretic peptide in the natriuretic response to central volume expansion induced by head-out water immersion in sodium-retaining cirrhotic subjects. *Am J Med* 85:375, 1988.

206. Koepke JP, Jones S, DiBona GF: Renal nerves mediate blunted natriuresis to atrial natriuretic peptide in cirrhotic rats. *Am J Physiol* 252:R1019, 1987.

207. Morali GA, Tobe SW, Skorecki KL, et al: Refractory ascites: Modulation of atrial natriuretic factor unresponsiveness by mannitol. *Hepatology* 16:42, 1992.

208. Zambraski EJ, Dunn MJ: Importance of renal prostaglandins in control of renal function after chronic ligation of the common bile duct in dogs. *J Lab Clin Med* 103:549, 1984.

209. Arroyo V, Planas R, Gaya J, et al: Sympathetic nervous activity, renin-angiotensin system and renal excretion of prostaglandin E2 in cirrhosis: Relationship to functional renal failure and sodium and water excretion. *Eur J Clin Invest* 13:271, 1983.

210. Boyer TD, Zia P, Reynolds TB: Effect of indomethacin and prostaglandin A1 on renal function and plasma renin activity in alcoholic liver disease. *Gastroenterology* 77:215, 1979.

211. Wong F, Massie D, Hsu P, et al: Indomethacin-induced renal dysfunction in patients with well-compensated cirrhosis. *Gastroenterology* 104:869, 1993.

212. Barnett HL, Forman CW, McNamara H, et al: The effect of adrenocorticotrophic hormone on children with the nephrotic syndrome: II. Physiologic observations on discrete kidney functions and plasma volume. *J Clin Invest* 30:227, 1951.

213. Brown EA, Markandu ND, Sagnella GA, et al: Evidence that some mechanism other than the renin system causes sodium retention in nephrotic syndrome. *Lancet* 2:1237, 1982.

214. Eisenberg MD: Postural changes in plasma volume in hypoalbuminemia. *Arch Intern Med* 112:140, 1963.

215. Yamauchi H, Hopper J Jr: Hypovolemic shock and hypotension as a complication in the nephrotic syndrome: Report of ten cases. *Ann Intern Med* 60:242, 1964.

216. Chamberlain MJ, Pringle A, Wrong OM: Oliguric renal failure in the nephrotic syndrome. *Q J Med* 35:215, 1966.

217. Anderson RJ, Taher MS, Cronin RE, et al: Effect of beta-adrenergic blockade and inhibitors of angiotensin II and prostaglandins on renal autoregulation. *Am J Physiol* 229:731, 1975.

218. Hooper J Jr, Ryan P, Lee JC, et al: Lipoid nephrosis in 31 adult patients: Renal biopsy study by light, electron, and fluorescence microscopy with experience in treatment. *Medicine* (Baltimore) 49:321, 1970.

219. Imai M, Sokabe H: Plasma renin and angiotensinogen levels in pathological states associated with edema. *Arch Dis Child* 43:475, 1968.

220. Kelsch RC, Light GS, Oliver WJ: The effect of albumin infusion upon plasma norepinephrine concentration in nephrotic children. *J Lab Clin Med* 79:516, 1972.

221. Krishna GG, Danovitch GM: Effects of water immersion on renal function in the nephrotic syndrome. *Kidney Int* 21:395, 1982.
222. McDonald KM, Rosenthal A, Schrier RW, et al: Effect of interruption of neural pathways on renal response to volume expansion. *Am J Physiol* 218:510, 1970.
223. Rahman SN, Abraham WT, Van Putten VJ, et al: Increased norepinephrine secretion in patients with the nephrotic syndrome and normal glomerular filtration rates: Evidence for primary sympathetic activation. *Am J Nephrol* 13:266, 1993.
224. Berlyne GM, Sutton J, Brown C, et al: Renal salt and water handling in water immersion in the nephrotic syndrome. *Clin Sci* 61:605, 1981.
225. Shapiro M, Nicholls K, Schrier RW: Mechanism of impaired water excretion in nephrotic syndrome. *Kidney Int* 27:154, 1985.
226. Usberti M, Gazzotti RM, Poiesi C, et al: Considerations on the sodium retention in nephrotic syndrome. *Am J Nephrol* 15:38, 1995.
227. Geers AB, Koomans HA, Boer P, et al: Plasma and blood volumes in the nephrotic syndrome. *Nephron* 38:170, 1984.
228. Meltzer JI, Keim HJ, Laragh JH, et al: Nephrotic syndrome: Vasoconstriction and hypervolemic types indication by renin-sodium profiling. *Ann Intern Med* 91:688, 1979.
229. Keller H, Noseda G, Morell A, et al: Analbuminemia. *Minerva Med* 63:1296, 1972.
230. Kalant N, Gupta DD, Despointes R, Giroud CJP: Mechanisms of edema in experimental nephrosis. *Am J Physiol* 202:91, 1962.
231. Bernard DB, Alexander EA, Couser WG, et al: Renal sodium retention during volume expansion in experimental nephrotic syndrome. *Kidney Int* 14:478, 1978.
232. Kuroda S, Aynedjian HS, Bank NA: A micropuncture study of renal sodium retention in nephrotic syndrome in rats: Evidence for increased resistance to tubular fluid flow. *Kidney Int* 16:561, 1979.
233. Grausz H, Lieberman R, Earley LE: Effect of plasma albumin on sodium reabsorption in patients with nephrotic syndrome. *Kidney Int* 1:47, 1972.
234. Usberti M, Federico S, Cianciaruso B, et al: Relationship between serum albumin concentration and tubular reabsorption of glucose in renal disease. *Kidney Int* 16:546, 1979.
235. Tobian L, Perry S, Mork J: The relationship of the juxtaglomerular apparatus to sodium retention in experimental nephrosis. *Ann Intern Med* 57:382, 1962.
236. Ichikawa I, Rennke HG, Hoyer JR, et al: Role for intrarenal mechanisms in the impaired salt excretion of experimental nephrotic syndrome. *J Clin Invest* 71:91, 1983.
237. Dusing R, Vetter H, Kramer HJ: The renin-angiotensin-aldosterone system in patients with nephrotic syndrome: Effects of 1-sar-8-ala-angiotensin II. *Nephron* 25:187, 1980.
238. Shapiro MD, Hasbergen J, Cosby R, et al: Role of aldosterone in the Na retention of patients with nephrotic syndrome. *Am J Kidney Dis* 8:81, 1986.
239. Hisanaga S, Yamamoto Y, Kida O, et al: Plasma concentration and renal effect of human atrial natriuretic peptide in nephrotic syndrome. *Jpn J Nephrol* 31:661, 1989.
240. Yokota N, Yamamoto Y, Iemura F, et al: Increased plasma levels and effects of brain natriuretic peptide in experimental nephrosis. *Nephron* 65:454, 1993.
241. Perico N, Remuzzi G: Renal handling of sodium in the nephrotic syndrome. *Am J Nephrol* 13:413, 1993.
242. Abassi Z, Shuranyi E, Better OS, et al: Effect of atrial natriuretic factor on renal cGMP production in rats with Adriamycin-induced nephrotic syndrome. *J Am Soc Nephrol* 2:1538, 1992.
243. Kleinknecht C, Broyer M, Gubler MC, et al: Irreversible renal failure after indomethacin in steroid resistant nephrosis. *N Engl J Med* 302:691, 1980.
244. Dorhout-Mees EJ, Roos JC, Boer P, et al: Observations on edema formation in the nephrotic syndrome in adults with minimal lesions. *Am J Med* 67:378, 1979.
245. Pedersen EB, Danielsen H, Madsen M, et al: Defective renal water excretion in nephrotic syndrome: The relationship between renal water excretion and kidney function, arginine-vasopressin, angiotensin II and aldosterone in plasma before and after water loading. *Eur J Clin Invest* 15:24, 1985.
246. Gur A, Adefuin PY, Siegel NJ, et al: A study of the renal handling of water in lipoid nephrosis. *Pediatr Res* 10:197, 1976.

247. Rascher W, Tulassay T, Seyberth HW, et al: Diuretic and hormonal responses to head-out water immersion in nephrotic syndrome. *J Pediatr* 109:609, 1986.
248. Tulassay T, Rascher W, Lang RE, et al: Atrial natriuretic peptide and other vasoactive hormones in nephrotic syndrome. *Kidney Int* 31:1391, 1987.
249. Usberti M, Federico C, Meccariello S, et al: Role of plasma vasopressin in the impairment of water excretion in nephrotic syndrome. *Kidney Int* 25:422, 1984.
250. Shapiro MD, Nicholls KM, Groves R, Schrier RW: Role of glomerular filtration rate in the impaired sodium and water excretion of patients with the nephrotic syndrome. *Am J Kidney Dis* 8:81, 1986.
251. Konstam MA, Dracup K, Baker DW, et al: *Heart Failure: Evaluation and Care of Patients with Left-Ventricular Systolic Dysfunction.* Clinical Practice Guideline Number 11. Rockville, Md, Agency for Health Care Policy and Research, 1994.
252. Taguma Y, Kitamoto Y, Futaki G, et al: Effect of captopril on heavy proteinuria in azotemic diabetics. *N Engl J Med* 313:1617, 1985.
253. Bjorck S, Nyberg G, Mulec H, et al: Beneficial effects of angiotensin converting enzyme inhibition on renal function in patients with diabetic nephropathy. *Br Med J* 293:471, 1986.
254. Gansevoort RT, De Zeeuw D, De Jong PE: Is the antiproteinuric effect of ACE inhibition mediated by interference in the renin-angiotensin system? *Kidney Int* 45:861, 1994.
255. Morgan T, Berliner RW: A study by continuous microperfusion of water and electrolyte movements in the loop of Henle and distal tubule of the rat. *Nephron* 6:388, 1969.
256. Birtch AG, Zakheim RM, Jones LG, et al: Redistribution of renal blood flow produced by furosemide and ethacrynic acid. *Circ Res* 21:869, 1967.
257. Giebisch G: Renal Potassium Excretion. In Rouiller C, Muller AF (eds): *The Kidney: Morphology, Biochemistry, Physiology.* New York, Academic, 1971, vol III, p 329.
258. Goldstein MH, Levitt MF, Hauser D, et al: Effect of meralluride on solute and water excretion in hydrated man: Comments on site of action. *J Clin Invest* 40:731, 1961.
259. Sit SP, Morita H, Vatner SF: Responses of renal hemodynamics and function to acute volume expansion in the conscious dog. *Circ Res* 54:185, 1984.
260. Forrest JN, Cox M, Hong C, et al: Demeclocycline versus lithium for inappropriate secretion of antidiuretic hormone. *N Engl J Med* 298:173, 1978.
261. Dikshit K, Vyden JK, Forrester JS, et al: Renal and extrarenal hemodynamic effects of furosemide in congestive heart failure after acute myocardial infarction. *N Engl J Med* 288:1087, 1973.
262. Johnston GD, Hiatt WR, Nies AS, et al: Factors modifying the early nondiuretic vascular effects of furosemide in man. *Circ Res* 53:630, 1983.
263. Francis GS, Siegel RM, Goldsmith SR, et al: Acute vasoconstrictor response to intravenous furosemide in patients with chronic congestive heart failure. *Ann Intern Med* 103:1, 1985.
264. Ikram H, Chan W, Espiner EA, et al: Haemodynamic and hormone responses to acute and chronic furosemide therapy in congestive heart failure. *Clin Sci* 59:443, 1980.
265. Bayliss J, Norell M, Canepa-Anson R, et al: Untreated heart failure: Clinical and neuroendocrine effects of introducing diuretics. *Br Heart J* 57:17, 1987.
266. Fett DL, Cavero PG, Burnett JC: Atrial natriuretic factor modulates the renal and endocrine actions of furosemide in experimental acute congestive heart failure. *J Am Soc Nephrol* 4:162, 1993.
267. Kaojarern S, Day B, Brater DC: The time course of delivery of furosemide into the urine: An independent determinant of overall response. *Kidney Int* 22:69, 1982.
268. Lahav M, Regev A, Ra'anani P, et al: Intermittent administration of furosemide vs continuous infusion preceded by a loading dose for congestive heart failure. *Chest* 102:725, 1992.
269. Van Meyel JJM, Smits P, Russel FGM, et al: Diuretic efficiency of furosemide during continuous administration versus bolus injection in healthy volunteers. *Clin Pharmacol Ther* 51:440, 1992.
270. Gabow PA, Moore S, Schrier RW: Spironolactone induced hyperchloremia acidosis in cirrhosis. *Ann Intern Med* 90:338, 1979.
271. Brickman AS, Massry SG, Coburn JW: Changes in serum and urinary calcium during treatment with hydrochlorothiazide: Studies on mechanisms. *J Clin Invest* 51:945, 1972.

272. Gabow PA, Hanson T, Popovtzer M, Schrier RW: Furosemide-induced reduction in ionized calcium in hypoparathyroid patients. *Ann Intern Med* 86:579, 1977.
273. Favere L, Glasson P, Reonad A, et al: Interacting diuretics and nonsteroidal antiinflammatory drugs in man. *Clin Sci* 64:407, 1983.
274. Lyons H, Pinn VW, Cortell S, et al: Allergic interstitial nephritis causing reversible renal failure in four patients with idiopathic nephrotic syndrome. *N Engl J Med* 288:124, 1973.
275. Stampfer M, Epstein SE, Beiser GD, et al: Hemodynamic effects of diuresis at rest and during intense upright exercise in patients with impaired cardiac function. *Circulation* 37:900, 1968.
276. Sherlock S: Ascites formation in cirrhosis and its management. *Scand J Gastroenterol [Suppl]* 7:9, 1970.
277. Shear L, Ching S, Gauzda GJ: Compartmentalization of ascites and edema in patients with hepatic cirrhosis. *N Engl J Med* 282:1391, 1970.
278. Gabuzda GJ, Hall PW III: Relation of potassium depletion to renal ammonium metabolism and hepatic coma. *Medicine* 45:481, 1966.
279. Gregory PB, Broekelschen PH, Hill MD, et al: Complications of diuresis in the alcoholic patient with ascites: A controlled trial. *Gastroenterology* 73:534, 1977.
280. Ginès P, Arroyo V, Quintero E, et al: Comparison between paracentesis and diuretics in the treatment of cirrhotics with tense ascites. *Gastroenterology* 93:234, 1987.
281. Ginès P, Tito LI, Arroyo V, et al: Randomized comparative study of therapeutic paracentesis with and without intravenous albumin in cirrhosis. *Gastroenterology* 94:1493, 1988.
282. Quintero E, Ginès P, Arroyo V, et al: Paracentesis versus diuretics in the treatment of cirrhotics with tense ascites. *Lancet* 1:611, 1985.
283. Salerno F, Badalamenti S, Incerti P, et al: Repeated paracentesis and i.v. albumin infusion to treat "tense" ascites in cirrhotic patients: A safe alternative therapy. *J Hepatol* 5:102, 1987.
284. Tito L, Ginès P, Arroyo V, et al: Total paracentesis associated with intravenous albumin management of patients with cirrhosis and ascites. *Gastroenterology* 98:146, 1990.

3

Pathogenesis and Management of Metabolic Acidosis and Alkalosis

Joseph I. Shapiro and William D. Kaehny

Acid-base disorders occur commonly in clinical medicine. Despite what appears at first glance to be a bewildering number of diagnostic considerations, the pathophysiology of these disorders can be approached quite logically with a minimum of laboratory and clinical data. An effective approach to clinical acid-base disorders is accomplished most easily with a stepwise, pathophysiologic approach.

Human acid-base homeostasis normally involves the tight regulation of CO_2 tension by respiratory excretion and plasma bicarbonate ($HCO_3{}^-$) concentration by renal elimination of protons (H^+) produced by metabolism. The pH of body fluids (which can easily be sampled) is determined by the CO_2 tension (in arterial blood, $PaCO_2$) and the $[HCO_3{}^-]$. Primary derangements of CO_2 tension are generally referred to as respiratory disturbances, whereas derangements of $[HCO_3{}^-]$ are called metabolic disturbances [1].

This chapter will review acid-base chemistry and physiology and then turn to a pathophysiologic approach to the diagnosis and management of metabolic acidosis and alkalosis.

Acid-Base Chemistry and Physiology

The chemistry of acids, bases, and buffers [2] and the normal physiology of acid and bicarbonate excretion [2, 3] are described in detail in several excellent reviews and will be summarized only briefly in this section.

Buffering

Clinical acid-base chemistry is basically the chemistry of buffers. For clinical purposes, an acid can be defined as a chemical that donates an H^+, and a base as an H^+ acceptor. For any acid (HA), its strength or tendency to donate H^+ can be defined by its dissociation constant K according to the relationship

$$[HA] = K_{eq} \times [H^+][A^-] \qquad (1)$$

Rearranging this equation and applying a log transformation results in the familiar

130

$$pH = pK + \log_{10} [A^-]/[HA] \tag{2}$$

Buffering refers to the ability of a solution containing a weak or poorly dissociated acid and its anion (a base) to resist change in pH when strong acid (i.e., highly dissociated acid) or alkali is added. To illustrate this important point, suppose 1 ml of 0.1M HCl was added to 9 ml of distilled water. The [H$^+$] would increase from 10^{-7}M to 10^{-2}M. In other words, the pH would fall from 7.0 to 2.0. However, if 1 ml of 0.1M HCl was added to 9 ml of a 1M phosphate buffer (pK = 6.9) at pH 7.0, most of the dissociated H$^+$ from HCl would combine with dibasic phosphate (HPO$_4^{2-}$) and only slightly change the ratio of dibasic to monobasic phosphate (H$_2$PO$_4^-$). In fact, the pH would fall by only about 0.1 pH units. The addition of acid has been buffered by the phosphate dissolved in water. Another way to think about this is that the pH was stabilized by substances that bound the free H$^+$ released by the HCl, in this case the phosphate. Such substances are called buffers [4].

Biochemical Determinants of pH

In humans, the bicarbonate buffer system is the most important buffer in the extracellular space. Proteins and inorganic phosphate are less important buffers. In the intracellular space, inorganic phosphate is probably the most important buffer, followed by bicarbonate and intracellular proteins. Although intracellular pH is probably more important in predicting physiologic and clinical consequences than extracellular pH [5], it is difficult to measure in vivo without using sophisticated investigational techniques such as ^{31}P nuclear magnetic resonance spectroscopy [6] that are not available for routine clinical application. Therefore, clinical efforts focus on classifying disease states based on what is measurable, that is, extracellular pH. In particular, attention is focused on the bicarbonate buffer system [2]. Because there is abundant carbonic anhydrase in blood, it can be assumed that equilibrium conditions apply. Therefore, the bicarbonate buffer system can be viewed as the equilibrium reaction:

$$H^+ + HCO_3^- \xrightarrow{K_{eq}} H_2CO_3 \quad \text{or} \tag{3}$$

$$[H^+] = K_{eq} \times [H_2CO_3]/[HCO_3^-] \tag{4}$$

Carbonic acid (H$_2$CO$_3$) is defined by the partial pressure of CO$_2$ and the solubility (S) of CO$_2$ in physiologic fluids, which is to all intents and purposes a constant S. The equation can therefore be rearranged as

$$[H^+] = K \times (S \times PCO_2)/[HCO_3^-] \tag{5}$$

which was attributed to Henderson in 1909. Taking the antilog of both sides results in

$$pH = pK + \log_{10} [HCO_3^-]/(S \times PCO_2) \tag{6}$$

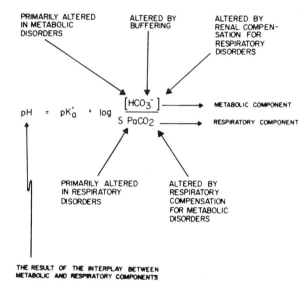

Fig. 3-1. Modified Henderson-Hasselbalch equation, portraying the interacting effects of the primary acid-base disturbance and the secondary mechanisms on the pH.

which is called the Henderson-Hasselbalch equation and was first described by Hasselbalch in 1916. In plasma at 37°C, the pK of this bicarbonate-PCO_2 buffer system is 6.1, and the solubility coefficient for CO_2 is 0.03. Therefore, this expression can be simplified to

$$pH = 6.1 + \log_{10}[HCO_3^-]/(0.03 \times PaCO_2) \tag{7}$$

This convenient expression allows us to view acid-base disorders as being attributable to the numerator of the ratio (metabolic processes), the denominator (respiratory processes), or both (mixed or complex acid-base disorders) [1] (Fig. 3-1).

Renal Acid Excretion

The kidneys regulate the $[HCO_3^-]$ at approximately 24 mM and the lungs control the $PaCO_2$ at about 40 mm Hg, thus producing an arterial pH of approximately 7.40. The kidneys regulate plasma $[HCO_3^-]$ and acid-base balance by reclaiming filtered HCO_3^- and generating new HCO_3^- to replace that lost internally in titrating metabolic acid and externally (e.g., from the gastrointestinal tract). A normal "western diet" generates approximately 1 mmol of acid/kg body weight per day. This acid load must be excreted by the kidney to maintain acid-base homeostasis. The easiest way to understand the molecular processes involved in renal acid excretion is to separate renal acid-base handling itself into two functions: bicarbonate reabsorption and net acid excretion [7].

Cellular Mechanisms of Proton Extrusion

In recent years, a number of renal cellular transport proteins that effect H^+ extrusion have been defined. These include the sodium-proton exchanger (Na^+/H^+ exchanger), which exchanges one H^+ for one sodium molecule [8, 9]; the sodium-phosphate symporter, which cotransports one sodium and one monobasic phosphate molecule; and the electrogenic H^+-ATPase, which directly pumps H^+ into the tubular lumen. It is important to realize that since the sodium-phosphate symporter transports monobasic phosphate ($H_2PO_4^-$), such transport is effective H^+ extrusion [10]. Other transport proteins that may be of importance to acid extrusion include the Na^+, K^+-ATPase, which is generally a basolateral protein [11], and the H^+/K^+ exchanger, which has been described on the apical side of collecting duct alpha intercalated cells [12].

The reclamation of HCO_3^- filtered from the blood occurs when HCO_3^- formed inside the renal tubular cells by either H^+ secretion or ammonium (NH_4^+) synthesis is transported back into the blood via the basolateral $Na^+(HCO_3^-)_3$ symporter [13] or a Cl_2^-/HCO_3^- antiporter [14]. Bicarbonate secretion can occur in several nephron segments [11].

Renal Acid-Base Metabolism

Bicarbonate Reabsorption. When plasma is filtered at the glomerulus, HCO_3^- enters the tubule lumen. Mechanistically, each HCO_3^- that is reclaimed requires the epithelial secretion of one H^+. This is accomplished largely by an Na^+/H^+ exchanger on the luminal membrane, although an electrogenic H^+-ATPase may also be involved. On an organ physiology level, we can think about HCO_3^- reabsorption in terms of the *plasma threshold* for bicarbonate, that is, the plasma HCO_3^- concentration at which HCO_3^- begins to appear in the urine. In terms of the maximal net activity of tubular HCO_3^- reabsorption (also called T_{max}), assuming glomerular filtration rate (GFR) of 100 ml/min and a plasma $[HCO_3^-]$ of 24 mM, the renal tubules must secrete about 2.4 mmol of H^+ per minute to reclaim all of the filtered HCO_3^-. Therefore, HCO_3^- reclamation by the tubules involves a tremendous amount of H^+ secretion. Bicarbonate reclamation is tightly coupled to sodium reabsorption and is also sensitive to a number of other influences. As the T_{max} for HCO_3^- increases, the plasma threshold for HCO_3^- increases. Conversely, decreases in T_{max} result in decreases in the plasma threshold. In particular, states of extracellular fluid (ECF) expansion and decreases in PCO_2 decreases the apparent T_{max} for HCO_3^-, whereas ECF contraction and increases in PCO_2 increase the apparent T_{max} for HCO_3^-. Parathyroid hormone inhibits proximal tubule HCO_3^- reabsorption and lowers the apparent T_{max} and plasma threshold for HCO_3^-. Most (but not all) of this HCO_3^- reabsorption (about 85–90%) occurs in the proximal tubule [3].

Carbonic anhydrase is present both intracellularly as well as on the tubular surface of the brush border of the proximal tubule cell and catalyzes the reversible reaction:

$$H_2O + CO_2 \longleftrightarrow H_2CO_3 \tag{8}$$

Protons secreted by proximal tubule cells combine with tubular fluid HCO_3^- in

Tubule Lumen   Proximal Tubule Cell   Peritubular Fluid

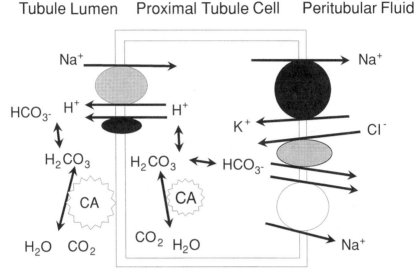

Fig. 3-2. Schematic depicting proximal tubule HCO_3^- reclamation process. Two vehicles for apical H^+ secretion—Na^+, H^+ exchanger (*lightly shaded ellipse*) and H^+-ATPase (*filled ellipse on apical side*)—are shown. Some basolateral ion pumps and exchangers including the Na^+, K^+-ATPase (*filled circle*) and $Na^+(HCO_3^-)_3$ symporter (*open circle*), and HCO_3^-/Cl^- exchanger (*lightly shaded ellipse*) are also shown. The role of carbonic anhydrase (CA) in both the tubular cell and on the brush border in HCO_3^- reabsorption is also depicted.

the tubular lumen to form H_2CO_3, which in the presence of the brush-border carbonic anhydrase readily dissociates to form H_2O and CO_2. Both H_2O and CO_2 can readily permeate proximal tubule cell membranes, and intracellularly they combine again in the presence of carbonic anhydrase to form H_2CO_3, which subsequently dissociates into HCO_3^- and H^+. Finally, HCO_3^- leaves the cell via several HCO_3^- transport proteins including the $Na^+(HCO_3^-)_3$ symporter as well as the Cl/HCO_3 exchanger. This process is shown schematically in Figure 3-2 [15].

Net Acid Excretion. Net acid excretion (NAE) is the net amount of H^+ eliminated from the body. If it is postulated that an excreted HCO_3^- molecule negates the value of an excreted H^+, then NAE by the kidney can be considered to be the amount of H^+ (both buffered and free) excreted in the urine minus the amount of HCO_3^- excreted in the urine. As discussed earlier, H^+ secretion into the tubule lumen mandates 1:1 stoichiometric HCO_3^- transport across the basolateral segment into the extracellular space; therefore, NAE represents the amount of new HCO_3^- generated by the kidneys and added to the body stores.

NAE is accomplished primarily through elimination of titratable acid (which is mostly phosphate) and nontitratable acid (in the form of NH_4^+) [7]. These terms refer to clinical chemistry titration techniques by which known amounts of alkali were added to urine until a color change with a pH indicator (e.g., phenolphthalein) occurred. This color change occurred above the pK for the phosphate buffer system but below the pK for ammonia-ammonium (about 9). The NAE is relatively insensitive to the urine pH. This concept is illustrated by the observation that addition of 1 mmol of HCl to 1 L of distilled water results in a pH of 3 (corresponding to an H^+ concentration of 10^{-3} M). Therefore in the extreme case (i.e., no buffers in the urine at all), one could envision extremely acid urine (i.e., a very low pH) that eliminated very few H^+ from the body. There are several clinical settings where acid urine is elaborated but NAE is insufficient. These will be discussed later. NAE requires the adequate function of both the proximal tubule to synthesize NH_4^+ (which generates an HCO_3^- molecule) as well as the distal tubule and collecting tubules, where H^+ and NH_4^+ secretion occur [15].

Proton secretion by the distal nephron involves the production of an electrogenic gradient that favors H^+ secretion. This gradient is produced by removal of sodium from the luminal fluid. In addition, there is a luminal H^+-ATPase, which directly pumps H^+ into the tubular lumen. Finally, the epithelial membrane must not allow backleak of H^+ or loss of the electrogenic gradient. Under normal circumstances, humans can elaborate a urine pH as low as 4.4, representing a $1000:1$ gradient of H^+ between tubular fluid and cells. NAE is sensitive to a variety of factors including the plasma K^+ concentration (increases in plasma K^+ decrease NH_4^+ excretion, whereas decreases in plasma K^+ enhance H^+ secretion by the distal nephron) and the effects of aldosterone. By stimulating the renin-angiotensin-aldosterone system, ECF contraction enhances distal acid secretion [11].

Ammonium Metabolism

The traditional view that NH_4^+ excretion was determined by simple passive trapping of NH_4^+ in the tubular lumen has been revised considerably. We now know that proximal tubule cells deaminate glutamine to form α-ketoglutarate and NH_4^+. Proximal tubule cells then secrete NH_4^+ into the lumen, probably via substitution for an H^+ using the luminal Na^+/H^+ antiporter. A key feature is that the further metabolism of α-ketoglutarate generates a new HCO_3^- molecule. Ammonium is later reabsorbed in the thick ascending limb of Henle (via substitution for K using the $Na^+/K^+/Cl^{2-}$ cotransporter), which ultimately increases medullary interstitial concentrations of NH_4^+. This NH_4^+ is later taken up by distal convoluted tubule and collecting duct cells, substituting for K^+ using the basolateral Na^+/K^+-ATPase, and ultimately is secreted into the tubular lumen, where it is excreted into the urine, possibly by substitution for H^+ in the apical Na^+/H^+ antiporter or H^+/K^+ exchanger [16, 17]. It is important to remember that the net return of a HCO_3^- molecule from α-ketoglutarate metabolism is dependent on the ultimate excretion of NH_4. This is because if this NH_4^+ molecule is not excreted in the urine, but rather is returned via the systemic circulation to the liver, it will be used to form urea at the expense of generating an H^+. Thus, the HCO_3^- molecule that was generated by the metabolism of the α-ketoglutarate will be neutralized, and no change in acid-base status will occur [7, 15].

Difficulties in the routine clinical measurement of urinary NH_4^+ concentrations have delayed appreciation of its importance in net acid-base balance during pathophysiologic conditions [18]. However, recent observations by Batlle and co-workers [19] suggest that the urinary $[NH_4^+]$ may be inferred fairly accurately by calculations based on urinary electrolyte concentrations. This will be discussed later in the chapter.

General Clinical Approach to Acid-Base Disorders

A relatively simple six-step method can be used to identify and treat acid-base disturbances. This approach presumes that the clinician has suspected an acid-base disturbance based on the history, physical examination, or other laboratory data. Once such suspicion exists, a blood gas (which gives pH, O_2 and CO_2 tensions, and a calculated $[HCO_3]$ value) and venous serum chemistry panel (which gives serum Na^+, K^+, Cl^-, and total CO_2 content $[TCO_2]$) are obtained, on which subsequent decisions are based. The remainder of this chapter and the subsequent chapter contain the information necessary to follow these steps successfully.

1. Examine the pH. Many students get confused by the potential complexity and forget this important and easy first step. Based on a normal sea level pH of 7.40 ± 0.02, a significant reduction in pH means that the major process ongoing is an acidosis. Conversely, an alkalemic pH means that the major process ongoing is an alkalosis.
2. Examine the directional changes of PCO_2 and $[HCO_3^-]$ from normal. If the pH is acid and the HCO_3^- is low, then metabolic acidosis must be present. Conversely, if the pH is alkalemic and the HCO_3^- is high, then a metabolic alkalosis must be present.
3. Assess the degree of compensation. Is this a simple (compensation appropriate) or mixed acid-base disorder? With metabolic acidosis, the PCO_2 (in millimeters of mercury) should decrease; conversely, with metabolic alkalosis, the PCO_2 should increase (Table 3-1). The rules of thumb for adequate compensation are presented in Table 3-2 and displayed graphically in Figure 3-3. Failure of respiratory compensation is equivalent to the presence of a primary respiratory acid-base disturbance. Note that one *never* gets to the normal initial pH for a given patient through compensation, although the pH value at times could reach the normal range.

Table 3-1. Simple acid-base disorders

Type of disorder	pH	PaCO$_2$	[HCO$_3^-$]
Metabolic acidosis	Decreased	Decreased*	Decreased
Metabolic alkalosis	Increased	Increased*	Increased
Respiratory acidosis	Decreased	Increased	Increased*
Respiratory alkalosis	Increased	Decreased	Decreased*

* Change due to compensation.

Table 3-2. Rules of thumb for bedside interpretation of acid-base disorders

Metabolic acidosis	$PaCO_2$ (in mm Hg) should fall by 1.0–1.5 × the fall in plasma $[HCO_3^-]$ (in mmol/L)
Metabolic alkalosis	$PaCO_2$ (in mm Hg) should increase by 0.25–1.0 × the rise in plasma $[HCO_3]$ (in mmol/L)
Acute respiratory acidosis	The plasma $[HCO_3]$ should rise by 0.1 × the increase in $PaCO_2$ (in mm Hg) ± 3 (in mmol/L)
Acute respiratory alkalosis	The plasma $[HCO_3]$ (in mmol/L) should fall by 0.1–0.3 × the increase in $PaCO_2$ (in mm Hg) but usually not to less than 18 mmol/L
Chronic respiratory acidosis	The plasma $[HCO_3]$ should rise by 0.4 × the increase in $PaCO_2$ (in mm Hg) ± 4 (in mmol/L)
Chronic respiratory alkalosis	The plasma $[HCO_3]$ (in mmol/L) should fall by 0.2–0.5 × the increase in $PaCO_2$ (in mm Hg) but usually not to less than 14 mmol/L

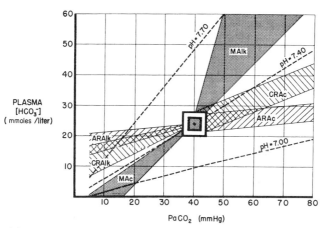

Fig. 3-3. Acid-base nomogram derived from Table 3-2 showing plasma HCO_3^- and $PaCO_2$ values seen with primary metabolic alkalosis (MAlk), metabolic acidosis (MAc), chronic respiratory acidosis (CRAc), chronic respiratory alkalosis (CRAlk), acute respiratory acidosis (ARAc), and acute respiratory alkalosis (ARAlk), and appropriate compensation.

4. Calculate the serum anion gap. The serum anion gap is discussed in detail later in this chapter. This useful calculation helps both in the differential diagnosis of metabolic acidosis and in identifying whether metabolic acidosis and alkalosis processes coexist.
5. Determine the underlying cause of the disturbance. Acid-base disorders are merely laboratory signs of an underlying disease. Once one has determined what the pathophysiologic nature of the acid-base disturbance is, the pathologic cause is often obvious.

6. Determine appropriate therapy. In some situations, the acid-base disturbance must be directly addressed. However, in all situations, treatment of the underlying causes is most advantageous.

Metabolic Acidosis

Causes of Metabolic Acidosis

Metabolic acidosis is a systemic disorder characterized by a primary decrease in $[HCO_3^-]$. This may occur in three ways:

1. The addition of strong acid that is buffered by (i.e., consumes) HCO_3^-.
2. The loss of HCO_3^- from body fluids, usually through the gastrointestinal tract or kidneys.
3. The rapid addition to the ECF of nonbicarbonate solutions (dilutional acidosis).

When HCO_3^- is lost or diluted, there is no organic anion that is generated. Reciprocal increases in the serum chloride concentration occur to preserve electroneutrality. Thus, these forms of metabolic acidosis are generally referred to as hyperchloremic or non–anion gap metabolic acidosis. When an organic acid consumes HCO_3^-, its organic anion is generated and may be retained in the ECF and serum. The serum chloride concentration does not increase with organic acidosis. An increase in the anion gap marks the existence and concentration of the organic anion [20].

Defense of Systemic pH During Metabolic Acidosis

Buffering

The hallmark of metabolic acidosis is a fall in plasma $[HCO_3^-]$. It should be stressed that the fall in $[HCO_3^-]$ is always mitigated by the participation of other buffers in both the ECF and intracellular fluid (ICF). Roughly one-half of an administered acid load is buffered by nonbicarbonate buffers [21]. Bone is an important buffer pool in states of chronic metabolic acidosis. In fact, the leaching of calcium salts from bone is one of the major deleterious effects of chronic metabolic acidosis [22–24].

Respiratory Compensation

With simple metabolic acidosis, a fall in $PaCO_2$ is a normal, compensatory response. Again, the failure of this normal adaptive response is equivalent to the diagnosis of respiratory acidosis in the setting of a complex or mixed acid-base disturbance. Conversely, an exaggerated fall in $PaCO_2$ producing a normal pH indicates the diagnosis of respiratory alkalosis in the setting of a complex or mixed acid-base disturbance [25] (see Chap. 4).

The mechanism by which metabolic acidosis induces hypocapnia appears to be mediated mostly by central nervous system pH receptors. This point is supported by the time course, specifically the temporal delay observed for respiratory compensation, seen in experimental metabolic acidosis [26].

The degree of compensation will vary from person to person. However, based on a large volume of clinical data, we can state with some confidence that the appropriate fall in $PaCO_2$ (in millimeters of mercury) should be between 1.0 and 1.5 times the fall in $[HCO_3^-]$ [25].

Correction

The kidney provides the mechanism for the third line of defense of pH. However, it must be stressed that this mechanism is rather slow compared to buffering (which begins immediately) and respiratory compensation (which begins within 15–30 minutes), taking up to 5 days to become maximal. Increases in NAE by the kidney develop in response to either metabolic acidosis (unless the kidney is the cause) or respiratory acidosis. This increase in NAE is due mostly to increases in NH_4^+ excretion, as titratable acid excretion is limited by the amount of excreted phosphate, which changes rather little. Of interest, the hypocapnia that occurs because of respiratory compensation actually limits renal correction in metabolic acidosis [27]. Note that renal correction also never restores the pH to the prior normal level until the disorder causing HCO_3^- loss or acid generation is halted.

Biochemical and Physiologic Effects of Metabolic Acidosis

Mild degrees of acidemia are generally well tolerated, at least acutely, and may even afford some physiologic advantages such as favorable oxygen delivery from hemoglobin. However, with marked acidemia (pH < 7.10), myocardial contractility is depressed, and peripheral resistance falls [28, 29]. These manifestations may be a result of the effect of acidosis to depress both vascular and myocardial responsiveness to catecholamines as well as innate myocardial contractility. Although the literature is somewhat confusing on this point, both myocardial β-receptor density as well as physiologic responses to β-agonists are decreased by metabolic acidosis [30, 31].

The intrinsic myocardial responses to metabolic acidosis have also received considerable attention in recent years. Clearly metabolic acidosis induces an intracellular acidosis in myocytes [30, 31]. This intracellular acidosis in turn impairs contractile responses to normal or even elevated cytosolic calcium concentrations [32, 33]. The mechanism by which this occurs appears to involve impairment of actin-myosin cross bridge cycling caused by increases in the concentration of inorganic phosphate in the monovalent form $H_2PO_4^-$ [34], a process that occurs in all striated muscle tissues. The increase in monovalent inorganic phosphate results both from the acidic environment, which increases the ratio of monovalent to divalent inorganic phosphate, and from an impairment of myocardial energy production, which increases the total intracellular concentration of inorganic phosphate [35, 36]. Metabolic acidosis and hypoxia appear to additively or synergistically impair myocardial function [37]. It is likely that the vasodepressor effect of acidosis has a similar metabolic mechanism [38].

Clinical Features of Metabolic Acidosis

With even mild degrees of acidosis, one can clinically observe an increase in ventilatory effort. With severe metabolic acidosis (e.g., pH < 7.20), respirations become extremely deep and rapid (Kussmaul's respiration). Mild degrees of acidosis do not appear to markedly impair hemodynamic stability, at least in subjects with otherwise normal cardiovascular function. However, severe metabolic acidosis may lead to hypotension, pulmonary edema, and ultimately, ventricular standstill [28, 39, 40]. Chronic metabolic acidosis, even if fairly mild, causes hypercalciuria and bone disease as bone buffering of acid leads to marked calcium losses from the bone [41]. This aspect is extremely important in determining treatment of renal tubular acidosis or the acidosis of chronic renal failure.

Laboratory Findings in Metabolic Acidosis

Simple metabolic acidosis is characterized by a decrease in blood pH, $[HCO_3^-]$, and PCO_2 (through compensation). Note that a failure to lower the PCO_2 by 1.0 to 1.5 times the fall in $[HCO_3^-]$ implies the coexistence of respiratory acidosis [25]. The clinical implications of this are quite profound, as this failure of compensation may signify impending severe respiratory failure. Serum electrolytes reveal a fall in total CO_2 content, which is simply the serum $[HCO_3^-]$ plus dissolved CO_2. The total CO_2 content traditionally has been used to represent the venous serum alkali or base content. The venous total CO_2 content is the sum of the HCO_3^- and the dissolved CO_2 and is usually 1 to 2 mmol/L higher than arterial $[HCO_3^-]$. Because acidosis tends to shift potassium out of cells in a rather complex manner [42] and renal potassium excretion tends to increase in many states of metabolic acidosis, normal or increased serum potassium in the face of decreased total body potassium stores occurs commonly in cases of metabolic acidosis [42] (see Chap. 5). Some metabolic acidosis states are characterized by the retention of an organic anion generated in concert with HCO_3^- consumption (organic acidosis), whereas other are not (hyperchloremic). As the screening of the plasma for such organic anions is not practical on a routine, immediate basis, a calculation performed on the serum electrolytes called the anion gap is employed [43].

Serum Anion Gap

The serum anion gap is a concept utilized in acid-base pathophysiology to infer whether an organic or mineral acidosis is present. The serum anion gap (SAG) is defined as follows [43]:

$$SAG = [Na^+] - [Cl^-] - [TCO_2] \tag{9}$$

Here, TCO_2 is used as an index of HCO_3^-. Unmeasured cations (UC) are defined as cations that are not Na^+ (e.g., K^+, Mg^{2+}, Ca^{2+}) and unmeasured anions (UA) as anions that are not Cl^- or HCO_3^- (e.g., SO_4^{2-}, $H_2PO_4^-$, HPO_4^{2-}, albumin, organic anions). Thus, electroneutrality demands that

$$[Na^+] + UC = [Cl^-] + [TCO_2] + UA \qquad (10)$$

where the [UA] and [UC] concentrations are expressed in milliequivalents per liter rather than millimoles per liter. Putting equations 9 and 10 together, we see that

$$SAG = UA - UC \qquad (11)$$

Normally, the serum anion gap is about 9 mEq/L (6–12 mEq/L), which is lower than the 12 mEq/L value originally reported due to more sensitive modern chloride measurements [44]. Although the serum anion gap is used routinely in the differential diagnosis of metabolic acidosis, it is a relative rather than absolute indicator of the underlying pathophysiology. Note that the maintenance of stoichiometry (i.e., 1 mEq increase in anion gap for every 1 mmol decrease in HCO_3^-) depends on the clearance mechanisms for the anion as well as the myriad factors that influence HCO_3^- concentration. Therefore, some organic acidoses may manifest trivial or even no increase in the serum anion gap, whereas some hyperchloremic acidoses may have serendipitous increases in the serum anion gap. This must be kept in mind when evaluating the differential diagnosis of metabolic acidosis. However, it can be stated with some assurance that a major increase in the anion gap (e.g., serum anion gap > 26 mEq/L) always implies the existence of an organic acidosis [45].

Urine Anion Gap

To address a different problem, urinary electrolytes have been used to estimate the quantity of NH_4^+ in the urine, a measurement that has been difficult to develop into a routine clinical test. The concept is quite similar to that described for the serum anion gap. In the urine, because of electroneutrality:

$$[Na^+] + [K^+] + UC = [Cl^-] + UA \qquad (12)$$

When urine pH is < 6, unmeasured anions do not include appreciable amounts of HCO_3^- but consist primarily of phosphate ($H_2PO_4^-$ more than HPO_4^{2-}) and, to a lesser degree, sulfate (SO_4^{2-}) and organic anions. Unmeasured cations are made up mostly of NH_4^+. Therefore, if the urine anion gap (UAG) is defined as

$$UAG = [Na^+] + [K^+] - [Cl^-] \qquad (13)$$

then the urine anion gap will be determined largely by the amount of NH_4^+ in the urine. In other words, the more NH_4^+ present, the more negative the urine anion gap. Batlle and co-workers have demonstrated that this holds true in clinical studies of metabolic acidosis [19]. In contrast to the serum anion gap, which is useful in many settings of clinical acid-base diagnosis and therapy, the urine anion gap has

Table 3-3. Differential diagnosis of metabolic acidosis

Normal anion gap (hyperchloremic)	Increased anion gap (organic)
Gastrointestinal loss of HCO_3^-	Increased acid production
Diarrhea	Lactic acidosis
Intestinal fistula or drainage	Diabetic ketoacidosis
Anion exchange resins	Starvation
Ingestion of $CaCl_2$ or $MgCl_2$	Alcoholic ketoacidosis
Renal loss of HCO_3^-	Inborn errors of metabolism
Renal tubular acidosis	Toxic alcohol ingestions
Carbonic anhydrase inhibitors	Salicylate intoxication
Hypoaldosteronism	Other intoxications
Potassium sparing diuretics	Failure of acid excretion
Miscellaneous	Acute renal failure
Recovery from ketoacidosis	Chronic renal failure
Dilutional acidosis	
Addition of HCl	
Parenteral alimentation	
Sulfur ingestion	

a very narrow clinical application in the differentiation of renal from nonrenal causes of non–anion gap metabolic acidosis.

Differential Diagnosis of Metabolic Acidosis

The differential diagnosis of metabolic acidosis is generally approached clinically by using the serum anion gap. Those acidosis states that are associated with retention of an organic anion are classified as increased anion gap or simply anion gap metabolic acidosis. Those acidosis states that are not associated with retention of an organic anion are classified as non–anion gap or hyperchloremic metabolic acidosis [43]. These disorders are listed in Table 3-3.

Causes of Hyperchloremic Metabolic Acidosis

Gastrointestinal Loss of HCO_3^-

Diarrhea. Diarrhea is the most common cause of hyperchloremic metabolic acidosis and should always be considered early in the differential diagnosis. The concentration of HCO_3^- in diarrheal fluid is generally greater than that of plasma. In the extreme case of cholera, patients may lose up to 20 L/day of fluid containing 30 to 50 mEq/L of HCO_3^- [46].

The diagnosis of diarrheal loss of HCO_3^-, however, may be difficult in the very young or very old. In the former, the distinction between diarrhea and an underlying renal tubular acidosis (RTA) is extremely important. In this setting, the urine anion gap may be very helpful. Patients with diarrhea as a cause of metabolic acidosis typically have a very negative urine anion gap (i.e., <10 mEq/L) reflecting the presence of ample urinary NH_4^+ concentrations, whereas patients with all forms of distal RTA have a positive urine anion gap reflecting the inadequate urinary NH_4^+ concentrations present [19].

Gastrointestinal Drainage and Fistulas. The succus entericus and pancreatic and biliary secretions are rich in HCO_3^- and poor in Cl^-. The succus entericus has a daily volume of 600 to 700 ml but may be increased in states of disease. Biliary secretions amount to more than 1 L/day of fluid, containing $[HCO_3^-]$ approaching 60 mmol/L. Pancreatic secretions may exceed 2 L/day, with HCO_3^- reaching 120 mmol/L. It is relatively obvious how such drainage or fistulas could cause significant metabolic acidosis [47].

Recently, the technique of combined pancreas-kidney transplantation has become popular for the treatment of type 1 diabetics with end-stage renal disease. Most often, urinary drainage of the HCO_3^--rich exocrine secretions of the pancreatic allograft is employed, which effectively limits the final NAE and thus may lead to significant metabolic acidosis [48, 49].

Urinary Diversion to Bowel. Patients may require urinary diversion from normal egress through the bladder for a variety of reasons. Approaches to this include the creation of an ileal loop conduit or, less commonly, drainage of the ureters into the sigmoid colon (ureterosigmoidostomy). Metabolic acidosis can develop with both procedures but is almost certain with ureterosigmoidostomy. The pathophysiology for both situations is the bowel mucosal secretion of HCO_3^- in exchange for Cl^- during water reabsorption, which may lead to significant HCO_3^- losses in the gastrointestinal tract effluent [47].

Chloride-Containing Anion Exchange Resins. Cholestyramine is a resin used to bind bile acids in the gut for a variety of purposes, including the treatment of obstructive liver disease as well as hypercholesterolemia. However, this resin has some affinity for HCO_3^- and may exchange Cl^- for HCO_3^- across the bowel mucosa. In conditions of renal insufficiency where new HCO_3^- generation is impaired, hyperchloremic metabolic acidosis has been reported [50].

$CaCl_2$ or $MgCl_2$ Ingestion. The divalent cations calcium and magnesium are absorbed incompletely in the gastrointestinal tract. If large amounts of these cations in soluble form (e.g., as the Cl_2 salts) are ingested, the unabsorbed Ca^{2+} or Mg^{2+} reacts with HCO_3^-, which has been exchanged across the gut mucosa for Cl^- to form an insoluble salt. Thus, plasma HCO_3^- falls to a moderate degree [51].

Renal Loss of HCO_3^-

Renal Tubular Acidosis. RTA refers to a group of functional disorders that are characterized by impairment of renal HCO_3^- reabsorption and H^+ excretion that is out of proportion to any reduction in GFR. In many cases, the RTAs exist in the presence of a completely normal GFR. Unfortunately, a nomenclature has evolved that confuses many experienced clinicians as well as trainees and students.

This section provides a pathophysiologic classification of these disorders while referring to this nomenclature.

RTAs can be divided into those characterized by impaired proximal HCO_3^- reabsorption and those due to disturbed distal nephron function (i.e., impaired NAE) [52]. The distal RTAs can be further divided into those that are associated with hypokalemia and those that are associated with hyperkalemia. The hyperkalemic type may be further subdivided into RTA due to hypoaldosteronism and RTA characterized by a general distal tubular defect [53].

Proximal RTA, also called type II RTA, is an uncommon but very instructional disorder [54, 55]. Basically, the acid-base disturbance is due to an impairment in proximal tubular reabsorption of HCO_3^-, the nephron site where 85 percent of HCO_3^- is usually reabsorbed. In this condition, the delivery of HCO_3^--rich fluid to distal nephron sites leads to substantial bicarbonaturia when plasma levels of HCO_3^- are normal and to urinary losses of potassium and sodium as well. Thus patients present with hypokalemia and hyperchloremic metabolic acidosis. When the plasma concentration of HCO_3^- is maintained at normal by administration of HCO_3^-, fractional HCO_3^- excretion (i.e., the fraction of filtered HCO_3^- that is excreted in the urine) exceeds 15 percent.

In physiologic terms, the apparent Tmax and plasma threshold for HCO_3^- are significantly reduced in patients with proximal RTA. However, once a level of plasma HCO_3^- is achieved that is below the patient's plasma threshold for HCO_3^-, renal acid handling is normal. In other words, NAE equals dietary and endogenous acid excretory needs, and the subject comes into a steady state of acid-base balance, albeit at a moderately reduced plasma HCO_3^- concentration (and a mild reduction in systemic pH). Because a steady state in acid handling is achieved, patients with proximal RTA have less severe acidosis as well as less nephrocalcinosis (which results from bone calcium mobilization from acidosis) than patients with distal RTAs.

A problem with proximal HCO_3^- reabsorption rarely may occur independently but more commonly coexists with other defects in proximal nephron function such as reabsorption of glucose, amino acids, phosphate, and uric acid. When general proximal nephron function is disturbed, the term *Fanconi's syndrome* is employed [56]. Patients with full-blown Fanconi's syndrome may have severe osteomalacia and malnutrition in addition to the mild metabolic acidosis associated with proximal RTA. Proximal RTA may occur as a primary disorder and present in infancy or may be acquired in the course of other diseases or as a result of exposure to substances toxic to this nephron segment. A list of causes of proximal RTA is shown in Table 3-4. Treatment of this condition is approached by addressing the underlying cause, but if this is ineffective, administration of large amounts of HCO_3^- (10–15 mmol/kg/day) and potassium to compensate for ongoing potassium losses in the urine caused by the bicarbonaturia is necessary. However, effective treatment markedly increases the ongoing urinary HCO_3^- and potassium losses and thus requires tremendous amounts of alkali (10–25 mmol/kg/day). This is necessary to avoid growth retardation and osteopenia in children, which may be produced by even mild degrees of acidemia.

Based on recent data, the distal RTAs all appear to be characterized primarily

Table 3-4. Causes of renal tubular acidosis

Proximal	Distal (hypokalemic)	Distal (hyperkalemic)
Primary	Primary	Hypoaldosteronism
Cystinosis	Hypercalcemia	Obstructive nephropathy
Wilson's disease	Nephrocalcinosis	Sickle cell disease/trait
Lead toxicity	Multiple myeloma	Lupus erythematosus
Cadmium toxicity	Lupus erythematosus	Analgesic nephropathy
Mercury toxicity	Amphotericin B	Renal transplant rejection
Amyloidosis	Toluene	Cyclosporine toxicity
Multiple myeloma	Renal transplant rejection	Other interstitial disease
Nephrotic syndrome	Medullary sponge kidney	
Medullary cystic disease		
Outdated tetracycline		
Injury from kidney preservation		

by impaired NAE, which is due, at least in part, to impaired NH_4^+ excretion. The central role of impaired NH_4^+ excretion in this disorder is highlighted by a recent clinical study in which all patients with either hypokalemic distal RTA (also called type I or classic distal RTA) or hyperkalemic distal RTA (previously referred to as type IV RTA) due to either hypoaldosteronism or a generalized tubular defect had a positive urine anion gap, reflecting decreased NH_4^+ excretion. How NH_4^+ excretion is impaired in this diverse set of clinical disorders is still incompletely understood [57].

Hypokalemic distal RTA has long been considered a disorder of the collecting duct where the quantity of H^+ secretion is inadequate to effect the necessary NAE for the subject to maintain acid-base balance. Clinically, patients with hypokalemic distal RTA present with hyperchloremic metabolic acidosis but are unable to acidify their urine (below pH 5.5 is commonly used) in response to an acid challenge. We stress that the failure to acidify the urine does not fully explain the defect in NAE, which is primarily due to an associated defect in NH_4^+ excretion [18, 58]. However, the failure to acidify the urine under conditions of systemic acidosis has historically been considered the clinical hallmark of hypokalemic distal RTA. The physiologic mechanisms for this impaired acidification have been a topic of interest for some time and are summarized with clinical examples in Table 3-5. Basically, four mechanisms have been suggested for impaired acidification by the distal nephron. These are (1) backleak through a leaky epithelium, (2) pump failure, where the H^+-ATPase cannot pump sufficient amounts of H^+, (3) voltage defect, where a favorable transepithelial voltage cannot be generated (e.g., decreased sodium delivery to the distal nephron or decreased sodium reabsorption in the distal nephron), and (4) rate defect/NH_4^+ defect, where urine pH is reduced but NH_4^+ excretion and NAE cannot be increased to normal amounts. Hypokalemic distal RTA appears to be caused by either backleak or pump failure. Hyperkalemic distal RTAs are probably caused by either voltage defect or rate defect/NH_4^+ defect.

Table 3-5. Examples of pathophysiologic mechanisms in clinical distal RTA

Physiological defect	Example
Backleak	Amphotericin B
Pump failure	Primary
Voltage defect	Amiloride
Rate defect/NH_4^+ defect	Hypoaldosteronism

A number of physiologic maneuvers have been used to examine these mechanisms clinically. The first and simplest test is that of a metered pH (i.e., using a pH meter rather than a dipstick) performed on urine collected under oil. In some cases, patients are able to maintain a normal plasma HCO_3^- concentration and systemic pH under most circumstances but do not respond normally to increases in acid generation by increasing NAE. This is called an incomplete distal RTA. If an incomplete distal RTA is suspected, ammonium chloride or calcium chloride is administered to induce a mild case of metabolic acidosis. This test basically screens for backleak, pump failure, or voltage defects. Infusion of sodium sulfate or sodium phosphate increases distal sodium delivery. The failure to lower urine pH after these maneuvers suggests pump failure or impaired voltage due to inadequate distal sodium reabsorption. Another maneuver is to determine the urine-to-blood PCO_2 gradient when the patient has bicarbonaturia (urine $[HCO_3^-] > 100$ mM) induced by HCO_3^- administration. Under conditions where bicarbonaturia is induced, H^+ secreted into the collecting duct lumen will combine with HCO_3^- to form H_2CO_3. Because carbonic anhydrase is absent in the lumen of this segment (as well as the bladder), conversion to CO_2 and water is slow and occurs largely in the urinary collecting system (i.e., renal pelvis, ureters, and urinary bladder) where the surface area for CO_2 absorption is small. This CO_2 is essentially trapped and, when normalized for the blood PCO_2 (i.e., the difference between urine and blood), is a marker for the rate of distal H^+ secretion. Patients with backleak or pump failure generally have a small difference between urine and blood PCO_2 (<20 mm Hg).

Hypokalemic distal RTA may be primary or associated with other diseases or toxin exposure. A list of causes appears in Table 3-4. Some of the causes also may result in a hyperkalemic distal RTA due to a generalized tubular defect. Urinary obstruction and some of the autoimmune disorders are examples of hyperkalemic distal RTA. Perhaps the best understood cause of hypokalemic distal RTA is that caused by amphotericin toxicity, which results (at least experimentally) in acidification failure due to backleak. In its primary form, hypokalemic distal RTA usually occurs in young children. Because the children never achieve a normal acid-base balance, they typically present with severe metabolic acidosis, growth retardation, nephrocalcinosis, and nephrolithiasis. Hypokalemia, which is usually present, is actually caused by the associated sodium depletion and stimulation of the renin-angiotensin-aldosterone axis. Therefore, renal potassium losses actually decrease considerably when appropriate therapy with sodium bicarbonate is instituted. This is, of course, quite different from patients with proximal RTA, in whom urinary potassium losses increase considerably during therapy because of the bicarbonaturia associated urinary K losses. Another contrasting point between proximal RTA and hypokalemic distal RTA is the amount of alkali therapy needed. Once the acute acidosis is corrected, patients with hypokalemic distal RTA only need enough alkali to account for the amount of acid generated from diet and metabolism. Therefore, 1 to 3 mmol/kg/day is generally sufficient.

Hyperkalemic distal RTA from hypoaldosteronism occurs in several settings, summarized in Table 3-4. Best described is the case of either selective aldosterone deficiency or complete adrenal insufficiency. Probably the most common form of RTA is the hyporeninemic hypoaldosteronism often seen in patients with diabetic nephropathy. In patients with this form of RTA, urinary acidification as assessed by urine pH appears normal, but the patients are unable to raise NAE to appropriate levels. The defect, at least in some of these individuals, can be traced to impaired NH_4^+ synthesis in the proximal nephron, resulting directly from the hyperkalemia. Treatment of the hyperkalemia in some individuals with this disorder is sufficient to correct the disturbance in NAE. In patients with pure primary aldosterone deficiency, replacement of physiologic amounts of mineralocorticoid results in correction of the disturbance in acid-base metabolism and is both logical and appropriate therapy. However, in patients with the hyporeninemic hypoaldosteronism form, the renal defect requires pharmacologic amounts of mineralocorticoid (i.e., 5–10 times the usually physiologic dose) for efficacy. Moreover, these patients often have mild renal failure and tend to have total body sodium excess rather than deficit (as is the case in the pure hypoaldosteronism form). Therefore, the use of mineralocorticoid in this setting may be harmful. Treatment of the hyperkalemia by increasing renal K^+ excretion (e.g., with loop diuretics) or K excretion through the gastrointestinal tract with potassium binding resins (Kayexalate) may be the preferred approach in patients with the hyporeninemic hypoaldosteronism form.

Hyperkalemic distal RTA from a generalized tubular defect is considerably more common than either classic distal RTA or proximal RTA. A list of causes appears in Table 3-4. Urinary obstruction may be the most common and important cause of this form of distal RTA. Other causes important in selected populations include cyclosporine nephrotoxicity and allograft rejection in the renal transplant patient, sickle cell nephropathy in patients homozygous and occasionally heterozygous for the sickle cell gene, and many autoimmune disorders such as lupus nephritis and Sjögren's syndrome. In contrast to the hypoaldosteronism form, urinary acidification is impaired, similar to the hypokalemic distal RTA patients. Also in contrast to the hypoaldosteronism form, the hyperkalemia plays a less significant role in the genesis of impaired NH_4^+ excretion, which is tied directly to the impaired distal nephron function.

Carbonic Anhydrase Inhibitors. Carbonic anhydrase inhibitors such as acetazolamide inhibit both proximal tubular luminal brush border and cellular carbonic anhydrase. The net effect is a pattern of impaired HCO_3^- reabsorption similar to that of proximal RTA. These drugs are commonly used topically to treat glaucoma, but their use may be complicated by systemic effects such as hyperchloremic metabolic acidosis [59, 60].

Hypoaldosteronism. Hypoaldosteronism is associated with a hyperkalemic distal RTA. This may be produced by pharmacologic antagonism of aldosterone action or by impaired aldosterone secretion. Impaired aldosterone secretion may be caused by hyporeninemia (e.g., the hyporeninemic hypoaldosteronism associated with diabetes mellitus) or may be part of adrenal insufficiency (e.g., Addison's disease). With hyporeninemic hypoaldosteronism, some workers have suggested that the disorder is, at least in part, an adrenal disorder because plasma potassium concentrations that typically would induce aldosterone secretion do not. However, more recent studies have underlined the importance of permissive amounts of angiotensin II in allowing potassium to be an effective aldosterone secretagogue [61, 62].

Potassium Sparing Diuretics. Potassium sparing diuretics, which either block aldosterone action such as spironolactone or impair distal nephron sodium reabsorption such as amiloride, may also produce a hyperchloremic acidosis in concert with hyperkalemia [63, 64].

Miscellaneous Causes of Hyperchloremic Acidosis

Recovery from Ketoacidosis. Although diabetic ketoacidosis (DKA) is one of the best described forms of increased anion gap metabolic acidosis, during recovery from DKA, many patients may eliminate the organic anions, possibly through renal clearance, faster than their acidosis resolves, leaving them with a non–anion gap or hyperchloremic metabolic acidosis [65].

Dilutional Acidosis. The rapid expansion of ECF volume with fluids that do not contain HCO_3^- will lead to a dilution of HCO_3^- and mild metabolic acidosis. The fall in HCO_3^- produced in this manner is typically quite small (e.g., 10%) and is usually corrected fairly rapidly by renal generation of HCO_3^- (e.g., by renal correction) [66].

Addition of HCl. Administration of HCl or congeners (e.g., ammonium chloride or lysine chloride) rapidly consumes an HCO_3^- molecule without generating an organic anion and thus causes a hyperchloremic metabolic acidosis [67].

Parenteral Alimentation. Amino acid infusions without concomitant administration of alkali (or alkali-generating precursors) may produce a hyperchloremic metabolic acidosis in a manner similar to addition of HCl. This problem can be avoided by replacing the chloride salt of these amino acids with an acetate salt. When the acetate is metabolized, HCO_3^- is generated, which replaces the HCO_3^- consumed in reaction with the H^+ released by amino acid metabolism [68].

Sulfur Ingestion. Ingested elemental sulfur or sulfur released during metabolism of sulfur-containing amino acids (e.g., methionine or cysteine) is oxidized to sulfate with accompanying H^+ production. Sulfate is excreted rapidly by the kidneys, usually accompanied by sodium, whereas the excretion of H^+ produced by sulfur metabolism lags, resulting in a hyperchloremic metabolic acidosis. Ingestion of 40 to 50 g/day of flowers of sulfur, a folk remedy for constipation, for several days has produced profound hyperchloremic metabolic acidosis [69].

Causes of Increased Anion Gap Metabolic Acidosis

Organic Acidosis Resulting from Increased Acid Production

Lactic Acidosis. Lactic acidosis is probably the best example of a clinical organic acidosis. Causes of lactic acidosis are summarized in Table 3-6. Lactic acid is the final product of mammalian anaerobic metabolism. In general, aerobic tissues metabolize carbohydrates to pyruvate, which then undergoes oxidative metabolism within mitochondria. This oxidative metabolism regenerates NAD^+ consumed at a more proximal site in the glycolytic pathway. When tissues must perform anaerobic glycolysis, to regenerate this NAD^+, the reaction catalyzed by lactate dehydrogenase occurs:

$$H^+ + pyruvate + NADH \rightarrow lactate + NAD^+ \tag{14}$$

Although this reaction consumes an H^+, the net effect of glycolysis is to produce lactic acid (which dissociates to H^+ and lactate at physiologic pH) from carbohydrates (which are not H^+ donors) and thus to generate H^+. Under normal conditions in humans, relatively small amounts of lactate, specifically the L-isomer, are formed during normal metabolism, which are metabolized by the liver, maintaining relatively low plasma and urine levels of this metabolite. Under pathologic conditions associated with either local or systemic decreases in oxygen delivery, impairments

Table 3-6. Causes of lactic acidosis

Primary decrease in tissue oxygenation
  Septic shock
  Cardiogenic shock
  Hypovolemic shock
  Mesenteric ischemia
  Hypoxemia
Excessive energy expenditures
  Seizures
  Extreme exertion
  Hyperthermia
Deranged oxidative metabolism
  Diabetic ketoacidosis
  Malignancy
  Intoxications (e.g., ethanol, iron, isoniazid, carbon monoxide, strychnine)
Impaired lactate clearance
  Liver failure
Miscellaneous
  D-Lactic acidosis

in oxidative metabolism, or impaired hepatic clearance, lactic acidosis may develop [70, 71].

The diagnosis of lactic acidosis must be considered in all forms of metabolic acidosis associated with an increased anion gap, particularly those cases occurring in the clinical circumstances detailed in the previous paragraph. Determination of the serum or plasma lactate level may confirm this diagnosis, although many clinical laboratories may not provide this information on an emergency basis [70, 71]. In cases of D-lactic acidosis (e.g., seen with blind intestinal loops colonized with D-lactate–producing organisms), the usual measurement of lactate performed in clinical laboratories using an enzymatic reaction will not detect this D-isomer. Special measurement techniques such as ^{1}H nuclear magnetic resonance (NMR) spectroscopy (which does not distinguish between D and L forms) or specific measurement of the D form with the appropriate enzymatic analysis may be necessary to document elevations of D-lactate in this unusual clinical circumstance [72, 73].

Treatment of lactic acidosis must be directed at the underlying pathophysiology. Although the degree of acidemia in this setting may become deleterious in its own right, therapy with $NaHCO_3^-$ to directly address the metabolic acidosis has not been found to be effective clinically [74] and is itself deleterious in several experimental models [28, 75–77]. Other treatments such as dichloroacetate, which shifts metabolism of pyruvate from lactate formation [78], and Carbicarb, an experimental buffer [79], may have some advantages over supportive care or HCO_3^- administration. However, these agents are still under investigation in the United States and are not yet approved for routine clinical use.

Diabetic Ketoacidosis. DKA results from lack of sufficient insulin necessary to metabolize glucose and short-chain fatty keto acids, specifically β-hydroxybutyric and acetoacetic acids. It is the buildup of these latter substances that causes the disturbance in acid-base metabolism. Both of these keto acids are relatively strong acids that dissociate almost completely at physiologic pH into H^+ and the keto anions and cause an anion gap metabolic acidosis. Interestingly, the amount of insulin needed for catabolism of short-chain fatty acids is significantly less than that necessary for glucose homeostasis. Therefore, while DKA is a common presentation in patients with insulin-dependent diabetes mellitus, it is quite uncommon in patients with non–insulin-dependent diabetes mellitus, who more commonly present with marked increases in serum glucose concentrations without ketosis (e.g., nonketotic hyperglycemic coma) [65, 80–82]. When patients with nonketotic hyperglycemic coma develop an anion gap metabolic acidosis, keto acids are not usually demonstrable.

Patients with DKA typically present with altered sensorium, deep respirations, and severe anion gap metabolic acidosis with HCO_3^- concentrations as low as 1 to 10 mmol/L and arterial pH values that may be less than 7.0. Initially, the increase in the anion gap above normal may parallel the decrease in HCO_3^-, but during therapy, a dissociation of the decrease in anion gap (ΔAG) and the decrease in HCO_3^- concentration ($\Delta [HCO_3^-]$) may develop. This is probably due to renal elimination of the keto anions as renal perfusion and clearance improve during therapeutic volume restoration, but it may also signify some degree of underlying distal RTA (e.g., hyporeninemic hypoaldosteronism) in some subjects [83].

The diagnosis of DKA is made by the combination of anion gap metabolic acidosis, hyperglycemia, and demonstration of serum (or urine) keto anions. At times this diagnosis may not be easy to make because the hyperglycemia may not be marked and, when the pH is low, the majority of keto acids circulating in the serum may not be detected by the Acetest assay. Specifically, the Acetest reaction measures acetoacetic acid but is rather insensitive to β-hydroxybutyric acid. When the serum pH is low, as might be the case with severe DKA, the proportion of β-hydroxybutyric acid increases. Conversely, the presence of serum and urine ketones is not specific for DKA but may also be present in other conditions in the differential diagnosis such as alcoholic ketoacidosis and starvation ketoacidosis [65].

Patients who present with DKA may be among the sickest that a physician can treat. With appropriate therapy, however, mortality is quite low. Insulin, volume repletion, and management of electrolyte disturbances are the mainstays of therapy. Most patients with DKA present with considerable total body deficits of potassium, magnesium, and phosphorus, even though serum levels, particularly of potassium, may actually be high on presentation [84]. Treatment of DKA with $NaHCO_3$ is, at best, quite controversial [85]. Hazards associated with $NaHCO_3^-$ in this setting include hyperosmolarity (as ampules of $NaHCO_3$ are quite hypertonic), overshoot alkalosis, and paradoxical intracellular acidosis (discussed later), which may further compromise central nervous system function and hemodynamic stability [85]. Although some experts have recommended sodium bicarbonate infusions in DKA at some critical levels of systemic pH [86], we stress that $NaHCO_3$ has not been found to improve outcome in limited clinical trials in this setting [87, 88]. We do not recommend $NaHCO_3$ infusions for DKA.

Starvation. Voluntary or involuntary abstinence from caloric intake produces some metabolic processes that are similar to those seen with DKA. Specifically, hepatic ketogenesis is accelerated, and tissue ketone metabolism is reduced. Thus, increases in the plasma and urine concentrations of keto acids occur. Moreover, with prolonged starvation, decreases in plasma HCO_3^- may occur, producing a mild anion gap metabolic acidosis. However, the plasma $[HCO_3^-]$ does not generally fall to less than 18 mmol/L [89].

Alcoholic Ketoacidosis. Alcoholic ketoacidosis is probably the result of the combination of alcohol toxicity and starvation. Serum glucose levels range from very low (i.e., <50 mg/dl) to modestly elevated (e.g., 250–275 mg/dl), where confusion with the diagnosis of DKA may occur. Typically, patients present not with simple metabolic acidosis but rather with a complex acid-base disturbance containing features of anion gap metabolic acidosis, metabolic alkalosis produced by vomiting, and respiratory alkalosis due to hyperventilation. A markedly increased serum anion gap is a hallmark of this disorder (see Chap. 4). Treatment consists of vigorous volume and glucose repletion with additional attention to repletion of potassium, magnesium, phosphorus, and vitamin deficits [90].

Nonketotic Hyperosmolar Coma. Some patients with nonketotic hyperosmolar coma with severe hyperglycemia may also present with anion gap metabolic acidosis. In most cases, the organic anion that accumulates has not been identified but does not appear to be either keto anions or lactate [91, 92].

Inborn Errors of Metabolism. The accumulation of organic acids in body fluids with a resultant metabolic acidosis may be seen in certain inborn errors of metabolism such as maple syrup urine disease, methylmalonicaciduria, propionicacidemia, and isovalericacidemia. The disorders generally present shortly after birth [93].

Toxic Alcohol Ingestions. Some of the most important causes of anion gap metabolic acidosis to consider are those due to toxic alcohol ingestions, specifically methanol and ethylene glycol. Early diagnosis of these ingestions allows for prompt and usually successful therapy, whereas delay in the diagnosis may be associated with considerable morbidity and mortality. Patients who ingest either methanol or ethylene glycol generally develop profound anion gap metabolic acidosis during the course of their illness, but their acid-base status may initially be normal if they present soon after ingestion. The serum osmolar gap, defined as the difference between the measured serum osmolarity and the calculated serum osmolarity, is generally elevated soon after ingestion because of the presence of the toxic alcohol in the serum [94–96].

$$\text{Calculated serum osmolarity} = 1.86 \, [Na^+] + [glucose]/18 + [urea \; nitrogen]/2.8 \qquad (15)$$

where [Na] is in millimolar and [glucose] and [urea nitrogen] are in milligrams per deciliter.

Further along the course of this disease, the osmolar gap tends to collapse while anion gap metabolic acidosis worsens. Although useful in suggesting this diagnosis, elevations in the serum osmolar gap are not specific for toxic alcohol ingestions, largely because ethanol is the most common cause of an elevated serum osmolar gap [97, 98]. A modified form of equation 15 that adds the term [*ethanol*]/4.6 may be used in cases of suspected toxic alcohol ingestion in the setting of ethanol use.

Patients who ingest methanol either as a suicide attempt or accidentally typically present with abdominal pain, vomiting, headache, and visual disturbances. Methanol intoxication characteristically produces severe retinitis, which may lead to blindness, and may be detectable on funduscopic examination. Methanol toxicity is generally believed to result from the metabolism of the methanol by alcohol dehydrogenase to formic acid. Ingestion of as little as 30 ml of methanol is toxic, and ingestion of 100 to 250 ml of methanol is usually fatal unless treated [96].

Ethylene glycol is the major osmolyte in most commercial antifreeze. Ingestion may occur as a suicide attempt, but because of its sweet taste, accidental ingestions are quite common. Ethylene glycol intoxication is similar to that of methanol in that both produce central nervous system disturbances and severe anion gap metabolic acidosis. In contrast to methanol, ethylene glycol does not usually produce retinitis but can cause acute and chronic renal failure. As is the case for methanol, the major toxicity of ethylene glycol is caused by its metabolism through alcohol dehydrogenase to glycolate, glyoxalate, and oxalate [99]. Detection of oxalate crystals in the urine may support the clinical impression of ethylene glycol ingestion. The lethal dose of ethylene glycol is believed to be as little as 100 ml [94, 95].

Because metabolism of methanol and ethylene glycol directly lead to their major toxicities, immediate prevention of this metabolism plays an important role in the therapy of these intoxications. Fortunately, the affinity of alcohol dehydrogenase for ethanol is considerably greater than for either methanol or ethylene glycol, and infusing ethanol to achieve concentrations exceeding 100 mg/dl effectively prevents alcohol dehydrogenase–mediated metabolism of both ethylene glycol and methanol. To facilitate nontoxic clearance of the parent compounds, hemodialysis is an effective procedure. However, during hemodialysis, adjustments in the dosage of ethanol (which is also cleared by hemodialysis) are necessary to maintain sufficient blood concentrations [100].

Salicylate Overdose. Ingestion of large amounts of aspirin or methylsalicylate may lead to serious and complex acid-base abnormalities. Symptoms correlate quite poorly with blood levels, especially in the elderly, but almost always accompany extremely elevated blood levels (plasma [salicylate] > 50 mg/dl). Salicylates affect the central nervous system to stimulate respiration and produce a component of respiratory alkalosis, especially early in the course of toxicity. Most adults with salicylate toxicity present with either respiratory alkalosis or a mixed anion gap metabolic acidosis and respiratory alkalosis. In children, the decreases in plasma [HCO_3^-] and increases in the anion gap develop more rapidly, and presentation with simple anion gap metabolic acidosis is most common. The acids responsible for the metabolic acidosis and increase in the anion gap include salicylic acid itself as well as endogenous acids whose metabolism is affected by the toxic amounts of salicylates. A blood salicylate concentration of 100 mg/dl contributes 7.3 mEq/L to the anion gap. Some component of lactic acidosis generally accompanies severe salicylate toxicity [101].

The diagnosis of salicylate toxicity is suggested by the history of aspirin use, nausea, and tinnitus. This is further supported by the clinical findings of unexplained hyperventilation, anion gap metabolic acidosis, noncardiogenic pulmonary edema, and an elevated prothrombin time. When salicylate toxicity occurs in younger adults, it is generally a result of a suicide attempt and is easily diagnosed. However, in older adults as well as children, the diagnosis may be more elusive. Advanced age and a delay in the diagnosis of salicylate toxicity are associated with significant mortality [102].

Treatment of salicylate toxicity generally should include alkalization of the blood and urine with sodium bicarbonate. Despite the potential negatives associated with sodium bicarbonate use in acute anion gap metabolic acidosis, alkalization of the plasma decreases the diffusion of salicylate into central nervous system sites, where it is toxic; sodium bicarbonate also improves renal excretion by producing an alkaline urine [103]. However, hemodynamic compromise and fluid overload must be carefully avoided, especially in older patients or patients with underlying heart disease [104]. Hemodialysis is quite effective at removing salicylate from the body and should be considered for patients with severely elevated plasma levels (e.g., >90

mg/dl), with evidence of severe toxicity, or at risk for complications of aggressive alkalization [101].

Other Intoxications. A variety of other agents may produce anion gap metabolic acidosis. These include strychnine, oral iron overdose, isoniazid, papaverine, out-dated tetracyclines, hydrogen sulfide, carbon monoxide, toluene, and paraldehyde. In general, these produce lactic acidosis [99]. An exception to this generalization is toluene, which produces a severe RTA (generally distal, but may include a proximal component) in concert with an elevation of serum hippurate (a metabolite of the toluene) concentration [105].

Failure of Acid Excretion

Acute or Chronic Renal Failure. The failure of the kidney to excrete the usual 1 to 3 mmol/kg of acid produced each day leads to metabolic acidosis. With both acute and chronic renal failure, some retention of anions occurs (including phosphate, sulfate, and some poorly characterized organic anions), which produces some increase in the serum anion gap. Metabolic acidosis in the setting of acute and chronic renal failure is generally not severe unless a markedly catabolic state occurs or other acidotic conditions (e.g., lactic acidosis) supervene.

With acute renal failure, the sudden loss of renal excretory function is invariably accompanied by a failure of acid excretion. In this setting, adaptation has no time to occur. With chronic renal failure, adaptation in remaining nephrons has time to occur. Specifically, the remaining nephron units markedly increase their NH_4^+ excretion. The pathogenesis of metabolic acidosis is a failure of the enhanced ammoniagenesis in remaining nephron units to achieve the total NH_4^+ excretion and thus the necessary NAE required for acid-base balance. Phosphate retention, which ultimately decreases urinary phosphate involved in the titratable acid component of NAE, may also contribute to this failure of acid-base balance. In addition, the high concentrations of circulating parathyroid hormone seen in chronic renal failure decrease proximal tubular HCO_3^- reabsorption and also participate in the pathogenesis of metabolic acidosis [106].

Treatment of Metabolic Acidosis

Although acidosis itself is deleterious to the function of many organs, the treatment of most conditions associated with metabolic acidosis is generally best accomplished by treatment of the underlying disease state. With most of the hyperchloremic states of metabolic acidosis, gradual correction of the acidosis with HCO_3^- administered either as sodium bicarbonate or a substrate metabolized to HCO_3^- (e.g., citrate) is quite rational, effective, and ultimately beneficial. Oral administration of these agents is preferred. One gram of sodium bicarbonate delivers about 12 mmol of HCO_3^-. Commercially available sodium or mixed sodium and potassium citrate solutions (e.g., Shohl's solution or Polycitra) contain 1 mmol of HCO_3^- equivalent per ml. Although citrate solutions are generally better tolerated than sodium bicarbonate tablets (which cause bloating when they produce CO_2 gas in the stomach), citrate may increase gastrointestinal absorption of aluminum and should not be administered along with aluminum-based phosphate binders, especially in the setting of chronic renal failure [107, 108].

It must be stressed that the acute treatment of metabolic acidosis with intravenous sodium bicarbonate may actually be deleterious, especially in conditions associated with impaired tissue perfusion. To understand how acute therapy with sodium bicarbonate may be deleterious, one must consider the fate of the administered HCO_3^- molecules. When sodium bicarbonate is given, a change in the serum HCO_3^- concentration results. The magnitude of this change in serum HCO_3^- for a given dose of bicarbonate is determined by the apparent volume of distribution for HCO_3^- ($Vd_{HCO_3^-}$), which is defined as follows:

$$Vd_{HCO_3^-} = \text{dose of } HCO_3^-/(\Delta \text{ serum } [HCO_3^-]) \tag{16}$$

This $Vd_{HCO_3^-}$ is not constant but increases with increasing severity of acidosis. This variation in $Vd_{HCO_3^-}$ probably results both from increased buffering from some extracellular and intracellular proteins as well as from alterations in intracellular pH homeostasis. We must also consider that the addition of HCO_3^- to blood (or an organism) produces CO_2 by mass action. Again, when metabolic acidosis is present, more CO_2 is produced for a given dose of sodium bicarbonate. In fact, recent studies performed in a closed, human blood model demonstrate that the production of CO_2 from administered HCO_3^- is directly dependent on the initial pH. Therefore, when ventilation is normal, this extra CO_2 is rapidly eliminated by the lungs, and a portion of the $Vd_{HCO_3^-}$ can be considered to be extracorporeal. However, when pulmonary ventilation or, more commonly, tissue ventilation is impaired (by poor tissue perfusion), this CO_2 generated by infused HCO_3^- may diffuse into cells (far more rapidly than the original HCO_3^- molecule) and paradoxically decrease the intracellular pH. This is shown schematically in Figure 3-4. Experimentally, administration of sodium bicarbonate in animal models of metabolic acidosis has been associated with a fall in intracellular pH in several organs as well as additional hemodynamic compromise. In addition to this paradoxical intracellular acidosis, administration of hypertonic sodium bicarbonate (as it is often given as 50-ml ampules of 1M $NaHCO_3$) may also be associated with development of hypertonicity. This hypertonicity itself may have deleterious effects on cardiac function, especially in the setting of cardiac arrest resuscitation [109]. In general, we do not advocate the emergency administration of intravenous sodium bicarbonate for acute anion gap metabolic acidosis.

To address the concerns regarding sodium bicarbonate therapy, alternatives are currently under development, including non–CO_2-generating buffers such as Carbicarb (a 1:1 mixture of disodium carbonate and sodium bicarbonate) as well as dichloroacetate, which has been specifically designed to decrease lactate production in lactic acidosis [110]. Our experimental experience has shown that Carbicarb is an effective alkalinizer of the intracellular space in models where sodium bicarbonate causes a paradoxical worsening of intracellular acidosis [28, 111, 112]. Moreover, we have demonstrated that Carbicarb improves cardiac function as well as other

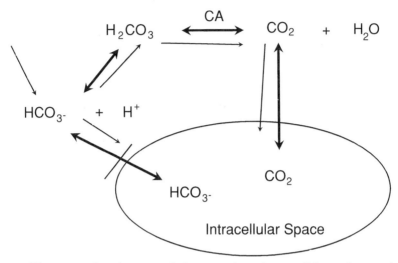

Fig. 3-4. Illustration of mechanism underlying paradoxical intracellular acidosis resulting from sodium bicarbonate administration. When additional HCO_3^- is added to the extracellular fluid (*narrow arrow*), HCO_3^- combines with H^+, and reaction is shifted by mass action to H_2CO_3, which results in increases in extracellular CO_2 tension. Because most cell membranes are more permeable to CO_2 than to HCO_3^-, this transiently causes the cellular CO_2 tension to rise more than the $[HCO_3^-]$, which results in decreases in intracellular pH.

physiologic parameters in experimental models of acidosis [28, 77]. We have recently observed that when Carbicarb is administered as an isotonic solution, improvement in cardiac function is more immediate and more pronounced than when it is administered as a hypertonic solution [113]. To date, however, only preliminary reports of the clinical use of this agent are available [114, 115].

Metabolic Alkalosis

Causes of Metabolic Alkalosis

Metabolic alkalosis is a systemic disorder caused by a process that leads to an increased pH due to a primary increase in the plasma $[HCO_3^-]$. This primary elevation of plasma $[HCO_3^-]$ may be caused by the following processes.

Net Loss of H^+ from the ECF

H^+ can be lost from the ECF externally through the gastrointestinal tract and the kidneys or can be shifted (at least theoretically) internally into cells. If H^+ losses exceed the daily H^+ load produced by diet and metabolism, increases in the plasma $[HCO_3^-]$ will occur. This is because the loss of H^+ at these sites mandates the generation of an HCO_3^- molecule. In the stomach, the gastric parietal cell secretion of H^+ by the luminal H^+-ATPase leaves an HCO_3^- to be reclaimed at the basolateral surface. In the kidney, H^+ secretion via the H^+-ATPase or Na^+/H^+ exchanger also leaves an HCO_3^- molecule for reclamation on the basolateral surface. Shifting of H^+ into cells has been postulated to accompany states of significant potassium depletion, thus increasing ECF $[HCO_3^-]$. Despite the appeal of this concept, evidence of intracellular acidosis developing during experimental potassium depletion has not been consistently observed [116].

Net Addition of Bicarbonate Precursors to the ECF

The administration of HCO_3^- or substances that generate HCO_3^- such as lactate, citrate, or acetate in a rate greater than that of metabolic H^+ production will also lead to a rise in ECF $[HCO_3^-]$. We stress that when renal function is normal, such increases in ECF $[HCO_3^-]$ will be offset by marked increases in renal HCO_3^- excretion as the plasma $[HCO_3^-]$ exceeds the plasma threshold for HCO_3^- reabsorption.

External Loss of Fluid Containing Chloride in Greater Concentration and Bicarbonate in Lesser Concentration than the Plasma

Loss of this type of fluid will lead to both a contraction of the ECF volume and a rise in the $[HCO_3^-]$. In this situation, H^+ is not lost externally, as in vomiting or nasogastric suction, but rather the remaining ECF $[HCO_3^-]$ increases as ECF volume contracts (contraction alkalosis) [66].

Pathophysiology of Metabolic Alkalosis

As discussed briefly, the normal kidney has a wonderful protective mechanism against the development of significant increases in ECF $[HCO_3^-]$, namely a threshold for tubular fluid $[HCO_3^-]$ above which proximal reabsorption ceases and HCO_3^- losses in the urine ensue. Therefore, in virtually all cases of metabolic alkalosis, the kidney must participate in the pathophysiology, at least at a passive level by not excreting the excess HCO_3^-.

A useful way to consider the pathogenesis of metabolic alkalosis is to separate factors that initiate or generate the metabolic alkalosis and those that maintain it.

Buffering

When HCO_3^- is added to the ECF, H^+ reacts with the HCO_3^- to produce CO_2, which is normally exhaled in expired gas. The increase in plasma and ECF $[HCO_3^-]$ is thus attenuated. This was discussed earlier in the section concerning the volume of distribution of HCO_3^-. Most of the H^+ used in this buffering comes from the intracellular fluid. A small increase in lactic acid production provides another source of H^+ [71].

Respiratory Compensation

The control of ventilation under normal conditions is apparently situated in the brain stem and is most sensitive to interstitial H^+ concentrations. However, when the O_2 tension in blood drops, hypoxia becomes an important stimulus of respiratory drive. Therefore, the respiratory compensation to metabolic alkalosis follows the same principles as respiratory compensation to metabolic acidosis, but in the opposite direction. Contraints regarding the oxygenation limit the magnitude of the hypoventilatory response to metabolic alkalosis. As a rule of thumb, the $PaCO_2$ should increase 0.25 to 1.0 times the increase in plasma $[HCO_3^-]$ during metabolic alkalosis. Failure to demonstrate such compensation in the setting of metabolic alkalosis defines the coexistence of primary respiratory alkalosis [25].

Renal Correction

The corrective response by the kidney to excrete excessive HCO_3^- in the urine will, under normal conditions, rapidly correct metabolic alkalosis. This is because once an initiating process increases the plasma $[HCO_3^-]$ so that it exceeds the plasma threshold for bicarbonate, the fall in plasma $[HCO_3^-]$ should follow a monoexponential decay whose time constant is determined by the volume of distribution for HCO_3^- and the GFR until it reaches the plasma threshold concentration. For example, if the GFR is 100 ml/min, the $Vd_{HCO_3^-}$ is 50 percent body water (or 21 L in a 70-kg man), and we assume that the $[HCO_3^-]$ is increased acutely by 10 mmol/L by some initiation process that does not affect the plasma threshold for bicarbonate, then within less than 4 hours, the $[HCO_3^-]$ will be only about 4 mmol/L above the plasma threshold. Therefore, we can see that it would be difficult to produce a significant increase in plasma $[HCO_3^-]$ without the participation of the kidney.

Factors in the Maintenance of Metabolic Alkalosis

Several factors tend to increase the apparent Tmax for HCO_3^- and thus increase net HCO_3^- reabsorption by the kidney.

Decreases in Effective Arterial Blood Volume

Absolute (e.g., volume losses through vomiting or bleeding) or effective (e.g., heart failure, nephrotic syndrome) arterial volume depletion will increase the Tmax and plasma threshold for HCO_3^-. This is accomplished both proximally (increased proximal tubule reabsorption of sodium and water) and distally (mineralocorticoid effect) in the nephron [117].

Chloride Depletion

Although chloride depletion occurs as part of the pathophysiology of decreases in ECF volume, detailed physiologic studies indicate that the chloride anion is independently involved in the process of HCO_3^- reabsorption. Specifically, even in the presence of expansion of the ECF, depletion of chloride leads to increases in the apparent Tmax and plasma threshold for HCO_3^- [118].

Aldosterone

An increase in distal sodium avidity resulting in increased renal HCO_3^- generation may occur in the absence of decreases in effective arterial blood volume if mineralo-corticoids are administered or produced locally [119].

Potassium Depletion

Potassium depletion is another factor that has been implicated for increasing the apparent Tmax and plasma threshold for HCO_3^- and maintaining metabolic alkalo-sis. One suggested explanation is that potassium depletion leads to a relative intra-cellular acidosis and this relative intracellular acidosis makes renal H^+ excretion more favorable [120]. Evidence against this concept includes the considerable con-centration differences involved in the preservation of electroneutrality by an ion that exists in nanomolar concentrations. In addition, renal intracellular pH mea-sured by ^{31}P NMR spectroscopy does not always decrease during experimental potas-sium depletion [121]. Moreover, in human studies, metabolic alkalosis can be cor-rected almost completely without correction of potassium depletion [122].

Hypercapnia

Increases in $PaCO_2$ are known to increase the apparent Tmax and plasma threshold for HCO_3^-. This may be mediated through decreases in intracellular pH (which have been documented during acute and chronic hypercapnia). Interestingly, the increases in $PaCO_2$ that occur during metabolic alkalosis as part of normal respira-tory compensation actually tend to impair renal correction through this mechanism [123].

Clinical Features of Metabolic Alkalosis

No specific symptoms or signs are pathognomonic of metabolic alkalosis. The dis-turbance should be suspected, however, in patients who have muscle cramps, weak-ness, arrhythmias, or seizures, especially if the appropriate clinical scenario (e.g., diuretic use, vomiting) is present. Some of these signs and symptoms may be related to alterations in ionized calcium because increases in pH cause plasma proteins to bind calcium more avidly, thus lowering ionized calcium concentrations. Severe alkalemia (pH > 7.6) may be associated with malignant arrhythmias (e.g., ventricu-lar tachycardia and fibrillation) as well as seizures [124, 125].

Laboratory Findings in Metabolic Alkalosis

Arterial blood gases reveal the diagnostic pattern, that is, an increased pH, increased $[HCO_3^-]$, and an increased $PaCO_2$. The increase in $PaCO_2$ is between 0.25 and 1.0 times the increase in $[HCO_3^-]$. The serum electrolytes demonstrate increased TCO_2 as well as decreased chloride and, usually, potassium concentrations. The hypokalemia results from both shifting of potassium into cells and increased renal losses. Potassium shifts into cells during metabolic alkalosis; however, the magnitude of such changes may be difficult to predict. Renal losses are enhanced throughout the course of metabolic alkalosis. The serum anion gap may be increased by up to 9 to 12 mEq/L with severe metabolic alkalosis. This is due to some small increases in lactate concentrations [71] but mostly to the increased electronegativity of albumin with elevated pH [126].

Urine electrolytes represent an important step in the classification of metabolic alkalosis. Specifically, they are used to determine whether decreases in effective arterial blood volume act as a maintenance factor in the pathogenesis of the metabolic alkalosis. Although the urinary sodium concentration may be inconsistent in this condition, especially if bicarbonaturia is present at the time that the urine sample is collected, the urinary chloride concentration allows one to classify patients into chloride-responsive and chloride-resistant categories of metabolic alkalosis. Chloride-responsive metabolic alkalosis resolves when volume expansion or improvement of hemodynamics occurs. Examples include patients who are vomiting or have received diuretics (but have discontinued them). Chloride-resistant metabolic alkalosis does not correct with these maneuvers. Examples are patients with primary mineralocorticoid excess or patients who are continuing to take diuretics. In patients with chloride-responsive metabolic alkalosis, the urinary chloride concentration usually will be less than 10 mmol/L, whereas patients with chloride-resistant metabolic alkalosis generally will have a urinary chloride concentration exceeding 20 mmol/L.

Differential Diagnosis of Metabolic Alkalosis

The differential diagnosis of metabolic alkalosis is generally approached by separating patients into those who have chloride depletion as a maintenance factor (e.g., chloride-responsive), those who do not have chloride depletion as a maintenance factor (chloride-resistant metabolic alkalosis), and those who have an unclassified (generally uncommon) form of metabolic alkalosis. As discussed previously, this differentiation is generally accomplished using the urinary chloride concentration (Table 3-7).

Chloride-Responsive Metabolic Alkalosis

Vomiting. Gastric secretory volume may exceed 1 to 2 L/day in patients with persistent vomiting. The gastric secretions may contain as much as 100 mmol/L of H^+, and since the gastric parietal cells generate an HCO_3^- molecule for each H^+ secreted, as much as 200 mmol of HCO_3^- may be generated in one day. Although this represents a significant initiation factor, the concomitant Na^+ and Cl^- losses (as much as 400 mmol/day), possibly along with the associated K^+ losses (more in the urine than in vomit, which generally has less than 15 mmol of potassium per liter), are the maintenance factors that allow metabolic acidosis to persist [127] (Fig. 3-5).

The degree of metabolic alkalosis associated with vomiting is generally mild; however, in conditions where gastric secretions are greatly stimulated (e.g., Zollinger-Ellison syndrome with gastric outlet obstruction), plasma $[HCO_3^-]$ may exceed 60 mmol/L [47].

Table 3-7. Differential diagnosis of metabolic alkalosis

Chloride-responsive metabolic alkalosis
    Vomiting
    Gastric drainage
    Villous adenoma
    Chloride diarrhea
    Diuretics
    Posthypercapnia
    Cystic fibrosis
Chloride-resistant metabolic alkalosis
    Hyperaldosteronism
    Cushing's syndrome
    Bartter's syndrome
    Licorice
    Profound potassium depletion?
Unclassified metabolic alkalosis
    Alkali administration
    Milk-alkali syndrome
    Transfusion of blood products
    Hypercalcemia
    Post-starvation
    Large doses of penicillin antibiotics

Gastric Drainage. The pathophysiology of gastric drainage, usually through a nasogastric tube, is essentially identical to that of vomiting [127].

Villous Adenoma of the Colon. Villous adenoma of the colon may result in profound diarrhea that is extremely rich in protein, sodium, potassium, and chloride. The losses of sodium, potassium, and chloride and the relatively low $[HCO_3^-]$ concentration in the diarrheal fluid in some patients may lead to metabolic alkalosis [128]. However, this condition more commonly causes HCO_3^- losses, which produce metabolic acidosis, as discussed earlier [47].

Chloride Diarrhea. Chloride diarrhea is a rare congenital syndrome arising from a defect in small- and large-bowel chloride absorption that leads to a chronic diarrhea with a stool fluid rich in chloride. Metabolic alkalosis develops through the mechanisms described for villous adenoma [47].

Diuretic Therapy. Diuretics that exert their effects either in the thick ascending limb of Henle (loop diuretics [e.g., furosemide, bumetanide]), or in the distal tubule (e.g., thiazide diuretics) may cause volume depletion as well as directly stimulate renin secretion (possibly through increases in distal tubular fluid sodium content), which leads to increases in aldosterone secretion, which stimulates distal nephron Na^+ reabsorption and K^+ and H^+ secretion. Thus, they both initiate metabolic alkalosis through H^+ losses and maintain metabolic alkalosis via volume depletion and ongoing H^+ losses by the kidney (if diuretics are continued). If the urinary

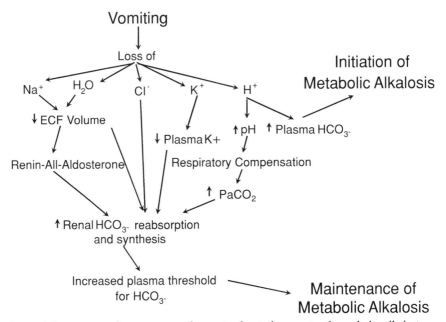

Fig. 3-5. Initiation and maintenance factors in the pathogenesis of metabolic alkalosis developing from vomiting are illustrated. Initial loss of H^+ from the stomach is the initiation factor where the concomitant loss of K^+, Na^+, Cl^-, and H_2O along with respiratory compensation set up the maintenance of the alkalosis by increasing renal HCO_3^- reabsorption and synthesis and the plasma threshold for HCO_3^-.

chloride is obtained while diuretic effects persist, it may be high, whereas if the urinary chloride is determined after sufficient time (generally >24–48 hours) has elapsed to eliminate diuretic effects, it should be low, reflecting volume depletion. Metabolic alkalosis along with hypokalemia is an extremely frequent complication of diuretic use. The possibility of diuretic use, even if such drugs are not prescribed, should be considered, especially in adolescents and adults. Diuretic abuse is seen commonly in patients suffering from anorexia nervosa [129].

Posthypercapnia. As discussed in Chapter 4, the renal compensation to chronic hypercapnia results in an elevation in plasma $[HCO_3^-]$. When hypercapnia is rapidly corrected (e.g., with intubation and mechanical ventilation), the patient is left with an elevated plasma $[HCO_3^-]$ until renal correction occurs, a process that generally takes at least several hours. If sufficient chloride is not provided to allow for renal correction, this metabolic alkalosis may persist [130].

Cystic Fibrosis. Several children with cystic fibrosis have been described in whom metabolic alkalosis developed due to marked loss of chloride in the sweat, which had relatively little HCO_3^-. The resultant volume depletion maintained the metabolic alkalosis in these patients [131].

Chloride-Resistant Metabolic Alkalosis

Primary Hyperaldosteronism. Aldosterone directly stimulates distal nephron H^+ secretion by several mechanisms, some of which are tied to sodium reabsorption and potassium secretion, whereas others appear to be independent of sodium or potassium transport. This increased H^+ secretion leads to either reclamation of filtered HCO_3^- destined for excretion or the generation of new HCO_3^-, which is ultimately retained in the ECF. Although the increase in ECF [HCO_3^-] produced by such distal nephron effects results in ECF volume expansion and secondary decrease in proximal tubule reabsorptive capacity for HCO_3^-, the distal processes are sufficient to maintain an elevated plasma threshold for HCO_3^-. Hence the clinical features of hypokalemic metabolic alkalosis are produced, often in concert with hypertension associated with the ECF volume expansion.

Such primary increase in mineralocorticoids may be caused by an adrenal tumor that selectively makes aldosterone (Conn's syndrome) or hyperplasia (usually bilateral) of the adrenal cortex. The diagnosis of such a primary mineralocorticoid excess state is dependent on the demonstration that volume expansion is present (e.g., unstimulatible plasma renin activity) and that aldosterone secretion is not suppressible by volume expansion [132].

Cushing's Syndrome. With adrenocorticotropic hormone–secreting tumors, primary adrenal cortical tumors, or hyperplasia due to congenital enzyme deficiencies, there may be an increase in corticosteroid synthesis. Many corticosteroids (specifically cortisol, deoxycorticosterone, and corticosterone) may also have considerable mineralocorticoid effects and produce hypokalemic metabolic alkalosis, sometimes accompanied by hypertension. Detailed metabolic analysis of the plasma and urine as well as imaging studies may be necessary to arrive at the precise diagnosis [119].

Bartter's Syndrome. Bartter's syndrome is a rare condition usually presenting in children that is characterized by hyperreninemia and hyperaldosteronemia in the absence of hypertension or sodium retention. Histologically, hyperplasia of the juxtaglomerular apparatus is noted, a finding that is not specific for this diagnosis [133, 134]. Functionally, the disorder is believed to be caused by a failure of chloride reabsorption in the thick ascending limb of Henle, a disturbance that results in a very high delivery of chloride and sodium to the distal nephron, activation of the renin-angiotensin-aldosterone system, and the production of hypokalemic metabolic alkalosis. Although the prostaglandin system has been suggested to participate in this disturbance, and sometimes prostaglandin synthesis inhibitors may be beneficial, it is likely that the increase in renal prostaglandins in this disorder is secondary. Clinically, it is extremely difficult to separate Bartter's syndrome from diuretic use, specifically those that inhibit chloride reabsorption in the thick ascending limb of Henle (e.g., furosemide, bumetanide). Surreptitious diuretic use must be considered foremost in adolescents or adults who present with unexplained hypokalemic metabolic alkalosis [129].

Licorice. A major component of "black" licorice, glycyrrhizic acid, may cause a hypokalemic metabolic alkalosis accompanied by hypertension and thus mimic primary hyperaldosteronism. The mechanism previously had been thought to be a primary mineralocorticoid effect of glycyrrhizic acid [135], but more recent data suggest that this substance actually causes up-regulation of renal mineralocorticoid receptors [136].

Profound Potassium Depletion. Several patients with profound hypokalemia (plasma $[K^+] < 2$ mmol/L) have had significant metabolic alkalosis associated with a urinary chloride concentration exceeding 20 mmol/L without evidence of mineralocorticoid excess. The alkalosis was not corrected during sodium repletion until the potassium deficit was also corrected [120]. This finding suggests that in some cases, potassium depletion may convert a chloride-responsive metabolic alkalosis to a chloride-resistant metabolic alkalosis. However, correction of metabolic alkalosis without repletion of large potassium deficits has been clearly demonstrated in humans [122].

Unclassified Metabolic Alkalosis

Alkali Administration. The kidney rapidly excretes alkali (as discussed earlier), and only if a maintenance factor supervenes or the administration of alkali continues will metabolic alkalosis be maintained. In some situations, however, alkali administration may generate metabolic alkalosis. This alkali load may be in the form of HCO_3^- or organic anions that are metabolized to HCO_3^- such as citrate or acetate. Specifically, in patients with chronic renal failure where the ability to excrete an HCO_3^- load is impaired (because GFR is reduced), administration of an alkali load may cause sustained metabolic alkalosis [137].

Milk-Alkali Syndrome. Milk-alkali syndrome is seen in patients with dyspepsia who consume moderate to large amounts of antacids containing calcium and absorbable alkali (e.g., calcium carbonate). Lack of ECF volume expansion along with hypercalcemia-mediated suppression of parathyroid hormone secretion contributes to the maintenance of metabolic alkalosis. Hypercalcemia also causes decreases in renal blood flow and glomerular filtration, which can further impair renal excretion of HCO_3^-. Alkalosis reduces calcium excretion and tends to potentiate associated hypercalcemia. Chronically, nephrocalcinosis may occur, which may ultimately decrease GFR, thus further reducing ability to excrete an alkali load [138].

Transfusion of Blood Products. Infusion of large amounts (>10 units) of blood products containing the anticoagulant citrate can produce moderate metabolic alkalosis. The production of HCO_3^- from citrate is totally responsible for the initiation of the metabolic alkalosis. In other situations, some degree of prerenal azotemia (e.g., administration of packed red blood cells to a patient with hemorrhagic shock) may supervene and maintain the metabolic alkalosis. Patients given parenteral hyperalimentation with excessive amounts of acetate or lactate may also develop metabolic alkalosis through an identical mechanism [137].

Hypercalcemia (Nonhyperparathyroid Etiology). Mild metabolic alkalosis has been associated with hypercalcemia that results from causes other than hyperparathyroidism (e.g., malignancy, sarcoid). This may be due to a suppression of parathyroid hormone, which then raises the plasma threshold for HCO_3^-, as discussed earlier [139].

Post-Starvation (Refeeding Alkalosis). Patients who break prolonged fasts with meals containing carbohydrates may develop a metabolic alkalosis that can persist for several weeks. The mechanism for the initiation of the metabolic alkalosis is unknown. Increases in renal sodium avidity (resulting from the ECF volume depletion occurring during starvation) appear to be the maintenance factor [89].

Large Doses of Penicillin Antibiotics. Intravenous administration of large doses of some penicillin antibiotics, specifically penicillin and carbenicillin, may result in hypokalemic metabolic alkalosis. The mechanism is believed to be the increase in delivery of poorly reabsorbable anions to the distal nephron with a resultant increase in H^+ and potassium secretion [140].

Treatment of Metabolic Alkalosis

The guiding principle for treating all acid-base disturbances is to address the underlying disease state. In some cases, however, the degree of acid-base abnormality itself becomes life-threatening, especially with mixed acid-base disturbances where the respiratory and metabolic components go in the same direction (e.g., respiratory alkalosis and metabolic alkalosis). When an elevated systemic pH becomes life-threatening (e.g., pH > 7.6 with seizures and ventricular arrhythmias), rapid reduction in systemic pH may be accomplished by control of ventilation. In such situations, intubation of the airway, sedation, and controlled hypoventilation with a mechanical ventilator (sometimes using inspired CO_2 and supplemental oxygen to prevent hypoxia) may be lifesaving [141].

Although historically administration of either HCl or its congeners (e.g., arginine chloride or ammonium chloride) had been advocated to correct metabolic alkalosis, we do not currently advocate such an approach. Our rationale is that these agents do have significant potential complications (e.g., hemolysis and tissue necrosis with HCl, ammonia toxicity with ammonium chloride) and simply do not work fast enough to prevent life-threatening complications such as seizures or arrhythmias. Therefore, for urgent intervention, we advocate the control of $PaCO_2$ outlined above. In less urgent settings, therapy of the metabolic alkalosis may be addressed after examining whether it is chloride-responsive or not. Chloride-responsive metabolic alkalosis responds quite well to volume repletion and improvement of renal hemodynamics. If hypokalemia is present, it should also be corrected. Treatment of the chloride-resistant metabolic alkalosis conditions generally mandates interference with the mineralocorticoid (or mineralocorticoid-like substance) that is maintaining renal H^+ losses. This can sometimes be accomplished pharmacologically (e.g., spironolactone or other distal potassium sparing diuretics like amiloride).

In some cases, the proximate cause of the metabolic alkalosis is necessary for the overall well-being of the patient. One example of this is a patient with severe heart failure who develops hypokalemic metabolic alkalosis as a result of loop diuretics, the continued use of which is mandated by the patient's congestive symptoms. In such cases, the proximal diuretic acetazolamide, which will decrease the plasma threshold for HCO_3^- by inhibiting proximal tubule HCO_3^- reabsorption, may be very effective [59]. In subjects who are undergoing persistent gastric drainage, administration of either an H_2 blocker or H^+-ATPase inhibitor to decrease gastric H^+ secretion may be advantageous [142]. In patients with advanced chronic renal failure in whom metabolic alkalosis has been induced (e.g., with antacid excess), hemodialysis may be necessary for correction.

References

1. Filley GF: *Acid-Base and Blood Gas Regulation*. Philadelphia, Lea & Febiger, 1971.
2. Stewart PA: *How to Understand Acid-Base: A Quantitative Primer for Biology and Medicine*. New York, Elsevier, 1981.
3. Alpern RJ, Warnock DG, Rector FCJ: Renal Acidification Mechanisms. In Brenner BM, Rector FC (eds), *The Kidney*. Philadelphia, Saunders, 1986, pp 206–250.
4. Lehninger AL: *Biochemistry*. New York, Worth, 1975.
5. Roos A, Boron WP: Intracellular pH. *Physiol Rev* 61:296–434, 1981.
6. Malhotra D, Shapiro JI: Nuclear magnetic resonance measurements of intracellular pH: Biomedical implications. *Con Magn Reson* 5:123–150, 1993.
7. Halperin ML, Jungas RL, Cheema-Dhadli S, Brosnan JT: Disposal of the daily acid load: An integrated function of the liver, lungs and kidneys. *Trends Biol Sci* 12:197–199, 1987.
8. Preisig PA, Alpern RJ: Chronic metabolic acidosis causes an adaptation in the apical membrane Na/H antiporter and basolateral membrane $Na(HCO_3)_3$ symporter in the rat proximal convoluted tubule. *J Clin Invest* 82:1445–1453, 1988.
9. Selvaggio AM, Schwartz JH, Bengele HH, Alexander EA: Kinetics of the Na^+-H^+ antiporter as assessed by the change in intracellular pH in MDCK cells. *Am J Physiol* 251:C558–C562, 1986.
10. Sabatini S: Distribution and function of the renal ATPase (H(+)-ATPase). *Semin Nephrol* 11:37–44, 1991.
11. Kurtzman NA: Disorders of distal acidification. *Kidney Int* 38:720–727, 1990.
12. Eiam-ong S, Dafnis E, Spohn M, et al: H-K-ATPase in distal renal tubular acidosis: Urinary tract obstruction, lithium, and amiloride. *Am J Physiol* 265:F875–F880, 1993.
13. Boron WF, Boulpaep EL: The electrogenic Na/HCO^3 cotransporter. *Kidney Int* 36:392–402, 1989.
14. Olsnes S, Ludt J, Tonnessen TI, Sandvig K: Bicarbonate/chloride antiport in Vero cells: II. Mechanisms for bicarbonate-dependent regulation of intracellular pH. *J Cell Physiol* 132: 192–202, 1987.
15. Halperin ML: How much new bicarbonate is formed in the distal nephron in the process of net acid excretion. *Kidney Int* 35:1277–1281, 1989.
16. Good DW, Dubose TDJ: Ammonia transport by early and late proximal convoluted tubule of the rat. *J Clin Invest* 79:684–691, 1987.
17. Good DW, Caflisch CR, Dubose TDJ: Transepithelial ammonia concentration gradients in inner medulla of the rat. *Am J Physiol* 252:F491–F500, 1987.
18. Carlisle EJ, Donnelly SM, Halperin ML: Renal tubular acidosis (RTA): Recognize the ammonium defect and pHorget the urine pH. *Pediatr Nephrol* 5:242–248, 1991.
19. Batlle DC, Hizon M, Cohen E, et al: The use of the urinary anion gap in the diagnosis of hyperchloremic metabolic acidosis. *N Engl J Med* 318:594–599, 1988.
20. Oh MS, Carroll HJ: The anion gap. *N Engl J Med* 297:814–822, 1977.
21. Schwartz WB, Orning KJ, Porter R: The internal distribution of hydrogen ions with varying degrees of metabolic acidosis. *J Clin Invest* 36:372–382, 1957.
22. Lemann J Jr, Litzow JR, Lennon EJ: The effects of chronic acid loads in normal man: Further

evidence for the participation of bone mineral in the defense against chronic metabolic acidosis. *J Clin Invest* 45:1608–1617, 1966.

23. Burnell JM: Changes in bone sodium and carbonate in metabolic acidosis and alkalosis. *J Clin Invest* 50:327–335, 1971.
24. Cunningham J, Fraher LJ, Clemens TL, et al: Chronic acidosis with metabolic bone disease: Effect of alkali on bone morphology and vitamin D metabolism. *Am J Med* 73:199–207, 1982.
25. Elkington JR: Clinical disorders of acid-base regulation: A survey of seventeen years diagnostic experience. *Med Clin North Am* (50)1325–1364, 1966.
26. Fencl V, Miller TB, Pappenheimer JR: Studies on the respiratory response to disturbances of acid-base balance, with deductions concerning the ionic composition of cerebral interstitial fluid. *Am J Physiol* 210:459–466, 1966.
27. Madias NE, Schwartz WB, Cohen JJ: The maladaptive renal response to secondary hypocapnia during chronic HCl acidosis in the dog. *J Clin Invest* 60:1393–1400, 1977.
28. Shapiro JI, Whalen M, Chan L: Hemodynamic and hepatic intracellular pH responses to bicarbonate and Carbicarb during acidosis. *Magn Reson Med* 16:403–410, 1990.
29. O'Brodovich HM, Stalcup SA, Pang LM, Mellins RB: Hemodynamic and vasoactive mediator response to experimental respiratory failure. *J Appl Physiol* 52:1230–1236, 1982.
30. Nimmo AJ, Than N, Orchard CH, Whitaker EM: The effect of acidosis on beta-adrenergic receptors in ferret cardiac muscle. *Exp Physiol* 78:95–103, 1993.
31. Davies AO: Rapid desensitization and uncoupling of human beta-adrenergic receptors in an in vitro model of lactic acidosis. *J Clin Endocrinol Metab* 59:398–405, 1984.
32. Orchard C: The effect of acidosis on excitation-contraction coupling in isolated ferret heart muscle. *Mol Cell Biochem* 89:169–173, 1989.
33. Allen DG, Orchard CH: The effects of pH on intracellular calcium transients in mammalian cardiac muscle. *J Physiol* 335:555–567, 1983.
34. Nosek TM, Fender KY, Godt RE: It is the diprotonated form of inorganic phosphate that causes force depression in skinned skeletal muscle fibers. *Science* 236:191–193, 1987.
35. Zhou HZ, Malhotra D, Shapiro JI: Contractile dysfunction during metabolic acidosis: Role of impaired energy metabolism. *Am J Physiol* 261:H1481–H1486, 1991.
36. Suleymanlar G, Zhou HZ, McCormack M, et al: Mechanism of impaired energy metabolism during acidosis: Role of oxidative metabolism. *Am J Physiol* 263:H1818–H1822, 1992.
37. Zhou HZ, Malhotra D, Doers J, Shapiro JI: Synergism between hypoxic injury and acidosis in the isolated heart. *Magn Reson Med* 29:94–98, 1993.
38. McGillivray-Anderson KM, Faber JE: Effect of acidosis on contraction of microvascular smooth muscle by alpha 1- and alpha 2-adrenoceptors: Implications for neural and metabolic regulation. *Circ Res* 66:1643–1657, 1990.
39. Russel CD, Illickal MM, Maloney JV Jr, Roeher HD, Deland EC: Acute response to acid-base stress in the dog. *Am J Physiol* 223:689–694, 1972.
40. Janusek LW: Metabolic acidosis: Pathophysiology, signs, and symptoms. *Nursing* 20:52–53, 1990.
41. Eiam-ong S, Kurtzman NA: Metabolic acidosis and bone disease. *Miner Electrolyte Metab* 20: 72–80, 1994.
42. Adrogue HJ, Madias NE: Changes in plasma potassium concentration during acute acid-base disturbances. *Am J Med* 71:456–467, 1981.
43. Emmett M, Narins RG: Clinical use of the anion gap. *Medicine* 56:(38)51, 1977.
44. Winter SD, Pearson JR, Gabow PA, et al: The fall of the serum anion gap. *Arch Intern Med* 150:311–313, 1990.
45. Gabow PA, Kaehny WD, Fennessey PV, et al: Diagnostic importance of an increased serum anion gap. *N Engl J Med* 303:854–858, 1980.
46. Wang F, Butler T, Rabbani GH, Jones PK: The acidosis of cholera: Contributions of hyperproteinemia, lactic acidemia, and hyperphosphatemia to an increased serum anion gap. *N Engl J Med* 315:1591–1595, 1986.
47. Phillips SF: Water and Electrolytes in Gastrointestinal Disease. In Maxwell MH, Kleeman CR (eds): *Clinical Disorders of Fluid and Electrolyte Metabolism*. New York, McGraw-Hill, 1980, pp 1267–1295.

48. Ketel B, Henry ML, Elkhammas EA, et al: Metabolic complications in combined kidney/pancreas transplantation. *Transplant Proc* 24:774–775, 1992.
49. Tom WW, Munda R, First MR, Alexander JW: Physiologic consequences of pancreatic allograft exocrine drainage into the urinary tract. *Transplant Proc* 19:2339–2342, 1987.
50. Kleinman PK: Cholestyramine and metabolic acidosis. *N Engl J Med* 290:861, 1974.
51. Haldane JBS, Hill R, Luck JM: Calcium chloride acidosis. *J Physiol* 57:20–37, 1923.
52. Lash JP, Arruda JA: Laboratory evaluation of renal tubular acidosis. *Clin Lab Med* 13:117–129, 1993.
53. Halperin ML, Goldstein MB, Richardson RM, Stinebaugh BJ: Distal renal tubular acidosis syndromes: A pathophysiological approach. *Am J Nephrol* 5:1–8, 1985.
54. Igarashi T, Ishii T, Watanabe K, et al: Persistent isolated proximal renal tubular acidosis—a systemic disease with a distinct clinical entity. *Pediatr Nephrol* 8:70–71, 1994.
55. Halperin ML, Kamel KS, Ethier JH, Magner PO: What is the underlying defect in patients with isolated, proximal renal tubular acidosis? *Am J Nephrol* 9:265–268, 1989.
56. Moss AH, Gabow PA, Kaehny WD, et al: Fanconi's syndrome and distal renal tubular acidosis after glue sniffing. *Ann Intern Med* 92:69–70, 1980.
57. Vasuvattakul S, Nimmannit S, Shayakul C, et al: Should the urine PCO_2 or the rate of excretion of ammonium be the gold standard to diagnose distal renal tubular acidosis? *Am J Kidney Dis* 19:72–75, 1992.
58. Richardson RM, Halperin ML: The urine pH: A potentially misleading diagnostic test in patients with hyperchloremic metabolic acidosis. *Am J Kidney Dis* 10:140–143, 1987.
59. DuBose TD Jr: Carbonic anhydrase-dependent bicarbonate transport in the kidney. *Ann NY Acad Sci* 429:528–537, 1984.
60. Maren TH: Carbonic anhydrase: Chemistry, physiology and inhibition. *Physiol Rev* 47:595–628, 1967.
61. Kurtzman NA, Gonzalez J, DeFronzo R, Giebisch G: A patient with hyperkalemia and metabolic acidosis. *Am J Kidney Dis* 15:333–356, 1990.
62. DeFronzo RA: Hyperkalemia and hyporeninemic hypoaldosteronism. *Kidney Int* 17:118–132, 1980.
63. Allen GG, Barratt LJ: An in vivo study of voltage-dependent renal tubular acidosis induced by amiloride. *Kidney Int* 35:1107–1110, 1989.
64. Garty H, Benos DJ: Characteristics and regulatory mechanisms of the amiloride-blockable Na^+. *Physiol Rev* 68:309, 1988.
65. Adrogue HJ, Wilson H, Boyd AEI, et al: Plasma acid-base patterns in diabetic ketoacidosis. *N Engl J Med* 307:1603–1610, 1982.
66. Garella S, Chang BS, Kahn SI: Dilution acidosis and contraction alkalosis: Review of a concept. *Kidney Int* 8:279–285, 1975.
67. Relman AS, Shelburne PF, Talman A: Profound acidosis resulting from excessive ammonium chloride in previously healthy subjects. *N Engl J Med* 40:1621–1627, 1961.
68. Heird WD, Dell RB, Driscoll JM Jr, et al: Metabolic acidosis resulting from intravenous alimentation mixtures containing synthetic amino acids. *N Engl J Med* 287:943–946, 1972.
69. Lemann J Jr, Relman AS: The relation of sulfur metabolism to acid-base balance and electrolyte excretion: The effects of DL-methionine in normal man. *J Clin Invest* 38:2215–2224, 1959.
70. Madias NE: Lactic acidosis. *Kidney Int* 29:752–774, 1986.
71. Kreisberg RA: Lactate homeostasis and lactic acidosis. *Ann Intern Med* 92:227–237, 1980.
72. Malhotra D, Shapiro JI, Chan L: NMR spectroscopy in the differential diagnosis of anion-gap acidosis. *JASN* 2:1046–1050, 1991.
73. Oh MS, Phelps KR, Traube M, et al: D-Lactic acidosis in a man with the short bowel syndrome. *N Engl J Med* 301:249–253, 1979.
74. Cooper DJ, Walley KR, Wiggs BR, Russell JA: Bicarbonate does not improve hemodynamics in critically ill patients who have lactic acidosis. *Ann Intern Med* 112:492–498, 1990.
75. Graf H, Leach W, Arieff AI: Evidence for a detrimental effect of bicarbonate therapy in hypoxic lactic acidosis. *Science* 227:754–756, 1985.
76. Graf H, Leach W, Arieff AI: Metabolic effects of sodium bicarbonate in hypoxic lactic acidosis in dogs. *Am J Physiol* 249:F630–F635, 1985.

77. Kucera R, Whalen M, Shapiro JI: Electroencephalographic consequences of alkalinization therapy during lactic acidosis: Different effects of sodium bicarbonate and Carbicarb. *J Crit Care* 6:71–84, 1991.
78. Stacpoole PW: The pharmacology of dichloroacetate. *Metabolism* 38:1124–1144, 1989.
79. Filley GF, Kindig NB: Carbicarb, an alkalinizing ion generating agent of possible clinical usefulness. *Trans Am Clin Climat Assoc* 96:141–153, 1984.
80. Brandt KR, Miles JM: Relationship between severity of hyperglycemia and metabolic acidosis in diabetic ketoacidosis. *Mayo Clin Proc* 63:1071–1074, 1988.
81. Paulson WD: Anion gap-bicarbonate relation in diabetic ketoacidosis. *Am J Med* 81: 995–1000, 1986.
82. Foster DW, McGarry JD: The metabolic derangements and treatments of diabetic ketoacidosis. *N Engl J Med* 309:159–165, 1983.
83. Oh MS, Carroll HJ, Godstein DA, Fein IA: Hyperchloremic acidosis during the recovery phase of diabetic ketosis. *Ann Intern Med* 89:925–927, 1978.
84. Soler NG, Bennett MA, Dixon K, et al: Potassium balance during treatment of diabetic ketoacidosis with special reference to the use of bicarbonate. *Lancet* 2:665–667, 1972.
85. Kaye R: Diabetic ketoacidosis—the bicarbonate controversy. *J Pediatr* 87:156–159, 1975.
86. Soler NG, Bennett MA, Fitzgerald MG, Malins JM: Successful resuscitation in diabetic ketoacidosis: A strong case for the use of bicarbonate. *Postgrad Med J* 50:465–468, 1974.
87. Matz R: Rationale for not using bicarbonate. *NY State J Med* 76:1299–1303, 1976.
88. Gamba G, Oseguera J, Castrejon M, Gomez-Perez FJ: Bicarbonate therapy in severe diabetic ketoacidosis: A double blind, randomized, placebo controlled trial. *Rev Invest Clin* 43: 234–238, 1991.
89. Stinebaugh BJ, Schloeder FX: Glucose-induced alkalosis in fasting subjects: Relationship to renal bicarbonate reabsorption during fasting and refeeding. *J Clin Invest* 51:1326–1332, 1972.
90. Halperin ML, Hammeke M, Josse RG, et al: Metabolic acidosis in the alcoholic: A pathophysiologic approach. *Metabolism* 32:308–315, 1983.
91. Arieff AI, Carroll HJ: Nonketotic hyperosmolar coma with hyperglycemia: Clinical features, pathophysiology, renal function, acid-base balance, plasma-cerebrospinal fluid equilibria and the effects of therapy in 37 cases. *Medicine* (Baltimore) 51:73–94, 1972.
92. Arieff AI, Carroll HJ: Hyperosmolar nonketotic coma with hyperglycemia: Abnormalities of lipid and carbohydrate metabolism. *Metabolism* 20:529–538, 1971.
93. Halperin ML: Metabolism and acid-base physiology. *Artif Organs* 6:357–362, 1982.
94. Gabow PA: Ethylene glycol. *Am J Kidney Dis* 11:277–279, 1988.
95. Gabow PA, Clay K, Sullivan JB, Lepoff R: Organic acids in ethylene glycol intoxication. *Ann Intern Med* 105:16–20, 1986.
96. McMartin KE, Ambre JJ, Tephly TR: Methanol poisoning in human subjects: Role for formic acid accumulation in the metabolic acidosis. *Am J Med* 68:414–418, 1980.
97. Schelling JR, Howard RL, Winter SD, Linas SL: Increased osmolal gap in alcoholic ketoacidosis and lactic acidosis. *Ann Intern Med* 113:580–582, 1990.
98. Sklar AH, Linas SL: The osmolal gap in renal failure. *Ann Intern Med* 98:481–482, 1983.
99. Streicher HZ, Gabow PA, Moss AH, et al: Syndromes of toluene sniffing in adults. *Ann Intern Med* 94:758–762, 1981.
100. Jacobsen D, Hewlett TP, Webb R, et al: Ethylene glycol intoxication: Evaluation of kinetics and crystalluria. *Am J Med* 84:145–152, 1988.
101. Hill JB: Salicylate intoxication. *N Engl J Med* 288:1110–1116, 1973.
102. Gabow PA, Anderson RJ, Potts DE, Schrier RW: Acid-base disturbances in the salicylate-intoxicated adult. *Arch Intern Med* 138:1481–1484, 1978.
103. Gordon IJ, Bowler CS, Coakley J, Smith P. Algorithm for modified alkaline diuresis in salicylate poisoning. *Br Med J* 289:1039–1040, 1984.
104. Anderson RJ, Potts DE, Gabow PA, Rumack BH, Schrier RW: Unrecognized adult salicylate intoxication. *Ann Intern Med* 85:745–748, 1976.
105. Batlle DC, Sabatini S, Kurtzman NA: On the mechanism of toluene-induced renal tubular acidosis. *Nephron* 49:210–218, 1988.
106. Halperin ML, Ethier JH, Kamel KS: Ammonium excretion in chronic metabolic acidosis: Benefits and risks. *Am J Kidney Dis* 14:267–271, 1989.

107. Molitoris BA, Froment DH, Mackenzie TA, et al: Citrate: A major factor in the toxicity of orally administered aluminum compounds. *Kidney Int* 36:949–953, 1989.
108. Froment DPH, Molitoris BA, Buddington B, et al: Site and mechanism of enhanced gastrointestinal absorption of aluminum by citrate. *Kidney Int* 36:978–984, 1989.
109. Kette F, Weil MH, von-Planta M: Buffer agents do not reverse intramyocardial acidosis during cardiac resuscitation. *Circulation* 81:1660–1666, 1990.
110. Stacpoole PW, Lorenz AC, Thomas RG, Harman EM: Dichloroacetate in the treatment of lactic acidosis. *Ann Intern Med* 108:58–63, 1988.
111. Shapiro JI, Whalen M, Kucera R, et al: Brain pH responses to sodium bicarbonate and Carbicarb during systemic acidosis. *Am J Physiol* 256:H1316–H1321, 1989.
112. Kucera RR, Shapiro JI, Whalen MA, et al: Brain pH effects of $NaHCO_3$ and Carbicarb in lactic acidosis. *Crit Care Med* 17:1320–1321, 1989.
113. Huntley JJA, McCormack M, Jin H, et al: Importance of the tonicity of Carbicarb on the functional and metabolic responses of the acidotic isolated heart. *J Crit Care* 8:222–227, 1993.
114. Shapiro JI, Mathew A, Whalen M, et al: Different effects of sodium bicarbonate and an alternate buffer (Carbicarb) in normal volunteers. *J Crit Care* 5:157–160, 1990.
115. Leung JM, Landow L, Franks M, et al: Safety and efficacy of intravenous Carbicarb in patients undergoing surgery: Comparison with sodium bicarbonate in the treatment of mild metabolic acidosis. SPI Research Group. Study of Perioperative Ischemia. *Crit Care Med* 22:1540–1549, 1994.
116. Adam WR, Craik DJ, Kneen M, Wellard RM: Effect of magnesium depletion and potassium depletion and chlorothiazide on intracellular pH in the rat, studied by 31P NMR. *Clin Exp Pharmacol Physiol* 16:33–40, 1989.
117. Shapiro JI, Anderson RJ: Sodium Depletion States. In Brenner BM, Stein J (eds): *Topics in Nephrology*. New York, Churchill Livingstone, 1985, pp 155–192.
118. Kassirer JP, Berkman PM, Lawrenz DR, et al: The critical role of chloride in the correction of hypokalemic alkalosis in man. *Am J Med* 38:172–181, 1965.
119. Melby JC: Assessment of adrenocortical function. *N Engl J Med* 285:735–739, 1971.
120. Garella S, Chazan JA, Cohen JJ: Saline-resistant metabolic alkalosis or "chloride-wasting nephropathy": Report of four patients with severe potassium depletion. *Ann Intern Med* 73:31–38, 1970.
121. Adam WR, Koretsky AP, Weiner MW: Measurement of renal intracellular pH by 31P NMR: Relationship of pH to ammoniagenesis. *Contrib Nephrol* 47:15–21, 1985.
122. Kassirer JP, Schwartz WB: Correction of metabolic alkalosis in man without repair of potassium deficiency: A reevaluation of the role of potassium. *Am J Med* 40:10–18, 1966.
123. Lucci MS, Tinker JP, Weiner IM, DuBose TD Jr: Function of proximal tubule carbonic anhydrase defined by selective inhibition. *Am J Physiol* 245:F443–449, 1983.
124. Greenbaum DM: Secondary cardiac dysrhythmias. *Heart Lung* 6:308–316, 1977.
125. Miller RB: Central nervous system manifestations of fluid and electrolyte disturbances. *Surg Clin North Am* 48:381–393, 1968.
126. Madias NE, Ayus JC, Adrogue HJ: Increased anion gap in metabolic alkalosis: The role of plasma-protein equivalency. *N Engl J Med* 300:1421–1423, 1979.
127. Kassirer JP, Schwartz WB: The response of normal man to selective depletion of hydrochloric acid: Factors in the genesis of persistent gastric alkalosis. *Am J Med* 40:10–18, 1966.
128. Babior BM: Villous adenoma of the colon: Study of a patient with severe fluid and electrolyte disturbances. *Am J Med* 41:615–622, 1966.
129. Jamison RL, Ross JC, Kempson RL, et al: Surreptitious diuretic ingestion and pseudo-Bartter's syndrome. *Am J Med* 73:142–150, 1982.
130. Brackett NC Jr, Wingo CF, Muren O, Solano JT: Acid-base response to chronic hypercapnia in man. *N Engl J Med* 280:124–130, 1969.
131. Gottleib RP: Metabolic alkalosis in cystic fibrosis. *J Pediatr* 79:930–938, 1971.
132. Kassirer JP, London AM, Goldman DM, et al: On the pathogenesis of metabolic alkalosis in hyperaldosteronism. *Am J Med* 49:306–312, 1970.
133. Bartter FC, Pronove P, Gill JR Jr: Hyperplasia of the juxtaglomerular complex with hyperaldosteronism and hypokalemic alkalosis. *Am J Med* 33:811–822, 1962.

134. Bartter FC: So-called Bartter's syndrome. *N Engl J Med* 281:1483–1484, 1969.
135. Blachley JD, Knochel JP: Tobacco chewer's hypokalemia: Licorice revisited. *N Engl J Med* 302:784–785, 1980.
136. Farese RV Jr, Biglieri EG, Shackleton CH, et al: Licorice-induced hypermineralocorticoidism. *N Engl J Med* 325:1223–1227, 1991.
137. Rahilly GT, Berl T: Severe metabolic alkalosis caused by administration of plasma protein fraction in end-stage renal failure. *N Engl J Med* 301:824–826, 1979.
138. Ohrwoll ES: The milk-alkali syndrome: Current concepts. *Ann Intern Med* 97:242–250, 1982.
139. Heinemann HO: Metabolic alkalosis in patients with hypercalcemia. *Metabolism* 14: 1137–1152, 1965.
140. Lipner HI, Ruzany F, Dasgupta M, et al: The behavior of carbenicillin as a non-reabsorbable anion. *JLCM* 86:183–185, 1975.
141. Morrison RS: Management of emergencies: 8. Metabolic acidosis and alkalosis. *N Engl J Med* 274:1195–1197, 1966.
142. Barton CH, Vaziri ND, Ness RL: Cimetidine in the management of metabolic alkalosis induced by nasogastric drainage. *Arch Surg* 114:70–72, 1979.

4

Pathogenesis and Management of Respiratory and Mixed Acid-Base Disorders

William D. Kaehny

Respiratory acid-base disorders are caused by primary changes from normal in excretion of carbon dioxide (CO_2) by the lungs. Primary means that the changes are not secondary to changes in pH caused by metabolic acid-base disorders. Under usual metabolic conditions, the body makes 13,000 to 15,000 mmol of CO_2 per day from the catabolism of carbohydrate, protein, and fat. If the lungs excrete this amount, the quantity of CO_2 in the body remains the same. This is reflected by the amount of CO_2 dissolved in blood and the partial pressure of the CO_2 gas in equilibrium with it (PCO_2). A small amount of the dissolved CO_2 reacts with water to form carbonic acid (H_2CO_3), the acid part of the Henderson-Hasselbalch acid-base equation discussed in Chapter 3 and in detail elsewhere [1]. It is simpler to use the PCO_2 in arterial blood ($PaCO_2$) to represent the respiratory or acid component of this equation:

$$pH \leftarrow \frac{[HCO_3{}^-]}{PaCO_2}$$

If the lungs fail to excrete the daily production or, for that matter, excrete more than the daily production of CO_2, the quantity of CO_2 in the body changes, and therefore the amount dissolved in the blood and the pressure it generates (PCO_2) change in the same direction. This change generates either of the two simple (or primary) respiratory acid-base disorders: Hypercapnia, or high CO_2 level, generates respiratory acidosis; hypocapnia, or low CO_2 level, generates respiratory alkalosis.

The whole body responds to this imbalance between CO_2 production (rarely inhalation) and CO_2 excretion via effective ventilation in a programmed fashion. In step 1, the pH change causes rapid chemical *buffering*. Buffers within cells either take up hydrogen ions (H^+), producing a bicarbonate ($HCO_3{}^-$) in the blood or give up H^+ to titrate (consume) $HCO_3{}^-$ in the blood. In step 2, the abnormal blood PCO_2 alters the renal tubular cell PCO_2, causing changes in H^+ secretion that result in changes in renal net acid excretion (NAE) that, in turn, raise or lower blood [$HCO_3{}^-$]. We call this process by its traditional name of *compensation*, but it is more of an *adaptation* to a new state of CO_2 balance. This process takes days to reach a new steady state. Thus, it occurs only in *chronic* respiratory acid-base disorders. In step 3, the respiratory system *corrects* the problem and restores the whole-body CO_2 content and the arterial PCO_2 ($PaCO_2$) to previously normal values. Obviously, this can occur only if the causative disorder is cured or corrected. Notably, changes in oxygen (O_2) supply and demand and the PaO_2 do not define respiratory acid-base disorders, but they can cause both respiratory acid-base disorders and metabolic acidosis through their effects on respiratory drive and lactic acid metabolism [2].

Respiratory Acidosis

Respiratory acidosis is a disorder caused by processes that increase PCO_2 and thereby lead to a decrease in the pH. The PCO_2 increases when the lungs fail to excrete metabolically produced CO_2. Since CO_2 production does not change significantly in most circumstances, a decrease in effective alveolar ventilation is the usual way that the PCO_2 is increased. Effective alveolar ventilation can be diminished in two major ways, namely, by decreased minute ventilation and ventilation-perfusion inequality [3].

With decreased effective alveolar ventilation, CO_2 excretion falls short of production, and the quantity of CO_2 carried per milliliter of blood increases, as reflected in an increased $PaCO_2$. When a steady state of hypercapnia is reached, the ventilatory excretion of CO_2 again equals production. This new state occurs because the quantity of CO_2 carried to the pulmonary vascular bed is increased to a degree sufficient to allow the CO_2 excretion to equal the rate of production despite decreased effective alveolar ventilation. In other words, with hypercapnia, the quantity of CO_2 per milliliter of exhaled gas is increased.

When the $PaCO_2$ rises, the amount of dissolved CO_2 increases and shifts the equilibrium reaction to favor the production of H_2CO_3; thus, $CO_2 + H_2O \rightleftharpoons H_2CO_3$. This increased acid results in a fall in pH or respiratory acidosis. This process can be visualized more simply as a rise in $PaCO_2$, which reduces the ratio of the HCO_3^- concentration to the $PaCO_2$, thereby causing a fall in pH:

$$\downarrow pH \leftarrow \frac{[HCO_3^-]}{\uparrow PaCO_2}$$

The chemistry of these reactions is discussed in Chapter 3 and in detail in standard physiology and acid-base texts [4].

Pathophysiology of Respiratory Acidosis

Buffering

The immediate response to the low pH generated by the increased $PaCO_2$ and H_2CO_3 is to buffer (or bind) hydrogen ions with nonbicarbonate buffers. Bicarbonate does not work as an effective buffer in this situation because it reacts with hydrogen ion to form H_2CO_3, which is the original culprit. In the extracellular fluid (ECF) space, proteins constitute the only buffer; while within the cells, hemoglobin, phosphate, proteins, and lactate are the major nonbicarbonate buffers; 97 percent of the buffering of H_2CO_3 derives from intracellular rather than ECF buffers [5].

Renal Compensation

The whole-body compensation for respiratory acidosis resides solely in the kidneys. The kidneys respond to the increased systemic PCO_2 by increasing the production and excretion of ammonium (NH_4^+). Through the process described in Chapter 3, this generates new HCO_3^-, which results in a rise in plasma $[HCO_3^-]$. The increased urinary NH_4^+ excretion is balanced by increased Cl^- excretion with resultant fall in plasma $[Cl^-]$. When a steady state of hypercapnia is reached, chloride excretion returns to normal and equals intake. NH_4^+ excretion also returns to normal, even though H^+ secretion remains increased. The persistently increased H^+ secretion is needed to reclaim the increased filtered HCO_3^- load that results from the increase in plasma concentration [6, 7]. The chemical buffering and renal compensation that occur with chronic respiratory acidosis are diagramed in Figure 4-1.

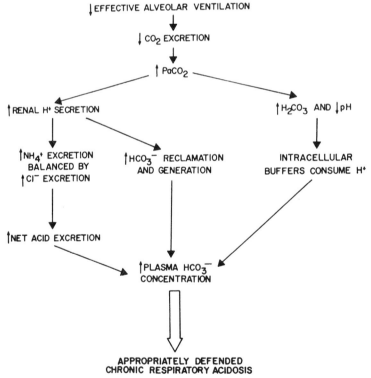

Fig. 4-1. Pathophysiology of chronic respiratory acidosis. Chemical buffering and renal compensation combine to elevate the plasma $[HCO_3^-]$. The renal mechanisms involve an adaptive increase in ammonium and chloride excretion until the new steady state is reached.

Correction of Respiratory Acidosis

The third, or corrective, response to respiratory acidosis is the restoration of effective ventilation. Correction or amelioration of an acute neurologic process causing hypoventilation, or of a ventilatory or gas-exchange defect, may be possible. Unfortunately, most processes that result in chronic hypercapnia are due to irreversible parenchymal lung damage and thus at best can be corrected only partially.

In metabolic acidosis, the corrective agent, the kidney, is sometimes a cause of the disorder, as in uremic acidosis, but other times is not, as in diabetic ketoacidosis. In respiratory acidosis, however, the respiratory system, which includes neural control, mechanical, circulatory, and membrane exchange components, always is involved as the cause of the disorder and is also the corrective agent.

Acute Respiratory Acidosis (Acute Hypercapnia)

Acute respiratory acidosis results from acute alveolar hypoventilation with a primary elevation of the $PaCO_2$, when only the buffering defense has had time to come into play. While buffering occurs almost immediately, the renal response does not exert a noticeable influence for 12 to 24 hours [8]. This is the period of time in which pure acute respiratory acidosis is observed. An appropriate defense of pH in acute respiratory acidosis is characterized by an elevation of the plasma $[HCO_3^-]$ by about 1 mmol/L (above 24) for each 10 mm Hg acute increment in $PaCO_2$ (above 40) [9]:

$$\Delta[HCO_3^-] = (\Delta PaCO_2/10) \pm 3$$

Clinical Features and Systemic Effects of Acute Respiratory Acidosis

The acute onset of hypercapnia invariably is accompanied by hypoxemia, which usually dominates the clinical picture. Depending on the underlying disorder and the state of consciousness, the patient may present with the signs and symptoms of acute respiratory distress, including marked restlessness, tachypnea, and marked dyspnea. As the process worsens, stupor and eventually coma develop. CO_2 has vasodilating properties, and thus hypercapnia is associated with increased cerebral blood flow. This increase in blood flow to the brain probably accounts for the headaches and occasional signs of increased intracranial pressure that can occur with both acute and chronic hypercapnia [10, 11]. Severe acute respiratory acidosis can cause refractory hypotension through two mechanisms [12]. First, cardiac contractility is reduced, and cardiac output falls. Second, peripheral arterial smooth muscle relaxes, causing vasodilation and decreased systemic vascular resistance. Modest acute increases in $PaCO_2$ (10–15 mm Hg) actually increase cardiac output as well as pulmonary artery pressure [13].

Laboratory Findings in Acute Respiratory Acidosis

The arterial blood reflects the pathophysiologic state with an elevated PCO_2, a moderately elevated plasma $[HCO_3^-]$ (<30 mmol/L), and a low pH. If the patient is breathing room air, the PaO_2 will be decreased. The venous serum electrolytes

Table 4-1. Causes of acute respiratory acidosis

Neuromuscular abnormalities
    Brain stem injury
    High cord injury
    Guillain-Barré syndrome
    Myasthenia gravis
    Botulism
    Narcotic, sedative, or tranquilizer overdose
    Status epilepticus
    Postoperative hyponatremia with herniation
Airway obstruction
    Foreign body
    Aspiration of vomitus
    Laryngeal edema
    Severe bronchospasm
Thoracic-pulmonary disorders
    Flail chest
    Pneumothorax
    Severe pneumonia
    Smoke inhalation
    Severe pulmonary edema
Vascular disease
    Massive pulmonary embolism
Respirator-controlled ventilation
    Inadequate frequency, tidal volume settings
    Large dead space
    Total parenteral nutrition (increased CO_2 production)

reveal a modestly elevated total CO_2 content, with usually normal plasma concentrations of sodium, potassium, and chloride [9].

Causes of Acute Respiratory Acidosis

Some of the causes of acute respiratory failure, which leads to acute CO_2 retention, are listed in Table 4-1.

Treatment of Acute Respiratory Acidosis

The key to treatment of acute respiratory acidosis is the restoration of effective ventilation. Modest amounts of sodium bicarbonate ($NaHCO_3$) may be given intravenously to mitigate severe acidosis; the latter is only a holding measure to prevent the serious cardiovascular effects of marked acidosis until definitive therapy is established [14]. Because equilibration of HCO_3^- across the blood-brain barrier is markedly slower than that of CO_2, a delay in the correction of the cerebral pH may occur, and cerebrospinal fluid pH falls initially [15].

Chronic Respiratory Acidosis (Chronic Hypercapnia)

Chronic respiratory acidosis is caused by chronic decreased effective alveolar ventilation with a primary elevation of the $PaCO_2$. The duration of the elevation of

PaCO$_2$ must be sufficient to permit adaptation of the renal mechanisms to be maximized. In the dog, a new steady state of blood acid-base values occurs 5 days after the onset of hypercapnia [8]. The exact time interval needed to establish "chronic" hypercapnia in humans has not been established. A quantitative relationship has been described between the steady-state PaCO$_2$ and the H$^+$ concentration in patients with chronic hypercapnia. This relationship is linear and is described by a slope of about 0.25 nmol of H$^+$ per 1 mm Hg increase in PaCO$_2$ [16, 17]. A clinical guide for bedside use expresses the relationship between PaCO$_2$ and plasma [HCO$_3$$^-$] in chronic hypercapnia as follows: For each increment of 10 mm Hg in PaCO$_2$, the plasma [HCO$_3$$^-$] rises by 4 mmol/L, with a range of 4 mmol/L in either direction. The following formula summarizes this rule of thumb:

$$\Delta \text{ plasma [HCO}_3{}^-] = 4 \times \frac{\Delta \text{PaCO}_2}{10} \pm 4 \text{ mmol/L}$$

Clinical Features and Systemic Effects of Chronic Respiratory Acidosis

Patients with chronic respiratory acidosis exhibit few if any signs or symptoms related directly to the CO$_2$ retention and acidosis. However, papilledema and other neurologic disturbances have been described in several patients [18, 19]. The signs and symptoms of the chronic pulmonary disease, with or without cor pulmonale, usually predominate. Chronic respiratory acidosis causes decreased bone mineralization, although to a lesser degree than does metabolic acidosis [20]. This effect does not appear to be mediated by altered function of bone osteoclasts or osteoblasts [21].

Laboratory Findings in Chronic Respiratory Acidosis

Arterial blood examination reveals a low pH (not less than 7.25 even with severe chronic CO$_2$ retention), an elevated PaCO$_2$, and an elevated plasma [HCO$_3$$^-$]. Plasma sodium and potassium concentrations are usually normal. Total plasma CO$_2$ content is elevated, and plasma chloride concentration is reciprocally decreased. The anion gap is usually normal [16]. The urine pH is usually acid.

Causes of Chronic Respiratory Acidosis

Chronic respiratory acidosis is seen most commonly in patients with chronic obstructive airway disease. However, any condition that can lead to chronic retention of CO$_2$ [22] will cause the same acid-base disturbance. Examples of such conditions are given in Table 4-2.

Treatment of Chronic Respiratory Disease

Chronic respiratory acidosis can be corrected effectively only by restoring or improving the ability of the respiratory system to excrete CO$_2$. This is often impossible because of an irreversible pathologic condition. However, adequate airway drainage, relief of bronchospasm, and treatment of pulmonary infections and congestive heart failure may lead to significant improvement. Because the arterial pH remains above 7.25 even with chronic PaCO$_2$ elevations to 110 mm Hg [23], the acidosis per se

Table 4-2. Causes of chronic respiratory acidosis

Neuromuscular abnormalities
    Chronic narcotic or sedative ingestion
    Primary hypoventilation
    Pickwickian syndrome
    Poliomyelitis
    Diaphragmatic paralysis
    Hypothyroidism
    Sleep apnea syndrome
Thoracic-pulmonary disorders
    Chronic obstructive airway disease
    Kyphoscoliosis
    End-stage interstitial pulmonary disease

is not dangerous, although the patient is at more risk for serious acidemia if metabolic acidosis occurs. Attention to the maintenance of adequate oxygen tension (PO_2) is the critical need. Acidosis does cause constriction of venous capacitance vessels, and thus any fluid administration may acutely expand central blood volume and cause cardiac decompensation and pulmonary edema. Utmost caution should therefore be taken during fluid administration to patients with any form of respiratory acidosis.

Acute Hypercapnia Superimposed on Chronic Respiratory Acidosis

When a patient in a steady state of chronic hypercapnia suffers a new insult to his or her ability to excrete CO_2, the $PaCO_2$ rises acutely to a new level. Thus the plasma [HCO_3^-] and blood pH will be lower than predicted for a given chronic level of $PaCO_2$. However, the change in pH is not as great as would be expected for a similar acute increment in $PaCO_2$ occurring in a previously normal person. That is, the pH is better protected against an acute rise in $PaCO_2$ when there is a background of chronic respiratory acidosis than it is with acute respiratory acidosis alone [24, 25]. The mechanism for this is not entirely clear but has been attributed partially to the physicochemical effect of the preexisting higher [HCO_3^-], which would reduce the fall in pH as compared with that seen for a similar increment in $PaCO_2$ in a patient with a normal [HCO_3^-]. In addition, the kidney rapidly increases H^+ excretion when an acute rise in PCO_2 is superimposed on chronic respiratory acidosis. This is in contrast to acute respiratory acidosis alone, in which renal acid excretion makes little quantitative contribution to H^+ balance.

    Treatment is directed toward correction of the acute disorder and providing supplemental oxygen. Doxapram hydrochloride may help patients with chronic CO_2 retention with an acute worsening to avoid mechanical ventilation until treatment of the underlying disorder can have effect. This agent works by stimulating both central and peripheral chemoreceptors to enhance respiratory rate and tidal volume. Case reports describe decreases in $PaCO_2$ of as much as 60 mm Hg [26].

Respiratory Alkalosis

Respiratory alkalosis is caused by a process that leads to a rise in pH due to a primary decrease in the $PaCO_2$. The $PaCO_2$ can fall only if the excretion of CO_2 by the lungs exceeds the production of CO_2 by metabolic processes. Because the production of CO_2 usually remains relatively constant, a negative CO_2 balance results primarily from increased alveolar ventilation. Hyperventilation can result from two processes: (1) increased neurochemical stimulation of ventilation by central or peripheral neural mechanisms and (2) ventilation physically increased, either artificially with mechanical ventilators or voluntarily with increased conscious effort. Alveolar hyperventilation produces increased CO_2 excretion, which reduces the $PaCO_2$ and H_2CO_3. This fall in $PaCO_2$ increases the ratio of the $[HCO_3^-]$ to $PaCO_2$, which results in a rise in the pH of the blood, that is, alkalemia.

$$\uparrow pH \leftarrow \frac{[HCO_3^-]}{\downarrow PaCO_2}$$

The buffering response constitutes the *acute* phase of respiratory alkalosis, whereas the renal response to hypocapnia defines the *chronic* stage of respiratory alkalosis.

Pathophysiology of Respiratory Alkalosis

Buffering

Buffering constitutes the first response in respiratory alkalosis. In order to return the pH toward normal in the face of the decreased H_2CO_3 or $PaCO_2$, the plasma $[HCO_3^-]$ must be decreased. Therefore, H^+ is released from body buffers, and the plasma $[HCO_3^-]$ is reduced by the following net reaction:

$$H^+ + HCO_3^- \rightarrow CO_2 + H_2O$$

Intracellular buffers supply about 99 percent of the H^+, while plasma proteins contribute about 1 percent to the buffering effort [5]. Cellular metabolism contributes by increasing the production of lactic acid and possibly of slight amounts of other organic acids. Lactate concentration increased by 0.5 mmol/L in a study in anesthetized patients; this represents about 10 percent of the total buffering effort. Buffering is completed within minutes, and the steady state persists for at least 2 hours [27]. The alacrity of the response is critical, since the $PaCO_2$ can decrease abruptly, and without buffering, life-threatening alkalemia would occur. The quantitative change in plasma $[HCO_3^-]$ is not great, however, and the pH therefore may rise markedly. The arterial $[HCO_3^-]$ fell to as low as 18 mmol/L at $PaCO_2$ levels of 15 to 20 mm Hg in anesthetized patients [27]. A rule of thumb for acute respiratory alkalosis is that the $[HCO_3^-]$ should decrease by 1 mmol/L for each 10 mm Hg decrement in $PaCO_2$:

$$\Delta[HCO_3^-] = 1 \times (\Delta PaCO_2/10) \pm 3$$

Renal Compensation

The second adaptive response in respiratory alkalosis is handled by a renal mechanism. The kidney attempts to lower the plasma [HCO_3^-] in either of two ways: by decreasing the reclamation of filtered HCO_3^-, thus leading to bicarbonaturia, or by reducing the generation of new HCO_3^- to replace that consumed in the daily buffering of the dietary metabolic acid load. In animals, the kidney appears to make the second choice, because a decreased NH_4^+ excretion without an increased HCO_3^- excretion occurs during the phase of adaptation to chronic hypocapnia. This reduction in excretion of NH_4^+, a cation, is balanced electrochemically by increased sodium or potassium excretion [28]. After a new steady state is reached, excretion of these electrolytes returns to normal. The process of renal adaptation appears to occur rapidly and is probably completed within 24 to 48 hours [28]. In humans, the early stage of renal adaptation for prolonged hypocapnia is characterized by bicarbonaturia, natriuresis, and decreased NH_4^+ and titratable acid excretion [29, 30]. The stimulus for this renal response appears to be independent of systemic pH changes but is a direct effect of the $PaCO_2$ level on renal reabsorption of anion, either HCO_3^- or chloride [31, 32]. The chemical buffering and proposed renal response in respiratory alkalosis are diagrammed in Figure 4-2.

The quantitative contribution of the kidney to pH defense is difficult to judge in humans. Subjects with hypocapnia due to voluntary hyperventilation or altitude hypoxemia had decreases in plasma [HCO_3^-] of 2.1 to 4.9 mmol/L per 10 mm Hg decrease in $PaCO_2$ during 1 to 11 days of hypocapnia [29, 30, 33, 39]. Their arterial pH remained frankly alkalemic. However, some studies of lifelong, high-altitude dwellers have shown decreased plasma [HCO_3^-] sufficient to produce pH values of 7.4 with $PaCO_2$ levels as low as 28 to 30 mm Hg [35–37]. For clinical purposes, a useful rule is to diagnose simple chronic respiratory alkalosis when plasma [HCO_3^-] is decreased 4 mmol/L below 24 for each 10 mm Hg chronic decrement below 40 in the $PaCO_2$.

$$\Delta[HCO_3^-] = 4 \times (\Delta PaCO_2/10) \pm 2$$

Correction of Respiratory Alkalosis

The third, or corrective, response in respiratory alkalosis entails correction of the hyperventilation that maintains the negative CO_2 balance. This, of course, is dependent on removal of the neurohumoral stimulus to the respiratory center or on cessation of mechanical or voluntary hyperventilation. The latter is easier to achieve since neural stimulation of ventilation often is due to pathophysiologic processes that are difficult to correct.

Clinical Features and Systemic Effects of Respiratory Alkalosis

Hypocapnia may be manifested by symptoms and signs of neuromuscular irritability. Patients may complain of perioral and extremity paresthesias, muscle cramps, and

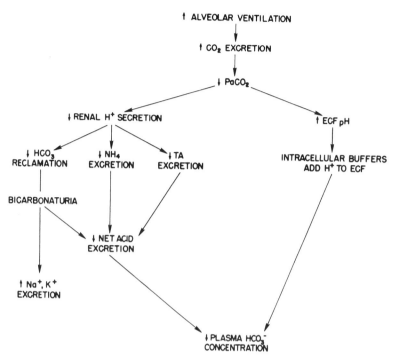

Fig. 4-2. Pathophysiology of chronic respiratory alkalosis. Intracellular buffers donate H+ to the ECF to produce a small decrease in plasma [HCO$_3$−] during acute hypocapnia. The net effect on renal function of prolonged hypocapnia is a decrease in H+ secretion, which results in a fall in net acid excretion below the level necessary to maintain acid balance. Thus plasma [HCO$_3$−] falls. Urinary acid and electrolyte excretion return to normal after steady-state PaCO$_2$ and [HCO$_3$−] are achieved.

even tinnitus. Hyperreflexia, tetany, and even seizures may occur [38, 39]. Hypocapnia causes cerebral vasoconstriction with reduced blood flow, which may have deleterious and even fatal effects on the brain, especially in patients with sickle cell disease [40–43]. Marked alkalemia may cause serious, refractory cardiac arrhythmias and electrocardiographic changes of ischemia [44–48].

Laboratory Findings with Respiratory Alkalosis

If arterial blood pH is increased, a decreased PaCO$_2$ and plasma [HCO$_3$−] are diagnostic of respiratory alkalosis. Venous serum total CO$_2$ content reflects the decrease in [HCO$_3$−], and chloride concentration is slightly increased. Serum potassium is increased by an average of 0.3 mmol/L in acute respiratory alkalosis. This effect appears to be stimulated by the buffering-induced fall in [HCO$_3$−], which activates the α-adrenergic system [49] (see also Chap. 5). Serum phosphorus concentration may decrease only slightly or to seriously low levels [50, 51] (see Chap. 6). Urine pH is not clinically informative. It may be relatively alkaline (>6.0) during the onset of acute hypocapnia but then fluctuate into the more acidic range, as in the eucapnic state [29].

Differential Diagnosis of Respiratory Alkalosis

Respiratory alkalosis is the most common acid-base disorder among seriously ill patients [52]. The reason for this is apparent from a review of the list of causes of respiratory alkalosis (Table 4-3).

Central stimulation of the medullary respiratory center occurs with anxiety, pain, pregnancy, febrile states, and salicylate intoxication. Mechanical irritation by brain trauma or tumor is another respiratory stimulant.

Stimulation of the peripheral pathways to the medullary respiratory center occurs in pulmonary-thoracic disorders that cause hypoxemia with relatively unimpaired CO_2 transport, in altitude hypoxemia, in asthma [53], and in disorders that decrease lung compliance (stiff lung) without necessarily causing hypoxemia.

Mechanical ventilation may produce respiratory alkalosis if the rate and tidal volume are set so that pulmonary excretion of CO_2 is allowed to exceed CO_2 production. However, increased minute ventilation is often necessary in order to deliver adequate quantities of oxygen to patients with severe pulmonary insufficiency.

Patients with hepatic cirrhosis often have respiratory alkalosis [54, 55]. The mechanism is probably multifactorial [56], although increased pulmonary shunting [57], hyponatremia [58], and increased blood ammonia levels [59] have been implicated. Respiratory alkalosis is an early manifestation of gram-negative sepsis and other

Table 4-3. Causes of respiratory alkalosis

Central stimulation of respiration
    Anxiety
    Head trauma
    Brain tumors or vascular accidents
    Salicylates
    Fever
    Pain
    Pregnancy
Peripheral stimulation of respiration
    Pulmonary emboli
    Congestive heart failure
    Interstitial lung diseases
    Pneumonia
    "Stiff lungs" without hypoxemia
    Altitude
    Asthma
Multiple mechanisms
    Hepatic insufficiency
    Gram-negative septicemia
Mechanical or voluntary hyperventilation

Table 4-4. Mixed acid-base disorders

Disorders	Adaptation	pH
Inadequate response		
Metabolic acidosis and respiratory acidosis	$PaCO_2$ too high and $[HCO_3^-]$ too low for simple disorders	↓↓
Metabolic alkalosis and respiratory alkalosis	$PaCO_2$ too low and $[HCO_3^-]$ too high for simple disorders	↑↑
Excessive response		
Metabolic acidosis and respiratory alkalosis	$PaCO_2$ too low and $[HCO_3^-]$ too low for simple disorders	Normal or slightly ↓ or ↑
Metabolic alkalosis and respiratory acidosis	$PaCO_2$ too high and $[HCO_3^-]$ too high for simple disorders	Normal or slightly ↑ or ↓
Triple disorders		
Metabolic alkalosis, metabolic acidosis, and either respiratory acidosis or alkalosis	$PaCO_2$ and $[HCO_3^-]$ not appropriate for simple disorders and anion gap >17 mEq/L	Variable

forms of shock, and the clinician should therefore suspect these processes in the appropriate clinical setting [60].

Treatment of Respiratory Alkalosis

The only definitive treatment is to correct or ameliorate the basic disorder responsible for the hyperventilation. Correcting significant hypoxemia is more critical for the patient's well-being than is correcting the acid-base disturbance.

If alkalemia is causing deleterious neuromuscular or cardiac rhythm problems in a patient on mechanical ventilation, decreasing the minute ventilation or increasing the dead space may be effective. If this cannot be done without compromising oxygenation, the use of an inhaled gas mixture containing 3% CO_2 may be helpful for short periods of time [61]. Use of morphine to decrease hyperventilation and alleviate anxiety is reasonable if adequate oxygenation is insured. The morphine effect can be rapidly reversed with naloxone.

Mixed Acid-Base Disorders

Mixed acid-base disorders occur when two or even three primary events act to alter the acid-base state at the same time. Five double and two triple mixed acid-base disorders can occur as listed in Table 4-4. The two primary respiratory acid-base disorders, respiratory acidosis and respiratory alkalosis, cannot coexist.

Diagnosis of Mixed Acid-Base Disorders

A mixed acid-base disorder can be suspected from the clinical setting (e.g., a patient with cor pulmonale on diuretics) and can be diagnosed from arterial blood studies.

The key to the diagnosis of a mixed disturbance is the clear understanding of the expected compensation in the primary, uncomplicated acid-base disorders. If the compensation is appropriate, the disorder is simple; if they are out of the expected range for an uncomplicated, primary disorder, a mixed disorder is suspected. To determine whether compensation is appropriate for a given disorder, it is essential to know the expected response. Table 3-1 shows the expected directional changes in pH, $PaCO_2$, and plasma $[HCO_3^-]$ for each simple disorder. Rules of thumb for estimating the expected changes in these values are listed in Table 3-2. If a given set of blood acid-base values does not fall within the range of the expected response for that acid-base disorder, a mixed disorder should be suspected.

Certain of the mixed acid-base disorders may cause dangerous deviations of pH from normal, whereas others may produce pH values within the normal range. The dangerous combinations are those in which the primary disorders block the compensation for each other. For example, the hypercapnia of respiratory acidosis prevents the adaptive hypocapnia of metabolic acidosis, and the hypobicarbonatemia of metabolic acidosis blocks the adaptive rise in plasma $[HCO_3^-]$ expected in respiratory acidosis. The dangerous disorders thus are characterized by *failure of compensation* (see Table 4-4).

The "benign" mixed acid-base disorders are those in which the primary disorders provide *excessive compensation* for each other (see Table 4-4). For example, salicylate intoxication may produce acidosis, such as a plasma $[HCO_3^-]$ of 10 mmol/L or a reduction of 14 mmol/L below normal sea-level values. Application of the rule of thumb for metabolic acidosis (see Table 3-2) predicts the maximum fall in $PaCO_2$ to be $1.5 \times 14 = 21$ mm Hg. Thus, a $PaCO_2$ of less than 19 mm Hg $(40 - 21)$ would not be appropriate for simple metabolic acidosis. Salicylate has a primary stimulating effect on ventilation, however, and may produce sufficient hyperventilation to lower the $PaCO_2$ to 14 mm Hg in this example. Thus, the primary hypocapnia would result in excessive compensation for the fall in $[HCO_3^-]$ and pH produced by salicylate intoxication. Reciprocally, the fall in $[HCO_3^-]$ would be greater than that predicted as appropriate for respiratory alkalosis (see Table 3-2).

A nomogram for interpreting acid-base variables is displayed in Figure 3-3. A point falling outside the indicated predictive bands suggests the presence of a mixed acid-base disorder. Since, however, a mixed disorder also may result in a set of acid-base variables falling within a band, as discussed in the figure legend, acid-base variables must be interpreted in light of the entire clinical circumstances and not as an isolated set of numbers.

Common Mixed Acid-Base Disorders

Respiratory Acidosis and Metabolic Alkalosis

Patients with chronic lung diseases that produce CO_2 retention and respiratory acidosis often develop congestive heart failure. If diuretics are used to treat the heart failure, the plasma $[HCO_3^-]$ may rise to levels greater than those appropriate for renal compensation in chronic respiratory acidosis (see Table 3-2 and Fig. 3-3). The pH may rise to the normal range or even to frankly elevated levels. These changes may finally result in a set of acid-base variables appropriate for simple metabolic alkalosis, for example, plasma $[HCO_3^-]$, 48 mmol; $PaCO_2$, 60 mm Hg; pH, 7.52. Clinical information indicated, however, that this particular set of laboratory values resulted from the coexistence of two primary acid-base disorders: chronic respiratory acidosis, with a primary increase in $PaCO_2$ and secondary compensatory rise in plasma $[HCO_3^-]$, and metabolic alkalosis, with a primary increase in $[HCO_3^-]$ above the expected level for chronic respiratory acidosis.

Difficulty in interpreting the acid-base variables may arise if clinical information is not available or not clear as to the existence of lung disease with chronic CO_2 retention. In that instance, it is helpful to observe the patient's response to the cessation of diuretics and administration of sodium and potassium chloride. This treatment will correct simple metabolic alkalosis (see Chap. 3) but achieve only some improvement in the $PaCO_2$ in the mixed disorder. A large alveolar-arterial PO_2 gradient (>15 mm Hg) indicates lung disease and is suggestive of some component of respiratory acidosis.

Although this mixed disorder is one of the excessive compensation variety in which pH does not deviate markedly from normal, it should be treated to maintain the PaO_2 at the best attainable level. The increase in plasma $[HCO_3^-]$ and concomitant rise in pH due to diuretic-induced metabolic alkalosis are sufficient to suppress ventilation in patients with chronic respiratory acidosis, thus causing a decrease in PaO_2 [62]. Treatment of this mixed disorder should be directed at lowering the plasma $[HCO_3^-]$ through sodium chloride and potassium chloride therapy, which best allows the kidney to excrete HCO_3^- retained as a result of diuretic-induced metabolic alkalosis (see Chap. 3). Of course, this therapy must be used with caution to avoid exacerbating the congestive heart failure. Although the pH will fall to acidemic levels, this is beneficial inasmuch as it stimulates ventilation, thus increasing PaO_2 and decreasing $PaCO_2$. In any event, pH in chronic respiratory acidosis is well defended and does not fall below 7.25, as discussed earlier [23].

Respiratory Acidosis and Metabolic Acidosis

Mixed respiratory and metabolic acidosis may develop in patients with cardiorespiratory arrest, in patients with chronic lung disease who are in shock, and in patients with metabolic acidosis of any type who develop respiratory failure. This mixed disorder is a failure of compensation (see Table 4-4). The respiratory disorder prevents the fall in $PaCO_2$ expected in the defense against metabolic acidosis. The metabolic disorder prevents the buffering and renal mechanisms from raising the plasma $[HCO_3^-]$ as expected in the defense against respiratory acidosis. In the absence of these responses the pH falls profoundly, even when the changes in plasma $[HCO_3^-]$ and $PaCO_2$ are only moderate.

If the respiratory acidosis is less severe than the metabolic acidosis, the $PaCO_2$ may be normal or even reduced, but not to the level appropriate for the respiratory response expected for the metabolic acidosis. If the respiratory acidosis predominates over the metabolic acidosis, plasma $[HCO_3^-]$ is normal or even increased but not to the level expected for the degree of CO_2 retention, thus indicating a mixed disturbance. This mixed acid-base disorder should be treated with attention to both the respiratory and the metabolic acidosis. Mechanical ventilation may be needed to reduce the $PaCO_2$. As respiratory treatment is instituted, $NaHCO_3$ may be administered intravenously to treat the metabolic component of the acidosis while the specific etiology and treatment are sought [14].

Respiratory Alkalosis and Metabolic Acidosis

The combination of respiratory alkalosis and metabolic acidosis is seen often in patients with hepatic failure. Such patients may have respiratory alkalosis due to hyperventilation and metabolic acidosis due to renal failure, renal tubular acidosis, liver failure with lactic acidosis, or any combination. Patients with chronic renal failure and metabolic acidosis are susceptible to bacteremia, which may cause increased ventilation and respiratory alkalosis. Salicylate intoxication may cause mixed metabolic acidosis and respiratory alkalosis [63]. This combination is a mixed disorder with excessive compensation (see Table 4-4). The respiratory alkalosis lowers the $PaCO_2$ beyond the appropriate range of the respiratory response for metabolic acidosis. The plasma $[HCO_3^-]$ also falls below the level expected in simple respiratory alkalosis. In a sense, the compensation for either disorder alone is enhanced; thus, the pH may be normal or close to normal, with a low $PaCO_2$ and a low plasma $[HCO_3^-]$. The primary therapeutic approach should be directed at treatment of the underlying disorders. The acid-base problem per se usually does not need treatment, since the pH is usually closer to normal than it is in either simple disorder alone.

Respiratory Alkalosis and Metabolic Alkalosis

The combination of respiratory and metabolic alkalosis probably is the most common mixed acid-base disorder. This is a mixed disorder with failure of compensation (see Table 4-4). It may be seen in patients with hepatic cirrhosis who hyperventilate, use diuretics, or vomit and in patients with chronic respiratory acidosis and appropriately elevated plasma $[HCO_3^-]$ who are placed on mechanical ventilators and undergo a rapid fall in $PaCO_2$ to hypocapnic levels. Each of the two disorders blocks the appropriate compensatory mechanism of the other; therefore, a marked rise in pH may occur. Depending on the severity of each disorder, the $PaCO_2$ may be normal, reduced, or even increased, while the plasma $[HCO_3^-]$ may be normal or elevated. Correction of the metabolic alkalosis by administration of sodium chloride and potassium chloride should be undertaken, and readjustment of the ventilator or treatment of an underlying disorder causing hyperventilation may correct or ameliorate the respiratory disorder.

Metabolic Acidosis and Metabolic Alkalosis

Metabolic acidosis and metabolic alkalosis may coexist in that two separate processes occur sequentially or simultaneously to exert opposing effects on the plasma $[HCO_3^-]$. This situation should be suspected in cases of metabolic acidosis associated with markedly increased anion gaps when the increments in anion gap are much greater than the decrements in plasma $[HCO_3^-]$. Such a picture suggests that the plasma $[HCO_3^-]$ was set at a value above normal at the time the metabolic acidosis developed.

Table 4-5. Example of a triple acid-base disorder

Clinical event	Vomiting	→ Hypovolemic shock	→ Hyperventilation
	↓	↓	↓
Acid-base disorder	Metabolic alkalosis	+ Metabolic acidosis	+ Respiratory alkalosis
pH	7.53	7.35	7.46
PaCO$_2$ (mm Hg)	44	30	20
[HCO$_3^-$] (mmol/L)	36	16	14
Anion gap (mEq/L)	12	30	32

"Triple" Acid-Base Disorders

The occurrence of a primary respiratory disorder in a patient with metabolic acidosis superimposed on metabolic alkalosis results in a "triple" acid-base disorder. That is, three primary processes have acted to alter the acid-base variables. An example is given in Table 4-5. Vomiting raised the plasma [HCO$_3^-$], which raised the pH, which suppressed ventilation, allowing the PaCO$_2$ to rise a bit. The patient became hypotensive and began to increase lactic acid production and decrease lactate catabolism, which lowered the [HCO$_3^-$] from its high level and increased the anion gap well above normal. The hypotension stimulated ventilation beyond that expected for the degree of acidemia, resulting in a further fall in PaCO$_2$, which raised the pH to the alkalemic range. Thus, the high pH and low PaCO$_2$ identify the presence of respiratory alkalosis. The anion gap greater than 27 mEq/L signals the presence of an organic metabolic acidosis. Adding the increase in anion gap above normal (32 − 9 = 23 mEq/L), which marks the replacement of a HCO$_3^-$ by a metabolic acid anion, to the observed [HCO$_3^-$] (23 + 14 = 37 mmol/L) indicates the presence of the metabolic alkalosis that raised the [HCO$_3^-$] in the first place. The serum anion gap is usually the key to the unraveling of triple acid-base disorders. Treatment should be directed at correcting the underlying diseases and replacing volume and electrolyte deficits.

Appendix: Calculation of Acid-Base Values

There are several methods for checking the mathematical integrity of a set of acid-base values or for calculating the third variable from two measured variables. Various nomograms have been developed for these purposes [64, 65]. If a nomograph is not readily available, a rapid arithmetic calculation based on the Henderson equation can be used.

$$\text{Henderson equation: } [H^+] = K \frac{[H_2CO_3]}{[HCO_3^-]}$$

$$\text{Substituting } S \cdot PaCO_2 \text{ for } H_2CO_3: [H^+] = K' \frac{S \cdot PaCO_2}{[HCO_3^-]}$$

$$K' \text{ for this system is approximately 800 and S is 0.03: } [H^+] = 800 \frac{0.03 \, PaCO_2}{[HCO_3^-]} \quad \text{or}$$

$$[H^+] = 24 \frac{PaCO_2}{[HCO_3^-]}$$

The use of this modified Henderson equation thus avoids the need to deal with logarithms.

It is necessary, however, to estimate $[H^+]$ from the pH or to calculate the pH from the $[H^+]$. Two methods are available. In the pH range between 7.28 and 7.45, $[H^+]$ equals 80 minus the decimal fraction of the pH; for example, at a pH of 7.29, $[H^+] = 80 - 29 = 51$ nmol/L. Beyond this range, the estimation becomes less accurate, but it is still useful for most clinical situations [66].

Another method provides more accurate estimates of $[H^+]$ at the extremes of the clinical range of pH:

At pH 7.0, $[H^+] = 100$ nmol/L

At pH 7.4, $[H^+] = 40$ nmol/L

At each increment of 0.1 unit in pH, $[H^+]$ is estimated as 80 percent of the previous value; for example, at pH 7.5, $[H^+] = 0.80 \times 40 = 32$ nmol/L; at pH 7.6, $[H^+] = 0.80 \times 32 = 25$ nmol/L. $[H^+]$ at interval pH values can be obtained by interpolation. For pH values of less than 7.0, $[H^+]$ is estimated as 125 percent of the next higher value; for example, at pH 6.9, $[H^+] = 1.25 \times 100 = 125$ nmol/L [67].

These calculations thus allow a check on the mathematical integrity of a set of acid-base values or the estimation of the third variable from the other two. In addition, the estimation of $[H^+]$ from the pH is useful, since many confidence bands for the appropriate response to the simple acid-base disorders are based on this value [9, 27].

References

1. Forster RE: Buffering in Blood, with Emphasis on Kinetics. In Seldin DW, Giebisch G (eds): *The Kidney: Physiology and Pathophysiology* (2nd ed). New York, Raven Press, 1992, pp 171–192.
2. Sapir DG, Levine DF, Schwartz WB: The effects of chronic hypoxemia on electrolyte and acid-base equilibrium: An examination of normocapneic hypoxemia and of the influence of hypoxemia on the adaptation to chronic hypercapnia. *J Clin Invest* 46:369–377, 1967.
3. Weinberger SE, Schwarzstein RM, Weiss JW: Hypercapnia. *N Engl J Med* 321:1223–1231, 1989.
4. Moe DW, Rector FC Jr, Alpern RJ: Renal Regulation of Acid-Base Metabolism. In Narins RG (ed): *Clinical Disorders of Fluid and Electrolyte Metabolism* (5th ed). New York, McGraw-Hill, 1994, pp 203–242.
5. Giebisch G, Berger L, Pitts RF: The extrarenal responses to acute acid-base disturbances of respiratory origin. *J Clin Invest* 34:231–245, 1955.
6. Krapf R: Mechanisms of adaptation to chronic respiratory acidosis in the rabbit proximal tubule. *J Clin Invest* 83:890–896, 1989.
7. Ruiz OS, Arruda JAL, Talor Z: Na-HCO$_3$ cotransport and Ns-H antiporter in chronic respiratory acidosis and alkalosis. *Am J Physiol* 256:F414–F420, 1989.
8. Schwartz WB, Brackett NC Jr, Cohen JJ: The response of extracellular hydrogen ion concentration to graded degrees of chronic hypercapnia: The physiologic limitation of the defense of pH. *J Clin Invest* 44:291–301, 1965.
9. Brackett NC Jr, Cohen JJ, Schwartz WB: Carbon dioxide titration curve of normal man: Effect of increasing degrees of acute hypercapnia on acid-base equilibrium. *N Engl J Med* 272:6–12, 1965.

10. Dulfano MJ, Ishikawa S: Hypercapnia: Mental changes and extrapulmonary complications. An expanded concept of the "CO_2 intoxication" syndrome. *Ann Intern Med* 63:829–841, 1965.
11. Epstein FH: Signs and Symptoms of Electrolyte Disorders. In Maxwell MH, Kleeman CR (eds): *Clinical Disorders of Fluid and Electrolyte Metabolism* (3rd ed). New York, McGraw-Hill, 1980, pp 499–516.
12. Potkin RT, Swenson ER: Resuscitation from severe acute hypercapnia: Determination of limits of tolerance and survival. *Chest* 102:1742–1745, 1992.
13. Chabot F, Mertes PM, Delorme N, et al: Effect of acute hypercapnia on alpha atrial natriuretic peptide, renin, angiotensin II, aldosterone, and vasopressin plasma levels in patients with COPD. *Chest* 107:780–786, 1995.
14. Lakshminarayan S, Sahn SA, Petty TL: Bicarbonate therapy in severe acute respiratory acidosis. *Scand J Respir Dis* 54:128–131, 1973.
15. Bulger RJ, Schrier RW, Arend WP, et al: Spinal-fluid acidosis and the diagnosis of pulmonary encephalopathy. *N Engl J Med* 274:433–437, 1966.
16. Brackett NC Jr, Wingo CF, Muren O, et al: Acid-base response to chronic hypercapnia in man. *N Engl J Med* 280:124–130, 1969.
17. Van Ypersele de Strihou C, Brasseur L, DeConinck J: The "carbon dioxide response curve" for chronic hypercapnia in man. *N Engl J Med* 275:117–122, 1966.
18. Manfredi F, Merwarth CR, Buckley CE III, et al: Papilledema in chronic respiratory acidosis. *Am J Med* 30:175–180, 1961.
19. Miller A, Bader RA, Bader ME: The neurological syndrome due to marked hypercapnia, with papilledema. *Am J Med* 33:309–318, 1962.
20. Bushinsky DA: The contribution of acidosis to renal osteodystrophy. *Kidney Int* 47:1816–1832, 1995.
21. Bushinsky DA: Stimulated osteoclastic and suppressed osteoblastic activity in metabolic but not respiratory acidosis. *Am J Physiol* 268:C80–C88, 1995.
22. Strumpf DA, Millman RP, Hill NS: The management of chronic hypoventilation. *Chest* 98:474–480, 1990.
23. Neff TA, Petty TL: Tolerance and survival in severe chronic hypercapnia. *Arch Intern Med* 129:591–596, 1972.
24. Goldstein MB, Gennari FJ, Schwartz WB: The influence of graded degrees of chronic hypercapnia on the acute carbon dioxide titration curve. *J Clin Invest* 50:208–216, 1971.
25. Ingram RJ Jr, Miller RB, Tate LA: Acid-base response to acute carbon dioxide changes in chronic obstructive pulmonary disease. *Am Rev Respir Dis* 108:225–231, 1973.
26. Hirshberg AJ, Dupper RL: Use of doxapram hydrochloride injections as an alternative to intubation to treat chronic obstructive pulmonary disease patients with hypercapnia. *Ann Emerg Med* 24:701–703, 1994.
27. Arbus GS, Hebert LA, Levesque PR, et al: Characterization and clinical application of the "significance band" for acute respiratory alkalosis. *N Engl J Med* 280:117–123, 1969.
28. Gennari FJ, Goldstein MB, Schwartz WB: The nature of the renal adaptation to chronic hypocapnia. *J Clin Invest* 51:1722–1730, 1972.
29. Gledhill N, Beirne GJ, Dempsey JA: Renal response to short-term hypocapnia in man. *Kidney Int* 8:376–386, 1975.
30. Krapf R, Beeler I, Hertner D, Hulter H: Chronic respiratory alkalosis: The effect of sustained hyperventilation on renal regulation of acid-base equilibrium. *N Engl J Med* 324:1394–1401, 1991.
31. Cohen JJ, Madias NE, Wolf CJ, et al: Regulation of acid-base equilibrium in chronic hypocapnia: Evidence that the response of the kidney is not geared to the defense of extracellular [H^+]. *J Clin Invest* 57:1483–1489, 1976.
32. Hilden SA, Johns CA, Madias NE: Adaptation of rabbit renal cortical Na^+-H^+ exchange activity in chronic hypocapnia. *Am J Physiol* 257:F615–F622, 1989.
33. Forster HV, Dempsey JA, Chosy LW: Incomplete compensation of CSF [H^+] in man during acclimatization to high altitude (4300 m). *J Appl Physiol* 38:1067–1072, 1975.
34. Severinghaus JW, Mitchell RA, Richardson BW, et al: Respiratory control at high altitude suggesting active transport regulation of CSF pH. *J Appl Physiol* 18:1155–1166, 1963.

35. Chiodi H: Respiratory adaptations to chronic high altitude hypoxia. *J Appl Physiol* 10:81–87, 1957.
36. Dill DB, Talbott JH, Consolazio WV: Blood as a physiochemical system: XII. Man at high altitudes. *J Biol Chem* 118:649–666, 1937.
37. Lahiri S, Milledge JS: Acid-base in Sherpa altitude residents and lowlanders at 4880 m. *Respir Physiol* 2:323–334, 1967.
38. Edmondson JW, Brashear RE, Li T: Tetany: Quantitative interrelationships between calcium and alkalosis. *Am J Physiol* 228:1082–1086, 1975.
39. Kilburn KH: Shock, seizures, and coma with alkalosis during mechanical ventilation. *Ann Intern Med* 65:977–984, 1966.
40. Arnow PM, Panwalker A, Garvin JS, et al: Aspirin, hyperventilation, and cerebellar infarction in sickle cell disease. *Arch Intern Med* 138:148–149, 1978.
41. Ayres SM, Grace WJ: Inappropriate ventilation and hypoxemia as causes of cardiac arrhythmias: The control of arrhythmias without antiarrhythmic drugs. *Am J Med* 46:495–505, 1969.
42. Kety SS, Schmidt CF: The effects of altered arterial tensions of carbon dioxide and oxygen on cerebral blood flow and cerebral oxygen consumption of normal young men. *J Clin Invest* 27:484–491, 1948.
43. Protass LM: Possible precipitation of cerebral thrombosis in sickle-cell anemia by hyperventilation. *Ann Intern Med* 79:451, 1973.
44. Jacobs WF, Battle WE, Ronan JA Jr: False-positive ST–T-wave changes secondary to hyperventilation and exercise: A cineangiographic correlation. *Ann Intern Med* 81:479–482, 1974.
45. Lawson NW, Butler CH III, Ray CT: Alkalosis and cardiac arrhythmias. *Anesth Analg* (Paris) 52:951–962, 1973.
46. Neill WA, Pantley GA, Nakomchai V: Respiratory alkalemia during exercise reduces angina threshold. *Chest* 80:144–153, 1981.
47. Weber S, Cabanes L, Simon J-C, et al: Systemic alkalosis as a provocative test for coronary artery spasm in patients with infrequent resting chest pain. *Am Heart J* 115:54–59, 1988.
48. Yakaitis RW, Cooke JE, Redding JS: Reevaluation of relationships of hyperkalemia and PCO_2 to cardiac arrhythmias during mechanical ventilation. *Anesth Analg* (Paris) 50:368–373, 1971.
49. Krapf R, Caduff P, Wagdi P, et al: Plasma potassium response to acute respiratory alkalosis. *Kidney Int* 47:217–224, 1995.
50. Knochel JP: The pathophysiology and clinical characteristics of severe hypophosphatemia. *Arch Intern Med* 137:203–220, 1977.
51. Mostellar ME, Tuttle EP Jr: The effects of alkalosis on plasma concentration and urinary excretion of inorganic phosphate in man. *J Clin Invest* 43:138–149, 1964.
52. Mazzara JT, Ayres SM, Grace WJ: Extreme hypocapnia in the critically ill patient. *Am J Med* 56:450–456, 1974.
53. Mountain RD, Heffner JE, Brackett NC Jr, et al: Acid-base disturbances in acute asthma. *Chest* 98:651–655, 1990.
54. Mulhausen R, Eichenholz A, Blumentals A: Acid-base disturbances in patients with cirrhosis of the liver. *Medicine* (Baltimore) 46:185–189, 1967.
55. Record CO, Iles RA, Cohen RD, et al: Acid-base and metabolic disturbances in fulminant hepatic failure. *Gut* 16:144–149, 1975.
56. Lange PA, Stoller JK: The hepatopulmonary syndrome. *Ann Intern Med* 122:521–529, 1995.
57. Wolfe JD, Tashkin DP, Holly FE, et al: Hypoxemia of cirrhosis: Detection of abnormal small pulmonary vascular channels by a quantitative radionuclide method. *Am J Med* 63:746–754, 1977.
58. Wilder CE, Morrison RS, Tyler JM: Relationship between serum sodium and hyperventilation in cirrhosis. *Am Rev Respir Dis* 96:971–976, 1967.
59. Wichser J, Kazemi H: Ammonia and ventilation: Site and mechanism of action. *Respir Physiol* 20:393–406, 1974.
60. Simmons DH, Nicoloff J, Guze LB: Hyperventilation and respiratory alkalosis as signs of gram-negative bacteremia. *JAMA* 174:2196–2199, 1960.
61. Trimble C, Smith DE, Rosenthal MH, et al: Pathophysiologic role of hypocarbia in post-traumatic pulmonary insufficiency. *Am J Surg* 122:633–638, 1971.

62. Bear R, Goldstein M, Phillipson E, et al: Effect of metabolic alkalosis on respiratory function in patients with chronic obstructive lung disease. *Can Med Assoc J* 117:900–903, 1977.
63. Yip L, Dart RC, Gabow PA: Concepts and controversies in salicylate toxicity. *Emerg Med Clin North Am* 12:351–364, 1994.
64. Cohen JJ: A new acid-base nomogram featuring hydrogen ion concentration: Henderson revisited. *Ann Intern Med* 66:159–164, 1967.
65. Singer RB, Hastings AB: An improved clinical method for the estimation of disturbances of the acid-base balance of human blood. *Medicine* (Baltimore) 27:223–242, 1948.
66. Kassirer JP, Bleich HL: Rapid estimation of plasma carbon dioxide tension from pH and total carbon dioxide content. *N Engl J Med* 272:1067–1068, 1965.
67. Fagan TJ: Estimation of hydrogen ion concentration (letter). *N Engl J Med* 288:915, 1973.

5

Disorders of Potassium Metabolism

Linda N. Peterson and Moshe Levi

Potassium is the most abundant cation in the body, with total body potassium stores in adults amounting to about 3000 to 4000 mmol. Yet, in contrast to sodium, less than 2 percent can be found in extracellular fluid (ECF). This striking compartmentalization of potassium in intracellular fluid and sodium in ECF is a condition established and maintained by the cells themselves. The membrane-bound Na,K-ATPase pump, expressed in virtually every cell in the body, transports potassium into cells while simultaneously extruding sodium. The energy in adenosine triphosphate is transformed into ion gradients for sodium and potassium. An intracellular negative voltage develops as a consequence of outward diffusion of potassium through selective channels. The negative potential inside the cell increases until the electrical force holding potassium in the cell is equal to the chemical force favoring potassium exit. This condition of electrochemical equilibrium for potassium is reached at about -90 mV. The steady-state resting membrane potential is about 15 mV less negative than this, due to the inward movement of sodium down its electrochemical gradient. In addition to the critical dependence of protein synthesis and consequent cell growth on intracellular potassium concentration, the electrochemical gradients for potassium and sodium drive or participate in a number of processes in the body. These include nerve conduction, synaptic transmission, muscle contraction, fluid transport, hormone release, and embryonic development.

Since the resting membrane potential depends primarily on the potassium gradient across the cell membrane, variations in extracellular potassium concentration* have the most profound effect on the excitability of neuromuscular tissue, particularly the heart. As a consequence, plasma potassium concentration is rigidly maintained between 3.5 and 5.0 mEq/L. *Hypokalemia* is defined as a reduction in plasma potassium below 3.5 mEq/L. *Hyperkalemia* is defined as a potassium concentration greater than 5.0 mEq/L. Both conditions are associated with potentially fatal cardiac arrhythmias.

If blood is drawn and stored carefully, the potassium concentration measured in

---

* The terms *extracellular* and *plasma* will be used interchangeably when referring to potassium concentration.

192

the sample will accurately estimate the existing plasma concentration in the patient. False hyperkalemia or pseudohyperkalemia is caused by the release of potassium from cells during or after the removal of the blood sample from the patient. A major cause of pseudohyperkalemia is hemolysis due to mechanical trauma during venipuncture or repeated clenching and unclenching of the hand after the tourniquet has been applied. In the latter case, there can be a 1- to 2-mEq/L artifactual increase in plasma potassium concentration. Pseudohyperkalemia can also occur in subjects with marked leukocytosis (white blood cell (WBC) count >100,000/mm^3) or increased platelet count greater than 400,000/mm^3. Pseudohyperkalemia can be avoided by minimizing trauma and hand clenching during venipuncture, by rapidly separating red cells, and by using plasma rather than serum for potassium measurements [1].

Pseudohypokalemia is caused by the uptake of potassium by metabolically active cells after the blood sample has been removed from the patient. This is likely to occur if the patient has an elevated WBC count (e.g., in acute myeloid leukemia) or if the blood stands for a long period of time at room temperature. Pseudohypokalemia can be avoided by immediately separating the cells from plasma or by storing the blood at 4°C [1]. The term *hypokalemia* applies only to a decrease in extracellular potassium concentration, while the term *potassium-depletion* refers to a reduction in cellular potassium stores. Potassium depletion is not always accompanied by hypokalemia if cellular uptake is simultaneously impaired. A reduction in intracellular potassium stores in the absence of hypokalemia does not disturb excitable tissue. Typical potassium deficits in adults amount to 200 to 300 mmol, which reduces intracellular potassium concentration by about 5 to 8 percent. Since the ratio of potassium concentration across the cell membrane barely changes from 37.5:1 (intracellular-extracellular, 150/4) to 36:1 (144/4), there is a minimal effect on resting membrane potential. However, if the extracellular compartment sustained the loss of only one-tenth of the above amount, that is, 20 to 30 mmol, plasma potassium concentration would be reduced by about 50 percent. The potassium concentration ratio changes from the normal of 37.5:1 (150/4) to 75:1 (150/2). Due to the reduction in extracellular potassium concentration, the driving force for outward potassium movement is increased and cells hyperpolarize. Although potassium depletion unaccompanied by hypokalemia does not disturb cardiac and skeletal muscle, it is vital to realize that these patients are at risk for developing sudden hypokalemia during the course of treatment. At that time, all of the disturbances in excitable tissue will be evident. The purpose of this chapter is to describe the regulation of plasma potassium concentration: the causes, effects, and treatment of hypo- and hyperkalemia.

Determinants of Plasma Potassium Concentration

The relation between intake, distribution, and excretion of potassium is illustrated in Figure 5-1. Normal individuals ingesting 100 mmol of potassium each day remain

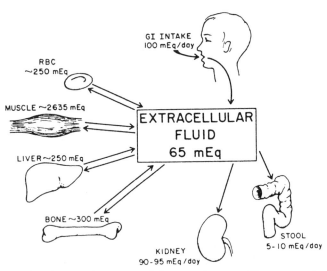

Fig. 5-1. External and internal potassium balance in humans. Plasma potassium concentration is affected by the relation between intake, distribution, and excretion of this ion. (From J. D. Smith, M. Bia, and R. A. DeFronzo, Clinical Disorders of Potassium Metabolism. In A. Arieff and R. A. DeFronzo [eds], *Fluid, Electrolyte, and Acid-Base Disorders.* New York: Churchill Livingstone, 1985.)

in balance by excreting 92 percent of the ingested potassium in the urine and the remaining 8 percent in the stool [2]. Within a 24-hour period, the kidneys will eliminate the daily dietary load of potassium; however, it should be noted that extrarenal mechanisms exist to buffer transient changes in plasma potassium. Following the ingestion of potassium, only half is excreted by the kidneys over the first 4 to 6 hours. The remaining 50 percent is taken up by peripheral tissues. For example, if all the potassium contained in two 10-ounce bags of potato chips (70 mEq) was ingested and distributed exclusively in the extracellular compartment, plasma potassium concentration would double. This degree of hyperkalemia would cause life-threatening electrical disturbances in the heart. It is also clear that redistribution of a very small fraction (1–2%) of intracellular potassium into extracellular fluid can easily increase plasma potassium concentration to a dangerous level.

The kidney is the major organ responsible for potassium excretion, and its role in maintaining potassium balance is obvious (see Fig. 5-1). To the extent that the kidney fails to excrete the daily intake, demands will be placed on the intestinal tract and intracellular buffering to offset increases in plasma potassium concentration. Extrarenal tissues have a limited capacity to increase potassium stores. On the other hand, the kidney can be the primary source of accelerated losses of potassium if excretion is inappropriately stimulated. This is often the cause of hypokalemia.

The gastrointestinal tract eliminates only 5 to 10 percent of the daily intake of potassium. Most of the excreted potassium is derived from colonic epithelial cell secretion. These cells respond to many of the factors that stimulate potassium-secreting cells of the kidney [3, 4]. In chronic renal failure, the colon may excrete more than 30 percent of the dietary burden [3]. Because of the capacity of the colon to secrete potassium, it can be useful in the elimination of excess potassium in hyperkalemic patients. Yet, it should not be forgotten that abnormal stimulation of colonic secretion can be a source of significant potassium loss. The concentration of potassium in lower gastrointestinal secretions can exceed 80 mEq/L [4]. Diarrhea due to a multitude of etiologies (e.g., colonic villous adenomas, cholera, Zollinger-Ellison syndrome, Verner-Morrison syndrome or vasoactive intestinal peptide tumor syndrome [pancreatic cholera], laxative and enema abuse) can be associated with excessive stool potassium losses and hypokalemia. Potassium concentration in gastric fluid is usually less than 10 mEq/L and only partially explains hypokalemia in patients with vomiting. Rather, increased renal losses and increased cellular uptake largely account for potassium depletion and hypokalemia in this setting.

Hypokalemia and hyperkalemia develop due to an imbalance between potassium intake, distribution, and/or excretion. These three variables must be analyzed in each patient to determine the underlying disturbance. Additionally, a thorough understanding of extrarenal and renal potassium homeostasis can be used to restore potassium balance and plasma potassium concentration to normal.

Intake of Potassium

North American diets supply about 60 to 100 mmol of potassium, primarily in the form of citrus fruits, vegetables, and meat [3, 5]. Since potassium is present in so many foods ingested in a normal diet, only inadequate food intake (e.g., anorexia, bulimia, alcoholism) will cause significant potassium depletion. The poor and the elderly tend to have lower potassium intake due to less than ideal diets. Net potassium intake may also be decreased by the ingestion of clay-containing soils that impair intestinal potassium absorption. This is more common in pediatric populations. Even in the face of reduced potassium intake, the contribution of increased loss should also be evaluated.

The minimum daily adult requirement is approximately 0.3 to 0.4 mmol/kg body weight [3]. In neonates and small infants, the value is given in proportion to caloric intake, that is, 2.4 mmol of potassium per 100 kcal [6]. Normal intracellular potassium concentration is required in protein synthesis and cellular growth. Studies in animals and humans have documented the dependence of normal growth on adequate potassium intake [7, 8]. Once intake falls below the minimum daily requirement, negative potassium balance ensues. Renal potassium conservation in humans requires about 1 to 2 weeks to fully activate, and during this time excretion will exceed intake by a significant degree [4, 5].

As long as potassium intake increases gradually over a period of days, balance can be maintained even at a potassium intake almost 10 times greater than normal. Prior to the Potato Famine of 1848, most of the caloric intake of the Irish population had been sustained by a diet consisting almost exclusively of potatoes, a high-potassium food. Adaptation to a high-potassium diet requires increased cellular buffering, elevated plasma potassium concentration, and marked stimulation of renal secretion by aldosterone [9, 10]. Accelerated intake from either exogenous or endogenous sources can cause a transient increase in plasma potassium concentration. However, sustained hyperkalemia usually indicates an underlying defect in renal potassium excretion or impaired potassium distribution. The most common exogenous source is KCl supplements or salt substitutes. Concomitant use of potassium sparing diuretics, underlying renal disease, advanced age, or diabetes mellitus is present in over 50 percent of patients who develop hyperkalemia while taking KCl supplements or salt substitutes. Other common sources of excess potassium are large doses of potassium pencillin (1.7 mEq K/million units) or administration of old stored blood that has a high potassium concentration [1]. In the case of massive transfusion of old stored blood, cardiac tolerance to hyperkalemia is decreased by hypocalcemia due to the presence of the anticoagulant citrate [3].

Distribution of Potassium

There are a number of factors that can affect the distribution of potassium between intracellular and extracellular compartments (Table 5-1). Insulin, exercise, and β-adrenergic catecholamines affect potassium distribution under normal physiologic circumstances. The other factors are capable of disturbing potassium distribution when the hormone or drug concentrations or parameters are outside the normal range. Although aldosterone receptors coupled to nongenomic signal transduction systems have been identified in nonrenal cells [11], this hormone does not play an important role in extrarenal potassium homeostasis. Maintenance of potassium distribution depends on the activity of the Na,K-ATPase pump to effect potassium movements into cells, the electrochemical gradient, and the status of potassium channels that normally allow potassium movement out of the cell.

Table 5-1. Major factors affecting potassium distribution between intracellular and extracellular fluid

Normal	Pathophysiologic
Insulin	Insulin excess or lack
Exercise	
Catecholamines	Catecholamines
β_2-Receptors	β_2-Receptors
	Stimulation or blockade
Metabolic alkalosis	Metabolic inorganic acidosis
	Necrosis or tissue injury
	Rapid cellular growth
	Genetic
	Thyrotoxicosis
	Hypertonicity
	Drugs/toxins

Normal

Insulin

A feedback loop has been identified establishing a role for insulin in the regulation of plasma potassium concentration. Increases in plasma potassium of only a few tenths of a millimole are sufficient to stimulate insulin release into the portal circulation [9, 12]. On the other hand, insulin stimulates potassium uptake in liver and muscle. The activated insulin receptor increases Na,K-ATPase activity, thus driving cellular potassium uptake via the pump and perhaps through potassium conductance channels, secondary to hyperpolarization.

Exercise

Muscular activity causes potassium accumulation in ECF due to potassium efflux during repolarization. The consequent increase in the conductance of potassium channels is beneficial in accelerating muscle repolarization and shortening the refractory period. The increase in extracellular potassium concentration also mediates vasodilatation, which increases muscle blood flow. Usually exercise is associated with increased sympathetic nervous system activity and release of adrenal medullary catecholamines. Catecholamines blunt the rise in plasma potassium concentration associated with vigorous exercise [13].

Catecholamines

As mentioned previously, circulating epinephrine stimulates potassium uptake in muscle. Activation of β_2-receptors increases cyclic adenosine monophosphate, which is associated with stimulation of Na,K-ATPase activity. Increased pump activity as well as hyperpolarization accounts for accelerated potassium uptake. This is a normal homeostatic mechanism to defend plasma potassium concentration [9, 12].

Pathophysiologic

Insulin

Insulin deficiency or excess is pathophysiologic and disturbs potassium distribution between intra- and extracellular fluids (see Table 5-1). Insulin deficiency, as in untreated diabetes mellitus, impairs cellular potassium uptake. Although patients have large potassium deficits due to accelerated renal losses, hypokalemia is masked. Unless potassium is administered simultaneously with insulin, severe hypokalemia will occur. As predicted, insulin excess will cause hypokalemia. This knowledge is utilized in clinical practice to move potassium into cells in patients with severe hyperkalemia. Glucose must be given with insulin to prevent hypoglycemia.

Facts: Insulin excess can cause hypokalemia; insulin deficiency can cause hyperkalemia.

Catecholamines

Increased activation of β_2-receptors will exaggerate potassium uptake following exercise and has been the cause of hypokalemia in patients taking β_2-agonists [1, 14,

15]. The clinical conditions that are associated with increased epinephrine release include hypoglycemia, coronary ischemia, delirium tremens, post–cardiopulmonary resuscitation, acute head trauma, acute theophylline intoxication, and during the induction phase of anesthesia. A similar effect in which plasma potassium concentration is lowered acutely is also induced by the administration of β-adrenergic agonists such as albuterol or terbutaline to treat asthma [16, 17] or dobutamine to treat heart failure. In heart failure patients, a rapid 0.4-mEq/L fall in plasma potassium concentration following the administration of dobutamine may exacerbate ventricular arrhythmias [18]. As predicted, blockade of β_2-receptors will predispose the patient to hyperkalemia during exercise and other times, if cellular potassium uptake is impaired for some other reason [1].

Facts: β-agonists can cause hypokalemia; β-antagonists can cause hyperkalemia.

Metabolic Alkalosis

Metabolic alkalosis stimulates cellular potassium uptake. As hydrogen ions leave cells to buffer extracellular alkalosis, inward movement of potassium is enhanced. The simultaneous existence of metabolic alkalosis in patients with increased potassium losses will exaggerate the resultant hypokalemia [3, 10]. In general, plasma potassium concentration falls less than 0.4 mEq/L per 0.1-unit increase in ECF pH. The effect of elevated plasma bicarbonate to enhance potassium movement into cells is utilized in the treatment of hyperkalemia. Bicarbonate is frequently administered with insulin and glucose in patients with life-threatening hyperkalemia to lower plasma potassium concentration into the normal range [19]. This provides the time required to initiate treatment to remove potassium from the body.

Fact: Metabolic alkalosis can cause hypokalemia.

Metabolic Inorganic Acidosis

The effect of metabolic acidosis on plasma potassium concentration depends on the accompanying anion (Fig. 5-2). If the acidosis is due to an inorganic acid such as hydrochloric (e.g., diarrheal illness, renal tubular acidosis), phosphoric, or sulfuric (renal failure), hydrogen ions enter cells alone due to cellular impermeability to these anions. The inward movement of solitary hydrogen ions causes potassium ions to leave the cell. Inorganic metabolic acidosis, by itself, in the absence of other disturbances, causes an elevation of plasma potassium concentration [1].

Fact: Metabolic inorganic acidosis can cause hyperkalemia.

Metabolic Organic Acidosis

Metabolic acidosis caused by organic acids such as lactic acid (cardiac arrest, metabolic poisons) or β-hydroxybutyric acid (diabetic ketoacidosis) is not associated with potassium movement out of cells [1] (see Fig. 5-2). Since cells are permeable to these anions, hydrogen ions enter with the accompanying anions such that outward potassium movement does not occur. Therefore, if plasma potassium concentration is elevated in a patient with metabolic organic acidosis, another cause should be sought for the hyperkalemia.

It is possible to predict whether potassium distribution across cell membranes is disturbed in inorganic acidosis. However, whether the patient will be hyperkalemic

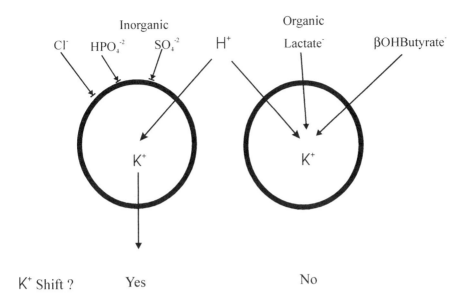

Inorganic

Cl^- HPO_4^{-2} SO_4^{-2} H^+

Organic

Lactate⁻ βOHButyrate⁻

K^+ K^+

K^+ Shift ? Yes No

Hyperkalemia ? It depends

Fig. 5-2. Effect of inorganic and organic metabolic acidosis on potassium movement out of cells. Potassium moves into extracellular fluid when the acid is inorganic. Although hyperkalemia would be expected, the resultant plasma potassium concentration will depend on intake, excretion, and other factors affecting distribution.

will depend on the other factors affecting plasma potassium concentration. For example, it is not uncommon for plasma potassium concentration to be normal in patients with metabolic inorganic acidosis due to diarrhea. These patients are actually potassium depleted due to accelerated gastrointestinal loss. The reduction in plasma potassium due to the deficit is offset by the effect of inorganic acidosis to increase movement of potassium out of cells. After the illness subsides and the acidosis is corrected, hypokalemia develops in many patients [20].
Fact: Metabolic organic acidosis does not disturb potassium distribution.

Necrosis or Tissue Injury

Destruction of cells by any means will result in potassium addition to ECF. This may occur in rhabdomyolysis, severe burns, hemolysis, tumor lysis (most common after chemotherapy in patients with malignant lymphomas), or patients with severe hypothermia. This type of internal transfusion can be the most difficult to manage clinically. Traumatic injury may be particularly difficult, since acute renal failure may also develop secondary to myoglobin exposure or ischemia associated with blood loss [3, 9].
Fact: Tissue injury by any means can cause hyperkalemia.

Rapid Cellular Growth

Normal cellular growth is impossible without adequate potassium intake; likewise, accelerated growth will demand increased potassium intake. If potassium is not provided during the treatment of pernicious anemia with vitamin B_{12}, hypokalemia will occur as developing erythrocytes remove potassium from ECF [21]. Plasma potassium concentration may decrease to 3.0 mEq/L or lower. A similar situation occurs when neutropenia is treated by the administration of granulocyte-macrophage colony-stimulating factor. Although not strictly related to growth, hypokalemia can occur following multiple transfusions of frozen, washed red cells. These cells lose up to 50 percent of intracellular potassium during storage and will lower plasma potassium concentration after reintroduction into the body [22].

Fact: Cell growth that is not matched by a corresponding increase in potassium intake can cause hypokalemia.

Genetic

Intrinsic defects in skeletal muscle ion channels that disturb potassium distribution have been identified [23]. These are the periodic familial hypo- and hyperkalemic paralyses. Patients suffer intermittent muscle paralysis associated with changes in plasma potassium concentration. Due to the profound effect of plasma potassium concentration on resting membrane potential, variations in plasma potassium concentration are usually the initiating stimulus provoking the attack, and plasma potassium concentration is consequently affected by the change in muscle function. Potassium channels are normal in these patients.

Hyperkalemic Periodic Familial Paralysis. A population of abnormal sodium channels that fail to inactivate normally has been identified in patients with the hyperkalemic disorder [23]. With this disorder, under resting conditions, inward sodium current is greater than normal. In these patients, if plasma potassium concentration increases (e.g., after a meal), the resultant depolarization increases conductance of all sodium channels. Inward sodium current persists because the abnormal channels do not inactivate. This causes further depolarization of the muscle. Normal sodium channels become inactivated due to the sustained subthreshold depolarization causing paralysis. Increased potassium efflux occurs secondary to cellular depolarization. It is important to note that (1) this defect is expressed only in skeletal muscle cells, (2) skeletal muscle paralysis is not due to hyperkalemia, and (3) hyperkalemia would be expected to adversely affect cardiac function. The disease is inherited as a single-gene autosomal dominant trait; hence, only half of the sodium channels are abnormal. It has been suggested that a disease in which all the sodium channels were affected would be nonviable. Treatment involves avoidance of situations that lead to skeletal muscle depolarization, such as increased plasma potassium concentration. Consistent with this view, agents that stimulate potassium uptake such as β_2-agonists are beneficial as well as acetazolamide [3, 24].

Fact: Inherited defects in skeletal muscle sodium channels cause periodic hyperkalemia paralysis.

Hypokalemic Familial Periodic Paralysis. A defect in skeletal muscle calcium channels exists in the more common hypokalemic disorders [23]. The disease is genetically linked to the voltage-sensitive calcium channel (dihydropyridine receptor), which participates in excitation-contraction coupling. Mutations in the affected gene cause calcium channels to become inactivated at lower membrane potentials [25]. The disease is inherited as a dominant trait, and the incidence in females is significantly less than in males. Attacks are precipitated by a reduction in plasma potassium concentration, such as after a carbohydrate-rich meal (insulin) or rest after vigorous exercise (catecholamines), factors that normally cause membrane hyperpolarization. In response to these stimuli, calcium current decreases, the muscle depolarizes, paralysis ensues, and extracellular potassium concentration decreases. The cause and effect relation between these changes is unknown. As in the hyperkalemic forms, (1) the defect resides only in skeletal muscle, (2) skeletal paralysis is not due to hypokalemia, and (3) cardiac disturbances are expected due to the hypokalemia. Treatment of the hypokalemic disorder includes ingestion of a high-potassium diet and/or potassium sparing diuretics, factors that would prevent hyperpolarization due to hypokalemia. Patients are cautioned to avoid high carbohydrate intake, since subsequent insulin release will increase potassium uptake. Acetazolamide has been found to be useful but not well tolerated in many patients [26].
Fact: Inherited defects in skeletal muscle calcium channels cause hypokalemic periodic paralysis.

Thyrotoxicosis
Periodic paralysis associated with hypokalemia is a common problem in thyroid hormone excess. It appears to be due to increased sensitivity to catecholamines and, unlike the genetic form of the disease, can be treated with β_2-blockers until thyrotoxicosis subsides [3].
Fact: Thyroid hormone excess can cause periodic hypokalemia and muscle paralysis.

Hyperosmolality
Increased osmolality of body fluids is associated with enhanced movement of potassium from intracellular fluid into ECF. This appears to be due to an increase in cell potassium concentration caused by water loss. The increased concentration gradient stimulates potassium efflux from cells. Hypertonicity probably contributes to some degree to the paradoxical elevation in plasma potassium concentration in diabetic ketoacidosis [3, 27].
Fact: Hyperosmolality can cause hyperkalemia.

Drugs/Toxins
It is not unexpected that severe inhibition of the Na,K-ATPase transport pump causes hyperkalemia. Hyperkalemia is perhaps the most serious problem associated with cardiac glycoside overdose. Treatment with digitalis antibodies (Fab fragment) has been found to be effective in reversing toxicity [28].

Barium poisoning causes hypokalemia and muscle paralysis [1, 3, 13]. Barium blocks potassium conductance channels, which are the major exit route for potassium. In the presence of barium, potassium uptake into cells by the Na,K-ATPase pump is unopposed, and consequently hypokalemia develops. The reduction in plasma potassium concentration then causes muscle paralysis, as described subsequently. Treatment involves increasing plasma potassium concentration to compete with barium for sites in the potassium channels.

The anesthetic succinylcholine depolarizes skeletal muscle, which increases potassium movement into ECF. In normal individuals, the increase in plasma potassium concentration is small. However, in patients in whom potassium efflux may be increased for other reasons (e.g., burns, trauma), severe hyperkalemia can be induced [29].

Facts: Treatment of some patients with muscle depolarizing agents (e.g., succinylcholine) and overdoses of Na,K-ATPase inhibitors (e.g., digitalis) cause hyperkalemia. Barium intoxication causes hypokalemia.

Renal Excretion of Potassium

This discussion will be limited to the effects of renal function and dysfunction on potassium homeostasis. Since the kidney is the major route of potassium elimination from the body, a disturbance in renal potassium handling can be the cause of excess potassium loss or retention. Depending on the magnitude of the potassium imbalance and the status of nonrenal tissue to buffer the change, the ability to regulate plasma potassium concentration may be severely impaired. It is important to understand renal potassium handling in order to evaluate and treat hypo- and hyperkalemic patients and, hopefully, to prevent these disorders by knowing which patients may be at risk.

Historical Notes

It was difficult to elucidate the mechanisms underlying potassium excretion because the amount of potassium excreted in the urine is only about 10 to 20 percent of the filtered amount. The amount of potassium filtered by the glomerulus can be roughly estimated by multiplying the glomerular filtration rate (GFR) by the plasma potassium concentration. The amount of potassium bound to albumin that cannot be filtered can be ignored. If the GFR is 173 L/day (120 ml/min), and plasma potassium is 4 mEq/L, the daily filtered load is 692 mEq (173 L $\times$ 4 mEq/L). Since only 100 mEq (dietary intake) is excreted in the urine, it was easy to deduce that there was extensive potassium reabsorption along the nephron. However, it was not known that the kidney could secrete potassium until the appearance of a report in 1937 that a renal failure patient excreted more potassium than was filtered [30]. Since that time until the present, intense investigative efforts have discerned the magnitude and direction of potassium movements along the nephron, which are depicted in Figure 5-3.

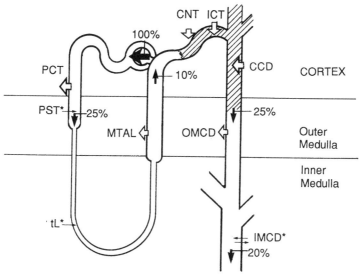

Fig. 5-3. Diagram of a mammalian nephron showing changes in the amount of potassium remaining as fluid moves from the glomerulus to the end of the collecting duct. Solid arrows and adjacent numbers indicate the percent of filtered potassium present at that site. Open arrows indicate magnitude and direction of potassium movement in designated locations. PCT = proximal convoluted tubule; PST = proximal straight tubule; tL = thin descending limb of Henle's loop; MTAL = medullary thick ascending limb; CNT = connecting tubule; ICT = initial collecting tubule; CCD = cortical collecting duct; OMCD = outer medullary collecting duct; IMCD = inner medullary collecting duct. *Indicates potential sites of secretion or reabsorption.

Potassium Transport Along the Nephron

Potassium is extensively reabsorbed in the proximal tubule. Only 25 percent of the filtered amount of potassium is present at the end of the proximal tubule. The proximal convoluted tubule is largely responsible for potassium reabsorption that is driven passively by the electrical gradient [10]. The proximal straight tubule normally secretes potassium at a low rate, but this can increase significantly when an excess of potassium must be excreted [10]. It is likely that the potassium secretion by the proximal straight tubule helps patients with chronic renal failure remain in potassium balance.

Potassium can be secreted passively into the thin descending limb in inner cortical nephrons that have loops of Henle penetrating into the inner medulla. This process undermines potassium reabsorption in the upstream segments to some extent but is a consequence of the permeability characteristics required for the urinary concentrating mechanism.

The thick ascending limb reabsorbs approximately 15 percent of the filtered potassium. Net reabsorption of sodium chloride is driven by the primary active transport of sodium and potassium across the basolateral membrane via the Na,K-ATPase pump coupled to electrically silent uptake of sodium, two chloride, and potassium by the furosemide sensitive luminal cotransporter [31]. Although the uptake step is electrically silent, a lumen-positive potential develops. The lumen-positive voltage is responsible for passive potassium reabsorption and drives approximately 50 percent of sodium chloride reabsorption between cells (paracellular pathway). The medullary thick ascending limb also reabsorbs ammonium ions, which compete with potassium for the same site on the luminal sodium chloride cotransporter [32]. This in part explains the relation between potassium metabolism and acid-base balance, which will be discussed later.

Under normal circumstances, urinary potassium excretion is determined primarily by potassium secretion along the distal nephron. The main sites of regulated potassium secretion are the connecting tubules, the initial collecting tubule, and the cortical collecting duct [10, 33–35] (see Fig. 5-3). For the purpose of simplification, this region will be referred to as the cortical collecting duct. Potassium secretion in the cortical collecting duct can increase dramatically to the point where the amount of potassium in luminal fluid exceeds the amount that was originally filtered. This region of the nephron and portions of the medullary collecting duct also contain potassium reabsorbing cells, which become active when potassium retention is required. Previously, one cell type was thought to be capable of secreting and reabsorbing potassium. However, it is now known that distinct cells resident in the cortical collecting duct are responsible for the variability of potassium transport. This discussion will focus on the potassium reabsorbing and secreting cells of the cortical collecting duct.

Intercalated Cells

The cortical collecting duct consists primarily of principal cells (60%), with the balance intercalated cells (40%). Potassium reabsorption by the cortical collecting duct is mediated by type A (alpha) intercalated cells in this segment. The membrane proteins involved in potassium transport in these cells are illustrated in Figure 5-4. They are distinguished by the absence of Na,K-ATPase activity, the expression of two luminal primary active acid secreting pumps, and a basolateral HCO_3^-/Cl^- antiporter [10]. One of the proton pumps is linked to the simultaneous reabsorption of potassium (H,K-ATPase) and shares considerable homology to that expressed by gastric epithelial cells [35]. The other pump transports solitary hydrogen ions. The type A cells work in unison with bicarbonate secreting type B (beta) intercalated cells. Under normal circumstances, it has been estimated that there is little or no movement of H^+ or HCO_3^- because the transport is antagonistic [34]. On the other hand, during dietary potassium depletion, the type A cells mediate active potassium reabsorption. In potassium-depleted animals, there is increased expression and activity of the H,K-ATPase pump in type A cells in the cortical collecting duct and in the outer medullary collecting duct [35]. When the kidney must conserve potassium, the activity of principal cells declines due to decreased aldosterone, and the activity of type A intercalated cells increases [34, 35]. During potassium conservation, increased H,K-ATPase activity is associated with enhanced potassium bicarbonate reabsorption, yielding luminal fluid more acidic. This effect increases retrapping of

ICT, CCD

Intercalated Cell
(A Type)

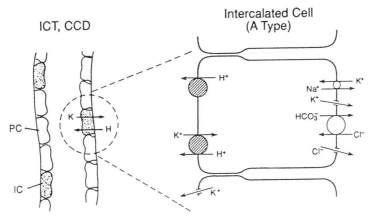

Fig. 5-4. Model for type A intercalated cells in the cortical collecting duct. These cells are the site of potassium reabsorption via the H,K-ATPase. Proton secretion is also driven by an H-ATPase. (From R. G. O'Neil, Aldosterone regulation of sodium and potassium transport in the cortical collecting duct. *Semin. Nephrol.* 10:365, 1990.)

NH_3 as NH_4^+ and ensures its ultimate excretion in the urine. In this way, the efficiency of renal bicarbonate production by ammoniagenesis, which is stimulated by potassium depletion, is further enhanced [32, 36]. The alkalosis that develops in severe potassium depletion is due to stimulation of ammoniagenesis by potassium depletion in the proximal tubule coupled to efficient excretion of ammonium in the urine. The latter process is enhanced by the action of type A intercalated cells of the outer medullary collecting duct.

Principal Cells

Potassium secretion by the cortical collecting duct is mediated by principal cells in this segment. The cotransporters and ion conductance channels involved in secretion are illustrated in Figure 5-5. Potassium secretion involves active uptake across the basolateral membrane by the Na,K-ATPase pump. Energy expended by the active transport pump is translated into the establishment of large concentration gradients for potassium and sodium across the luminal and peritubular membranes, respectively. Potassium preferentially exits across the luminal membrane through potassium conductance channels due to the favorable electrochemical concentration gradient. The electrical potential across the luminal membrane is depolarized due to inwardly directed sodium movement through sodium conductance channels. It is interesting to note that this is in contrast to the proximal nephron, in which sodium entry occurs through nonconductive cotransporters. The luminal membrane of the principal cell permits the inwardly directed sodium gradient to provide the electrical driving force for potassium secretion. Net secretion of potassium stops if sodium conductance channels in the luminal membrane are blocked, for example, by the potassium sparing diuretic amiloride. In the presence of this drug, the luminal membrane voltage increases to approximately -70 mV. Under these conditions, the chemical concentration gradient that favors potassium secretion is opposed

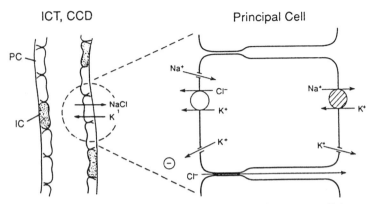

Fig. 5-5. Model for principal cells in the cortical collecting duct. Transcellular potassium secretion depends on potassium uptake by the Na,K-ATPase pump and movement through potassium channels or K/Cl cotransporter in the luminal membrane. Sodium reabsorption proceeds through luminal sodium channels and the basolateral Na,K-ATPase pump. (From R. G. O'Neil, Aldosterone regulation of sodium and potassium transport in the cortical collecting duct. *Semin. Nephrol.* 10:365, 1990.)

by an equivalent electrical gradient oriented in the opposite direction. There is uncertainty regarding the mechanism of chloride reabsorption. Most, but not all evidence is consistent with the view that chloride is reabsorbed passively between cells driven by the lumen negative potential [34]. However, it is possible that principal cells may have a thiazide-sensitive Na/Cl cotransporter. The mechanism by which sodium enters the principal cell will have an impact on potassium secretion. If sodium reabsorption does not involve passage through sodium conductance channels, potassium secretion will be reduced. Note in Figure 5-5 the presence of a cotransporter that mediates potassium and chloride secretion into the lumen of the cortical collecting duct. Normally this cotransporter is inactive due to the presence of chloride ions in luminal fluid. However, if chloride concentration in the lumen decreases, then the electrochemical driving forces will favor K/Cl cosecretion [10]. In theory, potassium secretion by principal cells can be modulated by factors affecting (1) the Na,K-ATPase pump, (2) plasma potassium concentration, (3) the potassium concentration gradient and the potassium conductance of the luminal membrane, (4) the sodium concentration gradient and the sodium conductance of the luminal membrane, and (5) the activity of the luminal potassium chloride cotransporter.

Factors Affecting Principal Cell Potassium Secretion

Several factors affect potassium secretion by the cortical collecting duct, some have direct effects on principal cells, while others exert indirect effects (Table 5-2).

Table 5-2. Factors affecting principal cell potassium secretion

Direct effects	Indirect effects
Aldosterone	Loop and thiazide diuretics
Sodium delivery—flow rate	Sodium intake
Antidiuretic hormone	
Chloride delivery—anion effect	
Plasma potassium concentration	
pH luminal fluid	
Potassium sparing diuretics	
Aldosterone antagonists	
Sodium channel blockers	

Direct Effects

Aldosterone

Aldosterone excess and deficiency always disturb potassium balance. Normal rates of potassium secretion do not occur in the absence of aldosterone. Adrenal insufficiency causes potassium retention and sodium wasting, which can be reversed by aldosterone, but not by glucocorticoid hormone [37]. On the other hand, excess mineralocorticoid hormone stimulates sodium reabsorption and potassium secretion. The role of plasma potassium concentration in the regulation of aldosterone has been established by identification of a feedback loop involving stimulation of aldosterone by increasing plasma potassium concentration.

Aldosterone plays an important regulatory role in the excretion of potassium after each meal. Investigations in humans have shown that the increase in plasma potassium concentration following a meal is sufficient to stimulate aldosterone release. These events occur with an appropriate time delay before the onset of increased potassium excretion [38, 39].

The principal cell is the major target of aldosterone in the kidney. Within an hour after introduction of aldosterone, sodium conductance of the luminal membrane increases, thus enhancing the driving force for potassium secretion. This involves unmasking or activation of previously existing sodium channels. After more prolonged exposure to aldosterone (i.e., 6–12 hours), there is increased synthesis and insertion of luminal sodium and potassium conductance channels and Na,K-ATPase pumps on the basolateral membrane [37, 40]. Activity of the Na,K-ATPase pump can be so great that the voltage across the basolateral membrane hyperpolarizes, which causes passive entry of potassium through basolateral potassium conductance channels [34]. Aldosterone produces its effects in principal cells by a genomic signal transduction system. Aldosterone enhances the intrinsic capacity of the principal cell to secrete potassium. Higher aldosterone concentrations are associated with greater stimulation of principal cells, which will persist as long as aldosterone concentration is above normal. The actual amount of potassium secreted, however, will depend on the status of the other factors that modulate potassium secretion. Integration of these responses will be discussed subsequently.

Sodium Delivery—Flow Rate

Potassium secretion will not occur if luminal sodium channels are closed. Continuous inward movement of sodium through channels is required to depolarize the luminal voltage to permit potassium secretion [10]. The major factor affecting the rate of inward sodium movement is the chemical concentration gradient for sodium across the luminal membrane of the principal cell. Thus, provided the channel is open, maintaining a high luminal sodium concentration will increase inward sodium movement and maximize depolarization of the luminal membrane. Normally, when fluid flow rate through the cortical collecting duct increases, a high luminal sodium concentration is maintained. At low flow rates in the cortical collecting duct, sodium concentration declines as sodium is reabsorbed (Fig. 5-6). At the end of the cortical collecting duct, there is no gradient for sodium entry into principal cells. In contrast, when flow rate increases, despite high rates of sodium reabsorption through sodium conductance channels, sodium concentration barely declines by the end of the cortical collecting duct. Therefore, a favorable gradient for sustained sodium reabsorption exists along the entire cortical collecting duct and stimulates potassium secretion continuously. This is the mechanism underlying increased potassium secretion associated with loop, thiazide, and proximally acting diuretics including osmotic diuresis (untreated diabetes mellitus, mannitol, and some antibiotics).

Antidiuretic Hormone

In addition to the effect of antidiuretic hormone (ADH), or vasopressin, on water permeability, this hormone increases the open state of the sodium channel [10, 33].

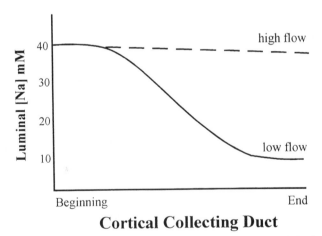

Cortical Collecting Duct

Fig. 5-6. Effect of flow rate on sodium concentration ([Na]) in luminal fluid measured along the length of the cortical collecting duct. At low flow rates, sodium concentration declines from 40 mm/L to about 10 mm/L by the end of the cortical collecting duct due to unsaturated sodium reabsorption. At high flow rates, however, sodium reabsorption is saturated, and sodium concentration remains at 40 mm/L along the entire length of the segment.

In the absence of ADH, most sodium channels are closed, and potassium secretion diminishes. The opposite occurs when ADH concentration increases. However, the magnitude of the effect of ADH on potassium secretion will depend on sodium delivery (i.e., flow rate) in the cortical collecting duct (assuming normal aldosterone). This dual effect of ADH on water permeability and on sodium reabsorption and potassium secretion allows regulation of water excretion without disturbing sodium and potassium excretion (balance). For example, during water conservation, ADH increases the water permeability of principal cells, causing approximately two-thirds of the water delivered to the collecting duct to be reabsorbed. A decrease in fluid delivery of this magnitude would, by itself, decrease potassium secretion. However, since ADH increases the open state of the sodium channel (increased conductance, i.e., permeability), sufficient numbers of sodium ions will traverse the channels, causing depolarization of the luminal membrane. Therefore, despite the lower flow rate through the cortical collecting duct in the presence of elevated ADH, normal rates of potassium secretion will prevail.

Chloride Delivery—Anion Composition

Administration of sodium with anions other than chloride (e.g., sulfate, bicarbonate, nitrate) can greatly augment renal potassium losses. This may be explained in whole, or in part, by the effect of decreased luminal chloride concentration rather than the presence of other anions. As mentioned earlier, experimental evidence supports the existence of a K/Cl cosecretion mechanism in the luminal membrane of the principal cell, which secretes potassium chloride when luminal chloride concentration is reduced below 15 mEq/L [10]. In most situations, increased delivery of nonchloride anions to principal cells is associated with reduced luminal chloride concentration.

In addition, an effect of nonchloride anions to increase sodium delivery should not be ignored. Most of these anions are poorly reabsorbed in the proximal tubule, if at all, and would be expected to interfere with water and sodium reabsorption in the proximal nephron segments. However, current knowledge of chloride reabsorption in the cortical collecting duct is insufficient to account completely for the effect of nonchloride anions on potassium secretion.

Plasma Potassium Concentration

Plasma potassium concentration, in addition to stimulating aldosterone synthesis and release, directly stimulates the Na,K-ATPase activity of principal cells [37, 40]. The increase in intracellular potassium concentration sustains greater rates of potassium secretion. At any aldosterone concentration, increments in plasma potassium concentration result in greater rates of principal cell potassium secretion. It is quite likely that increments in plasma potassium concentration that occur in chronic renal disease actually serve as an additional stimulus to maintain potassium secretion at near normal rates. Changes in potassium intake affect potassium secretion primarily by affecting plasma potassium concentration and consequently aldosterone level.

pH

Metabolic alkalosis stimulates principal cell potassium secretion and increases urinary potassium excretion [10, 33]. This is due in part to a direct effect of alkaline pH to increase basolateral potassium uptake and to increase the open state of the luminal potassium channel. The ultimate degree of principal cell potassium secretion therefore will depend on aldosterone and ADH levels, sodium delivery, and the extent to which chloride delivery is decreased (anion effect).

Although metabolic acidosis directly inhibits principal cell potassium secretion, urinary potassium excretion is usually markedly elevated under most conditions [3, 10]. This is particularly true in patients with untreated diabetes mellitus, in whom the largest potassium deficits have been observed [1, 41]. This can be understood in view of the other factors that are simultaneously affecting principal cell secretion. In most of these patients, aldosterone and ADH are elevated, sodium delivery is increased (osmotic diuresis), and chloride delivery is reduced (ketoanions). Thus, the direct inhibitory effect of acidosis can be overridden under these conditions.

Potassium Sparing Diuretics

Spironolactone, triamterene, and amiloride are weak natriuretic agents that promote the loss of only 2 to 3 percent of the filtered sodium while simultaneously reducing urinary potassium excretion. Spironolactone, but not triamterene and amiloride, is a steroid derivative that specifically antagonizes the effects of aldosterone in principal cells, thus accounting for its antikaliuretic activity. It competitively inhibits aldosterone binding to its nuclear receptor, thereby blocking the effects of the hormone. Spironolactone may be the diuretic of choice in some edematous patients because it enters principal cells from the basolateral side. When GFR is decreased in patients, delivery of other diuretics to luminal target sites may be difficult [10, 42].

Amiloride and triamterene impair potassium secretion in principal cells by blocking sodium conductance channels. In the presence of amiloride or triamterene, the luminal membrane hyperpolarizes, and potassium secretion ceases. These drugs prevent potassium secretion by principal cells in response to any stimulus [10]. Amiloride is frequently combined with thiazide or loop diuretics to prevent potassium loss that normally occurs [42]. Although the potassium sparing diuretics are useful in preventing diuretic-induced potassium deficiency, it should be remembered that their use may cause hyperkalemia in patients at risk or if taken inappropriately (see Decreased Urinary Excretion as a Cause of Hyperkalemia).

Recently, hyperkalemia in some patients with acquired immune deficiency syndrome (AIDS) was shown to be associated with the use of trimethoprim. This drug is administered for the treatment of *Pneumocystis carinii*. Subsequent investigations showed that trimethoprim has a similar mechanism of action in the cortical collecting duct as amiloride [43]. In the same study, trimethoprim caused a reversible elevation in plasma potassium concentration in AIDS patients. In half of the patients, plasma potassium concentration increased to values greater than 5 mEq/L. To avoid serious hyperkalemia, therefore, caution should be exercised when using this drug.

Indirect Effects

Loop, Thiazide, and Proximally Acting Diuretics

Loop, thiazide, and proximally acting diuretics are a frequent cause of increased potassium excretion in the clinical setting. Although diuretic agents with kaliuretic activity may decrease sodium and fluid reabsorption by different mechanisms, they probably all enhance secretion of potassium by increasing sodium delivery to the cortical collecting duct. Loop diuretics (e.g., furosemide, bumetanide) further promote potassium loss by directly inhibiting potassium reabsorption in the thick ascending limb and by promoting a small amount of potassium secretion [10, 31]. Also, since furosemide and its analogues abolish the medullary osmotic gradient, inhibition of fluid reabsorption in the descending limb contributes to further increases in sodium delivery to the cortical collecting duct. Lastly, almost all patients treated with diuretics develop a degree of effective circulating volume contraction. The consequent elevations of aldosterone and ADH potentiate flow-stimulated potassium secretion.

The magnitude of hypokalemia is greater with the longer-acting (>24 hours) diuretics, such as chlorthalidone, as compared with the short-acting (<6 hours) diuretics, such as furosemide. Potassium losses will reflect the magnitude of the diuresis and sodium intake. A low dose of hydrochlorothiazide (e.g., 12.5 mg/day) does not cause significant potassium depletion and usually is effective for the treatment of hypertension. Also, potassium loss can be minimized by sodium restriction. If diuretic dose and dietary potassium and sodium intake are relatively constant, most potassium loss will occur during the first 2 weeks of treatment [42]. At this time, a new steady state is reached in which intake and excretion are equal. If hypokalemia has not developed after this 2-week period, it is unlikely to be a concern in that patient. Elderly patients, especially women, are more at risk of diuretic-induced hypokalemia due to lower total body potassium [44].

Sodium Intake

The kaliuretic effect of the acute administration of sodium-containing salts is well documented and can be attributed to increased sodium delivery to the cortical collecting duct. Chronic high sodium intake does not disturb potassium balance, since aldosterone release is suppressed. Independent control of effective circulating volume and potassium balance will be discussed subsequently.

Dietary sodium restriction is associated with a reduction in renal potassium excretion. This is due to avid reabsorption of potassium by the collecting duct and because sodium reabsorption by principal cells is required for normal response to elevated aldosterone [40, 45]. Assembly and insertion of the Na,K-ATPase pump into the basolateral membrane is a sodium-dependent processes. When sodium chloride is administered acutely to sodium-deficient animals, an enhanced capacity of the cortical collecting duct to secrete potassium is revealed. Increased sodium delivery is responsible for the increase in potassium secretion.

Integrated Responses

The absence of aldosterone or ADH, the presence of potassium sparing diuretics, or insufficient sodium delivery will prevent potassium secretion. Although elevated aldosterone, increased sodium delivery, and reduced chloride delivery each can stimulate potassium secretion, the status of the other factors will determine the amount of potassium that is actually secreted. For example, potassium secretion may not increase when sodium delivery increases if aldosterone is reduced or ADH is absent. The necessary interplay between these factors allows independent regulation of effective circulating volume (ECV) and potassium balance by aldosterone and of water balance and electrolyte balance by ADH.

A review of the mechanisms by which ECV is regulated illustrates this point (see Chap. 2). If ECV is expanded or contracted, the kidney is able to excrete or conserve sodium chloride and water, without disturbing potassium balance. This can be attributed to inverse effects on sodium delivery and aldosterone on principal cell secretion. This is due to the integrated responses of renal sympathetic nerves and angiotensin II on the glomerulus and proximal tubule and of aldosterone action on principal cells. The following scenario involving significant loss or redistribution of ECF shows how ECV and potassium balance can be regulated independently.

When ECV decreases, renal sympathetic nerve activity increases due to baroreceptor responses. Renin release occurs, and angiotensin II is produced. Filtration rate decreases and proximal tubule sodium chloride reabsorption increases due to the combined action of catecholamines and angiotensin II. Simultaneously, in response to the increase in circulating angiotensin II, aldosterone concentration rises. Within a few hours, the intrinsic capacity of principal cells to secrete potassium is

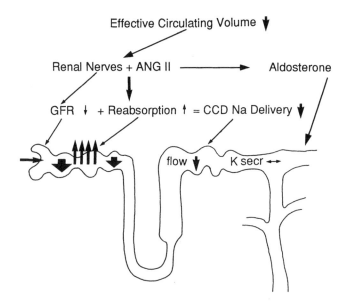

HIGH ALDO + LOW CCD NA DELIVERY = NORMAL CCD K SECRETION

Fig. 5-7. In response to a reduction in effective circulating volume, delivery of sodium to the cortical collecting duct (CCD) is reduced, and aldosterone (ALDO) is increased. Although aldosterone would enhance the capacity of principal cells to secrete potassium, the reduction in sodium delivery offsets this stimulation, and net potassium secretion (K secr) remains normal. See text for further explanation. Ang II = angiotensin II; GFR = glomerular filtration rate.

greatly enhanced (see Aldosterone). However, despite the marked stimulation of principal cells by aldosterone, renal potassium excretion does not increase. The reason for this paradox is that the decrease in sodium delivery to the collecting duct offsets the direct stimulation of aldosterone on potassium secretion (Fig. 5-7). The action of renal nerves and angiotensin II reduces the filtered load of sodium and enhances proximal reabsorption. This further decreases the amount of sodium delivered to the cortical collecting duct. In this way, ECV can be returned to normal by retention of sodium chloride and water by the proximal nephron, while aldosterone maintains normal rates of potassium secretion at a reduced sodium delivery in the cortical collecting duct.

In humans with a normal potassium intake, it is abnormal to have elevated aldosterone levels in combination with normal or increased sodium delivery to the cortical collecting duct. This combination is a common underlying cause of increased renal potassium losses encountered in the following pathophysiologic conditions.

Renal Causes of Accelerated Potassium Loss

Mineralocorticoid Excess

Regardless of the source, the presence of excess mineralocorticoid hormone in an otherwise normal individual results in increased sodium chloride and water retention, hypertension, and continuous stimulation of potassium secretion. Edema does not develop, since the expansion of ECV leads to the suppression of sodium-retaining mechanisms (see Fig. 5-7) and release of atrial natriuretic peptide [46, 47]. Filtration rate increases, and proximal salt and water reabsorption decreases, which combine to increase sodium delivery to the cortical collecting duct. In the setting of elevated aldosterone, principal cells are stimulated to secrete potassium, and increased sodium delivery adds to the stimulation. Although the kidney escapes from continued sodium reabsorption, it cannot escape from the potassium loss. Metabolic alkalosis develops due to enhanced proximal ammonium production secondary to potassium depletion.

Primary Hyperaldosteronism

The autonomous hypersecretion of aldosterone may result from a unilateral adrenal adenoma or carcinoma or from bilateral hyperplasia. An adenoma is responsible for about 60 percent of cases, with hyperplasia accounting for most of the remaining cases. The mechanism responsible for idiopathic adrenal hyperplasia is not well understood. The treatment of choice for adenoma, when possible, is surgical removal, whereas for hyperplasia it is medical, including treatment with amiloride or spironolactone, angiotensin-converting enzyme inhibitors, and calcium channel blockers.

Glucocorticoid-Remediable Hyperaldosteronism

Glucocorticoid-remediable hyperaldosteronism is a rare form of adrenal hyperplasia in which the hypersecretion of aldosterone can be reversed with glucocorticoid therapy. Normal subjects synthesize aldosterone in the zona glomerulosa, which lacks 17-hydroxylase required for cortisol synthesis, but not in the adrenocortico-tropic hormone (ACTH)–sensitive zona fasciculata, which lacks the enzymes required to add the necessary aldehyde to corticosterone at the 18-carbon position. Patients with glucocorticoid-remediable hyperaldosteronism have ACTH-sensitive aldosterone production occurring in the zona fasciculata. The primary defect is a chimeric gene on chromosome 8 that contains the regulatory region of 11β-hydroxylase and the coding sequences of the aldosterone synthase gene [48, 49].

Glucocorticoid-remediable hyperaldosteronism is inherited as an autosomal dominant trait. The presence of this rare disorder as the cause of primary hyperaldosteronism should be suspected from the positive family history and the typical onset of hypertension before age 21. The diagnosis can be confirmed by documenting the increased secretion of 18-carbon oxidation products of cortisol (18-hydroxycortisol and 18-oxocortisol) or by direct genetic analysis.

Treatment consists of administration of glucocorticoids, dexamethasone or prednisone, which corrects the overproduction of aldosterone by diminishing ACTH release and which usually also normalizes the blood pressure.

Congenital Adrenal Hyperplasia

17α-Hydroxylase deficiency impairs cortisol and androgen synthesis; the ensuing rise in ACTH release will increase the synthesis of the mineralocorticoids deoxycorticosterone and corticosterone, resulting in hypertension, hypokalemia, and metabolic alkalosis, but no virilization.

11β-Hydroxylase deficiency, like 17-hydroxylase deficiency, is associated with ACTH-induced overproduction of the mineralocorticoid deoxycorticosterone, leading to hypertension and hypokalemia. This disorder, however, is virilizing, since there is also hypersecretion of adrenal androgens.

Cushing's Syndrome (Glucocorticoid Excess)

Cortisol is synthesized in the zona fasciculata under the influence of ACTH. Cortisol binds as avidly as aldosterone to the mineralocorticoid receptor. Cortisol, however, normally has weak mineralocorticoid activity because it is inactivated to cortisone in the aldosterone-sensitive cells in the cortical collecting duct [50]. In spite of this, some patients with Cushing's syndrome develop hypokalemia and metabolic alkalosis. This most commonly occurs in patients with ectopic ACTH production who markedly oversecrete cortisol [51]. In addition to cortisol, other ACTH-dependent mineralocorticoids, including deoxycorticosterone and corticosterone, also may play an active role in Cushing's syndrome. Hypercortisolism can result from hypersecretion of ACTH, due to a pituitary adenoma or a nonendocrine ACTH-producing tumor, or from primary adrenal diseases (adenoma or carcinoma) [52, 53].

Treatment consists of transsphenoidal microsurgery for pituitary disease and removal of a unilateral adrenal lesion. Patients who are not surgical candidates can be treated with ketoconazole or metyrapone (both inhibit 11β-hydroxylase, which converts deoxycorticol to cortisol), aminoglutethimide (which inhibits the conversion of cholesterol to pregnenolone), or the adrenolytic agent mitotane.

Licorice and the Syndrome of Apparent Mineralocorticoid Excess

Subjects chronically ingesting about 100 g (four twists) of real licorice, licorice-containing chewing tobacco, or licorice-like compounds including carbonoxolone can develop a reversible syndrome that acts like primary hyperaldosteronism [54, 55]. Glycyrrhenitic acid, a steroid in licorice, has slight mineralocorticoid activity. In addition, this compound also impairs the action of the enzyme 11β-hydroxysteroid dehydrogenase that converts cortisol to cortisone in aldosterone target tissues such as the collecting tubules in the kidney [56]. Increased levels of cortisol therefore activate the mineralocorticoid receptors and produce a syndrome similar to primary hyperaldosteronism. Endogenous aldosterone secretion is appropriately suppressed in this setting.

In the syndrome of apparent mineralocorticoid excess, there is a genetic defect in which cortisol metabolism is impaired in the cortical collecting ducts [57, 58]. Administration of dexamethasone suppresses endogenous cortisol production and corrects the hypokalemia. Alternatively, amiloride or spironolactone and a low-sodium diet also correct the hypokalemia in the syndrome of apparent mineralocorticoid excess.

Bartter's Syndrome

Bartter's syndrome generally presents early in life and is associated with growth retardation, hypokalemia, metabolic alkalosis, hyperaldosteronism, hyperreninemia, marked hypertrophy and hyperplasia of the juxtaglomerular apparatus, normal blood pressure, insensitivity to exogenous angiotensin II, polyuria, polydipsia, increased renal prostaglandin E_2 production, and decreased concentrating ability. Urinary calcium excretion is increased, and the plasma magnesium concentration is either normal or mildly reduced in most patients [59,60].

In most families, transmission of the disease follows a pattern consistent with autosomal recessive inheritance. The urinary findings suggest, and recent genetic studies confirm, a primary defect in sodium chloride reabsorption in the thick ascending limb of the loop of Henle [60,61]. Activation of the renin-angiotensin-aldosterone system and increased sodium delivery due to the reabsorptive defect, enhance potassium secretion in the cortical collecting duct causing hypokalemia and consequent metabolic alkalosis [42,60].

Until genetic analysis becomes available, diagnosis depends on establishing renal potassium and Cl$^-$ wasting and the exclusion of other known causes [62]. Treatment consists of (1) replacement of potassium chloride, (2) correction of hypomagnesemia, (3) use of prostaglandin synthase inhibitors, and (4) use of potassium sparing diuretics, amiloride, spironolactone, or triamterene.

Gitelman's Syndrome

Gitelman's syndrome, once thought to be a variant of Bartter's syndrome, was known as the syndrome of tubular hypomagnesemia-hypokalemia with hypocalciuria [60,

63]. Gitelman's syndrome is a more benign condition that may not be diagnosed until late childhood or even adulthood. Reduced calcium excretion, magnesium wasting and hypomagnesemia are characteristic and patients may present with tetany [63]. Concentrating ability is unaffected. Inheritance of the disease follows the pattern of an autosomal recessive trait and has recently been found to be caused by mutations in the NaCl cotransporter in the distal convoluted tubule [64]. Impaired thiazide-sensitive NaCl transport can account for the decrease in Ca^{2+} excretion (in contrast to the hypercalciuria seen in Bartter's syndrome). Mg^{2+} wasting is secondary to enhanced Ca^{2+} reabsorption in the distal convoluted tubule, while hypokalemia is due to flow stimulated K secretion in the cortical collected duct.

Liddle's Syndrome

Liddle's syndrome is a rare autosomal dominant condition in which there is a primary increase in collecting tubule sodium reabsorption and, in most cases, potassium secretion. Correction of the hypokalemia and hypertension in one patient by renal transplantation suggested that enhanced activity of the luminal membrane sodium channels, rather than a circulating factor such as increased secretion of a nonaldosterone mineralocorticoid, is the underlying defect in this disorder [65]. Recently, Liddle's syndrome has been found to be caused by mutations in the β subunit of the epithelial sodium channel. Functionally these mutations result in constitutive activation of the amiloride-sensitive renal sodium channel [66].

Therapy in Liddle's syndrome consists of amiloride or triamterene, potassium sparing diuretics that directly inhibit the sodium channel. Interestingly, the mineralocorticoid antagonist spironolactone is ineffective, since the increase in sodium channel activity is not mediated by aldosterone.

Renal Tubular Acidosis

Hypokalemia secondary to excessive urinary potassium excretion is a common complication of both type 1 and type 2 renal tubular acidosis (RTA) [67].

In type 1 (distal) RTA, distal H^+ secretion is reduced. This is associated with increased sodium reabsorption coupled to potassium secretion. Severe potassium depletion with a plasma potassium concentration below 2.0 mEq/L may occur in this disorder [68]. One of the more common causes of type 1 RTA in adults is Sjögren's syndrome [69]. In most patients with distal RTA, potassium supplements are not required to maintain normokalemia when correction of acidosis is achieved. In some patients, however, potassium losses continue despite correction of the acidosis.

In type 2 (proximal) RTA, increased quantities of sodium and HCO_3^- are delivered to the cortical collecting duct, which enhances urinary potassium secretion. This effect becomes even more prominent after the institution of alkali therapy, which raises the filtered HCO_3^- load above proximal tubular reabsorptive capacity. These patients therefore require potassium as well as HCO_3^- replacement therapy.

Hypomagnesemia

Hypomagnesemia is a relatively common finding in hypokalemic patients. Hypomagnesemia of any cause can lead to potassium depletion and hypokalemia [4, 70]. In addition, in some cases the underlying abnormality, including thiazide or loop diuretics, cisplatin toxicity, or primary hyperaldosteronism, impairs both potassium and Mg^{2+} reabsorption by the kidney.

The mechanisms proposed for Mg^{2+} deficiency to cause increased potassium secretion include enhanced secretion of aldosterone and enhanced opening of potassium channels in the luminal membrane of the thick ascending limb of the loop of Henle.

Correction of the hypokalemia is usually not possible by potassium repletion alone, unless magnesium balance is also corrected at the same time [71]. Magnesium repletion in the presence of hypokalemia should preferably begin with magnesium oxide, as the use of magnesium sulfate can initially increase urinary potassium losses, since sulfate acts as a nonreabsorbable anion.

Antibiotics and Other Drugs

The majority of penicillin derivatives, including sodium penicillin and carbenicillin, have been implicated as causes of hypokalemia [72]. Potential mechanisms include the following: (1) Penicillin may act as an osmotic diuretic, and since it is a strong organic acid that is completely ionized at any urine pH, it may function as a nonreabsorbable anion, which reduces chloride delivery to the cortical collecting duct; and (2) the administration of these antibiotics, especially carbenicillin, is often associated with a large sodium load, which enhances cortical collecting duct flow rate. These factors combine to stimulate potassium secretion.

Hypokalemia is also commonly seen in patients treated with amphotericin B. Increased membrane permeability due to an interaction of amphotericin with membrane sterols promotes distal potassium secretion by increasing the potassium permeability of the luminal membrane. In addition, amphotericin also causes type 1 RTA, which further contributes to the potassium secretion. The tubular acidosis is probably related to increased membrane permeability to H^+ ions or to H_2CO_3, which allows the secreted acid to back-diffuse out of the tubular lumen [1].

Cis-dichlorodiamine platinum (cisplatin), a chemotherapeutic agent, has been associated with hypokalemia, as well as hypomagnesemia. In this case, the hypokalemia is usually resistant to potassium replacement therapy until the magnesium deficiency is corrected [73].

Toluene, an organic solvent inhaled for its effects on the central nervous system, can also cause severe hypokalemia [74]. Hypokalemia is due primarily to increased renal potassium loss secondary to increased excretion of hippurate.

Diagnostic Approach to the Hypokalemic Patient

The search for the etiology of hypokalemia should include an evaluation of intake, distribution, and excretion of potassium by the following: (1) a careful history, including use of drugs, medications, and presence of vomiting or diarrhea, (2) physical examination, including blood pressure and orthostatic changes in blood pressure and heart rate, (3) urine and plasma electrolytes and osmolality, (4) arterial blood gas, and (5) electrocardiogram (ECG).

The most useful tests to monitor the urinary potassium excretion include

1. The 24-hour potassium excretion rate: It should be less than 15 mmol/day in the presence of hypokalemia of extrarenal etiology. The disadvantage of this test is that it takes a long time before the clinician has access to the results.
2. Spot urine for [potassium] [creatinine] ratio: It should be less than 1 mmol of potassium per 1 mmol of creatinine in the presence of hypokalemia of extrarenal etiology. The advantage of this test is that it can be performed on a random urine sample, and the results are available within 1 to 2 hours.
3. Transtubular potassium gradient (TTKG), which is also performed on a spot urine:

$$TTKG = \frac{[K]_{urine}/[urine/plasma]_{osmolality}}{[K]_{plasma}}$$

TTKG is a test designed to reflect the driving force for potassium secretion in the cortical collecting tubule. TTKG should be less than 2 in the presence of hypokalemia of extrarenal origin. If hypokalemia is a result of renal losses, for example, secondary to hyperaldosteronism, then typical TTKG values are greater than 6 [41, 75].

A diagnostic approach to hypokalemia based on these criteria is given in Figures 5-8, 5-9, and 5-10.

Consequences of Potassium Depletion

Neuromuscular Effects

Potassium levels below 3.0 mEq/L are often associated with complaint of muscular weakness, generalized malaise, fatigue, the restless legs syndrome, and occasionally myalgias. Severe potassium depletion can result in two major neuromuscular complications: paralysis and rhabdomyolysis [13].

Hypokalemia, whether produced by transcellular shifts or potassium depletion, can alter the function of excitable tissues; the effect on muscle is most notable. The specific effects on cardiac muscle will be discussed subsequently. The increase in the intracellular to extracellular potassium ratio hyperpolarizes the membrane, which then increases the threshold for initiating an action potential. Even after an action potential has arisen at the neuromuscular junction, spread along the muscle fiber will be greatly impaired. As the degree of hypokalemia worsens, the decrease in the conductance of potassium channels allows the underlying sodium and calcium conductances to have a greater effect on the resting membrane potential. It is not uncommon for the resting muscle to depolarize, and inactivation of sodium channels can then be the primary cause of the paralysis.

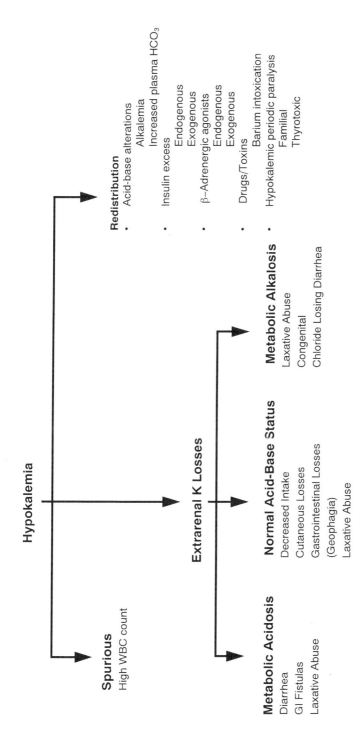

Fig. 5-8. Diagnostic approach to the patient with hypokalemia of extrarenal origin. WBC = white blood cell; GI = gastrointestinal.

220

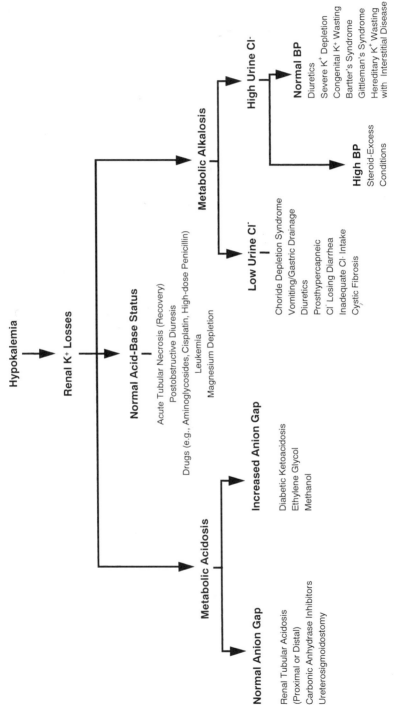

Fig. 5-9. Diagnostic approach to the normotensive or hypotensive patient with hypokalemia of renal origin. BP = blood pressure.

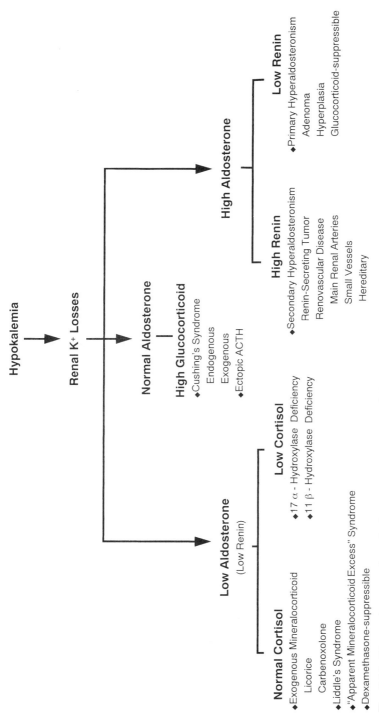

Fig. 5-10. Diagnostic approach to the hypertensive patient with hypokalemia of renal origin. ACTH = adrenocorticotropic hormone.

Skeletal muscle dysfunction can also be attributed to other defects associated with potassium depletion: (1) impaired muscle blood flow and absence of exercise-induced vasodilatation, (2) a depletion of energy (glycogen) stores, and (3) total loss of cellular integrity, which can result in muscle necrosis (rhabdomyolysis).

Involvement of smooth muscle in the gastrointestinal tract can produce a paralytic ileus and the symptoms of abdominal distention, anorexia, nausea, vomiting, and constipation. Urinary bladder mobility is also decreased as a result of potassium depletion.

Cardiac Effects

The cardiac effects are the most serious consequence of hypokalemia. Reductions in plasma potassium concentration are associated with characteristic changes in the ECG, which are shown in Figure 5-11. As plasma potassium concentration decreases, ventricular repolarization is strikingly delayed. Despite hyperpolarization of the resting membrane potential from -90 to about -100 mV, the rate of outward potassium movement decreases during the action potential. This is due to the decrease in potassium channel activity (conductance) caused by the reduction in plasma potassium concentration. The shoulder of the falling phase of the action potential becomes progressively less steep and is manifested in the ECG by the flattening of the T wave. Delayed repolarization contributes in a major way to the increased duration of the action potential. Normally the U wave represents repolarization of Purkinje fibers. In severe hypokalemia (1–2 mEq/L), the T wave and U wave combine, creating a wave with greater amplitude. ECG evidence of

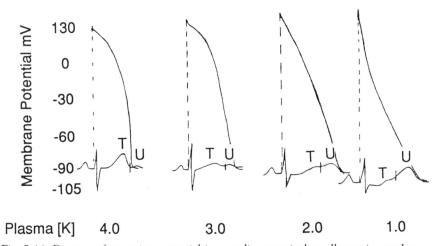

Fig. 5-11. Diagram of an action potential in a cardiac ventricular cell superimposed on the simultaneously recorded electrocardiogram for plasma potassium concentrations of 4.0, 3.0, 2.0, and 1.0 mEq/L. The left axis represents the ventricular cell membrane potential in millivolts (mV). See text for further information. (Adapted from B. Surawicz, Relationship between electrocardiogram and electrolytes. *Am. Heart J.* 73[6]:815, 1967.)

hypokalemia is primarily based on ST segment depression and abnormalities in T and U waves [76, 77].

The greatest cardiac risk in hypokalemia is the threat of reentry currents arising during the prolonged repolarization phase, leading to the development of arrhythmias [1, 76]. The increased incidence of arrhythmias in hypokalemia may also be related to the activation of sodium channels secondary to hyperpolarization of the resting membrane potential causing increased automaticity. Hypokalemia appears to predispose to serious ventricular ectopy such as ventricular tachycardia and fibrillation, particularly in the setting of coronary artery disease and acute myocardial infarction [1, 78, 79].

In the case of diuretic-induced hypokalemia, no large study has dealt with all the variables that may complicate the cardiac effects, that is, decreased cellular potassium concentration, decreased plasma and cellular magnesium concentration, increased systemic pH or concurrent use of other drugs, and underlying cardiac disease. Any one of these variables may alter the cardiac effects of hypokalemia. In the final analysis, a low level of plasma potassium concentration (particularly <3.0 mEq/L), the presence of underlying cardiac disease, and concomitant use of other drugs that can either lower plasma potassium concentration (e.g., β-agonists) or increase the risk of cardiac arrhythmias (e.g., digoxin) [11] should sway the clinician to avoid diuretics and to treat diuretic-induced hypokalemia. Although cardiac necrosis has been described in some hypokalemic individuals, other contributory factors cannot be eliminated [3].

Effects on Blood Pressure

Epidemiologic surveys suggest that populations ingesting diets low in potassium are more susceptible to the development of hypertension. Several clinical studies have demonstrated that potassium depletion is associated with an increase in blood pressure, while potassium supplementation exerts the opposite effect [80, 81]. The mechanism underlying the increase in blood pressure during potassium depletion is not well understood. Sodium retention, which accompanies potassium depletion, most likely plays an important role, as the hypertensive effect of potassium depletion fails to become manifest if sodium intake is curtailed.

Metabolic Effects

Carbohydrate intolerance is the most common metabolic disorder associated with potassium depletion [3]. Impairment in glucose tolerance during potassium K depletion is due to diminished insulin secretion secondary to diminished beta-cell response to glucose. Glucose intolerance in hyperaldosteronism or vigorous thiazide therapy is only observed in patients who are hypokalemic.

Potassium depletion stimulates renin production with a consequent increase in angiotensin II; however, aldosterone secretion decreases [3]. Potassium directly stimulates aldosterone synthesis and potentiates stimulation by angiotensin II and ACTH. With hypokalemia, the decline in aldosterone is beneficial in defending body stores of potassium during potassium depletion. The decrease in aldosterone augments stimulation of renin production, which is currently stimulated by potassium depletion itself.

Potassium deficiency affects protein metabolism, as manifested by a retarded rate of growth in young animals [7]. This effect probably contributes to failure to obtain positive nitrogen balance during potassium-deficient hyperalimentation [8] as well as failure to thrive in children with Bartter's syndrome. Growth retardation may be a consequence of impaired growth hormone release or altered protein synthesis due to relative insulin deficiency [82].

Renal Effects

Potassium depletion has both structural and functional effects on the kidney.

Morphologic Changes

In humans, the characteristic histologic finding is vacuolization of proximal and distal tubular cells. In chronic potassium depletion, diffuse chronic interstitial nephritis and scarring have been observed. Furthermore, chronic hypokalemia from hyperaldosteronism is associated with renal cyst formation and interstitial scarring. The numbers and size of cyst in these patients decrease following correction of hypokalemia.

Functional Effects

Potassium depletion is associated with several effects in renal function, including a decrease in renal blood flow, impaired urinary concentrating ability, increased ammonia production, increased bicarbonate reabsorption, increased sodium reabsorption, and impaired phosphate reabsorption [4, 83, 84].

The impaired urinary concentration is associated with polyuria and polydipsia. There are two components to the polydipsia: (1) a primary increase in thirst, possibly secondary to enhanced angiotensin II effect on the thirst center [85], and (2) diminished urinary concentrating ability, or nephrogenic diabetes insipidus, due to inhibition of thick ascending limb sodium chloride reabsorption [86].

Hypokalemia causes increased production of NH_3 and NH_4^+ by the proximal tubular cells, resulting in increases in urinary NH_4^+ excretion [3, 36]. In hypokalemia, the ensuing intracellular acidosis most likely is responsible for the increased NH_4^+ production. The increase in ammonia production may be clinically important in patients with severe hepatic disease, in whom hypokalemia can precipitate hepatic coma.

Treatment of Hypokalemia

The immediate objective of potassium replacement is to prevent life-threatening cardiac and muscular complications, and the ultimate objective is to replenish total body potassium stores.

The potassium deficit can only be approximated, since there is no definite correlation between the plasma potassium concentration and body potassium stores. A reduction in the plasma potassium concentration from 4.0 to 3.0 mEq/L represents a loss of 200 to 400 mEq of potassium. An additional 200- to 400-mEq deficit will lower plasma potassium concentration to 2.0 mEq/L. However, continued potassium losses may not produce much more hypokalemia, as the release of potassium from the cells is usually able to maintain the plasma potassium concentration near 2.0 mEq/L.

Transcellular shifts of potassium may further complicate the estimation of a given potassium deficit. In patients with periodic paralysis, body potassium stores are normal, as the hypokalemia is due to potassium movement into the cells. In states associated with acidosis (e.g., RTA) or hyperosmolality (e.g., diabetic ketoacidosis), the plasma potassium concentration may underestimate potassium losses. Initiation of bicarbonate therapy in RTA may rapidly lower serum potassium concentration by enhancing cellular potassium uptake. Initiation of therapy with saline and insulin in diabetic ketoacidosis may rapidly lower plasma potassium concentration by promoting urinary losses and cellular uptake of potassium.

Guidelines for Potassium Replacement

A variety of potassium preparations are available for oral and intravenous use, including the Cl^-, HCO_3^-, citrate, phosphate, and gluconate salts.

1. In patients with metabolic alkalosis, since there is also a simultaneous deficit in Cl^-, the administration of potassium with Cl^- is essential for correction of both the alkalosis and the potassium deficit.
2. In patients with metabolic acidosis, $KHCO_3$ or potassium citrate is the preferred form of potassium replacement therapy.
3. If equal doses of KCl and $KHCO_3$ are given, there will be a significantly greater increase in the plasma potassium concentration with KCl than with $KHCO_3$. This difference is probably related to the ability of HCO_3^- to enter the cells in comparison with that of Cl^-, which is mostly limited to the ECF.

When possible, it is preferable to replace potassium orally. The preferred preparations are KCl elixir (not very palatable), KCl tablets, and salt substitute, which comes in crystalline form. It should be noted that potassium replacement with potassium-rich foods such as bananas and orange juice may be less effective, since these foods contain citrate and phosphate rather than Cl^- and therefore are not as effective, especially in patients with hypokalemia in the presence of metabolic alkalosis.

In patients who are unable to eat, potassium must be given intravenously. It is important to administer potassium in solutions that do not contain dextrose, since the enhanced insulin secretion may result in a further lowering of plasma potassium concentration.

Rate of Potassium Repletion

In the majority of patients who have mild to moderate hypokalemia (plasma potassium concentration 3.0–3.5 mEq/L), unless the patients are on digitalis or have hepatic coma, the potassium can be replaced slowly by the oral route, at the rate of 30 to 60 mEq/day.

In patients with severe hypokalemia (usually plasma potassium <2.5 mEq/L), plasma potassium needs to be corrected rapidly, either by the oral route, 60 mEq of KCl every hour, or intravenously, at a maximum rate of 10 to 20 mEq/hr [87]. The key is to continuously monitor the ECG and to obtain frequent measurements of plasma potassium. Once again, since it is hard to estimate the exact degree of potassium deficit, it is difficult to calculate the precise amount of potassium that needs to be administered. The key to success is therefore frequent monitoring and assessment. It is also important to avoid overreplacement, which can result in hyperkalemia, a condition that is potentially as life threatening as severe hypokalemia.

Decreased Urinary Excretion as a Cause of Hyperkalemia

Inadequate sodium delivery to the cortical collecting duct secondary to effective circulating volume depletion (see Integrated Responses), renal failure, and hypoaldosteronism are the major causes of reduced urinary potassium excretion resulting in persistent hyperkalemia [10].

Inadequate Cortical Collecting Duct Sodium Delivery

Decreases in sodium delivery to cortical collecting duct principal cells secondary to a reduction in renal plasma flow and/or GFR or an increase in sodium and volume reabsorption by the proximal tubule or loop of Henle can result in hyperkalemia. The most common clinical situations in which decreased distal sodium delivery can lead to hyperkalemia include severe heart failure or acute pulmonary edema, hepatic cirrhosis with ascites, and patients with chronic renal disease who become intravascularly volume depleted [88]. In these cases, hyperkalemia is encountered, especially when urine flow rate is less than 600 ml/day.

Renal Failure

In patients who develop acute oliguric renal failure, hyperkalemia is very frequent and occurs as a result of several factors, including (1) markedly decreased cortical collecting duct sodium delivery, (2) GFR less than 10 ml/min, which becomes rate limiting for potassium excretion, (3) acute tubular necrosis and tubulointerstitial nephritis damage to nephron segments, which are primarily responsible for potassium secretion, (4) the acuteness of the renal failure and the tubular damage, which impair the usual tubular adaptive mechanisms for compensatory increase in urinary potassium excretion, and (5) metabolic acidosis, tissue catabolism, and acute renal failure associated with tissue necrosis, such as burns and rhabdomyolysis, when there is increased release of potassium into the ECF compartment [9].

In contrast, in patients with chronic renal failure, hyperkalemia does not occur unless the GFR is less than 10 ml/min or the patients have hypoaldosteronism or aldosterone resistance. In these patients, the potassium balance is maintained by increased potassium secretion per functioning nephron, which is mediated in part by aldosterone and enhanced Na,K-ATPase activity [89]. These adaptive mechanisms are effective in preventing hyperkalemia provided that urine output is in excess of 600 ml/day. Hyperkalemia, however, develops when there is increased oral potassium intake or increased cell potassium release as a result of tissue necrosis or if drugs are used that cause hypoaldosteronism or block the tubular secretion of potassium.

In chronic renal failure, in addition to the absolute decrease in urinary potassium excretion, potassium entry into the cells may also be impaired. The factors primarily responsible are the presence of inorganic metabolic acidosis (see Distribution of Potassium) and decreased skeletal muscle Na,K-ATPase activity [89].

Impaired Renin-Aldosterone Axis

Hypoaldosteronism may result from a variety of conditions that interfere with the production or the renal tubular effect of aldosterone. The most common causes are hyporeninemic hypoaldosteronism, primary adrenal insufficiency, and drugs in adults and adrenal enzyme deficiencies or pseudohypoaldosteronism in children.

In addition to hyperkalemia, hyponatremia, azotemia, and hyperchloremic metabolic acidosis are also present in hypoaldosteronism. The metabolic acidosis is due in part to the hyperkalemia, since when the plasma potassium concentration is normalized there is correction of the acidosis. This effect of hyperkalemia is mediated by reduced renal tubular HCO_3^- absorption and NH_4^+ secretion and recycling [36, 90, 91].

Addison's Disease

Patients with primary adrenal insufficiency, or Addison's disease, have decreases in both mineralocorticoid and glucocorticoid secretion. Tuberculosis and primary atrophy were once the most common causes, but presently autoimmune disease is the most common cause of this problem in adult patients.

Adrenal Enzyme Deficiencies

Signs of mineralocorticoid deficiency may result from reduced activity of enzymes involved in steps prior to the synthesis of deoxycorticosterone (3β-hydroxysteroid dehydrogenase and 21-hydroxylase) or in the conversion of corticosterone to aldosterone (corticosterone methyl oxidase or aldosterone synthase). Although 11β-hydroxylase deficiency also decreases aldosterone production by impairing the conversion of deoxycorticosterone to corticosterone, there is buildup of deoxycorticosterone, which results in signs of mineralocorticoid excess, including hypertension and hypokalemia.

21-Hydroxylase deficiency is the most common form of congenital adrenal hyperplasia. It is an autosomal recessive disorder involving different alterations on the short arm of chromosome 6. In addition to impairing mineralocorticoid synthesis,

21-hydroxylase deficiency also impairs the conversion of 17-hydroxyprogesterone to deoxycortisol, the precursor of cortisol. The concurrent cortisol deficiency stimulates the release of ACTH, resulting in enhanced adrenal androgen synthesis and virilization.

Children with the classic syndrome present in infancy with salt wasting, hyperkalemia, and virilization. There are additional clinical presentations as well that reflect different abnormalities in the 21-hydroxylase gene [92, 93]. Treatment of 21-hydroxylase deficiency consists of replacement therapy with cortisol and the synthetic mineralocorticoid fluorocortisone.

Hyporeninemic Hypoaldosteronism

In the absence of oliguric acute renal failure and drugs that interfere with aldosterone production or renal tubular secretion of potassium, the syndrome of hyporeninemic hypoaldosteronism accounts for the majority of patients with hyperkalemia. Most patients with this syndrome have mild to moderate renal insufficiency with a GFR of 20 to 60 ml/min. Almost all of the patients have diabetes mellitus or chronic interstitial nephritis.

The hypoaldosteronism appears to be mostly induced by reduced plasma renin and angiotensin II activity. In addition, there is also an intra-adrenal defect. This is suggested by the observations that some patients have a normal plasma renin activity and/or impaired aldosterone secretion in response to angiotensin II infusion [94]. Studies in diabetic animals have demonstrated that the impaired response of the zona glomerulosa cells to angiotensin II is due to a postreceptor defect. The aldosterone secretory defect is specific for angiotensin II as the aldosterone secretory response to ACTH is not diminished [95].

In addition to the hypoaldosteronism, the decrease in renal function is also an important factor in the genesis of the hyperkalemia. In spite of the decrease in urinary potassium excretion as a result of the hypoaldosteronism, patients with normal renal function could compensate, since the rise in plasma potassium concentration directly enhances distal tubular potassium secretion. Thus, the presence of hypoaldosteronism and the decrease in renal function have synergistic effects in impairing renal tubular potassium secretion.

Several factors have been proposed to cause both the renal and adrenal functional changes. These include a defect in prostaglandin production and/or presence of volume expansion. Prostaglandins promote renin secretion and facilitate aldosterone release by angiotensin II. Primary presence of prostaglandin deficiency or non-steroidal anti-inflammatory drugs that inhibit prostaglandin synthesis therefore result in hyperkalemia [96]. Volume expansion promotes the release of atrial natriuretic peptide, and atrial natriuretic peptide suppresses renin secretion and aldosterone release [97]. These changes can explain the presence of hyperkalemia in patients with acute glomerulonephritis and volume overload [98].

Adults with hyporeninemic hypoaldosteronism usually present with asymptomatic hyperkalemia; sodium wasting and volume depletion are generally not seen in the absence of concurrent glucocorticoid deficiency due to primary adrenal insufficiency or Addison's disease.

In addition to the measurement of plasma aldosterone concentration, determination of the TTKG also provides an estimate of cortical collecting duct potassium secretory response to circulating aldosterone [41, 75]. The TTKG in normal subjects on a regular potassium diet is 8 to 9 and rises above 11 in subjects on a high-potassium diet, indicating an appropriate increase in potassium secretion. A value below 5 to 7 in a hyperkalemic patient is highly suggestive of hypoaldosteronism or aldosterone resistance.

The treatment of hyporeninemic hypoaldosteronism consists of a low-potassium diet plus a loop or thiazide-type diuretic in combination with oral $NaHCO_3$ or sodium citrate, which increases urinary potassium losses. When necessary, patients can also be treated with the synthetic mineralocorticoid fluorocortisone. Although it corrects the mineralocorticoid deficiency and lowers plasma potassium concentration, fluorocortisone can worsen hypertension or edema, which is frequently present in these patients. Finally, if all measures fail, Kayexalate, 5 g given once to three times a day orally, can be used.

Drugs

Several drugs are known to be associated with hyperkalemia because they can either impair renin-aldosterone secretion, impair renal tubular potassium secretion, or alter transcellular potassium distribution.

Cyclosporine can cause a decrease in aldosterone release, and it can impair tubular potassium secretion [99, 100]. Cyclosporine inhibits Na,K-ATPase activity in the potassium secretory cells in the outer medullary and cortical collecting ducts, which would result in impaired intracellular potassium accumulation and cellular potassium secretion [101].

Heparin therapy reduces aldosterone secretion by a direct action on the adrenal gland. Even low-dose, subcutaneous administration of heparin can cause a major reduction in aldosterone production and hyperkalemia within 1 week of initiation of therapy [102, 103].

As discussed previously, potassium sparing diuretics and drugs that block sodium conductance channels impair cortical collecting duct potassium secretion (see Factors Affecting Principal Cell Potassium Secretion). Drug-induced hyperkalemia is specifically prevalent when patients are prescribed two or more drugs that impair renal tubular potassium secretion, when there is at least some impairment of renal function, and in the elderly [44].

Pseudohypoaldosteronism

In pseudohypoaldosteronism, there is aldosterone resistance in the target organs, including in the kidney, colon, and sweat glands. This disorder is associated with sodium wasting resulting in volume depletion, hyperkalemia, and increased plasma renin activity and plasma aldosterone concentration. The hereditary form is associated with generalized aldosterone resistance due to diminished numbers of mineralocorticoid receptors [104]. The acquired form is limited to the kidney and is seen primarily with tubulointerstitial diseases such as urinary tract obstruction, chronic pyelonephritis, and amyloidosis.

Renal Tubular Secretory Defect

In some patients, hyperkalemia occurs as a result of low urinary potassium excretion in spite of normal renin and aldosterone levels. The presence of a selective defect in potassium secretion has been described in subjects with renal transplant rejection and lupus nephritis.

A selective defect in urinary potassium secretion is also found in subjects with Gordon's syndrome. These subjects present with hyperkalemia, hypertension, and normal renal function. The primary defect in these subjects is enhanced distal nephron Cl^- reabsorption; sodium is reabsorbed with Cl^- by a mechanism that does not involve potassium or hydrogen ion secretion. The net effect is volume expansion and hypertension, with appropriate suppression of renin and aldosterone release [105–107]. Therapy consists of the administration of a thiazide diuretic (which decreases Na/Cl^- cotransport in the distal convoluted tubule) and, as necessary, a low-potassium diet.

Hyperkalemic Distal Renal Tubular Acidosis

Hyperkalemic distal RTA consists of the combination of hyperkalemia, impaired renal potassium excretion, hyperchloremic metabolic acidosis, and distal RTA. The patient with hyperkalemic distal RTA is readily distinguished from the person with classic distal RTA by the presence of hypokalemia in the latter. The response to sodium sulfate (Na_2SO_4) or furosemide also helps to differentiate these two groups and provides insights into the pathogenesis of these two forms of RTA. In normal subjects, administration of furosemide or Na_2SO_4 augments H^+ and potassium secretion in the cortical collecting duct, as a result of the increase in sodium delivery and a decrease in luminal chloride concentration. The net effect in normal subjects is a decrease in urine pH below 5.5 and an increase in urinary potassium excretion. In patients with classic distal RTA, Na_2SO_4 and furosemide fail to lower urine pH below 5.5 because of the impairment in H^+-ATPase pump in the intercalated cells, but potassium excretion is increased because sodium reabsorption and potassium secretion by principal cells are normal. In patients with hyperkalemic distal RTA, however, Na_2SO_4 and furosemide fail to increase either potassium or H^+ excretion, as the primary defect results from impaired distal nephron sodium reabsorption [108, 109].

Hyperkalemic distal RTA most often occurs in patients with obstructive uropathy and sickle cell disease. Treatment of hyperkalemia consists of alkali therapy ($NaHCO_3$ or sodium citrate), a low-potassium diet, and a diuretic to increase flow to the cortical collecting duct.

Diagnostic Approach to the Hyperkalemic Patient

The approach to the diagnosis of the etiology of hyperkalemia consists of determining whether the hyperkalemia is caused by increased potassium intake, potassium release from the cells or impaired cellular potassium uptake, or reduced urinary

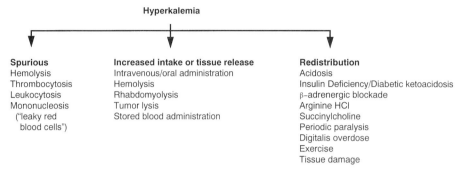

Fig. 5-12. Diagnostic approach to the patient with hyperkalemia of extrarenal origin.

potassium excretion. The search for the etiology of hyperkalemia should include (1) a careful history, including use of drugs, medications, dietary intake, and presence of renal disease or diabetes mellitus, (2) physical examination, including blood pressure, orthostatic changes in blood pressure and heart rate, and presence of edema, (3) urine and plasma electrolytes and osmolality, (4) arterial blood gas, and (5) ECG.

The most useful urine tests to monitor urinary potassium excretion include fractional excretion of potassium as a function of measured or estimated GFR and TTKG, which determines the degree of aldosterone effect on the cortical collecting duct (see Diagnostic Approach to the Hypokalemic Patient). A diagnostic approach to hyperkalemia of extrarenal or renal origin is presented in Figures 5-12 and 5-13.

Consequences of Hyperkalemia

Neuromuscular Effects

Hyperkalemia causes skeletal muscle weakness and paralysis [13]. An increased plasma potassium concentration causes sustained subthreshold depolarization, which adversely affects sodium channel activity. Subthreshold depolarization brings the membrane potential closer to the voltage required to generate an action potential (threshold), and a significant number of sodium channels open. Sodium channels are activated by depolarization; however, once opened, they close in a time-dependent manner, that is, they remain open for a fixed period of time. If threshold voltage is not reached rapidly, these sodium channels close (inactivate) and will not open again until the membrane hyperpolarizes. The number of sodium channels inactivated will be related to the magnitude of membrane depolarization (i.e., proximity to threshold), which is directly related to the increase in plasma potassium concentration. The extent of sodium channel inactivation can be so great that the muscle fiber can be depolarized above threshold and remain completely inexcitable. This phenomenon is called sodium inactivation. In hyperkalemia, despite normal synaptic transmission, the motor end plate and the entire muscle cell membrane can be inexcitable. Severe muscle paralysis in hyperkalemia will usually not be seen

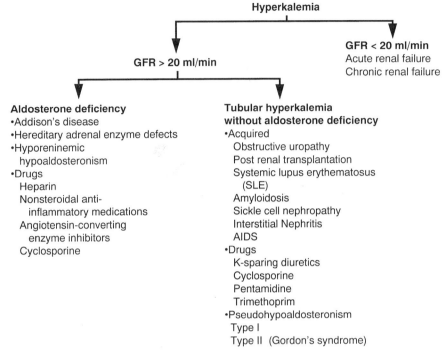

Fig. 5-13. Diagnostic approach to the patient with hyperkalemia of renal origin. GFR = glomerular filtration rate.

because of the fatality associated with cardiac arrhythmias, which begin to develop as plasma potassium concentration increases.

Cardiac Effects

The cardiac effects are the most serious consequence of hyperkalemia [76, 77]. Increases in plasma potassium concentration are associated with characteristic changes in the ECG, which are shown in Figure 5-14. As plasma potassium concentration increases to 12 mEq/L, resting membrane potentials in atrial and ventricular cells depolarize from −90 mV to about −75 mV. Sustained subthreshold depolarization causes the abnormal delay in atrial and ventricular depolarization during an action potential, manifested by the flattening and eventual loss of the P wave and progressive widening of the QRS complex. However, ventricular repolarization is enhanced, causing peaked T waves. This is due to an increase in the conductance of potassium channels caused by the increase in plasma potassium concentration. With severe hyperkalemia, the classic sine wave pattern is seen due to the merging of the widened QRS complex with the peaked T waves. Notice the decrease in the peak voltage of the action potential with increasing potassium concentration. This is due to the diminished number of active sodium channels. Ventricular arrhythmias

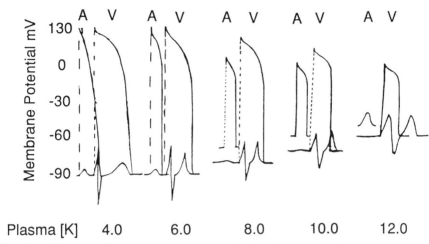

Fig. 5-14. Diagram of action potentials in atrial (A) and ventricular (V) cells superimposed on the simultaneously recorded electrocardiogram for plasma potassium concentrations of 4.0, 6.0, 8.0, 10.0, and 12.0 mEq/L. The left axis represents the muscle cell membrane potential in millivolts (mV). See text for further explanation. (Adapted from B. Surawicz, Relationship between electrocardiogram and electrolytes. *Am. Heart J.* 73[6]: 816, 1967.)

or cardiac arrest may occur at any point in this progression. Cardiac arrest is more common in hyperkalemia than in hypokalemia.

Treatment of Hyperkalemia

The treatment of hyperkalemia depends on the degree of the increase in the plasma potassium concentration and whether there are ECG changes or neuromuscular symptoms. A plasma potassium concentration above 7.5 mEq/L, severe muscle weakness, or marked ECG changes are potentially life-threatening and require immediate treatment using all the modalities listed in Table 5-3.

The cardiac and neuromuscular effects of hyperkalemia can be reversed by several mechanisms, including antagonism of membrane actions, increased potassium entry into the cells, and removal of the excess potassium.

Calcium

Calcium antagonizes the potassium-induced decrease in membrane excitability, restoring membrane excitability toward normal (Fig. 5-15). Muscle excitation is critically dependent on maintenance of the normal difference between the resting and threshold potentials, represented by the double-ended arrow on the far left of Figure 5-15. Plasma calcium concentration affects threshold potential, while plasma potassium concentration affects the resting membrane potential. Hyperkalemia causes

Table 5-3. Treatment of hyperkalemia

Medication	Mechanism of action	Dosage	Peak effect
Calcium gluconate	Antagonism of membrane actions	10–30 ml of 10% solution IV over 2 min	~5 min
Insulin and glucose	Increased K^+ entry into the cells	Insulin, 10 U IV bolus followed by 0.5 mU/kg of body weight per minute in 50 ml of 20% glucose	30–60 min
Sodium bicarbonate	Increased K^+ entry into the cells	44–50 mEq IV over 5 min; can be repeated within 30 min	30–60 min
Albuterol	Increased K^+ entry into the cells	20 mg in the nebulized form	30–60 min
Kayexalate	Removal of the excess K^+	20 g of resin with 100 ml of 20% sorbitol; can be repeated every 4–6 hr	2–4 hr
Hemodialysis	Removal of the excess K^+	Dialysis bath K^+ concentration variable	30–60 min

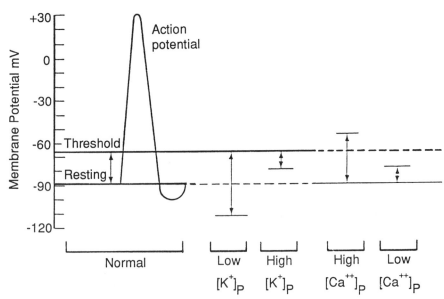

Fig. 5-15. Effect of plasma potassium concentration on resting membrane potential and of plasma calcium concentration on threshold potential in skeletal muscle. See text for further explanation. $[K^+]_p$ = plasma potassium concentration; $[Ca^{++}]_p$ = plasma calcium concentration ionized. (Adapted from A. Leaf and R. Cotran, *Renal Pathophysiology* [3rd ed.]. New York: Oxford University Press, 1985.)

sustained subthreshold depolarization, which inactivates sodium channels, rendering the membrane progressively less excitable (see Neuromuscular Effects). Elevation of plasma calcium concentration in this setting normalizes the difference between the resting and threshold potentials and restores sodium channel activity [110]. The protective effect of Ca^{2+} administration is quite rapid. The usual dose is 1 ampule (10 ml) of a 10% calcium gluconate solution infused over 2 to 3 minutes under ECG monitoring. This dose can be repeated after 5 minutes if the ECG changes persist. As predicted, toxicity of hyperkalemia is further enhanced in the presence of hypocalcemia.

Insulin and Glucose

Insulin lowers the plasma potassium concentration by driving potassium into cells. Insulin is administered as 10 units of regular insulin with 30 to 50 g of glucose to prevent hypoglycemia. This regimen lowers the plasma potassium concentration by 0.5 to 1.5 mEq/L. The effect of insulin is evident within 30 to 60 minutes and may last for 2 to 4 hours [14].

Sodium Bicarbonate

Raising the extracellular pH with $NaHCO_3$ drives potassium into the cells (see Distribution of Potassium). The usual dose is 44 to 50 mEq of $NaHCO_3$ infused over 5 minutes. The effect begins within 30 to 60 minutes and may persist for 2 to 4 hours [19].

β_2-Adrenergic Agonists

Activation of β_2-adrenergic receptors drives potassium into the cells (see Distribution of Potassium). Albuterol, 10 to 20 mg by nebulizer, can lower the plasma potassium concentration by 0.5 to 1.5 mEq/L within 30 to 60 minutes [14, 15].

The effects of calcium, insulin, $NaHCO_3$, and β_2-agonists are only transient. For the long-term achievement of normokalemia, these acute treatment modalities need to be followed by managements that remove the excess potassium from the body. These treatments include diuretics, cation-exchange resins, and dialysis.

Cation Exchange Resin

The cation exchange resin sodium polystyrene sulfonate (Kayexalate) takes up potassium in exchange for sodium in the gut. Each gram of Kayexalate binds 1 mEq of potassium and releases 1 to 2 mEq of sodium. When administered orally, 20 g of resin is given with 100 ml of a 20% sorbitol solution. Lower doses of 5 g once to three times a day can be used to treat chronic hyperkalemia. In patients who cannot take the oral solution, the resin can be given as a retention enema [111]. Cautions must be exercised in administering Kayexalate to postoperative patients, as intestinal necrosis has been reported to occur in this setting [112].

Dialysis

In patients with severe hyperkalemia, especially in the presence of advanced renal failure or when accompanied by a hypercatabolic state or severe tissue necrosis, dialysis will be needed to remove the excess potassium load. In this setting, hemodialysis is more effective than peritoneal dialysis.

References

1. Rose BD: *Clinical Physiology of Acid-Base and Electrolyte Disorders* (4th ed). New York, McGraw-Hill, 1994.
2. Smith JD, Bia M, DeFronzo RA: Clinical Disorders of Potassium Metabolism. In Arieff A, DeFronzo RA (eds): *Fluid, Electrolyte, and Acid-Base Disorders*. New York, Churchill Livingstone, 1985, pp 413–509.
3. Tannen RL: Potassium Disorders. In Kokko JP, Tannen RL (eds): *Fluids and Electrolytes*. Philadelphia, Saunders, 1986, pp 150–228.
4. Mujais SK, Katz AI: Potassium Deficiency. In Seldin DW, Giebisch G (eds): *The Kidney: Physiology and Pathophysiology* (2nd ed). New York, Raven Press, 1992, pp 2249–2278.
5. Lemann J Jr: Internal and External Solute Balance. In Seldin DW, Giebisch G (eds): *The Kidney: Physiology and Pathophysiology* (2nd ed). New York, Raven Press, 1992, pp 45–59.
6. *Nelson's Textbook of Pediatrics* (14th ed). Philadelphia, Saunders, 1992, pp 171–214.
7. Brokaw A: Renal hypertrophy and polydipsia in potassium deficient rats. *Am J Physiol* 172: 333–345, 1953.
8. Rudman D, Millikan WJ, Richardson TJ, et al: Elemental balances during intravenous hyperalimentation of underweight adult subjects. *J Clin Invest* 55:94–104, 1975.
9. DeFronzo RA: Clinical Disorders of Hyperkalemia. In Seldin DW, Giebisch G (eds): *The Kidney: Physiology and Pathophysiology* (2nd ed). New York, Raven Press, 1992, pp 2279–2337.
10. Wright FS, Giebisch G: Regulation of Potassium Excretion. In Seldin DW, Giebisch G (eds): *The Kidney: Physiology and Pathophysiology* (2nd ed). New York, Raven Press, 1992, pp 2209–2247.
11. Wehling M, Eisen C, Christ M: Aldosterone-specific membrane receptors and rapid nongenomic actions of mineralocorticoids. *Mol Cell Endocrinol* 90:C5–C9, 1992.
12. Rosa RM, Williams ME, Epstein FH: Extrarenal Potassium Metabolism. In Seldin DW, Giebisch G (eds): *The Kidney: Physiology and Pathophysiology* (2nd ed). New York, Raven Press, 1992, pp 2165–2190.
13. Knochel JP: Potassium Gradients and Neuromuscular Function. In Seldin DW, Giebisch G (eds): *The Kidney: Physiology and Pathophysiology* (2nd ed). New York, Raven Press, 1992, pp 2191–2208.
14. Allon M, Copkney C: Albuterol and insulin for treatment of hyperkalemia in hemodialysis patients. *Kidney Int* 38:869–872, 1990.
15. McClure RJ, Prasad VK, Brocklebank JT: Treatment of hyperkalemia using intravenous and nebulized salbutamol. *Arch Dis Child* 70:126–128, 1994.
16. Leikin JB: Hypokalemia after pediatric albuterol overdose: A case series. *Am J Emerg Med* 12:64–66, 1994.
17. Abdul RA, Rahman MB, McDevitt DG, et al: The effects of enalapril and spironolactone on terbutaline-induced hypokalemia. *Chest* 102:91–95, 1992.
18. Goldenburg IF, Olivari MT, Levine TB, et al: Effect of dobutamine on plasma potassium in congestive heart failure secondary to idiopathic or ischemic cardiomyopathy. *Am J Cardiol* 63:843–846, 1989.
19. Blumberg A, Weidmann P, Ferrari P: Effects of prolonged bicarbonate administration on plasma potassium in terminal renal failure. *Kidney Int* 41:369–374, 1992.
20. Magner PO, Robinson L, Halperin ML, et al: The plasma potassium concentration in metabolic acidosis: A re-evaluation. *Am J Kidney Dis* 11:220–224, 1988.

21. Lawson DH, Murray RM, Parker JL: Early mortality in the megaloblastic anaemias. *Q J Med* 41:1–14, 1972.
22. Rao TL, Marthru M, Salem MR, et al: Serum potassium levels following transfusion of frozen erythrocytes. *Anesthesiology* 52:170–172, 1980.
23. Hoffman EP, Lehmann-Horn F, Rudel R: Overexcited or inactive: Ion channels in muscle disease. *Cell* 80:681–686, 1995.
24. Ptacek LJ, Tawil RC, Griggs G, et al: Sodium channel mutations in acetazolamide-responsive myotonia congenita, paramyotonia congenita, and hyperkalemic periodic paralysis. *Neurology* 44:1500–1503, 1994.
25. Ptacek LJ, Rawil R, Griggs RC, et al: Dihydropyridine receptor mutations cause hypokalemic periodic paralysis. *Cell* 77:863–868, 1994.
26. Links TP, Smit AJ, Molenaar WM, et al: Familial hypokalemic periodic paralysis. *J Neurol Sci* 122:33–43, 1994.
27. Conte G, Dal Canton A, Imperatore P, et al: Acute increase in plasma osmolality as a cause of hyperkalemia in patients with renal failure. *Kidney Int* 38:301–307, 1990.
28. Smith TW, Butler VP, Haber E, et al: Treatment of life-threatening digitalis intoxication with digoxin-specific Fab antibody fragments. *N Engl J Med* 307:1357–1362, 1982.
29. Schwartz DE, Kelly B, Caldwell JE, et al: Succinylcholine-induced hyperkalemic arrest in a patient with severe metabolic acidosis and exsanguinating hemorrhage. *Anesth Analg* 75: 291–293, 1992.
30. McCance RA, Widdowson EM: Alkalosis with disordered kidney function. *Lancet* 2:247–249, 1937.
31. Reeves WB, Andreoli TE: Sodium Chloride Transport in the Loop of Henle. In Seldin DW, Giebisch G (eds): *The Kidney: Physiology and Pathophysiology* (2nd ed). New York, Raven Press, 1992, pp 1975–2001.
32. Good DW: Effects of potassium on ammonia transport by medullary thick ascending limb of the rat. *J Clin Invest* 80:1358–1365, 1987.
33. Schlatter E: Potassium transport in the cortical collecting duct. *Semin Renal Physiol* 65: 169–179, 1993.
34. Stokes JB: Ion transport by the collecting duct. *Semin Nephrol* 13:202–212, 1993.
35. Wingo CS, Armitage FE: Potassium transport in the kidney: Regulation and physiological relevance of H,K-ATPase. *Semin Nephrol* 13:213–224, 1993.
36. Halperin ML: Biochemistry and Physiology of Ammonium Excretion. In Seldin DW, Giebisch G (eds): *The Kidney: Physiology and Pathophysiology* (2nd ed). New York, Raven Press, 1992, pp 1471–1489.
37. Stanton BA: Regulation of Na and K transport by mineralocorticoids. *Semin Nephrol* 7:82–90, 1987.
38. Adam WR, Ellis AG, Adams BA: Aldosterone is a physiologically significant kaliuretic hormone. *Am J Physiol* 252:1048–1054, 1987.
39. Rabelink RJ, Koomans HA, Hene RJ, et al: Early and late adjustment to potassium loading in humans. *Kidney Int* 38:942–947, 1990.
40. O'Niel RG: Aldosterone regulation of sodium and potassium transport in the cortical collecting duct. *Semin Nephrol* 10:365–374, 1990.
41. Halperin ML, Goldstein MB: *Fluid, Electrolyte and Acid-Base Physiology* (2nd ed). Philadelphia, Saunders, 1994.
42. Rose BD: Diuretics. *Kidney Int* 39:336–352, 1991.
43. Velazquez H, Perazella MA, Wright FS, et al: Renal mechanism of trimethoprim-induced hyperkalaemia. *Ann Intern Med* 119:296–301, 1993.
44. Modest GA, Price B, Mascoli N: Hyperkalemia in elderly patients receiving standard doses of trimethoprim-sulfamethoxazole. *Ann Intern Med* 120:437, 1994.
45. Peterson LN, Wright FS: Effect of sodium intake on renal potassium excretion. *Am J Physiol* 233:F225–F234, 1977.
46. Romero JC, Knox FG, Opgenorth JP, et al: Contribution of sympathetic neural reflexes to mineralocorticoid escape. *Fed Proc* 44:2382–2387, 1985.
47. Yokota N, Bruneau BG, Kuroski-DeBold ML, et al: Atrial natriuretic factor significantly

contributes to the mineralocorticoid escape phenomenon: Evidence for a guanylate cyclase mediated pathway. *J Clin Invest* 94:1938–1946, 1994.

48. Rich GM, Ulick S, Cook S, et al: Glucocorticoid-remediable aldosteronism in a large kindred: Clinical spectrum and diagnosis using a characteristic biochemical phenotype. *Ann Intern Med* 116:813–820, 1992.
49. Lifton RP, Dluhy RG, Powers M, et al: A chimeric 11 beta-hydroxylase/aldosterone synthase gene causes glucocorticoid-remediable aldosteronism and human hypertension. *Nature* 355: 262–265, 1992.
50. Morris DJ, Souness GW: Protective and specificity-conferring mechanisms of mineralocorticoid action. *Am J Physiol* 263:759–768, 1992.
51. Ulick S, Wang JZ, Blumenfeld JD, et al: Cortisol inactivation overload: A mechanism of mineralocorticoid hypertension in the ectopic adrenocorticotropin syndrome. *Clin Endocrinol Metab* 74:963–967, 1992.
52. Kaye RB, Crapo L: The Cushing syndrome: An update on diagnostic tests. *Ann Intern Med* 112:434–444, 1990.
53. Klibanski A, Zervas NT: Diagnosis and management of hormone-secreting pituitary adenomas. *N Engl J Med* 324:822–831, 1991.
54. Blachley JD, Knochel JP: Tobacco chewer's hypokalemia: Licorice revisited. *N Engl J Med* 302:784–785, 1980.
55. Farese RV Jr, Biglieri EG, Shackleton CH, et al: Licorice-induced hypermineralocorticoidism. *N Engl J Med* 325:1223–1227, 1991.
56. Kenouch S, Country N, Farman N, et al: Multiple patterns of 11 beta-hydroxysteroid dehydrogenase catalytic activity along the mammalian nephron. *Kidney Int* 42:56–60, 1992.
57. Benediktsson R, Edwards CRW: Apparent mineralocorticoid excess. *J Human Hypertens* 8: 371–375, 1994.
58. New MI: Apparent mineralocorticoid excess: A personal history. *Steroids* 59:66–68, 1994.
59. Stein JH: The pathogenetic spectrum of Bartter's syndrome. *Kidney Int* 28:85–93, 1985.
60. Simon DB, Lifton RP: The molecular basis of inherited hypokalemic alkalosis Bartter's and Gitleman's syndrome. *Am J Physiol* 271:F961–F966, 1996.
61. Simon DB, Karet FE, Handan JM, et al: Bartter's syndrome, hypokalaemic alkalosis with hypercalcuria, is caused by mutations in the Na-K-2Cl cotransporter NKCC2. *Nature Genetics* 13:183–188, 1996.
62. Veldhuis JD, Bardin CW, Demers LM: Metabolic mimicry of Bartter's syndrome by covert vomiting: Utility of urinary chloride determinations. *Am J Med* 66:361–363, 1979.
63. Bettinelli A, Bianchetti MG, Girardin E, et al: Use of calcium excretion values to distinguish two forms of primary renal tubular hypokalemic alkalosis: Bartter and Gitelman syndromes. *J Pediatr* 120:38–43, 1992.
64. Simon DB, Nelson-Williams C, Ria MJ, et al: Gitelman's variant of Bartter's syndrome, inherited hypokalaemic alkalosis, is caused by mutations in the thiazide-sensitive Na-Cl cotransporter. *Nature Genetics* 24–30, 1996.
65. Botero-Velez M, Curtis JJ, Warnock DG: Brief report: Liddle's syndrome revisited—a disorder of sodium reabsorption in the distal tubule. *N Engl J Med* 330:178–181, 1994.
66. Shimkets RA, Warnock DG, Bositis CM, et al: Liddle's syndrome: Heritable human hypertension caused by mutations in the beta subunit of the epithelial sodium channel. *Cell* 79: 407–414, 1994.
67. Sebastian A, McSherry E, Morris RC Jr: Renal potassium wasting in renal tubular acidosis (RTA): Its occurrence in types 1 and 2 RTA despite sustained correction of systemic acidosis. *J Clin Invest* 50:667–678, 1971.
68. Hattori N, Hino M, Ishihara T, et al: Hypokalemic paralysis associated with distal renal tubular acidosis. *Intern Med* 30:662–665, 1992.
69. Poux JM, Peyronnet P, LeMeur Y, et al: Hypokalemic quadriplegia and respiratory arrest revealing primary Sjögren's syndrome. *Clin Nephrol* 37:189–191, 1992.
70. Ryan MP: Interrelationships of magnesium and potassium homeostasis. *Miner Electrolyte Metab* 19:290–295, 1993.
71. Whang R, Whang DD, Ryan MP: Refractory potassium depletion: A consequence of magnesium deficiency. *Arch Intern Med* 152:40–45, 1992.

72. Titanji R, Trofa A: Hypokalemia associated with ticarcillin-clavulanic acid. *Md Med J* 42: 1013–1014, 1993.
73. Bianchetti MG, Kanaka C, Ridolfi-Luthy A, et al: Chronic renal magnesium loss, hypocalciuria and mild hypokalaemic metabolic alkalosis after cisplatin. *Pediatr Nephrol* 4:219–222, 1990.
74. Carlisle EJF, Donnelly SM, Vasuvattakul S, et al: Glue-sniffing and distal renal tubular acidosis: Sticking to the facts. *J Am Soc Nephrol* 1:1019–1027, 1991.
75. Ethier JH, Kamel S, Magner PO, et al: The transtubular potassium concentration in patients with hypokalemia and hyperkalemia. *Am J Kidney Dis* 15:309–315, 1990.
76. Surawicz B: Relationship between electrocardiogram and electrolytes. *Am Heart J* 73(6): 814–834, 1967.
77. Surawicz B: Contributions of cellular electrophysiology to the understanding of the electrocardiogram. *Experientia* 43:1061–1068, 1987.
78. Podrid PH: Potassium and ventricular arrhythmias. *Am J Cardiol* 65:33E–44E, 1990.
79. Schulman M, Narins RG: Hypokalemia and cardiovascular disease. *Am J Cardiol* 65:4E, 1990.
80. Krishna GG, Kapoor SC: Potassium depletion exacerbates essential hypertension. *Ann Intern Med* 115:77–83, 1991.
81. Linas SL: The role of potassium in the pathogenesis and treatment of hypertension. *Kidney Int* 39:771–786, 1991.
82. Podolsky S, Melby JC: Improvement of growth hormone response to stimulation in primary aldosteronism with correction of potassium deficiency. *Metabolism* 25:1027, 1976.
83. Tizianello A, Garibotto G, Robaudo C, et al: Renal ammoniagenesis in humans with chronic potassium depletion. *Kidney Int* 40:772–778, 1991.
84. Agnoli GC, Borgatti R, Cacciari M, et al: Effects of angiotensin-converting enzyme inhibition on renal dysfunction induced by moderate potassium depletion in healthy women. *Clin Physiol* 14:205–222, 1994.
85. McKay AJ, Poirier CD, Peterson LN: Converting-enzyme inhibition abolishes polydipsia induced by dietary NaCl and K depletion. *Am J Physiol* 258(Regulatory Integrative Comp Physiol 27):F1164–F1172, 1990.
86. McKay AJ, Peterson LN: K infusion corrects thick ascending limb Cl reabsorption in K-depleted rats by an aldosterone-independent mechanism. *Am J Physiol* 264:F792–F799, 1993.
87. Kruse JA, Carlson RW: Rapid correction of hypokalemia using concentrated intravenous potassium chloride infusions. *Arch Intern Med* 150:613–617, 1990.
88. Popovtzer MM, Katz FH, Pingera WF, et al: Hyperkalemia in salt-wasting nephropathy: Study of the mechanism. *Arch Intern Med* 132:203–208, 1973.
89. Bonilla S, Geocke A, Bozzo S, et al: Effect of chronic renal failure on Na,K-ATPase alpha-1 and alpha-2 mRNA transcription in rat skeletal muscle. *J Clin Invest* 88:2137–2141, 1991.
90. DuBose TD Jr, Good DW: Effects of chronic hyperkalemia on renal production and proximal tubular transport of ammonium in rats. *Am J Physiol* 260:F680–F686, 1991.
91. DuBose TD Jr, Good DW: Chronic hyperkalemia impairs ammonium transport and accumulation in the inner medulla of the rat. *J Clin Invest* 90:1443–1449, 1992.
92. Ulick S, Wang JZ, Morton DH: The biochemical phenotypes of two inborn errors in the biosynthesis of aldosterone. *J Clin Endocrinol Metab* 74:1415–1420, 1992.
93. Speiser PW, Dupont J, Zhu D, et al: Disease expression and molecular genotype in congenital adrenal hyperplasia due to 21-hydroxylase deficiency. *J Clin Invest* 90:584–595, 1992.
94. Kigoshi T, Morimoto S, Uchida K, et al: Unresponsiveness of plasma mineralocorticoids to angiotensin II in diabetic patients with asymptomatic normoreninemic hypoaldosteronism. *J Lab Clin Med* 105:195–200, 1985.
95. Azukizawa S, Kaneko M, Nakano S, et al: Angiotensin II receptor and postreceptor events in adrenal zona glomerulosa cells from streptozotocin-induced diabetic rats with hypoaldosteronism. *Endocrinology* 129:2729–2733, 1991.
96. Nadler JL, Lee FO, Hsuch W, et al: Evidence of prostacyclin deficiency in the syndrome of hyporeninemic hypoaldosteronism. *N Engl J Med* 314:1015–1020, 1986.
97. Clark BA, Brown RS, Epstein F: Effect of atrial natriuretic peptide on potassium-stimulated aldosterone secretion: Potential relevance to hypoaldosteronism in man. *J Clin Endocrinol Metab* 75:399–403, 1992.

98. Don BR, Schambelan M: Hyperkalemia in acute glomerulonephritis due to transient hyporeninemic hypoaldosteronism. *Kidney Int* 38:1159–1163, 1990.
99. Kamel KS, Ethier J, Quaggin S, et al: Studies to determine the basis for hyperkalemia in recipients of a renal transplant who are treated with cyclosporine. *J Am Soc Nephrol* 2: 1279–1284, 1992.
100. Jones JW, Gruessner RW, Gores PF, et al: Hypoaldosteronemic hyporeninemic hyperkalemia after renal transplantation. *Transplantation* 56:1013–1014, 1993.
101. Tumlin JA, Sands JM: Nephron segment-specific inhibition of Na/K-ATPase activity by cyclosporin A. *Kidney Int* 43:246–251, 1993.
102. Edes TE: Heparin-induced hyperkalemia. *Postgrad Med* 87:104–106, 1990.
103. Siebels M, Andrassy K, Vecsei P, et al: Dependent suppression of mineralocorticoid metabolism by different heparin fractions. *Thromb Res* 66:467–473, 1992.
104. Kuhnle U, Nielsen MD, Teitze H-U: Pseudohypoaldosteronism in eight families: Different forms of inheritance are evidence for various genetic defects. *J Clin Endocrinol Metab* 70: 638–641, 1990.
105. Schambelan M, Sebastian R, Rector FC Jr: Mineralocorticoid-resistant renal hyperkalemia without salt-wasting (type II pseudohypoaldosteronism): Role of increased renal chloride reabsorption. *Kidney Int* 19:716–727, 1981.
106. Gordon RD: Syndrome of hypertension and hyperkalemia with normal glomerular filtration rate. *Hypertension* 8:93–102, 1986.
107. Take C, Ikeda K, Kurasawa T, et al: Increased chloride reabsorption as an inherited renal tubular defect in familial type II pseudohypoaldosteronism. *N Engl J Med* 324:472–476, 1991.
108. Kurtzman NA, Gonzalez J, DeFronzo RA, et al: A patient with hyperkalemia and metabolic acidosis. *Am J Kidney Dis* 15:333–356, 1990.
109. Schlueter W, Keilani T, Hizon M, et al: On the mechanism of impaired distal acidification in hyperkalemic renal tubular acidosis: Evaluation with amiloride and bumetanide. *J Am Soc Nephrol* 3:953–964, 1992.
110. Leaf A, Cotran R: *Renal Pathophysiology.* New York, Oxford University Press, 1976.
111. Burnett RJ: Sodium polystyrene-sorbitol enemas. *Ann Intern Med* 112:311–312, 1990.
112. Gerstman BB, Kirkman R, Platt R: Intestinal necrosis associated with postoperative orally administered sodium polystyrene sulfonate in sorbitol. *Am J Kidney Dis* 20:159–161, 1992.

6

Disorders of Calcium, Phosphorus, Vitamin D, and Parathyroid Hormone Activity

Mordecai M. Popovtzer, James P. Knochel, and Rajiv Kumar

Serum Calcium Concentration

The calcium ion is essential to many physiologic phenomena, including preservation of the integrity of cellular membranes, neuromuscular activity, regulation of endocrine and exocrine secretory activities, blood coagulation, activation of the complement system, and bone metabolism.

Total Serum Calcium Concentration

The normal range for total serum calcium must be established for each laboratory and varies according to the method used. Total serum calcium is divisible into protein-bound and ultrafiltrable (diffusible) calcium (Fig. 6-1).

Protein-Bound Calcium

Approximately 40 percent of total calcium is bound to serum proteins, and 80 to 90 percent of this calcium is bound to albumin. Variations in serum protein will alter proportionately the concentration of the protein-bound and total serum calcium. An increase in serum albumin concentration of 1 g/dl will increase protein-bound calcium by 0.8 mg/dl, while an increase of 1 g/dl of globulin will increase protein-bound calcium by 0.16 mg/dl. Thus it is obvious that changes in total serum calcium concentration cannot be used for the assessment of the effect on bound calcium concentration unless the changes in albumin and globulin concentrations also are determined. Marked changes in serum sodium concentration also affect the protein binding of calcium. Hyponatremia increases whereas hypernatremia decreases protein-bound calcium. Changes in pH will also affect protein-bound calcium, and an increase or decrease of 0.1 pH will respectively increase or decrease protein-bound calcium by 0.12 mg/dl. In vitro freezing and thawing serum samples may also decrease the binding of calcium.

Ultrafiltrable (Diffusible) Calcium

Serum ultrafiltrable calcium is obtained by applying pressure on serum against a semipermeable membrane. Serum water thus is forced across the membrane, and

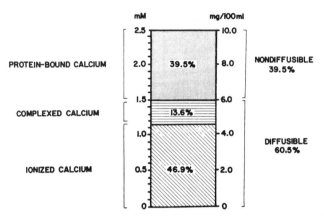

Fig. 6-1. Calcium fractions in the serum. (Adapted from E. W. Moore, Ionized calcium in normal serum, ultrafiltrates and whole blood determined by ion-exchange electrode. *J. Clin. Invest.* 49:318, 1970.)

the ultrafiltrate is analyzed for calcium concentration and then corrected for total serum solids. The samples must be handled anaerobically, since changes in pH may affect calcium binding. Under normal conditions, ultrafiltrable calcium constitutes 55 to 60 percent of the total serum calcium.

Free (Ionized) Calcium

The biologically active component of diffusible calcium is ionized calcium. Flow-through and static ion exchange electrodes, which function similarly to the conventional pH electrodes, are used. Serum ionized calcium concentration in normal subjects ranges from 4.0 to 4.9 mg/dl deciliter, or 47 percent of total serum calcium. Since changes in pH alter the concentration of ionized calcium, the samples have to be handled anaerobically. Determinations are best made on freshly separated serum, since heparin creates complexes with calcium, and the presence of fibrin may interfere with the structural integrity of the porous membrane used in the procedure. Storage of serum in oil does not prevent changes in pH, since carbon dioxide dissolves readily in oil. An increase in serum pH of 0.1 unit may cause a decrease in ionized calcium of 0.16 mg/dl [1, 2]. As with ultrafiltrable calcium, freezing and thawing of serum may alter the level of ionized calcium.

Complexed Calcium

The nonionized portion of diffusible or ultrafiltrable calcium is called complexed calcium. The calcium complexes are formed with bicarbonate, phosphate, and acetate. The amount of complexed calcium is measured indirectly by subtracting the ionized calcium (47%) from the ultrafiltrable calcium (60%) and thus equals about 13 percent of total serum calcium. The complexed calcium has been found to be increased twofold in patients with uremia.

Serum Phosphorus Concentration

Serum phosphorus occurs in two forms, organic and inorganic. Organic phosphorus is composed entirely of phospholipids bound to proteins. The inorganic fraction is the principal circulating form of phosphorus and is routinely assayed for clinical uses. About 90 percent of inorganic phosphorus is ultrafiltrable. About 53 percent of the ultrafiltrable inorganic phosphorus in serum is dissociated, with the ratio of $H_2PO_4^-$ to HPO_4^{2-} of $1:4$; the remainder of ultrafiltrable phosphate is in the form of salts of sodium, calcium, and magnesium. During marked hyperphosphatemia (8–10 mg/dl of serum), a significant portion of phosphate forms colloidal complexes with calcium that are rapidly removed from the circulation.

It has been proposed that an increase in serum phosphorus leads to a reciprocal fall in serum calcium, so that the product of both ions remains constant. The assumption was that a solubility equilibrium exists between the bone and the extracellular fluid (ECF). However, this appears to be an oversimplification of a more complex equilibrium. An inverse relationship between serum calcium and phosphorus is present only under extreme changes of serum phosphorus; for example, a decrease in serum calcium occurs following an acute rise in serum phosphorus. By contrast, this relationship does not hold for acute changes in serum calcium, since a rapid increase in calcium leads to a rise rather than a fall in serum phosphorus before any changes in urinary phosphorus occur [2]. This effect may be due to the release of phosphorus from cells.

Serum phosphorus concentration also is influenced by age. In adults the normal concentration ranges from 2.5 to 4.0 mg/dl, whereas in children it ranges from 4 to 6 mg/dl. The level of alkaline phosphatase in children is also higher than in adults. These age differences are probably related to different rates of skeletal growth. Serum phosphorus decreases during hyperventilation and alkalosis and increases during acidosis. Serum phosphorus also varies directly with its content in the diet. Administration of glucose causes a fall in serum phosphate due to the flux of phosphate into cells with the phosphorylation of glucose. The administration of insulin and epinephrine also reduces serum phosphorus concentration. Hypophosphatemia occurring in sepsis and acute myocardial infarction may result from the release of epinephrine into the circulation.

Calcium and Phosphorus Balance

Total body calcium ranges from 1.0 to 1.5 kg and that of phosphorus from 0.5 to 0.8 kg. Ninety-nine percent of total calcium and 85 percent of total phosphorus are stored in the skeleton. Only 0.1 percent of both is in the ECF, and the remainder is intracellular.

Dietary Calcium and Phosphorus

Dietary calcium and phosphorus intake varies considerably. In general, balanced diets provide from 800 to 1200 mg of calcium and from 800 to 1500 mg of phosphorus

Table 6-1. Calcium and phosphorus content in different foods

Food	Calcium (mg/100 g)	Phosphorus (mg/100 g)
Cow's milk	120	100
Hard American cheese	697	771
Cottage cheese	100	110
Eggs	54	205
Meat	13	200

per day. The minimum daily requirement of calcium is 400 to 500 mg, and an intake below this amount may cause a negative calcium balance. Dietary calcium can be reduced to about 200 mg by the exclusion of dairy products [3], and boiling of vegetables causes a loss of 25 percent of their calcium content. To increase the amount of calcium in the diet, it has become common to enrich bread with powdered milk. Drinking water is also a source of calcium; "soft" water has 1 to 3 mg/dl of calcium, and "hard" water has 3 to 10 mg/dl. Human diets, almost without exception, contain more phosphorus than calcium, since phosphorus is present in almost all foodstuffs. The amount of calcium and phosphorus in various foods is shown in Table 6-1.

Intestinal Absorption of Calcium

Calcium is absorbed along the small intestine, more in the duodenum and proximal jejunum than in the ileum [3–5]. The absorption of calcium is completed within 4 hours after its oral intake [5, 6].

Calcium absorption in the gastrointestinal tract occurs via two transport processes [7–10]. Transcellular calcium absorption, which is saturable and physiologically regulated, follows three steps: (1) luminal entry into mucosal cells through apical calcium channels, (2) binding to a protein carrier and transfer to the serosal side, and (3) extrusion from the cell by an active process. Increasing body demands for calcium activate maximally the transcellular transportation. Paracellular calcium absorption is nonsaturable and is driven by concentration gradients between luminal and serosal spaces. Thus, the rate of absorption primarily depends on calcium concentration in the lumen. This pathway of absorption predominates in distal small bowel. The paracellular absorption route traverses the apical tight junctions of the mucosal cells; therefore, changes in permeability in these sites may also affect the rate of transport.

Another transfer system is known as the vesicular transcellular calcium traffic. This proceeds by endocytosis of calcium at the luminal cell membrane and exocytosis at the serosal side. The importance of this pathway is under investigation.

With low calcium intake, the absorption of calcium becomes more efficient, thus ensuring that adequate amounts of calcium are delivered to the body. This process of adjustment to low calcium intake, which is not entirely understood, has been termed adaptation. Younger persons exhibit this phenomenon of adaptation better than do older ones. The absorption of calcium also increases in direct proportion to the requirements; for example, calcium absorption increases during pregnancy and during depletion of total body calcium.

Oral calcium may be complexed, chelated, or precipitated in the gastrointestinal tract by a variety of substances that render it unavailable for absorption. These substances include phytate, oxalate, and citrate. Certain drugs including colchicine, fluoride, theophylline, and glucocorticoids also interfere with calcium absorption. Rapid motility or shortening of the length of the gastrointestinal tract also may diminish the absorption of calcium. Decreased calcium absorption has been observed with protein depletion both in human subjects and in rats. A deficiency of the specific calcium binding protein in the intestinal mucosal cells has been proposed as the mechanism accounting for this failure of calcium transport.

In the absence of oral intake, calcium continues to be excreted in the feces, and a negative calcium balance ensues. Thus, it is apparent that some of the fecal calcium is derived from intestinal secretion. Using an intravenous tracer method, the daily calcium secretion has been estimated to be on the order of 150 mg/day. This amount does not change during an intravenous load of calcium.

Net calcium absorption (dietary calcium minus fecal calcium) can be determined by maintaining the patient on a constant diet and collecting stools. This balance method is time-consuming, since it requires an equilibration period of several days followed by a collection period of several days. The results may be expressed in absolute values, where the net calcium absorption is the difference between calcium intake and calcium fecal excretion. Alternatively, the results can be expressed as fractional calcium absorption, as shown in the following formula:

$$\text{Fractional calcium absorption} = \frac{\text{dietary calcium} - \text{fecal calcium}}{\text{dietary calcium} \times 100}$$

Intestinal Absorption of Phosphorus

About 50 to 65 percent of dietary phosphorus is absorbed, mostly in the jejunum. Evidence from in vitro studies indicates that phosphorus absorption is an active process. The active process is sodium-coupled and saturable. There is a linear correlation, however, between phosphorus intake and net absorption. The latter reflects the passive paracellular pathway of transport, which is determined by concentration gradients of phosphorus across the intestinal mucosa. In contrast to findings in animals, high phosphate intake in humans does not seem to cause a decrease in calcium absorption. However, the presence of phosphate in the diet is necessary for calcium absorption. Phosphate absorption may be decreased by a high calcium intake or by ingestion of aluminum hydroxide antacids, which bind phosphorus in the bowel, thereby inhibiting its absorption.

Urinary Excretion of Calcium

The urinary excretion of calcium varies considerably in normal subjects, but the oral intake only modestly affects the daily urinary excretion of calcium. The upper normal range of calcium excretion per day has been estimated to be less than 300 mg for men and less than 250 mg for women or 4 mg/kg body weight. Unlike the response to a low-sodium diet, institution of a diet very low in calcium does not lead immediately to a substantial reduction in urinary calcium. However, in clinical states of protracted calcium depletion, such as in patients with intestinal malabsorption and osteomalacia, urinary excretion of calcium may be reduced to 50 mg/day or less.

Only ultrafiltrable calcium crosses the glomerular capillary walls and is then partially reabsorbed by the tubular epithelial cells. In adults, 97 to 99 percent of filtered calcium is reabsorbed. The tubules reabsorb ionized calcium more easily than complexed calcium, which accounts for the fact that the proportion of ionized calcium in the urine is only 20 percent of the total, the remainder being complexed calcium. The calcium complexes contain many anions such as citrate, sulfate, phosphate, and gluconate. Citrates in the urine bind calcium most powerfully. At a neutral pH in a liter of urine containing 100 mg of calcium and 480 mg of citrate, 60 percent of calcium would be chelated with citrate, and this fraction would fall to 40 percent at a pH of 5.0.

Urinary excretion of calcium is influenced by oral intake and urinary excretion of sodium. Thus any attempt to assess urinary calcium excretion must take into account the oral intake and excretion of sodium. It also has been found that factors that affect the renal excretion of sodium, such as ECF volume expansion, will similarly alter the renal excretion of calcium. Chronic expansion of ECF volume with mineralocorticoid hormone also increases the urinary excretion of calcium.

Renal tubular calcium reabsorption occurs both by transcellular and paracellular pathways. Calcium enters the cells across the brush-border membrane passively, down its electrochemical gradient, partly through the calcium channels. It is extruded actively at the basolateral membrane by several putative mechanisms including $3Na^+/Ca^{2+}$ exchanger, adenosine triphosphate (ATP)–dependent calcium pumps, and ATP-dependent $2H^+/Ca^{2+}$ exchanger.

It has been estimated that 50 to 70 percent of filtered calcium is reabsorbed in the proximal nephron, 30 to 40 percent is reabsorbed between the end of the accessible part of the proximal tubule and the distal tubule, and the remaining 10 percent is reabsorbed in the distal nephron [10, 11]. Micropuncture studies have demonstrated that sodium and calcium exhibit very similar reabsorptive characteristics in the proximal tubule. In the thick ascending segment of the loop of Henle, the absorption of both ions follows the same direction. Lumen-positive voltage is the driving force for calcium reabsorption in this segment. Furosemide abolishes the transepithelial potential and therefore reduces calcium absorption in parallel with reduced sodium reabsorption. Parathyroid hormone (PTH) reduces urinary excretion of calcium but augments urinary excretion of sodium. Moreover, thiazide diuretics induce a natriuresis but cause urinary retention of calcium when they are administered on a chronic basis. Similarly, spironolactone, amiloride, and triamterene enhance natriuresis but decrease urinary calcium excretion. Thus sodium and calcium reabsorption in the distal nephron can be dissociated. It is of interest that the fine tuning of urinary calcium excretion occurs in the distal tubule by active transcellular mechanisms.

Changes in the filtered load of calcium also may affect the excretion of this ion. Thus hypocalcemia, regardless of its cause, is associated with a low urinary calcium excretion. A micropuncture study in dogs demonstrated that elevation of plasma calcium from a low to a normal level inhibits calcium reabsorption in the loop of Henle independent of PTH. This may be an important mechanism in determining calcium excretion rate [12].

Extracellular calcium ($Ca^{2+}o$)–sensing receptors represent a new concept in the physiology of signal transduction that is pertinent to the previous observations [13]. Accordingly, extracellular calcium and other cations (e.g., Mg^{2+}) activate mechanism(s) that control their tubular transport via cell-surface receptors that recognize those cations as their extracellular ligands. The $Ca^{2+}o$-sensing receptors are G protein–coupled receptors that by activation of phospholipase C, hydrolysis of phosphatidylinositol 4,5-biphosphate and increased formation of inositol triphosphate and diacylglycerol lead to a transient rise in intracellular calcium. It has been suggested that the renal $Ca^{2+}o$-sensing receptors are expressed by the cells of the thick ascending limb of Henle's loop and play a role in the normal regulation of calcium absorption in this nephron segment. Thus normal or high luminal calcium concentration is likely to be "sensed" by the $Ca^{2+}o$-sensing receptor, triggering activation of the signal transduction cascade, leading to physiologically reduced calcium reabsorption. Conversely, low luminal calcium concentration (as present in hypocalcemia) would likely fail to activate the signal transduction pathway, thus leading to abnormally avid calcium reabsorption and hypocalciuria. The latter is also the explanation for the hypocalciuria observed in patients with familial hypocalciuric hypercalcemia, in whom the gene that encodes the $Ca^{2+}o$-sensing receptor has undergone inactivating mutation, leading to a defective receptor [13].

The renal capacity to excrete calcium also may be severely compromised by a reduction in glomerular filtration rate (GFR) and volume depletion. The reduced absolute and fractional excretion of calcium in early chronic renal failure when the GFR is only moderately reduced is not well understood [14, 15]. Two factors might contribute to this observation: secondary hyperparathyroidism and abnormalities of vitamin D metabolism [14]. In more advanced renal failure, fractional excretion of calcium is enhanced and correlates with the fractional clearance of sodium, suggesting that at this stage of renal insufficiency the renal handling of both ions may be altered by a similar mechanism [14].

Acute and chronic loads of phosphorus may decrease urinary excretion of calcium. It has been proposed that this reduced urinary calcium excretion is due to an increased deposition of mineral, either in the bone or in other tissues. The hypocalciuria following oral phosphates has been utilized in the treatment of renal calculi.

Phosphate depletion leads to an increased urinary excretion of calcium; the mechanism for this effect remains to be defined. The possible role of secondary hypoparathyroidism was not supported by studies in animals in which parathyroidectomy did not alter substantially the hypercalciuric response to phosphate depletion. In rats, the hypercalciuric response to phosphate depletion is associated with increased intestinal absorption of calcium. A relevant finding is that phosphate depletion may enhance renal conversion of 25-hydroxyvitamin D_3 (25[OH]D_3) into 1,25-dihydroxyvitamin D_3 (1,25[OH]$_2D_3$) which stimulates intestinal absorption of calcium. Phosphate depletion also may be associated with the release of calcium from bone [16]. With phosphate depletion and the resultant hypercalciuria, osteomalacia may develop, with a subsequent decrease in calcium excretion.

Both metabolic and renal tubular acidosis are associated with an increased urinary excretion of calcium.

Urinary Excretion of Phosphorus

About 80 percent of serum inorganic phosphorus is filtered, and the ratio of $H_2PO_4^-$ to HPO_4^{2-} in the urine is dependent on the urine pH. The proximal convoluted and straight tubules are the major sites of phosphorus reabsorption. According to micropuncture studies, when glomerular filtrate reaches the late proximal tubule, 70 percent of filtered phosphorus is reabsorbed.

Phosphorus enters the brush-border membrane of the proximal tubule via sodium-phosphorus cotransport (sodium-phosphate symport) against a steep electrochemical gradient. This is energized by the sodium gradient generated by the basolateral sodium pump. Phosphorus moves out of the cell at the basolateral membrane mostly by a sodium-dependent transport (70%) and partly (30%) by a sodium-independent anion exchange system. Only the luminal cotransport is controlled by hormone factors (e.g., PTH).

The structure of a class of sodium-phosphate symporters in the brush-border membrane of the proximal tubule that facilitate the uptake of both sodium and phosphate in this segment of the nephron has now been elucidated. Many of the changes in the efficiency of phosphate transport are brought about by changes in the amount and activity of the sodium-phosphate symporter in this segment of the nephron. In addition, interesting new information has emerged concerning the control of phosphate reabsorption in the proximal tubule.

Urinary excretion of phosphorus depends to a great extent on oral phosphorus intake. Increased dietary phosphorus is associated with increased total and fractional urinary excretion of phosphorus. This may occur even in the absence of detectable changes in the serum level and filtered load of phosphorus. The state of parathyroid activity seems to play an important role in this phosphaturic response to a phosphate load, and in fact this response has been used as a diagnostic test for hyperparathyroidism. Oral intake of 3 g of elemental phosphorus has been reported to increase the excretion of phosphorus to the maximum of 35 percent of the filtered load in normoparathyroid subjects, but in hyperparathyroid patients the fractional phosphate excretion exceeds 35 percent. However, although the presence of parathyroid hyperactivity intensifies the phosphaturic response to phosphate load, the phosphaturic response also may be observed in hypoparathyroid patients.

Phosphate depletion resulting from phosphate-deficient diets or intestinal phosphate losses is associated with a decrease in urinary excretion of phosphate to negligible amounts. This avid reabsorption of phosphorus is reversed by fasting and acidosis. Animal experiments suggest that increased insulin secretion during phosphorus deprivation contributes to the decreased urinary excretion of phosphorus in the urine.

Growth hormone, thyroid hormone, insulin, and insulin-like growth factor increase phosphorus reabsorption.

Acute expansion of ECF volume with intravenous saline increases the urinary excretion of phosphorus; conversely, acute depletion of ECF volume tends to decrease urinary phosphorus [17]. However, the effect of chronically increased oral intake of sodium chloride on urinary phosphorus excretion and phosphorus balance is unknown. In this regard, patients with primary hyperaldosteronism showed no changes in urinary phosphorus excretion but exhibited hypercalciuria.

A high oral intake of calcium is associated with a decreased urinary excretion of phosphorus. Two possible factors may account for this observation. First, calcium may depress intestinal absorption of phosphorus by forming nonabsorbable complexes with phosphorus. Second, large amounts of oral calcium may suppress the secretion of PTH and reduce urinary excretion of phosphorus.

In contrast to its effect when given by the oral route, an intravenous load of calcium produces an acute increase in serum phosphorus concentration and augments excretion of phosphorus in the urine [2]. The rise in serum phosphorus has been attributed to a direct effect of hypercalcemia, namely, promotion of the release of intracellular phosphorus into the circulation [2]. This transient phosphaturia is followed by a substantial fall in urinary phosphorus excretion due to suppression of parathyroid activity [4]. In addition, hypercalcemia may exert a direct effect on the kidney, enhancing tubular reabsorption of phosphorus independently of parathyroid activity [18]. In contrast to this observation, however, is the finding that restoration of normocalcemia with intravenous calcium in patients with hypoparathyroidism is associated with increased urinary excretion of phosphorus. Likewise, the enhanced excretion of phosphorus that follows the administration of vitamin D to patients with hypoparathyroidism may be at least partly attributable to the restoration of the serum calcium level to normal.

Acute loads of phosphorus in parathyroidectomized animals produce a net decrease in tubular reabsorption of phosphorus despite markedly increased filtered load. This change has been linked with the attendant fall in serum calcium concentration and indeed may be reversed by maintaining a constant calcium level [19]. This and the foregoing observations show the dependence of renal handling of phosphorus on serum levels of calcium and emphasize the complexity of their interrelationship.

States of rapid catabolism with increased destruction of body tissues and metabolic acidosis are associated with hyperphosphatemia and phosphaturia. Similarly, cytolysis associated with the administration of cytotoxic agents to patients with neoplasms, especially neoplasms of lymphatic origin, is followed by severe hyperphosphatemia, phosphaturia, and hypocalcemia. Conversely, rapid regrowth of lymphatic tumors may lead to hypophosphatemia of marked degree because of incorporation of phosphorus in the tumor [20].

Intravenous administration of glucose has a dual effect on phosphorus metabolism. First of all, intravenous glucose tends to lower serum phosphorus, probably by incorporating phosphorus into the intracellular pool during the process of glucose phosphorylation. Second, glucose appears to have a direct renal effect in that it suppresses the reabsorption and increases the urinary excretion of phosphate. The competition of glucose and phosphate for transport across the epithelium of the proximal tubule has been demonstrated in studies with isolated renal tubules [21]. This competition may be most important in states of massive glucosuria with uncontrolled diabetes mellitus.

Most diuretic agents acutely increase urinary phosphorus excretion. However, with the development of ECF volume depletion, the phosphaturic response of diuretics is blunted and may be restored with replacement of urinary losses of sodium and water. Neither the phosphaturic effect of thiazides nor that of acetazolamide seems to be dependent on the presence of parathyroid glands. The phosphaturic effect of these diuretics is however linked to their ability to inhibit the enzyme carbonic anhydrase.

Denervation of kidneys leads to an increase in urinary excretion of phosphorus due to an increased production of dopamine and decreased α- and β-adrenergic renal receptor activity. This denervation phosphaturia may contribute to renal losses of phosphorus after kidney transplantation.

Acidosis increases and alkalosis reduces urinary excretion of phosphorus.

Regulation of Serum Calcium and Phosphorus Concentration by Hormonal Factors

Vitamin D and Its Metabolites

Vitamin D is the term that was first introduced by McCollum in 1922 for the antirachitic factor isolated from cod liver oil [22]. There are two naturally occurring sterol precursors of vitamin D, namely ergosterol, which is present in plants, and 7-dehydrocholesterol, which is found in animals and humans. Under exposure to ultraviolet irradiation, ergosterol is converted into ergocalciferol (calciferol), which is known as vitamin D_2. Vitamin D_1 is not one compound but a mixture of many sterols with antirachitic activity.

The main source of vitamin D in humans is endogenous vitamin D_3, produced by the ultraviolet irradiation of 7-dehydrocholesterol in the skin. Areas of skin in most adults contain 3 to 4 percent of 7-dehydrocholesterol, which is located beneath the stratum corneum. Excessive amounts of pigment in the skin therefore may interfere with the production of vitamin D_3. The cutaneous synthesis of vitamin D_3 is quite complex. Previtamin D_3 is formed from its precursor 7-dehydrocholesterol, also known as provitamin D_3. The above conversion depends on the levels of provitamin D_3, declines with age, and is mediated by initial exposure to ultraviolet light. Prolonged exposure, however, may inactivate previtamin D_3 and transform it to inert photoproducts, lumisterol and tachysterol. Vitamin D_3, also known as cholecalciferol, is formed from previtamin D_3 by thermal isomerization over 2 to 3 days in the skin and is also rapidly degraded by sunlight. Thus 10 to 15 minutes of exposure to sunlight can provide sufficient amounts of vitamin D_3 for several days' consumption.

The main source of exogenous vitamin D in the United States is milk, which contains about 400 units of vitamin D_2 in each quart. The daily requirement of vitamin D in infants is about 400 units; in older age groups, the requirement is much lower, as low as 70 units/day.

Metabolism of Vitamin D

Cholecalciferol is metabolized in the liver into 25-cholecalciferol (25-dihydroxyvitamin D_3 [25(OH)$_2D_3$]), which has a more potent antirachitic activity in vivo than the parent compound. Vitamin D undergoes 25-hydroxylation in the liver by 25-hydroxylase. 25-Hydroxylase is not a tightly regulated enzyme, but in animals receiving vitamin D, its activity is reduced by 50 percent. Phenobarbital, phenytoin, and rifampin in vivo alter the function of cytochrome P_{450} enzymes and the vitamin D–25-hydroxylase and bring about a decrease in the level of 25(OH)D_3 [23]. After enterohepatic circulation, 25(OH)D_3 is further metabolized in the kidney into 1,25-dihydroxycholecalciferol (1,25[OH]$_2D_3$), which is the most active known metabolite of vitamin D. On a weight basis, it is 10 times more effective than vitamin D_3 in curing rickets and 100 times more potent than 25(OH)D_3 in stimulating calcium mobilization from the bone. When plasma calcium and phosphate levels are normal, 25(OH)D–1α-hydroxylase activity is reduced, and instead 25(OH)D–24-hydroxylase activity prevails and metabolizes 25(OH)D_3 into 24,25(OH)$_2D_3$. Calcitriol is an important regulator of itself. It exerts a feedback inhibition through a genomic mechanism. Calcitriol suppresses 25(OH) D–1α-hydroxylase and activates the 25(OH)D–24-hydroxylase. In these circumstances, the production of 24,25(OH)$_2D_3$ prevails.

PTH seems to act as a tropic hormone in stimulating the production of 1,25(OH)$_2D_3$ in the kidney. Thus, with intact parathyroid glands, changes in serum calcium will indirectly regulate renal production of 1,25(OH)$_2D_3$ by altering the secretion of PTH. Specifically, hypocalcemia stimulates and hypercalcemia inhibits the synthesis of 1,25(OH)$_2D_3$. In addition, there is evidence that calcium acts directly to alter the renal synthesis of calcitriol. Low serum phosphorus stimulates and high serum phosphorus suppresses the renal synthesis of 1,25(OH)$_2D_3$ independently of PTH. Several other factors control the formation of 1,25(OH)$_2D_3$. Growth hormone via increased synthesis of insulin-like growth factor I stimulates the activity of 25(OH)D–1α-hydroxylase. Chronic metabolic acidosis in humans increases serum levels of calcitriol [24]. This effect could be mediated by acidosis-induced urinary losses of phosphate leading to cellular phosphate depletion. Once it is formed, 1,25(OH)$_2D_3$ is metabolized to several less active metabolites in target tissues [10, 25]. These transformations are enhanced by the hormone itself and may thus serve to decrease the biologic activity of the hormone once it has carried out its biologic functions. In addition, 1,25(OH)$_2D_3$ is excreted in bile as a monoglucuronide, other polar metabolites, and a 23-carbon acid, calcitroic acid [8, 10, 26]. 1,25(OH)$_2D_3$ undergoes an enterohepatic circulation in humans and various animal species. Proximal tubular cells are the major site of calcitriol formation. In addition, calcitriol may also be produced in decidual cells, keratinocytes, bone cells, endothelial cells, peripheral monocytes, and activated macrophages. (The various aspects of the metabolism of vitamin D are shown in Fig. 6-2.)

Dihydrotachysterol (DHT$_3$) is an analogue of vitamin D that was used in the

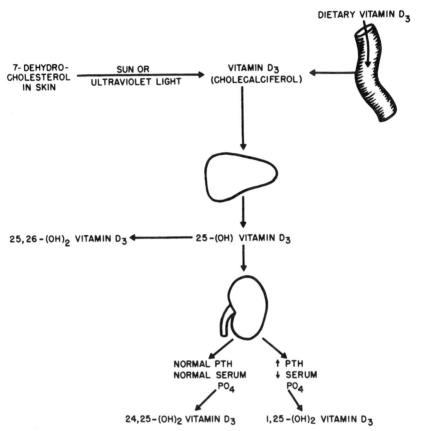

Fig. 6-2. Metabolism of vitamin D. The major source of vitamin D_3 is its production in the skin; the other important source is diet. PTH = parathyroid hormone.

treatment of hypoparathyroidism. At high doses it is more effective than vitamin D in mobilizing calcium from the bone, but in low doses it is less effective in curing rickets. DHT_3 undergoes hydroxylation in the liver to $25(OH)DHT_3$, which is the active form of DHT_3. Thus DHT_3 does not require the presence of the kidneys for the synthesis of its active metabolite. 1α-Hydroxycholecalciferol ($1\alpha[OH]D_3$) is a synthetic sterol that undergoes 25-hydroxylation in the liver to $1,25(OH)_2D_3$ and, like DHT_3, does not require the presence of renal tissue for its conversion into the active form of vitamin D_3. Calcitriol stimulates the metabolic clearance of $25(OH)D_3$. Increased calcitriol formation with increased serum concentration leads to a fall in the serum concentration of $25(OH)D_3$ [27].

Effect of Vitamin D on Intestinal Absorption

Vitamin D_3 stimulates intestinal absorption of calcium and of phosphorus.

The effect of vitamin D on calcium absorption becomes measurable several hours after its administration and is blocked by actinomycin D. Circulating calcitriol is a major regulator of intestinal calcium absorption. It exerts its effect mainly by a genomic mechanism mediated by binding to cytosolic vitamin D receptors. The calcitriol–vitamin D receptor complex interacts with specific DNA sequences of calcitriol-responsive genes and modulates transcriptional and post-transcriptional synthetic pathways. Vitamin D produces a cytosolic calcium binding protein. Calcium binding protein facilitates transcellular movement of calcium, which is the rate-limiting step in overall intestinal calcium absorption. In addition, vitamin D may act to enhance cellular calcium entry, possibly by increasing membrane fluidity (membranophilic effect) or by inducing calcium channels. The active extrusion of calcium at the basolateral side by plasma membrane-bound Ca, Mg-ATPase persists also in the absence of vitamin D. However, $1,25(OH)D_3$ has been shown to stimulate the activity and to promote the synthesis of the plasma membrane calcium pump in intestinal cells. The increased synthesis of calcium binding protein within the intestinal cell and the synthesis of an increased number of calcium pump units enhance the extrusion of calcium from within the intestinal cell into the ECF space. In addition to intestinal mucosa, calcitriol receptors are present also on osteoblasts, monocytes, human breast cancer cells, parathyroid gland, epidermal cells, and cerebellum [10, 25, 26].

Effect of Vitamin D on Bone Metabolism

Vitamin D promotes mineralization of the organic bone matrix. This action appears to be at least partly secondary to the effect of vitamin D on enhancing the intestinal absorption of calcium and phosphorus and thus maintaining their normal ECF concentrations. There is some evidence to support a direct role of vitamin D in bone accretion [28]. However, it has been shown that vitamin D–deficient osteomalacia may be cured with the intravenous administration of calcium and phosphorus despite persistence of a vitamin D deficiency state [29].

There is evidence that vitamin D and its metabolites $25(OH)D_3$ and $1,25(OH)_2D_3$ mobilize calcium and phosphorus from bone, an effect that has been demonstrated both in vivo and in vitro [30, 31]. This action of vitamin D therefore may increase serum calcium concentration independently of its enhancement of the intestinal transport of calcium. Studies in animals have shown that vitamin D stimulates both osteocytic and osteoclastic bone resorption, and this action does not require the presence of parathyroid hormone [30]. Calcitriol induces differentiation of monocytic cells into mature osteoclasts, and it increases the number of osteoclasts. Calcitriol increases osteoblast size and increases the synthesis of alkaline phosphatase and the blood level of osteocalcin. In vitro studies suggest that $1,25(OH)D_3$, but not other metabolites of vitamin D, may inhibit bone collagen synthesis [31].

The exact role of $24,25(OH)D_3$ in mineral metabolism is unknown. In animals, the hormone must be metabolized to $1,24,25(OH)_3D_3$ before it becomes active in intestinal absorption of calcium. In normal, hypoparathyroid, and anephric humans, however, $24,25(OH)D_3$ acts directly to increase intestinal absorption of calcium, even when given in relatively low doses [32]. This effect of $24,25(OH)D_3$ is associated with positive calcium balance without changes in serum concentration or urinary excretion. In view of this observation and the previously reported effect of

$24,25(OH)_2D_3$ to promote the synthesis of protein by chondrocytes, it has been proposed that $24,25(OH)D_3$ may be the metabolite that is directly involved in skeletal metabolism [32]. Furthermore, it has been reported that $1\alpha(OH)D_3$ alone does not prevent rickets in chicks, whereas $24,25(OH)D_3$ alone is effective [33]. Experimental studies have also demonstrated that $24,25(OH)_2D_3$ may play an important role in the suppression of bone resorption in rats after nephrectomy [34]. Recent in vitro studies demonstrated that $24,25(OH)D_3$ antagonizes the osseous calcium mobilizing effect of calcitriol [35].

Effect of Vitamin D on Renal Handling of Phosphorus and Calcium

The effect of vitamin D on renal handling of phosphorus has been the subject of numerous investigations. The main difficulty encountered in interpreting the changes in urinary excretion of phosphorus has been related to the calcemic actions of vitamin D, which, by suppressing PTH secretion, would indirectly alter renal handling of phosphorus. Thus the enhanced tubular reabsorption of phosphorus following the administration of vitamin D to patients with osteomalacia and rachitic animals with intact parathyroid glands could be accounted for either by inhibition of PTH secretion or by a direct tubular action of vitamin D. The results of studies in animals suggest that both $25(OH)D_3$ and $1,25(OH)_2D_3$ acutely enhance tubular reabsorption of phosphorus [36]; in rats, this effect requires the presence of either endogenous or exogenous PTH. The antiphosphaturic effect of minimal doses of $1,25(OH)D_3$ was demonstrated (in chronic studies) in vitamin D–deficient rats [37]. The effects of $1,25(OH)D_3$ are summarized in Figure 6-3.

Large doses of vitamin D cause hypercalciuria, possibly by increasing absorption of calcium from the intestine. In contrast, acute clearance studies in dogs showed an increased tubular absorption of calcium after intravenous administration of vitamin D [38]. Vitamin D, however, does not appear to be essential for the renal conservation of calcium, since urinary calcium excretion may be reduced to extremely low levels in osteomalacia resulting from vitamin D deficiency [29].

In addition to the effect of vitamin D on the intestine, bones, and kidney, vitamin D acts directly on parathyroid tissue to suppress secretion of PTH. Studies in rats in our laboratory demonstrated that physiologic amounts of $1,25(OH)D_3$ inhibit the levels of PTH messenger RNA (mRNA), independent of serum calcium levels [39]. This action of calcitriol is mediated by the vitamin D receptor. Calcitriol acts on at least two negative regulatory elements upstream in the 5' flanking region of the PTH gene to suppress transcription. Furthermore, calcitriol modulates secretion and synthesis of PTH by increasing gene expression of the vitamin D receptor in the parathyroid gland [27].

In view of this information, a feedback loop may be formulated that has the following sequence: PTH stimulates the formation of $1,25(OH)_2D_3$. $1,25(OH)D_3$ closes the feedback loop by suppressing secretion of PTH. Thus, among other functions, $1,25(OH)D_3$ may have a modifying effect on the secretion of PTH [27].

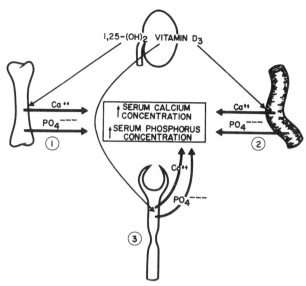

Fig. 6-3. Hypercalcemic and hyperphosphatemic effect of 1,25-(dihydroxy) vitamin D_3. Its actions are (1) mobilization of mineral from bone, (2) enhanced intestinal absorption of calcium and phosphorus, and (3) augmented tubular absorption of phosphorus and calcium. The net physiologic effect is the maintenance of a normal serum calcium and phosphorus product, which allows mineralization of bone.

Vitamin D activity in the serum and in other tissues may be measured by both bioassay and radioimmunoassay techniques. The radioreceptor assay can determine the serum levels of the various metabolites. These competitive protein binding assays have great potential importance in determining the mechanisms underlying clinical disorders secondary to abnormalities in vitamin D metabolism.

Parathyroid Hormone

PTH is a single-chain polypeptide of 84 amino acid residues (molecular weight [mol wt] 9500) with biologic activity in the N-terminal 1 to 34 region of the molecule.

The biosynthesis of the hormone starts with prepro-PTH, a 110 amino acid chain polypeptide, which is the translation product of PTH mRNA. Pro-PTH is produced after cleavage of 21 amino acids. PTH is produced after additional cleavage and is stored in secretory droplets. The amount of stored hormone is sufficient for basal secretion over 5 to 6 hours and for 2 hours of augmented secretion. Thus the synthesis is closely linked to secretory activity.

PTH plays a central role in the physiologic regulation of serum calcium concentration. Serum calcium concentration is maintained within a very narrow range, primarily due to a feedback mechanism in which minimal changes in ionized calcium alter the secretory rate of PTH, which then restores the ionized calcium to its initial normal concentration by its action on bone. Serum concentration of phosphorus is not feedback regulated, and it therefore varies over a relatively wide range. Recent studies, however, suggest that changes in serum phosphate may be involved in the regulation of PTH secretion. This effect appears to be independent of changes in serum calcium and vitamin D [40, 41].

It is apparent that serum ionized calcium is the single most important physiologic factor controlling the secretory rate of PTH. A sensitive inverse relationship has been demonstrated between ionized calcium and serum levels of PTH [8]. The parathyroid cells have a cell surface sensing mechanism to extracellular calcium concentration that also recognizes other divalent and polyvalent cations such as Mg^{2+} and neomycin. This mechanism is based on a calcium-sensing receptor. Calcium-sensing receptor is a member of the G protein–coupled receptor family that responds to increased extracellular calcium by triggering phospholipase C pathway and elevating intracellular calcium concentration. The increased intracellular calcium inhibits PTH secretion from parathyroid cells. The calcium-sensing receptor that is expressed in the parathyroid, in the thyroid, and in the kidney was recently cloned and characterized [13]. In addition to its acute effect on PTH secretion, chronic changes in serum ionized calcium concentration, both hypercalcemia and hypocalcemia, reduce or increase the steady-state level of PTH mRNA and thus reduce or increase respectively the synthesis of PTH. In vivo, calcitriol causes a 90 percent decrease in prepro-PTH mRNA at 48 hours; the effect starts after 2 hours. As opposed to calcium, which exerts both an acute and chronic effect on PTH secretion, calcitriol does not have an acute effect on calcium secretion, but after 12 to 24 hours there is a decrease in PTH secretion [27].

An increase in PTH secretion also has been observed in cows during the administration of epinephrine, raising the possibility that the autonomic nervous system may play a role in controlling PTH secretion [42]. The results of an in vitro study with bovine parathyroid cells suggest that at normal serum calcium concentration the synthesis of PTH is maintained at or very close to maximum capacity. Low calcium concentration stimulates secretion and decreases intracellular degradation. High calcium concentration over a short time suppresses secretion and augments degradation.

Peripheral Actions of Parathyroid Hormone and Parathyroid Hormone–Related Peptide

The peripheral actions of PTH and parathyroid hormone–related peptide (PTHrP) on bone and kidney involve binding to cell surface receptors followed by activation of two pathways of signal transduction. Thus, PTH stimulates both the adenylate cyclase–cyclic adenosine monophosphate (cyclic AMP)–protein kinase A pathway and phospholipase C, which in turn leads to activation of protein kinase C (by diacylglycerol) and an increase in intracellular calcium (by inositol triphosphate). The stimulation of these two signaling pathways is mediated by coupling of the hormone-occupied receptor with two distinct G proteins, which link the receptor to effector pathways [43, 44]. The gene for the human PTH receptor for bone and kidney has been cloned, sequenced, and expressed in African green monkey kidney cells (cos). The evaluation of the structure and function relationship of the receptor and PTH is of interest. It has been demonstrated that N-amino-terminal fragment PTH sequence 1 to 34 reproduces all physiologic effects of PTH sequence 1 to 84. It has been shown that the amino acid sequences 10 to 15 and 24 to 34 of PTH are necessary for binding to the receptor. With regard to the biologic effects of PTH, it has shown that the first two N-terminal amino acids 1 and 2 are required for the activation of adenylate cyclase–protein kinase A pathway, whereas the amino acids sequence 28 to 34 are required for the activation of phospholipase C–protein kinase C pathway. Indeed, in vitro experiments, the fragment PTH sequence 3 to 34 was shown to suppress phosphate transport without activation of adenylate cyclase–protein kinase A pathway [43–45].

Effect of Parathyroid Hormone on Bone

PTH plays a major role in bone remodeling. PTH increases bone turnover due both to increase in osteoclast number and resorption and to stimulation of bone formation by osteoblast activation. PTH receptors are expressed in bone-forming cells, osteoblasts, and pro-osteoblasts, but not in osteoclasts. Thus, although PTH acts to increase osteoclastic resorption, it appears that this effect is not mediated via receptors on osteoclasts but are indirect, occurring through interaction of PTH with receptors on osteoblasts. It is hypothesized that PTH-activated osteoblasts enhance recruitment and stimulation of osteoclasts.

PTH augments release of mineral from bone by stimulating both osteocytic and osteoclastic bone resorption and possibly by enhancing calcium transport from the skeletal ECF into the systemic ECF. There is experimental evidence that the latter is a direct effect. The resulting increase in serum calcium concentration may be preceded by a short period of decreasing concentration because of an initial enhanced entry of calcium into bone cells.

The calcemic effect of PTH on bone requires the presence of vitamin D [46, 47]. The impaired response to PTH hormone in vitamin D deficiency may be due either to some permissive action of the vitamin or to the mechanical blocking effect of the osteoid that coats the surface of the mineralized bone and thus prevents access of the PTH. Correction of hypocalcemia per se in rats has been shown to restore the responsiveness of the bone to the action of the PTH in states of vitamin D deficiency. This observation is consistent with the possibility that calcium is a cofactor in the skeletal action of PTH. It has been recently proposed that PTH acts on two distinct cellular systems in the bone: (1) the bone remodeling system and (2) the calcium mobilization or calcemic-homeostatic system. The remodeling system consists of osteoclasts that resorb old bone and osteoblasts that form new bone. In this system, bone resorption is balanced by bone formation, and therefore no mineral escapes into the circulation. The homeostatic system is based on the action of surface osteocytes and osteocytes occupying lacunar spaces that regulate the movement of calcium between the bone fluid and the ECF. This mineral-releasing system is important in everyday regulation of serum calcium and requires $1,25(OH)_2D_3$ in addition to PTH. Recent in vitro studies suggest that the calcium-mobilizing effect of PTH is mediated by activation of the phospholipase C–protein kinase C signal transduction system [48].

Effect of Parathyroid Hormone on the Kidney

The primary renal effect of PTH is to produce phosphaturia by depressing net phosphate reabsorption in the proximal tubule. This tubular effect involves PTH receptor–mediated intracellular formation of messengers cyclic AMP, inositol tri-phosphate, diacylglycerol, and free cytosolic calcium and activation of protein kinase A and protein kinase C. These inhibit brush-border transport systems including sodium-phosphate cotransport and sodium-proton antiport exchange [43]. The results of certain studies suggest additional effects of PTH in more distal parts of the nephron on phosphorus absorption [49]. Phosphate depletion produces resistance to the phosphaturic action of PTH in rats; however, this has not been shown yet in humans.

Even though the effect of PTH in the proximal tubule is to depress calcium reabsorption, its net effect is to decrease urinary calcium excretion in dogs, rats [50], and humans. The net increase in tubular reabsorption of calcium appears to be primarily due to a distal action of the hormone, where about 10 to 20 percent of filtered calcium is reabsorbed [11]. Thus it appears that both the renal and skeletal actions of PTH act jointly to increase serum concentrations of calcium. Since PTH may increase bicarbonate, sodium, and amino acid excretion, the hormone does not appear to increase the reabsorption of these substances in the distal nephron.

Effect of Parathyroid Hormone on Intestinal Absorption of Calcium

A role for PTH in the intestinal absorption of calcium has been suggested by several studies in both animals and humans. However, at present there is no evidence to support a direct action of PTH on calcium transport in the intestine. The fact that PTH enhances the conversion of $25(OH)D_3$ to $1,25(OH)_2D_3$, which directly acts on the intestinal transport of calcium, may explain the apparent effects of the hormone. Even so, it is obvious that in states of vitamin D deficiency, the elevated levels of circulating PTH fail to maintain normal absorption of calcium. Conversely, vitamin D may affect intestinal absorption in the absence of PTH in patients with hypoparathyroidism. The multiple actions of PTH are summarized in Figure 6-4.

Radioimmunoassay of Parathyroid Hormone

Radioimmunoassay for circulating PTH was introduced by Berson and Yalow [51] in 1963. Further studies led to the recognition of the heterogeneity of circulating PTH, which apparently represents various molecular species of the hormone. The glandular hormone (mol wt 9500) consists of 84 amino acids (1 to 84 sequence) and has two terminals, amino ($-NH_2$) and carboxy ($-COOH$). The circulating PTH consists of the glandular hormone and its fragments. At least two different molecular species of circulating PTH have been detected by different antisera, one with a molecular weight of 4500 to 5000 and one with a molecular weight of 7000 to 7500. Structurally, there are two major split products that can be characterized by their terminals. The first product has the amino terminal, is the biologically active fragment, and has an amino acid sequence of 1 to 34. The second product has the carboxy terminal, is the biologically inactive fragment, and has an amino

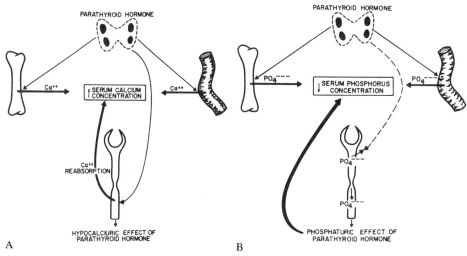

Fig. 6-4. (A) The hypercalcemic effect of parathyroid hormone is a summation of mineral mobilization from bone, calcium absorption from the bowel, and distal tubular reabsorption of calcium in the kidney. The effect on the bowel is probably related to parathyroid hormone–induced renal production of 1,25-(dihydroxy) vitamin D_3. (B) The hypophosphatemic effect of parathyroid hormone is based on its phosphaturic action, which supersedes its effect of mobilizing phosphorus from bone and enhancing phosphate absorption from the intestine. (Solid lines represent an enhancement of action; broken line represents an inhibition of action.)

acid sequence of 53 to 84. The level of total circulating immunoreactive PTH that reflects all molecular species appears to represent the chronic state of parathyroid function and is most useful in the diagnosis of parathyroid abnormalities. The level of the glandular (mol wt 9500) species represents acute changes in parathyroid activity, such as those that occur after calcium infusion. Although it has been suggested that the level of the carboxy terminal fragment provides the best differentiation between normal persons and patients with hyperparathyroidism, this seems paradoxic in view of the fact that the carboxy terminal is biologically inactive. It should be emphasized that radioimmunoassays that measure the carboxy terminal fragments do not provide a reliable estimate of parathyroid function in patients with renal insufficiency. This is because the clearance of C-terminal fragments is delayed in renal failure. Therefore their serum levels are determined not only by the secretory rate of parathyroid glands but also by the renal function. Thus, with renal failure, the radioimmunoassay of N-terminal species of PTH or of the intact hormone molecule provides a better indication of parathyroid function. The intact PTH assay employs two antibodies, one binding the N-terminal and the second binding the C-terminal. One antibody is fixed on beads that are then exposed to serum. After incubation with the tested serum, beads are separated and exposed to radiolabeled antibodies binding the opposite terminal. This is considered a most reliable assay.

Calcitonin

The discovery of calcitonin established the presence of a new regulatory system for calcium homeostasis. Calcitonin is a polypeptide with 32 amino acid residues and was isolated from the parafollicular cells of the thyroid gland or ultimobranchial body in a wide variety of species. Hypercalcemia stimulates release of calcitonin, which tends to lower serum calcium concentration [52].

Effect of Calcitonin on Bone

The major mechanism by which calcitonin lowers serum calcium and phosphorus concentrations is inhibition of bone resorption. This is associated with decreased osteoclastic activity and decreased urinary hydroxyproline excretion. In organ culture, after prolonged treatment with calcitonin, PTH may overcome the inhibitory effect of calcitonin and induce bone resorption. This phenomenon is termed escape and is also observed in vivo in animals with intact parathyroid glands chronically treated with calcitonin.

There is an antagonism between calcitonin and glucocorticoid hormones, since glucocorticoids interfere with the hypocalcemic action of calcitonin.

The receptors of calcitonin have been cloned from human giant cell tumor of bone, human ovary, and breast cell lines [44]. The calcitonin receptor is expressed by osteoclasts, as opposed to PTH and calcitriol receptors, which are expressed by osteoblasts, but not by osteoclasts. Similarly to PTH receptors, calcitonin receptors couple to two signal transduction pathways, adenylate cyclase–protein kinase A and phospholipase C–protein kinase C via linking with G proteins. Calcitonin acts directly to inhibit osteoclast action on the bone and inhibits osteoclast motility in isolated osteoclast preparations.

Effect of Calcitonin on the Kidney

Calcitonin increases urinary excretion of phosphorus, sodium, potassium, and calcium. This effect is independent of PTH. In fact, calcitonin acts to reverse the effect of PTH in two organs. It inhibits bone resorption and increases urinary calcium excretion; both actions tend to lower serum calcium. The phosphaturic action of calcitonin has been found to be associated with an increased urinary excretion of cyclic AMP.

Effect of Calcitonin on Intestinal Absorption

The effect of calcitonin on intestinal absorption has not been studied extensively. Preliminary reports indicate, however, that calcitonin has no effect on calcium absorption but may decrease the absorption of phosphorus, sodium, potassium, and chloride. The multiple actions of calcitonin are summarized in Figure 6-5.

The development of a sensitive radioimmunoassay for calcitonin has provided the means to study the control of secretion of this hormone. From a clinical standpoint, the radioimmunoassay serves as a valuable aid in the diagnosis of medullary carcinoma of thyroid, which is a calcitonin-secreting tumor.

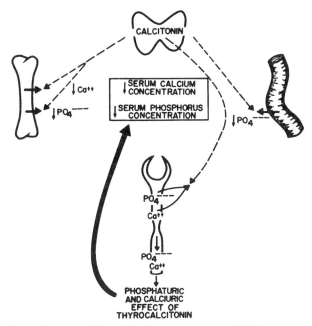

Fig. 6-5. The hypocalcemic and hypophosphatemic actions of calcitonin are based on inhibition of mineral mobilization from the bone, decreased tubular reabsorption and increased urinary excretion of calcium and phosphorus, and decreased intestinal absorption of phosphorus. (Solid lines represent an enhancing effect of the hormone, broken lines represent an inhibitory action.)

Disorders of Calcium and Phosphorus Metabolism Associated with Hypocalcemia

Vitamin D Deficiency

Hypocalcemia is a common feature of vitamin D deficiency. However, this disorder may be present with a normal serum calcium concentration. For example, vitamin D–deficiency rickets in children evolves in three stages. During the first stage, serum calcium concentration is low, serum phosphorus is normal, and immunoreactive PTH in the serum is normal [47, 53]. There is no satisfactory explanation for the normal PTH in the presence of hypocalcemia. During the second stage, there is a rise in PTH activity, and serum calcium concentration rises to a normal level as serum phosphorus concentration decreases. In the third stage, which is the most severe, both serum calcium and phosphorus concentrations are low [47]. It is unknown whether vitamin D–deficiency osteomalacia in adults shows a similar evolution.

The various common etiologies of vitamin D deficiency are listed in Table 6-2. As vitamin D is a fat-soluble vitamin, nutritional osteomalacia is usually associated with a deficient intake of food products containing fatty substances [47, 54]. Partial

Table 6-2. Common causes of vitamin D deficiency

Nutritional	Abnormal metabolism of vitamin D
Malabsorption	Vitamin D–dependent rickets
Following gastrectomy	Ingestion of barbiturates
Tropical and nontropical spure	Renal insufficiency
Chronic pancreatitis	Hepatic dysfunction
Biliary cirrhosis	Calcium deprivation
Ingestion of cathartics	
Intestinal bypass	
Anticonvulsant therapy	

gastrectomy may lead either to a simple dietary deficiency of vitamin D as a result of avoiding fatty foods or to malabsorption of vitamin D. Small-bowel disease may produce both malabsorption of vitamin D and mucosal resistance to its action. Bile salt deficiency interferes with vitamin D absorption, while hepatocellular failure may interfere with its metabolism. Factitious diarrhea due to prolonged ingestion of laxatives also may cause vitamin D deficiency. Likewise, nephrotic syndrome is associated with urinary losses and low circulating levels of $25(OH)D_3$ [55].

In addition to vitamin D deficiency resulting from nutritional and gastrointestinal causes, a group of disorders has been identified in which the deficiency is due to an abnormal metabolism of vitamin D. Vitamin D–dependent rickets is an inherited autosomal recessive disorder. It appears during early infancy and responds to pharmacologic doses of vitamin D and to physiologic doses of calcitriol. This disorder represents an inherited deficiency in the kidney of the enzyme $25(OH)_2D_3$ 1α-hydroxylase, which converts $25(OH)_2D_3$ into $1,25(OH)_2D_3$ [54].

Osteomalacia in patients ingesting phenobarbital is associated with low levels of circulating $25(OH)D_3$. It has been shown that the biologic half-life of vitamin D_3 and $25(OH)D_3$ is shortened in treated patients and that there is an accumulation of more polar metabolites, some of which are inactive [54]. This rapid turnover and the production of inactive forms of vitamin D have been attributed to induction of microsomal enzyme activity in the liver. Phenytoin does not interfere directly with vitamin D metabolism but can induce hypocalcemia through reduced intestinal absorption of calcium and decreased release from bone. Low circulating levels of $25(OH)D_3$ also have been observed in patients with chronic hepatic failure [27, 54].

Dietary calcium deprivation per se in rats increases the clearance and inactivation of $25(OH)D_3$ and leads to vitamin D deficiency. It has been suggested that this form of vitamin D deficiency is due to secondary hyperparathyroidism, which increases the renal production of calcitriol. The latter augments the degradation of $25(OH)D_3$ to inactive metabolites. Hypothetically, this mechanism may account for vitamin D deficiency observed in clinical states of calcium malabsorption including gastrointestinal diseases, resection, or bypass; chronic liver disease; anticonvulsant therapy; and morbid obesity [27, 56].

The clinical significance of abnormally low serum levels of $25(OH)_2D_3$ in patients with nephrotic syndrome due to excessive urinary losses of vitamin D–binding globulin has not yet been fully established. However, a study of bone histology in patients with nephrotic syndrome who had normal renal function revealed that the decrease in $25(OH)D_3$ level results in a decrease in ionized calcium, secondary hyperparathyroidism, and enhanced bone resorption as well as defective mineralization [55].

Understanding of the metabolic pathways of vitamin D may facilitate the investigation of various abnormalities. For example, low levels of $1,25(OH)_2D_3$ have been reported in patients with hypoparathyroidism. The lack of PTH and the presence of hyperphosphatemia may decrease the conversion of $25(OH)_2D_3$ into $1,25(OH)_2D_3$, which may explain the resistance to vitamin D in some patients with hypoparathyroidism. In support of this possibility is the finding of successful control of hypocalcemia with $1,25(OH)_2D_3$ in patients with hypoparathyroidism.

Hypoparathyroidism

Hypoparathyroidism is a common cause of hypocalcemia. Hypoparathyroidism may be secondary or idiopathic.

Secondary Hypoparathyroidism

Hypoparathyroidism may be caused by surgery. This variety of hypoparathyroidism may be due to accidental removal of parathyroids or traumatic interruption of their blood supply. Very often the parathyroid deficiency is transient in nature. Hypocalcemia that appears after excision of parathyroid adenoma results from functional suppression and hypofunction of the remaining normal glands. Hypoparathyroidism may be a component of multiple endocrine dysfunction, including adrenal insufficiency due to an autoimmune disorder. In hypoparathyroidism associated with pernicious anemia also, an autoimmune mechanism has been implicated. Hypoparathyroidism is a recognized complication of thalassemia occurring after multiple transfusions and also has been described in patients with Wilson's disease. Deposition of iron and copper, respectively, in the parathyroid glands is the likely mechanism of parathyroid hypofunction in these patients [54].

Hypocalcemia may occur with magnesium depletion. Hypomagnesemia has been reported to induce skeletal resistance to PTH. It has been proposed that low serum magnesium diminishes the synthesis of PTH. It is of interest that some patients with hypoparathyroidism who exhibit resistance to vitamin D will respond after administration of magnesium. Hypocalcemia associated with magnesium depletion responds poorly to intravenous calcium. Profound hypocalcemia may appear after therapeutic use of magnesium sulfate (e.g., in preeclampsia of pregnancy) due to suppression of PTH secretion. Certain drugs such as aminoglycosides and cytotoxic agents may have a direct toxic effect on parathyroid glands, leading to hypocalcemia. Irradiation of neck or administration of radioactive iodine may also affect parathyroid function [54].

Idiopathic Hypoparathyroidism

Idiopathic hypoparathyroidism may be sporadic or familial. The familial congenital type is associated with hypocalcemic seizures in infancy. Familial idiopathic hypoparathyroidism is a heterogenous group of disorders. It may result from a mutation of the prepro-PTH gene or mutations of currently unidentified loci that affect the development, structure, or regulation of function of parathyroid glands [57, 58].

The human PTH is encoded by a single gene that was mapped to the short arm of chromosome 11. Mutations in this gene may lead to familial hypoparathyroidism with autosomal dominant transmission. In the affected patients, the levels of PTH in serum may be low or undetectable [57, 58].

The DiGeorge syndrome consists of a congenital failure of development of the derivatives of the third and the fourth pharyngeal pouches, leading to absence of parathyroids and thymus. This syndrome may be inherited as an autosomal dominant disorder. It is associated with deletion of the long arm of chromosome 22.

X-linked recessive hypoparathyroidism, similarly to the DiGeorge syndrome, is associated with parathyroid agenesis and undetectable PTH levels in circulation. The X-linked recessive hypoparathyroidism gene was mapped to the distal long arm of the X chromosome [57, 58].

Recently autosomal dominant hypoparathyroidism was reported in families with activating mutations of the gene that encodes the extracellular calcium-sensing receptor in chromosome 3. In one family, missense mutation was found in the calcium-sensing receptor gene [13].

Pseudohypoparathyroidism

Pseudohypoparathyroidism is a rare inheritable disorder characterized by mental retardation, moderate obesity, short stature, brachydactyly with short metacarpal and metatarsal bones, exostoses, radius curvus, and expressionless face. The biochemical abnormalities are hypocalcemia and hyperphosphatemia [59, 60]. Some patients exhibit the biochemical abnormalities only. Thus the disorder may be subdivided into pseudohypoparathyroidism type IA, which is associated with both the somatic and the biochemical abnormalities, and type IB, which presents with the biochemical defect without the somatic abnormalities. In patients with pseudohypoparathyroidism, the administration of PTH fails to increase urinary cyclic AMP and is not associated with phosphaturia. It also has been shown that the response to the administration of exogenous dibutyryl cyclic AMP is intact in pseudohypoparathyroidism and causes pronounced phosphaturia. It has been proposed that the skeletal refractoriness to PTH shows a certain degree of selectivity. Accordingly, the bone responds to the remodeling action of the hormone but is resistant to its calcemic-homeostatic effect. Because of the hypocalcemic stimulus, secondary hyperparathyroidism may develop in some patients, leading to osteitis fibrosa cystica. Failure of the kidney to form $1,25(OH)_2D_3$ in response to PTH results in a low circulating level of this metabolite. This deficiency may be responsible, at least partly, for the skeletal refractoriness to the calcemic action of PTH that requires the presence of $1,25(OH)_2D_3$ [59].

Most patients with the type I form of pseudohypoparathyroidism manifest approximately 50 percent reduction in cellular activity of the α subunit of the G protein that stimulates adenylate cyclase (Gsα). Patients with type IA show a generalized Gsα deficiency and often manifest resistance to other hormones whose effects are mediated by Gsα-coupled receptors (e.g., calcitonin, glucagon, and thyroid-stimulating hormone). At variance with type IA, patients with pseudohypoparathyroidism type IB manifest a selective end-organ resistance to PTH alone [60].

In addition to the mechanism of target organ refractoriness, other mechanisms have been identified. In one patient, the administration of PTH was associated with a normal increase in urinary cyclic AMP but failed to produce phosphaturia [61]. Production of ineffective PTH, presumably because of a defect in the conversion of parathyroid prohormone into an active form, also was described in one patient [62]. The patient had normal to high levels of immunoreactive PTH, which was probably a biologically inactive hormone, since the patient readily responded to exogenous PTH.

Malignancy Associated with Hypocalcemia

Medullary carcinoma of the thyroid may present as a familial and autosomal dominant or as a sporadic disorder. The tumor is derived from parafollicular cells of ultimobranchial organ, which secrete calcitonin. Patients with this disorder have high levels of circulating calcitonin and exhibit an exaggerated increase of calcitonin in response to calcium infusion. Hypocalcemia has been reported to be present in some subjects. However, it is absent in others, and its absence despite very high levels of calcitonin is not well understood but has been attributed to a secondary increase in PTH. An "escape" from the effect of calcitonin, which has been observed in experimental conditions, is another possible factor. Elevated blood levels of calcitonin also have been reported in tumors other than medullary carcinoma of the thyroid, including carcinoma of the lung.

Hypocalcemia may develop in patients with malignant neoplasms in association with osteoblastic (bone-forming) metastases. These lesions may lead to rapid deposition of mineral in the newly formed matrix, thus causing hypocalcemia [63]. Such hypocalcemia has been described in patients with carcinoma of the prostate or carcinoma of the breast with osteoblastic metastases [63]. While most of these patients have shown osteoblastic lesions on radiologic examination, associated osteolytic lesions also have been present [63].

Hyperphosphatemia

The various causes of hyperphosphatemia that may lead to hypocalcemia are listed in Table 6-3. The oral or intravenous administration of phosphate lowers serum

Table 6-3. Hyperphosphatemia as a cause of hypocalcemia

Administration of phosphate	Renal disease
Oral phosphate	Acute renal failure
Cow's milk in infants	Chronic renal failure
Laxatives containing phosphate	Neoplasms treated with cytotoxic agents
Potassium phosphate tablets	Lymphomas
Phosphate-containing enemas	Leukemias
Intravenous phosphate	

calcium concentration in normal animals and in hypercalcemic human subjects. This observation formed the basis for the clinical use of phosphate administration in states of hypercalcemia. The association of hyperphosphatemia and hypocalcemia has been reported to occur in a variety of circumstances. Hyperphosphatemia has been observed in persons ingesting large quantities of phosphate-containing laxatives or receiving enemas with phosphate. Hyperphosphatemia and hypocalcemia with tetany may develop in babies fed cow's milk, which contains 1220 mg of calcium and 940 mg of phosphorus per liter (human milk contains 340 mg of calcium and 150 mg of phosphorus per liter).

The mechanism responsible for lowering serum calcium by the administration of phosphate is not entirely understood. One possibility is that the decrease in serum calcium concentration is due to deposition of calcium phosphate in the bone, in soft tissues, or in both. The results of animal studies do suggest that the administration of phosphate increases bone formation.

In chronic renal failure, a constant increase in serum phosphorus concentration is observed when GFR is 30 ml/min or less, and hyperphosphatemia is a common accompaniment of acute renal failure. It is important to emphasize, however, that in renal failure causes other than hyperphosphatemia may play an important role in hypocalcemia. An acquired resistance to vitamin D, which might represent a metabolic block in the 1α-hydroxylation of $25(OH)D_3$ to $1,25(OH)_2D_3$, or skeletal resistance to the calcium-mobilizing effect of PTH, or both, also is possibly involved [64].

In patients undergoing chemotherapy for neoplastic diseases, particularly of lymphatic origin, large quantities of phosphates may be released into the circulation as a result of the cytolysis. This sequence of events has been associated with acute hyperphosphatemia and hypocalcemia. Conversely, rapid regrowth of tumoral masses may lead to profound hypophosphatemia [20].

Acute Pancreatitis

The hypocalcemia associated with acute pancreatitis is not well understood. The precipitation of calcium soaps in the abdominal cavity, which results from the release of lipolytic enzymes and from fat necrosis, has been suggested as the mechanism of the hypocalcemia. Other studies implicate glucagon-induced hypersecretion of calcitonin as the mechanism of hypocalcemia in acute pancreatitis [54]. These latter results, however, have not been confirmed.

Even though it has been shown that hypocalcemia and urinary excretion of cyclic AMP respond to pharmacologic doses of PTH, one study suggests a relative peripheral resistance to appropriate levels of endogenous hormone and normal circulating $1,25(OH)_2D_3$. The cause of this refractoriness and its role in the hypocalcemia of acute pancreatitis are not apparent [65].

Neonatal Tetany

Neonatal tetany with hypocalcemia was first described in 1913. Several mechanisms have been suggested for the pathogenesis of this disorder, namely vitamin D deficiency, parathyroid hypofunction, and hyperphosphatemia due to a high content of phosphorus in the milk (cow's milk).

Congenital absence of the parathyroid glands, usually in association with other congenital anomalies, has been reported in neonatal tetany. Transient, idiopathic congenital hypoparathyroidism with hypoplasia or dysplasia of the parathyroid glands and with a subsequent compensatory hyperplasia has been described in infants with hypocalcemia [66]. In one study, low levels of circulating immunoreactive PTH were detected in a group of babies with hypocalcemia. This finding was attributed to possible immaturity of the parathyroid glands, which was usually transient [67].

Babies born to mothers with osteomalacia due to vitamin D deficiency have congenital rickets with hypocalcemia and tetany. In one study, serum levels of $25(OH)D_3$ were measured in 15 premature infants with neonatal hypocalcemia and in their mothers. In 11 of the 15 cases, plasma $25(OH)D_3$ was low in both mother and infant [68]. Babies born to mothers with hyperparathyroidism and hypercalcemia are at risk of hypocalcemia and tetany, probably due to suppression of their own parathyroid glands.

Osteopetrosis (Marble Bone Disease)

Osteopetrosis is a rare disease, with about 300 cases reported in the literature. The disease is characterized by abnormal bones that fracture easily, increased radiographic bone density, cranial nerve palsies because of compression of the nerves in their foramina, and mandibular osteomyelitis. There are two clinical forms of the disease. The first variant, malignant osteopetrosis, affects infants and usually is fatal. The second, benign osteopetrosis, may be recognized during any stage of adult life [69]. The inheritance of the malignant form of the disease is recessive; inheritance of the benign form is autosomal dominant. Hypocalcemia has been found only in a few cases and does not appear to be a constant feature of the disease [69].

The basic abnormality in osteopetrosis is not clear, but indirect evidence suggests that a defect in osteoclast function leading to uncoupling between bone formation and resorption with reduced osteoclastic activity is the underlying mechanism. Bone marrow transplantation and high doses of $1,25(OH)_2D_3$ with low calcium intake have been used in therapeutic trials. It has been demonstrated that the vitamin D derivative may enhance the bone-resorbing activity of osteoclasts that is impaired in osteopetrosis [70]. Recent trials of treatment with recombinant human interferon gamma are encouraging [71].

Administration of Phytate, Sodium Ethylenediaminetetraacetate, Citrate, and Mithramycin

Sodium phytate (sodium-inositol hexaphosphate) binds calcium in the intestine as calcium phytate and thereby inhibits calcium absorption. In normal subjects, the administration of phytate causes only a minimal drop in serum calcium, whereas in patients with latent hypoparathyroidism, it may precipitate hypocalcemia. Excessive dietary phytate (cereals) has been implicated as a possible cause of osteomalacia in certain ethnic groups in England [56]. Both citrate and sodium ethylenediaminetetraacetate (Na-EDTA), when given intravenously, bind ionized calcium and may induce hypocalcemia with low ionized calcium. Low serum ionized calcium may be a complication of ethylene glycol (antifreeze) poisoning. This is because calcium binding by oxalic acid, which is the metabolite of the poison, reduces serum ionized calcium.

Excessive intake of fluoride may induce hypocalcemia. This was reported recently in Alaska in connection with fluorosis that followed excessive addition of fluoride to drinking water [72]. Recently, drug-induced hypocalcemia was described in patients with acquired immune deficiency syndrome (AIDS). An analogue of pyrophosphate foscarnet that is used to treat cytomegalovirus infection caused hypocalcemia due to chelation of calcium and also due to concomitant hypomagnesemia [73]. Ketoconazole and pentamidine have been reported to cause hypocalcemia as well.

The association of low serum ionized calcium with essential hypertension and secondary hyperparathyroidism has been described and attributed to renal calcium leak [74]. This finding may be of clinical significance because a fall in serum ionized calcium may compromise myocardial performance and worsen the function of a failing heart in patients with hypertension.

Mithramycin is a potent inhibitor of RNA synthesis and has antitumor activity. It produces a decrease in serum calcium and phosphorus levels and in urinary hydroxyproline excretion. Mithramycin has been used to correct the hypercalcemia of various disorders, including malignancy with bone metastases. In experimental studies, mithramycin has been shown to inhibit the rate and magnitude of osteoclastic resorption induced by PTH; however, no demonstrable effect was found on normal bone formation or resorption in growing animals [75, 76].

Treatment of Hypocalcemia

Symptomatic hypocalcemia generally responds promptly to the intravenous administration of calcium. The commonly used preparations are 10% calcium gluconate (10-ml ampules containing 90 mg of elemental calcium) and 10% calcium chloride (10-ml ampules containing 360 mg of elemental calcium). The treatment should be instituted immediately, since delay may be associated with further aggravation of tetany and lead to generalized seizures and even cardiac arrest.

In patients with chronic hypocalcemia due to irreversible causes such as hypoparathyroidism, chronic treatment with oral calcium should follow the intravenous therapy. In mild cases, oral calcium administration constitutes the best initial therapy. The commonly used preparations are in tablet form: calcium lactate, 300 mg (60 mg of elemental calcium); chewable calcium gluconate, 1 g (90 mg of elemental calcium); and calcium carbonate (Os-Cal), 250 mg of elemental calcium. Oral calcium also may be used for patients for whom the diagnosis of irreversible hypoparathyroidism has not been established with absolute certainty. In patients who fail to respond to oral calcium, vitamin D in large doses is the only available treatment. The commonly used preparations are capsules containing 1.25 mg (50,000 units) of vitamin D_2 (ergocalciferol). The average dose ranges between 1.25 and 3.75 mg/day. DHT_3 is three times as potent as vitamin D_2 in raising serum calcium concentration. Each capsule contains 0.125 mg of DHT_3. The average daily dose ranges between 0.25 and 1.00 mg of DHT_3. Both vitamins also are available in liquid oil solutions. Both hypoparathyroidism and pseudohypoparathyroidism respond to physiologic doses of $1,25(OH)_2D_3$ and $1\alpha(OH)D_3$ with restoration of serum calcium to normal. Calcitriol is marketed as Rocaltrol and is dispensed in capsules containing 0.25 and 1.0 μg. Chlorothiazides may enhance the calcemic action of vitamin D and its analogues, whereas furosemide may aggravate the hypocalcemia through its hypercalciuric action.

Patients in whom hypocalcemia is associated with hypomagnesemia respond poorly to intravenous calcium, but with correction of the hypomagnesemia, serum calcium concentration is restored to normal levels.

Symptoms rarely develop in patients with chronic renal failure and hypocalcemia. However, very often reduction of elevated serum phosphorus with phosphate-binding antacids will cause an increase in serum calcium concentration.

Hypocalcemia associated with osteomalacia resulting from vitamin D deficiency is rarely symptomatic. It usually responds to physiologic doses of vitamin D and increased oral calcium intake.

Disorders of Calcium and Phosphorus Metabolism Associated with Hypercalcemia

Hypercalcemia presents a challenge to every clinician and diagnostician. In some instances, the cause of hypercalcemia is self-evident on the basis of the circumstantial clinical findings, while in other situations, extensive efforts are required to establish the etiology. The important causes of hypercalcemia are listed in Table 6-4.

Hyperparathyroidism

Primary hyperparathyroidism is present in 10 to 20 percent of all patients with hypercalcemia. The annual age-adjusted incidence is approximately 25 cases per 100,000. Because of this frequency and the amenability to surgical cure, making the diagnosis is very important. The disease is more common in females than in males; the incidence increases in women after menopause but is less frequent in older men. A single parathyroid adenoma is by far the most common cause of primary hyperparathyroidism. Carcinoma is very infrequent, occurring in less than 1 percent of all reported cases. Primary hyperplasia is found in less than 10 percent of all cases, but it is the most frequent cause in familial hyperparathyroidism.

The morphologic differentiation between adenomas and hyperplasia sometimes is very difficult. The presence of a capsule and a rim of compressed normal gland tissue around the periphery of an adenoma may be helpful in making a definitive diagnosis. The persistence or recurrence of hypercalcemia after surgery for a pur-

Table 6-4. Disorders associated with hypercalcemia

Primary hyperparathyroidism	Hypervitaminosis D
Adenoma and carcinoma	Hypervitaminosis A
Hyperplasia	Granulomatous diseases
Multiple endocrine adenomatosis	Sarcoidosis
Ectopic secretion of parathyroid hormone by	Tuberculosis
neoplasms (rare)	Histoplasmosis
Secondary hyperparathyroidism	Coccidioidomycosis
Malabsorption and vitamin D disease	Leprosy
Chronic renal failure	Foreign body granuloma
Following kidney transplantation	Hyperthyroidism
Familial hypocalciuric hypercalcemia	Adrenocortical insufficiency
Hypercalcemia associated with malignancy	Infantile hypercalcemia
Lytic bone metastases	Immobilization
Circulating tumor-secreted factors	Hypophosphatasia
Parathyroid hormone–related peptide	Milk-alkali syndrome
1,25-dihydroxyvitamin D_3–induced	Parenteral nutrition
hypercalcemia	Hypercalcemia associated with acute
Locally acting, noncirculating, tumor-	renal failure
secreted cytokines	Medications
Interleukin-1 and 6	Thiazides
Tumor necrosis factor-β	Lithium
Granulocyte macrophage	Theophylline
Colony-stimulating factor	Calcium ion exchange resins
Transforming growth factor-α	
Prostaglandins	
Hypercalcemia in patients with	
hyperabsorptive hypercalciuria	

ported adenoma warrants a more precise evaluation of the morphologic status of the parathyroid tissue removed. Also, with parathyroid hyperplasia, the quantity of parathyroid tissue to be removed—safely on the one hand, yet not allowing recurrence of the disease on the other hand—is a very difficult balance to achieve. If more than one gland shows histologic features of hyperplasia, removal of more than one gland is recommended; generally, approximately 200 mg of parathyroid tissue should remain.

In addition to the uncertainties related to morphologic differences between various forms of hyperparathyroidism, some of its functional characteristics also have been questioned. The widely accepted interpretation of the cause of the hypercalcemia in patients with parathyroid adenomas has been that the normal feedback regulation of PTH secretion is absent. That is, presumably the secreting cells of the adenoma were altered in such a way that their secretory function no longer responded to variations in serum calcium concentration; this state was defined as autonomy. The distinction between parathyroid adenoma and hyperplasia implied that the former is a primary disease rather than an adaptive response and that the latter represents a compensatory adaptation to low serum calcium concentration. The term *tertiary hyperparathyroidism* has been used to describe secondary hyperparathyroidism associated with an enormously enlarged mass of parathyroid tissue. Because of the inordinate number of secreting cells, large amounts of PTH enter the circulation despite the fact that each individual cell may respond normally to an elevation in serum calcium concentration by reducing the secretion of PTH from each cell. This is also supported by experimental studies [77]. Some patients with primary hyperparathyroidism have very pronounced hypercalciuria despite a very mild degree of hypercalcemia and minimal or no bone disease [78]. In patients with primary hyperparathyroidism, a very strong positive correlation was found between $1,25(OH)_2D_3$ in the serum and the urinary calcium excretion. Patients with nephrolithiasis and hypercalciuria had circulating levels of $1,25(OH)_2D_3$ higher than those present in hyperparathyroid patients without renal stones [79]. The reason for this difference in the $1,25(OH)_2D_3$ levels is unknown, but it stresses the importance of vitamin D metabolism in the clinical presentation of primary hyperparathyroidism.

The high incidence of parathyroid adenomas in association with various malignant neoplasms is not well understood but warrants consideration in every case in which a malignant tumor is accompanied by hypercalcemia [80].

Molecular biology provides the means to study the role of genomic aberrations as the underlying mechanism of primary hyperparathyroidism. In parathyroid adenomas, changes were reported to occur in the gene that encodes the PTH and that is located on chromosome 11 [81]. Likewise, alterations were identified in the X chromosome. The genomic abnormalities consist of loss of tumor-suppressor genes and/or overexpression of oncogenes on chromosome 11. Likewise inactivation of tumor-suppressor genes were found in the X chromosome. It is of interest that these genomic changes were found not only in patients with parathyroid adenoma but also in patients with parathyroid hyperplasia including hyperplasia secondary to chronic renal failure [82].

The familial occurrence of parathyroid adenomas with an autosomal dominant inheritance makes mandatory the biochemical screening of family members of patients with primary hyperparathyroidism. Establishing the diagnosis of familial hyperparathyroidism also may be important to the patient's surgeon, alerting him or her to the high incidence of hyperplasia and multiple adenomas in this group of patients. In some families, primary hyperparathyroidism also is associated with other endocrine tumors. The syndrome of hyperparathyroidism, medullary carcinoma of the thyroid with amyloid stroma, pheochromocytoma, and multiple neuromas is known as multiple endocrine neoplasia type II (MEN-II) or Sipple's syndrome. The syndrome described by Wermer consisted of hyperparathyroidism and tumors of the pituitary and of the pancreatic islet cells (MEN-I). Loss of alleles on chromosome 11 was described in patients with MEN-I [83].

Primary hyperparathyroidism can best be diagnosed by demonstrating persistent hypercalcemia with elevated serum PTH. Patients presenting with bone, renal, gastrointestinal, or neuromuscular symptoms are considered symptomatic and usually require surgery. Conversely, in asymptomatic patients, objective manifestations of primary hyperparathyroidism that are indications for surgery include markedly elevated serum calcium concentration, a previous episode of life-threatening hypercalcemia, a reduced creatinine clearance, presence of kidney stones, hypercalciuria, and substantially reduced bone density [84]. Imaging of the parathyroid glands before an initial neck exploration is not necessary. In contrast, operative exploration of the neck by experienced surgeons has a proved success rate of 95 percent [84].

Familial hypocalciuric hypercalcemia is an unusual form of parathyroid hyperplasia with autosomal dominant transmission. There is a high incidence of neonatal primary hyperparathyroidism among the offspring of the affected families. The clinical course is relatively benign with an absence of nephrolithiasis and an infrequent occurrence of pancreatitis and chondrocalcinosis. Mild parathyroid hyperplasia with modestly elevated levels of circulating PTH and increased urinary excretion of cyclic AMP have been reported in these patients. The unsatisfactory response to subtotal parathyroidectomy, however, suggests additional underlying abnormalities. The presence of hypocalciuria both before and after subtotal parathyroidectomy provides a strong argument that enhanced tubular reabsorption of calcium plays an important role in maintaining hypercalcemia. Hypermagnesemia, which appears to reflect increased tubular reabsorption of magnesium, is another unique feature of this hypercalcemic disorder. It has been proposed that a concurrence of defects in both the parathyroid glands and the kidneys in their response to serum calcium concentration is an explanation for this disorder [85].

Recent studies demonstrated that inactivating mutations in the human calcium-sensing receptor gene cause both familial hypocalciuric hypercalcemia (FHH) and neonatal severe hyperparathyroidism. The calcium-sensing receptor gene has been mapped to chromosome 3, the same chromosome to which the FHH disease locus was localized in the past. In most families with FHH, linkage to chromosome 3g predominates, although in one family linkage to chromosome 19f was demonstrated. Thus the disease exhibits genetic heterogeneity. Inheritance of a single copy of mutated gene causes FHH, whereas homozygous patients who inherit two inactive genes develop neonatal severe hyperparathyroidism. The latter is associated with severe hypercalcemia due to parathyroid hyperplasia that usually requires surgery. These mutations lead to a defective calcium-sensing receptor with a presumable impairment of signal transduction function possibly due to abnormal coupling with G protein. This in turn appears to lead to abnormally reduced parathyroid and renal responsiveness to changes in extracellular calcium, resulting in increased PTH secretion and avid tubular reabsorption of calcium. Thus the calcium-sensing receptor plays an important role in calcium-regulated secretion of PTH and in tubular reabsorption of calcium. The FHH-associated excessive reabsorption of calcium, probably in the thick ascending limb, that persists even after parathyroidectomy suggests that this abnormality is PTH independent [13, 86].

Malignancy Associated with Hypercalcemia

A malignant neoplasm is the single most common cause of hypercalcemia. Hypercalcemia is most commonly produced by tumors of lung, breast, kidney, and ovary and by hematologic malignancies. Very often the hypercalcemia is uncontrollable and thus is a harbinger of the patient's demise. Indeed, survival after the appearance of hypercalcemia is very poor, with a median of 3 months. Two main mechanisms are known to mediate the hypercalcemia of malignancy: local and humoral. The local mechanism is manifested by the presence of osteolytic lesions in the skeleton. The malignant cells may act to destroy the bone directly; however, even local osteolysis in most instances is mediated by activated osteoclasts. Many tumors may produce hypercalcemia by a dual mechanism, that is, both local and humoral. It has become apparent that humoral hypercalcemia of malignancy (HHM) is caused by a circulating factor that is secreted by the neoplasm [87]. This circulating substance acts on the bone to induce osteoclastic resorption and on the kidney to reduce phosphate reabsorption, to increase calcium reabsorption and to increase nephrogenous cyclic AMP excretion. All of these biochemical effects are characteristic of the actions of native PTH. However, only in two patients, one with small cell carcinoma of lung and the second with ovarian carcinoma, was the ectopic secretion of PTH demonstrated [88, 89]. In the vast majority of patients with HHM, the circulating factor was identified as PTHrP. PTHrP is a 141 amino acid protein that binds to the receptors common to the native PTH, but it is encoded by a distinct gene. Even though PTHrP shares structural homology of amino-terminal residues with PTH, immunoradiometric assay of PTH has been able to distinguish completely between patients with HHM and those with primary hyperparathyroidism [90, 91]. Thus hypercalcemia with absence of detectable PTH by radioimmunoassay and the presence of high urinary cyclic AMP supports the diagnosis of HHM. PTHrP was originally isolated from human malignant tumors associated with HHM. Subsequently, it was detected to be present in a variety of tissues including parathyroid adenoma, skin, breast, placenta, testis, pancreas, and brain [91]. With regard to the presence of PTHrP in parathyroid tissue, it has been suggested that PTH is produced by the chief cells (major component of parathyroid tissue), whereas PTHrP is produced by the oxyphil cells [91]. Accordingly, the detection of PTHrP in circulation per se does not rule out parathyroid adenoma. Rather, the absence of PTH and the presence of PTHrP by radioimmunoassays in fact rule out parathyroid adenoma and support the diagnosis of HHM.

In vitro PTHrP, similarly to native PTH, has been shown not only to stimulate renal adenylate cyclase and to increase the formation of cyclic AMP but also to activate the 1α-hydroxylase and to enhance the formation of $1,25(OH)_2D_3$. In vivo, however, contrary to patients with primary hyperparathyroidism who may have high levels of serum $1,25(OH)_2D_3$, patients with HHM have low serum levels of calcitriol. In this regard, it has been reported that certain solid neoplasms produce substances that may inhibit the activity of 1α-hydroxylase and suppress the formation of $1,25(OH)_2D_3$. This appears to be the most tenable explanation for the low calcitriol levels in patients with HHM [92].

Another interesting feature that distinguishes between patients with primary hyperparathyroidism and those with HHM are the findings of bone histomorphometry. Whereas in patients with primary hyperparathyroidism bone resorption is closely matched with bone formation, in patients with HHM bone resorption and formation are uncoupled; specifically in HHM, enhancement of bone resorption and suppression of bone formation occur. The cause of this discrepancy is not readily apparent. Additional studies will be necessary to determine whether malignancies produce factors that suppress bone formation [93].

High PTHrP levels are present in 80 percent of patients with bone metastases from breast cancer who present with hypercalcemia, whereas PTHrP was present only in 12 percent of patients with breast cancer and metastases at sites other than bone. These findings are consistent with the notion that PTHrP may promote the development and growth of metastases in the bones by its potent osteolytic activity, which provides the environment for the proliferation of malignant cells [94].

Hypercalcemia is a recognized complication of lymphoma including both Hodgkin's and non-Hodgkin's types. In many patients with lymphoma-associated hypercalcemia, serum levels of $1,25(OH)_2D_3$ are either elevated or inadequately suppressed by the hypercalcemia. The elevated $1,25(OH)_2D_3$ levels may play a role in the pathogenesis of hypercalcemia. In some cases, chemotherapy induced normalization of serum calcium and a concomitant fall in $1,25(OH)_2D_3$. Conversely, reappearance of hypercalcemia was associated with recurrent rise above normal of $1,25(OH)_2D_3$ levels. Human T-lymphotrophic virus-transformed lymphocytes are able to produce $1,25(OH)_2D_3$ from $25(OH)D_3$. Thus there is a possibility that in some cases of lymphoma, the malignant cells may have a similar capacity to produce $1,25(OH)_2D_3$, which may contribute to the development of hypercalcemia. It is, however, noteworthy that in a number of patients with lymphoma-associated hypercalcemia, the levels of PTHrP were elevated and were considered to be responsible for the rise in serum calcium. Obviously, both PTHrP and elevated $1,25(OH)_2D_3$ may act synergistically to cause hypercalcemia [92].

Hypercalcemia of Malignancy: The Role of Osteoclast-Activating Cytokines

Tumor cells in bone and tumor-associated macrophages release factors that are known as osteoclast-activating cytokines. These tumor-derived factors, implicated in the development of hypercalcemia of malignancy, are interleukin-1 (IL-1), interleukin-6 (IL-6), tumor necrosis factor-α (cachectin), tumor necrosis factor-β (lymphotoxin), transforming growth factor-α and arachidonic acid metabolites. In addition, tumor cells may produce mediators such as granulocyte-macrophage colony-stimulating factor that induce immune cells to produce tumor necrosis factor and IL-1. Cytokines are produced and act locally as osteolytic factors. In most instances, the osteoclast-stimulating activity of the cytokines requires the presence of osteoblastic cells. In animals, intravenous infusion of cytokines causes hypercalcemia; however, in clinical circumstances, these factors are believed to act locally in a paracrine fashion [94–97].

Hypercalcemia occurs in approximately one-third of patients with myeloma. Osteolytic bone lesions are the most common skeletal radiographic findings. The bone destruction in myeloma is mediated by osteoclasts that accumulate adjacent to the collections of myeloma cells. This association of myeloma cells with osteoclasts is most likely related to the osteoclast-activating effect of cytokines that are locally secreted by the malignant cells. Myeloma cells produce in vitro several osteoclast-activating factors, including lymphotoxin, IL-1, and IL-6. The increase in bone resorption in most cases is associated with a suppressed osteoblastic bone-forming activity. This explains the depressed skeletal uptake of bone-seeking radiolabeled elements in myeloma, resulting in negative bone scans in the vast majority of the affected patients. Myeloma cells exhibit a unique capability to grow rapidly in the bone. Myeloma cells secrete osteoclast-mobilizing and stimulating cytokines, whereas osteoclasts secrete IL-6, which is a major growth factor of the myeloma cells. This relationship between myeloma cells and osteoclasts explains the rapid destruction of bone in this malignancy [94–97].

Vitamin D Intoxication and Hypercalcemia

All patients receiving vitamin D, other than in small doses, for the treatment of hypoparathyroidism may develop hypercalcemia, with the attendant risk of renal failure. The appearance of hypercalcemia in hypoparathyroid patients receiving pharmacologic doses of either ergocalciferol (vitamin D_2) or DHT_3 is almost unpredictable, since the margin between normocalcemic and hypercalcemic doses of the vitamin is very narrow. Some episodes of hypercalcemia may pass unnoticed and yet may be the underlying cause of reduced renal function in these patients. The administration of thiazide diuretics also may be an aggravating factor in this situation, partly because it reduces the urinary excretion of calcium. The hypercalcemia associated with vitamin D intoxication may be present from 1 to 6 weeks after discontinuation of the treatment, and the normocalcemia may persist for an additional 4 months without any treatment. The toxic effect of vitamin D excess is associated with a high circulating level of $25(OH)D_3$, which is continuously produced by the liver from the adipose tissue stores of vitamin D. The serum level of $1,25(OH)_2D_3$ is generally not elevated and even may be reduced [98]. The hypercalcemia associated with $1,25(OH)_2D_3$ administration is, however, much more short-lived (3–7 days) [99].

Various factors may alter the response to vitamin D. After menopause, the inhibitory effect of estrogens on bone resorption may be absent, which would allow more calcium to be released from the bone for any given dose of vitamin D. The administration of corticosteroids may reduce the effect of vitamin D; in fact, corticosteroids may be used to treat vitamin D intoxication. The most important precaution in preventing the complications of vitamin D intoxication is to measure serum calcium concentrations frequently in these patients.

Vitamin A Intoxication and Hypercalcemia

Hypercalcemia associated with vitamin A intoxication has been much discussed [100, 101]. This condition has been associated with excessive intake of vitamin A, which is readily available for sale in various pharmaceutic preparations [101]. Isotretinoin, a derivative of vitamin D that is effective in the treatment of severe nodulocystic acne, has been reported as a cause of hypercalcemia [102]. The main symptom of vitamin A intoxication is painful swelling over the extremities. Prolonged hypercalcemia in this condition also has been associated with nephrocalcinosis and impairment of renal function [100]. In experimental animals, excessive amounts of vitamin A cause fractures, increased number of osteoclasts, and calcification of soft tissues [103]. In human subjects, periosteal bone deposition constitutes the typical radiographic feature [101].

Sarcoidosis and Hypercalcemia

Hypercalcemia in patients with sarcoidosis is associated with increased intestinal absorption of calcium and increased calcium release from the bone [104]; it is found in about 17 percent of all patients with sarcoidosis [105]. It is more frequent in males than in females [105]. In a small proportion of patients, very high serum calcium concentration leads to metastatic calcifications and eventual death due to uremia [105]. With the appearance of uremia, the hypercalcemia may disappear [106].

Seasonal incidence of hypercalcemia in sarcoidosis is directly related to the amount of sunlight exposure [107]. Plasma levels of $1,25(OH)_2D_3$ have been found to be increased in patients with sarcoidosis and hypercalcemia, a finding that accounts for the abnormal calcium metabolism in this disease [108]. In most of the patients, hypercalcemia may be corrected with the administration of glucocorticoids, which restores to normal both the elevated calcium and $1,25(OH)_2D_3$ concentrations in the serum [109]. Serum immunoreactive PTH has been found to be low in patients with sarcoidosis, regardless of the presence or absence of hypercalcemia.

In vitro studies demonstrated production of $1,25(OH)D_3$ by primary cultures of pulmonary alveolar macrophages harvested from patients with active sarcoidosis [110]. Thus the pathogenesis of hypercalcemia in sarcoidosis is extrarenal production of $1,25(OH)_2D_3$ by the macrophage, which is a major constituent of the sarcoid granuloma. A similar mechanism appears to be responsible for the hypercalcemia associated with other granulomatous diseases. Hypercalcemia has been reported in tuberculosis, leprosy, foreign body–induced granuloma, silicone-induced granuloma, disseminated candidiasis and coccidioidomycosis, histoplasmosis, berylliosis, granulomatous lipoid pneumonia, and eosinophilic granuloma [109, 110].

Hyperthyroidism, Hypothyroidism, and Hypercalcemia

The incidence of hypercalcemia in patients with hyperthyroidism varies from 10 to 22 percent in different reports [111]. This hypercalcemia may be reversed by antithyroid therapy [111]. Since the association of hyperthyroidism and hyperparathyroidism has been reported to be common, the therapeutic response of the hypercalcemia to the antithyroid therapy may be of some diagnostic significance [111]. The effect of thyroid hormone on calcium metabolism primarily consists of increased bone turnover, increased urinary calcium excretion, and decreased intestinal absorption of calcium, with a resultant negative calcium balance [112]. The action of thyroid hormone on bone is thus primarily responsible for the hypercalcemia. Thyroid hormone enhances the ability of PTH to increase bone reabsorption and also itself directly enhances bone reabsorption in vivo in the absence of PTH [113]. Serum phosphate may be elevated in hyperthyroidism, possibly due to suppression of parathyroid activity by the hypercalcemia and subsequent enhanced tubular reabsorption of phosphate.

In the vast majority of patients with hypothyroidism, serum calcium and phosphate levels are normal and alkaline phosphatase is low. Some patients, however, may manifest hypercalcemia. Calcium balance in patients with hypothyroidism tends to be positive as a result of increased intestinal absorption and reduced urinary excretion. Both changes predispose to the development of hypercalcemia. The bone turnover in hypothyroid patients is reduced.

Adrenal Insufficiency and Hypercalcemia

Hypercalcemia is a common abnormality in adrenal insufficiency [114, 115]. The mechanism of hypercalcemia in this clinical setting is not well understood. One study indicates that the increase in serum calcium concentration is due to an increase in the protein-bound fraction of serum calcium that results from accompanying volume depletion. The volume depletion also may cause an increase in the renal tubular reabsorption of calcium, and vitamin D's enhancement of calcium absorption from the intestine may be greater in the absence of glucocorticoid hormone.

Idiopathic Infantile Hypercalcemia

Idiopathic infantile hypercalcemia encompasses a group of disorders characterized by hypercalcemia during infancy, mostly of transient nature. According to the gravity of the clinical manifestation, it can be divided into benign and severe types. The benign type is associated with minimal symptomatology and has an excellent prognosis. The severe form is associated with serious somatic sequelae including mental deficiency, "elfin" face with depressed nasal bridge, epicanthal folds, supravalvular aortic stenosis, bladder diverticula, degenerative renal disease, occasionally pulmonic stenosis, ventricular septal defects, and dental abnormalities. These somatic distortions, which are known as Williams syndrome, are believed to reflect developmental defects resulting from hypercalcemia, probably already present in the fetal stage. The hypercalcemia is of limited duration; however, the somatic abnormalities are permanent. Thus many patients suffering from Williams syndrome who present with the clinical syndrome fail to show abnormalities in calcium metabolism.

Idiopathic infantile hypercalcemia has been attributed to hypersensitivity to vitamin D. In support of this possibility is the finding that hypercalcemia in this syndrome may occur with small doses of vitamin D, which are only two to three times larger than the physiologic dose [116]. The high incidence of this syndrome in a group of infants in England who were drinking milk fortified with excessive amounts of vitamin D, and its disappearance when vitamin D was eliminated from the diet, supported the possibility that the syndrome was due to hypersensitivity to vitamin D [117].

There is, however, no unifying pathogenesis underlying the abnormal calcium metabolism in idiopathic infantile hypercalcemia. Increased serum levels of $1,25(OH)_2D_3$ have been considered to be the mechanism of hypercalcemia by some investigators [118]. Others, however, have failed to show that abnormality even in the presence of hypercalcemia. Abnormalities in the regulation of calcitonin secretion with reduced stimulation by hypercalcemia were advanced as the possible mechanism by others.

A peculiar variant of the disease is hypercalcemia with fat necrosis. In this syndrome affecting infants, only hypercalcemia occurs, with areas of sclerosis of subcutaneous fat tissue [118]. In some cases, high levels of $1,25(OH)_2D_3$ were reported. Some investigators maintain that hypercalcemia is not a primary but rather a secondary phenomenon. In the latter instance, it has been proposed that the rise in $1,25(OH)_2D_3$ leading to hypercalcemia is secondary to the granulomatous inflammation of the fat necrosis. Irrespective of the mechanism, idiopathic infantile hypercalcemia is treated by dietary restriction of calcium and vitamin D.

Immobilization and Hypercalcemia

Immobilization may be associated with excessive loss of bone minerals, hypercalcemia, and rapidly developing osteoporosis. The lack of postural mechanical stimuli to the skeleton disturbs the balance between bone formation and reabsorption, thus leading to loss of bone mass and its minerals. Usually, the amount of calcium released from the bone is excreted in the urine and does not increase the serum calcium concentration [119]. However, in states of rapid bone turnover, which are present in normal children and adolescents and in patients with bone abnormalities such as Paget's disease, immobilization may result in overt hypercalcemia [119].

Hypophosphatasia

Hypophosphatasia is a syndrome characterized by low serum alkaline phosphatase, high serum levels of pyrophosphate, and skeletal abnormalities resembling osteomalacia [120]. The disorder may be associated with hypercalcemia, especially in infants.

Milk-Alkali Syndrome

Milk-alkali syndrome may occur in patients who ingest large amounts of milk and alkali as a therapy to relieve the symptoms of peptic ulcers. The syndrome is characterized by hypercalcemia, hyperphosphatemia, alkalosis, metastatic calcifications, and progressive renal failure. It has been shown that these abnormalities may be reversed by discontinuation of the therapy. Large doses of calcium carbonate seem to be the major factor in the development of this syndrome, since the use of antacids other than calcium carbonate do not lead to hypercalcemia [121]. It therefore appears that the hypercalcemia of milk-alkali syndrome results from high oral loads of calcium carbonate and causes renal retention of phosphate by suppressing PTH secretion. The resulting serum calcium-phosphorus product leads to metastatic calcification and impairment of renal function. Increased oral intake of calcium carbonate also has been reported to induce hypercalcemia in uremic patients. Similarly, the use of calcium-containing exchange resins for the treatment of hyperkalemia may cause hypercalcemia because of the release of calcium from the resin in the intestinal lumen [122]. Hypercalcemia has been described in patients recovering from acute renal failure. The etiology is not well understood, but in some patients it may be due to the combination of secondary hyperparathyroidism and released calcium from traumatized, necrotic muscle [123–125] and to high calcitriol levels produced by the traumatized muscles.

Thiazide Diuretics and Hypercalcemia

Chronic administration of thiazide diuretics may lead to hypercalcemia in patients treated with large doses of vitamin D (hypoparathyroid patients and patients with osteoporosis) and in patients with hyperparathyroidism. The mechanism of action may involve both (1) reduced urinary excretion of calcium due to a direct tubular effect, or ECF depletion with secondary increase in tubular reabsorption of sodium and calcium, or both, and (2) increased bone responsiveness to the resorptive actions of vitamin D and PTH [126, 127]. It has been demonstrated that thiazides may acutely enhance the skeletal response to PTH in the absence of changes in ECF volume, but there is no evidence for such an effect in hypoparathyroid patients receiving large doses of vitamin D [127].

Patients treated chronically with lithium may develop hypercalcemia with elevated PTH levels. Theophylline toxicity may also be associated with hypercalcemia, probably due to stimulation of β-receptors in the bone.

Treatment of Hypercalcemia

Lowering of serum calcium concentration can be produced by (1) inhibiting calcium release from the bone, or increasing its deposition in the bone and other tissues, or both; (2) increasing removal of calcium from the ECF or inhibiting its absorption in the bowel; and (3) decreasing the ionized fraction by complex formation with chelating substances.

Hypercalcemia augments urinary losses of sodium and water, resulting in the contraction of extracellular volume and reduced GFR. The latter leads to diminished urinary excretion of calcium and to further aggravation of hypercalcemia. Therefore, the first therapeutic goal is to restore the extracellular volume to normal by intravenous administration of normal saline. This usually requires 3 to 4 liters of saline. This therapeutic action per se will lower the serum calcium concentration, partly by the dilutional effect and partly by increased urinary excretion of calcium. During a rapid intravenous administration of saline, there is a risk of extracellular volume overload, which is particularly hazardous in elderly patients. Therefore, monitoring of central venous pressure in this situation may be very helpful. Likewise, the addition of loop diuretics as an adjunct therapy not only may minimize the risk of fluid overload but also may substantially increase the urinary excretion of calcium. The effect of loop diuretics as calciuretic agents requires prompt replacement of urinary losses of sodium and water. The use of loop diuretics may be particularly beneficial in patients who develop hypercalcemia as a result of excessive secretion and high serum levels of PTH, PTHrP, or both. In these circumstances, hormone-induced, excessive tubular reabsorption of calcium plays a major role in the development and maintenance of hypercalcemia [109].

Biphosphonates

Biphosphonates (formerly diphosphonates) represent a group of drugs with a high therapeutic potential for the treatment of hypercalcemia in general and that associated with malignancy in particular. Biphosphonates are related to an endogenous product of bone metabolism, pyrophosphate. The P—O—P bonds of pyrophosphate are cleaved by phosphatase in the process of bone mineralization and in the process of osteoclastic bone resorption. In the biphosphonates, carbon replaces the oxygen moiety, generating a bond P—C—P, which is resistant to hydrolysis by phosphatase. Biphosphonates have a great affinity for bone and bind tightly to calcified bone matrix, impairing both the mineralization and resorption of bone. In addition they interfere with the function of osteoclasts. They appear to have several direct effects on the osteoclast function, including prevention of osteoclast attachment to bone matrix and prevention of osteoclast differentiation and recruitment. Biphosphonates also inhibit the motility of isolated osteoclasts. Thus, they are very potent inhibitors of bone resorption. The first biphosphonate, ethane-hydroxybiphosphonate (etidronate [Didronel]) is now available for clinical use, but its potency as an antihypercalcemic is limited, at least when given orally. This is probably because its effect to reduce bone resorption is offset by its effect to inhibit bone mineralization. Reduction of serum calcium concentration has been achieved more successfully with the second generation of biphosphonates, including dichloromethylene biphosphonate (clodronate) and amino-hydroxypropylidene biphosphonate (pamidronate [ADP]), which causes a reduction in bone resorption with a dose that has a negligible effect on bone mineralization. Pamidronate and etidronate are currently approved for treatment of hypercalcemia of malignancy in the United States. In clinical trials, pamidronate and clodronate have been demonstrated to inhibit hypercalcemia, bone pain, and pathologic fractures in patients with malignancy-associated hypercalcemia. Pamidronate is most effective when given intravenously; a single infusion of 30 mg achieved normocalcemia in 90 percent of patients in one study. When compared, the effect of 30 mg of pamidronate is equal to 600 mg of clodronate and to 1500 mg of etidronate in controlling hypercalcemia. The third generation of biphosphonates, including alendronate, risedronate, and tiludronate, in preliminary studies is 500 times more efficient in inhibiting bone resorption than clodronate. Even though these compounds are more promising, not all are yet available for clinical use [97, 109].

Glucocorticoids

Glucocorticoids are effective in lowering serum calcium in states of vitamin D intoxication, sarcoidosis, and malignancy. The exact mode of their action is not well understood, but the possible mechanisms are suppression of bone resorption and decreased intestinal absorption. It has been pointed out that glucocorticoids are more effective in hypercalcemia associated with lymphoma, leukemia, and multiple myeloma than with other neoplasms. This effect of glucocorticoids might be related to a tumorlytic effect, to interference with the production of osteoclast-activating cytokines, or to both. The average effective dose is 3 to 4 mg/kg/day of hydrocortisone given intravenously or orally. The fall in serum calcium concentration occurs 1 to 2 days after starting the therapy [109].

Calcitonin

Calcitonin lowers serum calcium concentration by inhibiting bone resorption and by increasing urinary calcium excretion. The administration of calcitonin is associated with negligible toxicity; however, its therapeutic action has a limited duration because of the osteoclast escape phenomenon, which is apparent several days after starting therapy. Addition of glucocorticoids may be helpful to maintain efficacy.

Mithramycin (Plicamycin)

Mithramycin is a cytotoxic substance derived from an actinomycate of the genus *Streptomyces* and is used mainly in the treatment of testicular tumors. Mithramycin lowers serum calcium concentration by suppressing bone resorption. The dose, which is lower than the antitumor dose and has fewer side effects, is 25 μg/kg, given intravenously. The drug is available commercially as Mithracin. The effect starts 24 to 48 hours after injection and lasts several days. Side effects are suppression of bone marrow activity and hepatocellular and renal toxicity, which usually occur with repeated doses.

Phosphate

Oral and intravenous salts of phosphorus lower serum concentration and reduce urinary excretion of calcium. This effect has been variously attributed to (1) deposition of mineral in the bone, (2) increased deposition of calcium in soft tissues, and (3) suppression of bone resorption. The major untoward side effects of this therapy are extraskeletal calcifications, including nephrocalcinosis with resulting renal failure. Thus, the use of phosphates to treat hypercalcemia should be discouraged in patients with high serum phosphates and renal insufficiency. Phosphates may be given intravenously at a dose of 20 to 30 mg of elemental phosphorus per kilogram of body weight over 12 to 16 hours. Serum calcium concentration should be determined at close intervals. The commercially available preparation for intravenous use is InPhos; 40 ml of the solution contains 1000 mg of phosphorus, 65 mEq of sodium, and 8 mEq of potassium.

Other Therapies

Gallium nitrate has been approved by the Food and Drug Administration for therapy of hypercalcemia. It inhibits bone resorption by reducing the solubility of hydroxyapatite crystals. A major side effect of gallium nitrate is nephrotoxicity. The use of a somatostatin congener (lanreotide) has been reported to successfully inhibit hypercalcemia in a patient with a PTHrP-secreting pancreatic neoplasm. The calcium-lowering effect was associated with suppression of the serum levels of PTHrP [128].

The hypercalcemia associated with thyrotoxicosis and theophylline toxicity has been successfully treated with intravenous propranolol.

Intestinal absorption of calcium may be reduced by dietary restrictions and binding of calcium in the bowel with cellulose phosphate and sodium phytate to form nonabsorbable complexes.

Calcium also may be removed directly from the ECF with hemodialysis or peritoneal dialysis by employing calcium-free dialysate solution.

Reduction of serum ionized calcium may be accomplished with intravenous Na-EDTA, which is a chelating agent. The complexed calcium then is excreted in the urine. The main disadvantage of this therapy is the nephrotoxicity of EDTA.

Metabolic Bone Diseases

Rickets and Osteomalacia

Rickets and osteomalacia are metabolic disorders of the bone in which the mineralization process of the epiphyseal cartilage and organic bone matrix is impaired. This abnormality results in a decreased amount of mineralized bone (Fig. 6-6) and an increased amount of osteoid (or cartilage), which cause decreased mechanical strength of the bones. The bones therefore become soft, bend easily, and are liable to deformities and pseudofractures (Fig. 6-7). It should be mentioned that such an increase in the width of osteoid seams may be seen in conditions other than osteomalacia. With Paget's disease, the bone formation is rapid, and there may be a lag between the rate of apposition of bone matrix and its mineralization. This sequence therefore will lead to an increased width of osteoid seams. Histologically, however, the presence of a calcification front in bones from patients with Paget's disease and its absence in osteomalacia allow the distinction between these diseases. The calcification front may be demonstrated by specific histochemical staining techniques or by the administration of a tetracycline, which is incorporated specifically in the calcification front. During the healing of osteomalacia, the calcification front reappears.

The major symptoms of osteomalacia are diffuse bone and muscle pains, which cause disability and increasing needs for analgesic medication. The etiology of osteo-

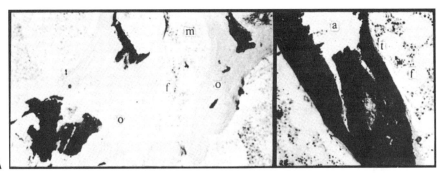

Fig. 6-6. (A) Osteomalacia. Bone trabeculae are calcified (*black stain*) only in the center, with a wide rim of osteoid tissue. (B) Normal bone. All bone trabeculae are calcified (*black stain*). a = artifact; f = fat; m = marrow; o = osteoid; t = trabeculae.

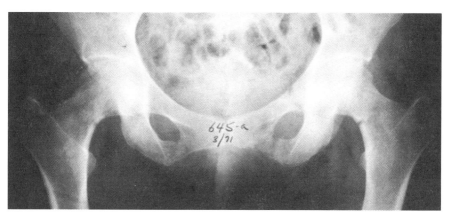

Fig. 6-7. Roentgenographic appearance of osteomalacia. The radiolucent lines on the necks of both femurs are pseudofractures.

malacia (Table 6-5) can be divided into two principal subgroups. The first group, which is the most common, is associated with abnormally low serum concentrations of phosphorus and calcium. In the second group, which is less common, the defect in mineralization is related in some way to abnormalities in the organic matrix and is not associated with a low serum calcium-phosphorus product.

Vitamin D deficiency causes osteomalacia primarily by decreasing the absorption of calcium and phosphorus from the intestine and thereby decreasing the serum concentrations of calcium and phosphorus. As previously mentioned, osteomalacia caused by vitamin D deficiency may be healed with the intravenous administration of calcium and phosphorus even without repletion of vitamin D [29]. It should be emphasized, however, that this finding does not exclude the possibility that vitamin D plays a direct role in the physiologic process of bone accretion. As already dis-

Table 6-5. Causes of rickets and osteomalacia

Group I: Low serum calcium-phosphorus product
   Vitamin D deficiency
   Vitamin D–dependent rickets, type I (1α-hydroxylase deficiency)
   Vitamin D–dependent rickets, type II (vitamin D resistance)
   Hypophosphatemia
      X-linked hypophosphatemic vitamin D–resistant rickets
      Hereditary hypophosphatemic rickets with hypercalciuria
      Fanconi's syndrome
      Oncogenic osteomalacia
      Excessive intake of phosphate-binding antacids
      Hypophosphatemic nonrachitic bone disease
   Renal tubular acidosis
Group II: Normal or high serum calcium-phosphorus product
   Renal osteomalacia
   Hypophosphatasia

cussed, vitamin D deficiency may result from either poor intake, decreased intestinal absorption, or lack of exposure to ultraviolet light.

Vitamin D–dependent rickets is an autosomal recessive disease featuring hypocalcemia and hypophosphatemia. It responds to vitamin D in pharmacologic doses only but does respond to physiologic doses of $1,25(OH)_2D_3$. On the basis of this observation, it has been proposed that the disorder is due to an enzymatic defect in the renal conversion of $25(OH)_2D_3$ into $1,25(OH)_2D_3$, which is the active form of vitamin D. In addition, hypocalcemia and rickets refractory to $1,25(OH)_2D_3$ were described as type II vitamin D–dependent rickets, also known as hereditary $1,25(OH)_2D_3$–resistant rickets. This familial disorder is inherited by autosomal recessive transmission and is characterized by rickets, impaired intestinal absorption of calcium, hypocalcemia, and alopecia, which may reflect a defect in the physiologic action of $1,25(OH)_2D_3$ in the skin. In contrast to vitamin D–dependent rickets type II, in type II serum $1,25(OH)_2D_3$ is elevated and the patients either respond to pharmacologic doses of $1,25(OH)_2D_3$ or do not respond at all. In some patients with this disorder, abnormal nuclear uptake, abnormal cystosol receptor binding of $1,25\text{-}(OH)_2D_3$, or both are present. These findings suggest that the mechanism of the end-organ resistance is a defect in the receptor. In other patients, however, this abnormality was not present, indicating a more distal postreceptor abnormality. In this regard, in one patient with type II vitamin D–dependent rickets with normal receptor function (receptor-positive resistance), failure of $1,25(OH)_2D_3$ to stimulate the enzyme $25(OH)_2D_3$–24-hydroxylase was demonstrated [129]. In normal people, $1,25(OH)_2D_3$ was shown to stimulate the formation of $24,25(OH)_2D_3$. The latter may represent a step in the physiologic action of $1,25(OH)_2D_3$ that is lacking in some patients with type II vitamin D–dependent rickets [130, 131]. Mutations of vitamin D–receptor genes have been identified in families with this abnormality. In one family, a nonsense mutation coding for a premature stop codon in exon 7 of the gene encoding vitamin D receptor was identified. In other families, the genetic abnormality consisted of a point mutation within the steroid binding domain of the vitamin D–receptor gene [132].

Hypophosphatemia due to excessive external losses of phosphorus may cause osteomalacia even in the presence of normal serum calcium concentration. Hypophosphatemic vitamin D–resistant rickets is a sex-linked dominant disorder in which both renal tubular and intestinal defects in phosphate reabsorption have been demonstrated [133, 134]. It has been proposed earlier that the initial abnormality in vitamin D–resistant rickets is a reduced gastrointestinal absorption of calcium that leads to parathyroid hyperactivity with increased renal losses of phosphorus. The question remains unresolved, since evaluation of parathyroid activity in these patients has been a subject of conflicting reports, indicating both high and normal levels of immunoreactive PTH. Thus at present there is no conclusive evidence available as to the exact mechanism of this disorder. Serum $1,25(OH)_2D_3$ levels in patients with vitamin D–resistant rickets are in the low normal or slightly below normal range. Because hypophosphatemia is expected to stimulate 1α-hydroxylase activity in the kidney, these relatively low values suggest that in addition to a defect in tubular phosphate absorption, the response of 1α-hydroxylase to low levels of serum phosphate is also impaired in hypophosphatemic vitamin D–resistant rickets. Hypophosphatemic vitamin D–resistant rickets occasionally may respond to treatment with large doses of oral phosphate as well as to pharmacologic doses of vitamin D.

The combined administration of oral phosphate supplements with $1,25(OH)_2D_3$ is better than the administration of either one alone for the cure of the bone disease. In hypophosphatemic mice, the animal model of the disease, the administration of phosphate cures the rickets but not the osteomalacia. The combined administration of phosphate supplements and $1,25(OH)_2D_3$ is necessary to achieve improvement of the osteomalacia as well [135]. Whether a similar therapeutic response applies to the human disease is unknown.

The presence of a tumor may be responsible for excessive urinary loss of phosphate and hypophosphatemic vitamin D–resistant rickets. The tumors that have been identified most frequently consist of mesenchymal and giant cells and are present in bones. In many patients, excision of the tumor has been associated with reversal of the tubular leak of phosphate and cure of the bone disease [136]. It has been proposed that the syndrome is the result of a release of phosphaturic substance by the tumor. Indeed, tumor extracts elicited phosphaturic cyclic AMP–independent effects when injected into animals [137, 138]. Likewise, in vitro, tumor extracts inhibited sodium-phosphate coupled uptake using opossum kidney cells [139].

Cai et al. [139] have recently performed studies on the biochemical properties of such a factor released by a tumor associated with oncogenic osteomalacia. This factor, now called "phosphatonin," is heat labile and has a molecular weight of between 8000 and 25,000 daltons. It inhibits sodium-dependent phosphate transport in cultured renal epithelia, without inhibiting sodium-dependent glucose or sodium-dependent amino acid transport. Unlike PTH, it does not cause an increase in the accumulation of cyclic AMP in renal cells, and its activity is not blocked by a PTH antagonist. This suggests that the factor is distinct from PTH.

Hypophosphatemic nonrachitic bone disease is an entity that resembles X-linked hypophosphatemia but is clinically less severe with regard to bone disease and gives no clear evidence of X-linked inheritance [140].

An additional form of hereditary hypophosphatemic rickets is the entity known as hereditary rickets with hypercalciuria. It differs from the classic form by presenting with high levels of $1,25(OH)_2D_3$ and hypercalciuria [141]. In this form, muscle weakness is the major clinical feature. Vitamin D metabolism appears to be normal, as reflected by an increased $1,25(OH)_2D_3$ in response to phosphate depletion.

Even though calcium deficiency per se has not been recognized as a cause of osteomalacia in humans, several reports suggest that this abnormality may cause rickets in babies and in children [142, 143]. It is possible that in these circumstances calcium deficiency–induced secondary hyperparathyroidism may lead to vitamin D deficiency. High circulating PTH levels stimulate renal 1α-hydroxylase, resulting in high $1,25(OH)_2D_3$ levels. Thus the proposed mechanism of this abnormality is increased breakdown of $25(OH)_2D_3$ by high levels of $1,25(OH)_2D_3$, causing a state of vitamin D deficiency [56].

Fanconi's syndrome is associated with multiple defects in tubular transport. The phosphaturia and renal tubular acidosis associated with this syndrome may be primarily responsible for the occurrence of the hypophosphatemic rickets [144]. The exact cause of osteomalacia in patients with renal tubular acidosis is not entirely clear, however. In animals, acidosis per se leads to the development of osteoporosis rather than osteomalacia. It has been proposed that hypercalciuria associated with renal tubular acidosis lowers serum calcium and stimulates the secretion of PTH, which in turn causes excessive urinary losses of phosphorus, with hypophosphatemia and osteomalacia. An alternative explanation for the phosphaturia is that acidosis directly increases urinary excretion of phosphorus. Osteomalacia also has been reported in patients with systemic acidosis following ureterosigmoidostomy some years earlier [145]. In this latter situation, the acidosis occurs as a result of fecal bicarbonate losses. The fact that osteomalacia associated with renal tubular acidosis may be cured in some patients with the correction of the acidosis emphasizes the potential role of acidosis in this disorder [146]. Osteomalacia also has been reported in patients with phosphate depletion due to excessive intake of phosphate-binding antacids and excessive use of laxatives.

All previously discussed disorders causing osteomalacia share one common feature, namely a reduced serum calcium-phosphorus product, which may be responsible for the failure of bone matrix to mineralize. However, osteomalacia in chronic renal failure develops in the presence of a high serum calcium-phosphorus product. In these patients, the mineralization defect may be related to intrinsic abnormalities of the organic matrix, to a circulating inhibitor of mineralization, or to deficiency of a specific metabolite of vitamin D. Aluminum toxicity causes a mineralization defect in some patients with hemodialysis-associated osteomalacia [147]. In osteomalacia associated with hypophosphatasia, the high concentration of pyrophosphates may block bone mineralization despite the presence of normal or high concentrations of serum calcium and phosphorus. Osteomalacia may also develop in association with the administration of biphosphonates, which share common chemical properties with pyrophosphates.

Osteomalacia may evolve in patients receiving long-term total parenteral nutrition. In this disorder, normal or slightly elevated serum concentration of calcium and phosphate has been reported. In one study, osteomalacia developed during supplementation with vitamin D. Associated abnormalities included hypercalciuria, exceeding the amount of calcium intake, mildly elevated concentrations of serum calcium and serum $25(OH)D_3$, and low serum $1,25(OH)_2D_3$ and serum PTH concentrations. Elimination of vitamin D supplements from the formula of parenteral nutrition reversed the biochemical and hormonal abnormalities and led to recovery from the bone disease [148]. This sequence suggests that either vitamin D toxicity or hypersensitivity to vitamin D with consequent loss of mineral in the urine was responsible for osteomalacia. The observed suppression of PTH secretion could play a role in the reduced bone turnover and increased losses of calcium in the urine, which could not be replaced because of the absence of the intestinal supply of calcium. Other studies proposed that either low $1,25(OH)_2D_3$ or aluminum toxicity could be causally related to the observed osteomalacia [149, 150]. Thus, the total parenteral nutrition–induced osteomalacia remains a poorly understood entity.

Table 6-6. Clinical forms of osteoporosis

Generalized, primary	Generalized, secondary
Type I: Postmenopausal	Corticosteroid therapy
Type II: Senile	Cushing's syndrome
Type III: Idiopathic	Hyperthyroidism
Juvenile	Rheumatoid arthritis
Adult	Long-term heparin administration
In pregnancy	Alcoholism
Local	Anorexia nervosa
Transitory migrant osteoporosis	Hypogonadism
Fracture and immobilization	Malabsorption
Neurogenic immobilization	Acidosis
Transient osteoporosis of the hip in	Cirrhosis of liver
pregnancy	Vitamin C deficiency
	Lactation-associated osteoporosis
	Space travel

Osteoporosis

Normal bone remodeling is based on matching of bone resorption with bone forma-tion. In adults, each year 25 percent of trabecular bone is resorbed and replaced. The turnover rate of cortical bone is substantially slower. Under normal conditions, the bone renewal process proceeds in cycles of resorption followed by formation. The quantitative coupling between resorption and formation helps maintain normal bone mass. The hallmark of osteoporosis is loss of bone mass caused by imbalance between bone resorption and formation. Loss of gonadal function and aging are the two most important conditions leading to osteoporosis. The former is known as postmenopausal osteoporosis and the latter as senile osteoporosis.

Peak Bone Mass

Osteoporosis is characterized by low bone mass and disrupted bone architecture, which lead to reduced bone strength and increase the risk of fractures (Table 6-6). Prevention of low bone mass is therefore of prime importance. One of the means of reaching this goal is to increase the peak bone mass buildup during adolescence. Adolescence is a crucial time for the development of bone mass. Bone mass increases with age throughout childhood, and it reaches its peak by late adolescence and early adulthood. Bone mass accretion during puberty appears to be critical in the development of peak bone mass. Peak bone mass is regarded as a major determinant of osteoporosis in later life [151].

Under normal conditions, after attainment of peak bone mass, the bone mass remains stable. An exception to this rule is the appearance of pregnancy-associated osteoporosis. It consists of four variants: idiopathic osteoporosis of pregnancy, tran-sient osteoporosis of the hip in pregnancy, postpregnancy spinal osteoporosis, and lactation-associated osteoporosis. Whether these are truly independent conditions or whether they relate specifically to pregnancy remains to be determined. The most important feature of all types of pregnancy-associated osteoporosis is complete recovery without residual damage. Heparin-induced osteoporosis in pregnancy is also reversible after discontinuation of heparin [152].

Starting during the fourth to fifth decade of life, an annual loss of 0.3 to 0.5 percent of bone mass may occur. After menopause, the rate of bone loss may increase tenfold. Loss of bone mass following menopause is characterized by increased bone turnover, featuring both increased bone resorption and increased bone formation. The osteoclastic resorbing activity, however, exceeds the osteoblastic bone-forming activity, resulting in net loss of bone mass. By contrast, the osteoporosis associated with aging, senile osteoporosis, is characterized by low bone turnover [153]. The major feature of aging osteoporosis is reduced osteoblastic activity with reduced supply of osteoblasts. Thus, the amount of bone formed during each remodeling cycle is reduced, leading to a net decrease in bone mass. Additional differences between the postmenopausal and senile osteoporosis are that in the former mainly the trabecular bone is affected whereas in the latter cortical and trabecular bones are affected equally. Estrogen deficiency is the underlying mechanism of postmenopausal osteoporosis. The deficiency of estrogen creates an imbalance in bone metabolism with at least two known abnormalities. First, in the absence of estrogen, the resorptive effect of PTH is augmented, with no change in bone forming. Second, estrogen suppresses the production of IL-6 by osteoblastic cells. IL-6 is an osteoclast-activating cytokine [154]. Thus, excessive formation of IL-6 leads to excessive bone loss in postmenopausal osteoporosis [153]. Serum levels of PTH and calcitriol are low in patients with postmenopausal osteoporosis. PTH levels are increased and calcitriol levels reduced in senile osteoporosis. In both conditions, there is reduced intestinal calcium absorption. Estrogen therapy in postmenopausal osteoporosis leads to an increase in plasma calcitriol levels and improves intestinal absorption of calcium [153, 154].

Low bone turnover, which is characteristic of senile osteoporosis, is also present in other types of secondary osteoporosis, including steroid-induced osteoporosis, alcohol-induced osteoporosis, osteoporosis associated with malabsorption and chronic liver disease, osteoporosis associated with anorexia nervosa, immobilization-induced osteoporosis, and idiopathic juvenile osteoporosis with and without hypercalciuria. On the other hand, osteoporosis associated with premature menopause, anovulatory cycles, primary hyperparathyroidism, secondary amenorrhea, and male hypogonadism is associated usually with high bone turnover. It is of interest that the two variants of osteoporosis differ also in the abnormalities in microarchitecture. In the high turnover type, the changes consist of thinning and loss of trabecular elements, reduced connectedness, erosions, and penetration of the trabecules with total disruption of the architecture; in the low bone turnover type, the only change is thinning of the trabecules with loss of horizontal trabecules.

Bone mass is strongly correlated with compressive strength. There is, however, a considerable overlap in bone density values between subjects with and without fractures. This emphasizes the importance of factors other than bone mass in the pathogenesis of fractures. These include bone microarchitecture, composition of bone matrix, composition of bone mineral, and other factors such as trauma.

Even though the vast majority of osteoporotic fractures occur in patients with postmenopausal osteoporosis and in the elderly, it is noteworthy, however, that the association of low bone mass with the occurrence of fractures has been also recorded in younger people. It has been shown that athletes with stress fractures had lower bone mineral than did well-matched control athletes. Likewise, there was a good correlation between menstrual irregularity, reduced bone mineral density, and stress fractures. A positive correlation between calcium intake and bone mineral density was demonstrated in young individuals.

Bone Densitometry

Bone densitometry represents a major advance in management osteoporosis. The introduction of advanced technology to assess the bone density has provided clinicians with a valuable tool to assess patients at risk of fractures and to monitor response to therapy. These methods include the utilization of dual energy x-ray absorptiometry (DXA), ultrasonic measurements (SOS), computerized x-ray tomography, and other methods. The indications for bone mineral density measurements recommended by the Scientific Advisory Board of the National Osteoporosis Foundation in the United State are (1) estrogen deficiency, (2) vertebral deformity and radiographic osteopenia, (3) asymptomatic primary hyperparathyroidism (reduced bone density is an indication for surgery), and (4) monitoring of therapy. Optional indications include the presence of several minor risk factors such as genetic factors, alcohol intake, high caffeine intake, smoking, and reduced physical activity.

It is of interest that in recent genetic studies, polymorphism of vitamin D–receptor gene has been linked with bone mineral density in twin studies. It has been shown, in postmenopausal women, that allelic variants in the gene encoding the vitamin D receptor can be used to predict differences in bone density. The molecular mechanism by which bone density is regulated by vitamin D receptor is not certain, although allelic differences in the three untranslated regions may alter mRNA levels. It has been proposed that the use of this genetic marker could allow earlier intervention in those with increased risk of osteoporosis [155]. In more recent reports, it has been emphasized that the vitamin D–receptor gene acts predominantly to determine peak bone mass, and other genes are likely to be involved in the regulation of bone loss after menopause [156].

Treatment of Osteoporosis

Undoubtedly, measures aimed at prevention of osteoporosis are most valuable, since in many cases the disease is irreversible and refractory to therapy. Achievement of adequate peak bone mass may be facilitated with adequate intake of calcium and vitamin D, good physical activity, and early detection and treatment of predisposing diseases. Nonsmoking and moderation in alcohol and caffeine intake should be recommended.

In established osteoporosis, the therapeutic goals are dual: to increase bone formation and to decrease bone resorption in order to maintain adequate bone mass and prevent osteoporotic fractures. There is a positive correlation between physical activity and bone density. Therefore, gravity exercises and muscle-strengthening exercises should be encouraged.

Estrogen inhibits bone resorption and therefore prevents bone loss and even may increase bone mass in postmenopausal women. The daily dose of conjugated estrogen is 0.625 mg; it may be given in conjunction with progesterone with good effect. Administration of estrogen not only prevents bone loss but also prevents vertebral and femoral fractures. It is recommended to treat with estrogen for at least 5 years. Recent reports on the incidence of breast cancer in estrogen-treated women need to be taken into consideration [157].

Biphosphonates and calcitonin reduce bone turnover and, like estrogens, may potentially lead to small increases in bone mass as a result of filling the remodeling space. Estrogens affect equally cortical and cancellous bone, whereas calcitonin and biophosphonates affect mainly cancellous bone [157–160].

Fluoride is used currently, and PTH may possibly be used in the future, to increase bone formation. Fluoride increases cancellous bone density. The quality of the bone may be abnormal with fluoride, resulting in reduced strength despite increased mass [160, 161].

Oral calcium supplements, with and without vitamin D including oral calcitriol, have been reported to be beneficial in certain studies.

Chronic Renal Disease

Hyperplasia of the parathyroid glands in autopsies of patients dying of uremia was reported in the early part of this century. In 1943, a form of rickets that failed to respond to physiologic doses of vitamin D but responded to pharmacologic doses was reported in children with renal insufficiency [162]. These preliminary observations stimulated the evaluation of two major skeletal abnormalities associated with chronic renal disease, osteitis fibrosa cystica and osteomalacia.

Both biochemical studies and measurements of circulating immunoreactive PTH suggest that hyperactivity of parathyroid glands is present in the early stage of chronic renal disease. Assuming that a decrease in serum calcium concentration is the stimulus for secondary hyperparathyroidism in chronic renal failure, several potential factors may cause the hypocalcemia. Loss of functioning nephrons with a decreased filtered load of phosphorus will lead to retention of phosphorus. The resulting increase in serum phosphorus concentration, with a reciprocal decrease in serum calcium concentration, will stimulate the secretion of PTH. The increase in parathyroid activity would correct the hyperphosphatemia by decreasing tubular phosphate reabsorption and increasing urinary excretion of phosphorus and return both serum phosphorus and calcium toward normal, but at the expense ("trade-off") of increasingly rising serum levels of PTH [163]. This hypothesis of the pathogenesis of secondary hyperparathyroidism in chronic renal failure has been supported by studies in chronically azotemic dogs in which phosphate restriction prevented the development of secondary hyperparathyroidism. The major assumptions, however, on which the "trade-off" hypothesis was based were not fulfilled entirely. First, no evidence was presented showing a rise in serum phosphorus in patients with early renal failure. In fact, these patients exhibit a normal or even low serum phosphate, with normal serum calcium. Likewise, sequential sampling of serum phosphate failed to demonstrate transient rises in serum phosphorus or decrements in serum calcium. Second, the patients with early renal failure do not show phosphate retention but rather have an increased ability to excrete phosphorus loads [163]. The fact that phosphate restriction was shown to reverse the rise in PTH cannot anymore be used as favoring the trade-off hypothesis. Phosphate levels per se, independent of serum calcium, have been shown to alter PTH secretion [40, 41].

Reduced intestinal absorption of calcium due to acquired resistance to vitamin D also has been proposed as a fundamental abnormality in chronic renal failure [164]. This possibility was supported by studies indicating that the conversion of $25(OH)_2D_3$ to $1,25(OH)_2D_3$ takes place in the kidney and that serum levels of $1,25(OH)_2D_3$ are reduced in patients with chronic renal failure [67]. It also has been reported that physiologic doses of $1,25(OH)_2D_3$ improve the abnormal gastrointestinal absorption of calcium in patients with chronic renal failure. These findings, however, apply to advanced renal disease. In early renal failure, intestinal absorption of calcium is normal, while serum PTH is already elevated.

Evidence has been advanced demonstrating a direct inhibitory effect of physiologic amounts of $1,25(OH)_2D_3$ on the synthesis of PTH in vivo at the genomic transcriptional level. Thus, reduced $1,25(OH)_2D_3$ levels in chronic renal failure could be responsible for the increased synthesis and secretion of PTH [39]. It is noteworthy, however, that in early renal failure serum levels of $1,25(OH)_2D_3$ are variable—normal, low, or even elevated. It has been claimed that the presumably "normal" $1,25(OH)_2D_3$ levels measured in early renal failure may in fact be abnormally low relative to the elevated PTH level. In this regard, it has been demonstrated that the administration of calcitriol or dietary phosphate restriction, in early renal disease, results in normalization of serum PTH levels. These observations do not necessarily prove conclusively that calcitriol deficiency is the mechanism of secondary hyperparathyroidism.

An additional proposed mechanism of evolution of secondary hyperparathyroidism is altered number or binding affinity of vitamin D receptors to $1,25(OH)_2D_3$, resulting in a blunted response of parathyroid glands to the inhibitory effect of $1,25(OH)_2D_3$ and uninhibited synthesis of PTH. Although reduced density and number of vitamin D receptors have been demonstrated in hyperplastic glands removed from uremic patients, this has not been demonstrated in patients with early renal failure as yet [165].

Parathyroid glands from uremic patients require higher ambient calcium concentrations than normal glands to suppress the secretion of PTH. Thus, the "set point" for calcium, that is, the concentration of calcium required to inhibit 50 percent of maximal PTH secretion, is shifted to the right. This abnormality of response to calcium can be partially corrected by treatment with calcitriol. The possibility that defects in the calcium-sensing receptor might be the mechanism of secondary hyperparathyroidism requires further evaluation.

The calcemic response to PTH in chronic renal failure is blunted. This could represent down-regulation of PTH receptors in the bone. It has been shown that this abnormality can be reversed after parathyroidectomy, suggesting that high PTH levels may play a role in the blunted calcemic response. The skeletal resistance to PTH has been demonstrated both in early and advanced renal insufficiency [163].

As renal failure advances, hyperphosphatemia develops and assumes a major role in the aggravation of secondary hyperparathyroidism. Likewise, the serum levels of $1,25(OH)_2D_3$ decrease, and the intestinal absorption of calcium is low. In many patients with advanced renal failure, the hyperplastic parathyroid glands do not respond anymore to physiologic regulation and become refractory to treatment. This sets the stage for the emergence of "tertiary" or "autonomous" hyperparathyroidism, which may require surgical removal of excessive parathyroid tissue. In these circumstances, hypercalcemia may develop as a result of loss of feedback regulation. The combined elevation of serum calcium and phosphorus levels with an increase in their product may lead to metastatic calcifications.

Recent studies have examined the clonality of hyperplastic parathyroid glands from patients with autonomous secondary uremic hyperparathyroidism. Tumor monoclonality was demonstrated in 64 percent of patients with uremic refractory hyperparathyroidism. Monoclonality implied that somatic mutation of certain genes controlling cell proliferation occurred in a single parathyroid cell, conferring a selective growth advantage to the transformed cell, leading to neoplastic transformation [166].

Renal Bone Disease

Secondary hyperparathyroidism causes the development of osteitis fibrosa cystica, which presents radiographically as subperiosteal bone resorption. These lesions are most commonly seen in the middle phalanges of the hands, distal ends of the clavicles, and proximal ends of the tibia.

Cystic lesions and brown tumors may be also a radiographic feature of hyperparathyroid bone disease.

Osteitis fibrosa cystica is the most common skeletal abnormality both in adults and in children with chronic renal failure. The hyperparathyroid osteodystrophy is characterized by rapid bone turnover, featuring both increased osteoclastic resorption and increased osteoblastic bone formation. The rapid bone turnover can be demonstrated by an increased number of double-tetracycline labels. The rapid bone turnover is also associated with marrow fibrosis and increased amounts of woven osteoid. It differs from normal lamellar osteoid in that there is a haphazard arrangement of collagen fibers. Although woven osteoid can be mineralized, the calcium is deposited as amorphous calcium phosphate instead of hydroxyapatite. The presence of woven bone is characteristic of states of active bone and is visualized with polarizing microscope. Advanced forms of osteitis fibrosa cystica present an abnormal bone architecture in which vast quantities of normal mineralized bone are replaced with fibrous tissue, with multiple cysts, and with woven bone that is mechanically defective. This leads to serious skeletal deformities and fractures.

Another interesting radiographic feature of renal osteodystrophy is osteosclerosis. This entity is associated with increased density of bone, as assessed by x-ray examination, and is most frequently observed in the vertebrae.

In many instances, the secondary hyperparathyroidism seen in advanced renal

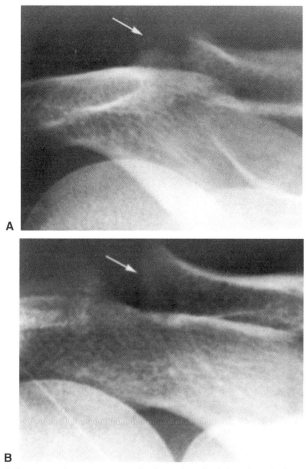

Fig. 6-8. (A) Subperiosteal resorption at the lateral end of the clavicle (*arrow*), with an irregular appearance and loss of cortical outline. (B) Healing of bone, with filling of the defect and reappearance of cortical outline after therapy with calcium carbonate and aluminum hydroxide. (*Arrow* indicates distal clavicle.)

insufficiency may be reversed with sustained control of serum calcium and phosphorus, which may be accomplished by the use of vitamin D, phosphate-binding antacids, and the administration of calcium carbonate. It has been shown that with continuous control of calcium and phosphorus levels in the serum, the level of circulating PTH decreases, and radiographically observed bone lesions may resolve [167] (Fig. 6-8). Metastatic calcifications also will resolve with this regimen [168]. In some patients, this therapeutic approach may not be successful because of extremely severe hyperplasia of the parathyroid glands, and subtotal parathyroidectomy is then the treatment of choice.

Intravenous use of pharmacologic doses of calcitriol, in intermittent doses, has been recommended as a highly efficient way to achieve better suppression of parathyroid hyperactivity in patients with chronic renal failure [169]. Indeed, many studies have confirmed the therapeutic efficacy of the intravenous intermittent administration in suppressing PTH levels. The effect of this form of therapy on bone histomorphometry is not entirely clear. In a limited number of studies, intravenous therapy with calcitriol led to marked suppression of bone turnover, with marked reduction in bone formation but with variable effect on osteoclastic resorption [170]. It is noteworthy that the initial clinical studies comparing the efficacy of the intermittent intravenous administration of calcitriol with the oral route of administration were uncontrolled. The results of a recent controlled randomized study comparing long-term oral administration of calcitriol with intermittent intravenous administration showed that they were equivalent in the treatment of secondary hyperparathyroidism. Additional observations of that study were that treatment of severe secondary hyperparathyroidism remains difficult regardless of the route of administration. Moreover, the dose of calcitriol was limited by side effects [171].

A recent clinical trial demonstrated a beneficial effect of oral administration of $24,25(OH)_2D_3$ when combined with $1\alpha(OH)D_3$ on hyperparathyroid bone disease in patients on chronic hemodialysis [172]. The potential therapeutic effect of this regimen requires further investigations.

Two additional distinct forms of bone disease in patients with chronic renal disease are osteomalacia and adynamic or aplastic bone disease.

A so-called vitamin D–refractory rickets was described in the 1940s in children with advanced renal insufficiency. This form of mineralization defect was most likely due to deficiency of calcitriol. Osteomalacia may be also present in predialysis patients with chronic renal failure. Most of these patients present with hypocalcemia and normophosphatemia, and their kidney disease is usually interstitial and/or obstructive uropathy. Many of them respond favorably to calcitriol administration.

Aluminum has been recognized as a toxic factor involved in the pathogenesis of uremic osteomalacia. The aluminum-related lesion is characterized by the presence of excessive amounts of inactive osteoid and very low bone turnover. In states of aluminum overload, the staining of bone for aluminum is usually strongly positive. Although this type of bone disease has been described mainly in patients undergoing chronic dialysis, it may also occur in uremic predialysis patients. Aluminum-associated osteomalacia is a very symptomatic bone disease manifested by severe skeletal pains and fractures [173]. Aluminum can be mobilized and removed with the use of the chelating agent deferoxamine mesylate, which binds aluminum. Removal of aluminum leads to recovery. With the restricted use of aluminum-based phosphate binders and the widespread employment of water treatment with reverse osmosis in dialysis units, aluminum-induced bone disease has become less frequent.

Adynamic bone at present is one of the enigmas in the spectrum of renal bone disease. It is characterized by very low bone turnover (low or absent tetracycline uptake) but with no obvious abnormalities in the static parameters of bone histomorphometry. This form of bone pathology has been variously attributed to suppression of parathyroid function by high calcium concentration in dialysate solution or by excessively high levels of circulating calcitriol such as those that follow the intravenous administration of pharmacologic doses of this metabolite of vitamin D [174].

It is of interest that patients with the aplastic bone lesion, similarly to those with osteomalacia, frequently develop hypercalcemia following oral or intravenous calcium loads. Thus, both aluminum-associated osteomalacia and adynamic bone are characterized by poor buffering capacity to exogenous calcium. Recent studies indicate that aplastic bone lesion is the prevalent bone abnormality in patients treated with chronic ambulatory peritoneal dialysis and in patients with diabetic end-stage renal disease [175]. In both groups, PTH levels are relatively low.

In addition to the discrete forms of bone disease outlined, there are also mixed types of renal osteodystrophy, which combine elements characteristic of more than one defined lesion. For example, the mixed form of uremic osteodystrophy consists of features typical of osteitis fibrosa; however, in addition, it is characterized by low forming activity with accumulation of excessive quantities of osteoid, as in osteomalacia. Another variant of mixed bone disease is similar to the aforementioned lesion, but the bone-forming parameters are normal. In the latter, the accumulation of osteoid has been attributed to a shortage in the supply of minerals and hence delayed mineralization of organic bone matrix. This lesion responds favorably to vitamin D therapy.

Tumoral Calcinosis

Extraskeletal calcifications with periarticular, vascular, and other soft tissue calcium deposits are present in patients with chronic renal failure. They are usually associated with advanced secondary hyperparathyroidism featuring high calcium $\times$ phosphate product. They may also occur without high calcium $\times$ phosphate product in selected uremic patients with preexisting collagen diseases including systemic lupus erythematosus, rheumatoid arthritis, and scleroderma.

Tumoral calcinosis in nonuremic patients with normal kidney function is a hereditary disorder with a renal tubular abnormality leading to excessive reabsorption and retention of phosphate. Recurrence of tumoral calcinosis after kidney transplantation suggests a deficiency of a systemic phosphaturic factor rather than an intrinsic tubular defect as an underlying mechanism [176].

β_2-Microglobulin Deposition

Skeletal disease due to the deposition of β_2-microglobulin is becoming very frequent now that patients are being maintained on hemodialysis for prolonged periods of time. β_2-Microglobulin is part of the major histocompatibility complex-1 and is produced by a large number of cells in the body. It can aggregate to form amyloid, which causes destructive arthropathy of various joints. It may accumulate around intervertebral articular spaces and produce spinal compression syndromes. Likewise, it can produce carpal tunnel syndrome. β_2-Microglobulin induces locally osteoclastic bone resorption. It remains to be established whether it may produce diffuse resorptive bone lesions similar to those present in uremic patients with severe secondary hyperparathyroidism [177].

Clinical Disorders of Hypophosphatemia

Hypophosphatemia is defined as an abnormally low concentration of inorganic phosphorus in serum or plasma. It often indicates phosphorus deficiency. However, hypophosphatemia may also occur under a variety of circumstances in which total body phosphorus stores are normal. Precisely defined, phosphorus deficiency means that the content of inorganic phosphorus in lean tissues (muscle) is below 28 mmol/kg of dry fat-free muscle. It may exist in the absence of hypophosphatemia.

There are many causes of moderate (1.5–2.5 mg/dl [Table 6-7]) and severe

Table 6-7. Causes of moderate hypophosphatemia

Pseudohypophosphatemia
  Mannitol
  Bilirubin
  Acute leukemia
Decreased dietary intake
Decreased intestinal absorption
  Vitamin D deficiency
  Malabsorption
  Steatorrhea
  Secretory diarrhea
  Vomiting
  PO_4^{3-} binding antacids
Shift from serum into cells
  Respiratory alkalosis
    Sepsis
    Heat stroke
    Neuroleptic malignant syndrome
    Hepatic coma
    Salicylate poisoning
    Gout
    Panic attacks
    Psychiatric depression
  Hormonal effects
    Insulin
    Glucagon
    Epinephrine
    Androgens
    Cortisol
    Anovulatory hormones
  Nutrient effects
    Glucose
    Fructose
    Glycerol
    Lactate
    Amino acids
    Xylitol

Cellular uptake syndromes
  Recovery from hypothermia
  Burkitt's lymphoma
  Histiocytic lymphoma
  Acute myelomonocytic leukemia
  Acute myelogenous leukemia
  Chronic myelogenous leukemia in blast crisis
  Treatment of pernicious anemia
  Erythropoietin therapy
  Erythrodermic psoriasis
  Hungry bone syndrome
    After parathyroidectomy
    Acute leukemia
Increased excretion into the urine
Hyperparathyroidism
Renal tubule defects
  Fanconi's syndrome
  X-linked hypophosphatemic rickets
  Hereditary hypophosphatemic rickets with hypercalciuria
  Polyostotic fibrous dysplasia
  Panostotic fibrous dysplasia
  Neurofibromatosis
  Kidney transplantation
  Oncogenic osteomalacia
  Recovery from hemolytic-uremic syndrome
Aldosteronism
Licorice ingestion
Volume expansion
Inappropriate secretion of antidiuretic hormone
Mineralocorticoid administration
Corticosteroid therapy
Diuretics
Aminophylline therapy

Table 6-8. Causes of severe hypophosphatemia

Acute renal failure
Chronic alcoholism and alcohol withdrawal
Dietary deficiency and PO_4^{3-} binding antacids
Hyperalimentation
Neuroleptic malignant syndrome
Recovery from diabetic ketoacidosis
Recovery from exhaustive exercise
Kidney transplantation
Respiratory alkalosis
Severe thermal burns
Therapeutic hyperthermia
Reye's syndrome
After major surgery
Periodic paralysis
Acute malaria
Drug therapy
  Ifosfamide
  Cisplatin
Acetaminophen intoxication
Cytokine infusions
  Tumor necrosis factor
  Interleukin-2

(<1.5 mg/dl [Table 6-8]) hypophosphatemia. Moderate hypophosphatemia is ordinarily benign but may indicate the presence of a disease such as hyperparathyroidism or osteomalacia. A fascinating cause of moderate hypophosphatemia is oncogenic osteomalacia, a disorder in which either benign tumors of mesenchymal origin or carcinoma of the breast or prostate produces a substance that partially blocks proximal tubular reabsorption of phosphate [178]. The result is hypophosphatemic myopathy characterized by myalgia and proximal muscle weakness with either a normal or only modestly elevated serum creatinine kinase value and osteomalacia characterized by pain in weight-bearing bones and fractures. New information on the nature of the putative "phosphaturic hormone" has recently been published by Cai et al. [139, 178]. Besides being the explanation for the paraneoplastic syndrome of oncogenic osteomalacia, this hormone may be the substance normally produced for the purpose of regulating phosphate excretion by the kidney. The work of Cai et al. [139, 178], using material from a patient with oncogenic osteomalacia, showed that this substance is not PTH or PTH-related peptide, since it is not dependent cyclic AMP hydrolysis for its action. Apparently, the substance reduces phosphorus reabsorption by interfering with sodium-phosphorus cotransport.

In nearly all instances of moderate hypophosphatemia in the absence of severe phosphorus deficiency, phosphorus has either been excreted into the urine as in a brisk diuresis or has been redistributed from the extracellular to the intracellular space. Thus, for example, cellular uptake of inorganic phosphorus occurs with glycolysis during administration of glucose, fructose, or insulin or from activation of phosphofructokinase during respiratory alkalosis.

Evidence available at this time indicates that severe hypophosphatemia in the presence of phosphorus deficiency may cause widespread disturbances of cellular function and structure. Similarly, if severe hypophosphatemia is superimposed on subtle cellular injury, such as may exist in chronic alcoholism, overt dysfunction or necrosis may follow. Fructose-induced cytosolic hypophosphatemia in liver cells in the absence of phosphorus deficiency or preexisting cellular injury might cause serious consequences [179]. However, in the absence of preexisting deficiency or injury, even severe hypophosphatemia, such as that induced by hyperventilation and glucose-insulin infusions [180], does not appear to be harmful. Such observations suggest that intracellular phosphorus deficiency plays a major role in cellular injury.

Etiology of Severe Hypophosphatemia

Pharmacologic Phosphate Binding in the Gut

Binding of phosphorus by large doses of aluminum hydroxide, magnesium hydroxide, or aluminum carbonate gels may cause severe hypophosphatemia when food intake of phosphorus is inadequate and also, at least conceivably, in the presence of a normal phosphorus intake if primary hyperparathyroidism coexists.

Thermal Burns

Severe hypophosphatemia is common in patients with extensive burns and usually appears within several days after the injury. Phosphorus is virtually undetectable in urine. Since burn patients nearly always hyperventilate, it seems likely that respiratory alkalosis and the resulting acceleration of glycolysis are responsible for the hypophosphatemia.

Hyperalimentation

In the setting of starvation and malnutrition, hyperalimentation without adequate phosphorus supplementation may cause severe hypophosphatemia [181]. It is important to emphasize that starvation per se does not cause severe hypophosphatemia. In experimental starvation, serum phosphorus concentration and muscle phosphorus content remain nearly normal. Refeeding with a high-calorie diet complete in all components except phosphorus causes muscle phosphorus content to fall rapidly in association with the development of hypophosphatemia. Indeed, in the latter circumstance, skeletal muscle appears to play the role of a reservoir, giving up its phosphorus so that vital organs such as brain and heart do not become phosphorus depleted [180]. Thus, tissue repair in one organ under conditions of phosphorus deprivation may create phosphorus deficiency in another.

Nutritional Recovery Syndrome

The nutritional recovery syndrome is a constellation of findings observed during refeeding of patients with severe protein-calorie malnutrition. In contrast to hyperalimentation, hypophosphatemia may occur during administration of calories in normally required quantities. Initial observations on this syndrome were made in prisoners during World War II. Refeeding, especially when overzealous and with simple carbohydrates, was sometimes followed by edema, ascites, hydrothorax, and death. Administration of thiamine did not consistently prevent these complications [180]. Refeeding with skim milk, however, was apparently associated with less morbidity, and the phosphorus provided in skim milk may have been important. Unfortunately, measurements of chemical composition of the blood or urine of those patients were not possible. In many respects, this syndrome can be reproduced in experimental animals that are starved and then refed [180].

This syndrome may be induced in virtually any patient who has lost substantial weight or who has severe protein-calorie malnutrition. Included are alcoholics, patients with severe gingival or dental disease who cannot eat, patients with anorexia nervosa, surreptitious vomiters, patients with malabsorption, and food fadists. A prerequisite is that their cells must be capable of anabolic response. Initial refeeding of severely wasted patients should be conducted with great caution, consisting of small quantities of calories and fluids, increased daily by small amounts to avoid acute derangements of serum composition.

Respiratory Alkalosis

Prolonged, intense hyperventilation may depress serum phosphorus to values of 0.3 mg/dl [182]. As will be explained, this could be very important in patients with alcoholic withdrawal. In contrast, a similar degree of alkalosis induced by infusing bicarbonate depresses serum phosphorus concentration to only 3.0 mg/dl. This difference in the hypophosphatemic effect of respiratory as compared to metabolic alkalosis is presumably related to the more pronounced intracellular alkalosis during hyperventilation. Carbon dioxide is readily diffusible across cellular membranes, but bicarbonate is not. Intracellular alkalosis activates phosphofructokinase, phosphorylation of glucose increases, and serum phosphorus is utilized. Urinary phosphorus excretion falls to zero. During bicarbonate infusion, intracellular alkalosis is either mild or nonexistent, glycolysis is not accelerated as it is in respiratory alkalosis, and consequently severe hypophosphatemia does not occur. During bicarbonate infusions, excretion of phosphorus into the urine increases.

Diabetic Ketoacidosis

Patients with adequately controlled diabetes mellitus generally have no recognizable disturbance of phosphorus metabolism. On the other hand, those who develop glycosuria, ketonuria, and polyuria almost invariably lose phosphate excessively into the urine [183]. This may be explained as follows: Acidosis decomposes organic compounds inside the cell, and inorganic phosphate moves into the plasma and is excreted in the urine. Osmotic diuresis due to coexistent glycosuria, ketonuria, and polyuria augments phosphaturia. Recent evidence suggests that insulin increases cellular uptake of phosphorus independently of glucose [184].

In untreated diabetic ketoacidosis, serum phosphorus may be normal or elevated, which contributes to excessive phosphaturia [185]. With insulin, fluids, and correction of the ketoacidosis, however, serum and urine phosphorus fall sharply. Despite the appearance of hypophosphatemia during treatment, previously well-controlled patients with diabetes ketoacidosis of only a few days' duration almost never have serious phosphorus deficiency [186]. On the other hand, if a patient with ketoacidosis has not been bothered by vomiting and has had a generous fluid intake so as to permit a sustained high rate of urine flow for many days or weeks, phosphorus deficiency may be severe. In such unusual circumstances, initial blood measurements may show hypophosphatemia despite acidosis. This pattern suggests severe phosphorus deficiency.

Alcoholic Withdrawal

In metropolitan charity hospitals, the most common cause of severe hypophosphatemia is alcoholism. Hypophosphatemia affects about 50 percent of patients with alcoholism requiring hospitalization [180]. Serum phosphorus may be normal, low, or high when the patient is first admitted to the hospital, but it falls rapidly during the first few hospital days.

A host of factors can be responsible for phosphate depletion in the alcoholic [180]. Among the obvious causes are poor intake, the use of antacids, and vomiting. Although diarrhea occurs commonly in alcoholics, fecal excretion of phosphorus does not increase substantially in diarrhea [180]. Ethanol per se has little effect on phosphorus excretion [187]. Chronic alcoholism, however, may cause magnesium deficiency and hypomagnesemia [188]. In turn, magnesium deficiency and hypomagnesemia may cause phosphaturia. Phosphaturia due to experimental magnesium deficiency [189] leads to phosphorus deficiency [190]. The degree of phosphaturia is related to the level of hyperphosphatemia [191].

A recent study of 61 chronic alcoholics showed evidence for renal tubular dysfunction that clearly could explain a number of the metabolic abnormalities observed in these patients [192], including phosphaturia. Each abnormality disappeared following abstinence from ethanol.

Ketoacidosis can be at least partially responsible for phosphate depletion in the patient with chronic alcoholism. Since such patients often eat poorly, ketonuria is common. Repeated episodes of ketoacidosis could decompose organic phosphates within cells and cause phosphaturia by mechanisms somewhat analogous to that in diabetic ketoacidosis. Notably, patients with alcoholic ketoacidosis often show disproportionately heavy phosphaturia when they are initially admitted to the hospital, even though they are severely phosphorus deficient. In most, as with diabetic ketoacidosis, the phosphaturia disappears rapidly after treatment is initiated.

Experimentally, administration of intoxicating quantities of ethanol to dogs for 2 months causes phosphorus deficiency in skeletal muscle despite ingestion of a highly nutritious diet containing abundant phosphorus. The mechanism by which ethanol causes phosphorus deficiency has not been elucidated [193].

Isolated instances of severe hypophosphatemia have been described in patients with chronic myelogenous leukemia undergoing blast crises [20, 194], erythropoietin therapy in patients with end-stage renal disease [195], psoriasis [196], reuptake into skeletal muscle following collapse in competitive runners [197, 198], rapidly growing tumors [20, 199], binge eating in children with anorexia nervosa [200], assisted ventilation in patients with asthma [201], patients recovering from hepatic trans-

Table 6-9. Consequences of severe hypophosphatemia

Definite
  Red cell dysfunction
  Leukocyte dysfunction
  Platelet dysfunction
  Central nervous system dysfunction
  Rhabdomyolysis
  Osteolysis
  Metabolic acidosis
  Cardiomyopathy
  Respiratory failure
Possible
  Hepatocellular dysfunction
  Renal dysfunction
  Ketoacidosis
  Peripheral neuropathy

plant [202], acute falciparum malaria [203], and secondary to ifosfamide therapy [204].

Consequences of Acute Hypophosphatemia

Current evidence suggests that there are at least eight definite and several possible effects of severe hypophosphatemia (Table 6-9).

Red Cell Dysfunction

The most important biochemical abnormalities of erythrocytes associated with hypophosphatemia are declines of 2,3-diphosphoglycerate (2,3-DPG) and ATP [180]. Hemoglobin and 2,3-DPG interact chemically so as to promote release of oxygen. This has been quantitated by means of the index P_{50}, which refers to the oxygen tension of mixed venous blood at 37°C, pH 7.4, when hemoglobin is 50 percent saturated. Low levels of 2,3-DPG may depress P_{50} values so that release of oxygen to peripheral tissues is diminished. Thus, acute hypophosphatemia may limit oxygen release at the cellular level and thereby cause tissue anoxia.

Structural defects of the red cell in hypophosphatemia include increased rigidity [205] and in rare instances hemolysis. Hemolysis has arisen in individuals who apparently have also sustained severe total body phosphorus depletion. It is usually provoked by an unusual stress on the metabolic requirements of the red cell, such as severe metabolic acidosis or infection. When hemolysis has occurred, ATP content invariably has been less than 15 percent of normal [205, 206].

Leukocyte Dysfunction

A serious complication of intravenous hyperalimentation therapy is systemic infection by bacterial and fungal organisms. This predisposition may be partly related to hypophosphatemia. Hypophosphatemic dogs show severe depression of the chemotactic, phagocytic, and bactericidal activity of granulocytes [207]. These abnormalities are reversed on correction of hypophosphatemia [207]. Similar observations have been made on a patient who became hypophosphatemic during hyperalimentation [180].

Respiratory alkalosis and hypophosphatemia may also occur in association with gram-negative bacteremia. Guinea pigs infected with *Salmonella* organisms became hypophosphatemic before death. When they were given phosphate, their mortality was significantly reduced, and the number of organisms found in their tissues were less [208].

Apparently, hypophosphatemia impairs granulocytic function by interfering with ATP synthesis. ATP provides energy for contraction of microfilaments, which in turn regulate the mechanical properties of leukocytes, that is, pseudopod and vacuole formation [180].

Platelet Dysfunction

Seven abnormalities of platelet function and structure have been observed in experimental hypophosphatemia [209]: (1) thrombocytopenia; (2) increase in platelet diameter, suggesting shortened platelet survival; (3) megakaryocytosis of the marrow; (4) marked acceleration of platelet disappearance from blood; (5) impairment of clot retraction; (6) a reduction in platelet ATP content; and (7) hemorrhage into the gut and skin. Although similar defects of platelet function seem likely to occur in clinical hypophosphatemia, conclusive proof for such an effect has not been obtained.

Central Nervous System Dysfunction

Some patients with severe hypophosphatemia display symptoms compatible with metabolic encephalopathy [210]. They show, in sequence, irritability, apprehension, weakness, numbness, paresthesias, dysarthria, confusion, obtundation, convulsive seizures, and coma. This clinical syndrome has been observed in patients without other apparent causes for encephalopathy who have been treated with intravenous hyperalimentation and also in patients during withdrawal from chronic alcoholism. Hallucinations occur but are uncommon. Obviously, delirium tremens and hypophosphatemic encephalopathy may coexist.

The relationship between hypophosphatemia and the decline of red cell 2,3-DPG becomes especially important in tissues where oxygen is necessary for energy metabolism. This may be true in the brain, where oxidation of glucose through the Krebs cycle is necessary for synthesis of ATP.

Patients who become hypophosphatemic during hyperalimentation may display paresthesias, mental obtundation, and hyperventilation. Those whose serum phosphorus values are severely depressed may show diffuse slowing of their electroencephalograms. Their electroencephalograms become normal on correction of hypophosphatemia. Perhaps the best evidence that hypophosphatemia plays a role in this encephalopathy has been the observation that it does not occur in patients receiving hyperalimentation with adequate phosphorus.

Rhabdomyolysis and Phosphate Depletion

An apparent relationship between hypophosphatemia and alcoholic myopathy has been observed in chronic alcoholism [211, 212]. When serum phosphorus concen-

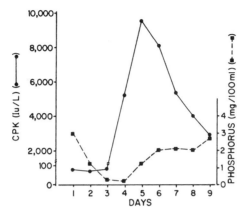

Fig. 6-9. Relationship between the onset of hypophosphatemia and elevation of creatine phosphokinase (CPK) activity. (From J. P. Knochel, The pathophysiology and clinical characteristics of severe hypophosphatemia. *Arch. Intern. Med.* 137:203, 1977.)

tration was less than 1 mg/dl and remained at that level for 1 to 2 days, serum creatine phosphokinase activity often rose sharply (Fig. 6-9). Total muscle phosphorus was markedly subnormal, averaging 13.2 mmol/100 g fat-free dry solids, compared to a normal value of 28 mmol/100 g. The resting muscle membrane potential was also subnormal, averaging − 70.4 mV, compared to a normal value of − 86.7 mV. The elevated tissue chloride level and sodium and water content and the subnormal resting membrane potential suggest that the bulk of the water, sodium, and chloride retained was inside the cells. Electromicroscopy shows focal myofibrillar damage and dissolution of Z bands [213].

To examine the possibility that phosphate deficiency itself might cause a myopathy, the effect of phosphorus deficiency was examined experimentally [214]. Resting muscle membrane potential fell; the sodium, chloride, and water content of the tissue increased, and potassium content decreased. These values returned to normal when phosphorus was replenished. It has been observed that administration of excessive calories to partially starved, phosphorus-deprived dogs results in pronounced hypophosphatemia, sharp elevation of creatine kinase, and frank rhabdomyolysis [215].

Osteolysis

Dietary deprivation of phosphorus in conjunction with administration of phosphate-binding antacids may cause severe hypophosphatemia, weakness, and bone pain. As serum phosphorus and phosphorus excretion into the urine decline, hypercalciuria appears. In children and growing animals, hypercalciuria may appear. In human volunteers, it has been found that hypercalciuria appears regularly in phosphorus-deficient women but may not occur in men [216].

Experimental phosphorus deficiency with hypophosphatemia increases synthesis of $1,25(OH)_2D_3$ by the kidney and decreases release of PTH. The elevated $1,25(OH)_2D_3$ will increase calcium and phosphorus absorption from the bowel.

Phosphorus deficiency causes mobilization of calcium and phosphorus from bone and muscle even before serum phosphorus falls. Indeed, one can postulate that a biologic response to such phosphorus deprivation may be mobilization of phosphorus from reservoirs in an attempt to forestall hypophosphatemia. In the process, calcium must also be mobilized, causing hypercalciuria. When calcium mobilization persists for a sufficient time, osteomalacia will occur.

Metabolic Acidosis

Excretion of hydrogen ions into the urine is for the most part facilitated by three processes. The first, simple lowering of urine pH, is important but of itself provides only a very small fraction of hydrogen ion excretion. The second process is production of ammonia by the renal tubular cell. A low urine pH is important to this process, since it increases trapping of ammonia in the tubular lumen by its conversion to ammonium, which is poorly diffusible. Ammonium ions in the urine may facilitate excretion of large quantities of hydrogen ion. Normally, an adult on a normal diet will excrete up to 1 mEq of acid per kilogram of body weight as ammonium per day. In severe diabetic ketoacidosis, ammonium excretion may reach values of 500 mEq/day.

The third process facilitating excretion of metabolic acid is phosphate buffer. By this mechanism, one sodium ion of the molecule Na_2HPO_4 is reabsorbed from tubular fluid in exchange for a hydrogen ion from the tubular cell, resulting in formation of NaH_2PO_4. This latter compound is usually measured as titratable acidity. Its availability as a mechanism for acid excretion is related to the quantity of phosphorus available for excretion into the urine.

Severe hypophosphatemia in association with phosphorus deficiency may result in metabolic acidosis through two important mechanisms. First, severe hypophosphatemia is generally associated with a proportionate reduction of phosphorus excretion into the urine, thereby limiting hydrogen excretion as titratable acid (NaH_2PO_4). If phosphate buffer is inadequate, the responsibility for acid excretion falls on production of ammonia and its conversion to ammonium. However, ammonia production becomes severely depressed in phosphorus deficiency. Experimental studies indicate that phosphorus deficiency may result in an elevation of intracellular pH [217]. Unfortunately, such changes have not been demonstrated in the kidney. However, if they do occur, the intracellular alkalosis could very well decrease ammonia production despite extracellular acidosis.

Metabolic acidosis associated with hypophosphatemia has been reported in children with diarrhea, inanition, and malnutrition resulting from lactase deficiency [218]. Upon refeeding without phosphorus supplementation, these children became hypophosphatemic. Excretions of phosphate, titratable acidity, and ammonium were abnormally low. Moderately severe metabolic acidosis supervened. Under the same conditions, when phosphorus supplementation was provided in sufficient quantity to prevent hypophosphatemia, phosphorus and ammonium excretion became normal, and acidosis was corrected.

In experimental and clinical phosphorus deficiency [219], metabolic acidosis does not generally occur. Excretion of both titratable acid and ammonium diminish, thereby preventing adequate excretion of acid into the urine. However, as calcium is motilized from bone, so is its anion, carbonate. Indeed, carbonate is released in sufficient quantity to buffer the retained H^+ so that metabolic acidosis does not occur. Experimentally, if bone dissolution is simultaneously inhibited by administration of colchicine, carbonate is no longer mobilized, and metabolic acidosis promptly supervenes.

Hypophosphatemic Cardiomyopathy

Steadily increasing clinical evidence indicates that phosphorus deficiency and hypophosphatemia are causes of congestive cardiomyopathy [180]. A patient observed by one of us is an impressive example. A 52-year-old woman with a long history of peptic ulcer disease had, during the year preceding admission, increased her antacid intake and eaten poorly. She was admitted to the hospital in frank biventricular failure with cardiomegaly, hydrothorax, pulmonary edema, hepatomegaly, and peripheral edema. Pulmonary artery wedge pressure was markedly elevated, and cardiac output was appreciably reduced. Conventional treatment for 2 to 3 days with thiamine, digitalis, diuretics, and bed rest was minimally effective, if at all. Serum phosphorus was 0.3 mg/dl on admission and fell to 0.2 mg/dl on day 2. Correction of hypophosphatemia with intravenous phosphate salts led to rapid improvement. After 6 weeks, the patient showed no signs and had no symptoms of heart disease. That phosphorus deficiency may cause myocardial insufficiency has also gained support from experimental work. Phosphorus-deficient dogs developed a low cardiac output, a decreased ventricular ejection velocity, and an elevated left ventricular end-diastolic pressure. Phosphorus repletion was followed by recovery [214].

Recognition of hypophosphatemic cardiomyopathy is especially important because preliminary observations suggest it may be one of the few types of congestive cardiomyopathy that may be completely reversible by appropriate treatment.

Respiratory Failure

Severe hypophosphatemia in hypercarbic patients treated for pulmonary insufficiency [220, 221] has been clearly recognized as a cause of diaphragm and intercostal muscle weakness. Such patients display delays in recovery and cannot tolerate cessation of ventilation therapy. Administration of phosphorus salts has produced rapid recovery. Hypophosphatemia also occurs in patients treated for severe asthma and has led to delays in recovery [222]. Patients with asthma and others with chronic obstructive pulmonary disease may become phosphorus deficient as a result of renal losses consequent to therapy with corticosteroids and aminophylline preparations [180]. Both of these agents may cause phosphorus deficiency independently of respiratory acidosis. In addition, chronic respiratory acidosis per se can cause phosphorus depletion by interfering with metabolism. Fiaccadori and his associates [223] have performed a series of studies on patients with hypercarbia and chronic obstructive pulmonary disease. They demonstrated severe reductions of phosphorus content in respiratory muscles and inappropriate phosphaturia, which they ascribe to corticosteroids, xanthine derivatives, loop diuretics, and β_2-adrenergic bronchodilators.

Possible Consequences of Hypophosphatemia

Hepatocellular Dysfunction

The first evidence that severe hypophosphatemia might cause hepatic dysfunction was offered by Frank and Kern [224]. Their patient was a 51-year-old woman with alcoholic cirrhosis whose serum phosphorus had fallen to 0.5 mg/dl in the wake of respiratory alkalosis. Bilirubin rose to 15.1 mg/dl and she became comatose. Over the following few days, serum phosphorus became normal spontaneously, and her neurologic findings cleared. We raise the possibility that spontaneous correction of hypophosphatemia via release of phosphorus from injured tissues such as skeletal muscle might be inadvertently lifesaving. Respiratory alkalosis has generally preceded the fall of serum phosphorus in our patients.

Such findings correspond to clinical observations in many patients with chronic alcoholism and hepatic disease, that is, that liver function often deteriorates after several days in the hospital at a time when hypophosphatemia becomes pronounced Obviously, this is another potentially important complication of hypophosphatemia that requires more detailed study [225].

Miscellaneous Defects

Suspected but unconfirmed are several additional defects possibly resulting from tissue anoxia. Renal bicarbonate wasting and renal glycosuria [217] have been reported and appear to reflect an impairment in the proximal tubular function of the kidney. Hypophosphatemia has also been considered to be a contributory factor in β-hydroxybutyric ketoacidosis in some patients with severe alcoholism [226]. Another report suggests that acute, severe hypophosphatemia may cause paralytic neuropathy [227].

Recapitulation

In patients undergoing treatment for diabetic ketoacidosis, the onset of hypophosphatemia seems related not only to rapid uptake of phosphorus by cells, a process that would be accelerated by administration of insulin and correction of acidosis. The appearance of hypophosphatemia after treatment is initiated does not imply a serious degree of phosphorus deficiency. Hypophosphatemia that is present before treatment is initiated, especially if it coexists with metabolic acidosis, suggests severe phosphorus deficiency.

In chronic alcoholics, the onset of hypophosphatemia may appear within 12 hours but tends to occur later, the nadir being observed on the second through the fourth days. Its onset probably varies directly with preexisting cellular deficiency and quantity of nutrients metabolized and is probably exaggerated by respiratory alkalosis. That the urine becomes virtually phosphorus free during this time would support this notion.

The onset of hypophosphatemia in patients who are receiving hyperalimentation is delayed for up to 10 days. This probably reflects the absence of tissue phosphorus deficiency before treatment begins.

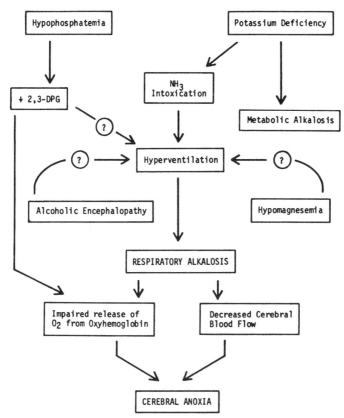

Fig. 6-10. Hypothetical explanation to interrelate hyperventilation, respiratory alkalosis, and phosphorus deficiency as causes of coma in alcoholic withdrawal. 2,3-DPG = 2,3-diphosphoglycerate.

In Figure 6-10, an attempt has been made to place much of the information already presented into a theoretical perspective. Hypophosphatemia (Fig. 6-10, upper left) may lead to a decline of 2,3-DPG content in the red cell. One possible consequence of this disturbance is impaired release of oxygen from erythrocytes. Another possible effect of abnormally low 2,3-DPG is that of hyperventilation due to anoxia of the respiratory center. In patients with alcoholic cirrhosis and portal hypertension, hypokalemia (Fig. 6-10, upper right) is common and may indirectly be responsible for ammonia intoxication [228]. Hypokalemia also has been associated with hyperventilation. Potassium deficiency would also tend to maintain metabolic alkalosis, which tends to favor the development of hypophosphatemia (see Chap. 3). In many patients with alcoholic withdrawal, hypomagnesemia has been cited as a possible cause of increased neuromuscular irritability and hyperventilation [229]. In such patients, metabolic encephalopathy due to alcoholic withdrawal per se could also cause hyperventilation. Hyperventilation and respiratory alkalosis play a central role in the scheme in Figure 6-10. When respirations become driven, as they often are in these patients, respiratory alkalosis and hypophosphatemia may become profound. Thus, if red cell 2,3-DPG is diminished by hypophosphatemia, the only remaining influence favoring release of oxygen into peripheral tissues would be acidosis (Bohr effect). Alkalosis, a more common finding, would further impair release of oxygen. It is of equal importance that profound respiratory alkalosis may sharply reduce cerebral blood flow. In the withdrawing alcoholic patient, whose red cell 2,3-DPG may be depressed because of phosphorus depletion, superimposed respiratory alkalosis also eliminates the Bohr effect. These influences acting together could seriously impair release of oxygen to the brain. If in addition there was a major decrease in cerebral blood flow resulting from respiratory alkalosis, it is not surprising that one would encounter paresthesias, aphasia, ataxia, mental obtundation, and seizures. The scheme in Figure 6-10 might also explain why major manifestations of hypophosphatemia are seldom observed in patients recovering from diabetic ketoacidosis. Not only is serious phosphorus deficiency rare in these patients, but also severe respiratory alkalosis is unusual.

Treatment of Hypophosphatemia

General principles of management for phosphorus deficiency in hypophosphatemia are similar to those for deficiency of many other ions or minerals. If an individual can tolerate oral administration of the supplement, it should be given by this route. Milk is an excellent source of phosphorus as well as potassium, calcium, and magnesium. Some patients with severe malnutrition may be unable to tolerate milk because of its content of lactose or fat. Skim milk may be tolerable, but in the event that it is not, one might attempt oral administration of Fleet enema solution, which is buffered sodium phosphate. The dosage is 15 to 30 ml three or four times daily. In most cases of severe hypophosphatemia, it is necessary to administer phosphate salts intravenously. One should select an intravenous preparation and become acquainted with its composition. Many commercial preparations are available (Table 6-10). The dosage should not be excessive, since hyperphosphatemia is a definite risk. Hypocalcemia and metastatic calcification with serious consequences are distinct hazards. In healthy subjects, a fall of calcium induced by phosphate infusion would

Table 6-10. Phosphate preparations for intravenous use

Preparation	Composition (mg/ml)	Phosphate (mmol/ml)	Sodium (mEq/ml)	Potassium (mEq/ml)
K phosphate	236 mg K_2HPO_4 224 mg KH_2PO_4	3.0	0	4.4
Na phosphate	142 mg Na_2HPO_4 276 mg $NaH_2PO_4 \cdot H_2O$	3.0	4.0	0
Neutral Na phosphate	10.0 mg Na_2HPO_4 2.7 mg $NaH_2PO_4 \cdot H_2O$	0.09	0.2	0
Neutral Na, K phosphate	11.5 mg Na_2HPO_4 2.6 mg KH_2PO_4	1.10	0.2	0.02

be in part corrected by release of PTH. However, if the patient also has hypomagnesemia, release of PTH would be suppressed, and in turn, hypocalcemia could conceivably become more severe and prolonged [230]. In any situation, alkalosis can potentiate the tendency for calcium phosphate formation and thereby enhance hypocalcemia.

Without phosphate treatment, approximately 73 percent of adults treated for diabetic ketoacidosis become hypocalcemic, and 55 percent become hypomagnesemic [231]. There is no evidence to indicate that the usual hypocalcemia becomes worse in patients given appropriate doses of phosphate salts. Thus, administration of intravenous phosphate in adults with diabetic ketoacidosis in doses ranging from 15 to 45 mmoles during the first 10 hours of treatment did not result in a significantly greater depression of serum calcium in those receiving phosphate than in those who did not. In a study by Keller and Berger [232], 40 to 100 mmoles of phosphate was administered to adult patients with diabetic ketoacidosis. The average serum calcium concentration fell from 9.4 to 8.3 mg/dl in those not treated with phosphate and from 8.7 to 7.8 mg/dl in those who were treated with phosphate. Based on such data, hypocalcemia occurs in the majority of patients during treatment of diabetic ketoacidosis whether phosphate is given or not. Notwithstanding this observation, large doses of phosphate supplements can aggravate hypocalcemia.

Treatment with phosphate salts in the management of diabetic ketoacidosis has become exceptionally popular in the United States. This is done because nearly all patients with diabetic ketoacidosis show a decline in serum phosphate following administration of fluids and insulin. Despite this, several studies indicate that the great majority of patients with diabetic ketoacidosis are not significantly phosphorus depleted. In addition, administration of phosphate salts to such individuals does not hasten repair of red cell metabolic compositional abnormalities [186], does not decrease insulin requirements, does not hasten recovery ketoacidosis, and finally, does not improve glucose utilization or decrease insulin requirements [232]. Clerbaux et al. [233] and Gustin et al. [234] propose that phosphate supplementation in patients with diabetic ketoacidosis may increase peripheral oxygen delivery independently of 2,3-DPG in erythrocytes. Quantitatively, the improvement was minimal. Most of these patients have been sick for only 2 or 3 days and have simply not had sufficient time to become phosphorus depleted. On the other hand, there is a small percentage of patients who experience weeks of polyuria who are able to consume large quantities of liquids because of an absence of vomiting, who because of prolonged ketoacidosis mobilize a significant portion of their cellular phosphorus content, which is then excreted into the urine. These patients may have important degrees of phosphorus deficiency at the time of admission to the hospital. They can be recognized by the combination of metabolic acidosis associated with hypophosphatemia and hypokalemia, since potassium is often lost in the urine with phosphorus. These patients can be expected to become severely hypophosphatemic, implying levels below 1 mg/dl, very promptly following initiation of fluid therapy and insulin. Such patients unquestionably require replacement of phosphate, potassium, and possibly magnesium very early in the course of their treatment to prevent complications related to specific deficiencies of these minerals and ions.

The necessity for phosphate therapy in patients undergoing long-term hyperalimentation should be determined by repeated measurements of serum phosphorus and accordingly increasing the quantity of supplemental phosphorus provided in their hyperalimentation mixture if necessary. Otherwise, such patients have been shown to become severely phosphorus depleted after a period of 8 to 12 days.

The recent demonstration by Michout and co-workers [235] and Friedlander et al. [236] that dipyridamole reduces phosphaturia in patients with proximal tubular defects possibly represents a major advance. By inhibiting adenosine uptake by proximal tubular epithelium, dipyridamole mitigates phosphaturia due to Na^+/Pi-cotransport.

References

1. Moore EW: Ionized calcium in normal serum, ultrafiltrates and whole blood determined by ion-exchange electrode. *J Clin Invest* 49:318, 1970.
2. Chen PS Jr, Neuman WF: Renal excretion of calcium by the dog. *Am J Physiol* 180:623, 1955.
3. Fordtran JS, Locklear TW: Ionic constituents and osmolality of gastric and small intestinal fluids after eating. *Am J Dig Dis* 11:503, 1966.
4. Popovtzer MM, Massry SG, Coburn WJ, et al: Calcium infusion test in chronic renal failure. *Nephron* 7:400, 1970.
5. Wills MR: Intestinal absorption of calcium. *Lancet* 1:820, 1973.
6. Wills MR, Zisman E, Worstman J, et al: The measurement of intestinal calcium absorption by external radioisotope counting: Application to study of nephrolithiasis. *Clin Sci* 39:95, 1970.
7. Borke JL, Caride A, Verma AK, et al: Cellular and segmental distribution of Ca^{++} pump epitopes in rat intestine. *Pflugers Arch* 417:120, 1990.
8. Borke JL, Penniston JT, Kumar R: Recent advances in calcium transport by the kidney. *Semin Nephrol* 10:15, 1990.
9. Gross MD, Kumar R: The physiology and biochemistry of vitamin D–dependent calcium binding proteins. *Am J Physiol* 259:F195, 1990.
10. Kumar R: Vitamin D metabolism and mechanisms of calcium transport. *J Am Soc Nephrol* 3:30, 1990.
11. LeGrimellec C, Roinel N, Morel F: Simultaneous Mg, Ca, P, K, Na and Cl analysis in rat tubular fluid: I. During perfusion of either insulin or ferrocyanide. *Pflugers Arch* 340:181, 1973.
12. Sutton RAL, Wong NLM, Quamme GA, et al: Renal tubular calcium transport: Effects of changes in filtered calcium load. *Am J Physiol* 245:515, 1983.
13. Brown EM, Pollak M, Hebert CH: Sensing of extracellular Ca^{2+} by parathyroid and kidney cells: Cloning and characterization of extracellular Ca^{2+}-sensing receptor. *Am J Kidney Dis* 25:506–513, 1995.
14. Popovtzer MM, Schainuck LI, Massry SG, et al: Divalent ion excretion in chronic kidney disease: Relation to degree of renal insufficiency. *Clin Sci* 38:297, 1970.
15. Popovtzer MM, Massry SG, Coburn JW, et al: The interrelationship between sodium, calcium and magnesium excretion in advanced renal failure. *J Lab Clin Med* 73:763, 1969.
16. Lotz M, Zisman E, Bartter FC: Evidence for a phosphorus depletion syndrome in man. *N Engl J Med* 278:409, 1968.
17. Steele TH: Dual effect of potent diuretics on renal handling of phosphate in man. *Metabolism* 20:749, 1971.
18. Lavender AR, Pullman TN: Changes in inorganic phosphate excretion induced by renal arterial infusion of calcium. *Am J Physiol* 205:1025, 1963.
19. Wong NLM, Quamme GA, Dirks JH, et al: Mechanism of the reduced proximal phosphate reabsorption during phosphate infusion. *Clin Res* 26:872A, 1978.

20. Matzner Y, Prococimer M, Polliack A, et al: Hypophosphatemia in a patient with lymphoma in leukemic phase. *Arch Intern Med* 141:805–806, 1981.
21. Dennis UW, Brazy PC: Sodium phosphate, glucose, bicarbonate and alanine interactions in the isolated proximal convoluted tubule of the rabbit kidney. *J Clin Invest* 62:387, 1978.
22. McCollum EV. The paths to the discovery of vitamins A and D. *J Nutr* 91(Suppl 1):11, 1967.
23. Brodie MJ, Boobis AR, Hillyard CJ, et al: Effect of rifampicin and isoniazid on vitamin D metabolism. *Clin Pharmacol Ther* 32:525, 1982.
24. Krapf R, Vetsch R, Netsch W: Chronic acidosis increases the serum concentration of $1,25(OH)_2$ vitamin D_3 in humans by stimulating its production. *J Clin Invest* 90:2456–2463, 1992.
25. Kumar R, Schnoes HK, DeLuca HF: Rat intestinal 25-hydroxyvitamin D_3 and $1\alpha,25$-dihydroxyvitamin D_3–24-hydroxylase. *J Biol Chem* 253:3804, 1978.
26. Kumar R: Hepatic and intestinal osteodystrophy and the hepatobiliary metabolism of vitamin D. *Ann Intern Med* 98:662, 1983.
27. Katz BS, Bell NH: The vitamin D endocrine system: Current concepts and unanswered questions. *Ital J Miner Electrol Metab* 7:231–236, 1993.
28. Matsumoto T, Igarashi C, Takenchi Y, et al: Stimulation of $1,25(OH)_2$ vitamin D_3 of in vitro mineralization by osteoblast-like (MC3T3-E) cells. *Bone* 12:27–32, 1991.
29. Popovtzer MM, Mathay R, Alfrey AC, et al: Vitamin D Deficiency Osteomalacia: Healing of the Bone Disease in the Absence of Vitamin D with Intravenous Calcium and Phosphorus Infusion. In Frame B, Parfitt AM, Duncan H (eds): *Clinical Aspects of Metabolic Bone Disease*. Amsterdam, Excerpta Medica, International Congress Series, 1973, p 382.
30. Baylink D, Wergedal J, Rich M, et al: Vitamin D–enhanced osteocytic and osteoclastic bone resorption. *Am J Physiol* 224:1345, 1973.
31. Raisz LG: Recent advances in bone cell biology: Interactions of vitamin D with other local and systemic factors. *Bone Miner* 9:191–197, 1990.
32. Russell RGG, Kanis JA, Smith R: Physiological and Pharmacological Aspects of 24,25-Dihydroxycholecalciferol in Man. In Massry SG, Ritz E, Rapado A (eds): *Homeostasis of Phosphate and Other Minerals*. New York, Plenum, 1978, pp 487–503.
33. Ornoy A: 24,25-Dihydroxyvitamin D is a metabolite of vitamin D essential for bone formation. *Nature* (London) 276:517, 1978.
34. Pavlovitch JH, Gournor-Witmer G, Bourdeau S, et al: Suppressive effects of 24,25-dihydroxycholecalciferol on bone resorption induced by acute bilateral nephrectomy in rats. *J Clin Invest* 68:803, 1981.
35. Yamato H, Matsumoto T, Okazaki R, et al: Effect of $24,25(OH)_2D_3$ on the formation and function of osteoclast. Proceedings of the 9th International Workshop of Calcified Tissues. Trends in Calcified Tissue Research. Jerusalem, 1991, p 11.
36. Popovtzer MM, Robinette JB, DeLuca HF, et al: Acute effects of 25-hydroxycholecalciferol on renal handling of phosphorus: Evidence for a parathyroid hormone dependent mechanism. *J Clin Invest* 53:913, 1974.
37. Brautbar N, Walling MW, Coburn JW: Interactions between vitamin D deficiency and phosphorus depletion in the rat. *J Clin Invest* 64:335, 1979.
38. Puschett JB, Moranz J, Kurnick WS: Evidence for a direct action of cholecalciferol and 25-hydroxycholecalciferol on the renal transport of phosphate, sodium, and calcium. *J Clin Invest* 51:373, 1972.
39. Silver J, Naveh-Many T, Mayer H, et al: Regulation by vitamin D metabolites of parathyroid hormone gene transcription in vivo in the rat. *J Clin Invest* 78:1296–1301, 1986.
40. Lopez-Hilker S, Duso AS, Rapp NS, et al: Phosphorus restriction reverses hyperparathyroidism in uremia independent of changes in calcium and calcitriol. *Am J Physiol* 28:F432–F437, 1990.
41. Aparicio M, Combe C, Lafage MH, et al: In advanced renal failure dietary phosphate restriction reverses hyperparathyroidism independent of changes in the levels of calcitriol. *Nephron* 63:122–123, 1993.
42. Fischer JA, Blum JW, Biswanger U: Acute parathyroid hormone response to epinephrine in vivo. *J Clin Invest* 52:2434, 1973.

43. Muff R, Fischer JA, Biber J, et al: Parathyroid hormone receptors in control of proximal tubule function. *Ann Rev Physiol* 54:67–79, 1992.
44. Goldring SR, Segre GV: Characterization of structural and functional properties of the cloned calcitonin and parathyroid hormone/parathyroid hormone related peptide receptors. *Ital J Miner Electrol Metab* 8:1–7, 1994.
45. Cole JA, Eber SL, Poelling RE, et al: A dual mechanism for regulation of kidney phosphate transport by parathyroid hormone. *Am J Physiol* 253:E221–E227, 1987.
46. Au WYW, Raisz LG: Restoration of parathyroid responsiveness in vitamin D–deficient rats by parenteral calcium or dietary lactose. *J Clin Invest* 46:1572, 1967.
47. Kruse K: Pathophysiology of calcium metabolism in children with vitamin D deficiency rickets. *J Pediatr* 126:736–741, 1995.
48. Sprague S, Popoutzer MM, Dranitzki-Elhalel M, et al: Parathyroid hormone induced calcium efflux from cultured calvaria is protein kinase C dependent. *Am J Physiol.* In press.
49. Amiel C, Huntziger H, Richet G: Micropuncture study of handling of phosphate by proximal and distal nephron in normal and parathyroidectomized rats: Evidence for distal reabsorption. *Pflugers Arch* 317:93, 1970.
50. Talmage RV, Kraintz RW, Buchanan GD: Effect of parathyroid extract and phosphate salts on renal calcium and phosphate excretion after parathyroidectomy. *Proc Soc Exp Biol Med* 88:600, 1955.
51. Berson SA, Yalow RS: Immunochemical heterogeneity of parathyroid hormone in plasma. *J Clin Endocrinol Metab* 28:1037, 1968.
52. Copp DH, Cockeroft DW, Kueh Y: Calcitonin from ultimobranchial glands of dogfish and chickens. *Science* 158:924, 1967.
53. Scriver CR: Rickets and the pathogenesis of impaired tubular transport of phosphate and other solutes. *Am J Med* 57:43, 1974.
54. Guise TA, Mundy GR: Clinical review 69: Evaluation of hypocalcemia in children and adults. *J Clin Endocrinol Metab* 80:1473–1478, 1995.
55. Malluche HH, Goldstein DA, Massry SG: Osteomalacia and hyperparathyroid bone disease in patients with nephrotic syndrome. *J Clin Invest* 63:494, 1979.
56. Smith R: Asian rickets and osteomalacia (editorial). *J Med* 76:899–901, 1990.
57. Arnold A, Horst SA, Gardella TJ, et al: Mutation of the signal peptide-encoding region in preproparathyroid hormone gene in familial isolated hypoparathyroidism. *J Clin Invest* 86:1084–1087, 1990.
58. Thakker RV, Davies KE, Whyte MP, et al: Mapping the gene causing X-linked recessive hypoparathyroidism to Xq26-Xq27 linkage studies. *J Clin Invest* 86:40–45, 1990.
59. Breslau NA, Moses AM, Pak CYC: Evidence for bone remodeling but lack of calcium mobilization response in parathyroid hormone in pseudohypoparathyroidism. *J Clin Endocrinol Metab* 57:638, 1983.
60. Schipani E, Weinstein LS, Bergwitz C, et al: Pseudohypoparathyroidism type Ib is not caused by mutations in the coding exons of the human parathyroid hormone (PTH)/PTH-related peptide receptor gene. *J Clin Endocrinol Metab* 80:1611–1621, 1995.
61. Drezner M, Neelon FA, Lebovitz HE: Pseudohypoparathyroidism type II: A possible defect in the reception of cyclic AMP signal. *N Engl J Med* 289:1056, 1973.
62. Nusynowitz ML, Klein MH: Pseudoidiopathic hypoparathyroidism: Hypoparathyroidism with ineffective parathyroid hormone. *Am J Med* 55:677, 1973.
63. Raskin P, McClain CJ, Medsger TA: Hypocalcemia associated with metastatic bone disease. *Arch Intern Med* 132:539, 1973.
64. Massry SG, Coburn JW, Lee DBN, et al: Skeletal resistance to parathyroid hormone in renal failure. *Ann Intern Med* 78:357, 1973.
65. Hauser CJ, Kamrath RO, Sparks J, et al: Calcium homeostasis in patients with acute pancreatitis. *Surgery* 94:830, 1983.
66. Fanconi G, Prader A: Transient congenital idiopathic hypoparathyroidism. *Helv Paediatr Acta* 22:342, 1967.
67. Fairney A, Jackson D, Clayton BE: Measurement of serum parathyroid hormone with particular reference to some infants with hypocalcemia. *Arch Dis Child* 48:419, 1973.

68. Rosen JF, et al: 25-Hydroxyvitamin D: Plasma levels in mothers and their premature infants with neonatal hypocalcemia. *Am J Dis Child* 127:220, 1974.
69. Johnston CC, Lavy N, Lord T, et al: Osteopetrosis: A clinical, genetic, metabolic and morphologic study of the dominantly inherited, benign form. *Medicine* (Baltimore) 47:149, 1968.
70. Key L, Carnes S, et al: Treatment of congenital osteopetrosis with high-dose calcitriol. *N Engl J Med* 310:409, 1984.
71. Key LL, Rodriguiz RM, Willi SM, et al: Long-term treatment of osteopetrosis with recombinant human interferon gamma. *N Engl J Med* 332:1594–1599, 1995.
72. Gessner BD, Beller M, Middaugh JL, et al: Acute fluoride poisoning from public water system. *N Engl J Med* 330:95–99, 1994.
73. Jacobson MA, Gambertoglio JG, Aweeka FT, et al: Foscarnet-induced hypocalcemia and effects of foscarnet on calcium metabolism. *J Clin Endocrinol Metab* 72:1130–1135, 1991.
74. McCarron DA: Low serum concentration of ionized calcium in patients with hypertension. *N Engl J Med* 307:226, 1982.
75. Minkin C: Inhibition of parathyroid hormone stimulated bone resorption in vitro by the antibiotic mithramycin. *Calcif Tissue Res* 13:249, 1973.
76. Robins PR, Jowsey J: Effect of mithramycin on normal and abnormal bone turnover. *J Lab Clin Med* 82:576, 1973.
77. Gittes RF, Radde IC: Experimental model for hyperparathyroidism: Effect of excessive numbers of transplanted isologous parathyroid glands. *J Urol* 95:595, 1966.
78. Lloyd HM: Primary hyperparathyroidism: An analysis of the role of the parathyroid tumor. *Medicine* (Baltimore) 47:53, 1968.
79. Broadus AG, Horst RL, Lang R, et al: The importance of circulating 1,25(OH)$_2$ vitamin D$_3$ in the pathogenesis of hypercalciuric and renal stone formation in primary hyperparathyroidism. *N Engl J Med* 302:421, 1980.
80. Krementz ET, et al: The first 100 cases of parathyroid tumor from Charity Hospital of Louisiana. *Ann Surg* 173:872, 1971.
81. Arnold A, Kim HG, Gaz RD, et al: Molecular cloning and chromosomal mapping of DNA rearranged within the parathyroid hormone gene in parathyroid adenoma. *J Clin Invest* 83:2034–2040, 1989.
82. Arnold A, Brown MF, Urena P, et al: Monoclonality of parathyroid tumors in chronic renal failure and in primary parathyroid hyperplasia. *J Clin Invest* 95:2047–2053, 1995.
83. Thakker RV, Boulox P, Wooding C, et al: Association of parathyroid tumors in multiple endocrine neoplasia type I with loss of alleles on chromosome 11. *N Engl J Med* 321:218–224, 1989.
84. Consensus Development Conference Panel. Diagnosis and management of asymptomatic primary hyperparathyroidism: Consensus Development Conference statement. *Ann Intern Med* 114:593–597, 1991.
85. Marx SJ, Spiegel AM, Levine ML, et al: Familial hypocalciuric hypercalcemia. *N Engl J Med* 307:416, 1982.
86. Janicic N, Pansova Z, Cole DEC, et al: Insertion of ALU sequence in the Ca^{2+}-sensing receptor gene in familial hypocalciuric hypercalcemia and neonatal severe hyperparathyroidism. *Am J Hum Genet* 56:880–886, 1995.
87. Broadus AE, Mangin M, Ikeda K, et al: Humoral hypercalcemia of cancer: Identification of a novel parathyroid hormone-like peptide. *N Engl J Med* 319:556, 1988.
88. Yoshimoto K, Yamasaki R, Sakai H, et al: Ectopic production of parathyroid hormone by small cell lung cancer in a patient with hypercalcemia. *J Clin Endocrinol Metab* 68:976–981, 1989.
89. Nusbaum SR, Gaz RD, Arnold A: Hypercalcemia and ectopic secretion of parathyroid hormone by an ovarian carcinoma with rearrangement of the gene for parathyroid hormone. *N Engl J Med* 323:1324–1329, 1990.
90. Bleizikian JP: Parathyroid hormone–related peptide in sickness and health. *N Engl J Med* 322:1151–1153, 1990.
91. Matsushita H, Hara M, Honda K, et al: Inhibition of parathyroid hormone–related protein release by extracellular calcium in dispersed cells from human parathyroid hyperplasia secondary to chronic renal failure and adenoma. *Am J Pathol* 146:1521–1528, 1995.

92. Cox M, Haddad JG: Lymphoma, hypercalcemia and the sunshine vitamin. *Ann Intern Med* 21:709–712, 1994.
93. Mundy GR: Hypercalcemia of malignancy revisited. *J Clin Invest* 82:1–6, 1988.
94. Walls J, Bundred N, Howell A: Hypercalcemia and bone resorption in malignancy. *Clin Orthop Rel Res* 312:51–63, 1995.
95. Mundy GR, Toshiyuki Y: Facilitation and suppression of bone metastasis. *Clin Orthop Rel Res* 312:34–44, 1995.
96. Orr FW, Sanchez-Sweatman OH, Kostenuik P, et al: Tumor-bone interactions in skeletal metastasis. *Clin Orthop Rel Res* 312:19–33, 1995.
97. Houston SJ, Rubens RD: The systemic treatment of bone metastases. *Clin Orthop Rel Res* 312:95–104, 1995.
98. Beckman MJ, Johnson JA, Goff JL, et al: The role of dietary calcium in the physiology of vitamin D toxicity: Excess dietary vitamin D_3 blunts parathyroid hormone induction of kidney 1-hydroxylase. *Arch Biochem Biophys* 319:535–539, 1995.
99. Berl T, Berns AS, Huffer WE, et al: 1,25-Dihydroxycholecalciferol effects in chronic dialysis. *Ann Intern Med* 88:774, 1978.
100. Fisher G, Skillern PG: Hypercalcemia due to hypervitaminosis A. *JAMA* 227:1413, 1974.
101. Frame B, Jackson CE, Reynolds WA, et al: Hypercalcemia and skeletal effects in chronic hypervitaminosis A. *Ann Intern Med* 80:44, 1974.
102. Valentic JP, Elias AN, Weinstein GD: Hypercalcemia associated with oral isotretinoin in the treatment of severe acne. *JAMA* 250:1899, 1983.
103. Jowsey J, Riggs BL: Bone changes in a patient with hypervitaminosis A. *J Clin Endocrinol Metab* 28:1833, 1968.
104. Renier M, Sjurdsson G, Nunziata V, et al: Abnormal calcium metabolism in normocalcemic sarcoidosis. *Br Med J* 2:1473, 1976.
105. Mayock RL, et al: Manifestations of sarcoidosis: Analysis of 145 patients with review of nine series selected from literature. *Am J Med* 35:67, 1963.
106. Bell NH, Bartter FC: Transient reversal of hyperabsorption of calcium and of abnormal sensitivity to vitamin D in a patient with sarcoidosis during episode of nephritis. *Ann Intern Med* 61:702, 1964.
107. Anderson J, Dent CE, Harper C, et al: Effect of cortisone on calcium metabolism in sarcoidosis with hypercalcemia: Possible antagonistic actions of cortisone and vitamin D. *Lancet* 2:720, 1954.
108. Bell NH, Stern PH, Pantzer E, et al: Evidence that increased circulating 1α,25-dihydroxyvitamin D is the probable cause for abnormal calcium metabolism in sarcoidosis. *J Clin Invest* 64:218, 1979.
109. Bleizikian JP: Management of acute hypercalcemia. *N Engl J Med* 326:1196–1203, 1992.
110. Adams JS, Sharma OP, Gacad MA et al: Metabolism of 25-hydroxyvitamin D_3 by cultured pulmonary alveolar macrophages in sarcoidosis. *J Clin Invest* 72:1856, 1983.
111. Occasional survey: Calcium metabolism and bone in hyperthyroidism. *Lancet* 2:1300, 1970.
112. Baxter JD, Bondy PK: Hypercalcemia of thyrotoxicosis. *Ann Intern Med* 65:429, 1966.
113. Adams P, Jowsey J: Bone and mineral metabolism in hyperthyroidism: An experimental study. *Endocrinology* 81:735, 1967.
114. Jorgensen H: Hypercalcemia in adrenocortical insufficiency. *Acta Med Scand* 193:175, 1973.
115. Pedersen KO: Hypercalcaemia in Addison's disease: Report on 2 cases and review of literature. *Acta Med Scand* 181:691, 1967.
116. Lightwood R: Idiopathic hypercalcemia with failure to thrive. *Proc R Soc Med* 45:401, 1952.
117. O'Brien D: Idiopathic hypercalcaemia of infancy. *Pediatrics* 23:640, 1959.
118. Garabedian M, Jacoz E, Guillozo H, et al: Elevated plasma $1,25(OH)_2$ vitamin D_3 concentration in infants with hypercalcemia and an elfin facies. *N Engl J Med* 312:948–952, 1985.
119. Winters JL, Kleinschmidt AG, Frensili JJ, et al: Hypercalcemia complicating imobilization in treatment of fractures. *J Bone Joint Surg [Br]* 48A:1182, 1966.
120. Russell RGG, Bisaz S, Donath A, et al: Inorganic pyrophosphate in plasma in normal persons and in patients with hypophosphatasia, osteogenesis imperfecta, and other disorders of bone. *J Clin Invest* 50:961, 1971.

121. McMillan DE, Freeman RB: The milk alkali syndrome: A study of the acute disorder with comments on the development of the chronic condition. *Medicine* (Baltimore) 44:485, 1965.
122. Sevitt LH, Wrong OM: Hypercalcemia from calcium resin in patients with chronic renal failure. *Lancet* 2:950, 1968.
123. Chertow BS, Plymate SR, Becker FO: Vitamin D resistant idiopathic hypoparathyroidism: Acute hypercalcemia during acute renal failure. *Arch Intern Med* 133:838, 1974.
124. deTorrente A, Berl T, Cohn PD, et al: Hypercalcemia of acute renal failure. *Am J Med* 61: 119, 1976.
125. Farfel Z, Bourne HR: Deficient activity of receptor-cyclase coupling protein in platelets of patients with pseudohypoparathyroidism. *J Clin Endocrinol Metab* 51:1202, 1980.
126. Parfitt AM: The interactions of thiazide diuretics with parathyroid hormone and vitamin D: Studies in patients with hypoparathyroidism. *J Clin Invest* 51:1879, 1972.
127. Popovtzer MM, Subryan VL, Alfrey AC, et al: The acute effect of chlorothiazide on serum ionized calcium: Evidence for a parathyroid hormone dependent mechanism. *J Clin Invest* 55:1295, 1975.
128. Anthony LB, May ME, Oates JA: Case report: Lanreotide in the management of hypercalcemia of malignancy. *Am J Med Sci* 309:312–314, 1995.
129. Griffin JE, Zerwekh, JE: Impaired stimulation of 25(OH) vitamin D–24-hydroxylase in fibroblasts from a patient with vitamin D–dependent rickets type II: A form of receptor positive resistance of 1,25-dihydroxyvitamin D$_3$. *J Clin Invest* 72:1190, 1983.
130. Eil C, Liberman UA, Rosen JF, et al: A cellular defect in hereditary vitamin D dependent rickets type II: Defective nuclear uptake of 1,25(OH)$_2$ vitamin D in cultured skin fibroblasts. *N Engl J Med* 304:1588, 1981.
131. Silver J, Popovtzer MM: Hypercalcemia with elevated dihydroxycholecalciferol levels and hypercalciuria. *Arch Intern Med* 194:162, 1984.
132. Malloy PJ, Hochberg Z, Tiosano D, et al: The molecular basis of hereditary 1,25(OH)$_2$ vitamin D$_3$ resistant rickets in seven families. *J Clin Invest* 86:2071–2079, 1990.
133. Glorieux F, Scriver CR: Loss of parathyroid hormone sensitive component of phosphate transport in X-linked hypophosphatemia. *Science* 175:997, 1972.
134. Short EM, Binder HJ, Rosenberg LE: Familial hypophosphatemic rickets, defective transport of inorganic phosphate by intestinal mucosa. *Science* 179:700, 1973.
135. Marie PJ, Travers R, Glorieux FH: Healing of rickets with phosphate supplementation in the hypophosphatemic male mouse. *J Clin Invest* 67:911, 1981.
136. Weidner N: Review and update: Oncogenic osteomalacia-rickets. *Ultrastruct Pathol* 15: 317–333, 1991.
137. Popovtzer MM: Tumor-induced hypophosphatemic osteomalacia: Evidence for a phosphaturic cyclic AMP independent action of tumor extract. *Clin Res* 29:418A, 1981.
138. Wilins GE, Granleese G, Hegele RG, et al: Oncogenic osteomalacia: Evidence for a humoral phosphaturic factor. *J Clin Endocrinol Metab* 80:1628–1634, 1995.
139. Cai Q, Hodgson SF, Kao PC, et al: Brief report: Inhibition of renal phosphate transport by a tumor product in a patient with oncogenic osteomalacia. *N Engl J Med* 330:1645–1649, 1994.
140. Scriver CR, McDonald W, Reade T: Hypophosphatemic nonrachitic bone disease: An entity distinct from X-linked hypophosphatemia in the renal defect, bone involvement and inheritance. *Am J Med Genet* 1:101, 1977.
141. Tieder M, Modai D, Samuel R, et al: Hereditary hypophosphatemic rickets with hypercalciuria. *N Engl J Med* 312:611–617, 1985.
142. Kooh SW, Fraser D, Reilly BJ, et al: Rickets due to calcium deficiency. *N Engl J Med* 297: 1264, 1977.
143. Marie PJ, Plettiform JM, Ross P, et al: Histological osteomalacia due to dietary calcium deficiency in children. *N Engl J Med* 307:584, 1982.
144. Fanconi G: Tubular insufficiency and renal dwarfism. *Arch Dis Child* 29:1, 1954.
145. Hossain M: The osteomalacia syndrome after colocystoplasty: A cure with sodium bicarbonate alone. *Br J Urol* 42:243, 1970.
146. Richard P, Chamberlain MJ, Wrong OM: Treatment of osteomalacia of renal tubular acidosis by sodium bicarbonate alone. *Lancet* 2:994, 1972.

147. Ott SM, Maloney NA, Coburn JW, et al: The prevalence of bone aluminum deposition in renal osteodystrophy and its relation to the response to calcitriol therapy. *N Engl J Med* 307: 709, 1982.

148. Shike M, Sturtridge WC, Taur CS, et al: A possible role of vitamin D in the genesis of parenteral-nutrition-induced metabolic bone disease. *Ann Intern Med* 95:560, 1981.

149. Klein GL, Horst RL, Norman AW, et al: Reduced serum level of 1-alpha, 25-dihydroxyvitamin D during long-term total parenteral nutrition. *Ann Intern Med* 94:638, 1981.

150. Ott SM, Maloney NA, Klein GL, et al: Aluminum is associated with low bone formation in patients receiving parenteral nutrition. *Ann Intern Med* 98:910, 1983.

151. Chestnut CH: Theoretical overview: Bone development, peak bone mass, bone loss and fracture risk. *Am J Med* 91:25–95, 1991.

152. Kohlmeier S, Marcus R: Calcium disorders of pregnancy. *Endocrinol Metab Clin North Am* 24:15–39, 1995.

153. Manolagas SC, Julka RL: Bone marrow, cytokines, and bone remodelling: Emerging insights into the pathophysiology of osteoporosis. *N Engl J Med* 332:305–311, 1995.

154. Girasole G, Jilka RL, Passeri G, et al: 17β-Estradiol interleukin-6 production by bone marrow–derived stromal cells and osteoblasts in vitro: A potential mechanism for the antiosteoporotic effect of estrogens. *J Clin Invest* 89:883–891, 1992.

155. Morrison NA, Qi JC, Tokita A, et al: Prediction of bone density from vitamin D receptor alleles. *Nature* 367:284–287, 1994.

156. Spector TD, Keen RW, Arden NK, et al: Vitamin D receptor gene alleles and bone density in postmenopausal women: A UK twin study. *J Bone Miner Res* 9:S143, 1994.

157. Belchetz PE: Hormonal treatment of postmenopausal women. *N Engl J Med* 15:1062–1071, 1994.

158. Rodan GA, Seedor JG, Balena R, et al: Preclinical pharmacology of alendronate. *Osteoporosis Int* 3(Suppl 3):S7–S12, 1993.

159. Carano A, Teitelbaum SL, Knosek JD, et al: Biphosphonates directly inhibit the bone resorption activity in isolated avian osteoclasts in vitro. *J Clin Invest* 85:456–461, 1990.

160. Kleerekoper M: Osteoporosis and the primary care physician: Time to bone up. *Ann Intern Med* 123:466–467, 1995.

161. Pak CYC, Sakhaee K, Adams-Huet B, et al: Treatment of postmenopausal osteoporosis with slow-release sodium fluoride. *Ann Intern Med* 123:401–408, 1995.

162. Liu SH, Chu HI: Studies of calcium and phosphorus metabolism with special reference to pathogenesis and effects of dihydrotachysterol (AT 10) and iron. *Medicine* (Baltimore) 22: 103, 1943.

163. Llach F: Secondary hyperparathyroidism in renal failure: The trade-off hypothesis revisited. *Am J Kidney Dis* 25:663–679, 1995.

164. Stanbury SW, Lumb GA: Metabolic studies on renal osteodystrophy. *Medicine* (Baltimore) 41:1, 1962.

165. Korkor AB: Reduced binding of [^{3}H]-1,25(OH)$_2$D$_3$ in parathyroid glands of patients with renal failure. *N Engl J Med* 316:1573–1577, 1987.

166. Arnold A, Brown MF, Urena P, et al: Monoclonality of parathyroid tumors in chronic renal failure and in primary hyperparathyroid hyperplasia. *J Clin Invest* 95:2047–2053, 1995.

167. Popovtzer MM, Pinggera WF, Robinette JB: Successful conservative management of the clinical consequences of uremic secondary hyperparathyroidism. *JAMA* 231:960, 1975.

168. Popovtzer MM, Pinggera WF, Hutt MP, et al: Serum parathyroid hormone levels and renal handling of phosphorus in patients with chronic renal disease. *J Clin Endocrinol Metab* 35: 213, 1972.

169. Slatopolsky E, Weerts C, Thielan J, et al: Marked suppression of secondary hyperparathyroidism by intravenous administration of 1,25(OH)$_2$ vitamin D$_3$ in uremic patients. *J Clin Invest* 74:2136–2143, 1984.

170. Andress DL, Norris KC, Coburn JW, et al: Intravenous calcitriol in the treatment of refractory osteitis fibrosa in chronic renal failure. *N Engl J Med* 321:274–279, 1989.

171. Quarles LD, Yohay DA, Carroll BA, et al: Prospective trial of pulse oral versus intravenous calcitriol treatment of hyperparathyroidism in ESRD. *Kidney Int* 45:1710–1721, 1994.

172. Popovtzer MM, Levi J, Bar-Khayim Y, et al: Assessment of combined $24,25(OH)_2D_3$ and $1\alpha(OH)D_3$ therapy for bone disease in dialysis patients. *Bone* 13:369–377, 1992.

173. Andress DL, Maloney NA, Endres DB, et al: Aluminum-associated bone disease in chronic renal failure: High prevalence in a long term dialysis population. *J Bone Miner Res* 1:391–398, 1986.

174. Hercz G, Pei Y, Greenwood C, et al: Aplastic osteodystrophy without aluminum: The role of "suppressed" parathyroid function. *Kidney Int* 44:860–866, 1993.

175. Goodman WG, Ramirez JA, Beilin TR, et al: Development of adynamic bone in patients with secondary hyperparathyroidism after intermittent calcitriol therapy. *Kidney Int* 46:1160–1166, 1944.

176. Popovtzer MM, Backenroth-Maayan R, Elhalel-Dranitzki M, et al: Recurrence of tumoral calcinosis after kidney transplantation: Evidence against an intrinsic defect of tubular phosphate reabsorption (abstract). *J Am Soc Nephrol* 6:954, 1995.

177. Sprague SM, Popovtzer MM: Is β_2-microglobulin a mediator of bone disease. *Kidney Int* 47:1–6, 1995.

178. Econs MJ, Drezman MK: Tumor-induced osteomalacia: Unveiling a new hormone (editorial). *N Engl J Med* 330:1679–1681, 1994.

179. Woods HF, Eggleston LV, Krebs HA: The cause of hepatic accumulation of fructose-1-phosphate on fructose loading. *Biochem J* 119:501, 1970.

180. Agarwal R, Knochel JP: Fluid and Electrolyte Disorders Associated with Chronic Alcoholism and Liver Disease. In Kokko JP, Tannen RL (eds): *Fluids and Electrolytes*. Philadelphia, Saunders, in press.

181. Silvis SE, Paragas PD: Paresthesias, weakness, seizures and hypophosphatemia in patients receiving hyperalimentation. *Gastroenterology* 62:513, 1972.

182. Mostellar ME, Tuttle EP Jr: Effects of alkalosis on plasma concentration and urinary excretion of inorganic phosphate in man. *J Clin Invest* 43:138, 1964.

183. Guest GM, Rapoport S: Rise of acid-soluble phosphorus compounds in red blood cells. *Am J Dis Child* 58:1072, 1939.

184. Taylor DJ, Cooper SW, Cadoux-Hudson TA: Effect of insulin on intracellular pH and phosphate metabolism in human skeletal muscle in vitro. *Clin Sci* 81:123–128, 1991.

185. Seldin DW, Tarail R: The metabolism of glucose and electrolytes in diabetic acidosis. *J Clin Invest* 29:552, 1950.

186. Kono N, Kuwajima M, Tarui S: Alteration of glycolytic intermediary metabolism in erythrocytes during diabetic ketoacidosis and its recovery phase. *Diabetes* 30:346–353, 1981.

187. Kalbfleisch JM, Lindeman RD, Ginn HE, et al: The effects of ethanol administration on urinary excretion of magnesium and other electrolytes in alcoholic and normal subjects. *J Clin Invest* 42:1471, 1963.

188. Flink EB: Mineral Metabolism in Alcoholism. In Kissin B, Gegleiter H (eds): *The Biology of Alcoholism*. Vol. 1, Biochemistry. New York, Plenum, 1971.

189. Peterson VP: Metabolic studies in clinical magnesium depletion. *J Clin Invest* 42:305, 1963.

190. Whang R, Welt LG: Observations in experimental magnesium depletion. *J Clin Invest* 42:305, 1963.

191. Shils ME: Experimental production of magnesium deficiency in man. *Ann NY Acad Sci* 162:846, 1969.

192. DeMarchi S, Cecchin E, Basile A, et al: Renal tubular dysfunction in chronic alcohol abuse: Effects of abstinence. *N Engl J Med* 329:1927–1934, 1993.

193. Blachley JD, Ferguson ER, Carter NW, et al: Chronic alcohol ingestion induces phosphorus deficiency and myopathy in the dog. *Trans Assoc Am Physicians* 93:110, 1980.

194. Ra'anani P, Lahav M, Prokocimer M, et al: Life threatening hypophosphataemia in a patient with Philadelphia chromosome–positive chronic myelogenous leukaemia in acute blastic crisis. *Postgrad Med J* 68:283–286, 1992.

195. Kajikawa M, Nonami T, Kurokawa T, et al: Recombinant human erythropoietin and hypophosphatemia in patients with cirrhosis. *Lancet* 341:503–504, 1993.

196. McElhenny BE, Todd DJ, McCance D, et al: Erythrodermic psoriasis: Report of a case associated with symptomatic hypophosphataemia. *Clin Exp Dermatol* 18:167–168, 1993.

197. Wilkie DR: Profound hypophosphatemia in patients collapsing after a "fun run." *Br Med J* 292:692, 1986.
198. Dale G, Fleetwood JA: Profound hypophosphatemia in patients collapsing after a "fun run." *Br Med J* 292:447–448, 1986.
199. D'Erasmo E, Acca M, Celi FS: A hospital survey of hypocalcemia and hypophosphatemia in malignancy. *Tumor* 177:311–314, 1991.
200. Kaysar N, Kronenberg J, Polliack M, et al: Severe hypophosphataemia during binge eating in anorexia nervosa. *Arch Dis Child* 66:138–139, 1991.
201. Srinivasagam D, Seshadri MS, Peter JV, et al: Prevalence and pathogenesis of hypophosphatemia in ventilated patients. *Indian J Med Res* 96:87–90, 1992.
202. George R, Shiu MH: Hypophosphatemia after major hepatic resection. *Surgery* 111:281–286, 1992.
203. Davis TM, Pukrittayakamee S, Woodhead JS, et al: Calcium and phosphate metabolism in acute falciparum malaria. *Clin Sci* 81:217–304, 1991.
204. Sweeney LE: Hypophosphataemic rickets after ifosfamide treatment in children. *Clin Radiol* 47:345–347, 1993.
205. Jacob HS, Amsden P: Acute hemolytic anemia with rigid red cells in hypophosphatemia. *N Engl J Med* 285:1446, 1971.
206. Klock JC, Williams HE, Mentzer WC: Hemolytic anemia and somatic cell dysfunction in severe hypophosphatemia. *Arch Intern Med* 134:360, 1974.
207. Craddock PR, Yawata Y, Van Santen L, et al: Acquired phagocyte dysfunction: A complication of the hypophosphatemia of parenteral hyperalimentation. *N Engl J Med* 290:1403, 1974.
208. Garner GB, Heubner PF, O'Dell BL: Dietary phosphorus and salmonellosis in guinea pigs. *Fed Proc* 26:799, 1967.
209. Yawata Y, Hebbel RP, Silvis S, et al: Blood cell abnormalities complicating the hypophosphatemia of hyperalimentation: Erythrocytes and platelet ATP deficiency associated with hemolytic anemia and bleeding in hyperalimented dogs. *J Lab Clin Med* 84:643, 1974.
210. Knochel JP, Montanari A: Central Nervous System Manifestations of Hypophosphatemia and Phosphorus Depletion. In Arieff A, Griggs RC (eds): *Metabolic Brain Dysfunction in Systemic Disorders.* Boston, Little, Brown, 1992, pp 183–204.
211. Knochel JP, Bilbrey GL, Fuller TJ, et al: The muscle cell in chronic alcoholism: The possible role of phosphate depletion in alcoholic myopathy. *Ann NY Acad Sci* 252:274, 1975.
212. Knochel JP: Hypophosphatemia and rhabdomyolysis. *Am J Med* 92:455–477, 1992.
213. Ferguson ER, Blachley JD, Carter NW, et al: Derangements of muscle composition, ion transport and oxygen consumption in chronically alcoholic dogs. *Am J Physiol* 246(Renal Fluid Electrolyte Physiol):F700–F709, 1984.
214. Fuller TJ, Nochols WW, Brenner BJ, et al: Reversible depression in myocardial performance in dogs with experimental phosphorus deficiency. *J Clin Invest* 62:1194, 1978.
215. Knochel JP, Barcenas C, Cotton JR, et al: Hypophosphatemia and rhabdomyolysis. *J Clin Invest* 63:1240, 1978.
216. Dominguez JH, Gray RW, Lemann J Jr: Dietary phosphate deprivation in women and men: Effects on mineral and acid balances, parathyroid hormone and the metabolism of 25-OH-vitamin D. *J Clin Endocrinol Metab* 43:1056, 1976.
217. Gold LW, Massry SG, Arieff AI, et al: Renal bicarbonate wasting during phosphate depletion: A possible cause of altered acid-base homeostasis in hyperparathyroidism. *J Clin Invest* 52:2556, 1973.
218. Kohaut EC, Klish WJ, Beachler CW, et al: Reduced renal acid excretion in malnutrition: A result of phosphate depletion. *Am J Clin Nutr* 30:861, 1977.
219. Emmett M, Goldfarb S, Agus ZS, et al: The pathophysiology of acid-base changes in chronically phosphate-depleted rats: Bone-kidney interactions. *J Clin Invest* 59:291, 1977.
220. Aubier M, Murciano D, Lecogguic Y, et al: Effect of hypophosphatemia on diaphragmatic contractility in patients with acute respiratory failure. *N Engl J Med* 313:420–423, 1985.
221. Newman JH, Neff TA, Ziporin P: Acute respiratory failure associated with hypophosphatemia. *N Engl J Med* 296:1101–1103, 1973.
222. Laaban JP, Grateau G, Psychoyos I, et al: Hypophosphatemia induced by mechanical ventila-

tion in patients with chronic obstructive pulmonary disease. *Crit Care Med* 17:1115–1120, 1989.

223. Fiaccadori E, Coffrini E, Frachia C, et al: Hypophosphatemia and phosphorus depletion in respiratory and peripheral muscles of patients with respiratory failure due to COPD. *Chest* 105:1392–1398, 1994.

224. Frank BW, Kern F Jr: Serum inorganic phosphorus during hepatic coma. *Arch Intern Med* 110:865, 1962.

225. Knochel JP: Does hypophosphatemia play a role in acute liver failure? (editorial). *Hepatology* 9:504–505, 1989.

226. Miller PD, Heinig RE, Waterhouse C: Treatment of alcoholic acidosis: The role of dextrose and phosphorus. *Arch Intern Med* 138:67, 1978.

227. Weintraub MI: Hypophosphatemia mimicking acute Guillain-Barré-Strohol syndrome: A complication of parenteral hyperalimentation. *JAMA* 235:1040, 1972.

228. Baertl JM, Sancetta SM, Gabuzda GJ: Relation of acute potassium depletion to renal ammonium metabolism in patients with cirrhosis. *J Clin Invest* 42:696, 1963.

229. Victor M: The role of hypomagnesemia and respiratory alkalosis in the genesis of alcohol-withdrawal symptoms. *Ann NY Acad Sci* 215:235, 1973.

230. Rude RK, Oldham SB, Singer FR: Functional hypoparathyroidism and parathyroid hormone end-organ resistance in human magnesium deficiency. *Clin Endocrinol* 5:209, 1976.

231. Zipf WB, Bacon GE, Spencer ML, et al: Hypocalcemia, hypomagnesemia, and transient hypoparathyroidism during therapy with potassium phosphate in diabetic ketoacidosis. *Diabetes Care* 2:264, 1979.

232. Keller U, Berger W: Prevention of hypophosphatemia by phosphate infusion during treatment of diabetic ketoacidosis and hyperosmolar coma. *Diabetes* 29:87, 1979.

233. Clerbaux T, Reynaert M, Willems E, et al: Effect of phosphate on oxygen-hemoglobin affinity, diphosphoglycerate and blood gases during recovery from diabetic ketoacidosis. *Intens Care Med* 15:195–498, 1989.

234. Gustin P, Detry B, Cao ML, et al: Chloride and inorganic phosphate modulate binding of oxygen to bovine red blood cells. *J Appl Physiol* 77:202–208, 1994.

235. Michout P, Prie D, Amiel C, et al: Dipyramidole for renal phosphate leak? (letter). *N Engl J Med* 331:58–59, 1994.

236. Friedlander G, Couette S, Coureau C, et al: Mechanisms whereby extracellular adenosine 3′,5′-monophosphate inhibits phosphate transport in cultured opossum kidney cells and in rat kidney. *J Clin Invest* 90:848–858, 1992.

7

Normal and Abnormal Magnesium Metabolism

Allen C. Alfrey

Magnesium is the fourth most common cation in the human body, and it plays a critical role in many metabolic processes, including production and utilization of the energy that is essential in the maintenance of normal intracellular electrolyte composition. Magnesium is also necessary for a large number of enzymatic actions relating to the basic protein-synthesizing mechanisms. Extracellular magnesium is also broadly implicated in neuromuscular transmission and cardiovascular tone.

Cellular and extracellular magnesium concentrations are carefully regulated by the gastrointestinal tract, kidney, and bone. Several clinical disorders of magnesium metabolism have been well defined during the last two decades. Gastrointestinal losses and renal magnesium wasting constitute the major general causes of magnesium deficiency and hypomagnesemia. Hypermagnesemia occurs with excessive magnesium administration, particularly when renal function is reduced. In spite of the fact that a number of clinical disorders of magnesium metabolism have been well defined, these disturbances are still commonly overlooked. Whang and Ryder [1] found that of 1033 serum samples submitted for electrolyte determinations, only on 7.4 percent of the samples were magnesium determination requested. Furthermore, on analyzing all of these samples for magnesium levels, it was found that only 10 percent of hypomagnesemic and 13 percent of hypermagnesemic samples were identified by physician-initiated requests for this analyte.

Normal Magnesium Metabolism

The average daily diet in North America contains approximately 20 to 30 mEq (240–360 mg) of elemental magnesium [2]. The requirement for magnesium is considered to be about 18 to 33 mEq/day for young men and 15 to 28 mEq/day for women. This suggests that the average North American diet is only marginally adequate for maintenance of magnesium levels in healthy adults. Moreover, the requirements are higher during the rapid growth in infancy and adolescence and during pregnancy and lactation. Magnesium is ubiquitous in our diet and is especially abundant in green vegetables rich in chlorophyll (a chelator of magnesium), as

320

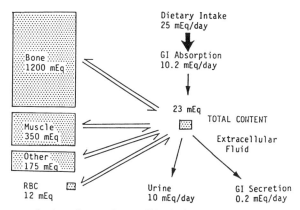

Fig. 7-1. Schematic display of normal overall body homeostasis of magnesium, including an approximate distribution in different tissues. GI = gastrointestinal; RBC = red blood cells.

well as in seafood, grains, nuts, and meats [2]. Under normal circumstances, the gastrointestinal tract and the kidney closely maintain magnesium balance (Fig. 7-1). It has been suggested that a minimum intake of magnesium required to maintain a positive balance in the body is approximately 0.3 mEq/kg/day.

Serum magnesium in healthy persons is closely maintained within a normal range of 1.40 to 1.75 mEq/L (0.8–0.9 mmol/L). Only 20 percent of the serum magnesium is protein-bound, in contrast to calcium, which is 40 percent bound to serum proteins. Variations of plasma protein concentration therefore have less effect on serum magnesium than on calcium concentration.

Only about 2 percent of the 21 to 28 g (1750–2400 mEq) of magnesium present in the adult human body is in the extracellular fluid (ECF) compartment [3]. The principal cellular stores of magnesium in the body are bone (67%) and muscle (20%) (see Fig. 7-1). Normal muscle has 76 mEq of magnesium per kilogram of fat-free solids, and much of this is complexed to intracellular organic phosphate and proteins [3]. The normal magnesium level in red blood cells is about 4.6 mEq/L, of which 84 percent is thought to be complexed to adenosine triphosphate (ATP). The magnesium content of erythrocytes appears to be inversely related to the age of the cell, with the reticulocytes containing about two times more magnesium than older red blood cells. As noted, bone is the principal source of magnesium. The normal calcium-to-magnesium ratio in bone is 50:1, with the ratio in trabecular bone being consistently higher than that in cortical bone. The major portion of magnesium is complexed with apatite crystal rather than bone matrix. Approximately 30 percent of bone magnesium is present as a surface-limited ion on the bone crystal, and this is freely exchangeable [4, 5]. However, considerable uncertainty exists with regard to the ease of exchangeability of magnesium with its cellular source [4]. Intracellular to extracellular distribution of magnesium is dissimilar to that of potassium. Minute changes in extracellular potassium rapidly result in changes in intracellular potassium concentration in muscle. Such shifts do not occur with magnesium, as magnesium is bound to intracellular ligands and is not readily available for exchange in muscle. Less than 15 percent of muscle and erythrocyte magnesium is thought to be exchangeable [6].

In summary, bone and muscle cells are the major intracellular magnesium pools in humans, of which only a small fraction is exchangeable with the ECF.

Gastrointestinal Absorption of Magnesium

About 30 to 40 percent of the normal dietary intake of magnesium is absorbed by the gastrointestinal tract. The fraction of magnesium absorbed may increase to as high as 80 percent when the dietary magnesium intake is restricted to as low as 2 mEq/day and may decrease to 25 percent at high magnesium intakes of 45 mEq/day or greater. Thus, magnesium absorption by the gut varies inversely with intake. Magnesium absorption in humans and animals occurs primarily in the more distal portion of the small intestine, namely the jejunum and ileum [7]. The intestinal magnesium absorption appears to occur down an electrochemical gradient through either transcellular or paracellular pathways. In the transcellular absorption, magnesium crosses the brush border of the intestinal cell down an electrochemical gradient; this appears to be facilitated by a carrier with a limited transport rate. The movement across the basolateral membrane involves an active transport system. In the paracellular pathway, magnesium is absorbed because of the positive magnesium chemical gradient across the paracellular channels. Magnesium absorption is also affected by paracellular water reabsorption. Bowel water absorption will affect magnesium concentration and absorption, and prolonged diarrhea results in an intestinal malabsorption of magnesium.

The control of intestinal magnesium absorption is not well understood. Most studies have suggested that vitamin D has little effect on magnesium absorption [8]. A study carried out in vitamin D–deficient patients showed that magnesium absorption was only minimally reduced prior to vitamin D repletion, and even following repletion it was increased only slightly in contrast to the large change in calcium absorption [9]. Similarly, Schmulen et al. [10] found that physiologic doses 1, 25-dihydroxyvitamin D_3 (1,25[OH]$_2$D$_3$) normalized the modest defect in jejunal magnesium absorption in uremic patients. This might imply that although vitamin D may have a small effect on proximal absorption of magnesium, it has little effect on the more distal sites for magnesium absorption in the small bowel. Unlike in the kidney, the basic absorptive systems of calcium and magnesium are independent of each other in the intestinal tract; calcium flux is normally twice that of the magnesium flux at similar luminal concentrations. It is probable that only ionized magnesium is available for absorption, and the amount available is affected by progressive precipitation of magnesium as insoluble phosphates, carbonates, and soaps beginning in the ileum, in the colon, and ultimately in the stool. Alterations of luminal concentrations of calcium and phosphate also indirectly affect magnesium absorption. Conversely, the elevation of intraluminal magnesium concentration may precipitate phosphate and thereby allow for greater calcium absorption. Steatorrhea may potentiate magnesium malabsorption through formation of nonabsorbable magnesium-lipid salts [11].

The major portion of magnesium found in the stool is derived from the diet. The magnesium concentration in saliva, gastric secretions, bile, and pancreatic and intestinal secretions ranges from 0.3 to 0.7 mmole and amount to only about 1 percent of the daily fecal output. Taken together, overall knowledge of the precise control of magnesium absorption in the intestinal tract is still lacking.

Renal Excretion of Magnesium

The status of body magnesium balance and particularly ECF magnesium concentration is largely determined by the renal excretion of magnesium. On a normal dietary intake of magnesium, urinary magnesium excretion averages 100 to 150 mg/day or 8 to 12 mEq/day. In patients receiving supplementary oral magnesium-containing antacids, urinary magnesium excretion can increase to 500 to 600 mg/day or more with little change in serum magnesium levels. Similarly, when dietary magnesium restrictions are imposed, 24-hour urinary magnesium excretion decreases in 4 to 6 days to as low as 10 to 12 mg (1 mEq) [13]. Thus, the ability of the kidney to conserve magnesium is excellent when it is needed. Glomerulotubular balance for magnesium seems to exist so that excretion varies minimally but appropriately as glomerular filtration rate (GFR) is altered. This is exemplified in chronic renal failure where the fractional excretion of magnesium rises sharply as GFR progressively falls, thus protecting against the development of significant hypermagnesemia. The most striking change in magnesium excretion occurs in response to alterations in plasma magnesium concentration. With marked hypermagnesemia secondary to high dietary intake or intravenous magnesium infusion, urinary magnesium excretion can approximate the filtered load of magnesium. Studies in several species have shown that there is a threshold value for magnesium excretion, close to the normal magnesium concentration, varying between 1.5 and 2.0 mg/dl of blood. Thus, when serum magnesium concentration falls slightly, urinary magnesium excretion rapidly decreases to very low values. Conversely, when serum magnesium rises slightly above normal, magnesium excretion rapidly increases. This is consistent with a tubular maximum (T_m) for the overall kidney reabsorption for magnesium [13]. Micropuncture studies in dogs subjected to progressive hypermagnesemia indicate that the apparent T_m of magnesium reflects a fortuitous composite of events in various parts of the nephron [14]. The concept of a T_m remains operationally useful in describing overall renal magnesium reabsorption under different circumstances.

Renal magnesium excretion is primarily determined by glomerular filtration and tubular reabsorption. Experimental support for magnesium secretion remains unconvincing [13]. The ultrafiltrable portion of plasma magnesium is 70 to 80 percent as determined by direct sampling of fluid from surface glomeruli of Munich-Wistar rats and by the use of artificial membranes. In the proximal tubule, some 20 to 30 percent of the filtered magnesium is reabsorbed. Luminal magnesium concentrations rise along the length of the proximal convoluted tubule to a value as high as 1.5 times greater than that of the ultrafiltrable magnesium in glomerular filtrate [15] (Fig. 7-2). This is unlike sodium and calcium, whose proximal tubule fluid concentrations remain nearly identical to their concentration in the glomerular filtrate. Recent studies of the straight portion of the proximal tubule have indicated a similar

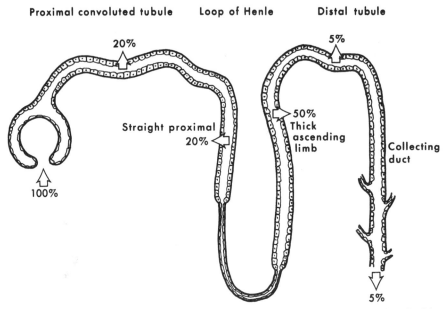

Proximal convoluted tubule   **Loop of Henle**   **Distal tubule**

Fig. 7-2. Normal distribution of magnesium reabsorption as a percent of the ultrafiltrable magnesium at the glomerulus.

magnesium transport system as in the superficial proximal convoluted tubule but at a lower rate of transport, a situation similar to that for sodium chloride. The major influence on proximal magnesium reabsorption is the status of the ECF volume. In states of volume depletion, absorption is enhanced; whereas in expanded states, absorption is decreased.

The early micropuncture studies of Morel and colleagues [15] indicated that the loop of Henle is the major site of magnesium reabsorption. Magnesium concentration in the early distal tubule fluid is only 60 to 70 percent of the ultrafiltrable magnesium concentration. This represents that some 50 to 60 percent of the filtered magnesium is reabsorbed in the loop of Henle, primarily in the thick ascending limb (see Fig. 7-2). This is also the site where most of the alterations in magnesium reabsorption occur, thereby determining the actual amount of magnesium excreted in the urine. There is both passive and active transport of magnesium through the paracellular and transcellular pathways. In hypermagnesemic states, magnesium reabsorption in the loop of Henle approaches zero [16]. Conversely, in hypomagnesemic states, the loop of Henle more avidly reabsorbs magnesium than normally, allowing only minimal amounts, less than 3 percent, of the filtered load to reach the distal tubules and be excreted in the urine [17].

An important interaction between calcium and magnesium has also been observed in the thick ascending limb. It is well known that hypercalcemia [16] or hypermagnesemia inhibits both magnesium and calcium reabsorption [18, 19]. This appears to occur on the basolateral side of the ascending limb cells, as elevating magnesium on the luminal side alone progressively increases magnesium reabsorption, while infusing magnesium to cause hypermagnesemia progressively reduces magnesium reabsorption [16]. Besides this influence on magnesium reabsorption, recent observations suggest that magnesium reabsorption is closely controlled in the thick ascending limb. Parathyroid hormone, calcitonin, glucagon, and antidiuretic hormone act through a common second messenger, adenosine 3',5'-cyclic monophosphate (cyclic AMP), to enhance magnesium transport and modulate magnesium excretion at that nephron site [20, 21].

In the distal convoluted tubule, magnesium concentrations rise along the length of the distal tubule, and only some 2 to 5 percent of the filtered magnesium is reabsorbed in this segment of the nephron. Distal magnesium reabsorption is readily saturated as distal magnesium delivery is increased [16]. Chronic mineralocorticoid administration leads to slight increases in magnesium excretion. However, this probably results from a modest degree of volume expansion rather than a direct effect of aldosterone on the distal tubule [22]. The collecting ducts play a very limited role in magnesium transport and may account for 1 to 3 percent of the reabsorption of the filtered magnesium load.

Physiologic and Pharmacologic Effects

Magnesium plays a critical and necessary role in intracellular metabolism. Magnesium is necessary for a wide spectrum of enzymatic reactions including various phosphokinases and phosphatases [23], which are involved in energy storage and utilization. Phosphatases are particularly important, as magnesium functions primarily to form magnesium-ATP, which is a substrate for these enzymes. Accordingly, these specific ions activate these ATPases, resulting in hydrolysis of ATP and the net transport of ions from one compartment to another. The ion-sensitive ATPases are situated in the intracellular compartments and membranes to regulate the flow of potential energy from the mitochondria and from the cytoplasm. Recognized magnesium ATPases include ouabain-sensitive Mg^{2+},Na^+,K^+-ATPase, ouabain-insensitive Mg^{2+},HCO_3^--ATPase, and Mg^{2+},Ca^{2+}-ATPase, which are associated with the sodium, proton, and calcium pumps, respectively. They are all essential for ionic control of the cell composition [24]. Magnesium is also involved in protein synthesis through its action on nucleic acid polymerization, its role in ribosomal binding to ribonucleic acid (RNA), and in the synthesis and degradation of deoxyribonucleic acid (DNA). In addition to its role in phosphorylation of glucose, magnesium may also control mitochondrial oxidative metabolism [25]. Adenylate cyclase, critical in the generation of intracellular secondary messenger cyclic AMP, has also been shown to be dependent on magnesium [26]. More recently, intracellular magnesium has been shown to have an important regulatory function on both K^+ and Ca^{2+} channels [27]. Magnesium is essential for activation of the K^+ channel by acetylcholine, guanosine triphosphate (GTP), and GTPase [28].

Intracellular magnesium is found in the free ion form or complexed to proteins or organophosphates. The free magnesium concentration determines the effect of concentrations of the high-energy nucleotide complex magnesium-ATP^2. Knowledge of the true ionic concentration of magnesium in the cell is important but difficult to measure. It is thought that only about 5 to 15 percent of cellular magnesium is truly ionized [29].

Magnesium Deficiency

Since magnesium is an essential element for both plants and animals, it exists almost everywhere in our environment. Thus it is rare to see spontaneous magnesium depletion from dietary indiscretion unless it is severe. Still, it has been suggested that the normal dietary intake of magnesium is marginal.

The essentiality of magnesium for animals was first shown by Kruse and associates [30] in 1932. During the same year, a spontaneous form of magnesium depletion was recognized in cattle [31]. This disease is called "grass staggers" (locoism) and is of considerable economic importance [32]. The disease closely resembles the magnesium depletion syndrome in humans [32]. It typically occurs within 1 to 2 weeks after cattle have been allowed to graze on the early spring pastures but may be observed as early as 2 days after such grazing. The disease is characterized by nervousness, anorexia, muscular twitching, unsteady gait, and convulsions that may lead to death. The animals are found to have severe hypomagnesemia, frequently in association with hypokalemia and hypocalcemia. Although the mechanism responsible for causing the magnesium depletion has not been clearly defined, it would appear that the excess ammonium content in spring grass results in the formation of magnesium ammonium phosphate, struvite, in the bowel. This magnesium compound is insoluble and poorly absorbed, thus explaining the magnesium depletion that occurs despite a normal magnesium content of the foliage ingested by the animals.

It was not until 1960 that Vallee and co-workers [33] described five patients with hypomagnesemia and symptoms and signs that are now felt to be classic for magnesium depletion. These patients had carpopedal spasms with positive Chvostek's and Trousseau's signs, and three also had convulsions. All patients' symptoms and signs abated following magnesium administration. Several investigators have attempted to produce magnesium depletion in humans by placing subjects on a low magnesium intake. In most studies, only minimal magnesium depletion has been induced. Shils [34], however, was able to cause severe magnesium depletion in seven patients who were placed on diets extremely low in magnesium for an extended period of time. Symptoms that appeared to be related to magnesium depletion developed in six of the seven patients; five had positive Trousseau's sign, and two of these patients also had a positive Chvostek's sign. All patients became lethargic and showed generalized weakness, anorexia, nausea, and apathy. Biochemical abnormalities included hypomagnesemia, hypocalcemia, hypokalemia, and decreased total-body exchangeable potassium. All abnormalities reverted to normal with replacement of magnesium alone.

Table 7-1. Causes of hypomagnesemia

Gastrointestinal
  Inadequate intake
  Steatorrheic states
  Severe diarrhea
  Familial magnesium malabsorption
Renal
  Intrinsic
    Familial or sporadic renal magnesium wasting
    Bartter's syndrome
    Aminoglycosides
    Cis-diaminedichloro platinum
    Cyclosporine
    Pentamidine
  Extrinsic (intrarenal)
    Volume expansion
    Hypercalciuria
    Sodium loads
    Diabetic ketoacidosis
    Diuretics
    Hyperaldosteronism
    Antidiuretic hormone secretion syndrome
Miscellaneous
  Alcoholism
  Thyrotoxicosis
  Burns

Clinical Conditions Associated with Magnesium Depletion

Defective Gastrointestinal Absorption of Magnesium

Gastrointestinal causes of magnesium depletion can be divided into four categories: decreased intake, steatorrheic states, severe diarrheal states, and selective magnesium malabsorption (Table 7-1). Caddell and Goddard [35] found serum magnesium to be subnormal in 19 of 28 children with protein-calorie malnutrition (kwashiorkor). This was felt to have resulted from the combination of poor intake of magnesium, vomiting, and diarrhea. Similarly, magnesium depletion has been described in hospitalized patients who have been maintained on parenteral nutrition for prolonged periods of time [36, 37].

Steatorrheic State. Hypomagnesemia has been described in a number of patients with small-bowel disease. Booth and colleagues [11] found that 15 of 42 patients with malabsorption syndromes had subnormal serum magnesium levels. They were able to show a rough correlation between serum magnesium levels and degree of steatorrhea, suggesting that the magnesium malabsorption might be a consequence of the formation of insoluble magnesium soaps. Supporting this possibility is the finding that magnesium absorption was improved when the patients were placed on a low-fat diet. The small-bowel diseases with the highest incidence of hypomagnesemia are idiopathic steatorrhea and disease of the distal ileum.

Diarrheal States. Besides the steatorrheic states, magnesium depletion can occur in any severe diarrheal state [38, 39]. As with potassium, fecal magnesium excretion is related to the total water content where the stool magnesium concentration is approximately 6 mEq/L [39]. Magnesium depletion has also been described in patients following jejunoileal bypass surgery for the treatment of morbid obesity, probably from a combination of factors including malabsorption, shortened transit time, and diarrhea [40].

Hereditary Magnesium Absorptive Defect. Several patients have been described who have an isolated defect in the gastrointestinal absorption of magnesium [41, 43]. Profound hypomagnesemia develops in these patients when they consume a standard dietary intake of magnesium. The absorptive defect can be overcome, however, by increasing the oral intake of magnesium. Most of these patients have had severe hypomagnesemia in association with reduced urinary magnesium excretion, hypocalcemia, and tetany.

The preponderance of males in the reported cases of this defect as well as its occurrence in male siblings has prompted Teebi [44] to suggest that it is a rare X-borne allele. However, more recent reports describing this condition in two sisters [45] and in a sister whose brother also had this disease would suggest it may be an autosomal recessive condition [41].

Renal Magnesium Wasting

Renal magnesium wasting can be of two distinct types. One represents a primary renal defect, whereas the second represents the kidney's responding in a normal manner to a variety of systemic and local factors that increase magnesium losses (see Table 7-1). Symptomatic hypomagnesemia is much more likely to be seen in the state of primary renal magnesium wasting. The hallmark of both of these states is a disproportionately elevated urinary magnesium excretion in association with hypomagnesemia. Normally, when serum magnesium falls only slightly due to extrarenal causes, urinary magnesium falls to less than 1 mEq/day (12 mg/day); whereas, if the kidney is responsible for the magnesium losses, urinary magnesium is increased relative to the hypomagnesemic state (>4 mEq/day). Thus, prior to magnesium replacement, urinary magnesium should be measured to determine whether the hypomagnesemic state resulted from renal or extrarenal causes.

Primary Renal Magnesium Wasting. Primary renal magnesium wasting can occur from either congenital or acquired causes. Congenital renal magnesium wasting is unusual, and to date less than 20 cases have been reported [46, 47]. Of interest, 10 of these cases were described in pairs of siblings [47]. Besides hypomagnesemia and renal magnesium wasting, other findings include nephrocalcinosis, hypokalemia, and hypocalcemia. Decreased renal concentrating ability and distal renal tubule acidosis may also be present. The most common presenting symptom is tetany.

The acquired forms of renal magnesium wasting are largely drug induced. Renal magnesium wasting has been well documented in a number of patients receiving aminoglycosides [48, 49]. More recently, renal magnesium wasting has been described in patients receiving *cis*-diaminedichloro platinum (*cis*-DDP) [50]. In one series, 23 of 44 patients treated with *cis*-DDP developed hypomagnesemia. Two of these patients required hospitalization because of severe symptomatic magnesium depletion. In an additional report of 50 patients treated with multiple courses of combined chemotherapy with *cis*-DDP, 76 percent developed hypomagnesemia [50]. This defect in renal magnesium handling can persist for months after the *cis*-DDP has been discontinued [50, 51]. Another drug that commonly causes hypomagnesemia is cyclosporine [52]. In contrast to other hypomagnesemic states, which are usually accompanied by hypokalemia, cyclosporine-induced hypomagnesemia is usually associated with either normokalemia or at times hyperkalemia [52]. On discontinuation of cyclosporine, the hypomagnesemia rapidly abates. More recently, renal magnesium wasting has been described in patients with acquired immune deficiency syndrome (AIDS) undergoing treatment with pentamidine for *Pneumocystis carinii* pneumonia [53]. Symptomatic hypomagnesemia can develop up to 2 weeks after cessation of therapy with this agent.

Secondary Forms of Renal Magnesium Wasting. Tubular reabsorption of magnesium is linked to a variety of other cations. Both sodium and calcium infusions can markedly increase urinary magnesium [54]. Usually because of the modest nature and short duration of infusions, magnesium depletion does not develop. However, when large saline infusions are given in association with diuretics, as are utilized in the treatment of hypercalcemia, hypomagnesemia may develop. Any chronic hypercalciuric state, such as seen with vitamin D therapy, can also cause magnesium wasting [55, 56].

Virtually all diuretics, with the exception of acetazolamide, can increase magnesium excretion, but only modestly, and magnesium supplementation is usually not required.

Another cause of renal magnesium wasting is ketoacidosis. Hypomagnesemia secondary to starvation was first recognized during World War II [57]. Jones et al. [58] subsequently showed that patients undergoing total starvation had an average magnesium loss of 10 mEq/day in their urine and suggested that ketoacidosis was responsible for this loss. Similarly, in patients with untreated diabetic ketoacidosis, there is marked renal magnesium wasting in the acidotic period as well as during early treatment [59]. Following insulin and fluid therapy, serum magnesium may fall precipitously, and tetany may occur [59, 60]. Phosphate replacement therapy in patients with diabetic ketoacidosis has also been associated with the induction of hypomagnesemia [61]. In view of these findings, Butler et al. [59, 60] have suggested that in addition to the other cations commonly given, magnesium replacement should be included in the management of diabetic ketoacidosis. However, the American Diabetic Association recommends magnesium supplementation only in those patients who have documented hypomagnesemia [62].

A number of other conditions are associated with increased urinary magnesium excretion such as Bartter's syndrome [63], primary and secondary hyperaldosteronism [22, 64], and inappropriate secretion of antidiuretic hormone [65]. The renal magnesium wasting in these settings, however, is usually not severe enough to cause clinically significant magnesium depletion.

Miscellaneous Causes of Hypomagnesemia

Hypomagnesemia has been a common finding in patients with chronic alcoholism [66]. Ethanol has been shown to increase urinary magnesium excretion acutely [67, 68]; however, this occurs only when the blood alcohol levels are rising. Furthermore, Dunn and Walser [69] showed that alcohol does not increase urinary magnesium excretion in patients maintained on a low-magnesium diet. It thus appears that alcohol-induced renal magnesium wasting is probably not the major mechanism responsible for magnesium depletion. A very important cause for the magnesium depletion in alcoholic patients may be the profound reduction in dietary intake of this cation. In view of the frequency with which hypophosphatemia is associated with hypomagnesemia in alcoholic patients, it seems possible that the magnesium depletion is in part a result of phosphate depletion. A number of investigators have reported increased urinary magnesium excretion in rats [70], dogs [71], and humans [72] during phosphorus depletion, although the mechanism of this phenomenon has not been defined.

Hypomagnesemia has also been observed in patients with hyperthyroidism [73, 74]. This hypomagnesemic state is associated with an increased exchangeable magnesium pool, suggesting that thyroid hormone has a direct stimulatory effect on the transport of magnesium into cells. The degree of hypomagnesemia has been correlated with the severity of the hyperthyroid state, with the lowest values found in apathetic thyrotoxicosis [74].

Hypomagnesemia has also been described in patients with severe burns. This probably results from a combination of factors including lack of oral intake and losses through the denuded skin [75].

Following parathyroidectomy, especially in patients with severe bone disease, serum magnesium may fall to subnormal levels [76]. The most apparent reason for this reduction in the serum magnesium concentration is the rapid deposition of magnesium in the newly formed bone salts.

Neonatal Hypomagnesemia

Hypomagnesemia can also occur in infants. Normally, there is a magnesium gradient between the blood of the mother and fetus, with magnesium being slightly higher in fetal blood. However, this gradient is not great enough to protect the fetus if the mother is magnesium depleted [77]. Hypomagnesemia has been described in newborns whose mothers have had malabsorption syndromes, have chronically ingested stool softeners, or have had hyperparathyroidism [78]. In a series of 20 children with magnesium depletion, the most common cause was the repeated passage of watery stools regardless of the specific cause [79]. A contributory factor was felt to be starvation, which was present in these children. In addition, hypomagnesemia has occurred in association with exchange transfusions, neonatal hepatitis, and polycythemia in infancy [80]. Offspring of diabetic mothers have also been reported to have hypomagnesemia [81].

Clinical Consequences of Magnesium Depletion

With the development of atomic absorption spectrophotometry, which made possible the accurate determination of plasma magnesium levels in hospital laboratories, it became apparent that hypomagnesemia is not an uncommon finding, especially in some hospital populations. Patients may have severe hypomagnesemia in the absence of any recognizable symptoms. When symptoms do occur, they are largely confined to the neuromuscular system. These symptoms include weakness, muscle fasciculation, tremors, and positive Chvostek's and Trousseau's signs. Generalized tetany occasionally may occur [33, 34]. The mechanism responsible for the development of tetany is poorly understood, but it is clear that tetany can occur in the absence of either hypocalcemia or alkalosis. A decreased concentration of either magnesium or calcium will lower the threshold to stimulation of a nerve, with resulting increased irritability [82, 83]. In muscle, however, their effects are antagonistic. A low concentration of magnesium enhances muscle contraction, whereas a low concentration of calcium inhibits it [84]. It has been suggested that the ECF magnesium depletion may increase acetylcholine action at the nerve ending, which then would lower the threshold of the muscle membrane [33].

In addition to the symptoms mentioned, patients with magnesium depletion may also have disturbances of the central nervous system, manifested by marked changes in their personality, including excessive anxiety and, at times, delirium and frank psychoses [85].

Although it is well recognized that hypomagnesemia can be associated with clinical symptomatology, the clinical importance of reduced tissue stores of magnesium is much less clear. Intracellular magnesium depletion with its effect on intracellular potassium may have an adverse effect on myocardial function and its electrophysiologic response.

Biochemical Consequences of Magnesium Depletion

The earliest biochemical alteration during magnesium depletion is a fall in serum magnesium concentration. In growing animals, serum magnesium falls during the first day the animal is on a magnesium-deficient diet [86]. Even humans have been shown to have a significant reduction in serum magnesium concentration within 5 to 7 days after being placed on a diet deficient in magnesium [12].

Erythrocyte magnesium concentration also has been measured during experimentally induced magnesium depletion in humans and has been found to fall, but less rapidly than the plasma magnesium concentration. Since factors other than the status of the body magnesium stores, such as erythrocyte age, also influence erythrocyte magnesium concentration, this determination cannot be used as a valid index of the body magnesium content [87].

A more uniform correlation between total-body magnesium and bone magnesium concentration has been found. In almost every study in which bone magnesium concentration has been measured during magnesium depletion, it has been found to be decreased [4, 5]. The surface-limited magnesium pool on bone seems to

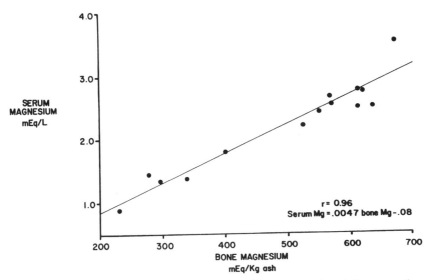

Fig. 7-3. Correlation between serum magnesium and bone magnesium in human and animal studies. (From A. C. Alfrey, N. Miller, and R. Trow, Effect of age and magnesium depletion on bone magnesium pools in rats. *J. Clin. Invest.* 54:1074, 1974. Reproduced by copyright permission of the American Society for Clinical Investigation.)

be readily available during magnesium depletion and is rapidly utilized to replace other body magnesium deficits. In addition, bone magnesium concentration has been shown to strongly correlate with serum magnesium levels in normal, magnesium-deficient, and magnesium-overloaded animals [5] and human subjects [4] (Fig. 7-3).

In contrast to bone, there is a poor correlation between plasma magnesium levels and muscle and cardiac magnesium levels [4]. However, a reasonably good correlation has been found between mononuclear blood cell magnesium and muscle and heart magnesium [88]. Most confusion regarding evaluation of the status of the body magnesium resides around the measurement of muscle magnesium concentrations. Muscle magnesium has been found to be decreased in magnesium-depleted animals [89] but to a lesser extent than bone magnesium. In addition, in a variety of conditions, muscle magnesium has been found to be reduced in association with normal or even increased plasma and bone magnesium levels [4, 90, 91]. There is a close interrelationship between muscle potassium and magnesium levels. During magnesium depletion, in association with the fall in muscle magnesium, there is also a decrease in muscle potassium concentration [4, 92]. This change in muscle potassium during magnesium depletion may result from an inability of the muscle to maintain an appropriate gradient for potassium, possibly as a consequence of reduced magnesium-dependent Na,K-ATPase activity and magnesium's effect on potassium channels [93]. A number of investigators have shown that muscle magnesium and potassium concentrations are affected similarly and to a larger extent in primary potassium depletion [4, 92] and malnutrition [94], showing that these changes in muscle cation composition are not necessarily characteristic of primary magnesium depletion. It has been found that muscle magnesium falls 0.5 mmole for every 10-mmole fall in muscle potassium during potassium depletion [4]. A similar relationship between these two ions exists in the myocardium [95]. Because muscle potassium is readily exchangeable and reflects total-body potassium, the most likely cause for the reported reduced muscle magnesium levels in patients with a variety of clinical disorders who have normal plasma magnesium levels [90, 91] would appear to be primary potassium depletion with secondary muscle magnesium depletion.

Bone and ECF magnesium are therefore the available magnesium pools that are utilized to replenish soft-tissue magnesium deficits during magnesium depletion. Furthermore, serum magnesium concentration, but not muscle, adequately reflects bone magnesium content and can be used as an indicator of total-body magnesium stores.

Besides the measurement of magnesium concentration in biologic tissues and fluids, the retention of magnesium following an acute intravenous infusion of magnesium has also been used to estimate the status of the body magnesium stores. Normal individuals in magnesium balance will excrete the majority of a systemically administered magnesium load in 24 to 48 hours. In contrast, individuals with magnesium deficits will retain a significant fraction of the injected magnesium [88, 96].

Effect of Magnesium on Calcium Metabolism

Severe magnesium depletion has been found to alter calcium metabolism significantly in animals as well as in humans. Studies in cattle [97], sheep [98], pigs [99], dogs [100], monkeys [101], rats [102], and humans [34] have shown that severe magnesium depletion is associated with hypocalcemia in all these species. Subsequently, calcium balance studies in animals, as well as in humans, have shown that with the development of hypocalcemia during magnesium depletion, external calcium balances remain unchanged or actually become more positive. Thus, the hypocalcemia results from alterations in internal control mechanisms for calcium. The interrelationship between magnesium and parathyroid hormone (PTH) is quite complex. Acutely magnesium appears to have a direct effect on PTH secretion [103]. Perfusion studies of goat and sheep parathyroid glands have shown that low magnesium concentration acutely stimulates the release of PTH. In vitro studies [104] showed a first-order relationship between PTH release and the combined concentrations of calcium and magnesium. That these divalent cations had an equivalent effect on hormone release was shown by the finding that when either cation was decreased in association with a corresponding increase of the other cation, PTH secretion was unchanged.

Parathyroid function appears to be affected in an opposite direction during chronic magnesium depletion. Immunoreactive PTH levels usually have been found to be normal, which is inappropriately low for the hypocalcemic and hypomagnesemic state, or actually low [105–107]. Recent studies provide support for an abnormality in PTH release in chronic magnesium depletion. Anast and colleagues [108] found that PTH levels increased within 5 minutes of administration of magnesium intravenously. Mennes and associates [109] also found that PTH levels rapidly increased in hypomagnesemic patients following intravenous administration of magnesium. Thus, it would appear that chronic magnesium depletion is associated with suppression of PTH release from the parathyroid glands rather than a direct effect on decreasing synthesis of this hormone. In further support of this is a recent finding of suppression of PTH secretion by magnesium depletion in a patient with pseudohypoparathyroidism, with subsequent elevated PTH levels noted following magnesium repletion [110]. It is of interest that although chronic magnesium depletion suppresses PTH release, it has little effect on other endocrine glands. Cohan and associates [111] showed normal responsiveness of the adrenal cortex, thyroid, gonads, and liver to their respective trophic hormones in hypomagnesemic patients.

A number of studies have suggested that the hypomagnesemia-induced hypocalcemia also results from skeletal resistance to PTH. Through in vitro techniques [112], it was found that PTH caused less calcium release from fetal rat bone when the medium was low in magnesium. Similarly, bones from magnesium-depleted animals were found to release less calcium and cyclic AMP when exposed to PTH than control bones [113].

Data obtained from in vivo studies have yielded conflicting results. Studies in magnesium-deficient dogs [114], rats [115], and monkeys [101] have shown a normal calcemic response to PTH. In contrast, PTH resistance was found in magnesium-deficient chicks as assessed by the hypercalcemic response [116, 117].

Studies in humans have also yielded conflicting results. The earliest studies performed by Estep and associates [118] in hypomagnesemic alcoholics, and Muldowney and co-workers [119] in patients with hypomagnesemia secondary to malabsorption syndromes, and Woodard et al. [120] in patients with diarrhea showed an impaired calcemic response from PTH. However, Chase and Slatopolsky [105] found a normal calcemic response from PTH in two hypocalcemic hypomagnesemic adults. A normal calcemic response from PTH has been found in the majority of hypomagnesemic children studied [121].

In human studies [122] as well as some animal studies [123], $1,25(OH)_2D_3$ levels have been found to be low during magnesium-induced hypocalcemia. However, the hypocalcemia does not appear to be related to the low $1,25(OH)_2D_3$ levels, since the hypocalcemia responds to magnesium replacement and the replacement has no effect on vitamin D levels.

It can therefore be concluded that several factors may be involved in the pathogenesis of magnesium depletion–induced hypocalcemia. Abnormal PTH release in response to a hypocalcemic stimulus has been well established. There also appears to be altered bone solubility, possibly as a result of loss of magnesium ions from the crystal surface and hydration shell, with replacement by calcium ions by heteroionic exchange. This could render the bone resistant to PTH as well as other factors that tend to solubilize bone salts. It is possible that early in the course of magnesium depletion PTH secretion is impaired, whereas later in the course of magnesium depletion there is a combination of suppression of PTH release and bone resistance to PTH. This might explain the discrepancies noted in the preceding studies, with the difference in bone response to PTH related to the duration and magnitude of magnesium depletion.

Effect of Magnesium Depletion on Potassium and Other Intracellular Constituents

Wang et al. [124], in studying 106 patients with hypokalemia, found that 42 percent were also hypomagnesemic. Similarly, Boyd et al. [125] reported a 38 percent incidence of coexisting hypomagnesemia in hypokalemic patients. However, Watson and O'Kell [126] found a much lower incidence, with only 7.4 percent of 136 hypokalemic patients also hypomagnesemic. This difference can possibly be explained by the type of patient population studied. The patients studied by Whang et al. [124] were from a University and Veterans Administration hospital, whereas Watson and O'Kell [126] studied patients hospitalized at a tertiary community hospital. From these studies, it would appear that in certain patient populations, such as alcoholics and diabetics with ketoacidosis, the combined disturbance of hypokalemia and hypomagnesemia may occur quite commonly.

Whang et al. [127] have suggested that two types of potassium depletion coexist with magnesium depletion. The first represents a combination of intracellular and extracellular potassium and magnesium depletion, whereas the second type represents only intracellular depletion of these two cations. Irrespective of the type of depletion, repletion of potassium frequently cannot be accomplished without the concomitant administration of magnesium. Whang et al. [127] and Rodriguez et al. [128] have used the terminology *refractory potassium repletion states* to describe this condition. The most common cause has been the use of diuretics to treat edematous disorders. In a review by Whang et al. [127], diuretic therapy was responsible for 63 percent (46 of 73) of the patients reported who had potassium depletion refractory to only potassium replacement. In the remaining patients, it resulted from a variety of disorders including Bartter's syndrome, familial hypokalemic alkalosis, burns, and alcoholism. Whang et al. [127] and Dyckner and Webster [129] have also found that potassium replacement alone may not increase muscle potassium and that a combination of potassium and magnesium replacement is required to normalize muscle potassium and magnesium. Animal studies would add additional support to this contention. Whang and Welt [130] showed that potassium losses from the rat diaphragm maintained in a low-magnesium bath could be prevented by adding more magnesium to the bath. Studies using the isolated rat interventricular septa have shown that increasing extracellular magnesium abruptly decreases ^{42}K efflux [131]. Magnesium has also been shown to reduce or prevent the net potassium loss from the heart induced by glycosides [132]. This was further supported by showing that a magnesium infusion in animals receiving acetylstrophanthidin prevented potassium loss from the myocardium as determined by measuring arterial and coronary sinus potassium concentrations [133]. It has been suggested that this effect of magnesium on intracellular potassium is a result of magnesium enhancing Na,K-ATPase activity [134]. However, this has been criticized by Shine [132], who suggests as an alternative that there might be a direct effect of magnesium on potassium channels in the sarcolemmal membrane or that magnesium's effect might be one of competing with calcium for cellular uptake. An additional factor that may be involved in magnesium-induced potassium depletion is aldosterone. During experimental magnesium depletion–induced kaliuresis, aldosterone levels have been found to be in-

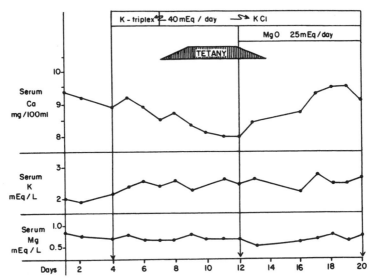

Fig. 7-4. An example of potassium replacement associated with the development of tetany in a patient with hypomagnesemia. Tetany developed in association with a slight rise in serum potassium and a gradual fall in serum calcium without a detectable change in serum magnesium.

creased, and the kaliuresis can be abolished with spironolactone [135]. However, somewhat at variance with this is the finding that magnesium infusion decreases urinary potassium excretion in patients with Bartter's syndrome without effecting plasma renin and aldosterone levels [136]. This suggests that magnesium repletion may modify kaliuresis by means other than or in addition to its effect on the renin-aldosterone system.

Although most investigators have felt the intracellular alteration in potassium and magnesium to be a result of magnesium depletion, it seems equally as likely, if not more likely under some conditions, that the disturbances are a consequence of primary potassium depletion with secondary magnesium depletion. Studies have shown that potassium can affect the cellular concentration of magnesium. House and Bird [137] showed that goats placed on a high-potassium diet retained more magnesium than goats maintained on a normal potassium intake given a similar intravenous magnesium load. In addition, as stated earlier, it has been well documented that in primary potassium depletion, intracellular magnesium is also reduced [4, 92]. This interrelationship between magnesium and potassium could have considerable clinical importance. Under a variety of conditions, it is impossible to replete intracellular deficits of magnesium and potassium without giving both of these cations together, whether the deficiency resulted from either primary potassium or magnesium depletion. In addition, a small number of patients have been reported who have developed tetany following potassium supplementation [138]. Although magnesium levels have not been measured in all of these patients, it seems likely in view of their underlying diseases that magnesium deficiency was also present. An example of potassium replacement inducing tetany is shown in Figure 7-4. This patient had renal magnesium and potassium wasting. He was maintained on a regular diet and was free of tetany. However, with potassium supplementation, serum magnesium and calcium fell, in association with a small rise in serum potassium, and the patient developed tetany. This was reversed with magnesium supplementation. It is suggested that potassium supplementation resulted in the intracellular movement of a small amount of potassium and magnesium, which reduced extracellular magnesium to a critical level, with resulting tetany and hypocalcemia.

Further support for the relationship between these two cations comes from the finding that increased extracellular magnesium causes an abrupt decrease in potassium efflux from the rat intraventricular septa [131]. Magnesium also decreased glycoside-induced potassium loss from the myocardium [132]. One mechanism by which magnesium may enhance intracellular potassium is by stimulating Na,K-ATPase activity, thus allowing the cell to maintain a potassium gradient [134].

Besides its effect on intracellular potassium, magnesium depletion also causes intracellular phosphorus depletion in muscles. Cronin and co-workers [139] described rhabdomyolysis in magnesium-depleted dogs and suggested that this resulted from magnesium depletion–induced intracellular phosphate depletion.

Effect of Magnesium on Cardiovascular Function

The effect of magnesium on cardiovascular function has received increasing attention during the last decade. Extracellular and/or intracellular magnesium depletion has been implicated in a variety of cardiovascular disturbances including ventricular arrhythmias, digitalis intoxication, modulation of vascular tone, and atherogenesis.

Cardiac arrhythmias are an important complication of magnesium depletion, especially in patients on digitalis. Magnesium depletion has been associated with a prolonged Q–Tc interval [140]. In addition, magnesium supplementation has been shown to reduce the Q–Tc intervals even in patients with normal serum magnesium levels [141, 142]. Torsades de pointes is a repetitive polymorphous ventricular tachycardia that occurs in the presence of Q–T prolongation, which is usually induced by drugs that prolong the Q–T interval. Because of its effect on prolonging the Q–T interval, magnesium depletion has also been implicated in the pathogenesis of torsades de pointes, although such a relation has rarely been shown [143]. Because of its ability to shorten the Q–T interval, magnesium supplementation has been used with some success in treating torsades de pointes [144].

In regard to cardiac function, there is a close association between magnesium and potassium. Magnesium has been shown to attenuate the electrophysiologic effects of hyperkalemia [145]. Furthermore, in view of the relationship between magnesium and intracellular and extracellular potassium depletion, magnesium depletion has been implicated as a potential cause of digitalis intoxication [146]. This is supported by the finding that an acute induction of hypomagnesemia in dogs with dialysis facilitates the development of digitalis intoxication and arrhythmias [134]. Moreover, ventricular arrhythmias, including those induced by digitalis, are sensitive to magnesium therapy [147]. However, it is unclear how much of these cardiovascular alterations are a direct result of magnesium depletion or else a consequence of the associated intracellular potassium depletion.

Some evidence has also been presented that subclinical magnesium depletion might predispose patients with acute myocardial infarction to develop arrhythmias [96]. Finally, magnesium depletion has been implicated in the pathogenesis of ischemic heart disease as a result of altering blood lipid composition [148] and accelerating atherogenesis, and causing coronary artery spasm [149]. However, the evidence supporting the role of magnesium in the pathogenesis of ischemic heart disease is at this time not very convincing.

Therapy of Magnesium Deficiency

Magnesium replacement is indicated in all patients with hypomagnesemia whether symptomatic or not. Symptoms are unusual unless serum magnesium levels are less than 1 mg/dl. Adequate replacement of magnesium deficits can usually be accomplished through dietary sources alone in patients with mild asymptomatic hypomagnesemia. Patients with severe symptomatic hypomagnesemia usually require parenteral replacement of magnesium deficits. A more controversial area concerns magnesium supplementation in the prevention and management of cardiac arrhythmias and the replacement of isolated intracellular magnesium depletion (i.e., myocardial and muscle) to enhance replacement of potassium deficits. Magnesium appears to have favorable effects on coronary blood flow, cardiac arrhythmias, and myocardial metabolism. One relatively large trial and a meta-analysis of many smaller trials suggest that magnesium can reduce arrhythmias and total mortality after acute myocardial infarction [150, 151]. However, a more definitive study involving over 50,000 patients failed to show any benefits of magnesium in the management of acute myocardial infarction [152]. Magnesium may be useful, at least as adjuvant therapy, in treating a variety of tachyarrhythmias including torsades de pointes and some associated with digitalis toxicity. As stated earlier, uncorrected intracellular magnesium deficiency can impair repletion of cellular potassium. At this time, it cannot be recommended that all patients with potassium depletion be repleted with both potassium and magnesium. However, patients with potassium depletion in association with any documented amount of hypomagnesemia should receive combined replacement with both of these cations. In addition, magnesium supplementation should be strongly considered in patients with severe potassium depletion or in those who appear to be resistant to potassium replacement.

Since the kidneys have a marked capability for excretion of magnesium, excessive magnesium treatment usually results in only temporary hypermagnesemia. However, when a patient has compromised renal function, magnesium should be administered cautiously and with close monitoring of the plasma magnesium levels. The different compounds commonly used for magnesium replacement, including their molecular weights and milliequivalents and milligrams of magnesium contained in 1 g, are listed in Table 7-2.

The magnesium deficit can be roughly calculated by assuming that the space of distribution is slightly larger than the ECF volume. This assumption seems to be valid, since during magnesium depletion soft-tissue magnesium stores are affected little, if at all, and only the surface-limited pool of magnesium on bone would equilibrate during repletion. Therefore, it appears that replacement therapy may be

Table 7-2. Magnesium salts used for replacement

Compound	Molecular weight	mEq/g	mg/g
$MgCl_2 \cdot 6H_2O^a$	203.23	9.75	116
$MgSO_4 \cdot 7H_2O^b$	246.50	8.13	97.6
$Mg(C_2H_3O_2)_2 \cdot 4H_2O^c$	214.47	9.35	112.1
MgO^d	40.0	46.0	550

[a] Magnesium chloride.
[b] Magnesium sulfate.
[c] Magnesium acetate tetrahydrate.
[d] Magnesium oxide.

adequate for a number of hypomagnesemic patients if only 30 percent as much magnesium as recommended by Flink [153] is used. However, in some conditions, the magnesium deficit may be in excess of this amount. It has been estimated that patients with diabetic ketoacidosis may retain 40 to 80 mEq (480–960 mg) of magnesium over 2 to 6 days following recovery [60, 154]. In some alcoholics, deficits of up to 1 mEq/kg have been found [155].

Whenever possible, intravenous magnesium replacement should be avoided in small children because of the danger of hypotension. For children weighing 4 to 7 kg, a safe initial dose is 0.5 ml of 50% $MgSO_4$ (2 mEq of magnesium), given intramuscularly. For heavier children, 1.0 ml of 50% $MgSO_4$ may be given intramuscularly [156].

For adults with normal renal function, suggested magnesium replacement is given in Table 7-3 [153, 157]. Oral replacement therapy is limited by the amount of magnesium administration that causes diarrhea. Oral replacement can also be made with antacids that contain both magnesium and aluminum salts (e.g., Maalox, Gelusil) in patients who develop diarrhea from magnesium oxide replacement. Patients

Table 7-3. Magnesium replacement

Intramuscular route (50% $MgSO_4$):
    Day 1: 4 ml (16.3 mEq of Mg) q2h for 3 doses and then q4h for 4 doses
    Day 2: 2 ml (8.1 mEq of Mg) q4h for 6 doses
    Days 3–5: 2 ml (8.1 mEq of Mg) q6h
Intravenous administration (50% $MgSO_4$):
    Nonemergent
        Day 1: 12 ml (49 mEq of Mg) in 1000-ml solution containing glucose infused over a 3 h; followed by 10 ml (40 mEq of Mg) in each of two 1-L solutions administered throughout the day
        Day 2: 12 ml (49 mEq of Mg) distributed equally in total daily IV fluids
        Days 3–5: The same as day 2
    Emergent (seizures) (50% $MgSO_4$)
        4 ml (16.3 mEq of Mg) diluted to 100 ml infused over a 10-min period
Oral therapy (MgO):
    250–500 mg (12.5–25.0 mEq of Mg) qid

maintained only on intravenous therapy for periods in excess of 5 to 7 days may require some magnesium supplementation to prevent the development of magnesium depletion. This can be accomplished by giving 100 mg (8 mEq) of magnesium daily if there are not excessive losses of this cation through the kidneys and gastrointestinal tract. Suggested prophylaxis therapy for acute myocardial infarction has been immediate intravenous loading injection of 8 mmol (16 mEq) followed by administration of 65 mmol of magnesium over the ensuing 24-hour period [150, 151]. For management of arrhythmias, it has been suggested that 8 mmol of magnesium sulfate be administered intravenously over 1 minute or that as much as 1.5 mmol/kg be given over a 10-minute period [158, 159].

Hypermagnesemia

Normally, plasma magnesium concentration increases in the hibernating animal [160] and during hypothermia [161]. Magnesium is commonly given parenterally for the treatment of eclampsia. Blood levels of magnesium usually are increased to 6 to 8 mEq/L but occasionally may be as high as 14 mEq/L [162]. This may result in neonatal hypermagnesemia, but in general, blood levels tend to be lower in the infant than in the mother. Other states in which hypermagnesemia has been described with some frequency are in patients with renal failure [163] and adrenocortical insufficiency [164]. The majority of patients with far-advanced renal failure have a modest elevation of serum magnesium levels [165]. Severe hypermagnesemia occurs most frequently in patients with marked renal failure who are given large amounts of oral magnesium salts, usually in the form of magnesium-containing antacids [166, 167]. Although the normal kidney has a great ability to excrete magnesium, magnesium intoxication can occur in patients with normal renal function [168, 169]. This usually results from an individual inadvertently receiving a large oral load of hypertonic magnesium salts. This results in two phenomena that can cause life-threatening hypermagnesemia. First, excessive magnesium is absorbed. Second, and possibly of greater importance, the hypertonic solution pulls fluid from the extracellular space into the gastrointestinal tract, which causes volume depletion and decreases renal function, which in turn compromises the excretion of the absorbed magnesium. Hypermagnesemia is being seen with increasing frequency in patients with drug overdoses due to the magnesium-containing laxatives commonly used to treat this condition [170]. Another group of patients at risk of developing hypermagnesemia are elderly patients with gastrointestinal disorders receiving magnesium-containing compounds [171].

Symptoms of Acute Magnesium Intoxication

Acute elevations of the serum magnesium levels depress the central nervous system as well as the peripheral neuromuscular junction. Magnesium in pharmacologic doses has a curare-like action on neuromuscular function. This is probably caused by inhibition of the prejunctional release of acetylcholine due to displacement of membrane-bound calcium at the neuromuscular junction, which then decreases the depolarizing action of acetylcholine [172]. Magnesium also increases the stimulus threshold in nerve fibers, and direct application of magnesium to the central nervous system blocks synaptic transmission. Electrophysiologic studies demonstrate reduced compound muscle action potential amplitudes, decremental amplitude responses to repetitive stimulation at low rates, and a marked amplitude increment following brief exercise [173].

When serum magnesium levels exceed 4 mEq/L, the deep tendon reflexes are depressed. At magnesium levels greater than 8 to 10 mEq/L, a flaccid quadriplegia may develop in the patient. At this stage, deep tendon reflexes are absent. The patient is typically conscious and reasonably alert. However, because of marked muscle weakness, there is difficulty talking and swallowing, and respiratory paralysis is a real hazard [85, 166]. Other symptoms include lethargy, nausea, dilated pupils, and respiratory depression [85, 167]. There may also be smooth-muscle paralysis, resulting in difficulty in micturition and defecation [166]. Hypotension and brady-cardia are common, and in rare cases, cardiac arrhythmias consisting of complete heart block and cardiac arrest have been observed [166].

Treatment of Acute Magnesium Intoxication

Treatment of hypermagnesemia is primarily directed at reducing the serum magne-sium levels. However, calcium acts as a direct antagonist to magnesium, and the injection of as little as 5 to 10 mEq of calcium may readily reverse a potentially lethal respiratory depression or cardiac arrhythmia [85]. Thus, intravenous calcium should be used as the initial treatment modality when life-threatening complications of magnesium intoxication are present.

Any parenteral or oral magnesium salt the patient has been taking should be discontinued immediately. If renal function is adequate, intravenous furosemide should be administered and urine volume replaced with 0.5 N saline. This approach ensures continuing urine output and prevents volume depletion. Calcium gluconate (15 mg of calcium per kilogram), given over a 4-hour period, can also be used to increase urinary calcium excretion and, in turn, magnesium excretion. In patients with severe impairment of renal function, dialysis may be required. This should be carried out with a dialysate free of magnesium. The serum magnesium usually can be decreased to a safe level in 4 to 6 hours of dialysis [167].

Chronic Magnesium Excess

The only state thus far described in which there is chronic excess of total body magnesium is chronic renal failure [163]. The only body magnesium pools increased during magnesium excess are ECF magnesium and bone magnesium [163]. The possible clinical importance of chronic magnesium excess has not been well defined. Magnesium has been shown to be an integral part of the soft-tissue calcium phos-phate deposits found in uremic patients [174], suggesting that this cation might in part be responsible for this complication. Additional studies are necessary to determine whether the magnesium excess in patients with chronic renal failure plays any role in the pathogenesis of renal osteodystrophy.

In summary, since magnesium determinations have become a routine procedure in most hospital laboratories, it has become apparent that disorders of magnesium metabolism occur with a frequency almost as great as those noted for the other major body elements. Furthermore, since serum magnesium reflects body stores of this cation, under most conditions disorders of magnesium metabolism are relatively easy to diagnose. Hypomagnesemia is found with some frequency in a variety of conditions including small-bowel disease, chronic alcoholism, malnutrition, endocrine abnormalities, and certain renal diseases. At times, the severity of magnesium depletion may be so great that such symptoms as tetany, delirium, frank psychosis, or even convulsions may occur.

Although acute magnesium intoxication has been repeatedly observed and can lead to death as a result of arrhythmias and respiratory arrest, the consequences of chronic magnesium excess have not been well defined and clearly deserve further study.

References

1. Whang R, Ryder KW: Frequency of hypomagnesemia and hypermagnesemia. JAMA 263: 3063–3064, 1990.
2. Seelig MS: The requirement of magnesium by the normal adult: Summary and analysis of published data. *Am J Clin Nutr* 14:212–218, 1964.
3. Walser M: Magnesium metabolism. *Ergeb Physiol* 59:185–296, 1967.
4. Alfrey AC, Miller NL, Butkus D: Evaluation of body magnesium stores. *J Lab Clin Med* 84: 153–162, 1974.
5. Alfrey AC, Miller NL, Trow R: Effect of age and magnesium depletion on bone magnesium pools in rats. *J Clin Invest* 54:1074–1086, 1974.
6. Alfrey AC, Miller NL: Bone magnesium pools in uremia. *J Clin Invest* 52:3019–3027, 1973.
7. MacIntyre I, Robinson CG: Magnesium and the gut: Experimental and clinical observations. *Ann NY Acad Sci* 162:865–873, 1970.
8. Miller ER, Ullrey DE, Zutaut CL, et al: Mineral balance studies with the baby pig: Effect of dietary vitamin D_2 levels upon calcium, phosphorus and magnesium balance. *J Nutr* 85: 255–259, 1965.
9. Hodgkinson A, Marshall DH, Nordin BEC: Vitamin D and magnesium absorption in man. *Clin Sci Mol Med* 57:121–123, 1979.
10. Schmulen AC, Lerman M, Pak CYC, et al: Effect of 1,25-$(OH)_2D_3$ on jejunal absorption of magnesium in patients with chronic renal disease. *Am J Physiol* 238:G349–G352, 1980.
11. Booth CC, Babouris N, Hanna S, et al: Incidence of hypomagnesaemia in intestinal malabsorption. *Br Med J* 2:141–144, 1963.
12. Gitelman HJ, Graham JB, Welt LG: A new familial disorder characterized by hypokalemia and hypomagnesemia. *Trans Assoc Am Physicians* 79:221–235, 1966.
13. Massry SG, Coburn JW, Kleeman CR: Renal handling of magnesium in the dog. *Am J Physiol* 216:1460–1467, 1969.
14. Wong NLM, Dirks JH, Quamme GA: Tubular maximum reabsorptive capacity for magnesium in the dog kidney. *Am J Physiol* 244:F78–F83, 1983.
15. Morel F, Roninel N, LeGrimellec, C: Electron probe analysis of tubular fluid composition. *Nephron* 6:350–364, 1969.
16. Quamme GA, Dirks JH: Effect of intraluminal and contraluminal magnesium on magnesium and calcium transfer in the rat nephron. *Am J Physiol* 238:187–198, 1980.

17. Carney SL, Wong NLM, Quamme GA, et al: Effect of magnesium deficiency on renal magnesium and calcium transport in the rat. *J Clin Invest* 65:180–188, 1980.
18. LeGrimellec C, Roinel N, Morel F: Simultaneous Mg, Ca, P, K, Na and Cl analysis in rat tubular fluid: II. During acute Mg plasma loading. *Pflugers Arch* 340:197–210, 1973.
19. LeGrimellec C, Roinel N, Morel F: Simultaneous Mg, Ca, P, K, Na and Cl analysis in rat tubular fluid: III. During acute Ca plasma loading. *Pflugers Arch* 346:171–189, 1974.
20. Quamme GA: Control of magnesium transport in the thick ascending limb. *Am J Physiol* 256:F197–F210, 1989.
21. De Rouffignac C, Di Stefano A, Wittner M, et al: Consequences of differential effects of ADH and other peptide hormones on thick ascending limb of mammalian kidney. *Am J Physiol* 260:R1023–R1035, 1991.
22. Horton R, Biglieri EG: Effect of aldosterone on the metabolism of magnesium. *Clin Endocrinol Metab* 22:1187–1192, 1962.
23. Lehninger AL: *Bioenergetics.* New York, Benjamin, 1965.
24. Kinne-Suffren E, Kinne R: Localization of a calcium-stimulated ATPase in the basolateral plasma membrane of the proximal tubule rat kidney cortex. *J Membr Biol* 17:264–274, 1974.
25. Humes HD, Weinberg JM, Knauss TC: Clinical and pathophysiologic aspects of aminoglycoside nephrotoxicity. *Am J Kidney Dis* 2:5–29, 1982.
26. Bellorin-Font E, Martin KJ: Regulation of PTH-receptor-cyclase system of canine kidney: Effects of calcium, magnesium and guanine nucleotides. *Am J Physiol* 241:F364–F373, 1981.
27. Kurachi Y, Nakajima T, Sugimoto T: Role of intracellular Mg^{2+} in the activation of muscarinic K^+ channel in cardiac atrial cell membrane *Pflugers Arch* 407:572–574, 1986.
28. Brown AM, Birnbaumer L: Direct G protein gating of ion channels. *Am J Physiol* 254:H401–H410, 1988.
29. Brinley FJ Jr, Scarpa A, Tiffert T: The concentration of ionized magnesium in barnacle muscle fibers. *J Physiol* (Lond) 266:545–565, 1977.
30. Kruse HD, Orent ER, McCollum EV: Studies on magnesium deficiency in animals: Symptomatology resulting from magnesium deprivation. *J Biol Chem* 96:519–539, 1932.
31. Sjollema D: Nutritional and metabolic disorders in cattle. *Nutr Abstr Rev* 1:621–632, 1932.
32. Blaxter KL, Cowlishaw B, Rook JAF: Potassium and hypomagnesemic tetany in calves. *Anim Prod* 2:1–15, 1960.
33. Vallee B, Wacker WE, Ulmer DD: The magnesium deficiency tetany syndrome in man. *N Engl J Med* 262:155–161, 1960.
34. Shils ME: Experimental human magnesium depletion: I. Clinical observations and blood chemistry alterations. *Am J Clin Nutr* 15:133–143, 1964.
35. Caddell JL, Goddard DR: Studies in protein-calorie malnutrition: 1. Chemical evidence for magnesium deficiency. *N Engl J Med* 276:533–535, 1967.
36. Baron DN: Magnesium deficiency after gastrointestinal surgery and loss of excretions. *Br J Surg* 48:344–346, 1960.
37. Flink EB, Stutzman RL, Anderson AR, et al: Magnesium deficiency after prolonged parenteral fluid administration and after chronic alcoholism, complicated by delirium tremens. *J Lab Clin Med* 43:169–183, 1954.
38. Heaton FW, Fourman P: Magnesium deficiency and hypocalcemia in intestinal malabsorption. *Lancet* 2:50–52, 1965.
39. Thoren L: Magnesium deficiency in gastrointestinal fluid loss. *Acta Chir Scand [Suppl]* 306:1–65, 1963.
40. Van Gaal L, Delvigne C, Vandewoude M, et al: Evaluation of magnesium before and after jejuno-ileal versus gastric bypass surgery for morbid obesity. *J Am Coll Nutr* 6:397–400, 1987.
41. Abdulrazzaq YM, Smigura RC, Wettrell G: Primary infantile hypomagnesemia: Report of two cases and review of literature. *Eur J Pediatr* 148:459–461, 1989.
42. Stromme JH, Nesbakken R, Normann T, et al: Familial hypomagnesemia: Biochemical, histological and hereditary aspects studied in two brothers. *Acta Paediatr Scand* 58:433–444, 1969.
43. Suh SM, Tashjian AH, Matsuo N, et al: Pathogenesis of hypocalcemia in primary hypomagnesemia: Normal end organ responsiveness to parathyroid hormone, impaired parathyroid gland function. *J Clin Invest* 52:153–160, 1973.

44. Teebi AS: Primary hypomagnesaemia: An X-borne allele? *Lancet* 1:701, 1983.
45. Milla PJ, Aggett PJ, Wolff OH, et al: Studies in primary hypomagnesaemia: Evidence for defective carrier-mediated small intestinal transport of magnesium. *Gut* 20:1028–1033, 1979.
46. Michelis MF, Drash AL, Linarelli LG, et al: Decreased bicarbonate threshold and renal magnesium wasting in a sibship with distal renal tubular acidosis (evaluation of the pathophysiologic role of parathyroid hormone). *Metabolism* 21:905–920, 1972.
47. Evans RA, Catter JM, George CRP, et al: The congenital magnesium-losing kidney: Report of two patients. *Q J Med* 1(197):39–52, 1981.
48. Bar RS, Wilson HE, Mazzaferri EL: Hypo-magnesemia hypocalcemia secondary to renal magnesium wasting. *Ann Intern Med* 82:646–649, 1975.
49. Keating MJ, Sethi MR, Bodey GP, et al: Hypocalcemia with hypoparathyroidism and renal tubular dysfunction associated with aminoglycoside therapy. *Cancer* 39:1410–1414, 1977.
50. Schilsky RL, Anderson T: Hypomagnesemia and renal magnesium wasting in patients receiving cisplatin. *Ann Intern Med* 90:926–928, 1979.
51. Buckley JE, Clark VL, Meyer TJ, et al: Hypomagnesemia after cisplatin combination chemotherapy. *Arch Intern Med* 144:2347–2348, 1984.
52. Wong NLM, Dirks JH: Cyclosporin-induced hypomagnesaemia and renal magnesium wasting in rats. *Clin Sci* 75:505–514, 1988.
53. Shah GM, Alvarado P, Kirschenbaum MA: Symptomatic hypocalcemia and hypomagnesemia with renal magnesium wasting associated with pentamidine therapy in a patient with AIDS. *Am J Med* 89:380–382, 1990.
54. Wesson LG Jr: Magnesium, calcium and phosphate excretion during osmotic diuresis in the dog. *J Lab Clin Med* 60:422–432, 1962.
55. George WK, George WD, Haan CL, et al: Vitamin D and magnesium. *Lancet* 1:1300–1301, 1962.
56. Richardson JA, Welt LG: The hypomagnesemia of vitamin D administration. *Clin Res* 11:250, 1963.
57. Mellinghoff K: Magnesium Stoffwechselstorungen bei Inanition. *Deutsche Arch Klin Med* 95:475–484, 1949.
58. Jones JE, Albrink MJ, Davidson PD, et al: Fasting and refeeding of various suboptimal isocaloric diets. *Am J Clin Nutr* 19:320–328, 1966.
59. Butler AM, Talbot NB, Burnett CH, et al: Metabolic studies in diabetic coma. *Trans Assoc Am Physicians* 60:102–109, 1947.
60. Butler AM: Diabetic coma. *N Engl J Med* 243:648–659, 1950.
61. Winter RJ, Harris CJ, Phillips LS, et al: Diabetic ketoacidosis induction of hypocalcemia and hypomagnesemia by phosphate therapy. *Am J Med* 67:897–904, 1979.
62. White JR, Campbell RK: Magnesium and diabetes: A review. *Ann Pharmacother* 27:775–780, 1993.
63. Bartter FC: So-called Bartter's syndrome (editorial). *N Engl J Med* 281:1483–1494, 1969.
64. Cohen MI, McNamara H, Finberg L: Serum magnesium in children with cirrhosis. *J Pediatr* 76:453–455, 1970.
65. Hellman ES, Tschudy DP, Bartter FC: Abnormal electrolyte and water metabolism in acute intermittent porphyria: Transient inappropriate secretion of antidiuretic hormone. *Am J Med* 32:734–746, 1962.
66. Heaton FW, Pyrah LN, Beresford LC, et al: Hypomagnesemia in chronic alcoholism. *Lancet* 2:802–805, 1962.
67. Kalbfleish JM, Lindeman RD, Ginn HE, et al: Effects of ethanol administration on urinary excretion of magnesium and other electrolytes in alcoholic and normal subjects. *J Clin Invest* 42:1471–1475, 1963.
68. McCollister RJ, Flink EB, Lewis MD: Urinary excretion of magnesium in man following the ingestion of ethanol. *Am J Clin Nutr* 12:415–420, 1963.
69. Dunn MJ, Walser M: Magnesium depletion in normal man. *Metabolism* 15:884–895, 1966.
70. Kreusser WJ, Kurokawa K, Aznar E, et al: Effect of phosphate depletion on magnesium homeostasis in rats. *J Clin Invest* 61:573–581, 1978.
71. Coburn JW, Massry SG: Changes in serum and urinary calcium during phosphate depletion. *J Clin Invest* 49:1073–1087, 1970.

72. Domingues JH, Gray RW, Lemann J Jr: Dietary phosphate deprivation in women and men: Effect on mineral and acid balance, parathyroid hormone and metabolism of 25-OH-vitamin D. *J Clin Endocrinol Metab* 43:1056–1068, 1976.

73. Tibbets DM, Aub JC: Magnesium metabolism in health and disease: III. In exophthalmic goiter, basophilic adenoma, Addison's disease and steatorrhea. *J Clin Invest* 16:511–515, 1937.

74. Marks P, Ashraf H: Apathetic hyperthyroidism and hypomagnesaemia and raised alkaline phosphatase concentration. *Br Med J* 1:821–822, 1978.

75. Broughton A, Anderson IRM, Bowden CH: Magnesium deficiency syndrome in burns. *Lancet* 2:1156–1158, 1968.

76. Heaton FW, Pyrah LN: Magnesium metabolism in patients with parathyroid disorders. *Clin Sci Mol Med* 25:475–485, 1963.

77. Dancis J, Springer D, Cohlan SA: Fetal homeostasis in maternal malnutrition: 1. Magnesium deprivation. *Pediatr Res* 5:131–136, 1971.

78. Schindler AM: Isolated neonatal hypomagnesaemia associated with maternal overuse of stool softener. *Lancet* 2:822, 1984.

79. Harris I, Wilkinson AW: Magnesium depletion in children. *Lancet* 2:735–736, 1971.

80. Tsang RC: Neonatal magnesium disturbances. *Am J Dis Child* 124:282–293, 1972.

81. Clark PCN, Carrel IJ: Hypocalcemic, hypomagnesemic convulsions. *J Pediatr* 70:806–809, 1967.

82. Frankenhaeuser B, Meves H: Effect of magnesium and calcium on frog myelinated nerve fiber. *J Physiol* (Lond) 142:360–365, 1958.

83. Gordon HT, Welsh JH: Role of ions in axon surface reactions to toxic organic compounds. *J Cell Physiol* 31:395–419, 1948.

84. Perry SV: Relation between chemical and contractile function and structure of skeletal muscle cell. *Physiol Rev* 36:1–76, 1956.

85. Welt LG, Gitelman H: Disorders of magnesium metabolism. *DM* 1:1–32, 1965.

86. Chutkow JG: Studies on the metabolism of magnesium in the magnesium deficient rat. *J Lab Clin Med* 65:912–926, 1965.

87. Wallach S, Cahill LN, Rogan FH, et al: Plasma and erythrocyte magnesium in health and disease. *J Lab Clin Med* 59:195–210, 1962.

88. Elin RJ: Assessment of magnesium status. *Clin Chem* 33:1965–1970, 1987.

89. Forbes RM: Effect of magnesium, potassium and sodium nutriture on mineral composition of selected tissues of the albino rat. *J Nutr* 88:403–410, 1966.

90. Lim P, Jacob E: Magnesium deficiency in liver cirrhosis. *Q J Med* 41:291–300, 1972.

91. Lim P, Jacob E: Tissue magnesium level in chronic diarrhea. *J Lab Clin Med* 80:313–321, 1972.

92. Baldwin D, Robinson PK, Zierler KL, et al: Interrelations of magnesium, potassium, phosphorus and creatinine in skeletal muscle of man. *J Clin Invest* 31:850–858, 1952.

93. Skou JC: The (Na$^+$ + K$^+$) activated enzyme system and its relationship to the transport of sodium and potassium. *Q Rev Biophys* 7:401–434, 1974.

94. Alleyne GA, Millward DJ, Scullard GH: Total body potassium muscle, electrolytes and glycogen in malnourished children. *J Pediatr* 76:75–81, 1970.

95. Johnwon CJ, Peterson DR, Smith EK: Myocardial tissue concentrations of magnesium and potassium in men dying suddenly from ischemic heart disease. *Am J Clin Nutr* 32:967, 1979.

96. Rasmussen HS, McNair P, Goransson L, et al: Magnesium deficiency in patients with ischemic heart disease with and without acute myocardial infarction uncovered by an intravenous loading test. *Arch Intern Med* 148:329–332, 1988.

97. Smith RH: Calcium and magnesium metabolism in calves: 4. Bone composition in magnesium deficiency and the control of plasma magnesium. *Biochem J* 71:609–615, 1959.

98. L'Estrange JL, Axford RFE: A study of magnesium and calcium metabolism in lactating ewes fed a semi-purified diet low in magnesium. *J Agric Sci* 62:353–368, 1964.

99. Miller ER, Ullrey DE, Zutaut CL, et al: Magnesium requirement of the baby pig. *J Nutr* 85:13–20, 1965.

100. Chiemchaisri H, Phillips PH: Certain factors including fluoride which affect magnesium calcinosis in the dog and rat. *J Nutr* 86:23–28, 1965.

101. Dunn MJ: Magnesium depletion in the rhesus monkey: Induction of magnesium-dependent hypocalcaemia. *Clin Sci Mol Med* 41:333–344, 1971.
102. MacManus J, Heaton FW: The effect of magnesium deficiency on calcium homeostasis in the rat. *Clin Sci Mol Med* 36:297–306, 1969.
103. Buckle RM, Care AD, Cooper CW, Gitelman HJ: The influence of plasma magnesium concentration on parathyroid hormone secretion. *J Endocrinol* 42:529–534, 1968.
104. Targounik JH, Rodman JS, Sherwood LM: Regulation of parathyroid hormone secretion in vitro: Quantitative aspects of calcium and magnesium ion control. *Endocrinology* 88: 1477–1482, 1971.
105. Chase LR, Slatopolsky E: Secretion and metabolic efficiency of parathyroid hormone in patients with severe hypo-magnesemia. *J Clin Endocrinol Metab* 28:363–371, 1974.
106. Connor TB, Toskes P, Mahaffey J, et al: Parathyroid function during chronic magnesium deficiency. *Johns Hopkins Med* 131:100–117, 1972.
107. Wiegmann T, Kaye M: Hypomagnesemic hypocalcemia: Early serum calcium and late parathyroid hormone increase with magnesium therapy. *Arch Intern Med* 137:953–955, 1977.
108. Anast CS, Winnacker LL, Forte LR, et al: Impaired release of parathyroid hormone in magnesium deficiency. *J Clin Endocrinol Metab* 42:707–713, 1976.
109. Mennes P, Rosenbaum R, Martin K, et al: Hypomagnesemia and impaired parathyroid hormone secretion in chronic renal failure. *Ann Intern Med* 88:206–209, 1978.
110. Allen DB, Friedman AL, Greer FR, et al: Hypomagnesemia masking the appearance of elevated parathyroid hormone concentrations in familial pseudohypoparathyroidism. *Am J Med Genet* 31:153–158, 1988.
111. Cohan BW, Singer FR, Rude RK: End-organ response to adrenocorticotropin, thyrotropin, gonadotropin-releasing hormone, and glucagon in hypocalcemic magnesium deficient patients. *J Clin Endocrinol Metab* 54:975–979, 1982.
112. Raisz LG, Niemann I: Effect of phosphate, calcium, and magnesium on bone resorption and hormonal responses in tissue culture. *Endocrinology* 85:446–452, 1969.
113. Freitag JJ, Martink KL, Comrades MB, et al: Skeletal-resistance to parathyroid hormone in magnesium deficiency: Studies in isolated perfused bone. *J Clin Invest* 64:1238–1244, 1979.
114. Suh SM, Csima A, Fraser D: Pathogenesis of hypocalcemia in magnesium depletion: Normal end-organ responsiveness to parathyroid hormone. *J Clin Invest* 50:2668–2673, 1971.
115. Hahn TJ, Chase LR, Avioli LV: Effect of magnesium depletion on responsiveness to parathyroid hormone in parathyroidectomized rats. *J Clin Invest* 51:886–891, 1972.
116. Breitenbach RP, Gonnerman WA, Erfling WL, et al: Dietary magnesium, calcium hormostasis and parathyroid gland activity of chickens. *Am J Physiol* 225:12–17, 1973.
117. Reddy CR, Coburn JW, Hartenbower DL, et al: Studies on mechanisms of hypocalcemia of magnesium depletion. *J Clin Invest* 52:3000–3010, 1973.
118. Estep H, Shaw WP, Watlington C, et al: Hypocalcemia due to hypomagnesemia and reversible parathyroid hormone unresponsiveness. *J Clin Endocrinol Metab* 29:942–948, 1969.
119. Muldowney FP, McKenna TJ, Kyle LH, et al: Parathormone-like effects of magnesium replenishment in steatorrhea. *N Engl J Med* 282:61–68, 1970.
120. Woodard JC, Webster PD, Carr AA: Primary hypomagnesemia with secondary hypocalcemia, diarrhea and insensitivity to parathyroid hormone. *Am J Dig Dis* 17:612–618, 1972.
121. Skyberg D, Stromme JH, Nesbakken HK, et al: Neonatal hypomagnesemia with selective malabsorption of magnesium: A clinical entity. *Scand J Clin Lab Invest* 21:355–363, 1968.
122. Fuss M, Cogan E, Gillet G, et al: Magnesium administration reverses the hypocalcaemia secondary to hypomagnesaemia despite low circulating levels of 25-hydroxyvitamin D and 1,25-dihydroxyvitamin D. *Clin Endocrinol* (Oxf) 22:807–815, 1985.
123. Carpenter TO, Carnes DL, Anast CS: Effect of magnesium depletion on metabolism of 25-hydroxyvitamin D in rats. *Am J Physiol* 253:E106–E113, 1987.
124. Whang R, Oei TO, Hamiter T: Frequency of hypomagnesemia associated with hypokalemia in hospitalized patients. *Am J Clin Pathol* 71:610, 1979.
125. Boyd JC, Bruns DE, Wills MR: Occurrence of hypomagnesemia in hypokalemic states. *Clin Chem* 29:178–179, 1983.
126. Watson KR, O'Kell RT: Lack of relationship between Mg^{2+} and K^+, concentration in serum. *Clin Chem* 26:520–521, 1980.

127. Whang R, Flink EB, Dyckner T, et al: Magnesium depletion as a cause of refractory potassium repletion. *Arch Intern Med* 145:1686–1689, 1985.
128. Rodriquez M, Solanki DL, Whang R: Refractory potassium repletion due to cisplatin-induced magnesium depletion. *Arch Intern Med* 149:2592–2594, 1989.
129. Dyckner T, Webster PO: Ventricular extrasystoles and intracellular electrolytes before and after potassium and magnesium infusions in patients on diuretic therapy. *Am Heart J* 97: 12–18, 1979.
130. Whang R, Welt LG: Observations in experimental magnesium depletion. *J Clin Invest* 42: 305–313, 1963.
131. Shine KI, Douglas AM: Magnesium effects on ionic exchange and mechanical function in rat ventricle. *Am J Physiol* 227:317–324, 1974.
132. Shine KI: Myocardial effects of magnesium. *Am J Physiol* 237:H413–H423, 1979.
133. Neff MS, Mendelsohn S, Kim KE, et al: Magnesium sulfate in digitalis toxicity. *Am J Cardiol* 79:57–68, 1972.
134. Seller RH, Cangiano J, Kim EE, et al: Digitalis toxicity and hypomagnesemia. *Am Heart J* 79:57–68, 1970.
135. Francisco LL, Sawin L, Dibona GF: Mechanism of negative potassium balance in the magnesium-deficient rat. *Proc Soc Exp Biol Med* 168:382–388, 1981.
136. Baehler RW, Work J, Kotchen TA, et al: Studies on the pathogenesis of Bartter's syndrome. *Am J Med* 69:933–939, 1980.
137. House WA, Bird RJ: Magnesium tolerance in goats fed two levels of potassium. *J Anim Sci* 41:1134–1140, 1975.
138. Engel FL, Martin SP, Taylor H: On the relation of potassium to the neurological manifestations of hypocalcemic tetany. *Johns Hopkins Med J* 84:285–301, 1949.
139. Cronin RE, Ferbuson ER, Shannon WA, et al: Skeletal muscle injury after magnesium depletion in the dog. *Am J Physiol* 243:F113–F120, 1982.
140. Seelig MS: Electrocardiographic patterns of magnesium depletion appearing in alcoholic heart disease. *Ann NY Acad Sci* 162:906–917, 1969.
141. Krasner BS, Girdwood R, Smith H: The effect of slow releasing oral magnesium chloride on the QTC interval of the electrocardiogram during open heart surgery. *Can Anaesth Soc J* 28: 329–333, 1981.
142. Davis WH, Ziady F: The effect of oral magnesium chloride therapy on the PTC and QUC intervals of the electrocardiogram. *S Afr Med J* 53:591–593, 1978.
143. Topol EJ, Lerman BB: Hypomagnesemic torsades de pointes. *Am J Cardiol* 52:1367–1368, 1983.
144. Tzivoni D, Keren A, Cohen AM, et al: Magnesium therapy for torsades de pointes. *Am J Cardiol* 53:528–530, 1984.
145. Kraft LE, Katholi RE, Woods WT, et al: Attenuation by magnesium of the electrophysiologic effects of hyperkalemia on human and canine heart cells. *Am J Cardiol* 45:1189–1195, 1980.
146. Seller RH: The role of magnesium in digitalis toxicity. *Am Heart J* 82:551–556, 1971.
147. Roden DA: Magnesium treatment of ventricular arrhythmias. *Am J Cardiol* 63:43G–46G, 1989.
148. Rayssiguier Y, Gueux E: Magnesium and lipids in cardiovascular disease. *J Am Coll Nutr* 5: 507–519, 1986.
149. Altura BM: Sudden-death ischemic heart disease and dietary magnesium intake. *Med Hypotheses* 5:843–848, 1979.
150. Woods KL, Fletcher S: Long-term outcome after intravenous magnesium sulphate in suspected acute myocardial infarction: The second Leicester Intravenous Magnesium Intervention Trial (LIMIT-2). *Lancet* 343:816–819, 1994.
151. Horner SM: Efficacy of intravenous magnesium in acute myocardial infarction in reducing arrhythmias and mortality. *Circulation* 86:774–779, 1992.
152. ISIS-4: A randomized factorial trial assessing early oral captopril, oral mononitrate and intervenous magnesium sulfate in 58,050 patients with suspected acute myocardial infarction. *Lancet* 345:669–685, 1995.
153. Flink EB: Therapy of magnesium deficiency. *Ann NY Acad Sci* 162:901–905, 1969.

154. Nabarro JDN, Spencer AGD, Stowers JM: Metabolic studies in severe diabetic ketosis. *Q J Med* 21:225–248, 1952.
155. Jones JE, Shane SR, Jacobs WH, et al: Magnesium balance studies in chronic alcoholism. *Ann NY Acad Sci* 162:934–946, 1969.
156. Caddell JL: Magnesium deficiency . . . in extremis. *Nutr Today* 2:14–20, 1967.
157. Parfitt AM, Kleerekiper M: Clinical Disorders of Calcium, Phosphorus and Magnesium Metabolism. In Maxwell MH, Kleeman CR (eds), *Clinical Disorders of Fluid and Electrolyte Metabolism.* New York, McGraw-Hill, 1980, p 1110.
158. Allen BJ, Brodsky MA, Capparelli EV, et al: Magnesium sulfate therapy for sustained monomorphic ventricular tachycardia. *Am J Cardiol* 64:1202–1204, 1989.
159. Sager PT, Widerhorn J, Petersen R, et al: Prospective evaluation of parenteral magnesium sulfate in the treatment of patients with reentrant AV supraventricular tachycardia. *Am Heart J* 119:308–316, 1990.
160. Riesdesel ML, Folk GE: Serum magnesium and hibernation. *Fed Proc* 15:151, 1956.
161. Hannon JP, Larson AM, Young DW: Effect of cold acclimatization on plasma electrolyte levels. *J Appl Physiol* 13:239–240, 1958.
162. Pritchard JA: The use of magnesium ion in the management of eclamptogenic toxemias. *Surg Gynecol Obstet* 100:131–140, 1955.
163. Contiguglia SR, Alfrey AC, Miller N, et al: Total body magnesium excess in chronic renal failure. *Lancet* 1:1300–1302, 1972.
164. Wacker WE, Parisi AE: Magnesium metabolism. *N Engl J Med* 278:658–663, 712–717, 772–776, 1968.
165. Spencer H, Lesniak M, Gatzo CA, et al: Magnesium absorption and metabolism in patients with chronic renal failure and in patients with normal renal function. *Gastroenterology* 79:26–34, 1980.
166. Randall RE Jr, Chen MD, Spray CC, et al: Hypermagnesemia in renal failure. *Ann Intern Med* 61:73–88, 1949.
167. Alfrey AC, Terman DS, Brettschneider L, et al: Hypermagnesemia after renal homotransplantation. *Ann Intern Med* 73:367–371, 1970.
168. Ditzler JW: Epsom salts poisoning and a review of magnesium-ion physiology. *Anesthesiology* 32:378–380, 1970.
169. Stevens AR, Wolff HG: Magnesium intoxication: Absorption from the intact gastrointestinal tract. *Arch Neurol* 63:749–759, 1950.
170. Weber CA, Santiago RM: Hypermagnesemia, a potential complication during treatment of theophylline intoxication with oral activated charcoal and magnesium-containing cathartics. *Chest* 95:56–59, 1989.
171. Clark BA, Brown RS: Unsuspected morbid hypermagnesemia in elderly patients. *Am J Nephrol* 12:336–343, 1992.
172. Ghoneim MM, Long JP: The interaction between magnesium and other neuromuscular blocking agents. *Anesthesiology* 32:23–27, 1970.
173. Swift TR: Weakness from magnesium-containing cathartics: Electrophysiologic studies. *Muscle Nerve* 2:295–298, 1979.
174. LeGeros RZ, Contiguglia SR, Alfrey AC: Pathological calcification associated with uremia. *Calcif Tissue Res* 13:173–185, 1973.

8

Disorders of the Renin-Angiotensin-Aldosterone System

Paul R. Conlin, Robert G. Dluhy, and Gordon H. Williams

The circulating renin-angiotensin-aldosterone system is an array of components that interact in sequence to produce vasoactive substances that function to maintain salt and water homeostasis and blood pressure regulation. The system forms a feedback loop whose level of activity can be suppressed or enhanced at a number of steps by intervening factors as well as interacting systems (Fig. 8-1). Disorders of this tightly regulated system either resulting from abnormalities of its primary components or due to the influence of secondary factors can lead to aberrations of fluid and electrolyte metabolism as well as disturbances in blood pressure. This chapter will focus first on the role of the renin-angiotensin-aldosterone system in normal physiology and then consider its involvement in various pathophysiologic states.

Physiology of the Renin-Angiotensin-Aldosterone System

In 1898, Tigerstedt and Bergman [1] noted that a saline extract of renal tissue produced a sustained rise in blood pressure. This was the initial discovery that suggested the presence of a circulating renin-angiotensin-aldosterone system as it is known today: Renin released by the kidney cleaves circulating angiotensinogen to form angiotensin I, which on passing through the pulmonary vascular bed is converted to angiotensin II by angiotensin-converting enzyme (ACE). For many years, this endocrine role of the system has served as the sole paradigm for renin-angiotensin system involvement in cardiovascular homeostasis. However, evidence is accumulating that all components of the renin-angiotensin system are also produced in many individual tissues and act as paracrine factors, possibly regulating cardiac and vascular remodeling and changes in adrenal glomerulosa sensitivity to agonists.

Renin

Renin is a peptide with molecular weight of 37,000 to 40,000. The finding that renin could be irreversibly inhibited by covalent modification of amino acids at the

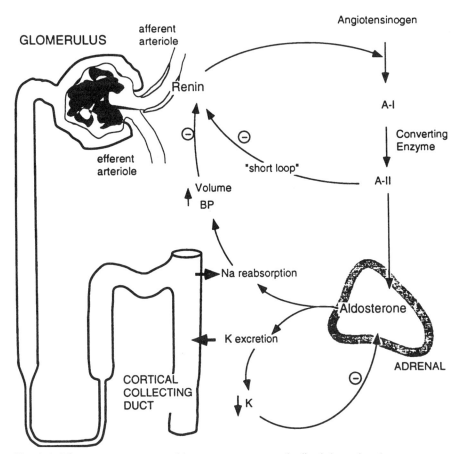

Fig. 8-1. The renin-angiotensin-aldosterone system is a feedback loop that functions to maintain circulating blood volume. It can be enhanced or suppressed at various steps by other volume-regulating factors. A = angiotensin; BP = blood pressure. (From R. M. Mortensen and G. H. Williams, Aldosterone Action. In L. J. DeGroot, et al. [eds.], *Endocrinology* [3rd ed.]. Philadelphia: Saunders, 1995. P. 1669.)

active site led to its inclusion in the aspartyl protease superfamily, which includes proteases such as pepsin, cathepsin D, and chymosin [2]. However, unlike these other proteases, renin is active at neutral pH and has high specificity for its substrate, angiotensinogen.

The renin gene has been cloned and sequenced and is composed of 10 exons separated by 9 introns spanning 11 kb of DNA [3]. Restriction fragment-length polymorphisms have been identified in the renin gene and its flanking regions but have not been linked to altered regulation of the renin gene [4].

The product of the renin gene when translated results in preprorenin. The subsequent removal of a 23-amino-acid signal pro-sequence and glycosylation during transfer to the endoplasmic reticulum result in the 47-kDa prorenin molecule [5].

Prorenin is largely devoid of renin catalytic activity due to inhibition of the active site by the pro-segment. This prorenin is packaged into secretory granules where it is either secreted constitutively or further processed to active renin, which is secreted in a regulated manner. Circulating prorenin remains largely unchanged, although some have suggested that it can serve as a reservoir for the generation of active renin in peripheral tissues [6]. Its role in volume homeostasis remains to be elucidated.

Regulation of Renin Secretion

Although the major site of renin gene expression is in the juxtaglomerular (JG) cells of the kidney, other tissues such as adrenal, vascular smooth muscle, testis, ovary, and pituitary have been reported to express renin, albeit at lower levels [7]. In the kidney, the secretion of renin by JG cells is controlled by both signals generated intrarenally, such as perfusion pressure and tubular fluid composition, and extrarenally, due to changes in sodium, potassium, or calcium intake and sympathetic nervous system activity (Table 8-1). Therefore, renin secretion reflects the input of these numerous signals, which are integrated by the JG cells through the influence of various intracellular second messengers (e.g., adenosine 3',5'-cyclic monophosphate [cyclic AMP], calcium).

The JG cells, located near the afferent arteriole of the glomerulus, have the ability to sense changes in perfusion pressure through changes in stretch of the arteriolar wall. They function as an intrarenal baroreceptor. In the setting of a reduced perfusion pressure, JG cells increase renin release, and following an increase in perfusion

Table 8-1. Factors regulating renin secretion

Factor	Effect
Renal perfusion pressure	
Increase	Inhibit
Decrease	Stimulate
Sodium chloride delivery at the macula densa	
Increase	Inhibit
Decrease	Stimulate
Angiotensin II	Inhibit
Plasma electrolytes	
Potassium	Inhibit
Calcium	Inhibit
Prostaglandins (PGI_2)	Stimulate
Sympathetic nervous system	
β-Adrenergic stimulation	Stimulate
α-Adrenergic stimulation	Inhibit
Natriuretic factors	
Dopamine	Inhibit
Atrial natriuretic hormone	Inhibit
Other factors	
Vasopressin	Inhibit
Adrenocorticotropic hormone	Stimulate

pressure, renin secretion is inhibited. The mechanism whereby JG cells note these changes and respond accordingly appears to be mediated through changes in cytosolic calcium [8]. The myoepithelial origin of JG cells likely contributes to their ability to sense intraluminal pressure changes.

Other circulating factors and signals generated through changes in dietary electrolyte consumption can affect renin release. Included in this are a variety of peptide hormones that have been shown to affect renin secretion. Angiotensin II has the ability to inhibit renin secretion while also vasoconstricting the renal blood supply. Conversely, when levels of angiotensin II are reduced by treatment with a converting enzyme inhibitor, renin secretion is markedly enhanced [9]. This regulation of renin secretion by angiotensin II has been termed the short feedback loop, since it provides a mechanism for control of renin release independently of other factors regulated by angiotensin II (e.g., increased aldosterone secretion and elevated blood pressure) that may provide feedback to alter renin secretion. As with renin inhibition by increased perfusion pressure, these inhibitory effects of angiotensin II on JG cells appear to be mediated through increases in cytosolic calcium [10]. As such, the stimulus-secretion paradigm involving a rise in cytosolic calcium as a stimulus to secretion that is typical in most endocrine tissues is reversed in the JG cell.

Other peptide hormones such as atrial natriuretic hormone (ANH), arginine vasopressin (AVP), and adrenocorticotropic hormone (ACTH) can also affect renin release. ANH has been shown to inhibit renin secretion. This has been demonstrated by ANH infusion to produce levels that mimic physiologic concentrations of the hormone [11]. Increased ANH levels may contribute to the suppression of renin secretion that occurs with volume expansion. Similarly, a role for AVP as an inhibitor of renin release has been suggested [12]. Limited data suggest that ACTH can stimulate renin secretion. This observation may be linked to the diurnal variation in renin levels, with higher morning levels declining during the day, which correlates with a similar diurnal rhythm of ACTH and cortisol secretion.

Additional factors that can directly regulate renin secretion include serum potassium and calcium. Changes in dietary potassium have been shown to have inverse effects on renin release: Increased potassium intake inhibits renin, whereas decreased intake stimulates renin secretion. These responses have been reproduced in vitro and interpreted to be due to direct effects of potassium on JG cells and independent of potassium effects on aldosterone secretion (see Aldosterone, P 356). Extracellular calcium likewise may have direct effects on JG cells to inhibit renin secretion both in vivo and in vitro. Studies of isolated perfused kidneys have shown that increasing the extracellular calcium concentration inhibits renin release, whereas removal of calcium stimulates renin release [14, 15].

Renal production of prostaglandins, particularly PGI_2, has been shown to increase renin secretion [16] and may be important in mediating the response to changes in renal perfusion pressure [17]. The source of renal prostaglandin synthesis appears to reside in preglomerular vascular endothelial cells. Inhibition of prostaglandin synthesis by agents such as indomethacin leads to a reduction in renin secretion both basally and following sodium depletion [18].

A major influence on renin secretion is exerted by the macula densa, a special group of distal tubular cells located in proximity to the JG cells that provide input to the JG cells regarding tubular fluid composition. Presumably functioning as "chemoreceptors," these cells sense changes in tubular fluid volume and electrolytes, particularly sodium and chloride, thus affecting renin release. As evidence for this, acutely infusing a small volume (100 ml) of sodium chloride leads to a prompt reduction in plasma renin activity (PRA), which is not seen following infusion of a similar volume of dextran, a non-salt-containing solution [19]. This has supported a role for ion sensing in the control of renin secretion presumably by macula densa mechanisms. Controversy exists as to whether the source of this inhibitory signal may be mediated through changes in tubular sodium or chloride concentrations. An important role of chloride is supported by evidence showing inhibition of renin by non-sodium-containing chloride solutions and the lack of effect of infusing non-chloride-containing sodium solutions [20]. Independent of the initiating signal, the resulting inhibition of renin secretion in the setting of an increased filtered load of sodium or chloride provides a mechanism for reduced angiotensin II and aldosterone production and, therefore, less salt and water retention.

Sympathetic nervous system activity can stimulate renin release either through intrarenal activation of renal sympathetic nerves or through catecholamines secreted by the adrenal medulla [21]. This mechanism contributes to the rise in renin secretion that occurs with assumption of upright posture. The transduction mechanism for this effect appears to be through interactions with β-adrenergic receptors on JG cells, which generate cyclic AMP as their second messenger. Agents that block β-receptors lead to a reduction in renin secretion. However, the catecholamine dopamine appears to have inhibitory effects on renin secretion independent of effects on vasodilating the renal vasculature and increasing tubular sodium handling [22]. The kidney is a major site of dopamine generation, and the production rate increases with salt loading.

Thus, renin production and secretion are tightly regulated by numerous bloodborne and intrarenally generated factors. The level of renin secretion and its subsequent effects on the other components in the cascade to angiotensin II generation are determined through complex integration of these various signals by the JG cells.

Angiotensinogen

Angiotensinogen is a peptide of 62,000 to 65,000 molecular weight that is largely of hepatic origin and circulates in the α_2-globulin fraction of serum. The 14 N-terminal amino acids serve as the sole substrate for renin catalytic activity. The decapeptide that results from renin catalysis of angiotensinogen is termed angiotensin I. This peptide is largely devoid of biologic activity until acted upon by ACE to form angiotensin II.

Hepatic angiotensinogen production can be stimulated by a variety of factors including glucocorticoids, estrogens, thyroxine, and angiotensin II [23]. Increased angiotensinogen production under the influence of these factors may contribute to the increased prevalence of hypertension noted in hyperthyroidism, Cushing's syndrome, and oral contraceptive use.

Levels of circulating angiotensinogen are much lower than the K_m of renin for its substrate; therefore, the level of angiotensinogen is rate limiting in this reaction.

When levels of angiotensinogen are increased, angiotensin II production likewise increases. The role of angiotensinogen per se in blood pressure regulation may assume its importance as it correlates with the amount of angiotensin II that is generated in plasma.

As with local production of renin, many tissues possess the ability to express the angiotensinogen gene. Although the liver is the major site of expression, adrenal, kidney, heart, and vascular tissue are rich in angiotensinogen messenger RNA (mRNA) [24]. Not surprisingly, those tissues that change their responsiveness with changes in salt intake (i.e., kidney, adrenal, and vasculature) also show similar changes in levels of angiotensinogen mRNA, whereas hepatic synthesis of angiotensinogen appears to be independent of dietary sodium intake [25].

Angiotensins

Angiotensin II is one of the most potent vasoconstrictors in the human body, having physiologic effects at subnanomolar concentrations. The octapeptide is formed by the action of ACE on angiotensin I, by cleaving of the two C-terminal amino acids. Angiotensin I has little known biologic activity prior to conversion to angiotensin II, which occurs predominantly in the pulmonary vasculature. A single pass through the lung converts nearly all of the entering angiotensin I [26]. Alternative pathways for generating angiotensin II from angiotensinogen or angiotensin I without involving ACE have been suggested, although their physiologic relevance remains to be elucidated.

ACE is a metalloprotease and requires the presence of zinc in the active site for functioning [27]. In addition to its activating effects on angiotensins, ACE is also involved in the degradation of other peptides such as bradykinin and enkephalins [28]. In some pathologic conditions such as hyperthyroidism [29], diabetes mellitus [30], sarcoidosis [31], and other granulomatous diseases, circulating levels of ACE are increased, although the mechanisms and significance of this finding remain obscure.

Once generated, angiotensin II has numerous sites of action and multiple effects. Nonpeptide receptor antagonists and molecular biology tools have revealed that angiotensin II binds to receptors, termed AT-1 and AT-2 receptors. Most, if not all of the described effects of angiotensin II are mediated by AT-1 receptors based on evidence that losartan, a nonpeptide AT-1 receptor inhibitor, blocks these effects. Little is known of the actions of AT-2 receptors except that their expression is widespread during fetal development. Angiotensin II has potent vasoconstrictive properties, and its role in glomerular hemodynamics and renal tubular sodium reabsorption is well described. It is a major stimulus for aldosterone secretion by the adrenal glomerulosa. Angiotensin II can also stimulate synthesis and release of nonrepinephrine from central and peripheral sympathetic nerve terminals [32]. In the central nervous system, angiotensin II can stimulate thirst, raise blood pressure, and enhance AVP secretion. The N-terminal aspartyl residue of angiotensin II can be removed by tissue aminopeptidases to yield the heptapeptide angiotensin III. This peptide is a potent secretagogue of aldosterone secretion and can induce renal vasoconstriction, although it is not known whether these effects are mediated by one of the described angiotensin II receptor subtypes or a separate receptor [33]. The physiologic role of these effects of angiotensin III remains unclear. The action

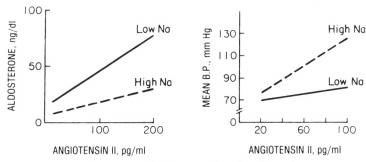

Fig. 8-2. Sodium intake has reciprocal effects on adrenal and vascular responses to angiotensin II. With sodium restriction, aldosterone responsiveness is enhanced, whereas vascular responses are reduced. B.P. = blood pressure. (From N. K. Hollenberg et al., Reciprocal influence of salt intake on adrenal glomerulosa and renal vascular response to angiotensin II in normal man. *J. Clin. Invest.* 54:34, 1974. Reproduced by copyright permission of the American Society for Clinical Investigation.)

of this and other aminopeptidases to cleave angiotensin II also serves as the major source of degradation of the peptide such that the intact peptide has a half-life in tissues of 1 to 2 minutes.

The physiologic response of target tissues to angiotensin II is modulated in response to sodium intake (Fig. 8-2). On a low-sodium diet, adrenal responsiveness to angiotensin II is enhanced, whereas vascular responsiveness is diminished. On a high-sodium diet, these response patterns are reversed [34]. In part, the vascular effects parallel changes in circulating angiotensin II levels (i.e., angiotensin II levels are increased on a low-sodium diet and decreased on a high-sodium diet), which may be the primary determinant of this vascular responsiveness. However, the adrenal does not appear to be driven by the same stimulus, as changes in angiotensin II levels per se do not affect the sensitivity of aldosterone secretion to angiotensin II [35]. Once sensitized by sodium restriction, angiotensin II–stimulated aldosterone secretion is enhanced even when angiotensin II levels are reduced by treatment with an ACE inhibitor.

ACE resides on the luminal surface of pulmonary capillary endothelial cells but has also been found in kidney, adrenal, brain, and other vascular tissue [36]. As with renin and angiotensinogen, which are generated in a variety of tissues, the presence of ACE in these same sites suggests that this local renin-angiotensin system may function in some organs as a paracrine/autocrine system. Production of ACE has been clearly shown in kidney, adrenal, heart, and vascular tissue. Local production of angiotensin II is thought to be involved in vascular and cardiac remodeling that occurs under physiologic conditions. Likewise, increased vascular resistance and vascular and cardiac hypertrophy seen in patients with hypertension may also be linked to abnormal regulation of these pathways. Some of the clinical effects of ACE inhibition such as improvement in cardiac function in patients with hypertension and congestive heart failure may be mediated through inhibition of these local renin-angiotensin systems. The understanding of these local systems, their regulation, and their participation in tissue responsiveness to angiotensin II remain to be elucidated.

Table 8-2. Factors regulating aldosterone secretion

Factor	Effect
Angiotensin II	Stimulate
Plasma electrolytes	
Potassium	Stimulate
Calcium	Inhibit
Pituitary-derived factors	
ACTH	Stimulate
Other non-ACTH pituitary hormones	Permissive
β-Endorphin	Stimulate
Natriuretic factors	
Dopamine	Inhibit
Atrial natriuretic hormone	Inhibit
Other factors	
Serotonin	Stimulate
Vasopressin	Stimulate
Endothelin	Stimulate

ACTH = adrenocorticotropic hormone.

Aldosterone

Aldosterone is the major mineralocorticoid produced by the external zone of the adrenal cortex, the zona glomerulosa. Other weak mineralocorticoids are produced by both the zona glomerulosa and the zona fasciculata but assume far less importance than aldosterone in volume homeostasis. As with renin secretion, the control of aldosterone production is complex because numerous factors can affect adrenal responsiveness (Table 8-2). The acute production of aldosterone is regulated by a variety of factors similar to those agents that affect renin release. However, other mechanisms acting chronically, particularly the state of sodium or potassium balance, also can affect the ability of the adrenal to produce aldosterone.

Like other steroid hormones, aldosterone is produced from cholesterol via a pathway of sequential steps involving molecular rearrangements and hydroxylations (Fig. 8-3). Unlike peptide hormones, which may be synthesized and stored for later secretion, aldosterone is synthesized and secreted immediately when glomerulosa cells

Fig. 8-3. The biosynthesis of adrenal steroids involves pathways to mineralocorticoids, glucocorticoids, and androgens. Enzyme defects in the steps to cortisol or aldosterone production typically result in glucocorticoid deficiency. However, depending on the site of the block, precursor steroids that are secreted in excess may result in either deficient or excessive mineralocorticoid function. Circled letters or numbers denote the specific enzymes: DE = cholesterol side-chain cleavage enzyme (desmolase); 3β = 3β-ol-dehydrogenase; 17 = 17α-hydroxylase; 11 = 11β-hydroxylase; 21 = 21-hydroxylase. (From G. H. Williams and R. G. Dluhy, Diseases of the Adrenal Cortex. In K. J. Isselbach et al. [eds.]: *Harrison's Principles of Internal Medicine* [13th ed]. New York: McGraw-Hill, 1994. P. 1954.)

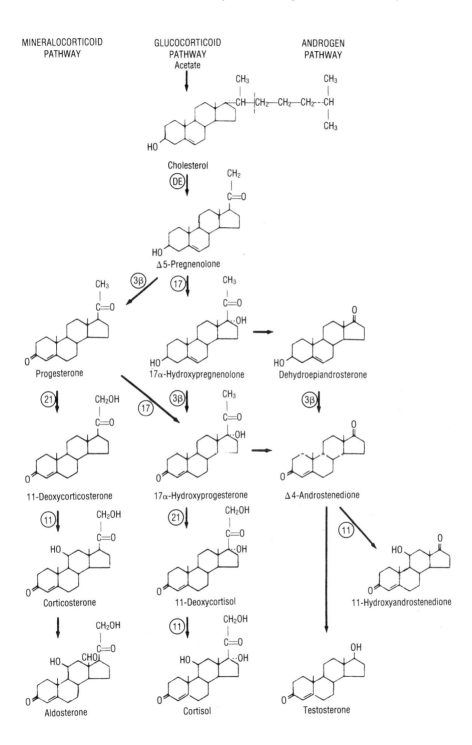

are stimulated. There is little if any storage of preformed hormone. The major common pathway for various secretagogues to influence aldosterone secretion is at the initiating step of cholesterol modification by the side-chain cleavage enzyme, termed the early pathway. All of the major stimulants and inhibitors of aldosterone secretion act to modify the function of this enzyme and do so acutely. The final step in aldosterone production involves the conversion of corticosterone to aldosterone, termed the late pathway, which can be regulated by some of these same agents and by other unidentified ones. This more chronic means of regulating aldosterone production provides a mechanism whereby the adrenal can enhance or reduce its responsiveness ("remodel") depending on the exposure to a sustained signal such as alterations in dietary sodium or potassium intake.

Aldosterone exerts its effects in target tissues (predominantly in the distal tubule of the kidney) by combining with high-affinity cytoplasmic receptors possessing a DNA binding domain, which becomes functional on binding the steroid. This subsequent active receptor-DNA interaction leads to an increase in the expression of an epithelial sodium channel. The mineralocorticoid receptor has been cloned and sequenced and has numerous similarities to the superfamily of steroid/thyroid hormone receptors, which act similarly on binding their specific ligand [37]. While the kidney is a major site of mineralocorticoid receptor expression, it is also expressed in other sites such as the hippocampus, heart, salivary gland, and colon.

In addition to structural similarity to glucocorticoid receptors, mineralocorticoid receptors in the kidney possess the ability to bind both cortisol and aldosterone. However, the selectivity of the mineralocorticoid receptor for aldosterone appears to be maintained by the intrarenal degradation of cortisol to the biologically inactive cortisone by the enzyme 11β-hydroxysteroid dehydrogenase. Cortisone is unable to bind to mineralocorticoid receptors. Therefore, aldosterone is allowed to exert its physiologic effects when competitive binding by cortisol to the receptors has been prevented. Abnormalities in this cortisol degradation pathway in which cortisone production is impaired may lead to excess mineralocorticoid effects mediated by cortisol binding to mineralocorticoid receptors (see Other Mineralocorticoid Excess States, p. 375).

The mechanisms by which aldosterone induces its mineralocorticoid effects are not well understood. Aldosterone serves two important functions: regulation of extracellular fluid volume and potassium homeostasis. Aldosterone acts primarily in the distal renal tubule and produces a net increase in sodium by increasing the membrane occupancy of specific sodium channels. As sodium reabsorption increases, potassium reabsorption is simultaneously reduced, largely through the maintenance of electroneutrality. Aldosterone may also have similar effects on gastrointestinal epithelium, salivary glands, and sweat glands, resulting in reabsorption of sodium and secretion of potassium. The reabsorbed sodium ions are transported into the interstitial fluid with passive diffusion of water.

In contrast to the acute effects, chronic exposure to mineralocorticoid results in initial expansion of the extracellular volume, which becomes limited due to "escape" from the sodium-retaining effects [38]. Thus, despite the continued presence of mineralocorticoid, further elevation of extracellular fluid volume is blunted; however, the kaliuretic effects of the mineralocorticoids remain. The mechanisms for this "escape" have been postulated to involve an increase in pressure natriuresis and elevations in ANH levels in response to volume expansion [39]. Other modulators of this effect may likewise be operative. Recent evidence suggests that chronic aldosterone excess also interacts with mineralocorticoid receptors in the heart, leading to accumulation of collagen, interstitial fibrosis, and cardiac hypertrophy. This effect of aldosterone is blocked by spironolactone, an aldosterone antagonist, at doses that do not change blood pressure, which suggests a specific direct role for aldosterone on cardiac tissue [40]. This potentially important extrarenal role of aldosterone is the subject of active investigation.

Regulation of Aldosterone Secretion

Agonists. Angiotensin II is a major stimulant of aldosterone secretion and, by producing aldosterone-induced sodium retention, closes the renin-angiotensin-aldosterone negative feedback loop. Thus, during periods of volume depletion, activation of the renin-angiotensin system leads to increased aldosterone production, whereas when volume is repleted, the system is suppressed, with a reduction in renin release leading to a decrease in aldosterone secretion.

The initial event in angiotensin II–stimulated aldosterone production involves the binding of angiotensin II to specific membrane receptors. While subtypes of angiotensin II receptors (AT-1 and AT-2 receptors) have been identified in the adrenal glomerulosa, the majority of angiotensin II binding (approximately 80%) is to AT-1 receptors. Through the use of specific nonpeptide inhibitors of these receptor subtypes, it has been shown that AT-1 receptors mediate all of the acute effects of angiotensin II on the adrenal glomerulosa. No specific role for AT-2 receptors has been identified. The level of sodium intake can modify receptor number in the rat, with salt restriction increasing receptor density [41]. In primates, however, salt restriction reduces receptor number. Angiotensin II interaction with adrenal glomerulosa cells produces a rise in cytosolic calcium along with the hydrolysis of membrane lipids, mainly phosphatidylinositol and phosphatidylcholine [42, 43]. This cascade provides the initial intracellular signal for the stimulation of aldosterone production. The responsiveness of aldosterone production to angiotensin III is equipotent to its responsiveness to angiotensin II, although it is unclear whether angiotensin III interacts with receptors for angiotensin II or with a separate receptor [44]. The role of angiotensin III in normal physiology remains to be elucidated.

Extracellular potassium also serves as a major regulator of aldosterone secretion independently of its effects on the renin-angiotensin system. As with angiotensin II, the potassium effects on adrenal glomerulosa cells involve increases in cytosolic calcium [45]. In humans, potassium loading either through diet or by infusion leads to a marked increase in aldosterone secretion [46]. This mechanism appears to be exquisitely sensitive to changes in extracellular potassium, as changes of 0.1 mEq/L can lead to a significant increase in aldosterone. This direct effect of potassium on adrenal secretion is in contrast to potassium effects on renin secretion in which renin is inhibited by increases in serum potassium. Since aldosterone facilitates potassium excretion by the kidney, this effect on aldosterone secretion provides an important negative feedback for the maintenance of normal potassium homeostasis.

ACTH has significant acute effects on aldosterone secretion similar to its effects on the zona fasciculata steroid cortisol. It interacts with specific membrane receptors and stimulates the production of cyclic AMP in glomerulosa cells [47]. However, when ACTH is infused chronically, aldosterone secretion is not maintained at its stimulated level beyond 24 hours despite maintenance of enhanced cortisol secretion [48]. This response is unlike that seen during chronic angiotensin II infusion, where aldosterone secretion remains stimulated [49]. The mechanisms for this apparent down-regulation of responsiveness of the zona glomerulosa to chronic ACTH are poorly understood. Pulsatile administration of ACTH may preserve aldosterone responsiveness, suggesting that the period of exposure to ACTH may be important. It has been suggested that during chronic ACTH the glomerulosa cells develop features similar to fasciculata cells and convert their steroid output to glucocorticoids [50]. Such a mechanism may be permissive in the adaptation to chronic stress and may explain the observation of impaired aldosterone secretion in critically ill patients.

Although ACTH mediates acute stress-induced rises in aldosterone production, its importance is likely minor in the normal regulation of aldosterone. In patients with hypopituitarism who have received glucocorticoid replacement therapy or in patients on chronic supraphysiologic doses of steroids, aldosterone secretion remains intact despite an absence of pituitary ACTH secretion [51]. Likewise, although mineralocorticoid receptors are present in the normal pituitary, no negative feedback loop between aldosterone and ACTH has been documented [52].

Other aldosterone secretagogues have been identified; however, their physiologic importance in regulating secretion has yet to be clarified. Serotonin (5-hydroxytryptamine [5-HT]) is a potent stimulator of aldosterone secretion both in vivo and in vitro [53]. However, this effect in vivo may be in part mediated by changes in renin secretion. The enhanced aldosterone secretion can be inhibited by the serotonin antagonist cyproheptadine, suggesting that there is a specific effect of serotonin on the adrenal. Experiments with the serotonin receptor antagonist cisapride suggest that this effect is mediated through the $5\text{-}HT_4$ receptor subtype [54]. Other agents such as β-endorphin, α-melanocyte-stimulating hormone, and endothelin have been suggested to increase aldosterone production. The regulation of these substances in regard to changes in volume or blood pressure remains to be determined; therefore, their importance in the overall regulation of aldosterone secretion is unclear.

Inhibitors. A variety of agents can inhibit aldosterone secretion and may serve as physiologic modulators of adrenal output. The catecholamine dopamine has been shown to have inhibitory effects on both aldosterone secretion and renin secretion. It is not known whether the adrenal glomerulosa possesses direct innervation by dopaminergic neurons or whether dopamine gains access to the adrenal glomerulosa from the adrenal medulla or from changes in circulating blood levels. Serum and urinary dopamine levels are increased in the setting of salt loading. Dopamine's role as a natriuretic substance is likely related to its inhibition of aldosterone secretion and its renal vasodilatory properties. In normal subjects on a high-salt diet, infusion of the dopamine antagonist metoclopramide produces an increase in aldosterone levels [22], suggesting that dopaminergic tone participates in the dampening of aldosterone secretion during high salt intake. These effects of endogenous dopamine appear to function at near maximal levels during high salt intake; dopamine infusion into sodium-replete subjects does not produce any further reduction in basal or angiotensin II–stimulated aldosterone secretion [55]. Thus, dopamine may be an important modulator of aldosterone secretion following increases in dietary sodium intake.

The other major catecholamines, epinephrine and norepinephrine, appear to have little effect on aldosterone secretion. Acute infusion of norepinephrine stimulates aldosterone secretion, but it has not been shown that this effect is dissociated from the profound effects of norepinephrine on renin secretion [56]. Norepinephrine has little effect on zona glomerulosa cells in vitro. Chronic reduction of sympathetic activity through the use of a sympatholytic agent may modestly shift the dose-response relationship of aldosterone secretion to angiotensin II but has little effect by itself on basal secretion [57].

ANH has potent inhibitory effects on aldosterone secretion. ANH exhibits its most marked effects as a suppressor of aldosterone secretion in sodium-depleted subjects or when administered with secretagogues (i.e., angiotensin II or potassium) [11]. As with dopamine, infusion of ANH into sodium-replete subjects has minimal effects on aldosterone secretion. Like dopamine, the effects of ANH on the adrenal are assumed to be part of the modulation of response to changes in dietary sodium. However, the physiologic role of ANH in the regulation of aldosterone secretion still remains to be elucidated.

As with renin secretion, increases in extracellular calcium have been noted to inhibit aldosterone secretion, particularly when serum calcium is raised acutely by calcium infusion. The mechanism of this inhibition is unclear. In addition, the adrenal's dependence on extracellular calcium is evident by inhibitory effects of calcium channel antagonists on aldosterone secretion both in vivo [58] and in vitro [47]. The effects of calcium channel antagonists are likely mediated by inhibition of calcium entry through voltage-sensitive calcium channels. Due to their dependence on cytosolic calcium, both potassium and angiotensin II stimulation of aldosterone are particularly sensitive to these agents.

Effects of Changes in Dietary Sodium or Potassium Intake

Changes in sodium or potassium intake can have dramatic effects on the sensitivity of the adrenal to stimulation by agonists. Both sodium restriction and potassium loading lead to an increase in adrenal responsiveness. The increased aldosterone production likely occurs as a result of increased activity of the late pathway of aldosterone biosynthesis as well as growth of the zona glomerulosa. During increased sodium intake or potassium restriction, adrenal responsiveness is reduced. The mechanisms for this change in response to alterations in dietary intake have not been identified. However, this change in the adrenal sensitivity to agonists is crucial to the maintenance of normal volume and potassium homeostasis. In the setting of increased potassium intake, the enhancement in aldosterone secretion facilitates renal potassium excretion. During high-salt intake, suppression of renin and angiotensin II formation and aldosterone secretion leads to increased renal sodium excretion and prevents excessive volume expansion and increased blood pressure.

Disorders of the Renin-Angiotensin-Aldosterone System

As described previously, the renin-angiotensin-aldosterone system's major function is to maintain normal extracellular volume and blood pressure regulation. In normal individuals, the system is activated in states characterized by hypotension or volume depletion, whereas the system is suppressed by volume repletion and a rise in blood pressure. This relationship between PRA and aldosterone secretion can serve as the basis for identifying a broad range of disorders of the renin-angiotensin-aldosterone system (Fig. 8-4). Pathologic states that produce any of these aberrations in volume

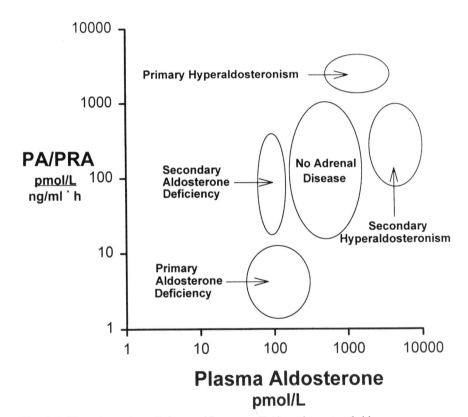

Fig. 8-4. The relationship of plasma aldosterone (PA) to the ratio of aldosterone to plasma renin activity (PRA) is shown during various states of aldosterone excess or deficiency. (Adapted from T. J. McKenna et al., Diagnosis under random conditions of all disorders. *J. Clin. Endocrinol. Metab.* 73:952, 1991, © The Endocrine Society.)

or blood pressure homeostasis can affect the activity of the system and in some cases reset the threshold of its activation. However, in some pathologic conditions (e.g., congestive heart failure), activation of the renin-angiotensin-aldosterone system may contribute further to the pathology rather than restoring normal volume regulation. In addition, abnormalities in the renin-angiotensin-aldosterone system may primarily contribute to a rise in blood pressure or an expansion of extracellular volume.

The Renin-Angiotensin-Aldosterone System in Hypertension

Essential Hypertension

Many groups have attempted to identify a pathogenetic role for the renin-angiotensin-aldosterone system in essential hypertension. Despite these efforts, considerable controversy still exists. Early reports identified the increased secretion of renin and aldosterone secretion in malignant hypertension [59]. However, in the vast majority of individuals with essential hypertension, renin and aldosterone secretion can be found within the spectrum of the responses of normotensive subjects.

Recent studies on the genetics of hypertension have revealed genotypic differences in some patients with moderately elevated blood pressure. For example, a variant of the gene encoding angiotensinogen—a threonine substituting for methionine at position 235—has been linked to patients with essential hypertension [60]. While this change in peptide structure does not occur in the region of the molecule responsible for the generation of angiotensin peptides, it has been shown that such patients do have elevated levels of angiotensinogen in peripheral plasma. The exact role for this genotypic abnormality as a contributor to high blood pressure in these subjects remains to be elucidated. However, it takes us one step closer to understanding the pathophysiology of hypertension in these patients.

Low-Renin Essential Hypertension. Profiling of the plasma renin response to stimulation has been frequently used to characterize hypertensive subjects (Fig. 8-5). Initial reports on renin activity in hypertension revealed that 25 to 33 percent of subjects had PRA below the levels found in normal subjects. Thus, the term *low renin* has been used to categorize this group of subjects with essential hypertension. Subjects with low-renin essential hypertension tend to be older than hypertensive subjects with normal- or high-renin essential hypertension. This in part may reflect the decline in renin secretion that is seen as a normal accompaniment of aging [55]. Many studies have also found a higher incidence of low-renin essential hypertension among black subjects. However, other studies have noted a lower "normal range" of PRA among normotensive blacks [56]. One unexplained but interesting observation of low-renin essential hypertension is that the incidence of stroke and myocardial infarction tends to be lower than in patients with normal- or high-renin essential hypertension.

Numerous attempts have been made to identify a single cause for low-renin essential hypertension, without success. The suppressed renin activity has been

364

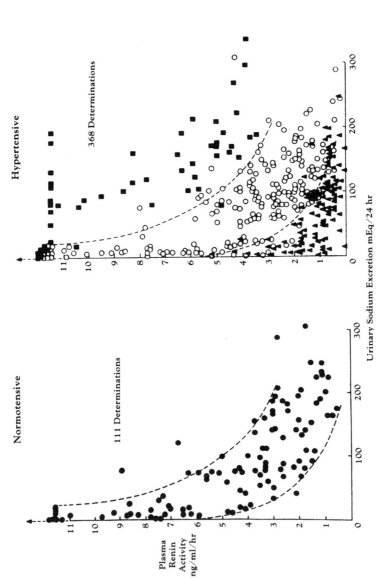

Fig. 8-5. The relationships of plasma renin activity to 24-hour urinary sodium excretion in normal subjects (*left panel*) and hypertensive individuals (*right panel*) are depicted. Low-renin (△), normal-renin (○), and high-renin essential hypertension (■) are shown as they compare to the renin responses in normal subjects (*dashed lines*). Note that approximately 30 percent of hypertensive subjects had low renin levels. (From H. R. Brunner et al., Essential hypertension: renin and aldosterone, heart attack and stroke. *N. Engl. J. Med.* 286:441, 1972.)

interpreted by some to involve a normal inhibition of renin secretion by the elevated blood pressure. Others have incriminated the presence of excess circulating mineralocorticoids, resulting in volume expansion and suppression of renin secretion, as is seen in primary hyperaldosteronism. Several aldosterone precursors such as 11-deoxycorticosterone (DOC) and 18-hydroxy-11-deoxycorticosterone have been found elevated in patients with low-renin essential hypertension [57, 61]. Despite these findings, other reports have found similar or lower levels of these and other mineralocorticoids when compared to patients with normal-renin essential hypertension [62].

The suggestion that low-renin essential hypertension is a volume-expanded state has not been proved. Such patients do not typically have higher blood volumes or lower serum potassium levels (signs of mineralocorticoid excess) than other patients with essential hypertension. However, it has been suggested that some low-renin hypertensives have abnormal aldosterone suppressibility. An interesting observation that may explain the supressed renin levels is that subjects with low-renin essential hypertension may have increased adrenal sensitivity to angiotensin II [63]. Thus, for a given level of angiotensin II, aldosterone secretion is greater than in normal-renin essential hypertension. In this setting, volume regulation resulting from increased aldosterone secretion would occur at lower levels of renin activity, and therefore the renin-angiotensin-aldosterone system would function at a lower set point. This finding may provide a mechanism whereby such patients have lower renin activity but may not completely explain the pathophysiology of their hypertension.

Normal- and High-Renin Essential Hypertension. The finding that renin secretion is normal or even increased in the setting of hypertension, which should normally suppress renin, has led many to the conclusion that the renin-angiotensin-aldosterone system contributes to the pathogenesis of hypertension. Explanations for this seemingly inappropriate renin secretion have speculated on increased sympathetic activity as a driving force to renin secretion or defective negative feedback mechanisms. In this latter regard, several studies have noted an impaired aldosterone secretion in response to volume depletion or sodium restriction in some hypertensive subjects. This defect appears to be present in 33 to 50 percent of normal- and high-renin essential hypertensives [64]. It has been hypothesized that the modulating effect of sodium intake on adrenal and vascular responsiveness to angiotensin II is abnormal in some hypertensive subjects.

A number of studies have evaluated this hypothesis in subjects with essential hypertension. Based on their responsiveness to changes in dietary sodium intake and angiotensin II infusion, patients with normal- and high-renin essential hypertension demonstrate two different response patterns. The majority show responsiveness similar to normal subjects. In the other group, however, following sodium restriction, the normal increase in adrenal sensitivity to angiotensin II does not occur. As well, the normal rise in renal blood flow and renal vascular sensitivity to angiotensin II during high sodium intake does not occur [65]. Due to this lack of modulating effects of sodium intake on angiotensin II responsiveness, this subgroup has been termed nonmodulating hypertension. It appears that nonmodulating hypertension represents a distinct subgroup rather than one end of a spectrum of disease [66].

The pathogenesis of the hypertension in nonmodulators during sodium depletion and sodium repletion has been suggested to be due to dual mechanisms (Figs. 8-6 and 8-7). When sodium is depleted, impaired aldosterone secretion in nonmodulators results in increased renin and angiotensin II generation to close the renin-angiotensin-aldosterone volume feedback loop. The vascular response to the increased angiotensin II could then lead to hypertension during sodium depletion. While on a sodium-replete diet, the abnormal renal sodium handling that results from a reduced renal blood flow response to the salt load may contribute to a sodium-mediated hypertension. Which mechanism is responsible for the hypertension then is dependent on the individual's sodium intake.

Although the pathophysiology of this syndrome remains unclear, a pathologic role for angiotensin II itself has been implicated. In response to treatment with an ACE inhibitor, the abnormal adrenal and renovascular responsiveness returns toward normal, whereas in normotensive and normal-responding hypertensive subjects there is no effect of ACE inhibition on angiotensin II responsiveness [67, 68]. This suggests that nonmodulators possess an abnormality in the regulation of responsiveness to angiotensin II or in the tissue angiotensin II receptors.

Among those hypertensive subjects who respond normally to changes in dietary sodium intake and angiotensin II responsiveness, it remains to be proved that the

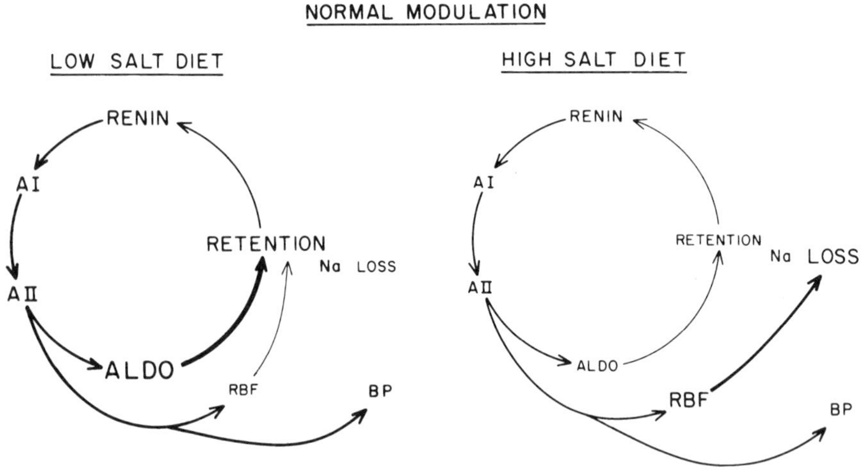

Fig. 8-6. Normal modulation of adrenal, renal, and blood pressure responses to angiotensin II (AII) during changes in salt intake is depicted. During low salt intake, the enhanced aldosterone (ALDO) response leads to volume retention and blunting of further increases in angiotensin II levels. Likewise, during high salt intake, increased renal blood flow (RBF) leads to natriuresis. Both mechanisms function to prevent a rise in blood pressure (BP) during changes in salt intake. AI = angiotensin I. (From G. H. Williams and N. K. Hollenberg, "Sodium-Sensitive" Essential Hypertension: Emerging Insights into Pathogenesis and Therapeutic Implications. In S. Klahr and S. G. Massry [eds.], *Contemporary Issues in Nephrology* [4th ed.]. New York: Plenum, 1985. P. 303.)

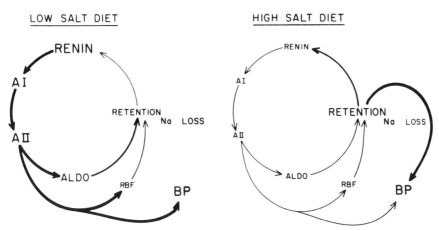

Fig. 8-7. Nonmodulation of adrenal, renal, and blood pressure responses to angiotensin II is depicted. During low salt intake, failure to enhance aldosterone (ALDO) production leads to an inappropriate rise in angiotensin II (AII) levels. During high salt intake, failure to increase renal blood flow (RBF) leads to inappropriate sodium retention. Both mechanisms can lead to a rise in blood pressure (BP). AI = angiotensin I. (From G. H. Williams and N. K. Hollenberg, "Sodium-Sensitive" Essential Hypertension: Emerging Insights into Pathogenesis and Therapeutic Implications. In S. Klahr and S. G. Massry [eds.], *Contemporary Issues in Nephrology* [4th ed.]. New York: Plenum, 1985. P. 303.)

renin-angiotensin-aldosterone system contributes to their pathophysiology. It is likely that this group is heterogeneous, with more than one pathogenetic factor responsible for the hypertension. The role of other factors such as ANH, catecholamines, AVP, or prostaglandins has been suggested to be involved in the hypertensive process; however, the data to support pathophysiologic effects of these substances in hypertension are still modest and controversial.

Renovascular Hypertension

The pathologic role of excess renin secretion in hypertension was first appreciated by Goldblatt et al. [69] with the observation that, in dogs, constriction of both renal arteries was associated with the development of hypertension. As is now appreciated, the release of renin is dependent on a decreased perfusion pressure to the affected kidney. When present unilaterally, increased renin secretion from the ischemic kidney results in suppression of renin release from the contralateral kidney. In the setting of bilateral disease, similar pathophysiology occurs, with the more ischemic kidney providing the major stimulus to renin secretion. The hypersecretion of renin thus results not only in increased angiotensin II generation but also increased aldosterone secretion, with ensuing sodium and water retention. Depending on the status of the contralateral kidney, the increased volume retention stimulated by angiotensin II and aldosterone is either excreted by the nonaffected kidney (as in unilateral renal artery stenosis) or is retained and contributes to the hypertension (as in bilateral renal artery stenosis or stenosis in a solitary kidney). As a result, the mechanisms causing the hypertension in the presence of renal hypoperfusion are multiple, with increased peripheral vascular resistance and, in part, increased extracellular fluid volume. The angiotensin-dependent nature of the hypertension is in some respects dependent on the pathophysiology as well as the individual's sodium intake. Unilateral renal artery stenosis, which is seen most commonly, is associated with greater renin-angiotensin dependency, as proved by the favorable blood pressure effects of administering angiotensin II receptor antagonists or ACE inhibitors [70].

Renovascular hypertension is a disease of all age groups; however, the pathophysiology of the vascular lesions may differ. Among younger individuals (<40 years of age), fibromuscular dysplasia of the arterial wall is most common and tends to occur more commonly in women. In older individuals, atherosclerotic disease tends to predominate, although this form of the disease may also be seen in younger individuals at risk for atherosclerosis. Other less common causes for the syndrome are thromboembolic occlusion or extrinsic compression of the renal artery, especially by a retroperitoneal tumor. In all of these entities, the final result is renal ischemia and enhanced renin secretion.

The diagnosis of renovascular hypertension requires two criteria: (1) the identification of an anatomic lesion (vascular obstruction) that is associated with excessive renin secretion by the affected kidney and (2) correction of the renal ischemia alleviates or improves the hypertension. This latter criterion is especially important, since the chronic phase of renovascular hypertension may be renin independent and unremediable to removal of the stenosis. In this setting, it is presumed that the persistent hypertension has resulted in structural damage to the contralateral kidney as well as other vascular tissues and allows persistence of hypertension after correction of the offending lesion.

Deciding on the appropriate tests to evaluate patients in whom renovascular hypertension is suspected remains controversial, as none is sufficiently sensitive and specific to serve as a screening test. Numerous imaging techniques have been employed to detect vascular obstruction to the kidney. Most notably, intravenous pyelography (IVP) and radioisotopic renograms have proved to be unhelpful because of their relatively high false-positive rates (15–20%) as well as similar false-negative rates. In combination, these procedures may improve the accuracy of diagnosis to greater than 85 percent but not without significant expense. The use of an ACE inhibitor in conjunction with isotope renograms has been shown to improve diagnostic capability [71]. In patients with significant renal artery stenosis, acute administration of an ACE inhibitor induces a fall in glomerular filtration rate (GFR) in the affected kidney. This is presumed to be due to reduction of angiotensin II effects on glomerular efferent arteriolar tone, which is important in the maintenance of GFR in the kidney with the arterial stenosis. The use of this test in patients on chronic ACE inhibitors does not have the same sensitivity as when the study is done with acute administration of the ACE inhibitor. Withdrawal of short-acting ACE inhibitors for greater than 24 hours or long-acting ACE inhibitors for greater than 72 hours followed by reintroduction on the day of study may restore sensitivity.

Intravenous and intra-arterial digital subtraction angiography (DSA) and arteriography remain the most useful techniques for imaging the renal arteries. DSA offers the advantage of intravenous dye injection and outpatient investigation. The reliability of intravenous DSA in comparison to other imaging techniques shows it to be more sensitive and specific than IVP. However, because of the sizable number of uninterpretable studies (15–20%), the overall utility of intravenous DSA compared to IVP is only marginally better. Furthermore, it possesses about 80 percent concordance with arteriography [72], which remains the gold standard for imaging the renal arteries. The use of intra-arterial DSA offers improved sensitivity over intravenous DSA, with the advantage of requiring a smaller dye load. This option is particularly attractive for patients at risk for contrast-induced nephropathy. Magnetic resonance imaging (MRI) angiography also shows promise in evaluating patients for renovascular disease in whom significant risk for contrast administration exists. Widespread experience with this approach is limited.

Once renal artery stenosis has been demonstrated, its functional significance must be proved, since greater than 75 percent of the luminal diameter must be obstructed before hemodynamic compromise will occur. Again, a variety of tests have been advocated as providing an assessment of function, most of which involve measurement of PRA either peripherally or from renal venous effluent. Measurement of peripheral PRA may be helpful if the level is high; however, changes in dietary salt intake and medication use can have profound effects on renin secretion independent of renal pathology, thus making this random measurement less helpful. It has been advocated that the administration of an ACE inhibitor prior to measurement increases renin activity more markedly in patients with renovascular hypertension than in those with essential hypertension [73].

Ultimately, measurement of increased renin secretion by the affected kidney with suppression of renin in the contralateral kidney confirms the diagnosis. A commonly used benchmark is the finding of renin activity from the renal vein of the affected kidney that is greater than 1.5 times that of the nonaffected kidney. With this method, patients with abnormal ratios will typically have a favorable response to correction of the vascular lesion. However, a significant number of patients with ratios below 1.5 have responded to correction of the vascular obstruction, suggesting that in the setting of a significant (>75%) obstruction, intervention may still be warranted. It has been suggested that some of these patients with "normal" ratios may have been studied under suboptimal conditions, such as in the presence of renin-inhibiting agents (e.g., β-blockers). As with the measurement of peripheral PRA, it has been proposed that administration of an ACE inhibitor prior to renal vein renin measurement enhances lateralization and increases the accuracy of diagnosis [74].

The treatment of renovascular hypertension focuses on correcting the inciting event or blunting the effects of hyperreninemia. The advent of percutaneous transluminal angioplasty has revolutionized the treatment and made the need for vascular reconstructive surgery much less necessary. The results of this procedure reveal a very high likelihood of achieving a successful dilatation of the offending renal artery; however, the incidence of cure or recurrence differs based on the underlying pathophysiology. Lesions due to fibromuscular dysplasia are typically responsive to angioplasty with either cure or significant improvement in the hypertension in 90 percent of patients. Restenosis is uncommon. Patients with atherosclerosis have much more varied responses to angioplasty, since many atheromatous lesions are extensions of aortic plaques, making correction of the stenosis difficult. Likewise, the events leading to atherosclerosis (e.g., preexisting essential hypertension, hypercholesterolemia) may continue to exist after removal of the vascular lesion, making the likelihood of restenosis greater [75].

Medical management may be considered for patients either who are not candidates for angioplasty or surgery or in whom these procedures have failed. The major concerns remain the effects of ischemia on renal function and proper control of the hypertension. Various agents have been used to treat such patients including β-blockers, calcium channel antagonists, and ACE inhibitors. The use of ACE inhibitors has represented a major advance in the medical management of renovascular hypertension. Use of an angiotensin II receptor antagonist (e.g., losartan) would potentially also be beneficial, although a significant clinical experience with losartan in this setting is lacking. By interrupting the generation of angiotensin II or blocking its effects, ACE inhibitors and angiotensin II receptor antagonists reduce the major driving force for hypertension in unilateral renal artery stenosis. They have also shown long-term benefits in control of the hypertension. Caution must be used in that patients with bilateral renal artery stenosis or stenosis in a solitary kidney may show a marked decrease in renal function on treatment with ACE inhibitors [76]. This adverse event has been presumed to be due to loss of angiotensin II effects on glomerular efferent arterioles, which serve to maintain glomerular filtration in the setting of reduced perfusion pressure. The reversibility of this loss of renal function remains unclear.

Surgical revascularization provides the best chance for restoring normal renal blood flow and improving renal function if angioplasty is unsuccessful, particularly when renal artery stenosis is due to atherosclerosis. Surgical risk is comparable to that of other vascular surgery repairs, and coexisting coronary and carotid disease may complicate risk. While some authors favor bypass grafting either from nondiseased aorta or hepatic/splenic arteries, recent results with endarterectomy of the renal artery show this procedure to be very useful.

Primary Reninism

Renin-dependent hypertension may be produced by rare tumors of the JG cells that produce and secrete renin excessively [77]. Most patients reported with this syndrome are young, generally less than 25 years old, and malignant hypertension has been observed. The disorder presents biochemically identical to renal artery stenosis, including the presence of renin hypersecretion and profound hypokalemia (due to secondary hyperaldosteronism). In many cases, prorenin secretion is also quite elevated. Tumors are mainly of renal origin. Rarely, ectopic renin-secreting cancers have been described. Some tumors may arise from the surface of the kidney and do not produce and secrete renin into the renal venous effluent. For this reason, radiographic evaluation with computed tomography (CT) scanning may be complementary to renal arteriography with renal vein sampling for renin secretion. The diagnosis is confirmed by finding renin hypersecretion in the absence of significant renal artery stenosis with radiographic evidence of a renal/extrarenal mass. Surgical removal of tumors cures the hyperreninemia and hypertension [78].

Primary Hyperaldosteronism

The observations by Conn [79] that hypertension, hypokalemia, and metabolic alkalosis occurred in a patient with an adrenal adenoma led to the identification of hyperaldosteronism as a secondary cause of hypertension. The hyperaldosteronism syndrome occurs in approximately 1 percent of patients with hypertension; however, its true prevalence may be greater, since the diagnosis is usually limited to the more symptomatic patients. Making the diagnosis is important, as it may lead to marked improvement or cure of the blood pressure and metabolic abnormalities with the institution of specific therapy.

Primary hyperaldosteronism has been found to be caused by three pathologic processes of the adrenal. Aldosterone-producing adenomas result from a single, usually benign tumor of the adrenal cortex that hypersecretes aldosterone. Bilateral adrenal hyperplasia results in idiopathic hyperaldosteronism with bilateral overproduction of aldosterone in the absence of a solitary adenoma. Speculation on the cause of this entity has included the presence of hypersecretion of an aldosterone-stimulating factor of pituitary origin [80] or the loss of normal dopaminergic inhibition [81]. Glucocorticoid-remediable hyperaldosteronism is a much less common form of hyperaldosteronism that occurs in an autosomal dominant pattern in which the hyperaldosteronism is reversible with glucocorticoids.

Most patients with primary hyperaldosteronism have mild to moderate hypertension, and it is uncommon to see malignant hypertension as a presenting sign. Hypertensive retinopathy can occur in patients with primary hyperaldosteronism, and it correlates with the severity and duration of the elevated blood pressure as with essential hypertension. Despite the continuous high levels of aldosterone, patients rarely exhibit edema, presumably because of the escape phenomenon described previously whereby the sodium-retaining effects of chronic mineralocorticoid excess are lost. Although extracellular fluid volume is expanded, there is no escape from the kaliuretic effects of aldosterone. Thus, many of the signs and symptoms that result are due to the potassium depletion. Serum potassium levels are typically less than 3.5 mEq/L and more commonly are at or below 3 mEq/L [82]. Muscle fatigue or cramping may be prominent. Electrocardiographic signs of hypokalemia may also be present. Serum sodium may be mildly elevated, and serum bicarbonate is likewise increased. Hypomagnesemia may also be present and may perpetuate the renal potassium wasting.

The hallmarks of primary hyperaldosteronism are renal potassium wasting, hypertension, and hypokalemia (Fig. 8-8). To confirm the diagnosis, it must be shown that the urinary potassium losses are independent of other known causes (especially diuretics). This is important to document, since the use of diuretics in the treatment of hypertension is so common, as is the ensuing mild hypokalemia. However, the use of diuretics in patients with primary hyperaldosteronism often results in marked hypokalemia (serum potassium < 3 mEq/L), and this may serve as a clue to the diagnosis. In the setting of hypokalemia, urinary potassium losses exceeding 30 to

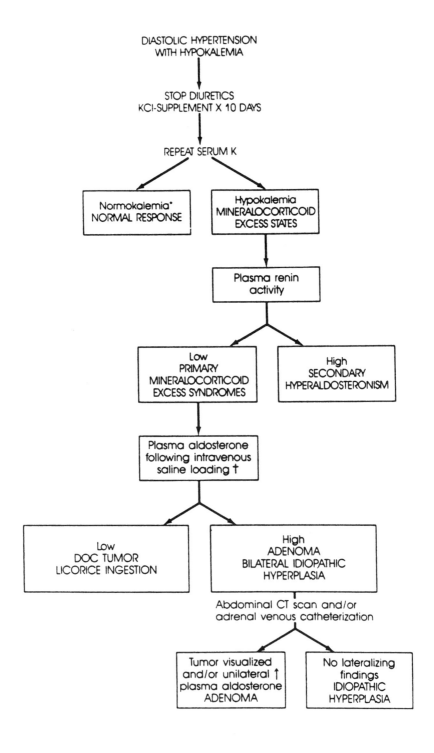

40 mEq/24 hours suggest impaired renal conservation of potassium consistent with increased mineralocorticoid effects.

After demonstration of inappropriate mineralocorticoid effects in the presence of hypertension, documentation of unregulated overproduction of aldosterone confirms the syndrome. An associated finding is the presence of suppressed renin production. Measuring the ratio of plasma aldosterone (measured in nanograms per deciliter) and PRA (measured in nanograms per milliliter per hour) in patients with hypertension and hypokalemia suggests primary hyperaldosteronism when the ratio exceeds 30 (see Fig. 8-4). The failure of PRA to rise normally after volume depletion through maneuvers such as dietary sodium restriction and assumption of upright posture is an important clue and distinguishes this diagnosis from those syndromes that may have secondary hyperaldosteronism as a feature (e.g., renovascular hypertension). As previously described, suppressed renin also occurs in patients with low-renin essential hypertension; therefore, this finding by itself does not distinguish between primary hyperaldosteronism and other causes of hypertension.

Various maneuvers have been proposed to demonstrate abnormal, autonomous aldosterone secretion, but those most commonly used involve volume expansion with sodium chloride as a test of normal suppression. Acute infusion of saline [83] or ingestion of a high-salt diet for 5 days suppresses aldosterone secretion in normal individuals but has limited effects on aldosterone secretion in primary hyperaldosteronism. The failure to normally suppress aldosterone secretion in response to this volume expansion confirms the diagnosis. A caveat to these maneuvers is that the volume expansion also results in enhanced sodium delivery to the distal tubule (the site of action of aldosterone on sodium and potassium transport), which can result in a precipitous fall in serum potassium.

Since the syndrome of primary hyperaldosteronism may be caused by different entities, it is important to identify the appropriate cause, as treatment options will differ based on the pathogenesis. The aldosterone response to upright posture is often helpful in discriminating aldosterone-producing adenomas from idiopathic hyperaldosteronism. Since idiopathic hyperaldosteronism typically retains responsiveness to angiotensin II, patients with this entity will have a rise in plasma aldosterone with assumption of upright posture. This maneuver activates angiotensin II generation in patients with idiopathic hyperaldosteronism, since their renin secretion is usually not profoundly suppressed as in aldosterone-producing adenomas. In contrast, aldosterone-producing adenomas are commonly responsive to ACTH and

◄────────────────────────────────────

Fig. 8-8. Diagnostic flow chart for evaluating the patient with suspected hyperaldosteronism.

* Serum potassium may be normal in some patients with mineralocorticoid excess who are consuming a low-salt–high-potassium diet or taking potassium sparing diuretics.

† This step should be avoided if severe hypertension (diastolic pressure > 115 mm Hg) or heart failure is present. Potassium should be repleted prior to saline infusion to avoid profound hypokalemia due to the kaliuresis induced by elevated aldosterone levels. (From G. H. Williams and R. G. Dluhy, Diseases of the Adrenal Cortex. In K. J. Isselbach et al. [eds.], *Harrison's Principles of Internal Medicine* [13th ed.]. New York: McGraw-Hill, 1994. P. 1966.)

thus will demonstrate a fall in plasma aldosterone following assumption of upright posture due to the normal diurnal variation of ACTH. Recently, some patients have been described with angiotensin II–responsive aldosterone-producing adenomas who have a rise in aldosterone levels with upright posture. Therefore, the utility of this test as the sole means for diagnosing the cause of hyperaldosteronism is limited. Biochemical studies may also assist in evaluating patients with hyperaldosteronism. Measurement of plasma 18-hydroxycorticosterone (levels > 100 ng/dl) or urinary 18-hydroxycortisol (levels > 60 μg/24 hr) can be indicative of aldosterone-producing adenomas [84].

Aldosterone-producing adenomas can be identified by abdominal CT scanning or MRI, which demonstrate an adrenal adenoma, although these tumors can sometimes be smaller than the resolution of these imaging techniques. In the absence of radiographic evidence of a tumor or to confirm the diagnosis, bilateral adrenal vein catheterization may be required. Under these conditions, simultaneous sampling of adrenal venous effluent for aldosterone and cortisol (to confirm appropriate catheter placement) will determine the unilateral or bilateral production of aldosterone, thus differentiating between aldosterone-producing adenomas and idiopathic hyperaldosteronism with bilateral adrenal hyperplasia [82].

Hyperaldosteronism due to aldosterone-producing adenomas is typically cured or significantly improved by surgical removal of the pathologic adrenal. One year postoperatively, 70 percent of patients are normotensive, but this rate drops to 53 percent after 5 years. Patients with idiopathic hyperaldosteronism have variable and usually negligible change in blood pressure after bilateral adrenalectomy. For this reason, it is important to clearly identify the etiology for hyperaldosteronism prior to referring for adrenalectomy. For those patients whose hyperaldosteronism is not remediable by surgery, use of the aldosterone antagonist spironolactone in conjunction with a low-salt diet may ameliorate much of the renal potassium wasting and improve the hypertension. Other potassium sparing diuretics, such as amiloride and triamterene, have also been used successfully [85].

Glucocorticoid-remediable aldosteronism was previously thought to be a very rare form of hyperaldosteronism, but recent advances suggest that it may not be as uncommon as first thought. It is important not to overlook the possibility of glucocorticoid-remediable aldosteronism in patients who present with clinical evidence of hyperaldosteronism, particularly at a young age. Important clues in diagnosing this entity are often obtained from a careful family history. The autosomal dominant inheritance pattern results in numerous family members affected commonly with early death due to hypertensive complications, primarily cerebral hemorrhage. Unlike other forms of hyperaldosteronism, glucocorticoid-remediable aldosteronism does not always present with overt signs and symptoms of mineralocorticoid excess. However, a hallmark of the syndrome is that patients with glucocorticoid-remediable aldosteronism will show profound suppression of aldosterone and lowering of blood pressure with dexamethasone, especially when treated early in the course of their disease. Other causes of hyperaldosteronism will be unaffected by exogenous steroids.

Much has been learned recently about the pathogenesis of this entity through the study of molecular genetics [86]. Patients with glucocorticoid-remediable aldo-

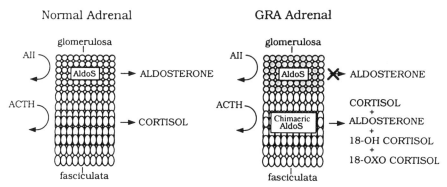

Fig. 8-9. In the normal adrenal, adrenocorticotropic hormone (ACTH) and angiotensin II (AII) are the major regulators of cortisol and aldosterone in the zona fasciculata and zona glomerulosa, respectively. Ectopic expression of the chimaeric gene with aldosterone synthase enzymatic activity in glucocorticoid-remediable aldosteronism results in aldosterone synthesis stimulated by ACTH. (From R. P. Lifton, R. G. Dluhy, M. Powers, et al., The molecular basis of a hypertensive disease: Chimaeric gene duplications result in ectopic expression of aldosterone synthase and glucocorticoid-remediable hyperaldosteronism. *Nature Genetics* 2:66, 1992.)

steronism have been discovered to have a gene duplication that results in aldosterone production by a hybrid gene containing elements of 11β-hydroxylase and aldosterone synthase expressed in the zona fasciculata under the stimulation of ACTH (Fig. 8-9). Genetic screening of at-risk individuals using the abnormal gene as the marker of disease presence has allowed identification of numerous individuals in families with an identified proband. Children less than 1 year of age can be diagnosed by this method. Most intriguing is that the phenotype is quite variable. Whereas all patients with glucocorticoid-remediable aldosteronism have the abnormal aldosterone synthase gene, not all have markedly elevated blood pressure or significant hypokalemia. In some patients, blood pressure and potassium levels are normal.

Treatment of patients with glucocorticoid-remediable aldosteronism depends largely on the severity of blood pressure elevation. Whereas patients with a very mild phenotype may not require treatment, those with more severe forms may require glucocorticoids, potassium sparing diuretics, and other antihypertensive therapy. Rarely, adrenalectomy may be required to control blood pressure.

Other Mineralocorticoid Excess States

After evaluating the patient with hypertension and signs of mineralocorticoid excess, despite the presence of a suppressed renin-angiotensin system, occasionally hypoaldosteronism will be found consistent with the presence of overproduction of another mineralocorticoid. Rarely DOC-producing adenomas of the adrenal have been found to produce the syndrome of hypertension, metabolic alkalosis, and hypokalemia. Also occurring rarely is the syndrome of mineralocorticoid excess due to defects in cortisol biosynthesis resulting in adrenal hyperplasia. Defects in 11β- or 17α-hydroxylation result in impaired cortisol production and a resultant increase

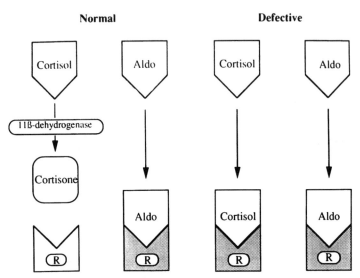

Fig. 8-10. The enzyme 11β-dehydrogenase converts cortisol to inactive cortisone and thereby allows aldosterone (Aldo) to bind to the mineralocorticoid receptor (R). When the enzyme is defective or inhibited, cortisol can bind to the receptor and produce mineralocorticoid effects. (From B. R. Walker and C. R. W. Edwards, Licorice-induced hypertension and syndromes of apparent mineralocorticoid excess. *Endocrinol. Clin. North Am.* 23:359, 1994.)

in ACTH secretion. Under the stimulation of ACTH, the adrenal becomes hyperplastic and hypersecretes cortisol precursors, particularly DOC, thus resulting in the syndrome of mineralocorticoid excess. The demonstration of increased production of these precursors confirms the diagnosis. Specific therapy involving cortisol replacement corrects the metabolic and blood pressure abnormalities (see Congenital Adrenal Hyperplasia).

A syndrome that occurs uncommonly is due to ingestion of compounds in chewing tobacco or licorice, specifically glycyrrhizic acid, which can produce the signs and symptoms of mineralocorticoid excess. This compound has been shown to inhibit the inactivation of cortisol to cortisone in the kidney by the enzyme 11β-hydroxysteroid dehydrogenase [87]. Therefore, cortisol is allowed to bind to renal mineralocorticoid receptors and exert mineralocorticoid effects (Fig. 8-10). A careful history establishes this diagnosis.

A congenital syndrome of increased mineralocorticoid activity, described by Ulick et al. [88], has been presumed to be due to deficiency of the enzyme 11β-hydroxysteroid dehydrogenase [89]. Similar to that seen with ingestion of glycyrrhizic acid, the absence of this functional enzyme results in impaired clearance of cortisol and thus exposes the kidney to excessive mineralocorticoid activity due to occupancy of the mineralocorticoid receptor by cortisol. An increased ratio of urinary cortisol metabolites to cortisone metabolites suggests this diagnosis.

Liddle's syndrome is a rare entity that was originally described in a family with signs of mineralocorticoid excess in the absence of hyperaldosteronism or hyperreninemia. The renal potassium wasting proved to be responsive to the potassium sparing diuretic triamterene. The genetic abnormality responsible for this syndrome has been recently identified. A subunit of the epithelial sodium channel, which is normally activated by aldosterone in the renal distal tubule, is abnormal in these patients [90]. This abnormality results in constitutive activity of the channel, thus resulting in unregulated sodium retention and potassium loss (due to maintenance of electroneutrality), which clinically appear as mineralocorticoid excess.

The Renin-Angiotensin-Aldosterone System in Edematous Disorders

The pathophysiologic factors responsible for edema formation can be varied; however, activation of the renin-angiotensin-aldosterone system is a common accompaniment often due to reduced effective arterial circulating volume. The resulting salt and water retention attempts to restore the arterial blood volume to normal but in so doing often exacerbates the underlying disease process. In these various states, numerous other neurohumoral responses are activated and also contribute to the increase in extracellular volume. Discussion of the multiple causes of edema formation in these pathologic states is beyond the scope of this discussion but has been reviewed elsewhere [91]. The following summarizes the more common edema-forming states and the role of the renin-angiotensin-aldosterone system in their pathogenesis.

Congestive Heart Failure

Congestive heart failure is characterized by either a low cardiac output (low-output failure) or low peripheral resistance (high-output failure) in conjunction with activation of neurohumoral systems including sympathetic activity, AVP secretion, and the renin-angiotensin-aldosterone system. Although these neurohumoral responses function predominantly to maintain cardiac output and perfusion pressure, they also increase ventricular afterload, salt and water retention, and edema formation. The "sensing" of a reduction in effective arterial blood volume in both high- and low-output states appears to be the initial event in stimulating salt and water retention. Following this event, the systemic response is similar regardless of the initial cardiac output.

Patients with congestive heart failure have been shown to have elevated levels of AVP, norepinephrine, ANH, renin, and aldosterone [92–94], particularly during the early decompensated stages. Levels of these factors, in general, return toward normal on correction of the decompensated state. Based on these observations, levels of these factors have been used as markers of the severity of the heart failure. However, it has also been recognized that the level of activation of the renin-angiotensin-aldosterone and sympathetic nervous systems varies widely in patients with congestive heart failure, particularly after therapy has been introduced.

Activation of renin secretion in congestive heart failure is probably secondary to both a decreased renal perfusion pressure and an enhanced sympathetic nervous system activity. The resulting angiotensin II generated not only increases perfusion pressure but also increases peripheral vascular resistance and stimulates aldosterone secretion in an attempt to restore effective blood volume. The role of angiotensin II as a pathogenic factor in the maintenance of a low cardiac output is underscored by the observations that interruption of angiotensin II generation by ACE inhibition results in a marked drop in peripheral resistance and cardiac afterload and an increase in cardiac output [95]. In patients with more marked cardiac failure manifested by hyponatremia and hyperreninemia, ACE inhibitors appear to have their most dramatic effects. In such patients, however, angiotensin II also serves a major role in blood pressure regulation such that judicious dosing of ACE inhibitors is warranted to avoid marked hypotension. The pathogenetic role of high angiotensin II levels in chronic congestive heart failure is underscored by the marked clinical improvement observed in patients treated with ACE inhibitors. Significant mortality benefit has been shown in patients with diminished left ventricular function who receive ACE inhibitors.

While the role of angiotensin II in congestive heart failure appears prominent, that of aldosterone is less evident. Treatment of patients with the aldosterone antagonist spironolactone results in a modest increase in urinary sodium excretion. In addition, ACE inhibition alone lowers aldosterone levels but does not necessarily increase urinary sodium excretion [95]. Part of this lack of effect may be secondary to the simultaneous drop in blood pressure induced by declining angiotensin II levels. In animal models of heart failure, it appears that aldosterone exerts its effects on sodium retention predominantly during the early stages of decompensation; later there is enhanced proximal tubule sodium reabsorption and a decline in sodium delivery to the site of aldosterone action in the distal tubule. Clinically, this is evident by the observation that ACE inhibition exerts its most dramatic effects on urinary sodium excretion in the setting of simultaneous diuretic administration.

Nephrotic Syndrome

The nephrotic syndrome results from glomerular basement membrane injury, which allows excessive quantities of serum proteins to be lost into the renal tubules and eventually excreted. As a result of this loss of serum proteins, which by definition exceeds 3 g daily, the plasma oncotic pressure is reduced, and transudation of intravascular fluid into the extracellular space occurs. The causes of nephrotic syndrome are many; however, each results in the presence of profound proteinuria and edema formation.

It was originally assumed that the loss of intravascular fluid would be the stimulus for activation of the various neurohumoral systems responsible for maintenance of volume homeostasis, including the renin-angiotensin-aldosterone system. However, some studies have suggested that patients with nephrotic syndrome who are actively retaining sodium may have normal or even increased blood volumes [96]. Thus, the mechanisms of sodium and volume retention and edema formation may be dissociated in some patients with nephrotic syndrome in comparison to those with congestive heart failure. It has been postulated that altered intrarenal mechanisms may be most important in these patients.

Despite these observations, many patients with the nephrotic syndrome truly have reductions in effective arterial blood volume, shown particularly in those with minimal change disease. Stimulation of the renin-angiotensin-aldosterone system occurs as a result of a reduced renal perfusion pressure and sympathetic stimulation. An important role for aldosterone in the fluid retention of the nephrotic syndrome has been suggested by the fact that treatment of such patients with spironolactone results in sodium and volume excretion and improvement of edema. In contrast, similar patients treated with an ACE inhibitor show reductions in aldosterone levels but little increase in natriuresis [97]. This treatment also results in a reduction of angiotensin II effects on vascular beds and glomerular hemodynamics, which may be important factors in maintaining glomerular filtration and delivery of sodium to the site of aldosterone action. Therefore, any natriuretic effect of reduced aldosterone levels may be obscured by sodium-retaining effects of a reduction in blood pressure and GFR induced by ACE inhibition.

Hepatic Cirrhosis

Hepatic fibrosis and scarring result from chronic insults to the liver induced by such offending agents as excess alcohol ingestion, viral infection, or toxin exposure. Complicating this loss of hepatic function are the resulting reduction in synthesis of plasma factors (e.g., albumin), portal hypertension, and ascites and edema formation. Theories on how sodium and water retention is enhanced in patients with cirrhosis are varied and in some respects invoke hemodynamic changes that fall on opposite ends of the spectrum. The role of the renin-angiotensin-aldosterone system in the pathogenesis of edema formation has been appreciated; however, the mechanisms of its activation remain somewhat speculative.

As in the nephrotic syndrome, a reduction in plasma oncotic pressure due to hypoalbuminemia (in this case resulting from impaired hepatic synthesis) can result in stimulation of renin secretion by increased sympathetic nervous system activity, reduced renal perfusion pressure, and a reduction in sodium delivery to the macula densa. Despite an enhancement in sodium and water retention, intravascular volume may remain low due to continued transudation of fluid into extravascular compartments, particularly the lower extremities and the abdominal cavity. Based on this hypothesis, the resulting hypovolemia would provide an appropriate stimulus for renin secretion.

Other data show that blood volume in cirrhotic patients may actually be increased and that renal sodium and water retention may be enhanced by other mechanisms. Supporting this concept is the observation that in experimentally induced cirrhosis, renal sodium and water retention can occur prior to the development of hypoalbuminemia. Likewise, extrahepatic obstruction of the portal vein, which results in splanchnic hypertension, can also produce enhanced renal sodium retention [98]. These data would suggest that a communication exists (either neural or humoral) between the liver/splanchnic circulation and the kidney that can enhance renal sodium conservation. Numerous attempts to identify this hepatorenal reflex have been unsuccessful. Supporting this concept is the observation that renal denervation abolishes this mechanism. Although this hypothesis is attractive based on experimental data, studies in humans have not confirmed a role for hepatorenal communication as the major stimulus for renal sodium retention.

In humans with cirrhosis and ascites, activation of the renin-angiotensin-aldosterone system is often present even prior to decompensation. Often cardiac output is normal or increased, with a reduction in peripheral resistance and blood pressure. A third hypothesis assumes that it is through this latter mechanism of reduced blood pressure due to peripheral vasodilation that renin secretion may be enhanced [99]. Thus, the peripheral vasodilation in cirrhosis per se may be pathophysiologic in the induction of fluid retention. Peripheral vasodilation in patients with cirrhosis has been described and is presumably due primarily to splanchnic vasodilation. Identification of the mechanisms responsible for these changes in vascular responsiveness may prove helpful in understanding the pathogenesis of edema formation in patients with cirrhosis.

Involvement of angiotensin II in blood pressure regulation in cirrhosis has been noted based on the hypotensive response to infusion of the angiotensin II antagonist saralasin [100]. Such patients are also typically sensitive to adrenergic blockade as well. Clinical results with ACE inhibition have shown a similar outcome. Likewise, aldosterone clearly participates in the sodium retention of cirrhosis as evidenced by enhanced sodium and water excretion following administration of spironolactone [101]. The diuresis that occurs is generally modest, suggesting that other sodium-retaining factors are likewise operative. As seen in patients with congestive heart failure, addition of more proximally acting diuretics, such as furosemide, may improve the diuresis.

Idiopathic Edema

The disorder entitled idiopathic (cyclic) edema represents a diagnosis of exclusion when edema formation occurs in otherwise healthy patients in the absence of known renal, cardiac, hepatic, or endocrine disease. The edema formation appears to be worsened by obesity and upright posture. Its occurrence has been noted predominantly in women, in whom edema formation will increase premenstrually.

Levels of PRA and aldosterone have been noted to be increased in many of these patients during upright posture [102]. Whether these changes are primary or secondary to some other underlying defect remains uncertain. Alterations in renal dopamine formation [103] and hepatic albumin synthesis [104] have also been reported. There appears to be no association with impaired ANH secretion as a cause for the fluid retention [105].

The clinical course of patients with idiopathic edema is typically benign, with periods of improved or worsened edema. Treatment, when applied, is typically for cosmetic reasons. When patients are upright for prolonged periods of time, application of support stockings is probably the most effective and least harmful form of therapy and has proved to be successful. Diuretics, including hydrochlorothiazide and spironolactone, have been used to reduce the edema. However, their excessive use should be discouraged, as it has been associated with electrolyte abnormalities and secondary hyperaldosteronism, which may worsen the underlying disorder (i.e., diuretic-induced edema). Finally, sympathomimetic agents have also been used, with varying success.

Other Disorders of the Renin-Angiotensin-Aldosterone System

Bartter's Syndrome

The syndrome of hypokalemic alkalosis, JG cell hyperplasia, and normal blood pressure in the absence of adrenal tumor was originally described by Bartter et al. in 1962 [106]. Although rare, the syndrome has been identified in additional patients, many of whom have displayed growth or developmental delay [107]. In addition to the metabolic abnormalities, Bartter's syndrome is associated with activation of the renin-angiotensin system, secondary hyperaldosteronism, and renal potassium wasting. An identifying characteristic of Bartter's syndrome is a reduced pressor response to angiotensin II but not norepinephrine, which may be explained by the high endogenous levels of angiotensin II generated by the hyperreninemia.

Numerous theories have been postulated to explain the pathophysiology of Bartter's syndrome. However, it is likely that this rare syndrome consists of a number of related causes resulting in a similar phenotype. Abnormal chloride transport in the renal proximal tubule has been identified in some but not all patients with Bartter's syndrome [108]. Likewise, sodium transport defects have been suggested [109]. The observation that patients with Bartter's syndrome hypersecrete prostaglandin metabolites led to the assumption that excessive renal prostaglandin synthesis may participate in the pathogenesis of the syndrome [110]. It followed that patients treated with indomethacin showed marked improvement in hyperreninemia, secondary hyperaldosteronism, and hypokalemia (presumably by inhibition of renin release secondary to the inhibition of prostaglandin synthesis).

It is important to identify alternative and likely more frequent causes of hypokalemic alkalosis and hyperreninemia, which would include surreptitious diuretic use and bulemic syndromes of frequent vomiting. Careful history taking and appropriate laboratory investigation including urinary screening for diuretics may be necessary. Also, in patients with frequent vomiting, a low urinary chloride level is typically seen and can be a useful adjunct in determining that diagnosis.

Treatment of patients with Bartter's syndrome is not universally successful. As previously mentioned, indomethacin may improve the hypokalemia and hyperreninemia. Supplementation with potassium alone may yield little benefit, as the hyperresponsive adrenal gland further enhances aldosterone production, thus blunting any significant change in potassium balance. In some cases, treatment with potassium sparing diuretics, such as spironolactone or amiloride, has yielded additional benefits.

Hypoaldosteronism

A variety of syndromes have been described with hypoaldosteronism either resulting from reduced adrenal stimulation due to impaired renin production or due to a primary defect in aldosterone production by the adrenal. Most cases are associated with clinical manifestations of mineralocorticoid deficiency including vascular and electrolyte abnormalities. In some cases, aldosterone levels may be low without clinical manifestations. Identification of the etiology of the hypoaldosteronism with institution of appropriate treatment can often lead to prompt resolution of life-threatening metabolic aberrations.

Primary Adrenal Insufficiency. Partial or complete destruction of the adrenal glands produces the classic example of aldosterone deficiency. In this setting, adrenocortical function is absent or severely impaired, producing a deficiency state of cortisol and aldosterone. It is this loss of mineralocorticoid function that likely contributes to the volume depletion, hyperkalemia, and metabolic acidosis that commonly accompany primary adrenal failure. The causes for primary adrenal insufficiency fall into the major categories of idiopathic atrophy (presumably autoimmune), infection (e.g., tuberculosis), hemorrhage, and infiltration by pathologic processes. Recently, the acquired immune deficiency syndrome (AIDS) has been added to this list of potential causes of adrenal insufficiency due to both infectious (cytomegalovirus) and infiltrative disease [111]. A complete review of adrenal insufficiency is beyond the scope of this discussion, but more detail is available elsewhere [112].

In the setting of aldosterone deficiency, the resulting volume depletion due to impaired renal sodium conservation leads to markedly elevated levels of PRA and angiotensin II. In the absence of glucocorticoid, however, vascular responsiveness to vasopressors, including angiotensin II and norepinephrine, is reduced, resulting in a reduction in blood pressure and particularly orthostatic hypotension. The hyponatremia that occurs is not simply explainable by mineralocorticoid deficiency. Increased secretion of AVP in response to the volume depletion leads to impaired solute-free water clearance. In addition, cortisol deficiency alone may lead to inappropriate secretion of AVP, with resulting hyponatremia that is correctable by glucocorticoid replacement [113].

Treatment of adrenal insufficiency involves replacement of physiologic levels of both glucocorticoid and mineralocorticoid. In the acute setting, supraphysiologic doses of glucocorticoids are typically required and may obviate the need for mineralocorticoids unless steroids with minimal mineralocorticoid effects (such as dexamethasone or methylprednisolone) are used. In the chronic management of such patients, glucocorticoid replacement is often supplemented with administration of fludrocortisone, a potent mineralocorticoid. PRA and angiotensin II levels are typically elevated in patients receiving inadequate mineralocorticoid replacement and can be used as a means of monitoring replacement doses. However, clinical evaluation, including postural blood pressure measurement, usually suffices in determining adequacy of treatment.

Congenital Adrenal Hyperplasia. Various enzyme defects in the pathway of adrenal steroidogenesis have been identified in patients, particularly children, who present with disorders of sexual differentiation or abnormal cortisol and aldosterone production. Since the end product of zona fasciculata steroid production, cortisol, is the only adrenal product providing negative feedback to pituitary secretion of ACTH, a defect in cortisol production results in ACTH hypersecretion with resulting adrenal hyperplasia. With continued stimulation of steroid precursors, those substances preceding the defective enzyme are released in excess into the circulation and can exert physiologic effects (see Fig. 8-3). Enzyme defects involving each of the steps of steroid production have been described, and each results in deficiencies of both cortisol and aldosterone. Either sodium wasting or retention can occur, depending on the precursors that are produced in excess.

The most common syndromes in which renal sodium wasting occurs are those due to deficiency of 21-hydroxylase, 3β-hydroxysteroid dehydrogenase, or corticosterone methyl oxidase (18-hydroxylase). In these settings, inadequate amounts of cortisol, aldosterone, or both are produced, and the immediate precursors, which are produced in excess, also lack mineralocorticoid effect. The diagnosis is typically made at birth or in early childhood, when excessive salt losing, hypotension, disordered sexual differentiation (in female infants), and occasionally hyperkalemia are noted. Documentation of excess secretion of the steroid precursors preceding the enzyme block confirms the site of the defect. Cortisol replacement restores the impaired negative feedback to ACTH secretion, and mineralocorticoid treatment corrects the salt wasting.

The autosomal recessive syndromes of corticosterone methyl oxidase deficiency produce selective aldosterone deficiency, since cortisol production does not require 18-hydroxylation. Two forms of this syndrome have been described. In the type I syndrome, aldosterone production is absent, but low levels of the aldosterone precursor 18-hydroxycorticosterone are present (probably of zona fasciculata origin), suggesting the presence of a selective deficiency of corticosterone methyl oxidase in the zona glomerulosa [114]. In the type II form of the syndrome, 18-hydroxycorticosterone levels are high and accompanied by low levels of aldosterone such that the ratio of these two substances in peripheral blood provides evidence for the diagnosis [115, 116]. In this syndrome, it is apparent that the zona glomerulosa possesses the ability to produce 18-hydroxylate corticosterone but is unable to convert this intermediate to the aldehyde product, aldosterone. This is associated with a mutation in the aldosterone synthase gene. In the type I syndrome, aldosterone synthase is inactive, whereas in the type II form, the enzyme remains capable of 11β-hydroxylation but not 18-oxidation. Based on these and other data, it has now been concluded that the enzyme that subserves 18-hydroxylation is different between zona glomerulosa and zona fasciculata. In support of this possibility is the observation that two 11β-hydroxylase genes that possess corticosterone methyl oxidase function are expressed in the rat glomerulosa cell, but only one is expressed in the zona fasciculata [117]. The enzyme that is expressed in zona fasciculata is able to perform the initial 18-hydroxylation but is incapable of completing the two-step oxidation to aldosterone. The additional isoform of the enzyme present in the zona glomerulosa (aldosterone synthase) possesses complete corticosterone methyl oxidase function, thus producing aldosterone.

The enzyme defects 11β-hydroxylase and 17α-hydroxylase also result in impaired cortisol and aldosterone secretion. However, the immediate precursors to these enzyme blocks allow for the excessive production of DOC, which possesses potent mineralocorticoid effects. The clinical manifestations of these enzyme deficiencies result in the syndrome of mineralocorticoid excess (as previously described), with volume expansion, suppressed PRA, hypertension, and hypokalemia. Many patients may escape diagnosis until adolescence or adulthood, when in addition to manifesting mineralocorticoid excess, female patients with 11β-hydroxylase deficiency may present with hirsutism and menstrual disturbances due to adrenal androgen excess. Those with 17α-hydroxylase deficiency of both sexes usually have primary hypogonadism. Cortisol replacement typically corrects the ACTH hyperstimulation of precursor substances and often cures the hypertension. A more extensive review of this topic has been reported elsewhere [118].

Hyporeninemic Hypoaldosteronism. The clinical findings of hyperkalemia, metabolic acidosis, and renal sodium wasting in patients with mild renal insufficiency have been associated with hyporeninemia and hypoaldosteronism. Tests of adrenal cortical function show a normal cortisol response to ACTH stimulation; however, the aldosterone response to either angiotensin II infusion or sodium restriction is blunted [119]. In addition, the normal postural rise in renin secretion is reduced. In these patients, the level of hyperkalemia is typically out of proportion to the degree of renal insufficiency. It is also not uncommon for such patients to be older and to have diabetes mellitus.

It is unclear why this syndrome should occur more frequently in patients with diabetes. Patients with diabetes commonly develop autonomic dysfunction and impaired renal sympathetic activity, which may lead to a reduction in renin secretion. Also, the role of insulin in transmembrane movement of potassium may in some way be involved. Hyporeninemic hypoaldosteronism has also been described in patients with AIDS, in patients with other renal disorders including obstructive uropathy [120], and in patients on chronic nonsteroidal anti-inflammatory drugs [121], in which inhibition of renal prostaglandin synthesis impairs renin secretion. The final common pathway for each of these etiologies to cause the syndrome is through the induction of hyporeninemia, leading to reduced angiotensin II generation and resulting atrophy of the zona glomerulosa. Once initiated, the resulting hyperkalemia may further reduce renin secretion, although correction of the hyperkalemia does not restore normal renin secretion. Some investigators have suggested that a separate adrenal defect needs to be implicated to explain the blunted aldosterone response to the hyperkalemic stimulus. However, evidence would suggest a primacy of angiotensin II in the maintenance of normal zona glomerulosa function. As an example of such, patients with hyperaldosteronism due to an adrenal adenoma typically have marked hyporeninemia and suppression of the contralateral adrenal zona glomerulosa due to the aldosterone-induced volume expansion. Following removal of the adenoma, it is not unusual for hypoaldosteronism with its clinical sequelae of hyperkalemia to persist for up to 6 months while the normal adrenal recovers its responsiveness [122].

While patients with AIDS have been described with hyporeninemic hypoaldosteronism [123], a more recently described abnormality that results in mild to moderate hyperkalemia is due to antikaliuretic properties of trimethoprim. This drug is an integral component of the combination sulfamethoxazole-trimethoprim commonly used as prophylaxis and treatment of pneumocystis pneumonia. It has been shown that trimethoprim inhibits sodium transport in the distal nephron in a manner similar to amiloride [124]. This hyperkalemia-inducing effect of trimethoprim can be distinguished from hyporeninemic hypoaldosteronism, since levels of PRA and aldosterone are not low.

Treatment of hyporeninemic hypoaldosteronism involves either removal of the offending agent or replacement with exogenous mineralocorticoid, usually fludrocortisone. Some patients require supraphysiologic doses of fludrocortisone, suggesting a renal resistance to mineralocorticoid. In some patients, furosemide may also be used to induce a kaliuresis.

Hyperreninemic Hypoaldosteronism During Critical Illness. A syndrome of increased PRA in the setting of relative hypoaldosteronism has been described in patients with serious medical illness [125]. Despite the hypoaldosteronism, patients will typically have normal serum potassium (due to frequent monitoring in the intensive care unit setting), appropriate elevations of cortisol, and decreased levels of 18-hydroxycorticosterone, which suggest that the site of the defect in aldosterone production is due to impaired zona glomerulosa function. Since the syndrome does not result in clinical evidence of mineralocorticoid deficiency, it has been assumed that the hypoaldosteronism is masked by the presence of appropriate hypercortisolism, which at high levels may exert renal mineralocorticoid effects.

The cause of hyperreninemic hypoaldosteronism remains elusive, although various factors have been evaluated. Excessive dopaminergic tone does not appear to be associated with the hypoaldosteronism, and increased levels of ANH have been found equally among patients with the syndrome and those with critical illness and normal aldosterone levels [126]. An interesting speculation is that the chronic high levels of ACTH present during serious illness result in an adrenal adaptation where cortisol production is preferentially spared while adrenal androgens and mineralocorticoids are lost. This has been based on experiments in which chronic ACTH infusion in humans results in a reduction in aldosterone secretion despite maintenance of cortisol secretion [127]. Following this fall in aldosterone, stimulation with other secretagogues such as potassium and angiotensin II has been shown to result in a blunted aldosterone response. In patients with the hyperreninemic hypoaldosterone syndrome, ACTH or angiotensin II infusion produces very little rise in aldosterone secretion despite maintenance of the vascular response to angiotensin II [125]. Similar experiments performed in sheep show that chronic high levels of ACTH produce hypertrophy of the zona fasciculata and atrophy of the zona glomerulosa.

Because of the absence of clinical manifestations of mineralocorticoid deficiency, the syndrome itself does not result in a pathophysiologic state per se. However, its presence has been associated with increased mortality. It is of note that one patient diagnosed with the syndrome demonstrated transient hyperkalemia during recovery from the illness [128], suggesting that hypoaldosteronism may be slow to recover. Treatment, therefore, relies on correction of the underlying condition leading to the critical illness.

Other Causes of Hypoaldosteronism. Less commonly encountered conditions associated with hypoaldosteronism include heparin administration [13,129], chronic potassium depletion, and hypopituitarism [51]. During heparin administration, aldosterone production may be depressed by an unknown but direct effect on the zona glomerulosa. This inhibition of aldosterone synthesis is reversed on withdrawal of heparin, typically within 3 to 5 days. Doses as low as 10,000 units/day have been shown to produce aldosterone deficiency. Patients who present with signs and symptoms of aldosterone deficiency while receiving heparin should also be carefully evaluated for evidence of adrenal hemorrhage, which produces glucocorticoid and mineralocorticoid deficiency. Chronic potassium depletion impairs aldosterone production and can lead to reduced responsiveness of the zona glomerulosa to other secretagogues. Such patients may develop hyperkalemia if potassium repletion is too rapid. Patients with hypopituitarism may have a reduced aldosterone response to sodium restriction and ACTH stimulation. Subjects with isolated ACTH deficiency (e.g., patients on chronic supraphysiologic doses of glucocorticoids) do not appear to have disordered aldosterone secretion. The patients with hypopituitarism lack a variety of hormones including cortisol, thyroid hormone, and growth hormone, which may be important in the maintenance of adrenal growth and function. Appropriate hormone replacement with cortisol and thyroid hormone leads to restoration of normal responsiveness.

Pseudohypoaldosteronism

Pseudohypoaldosteronism is a rare familial disorder that is manifested by renal salt wasting, hyperkalemia, and metabolic acidosis. Levels of PRA and aldosterone are markedly elevated, and cortisol levels are normal. Such patients are also resistant to the effects of exogenous mineralocorticoids. Originally described in 1958 [130], a number of cases have since been identified with familial clustering [131].

The pathogenesis of the pseudohypoaldosteronism syndrome appears to be due to a defective mineralocorticoid receptor [132], although no mutations affecting aldosterone action have been identified. As previously described, interaction of aldosterone with its receptor is necessary for DNA binding and the resulting effects on protein synthesis, which allow for the manifestation of mineralocorticoid effects. There are different forms of inheritance of the syndrome, with autosomal dominant and recessive forms present among different families [132]. Biochemical evidence of impaired receptor function has been demonstrated in relatives of affected individuals despite their lack of clinical symptoms. Thus, the syndrome appears to be due to different genetic defects, each resulting in impaired mineralocorticoid receptor function.

An additionally rare syndrome, termed pseudohypoaldosteronism type II, is characterized by hyperkalemia without renal sodium wasting with elevated aldosterone levels. However, the etiology of this syndrome may not necessarily involve resistance to mineralocorticoid effects on potassium secretion, as implicated by its name. In such patients, it has been demonstrated that an abnormal increase in potassium reabsorption occurs in conjunction with chloride reabsorption, thus leading to hyperkalemia and hyperaldosteronism [133].

The renin-angiotensin-aldosterone system maintains sodium and potassium balance as a means of preserving intravascular volume homeostasis and blood pressure. Disorders of the renin-angiotensin-aldosterone system can result from either abnormalities in the factors that regulate the system or primary abnormalities of renin, angiotensins, or aldosterone production. While this discussion is not meant to be exhaustive, it is clear that many disorders of salt and water metabolism or blood pressure regulation encountered in clinical practice involve the renin-angiotensin-aldosterone system. Understanding the normal physiology of this system allows for appreciation of how primary or secondary involvement of the renin-angiotensin-aldosterone system in various disease states contributes to their pathophysiology.

References

1. Tigerstedt R, Bergman PG: Niere and kreislauf. *Skand Arch Physiol* 8:223, 1898.
2. Misono KS, Inagami TT: Characterization of the active site of mouse submandibular gland renin. *Biochemistry* 19:2616, 1980.
3. Hobart PM, Fogliano M, O'Connor BA, et al: Human renin gene: Structure and sequence analysis. *Proc Natl Acad Sci USA* 81:5026, 1984.
4. Naftilan AJ, Burt D, Paul RE, et al: Identification and localization of four restriction fragment linked polymorphisms (RFLP) in the human renin gene. *Clin Res* 35:445, 1987.
5. Pratt RE, Carleton JE, Richie JP, et al: Human renin synthesis and secretion in normal and ischemic kidneys. *Proc Natl Acad Sci USA* 84:7837, 1987.
6. Dzau VJ: Possible prorenin activating mechanisms in the blood vessel wall. *J Hypertens* 5(Suppl 2):515, 1987.
7. Dzau VJ, Ellison KE, Brody T, et al: A comparative study of the distribution or renin and angiotensin messenger ribonucleic acids in rat and mouse tissues. *Endocrinology* 120:2334, 1987.
8. Fray JCS, Lush DJ, Park CS: Interrelationship of blood flow, juxtaglomerular cells, and hypertension: Role of physical equilibrium and Ca. *Am J Physiol* 251:R643, 1986.
9. Goldstone R, Horton R, Carlson EJ, Hsueh WA: Reciprocal changes in active and inactive renin after converting enzyme inhibition in normal man. *J Clin Endocrinol Metab* 56:264, 1983.
10. Churchill PC: Second messengers in renin secretion. *Am J Physiol* 249:F175, 1985.
11. Shenker Y: Atrial natriuretic hormone effect on renal function and aldosterone secretion in sodium depletion. *Am J Physiol* 255:R867, 1988.
12. Keeton TK, Campbell WB: The pharmacologic alteration of renin release. *Pharmacol Rev* 32:81, 1980.
13. Conn JW, Rovner DR, Cohen EL, et al: Inhibition by heparinoid of aldosterone biosynthesis in man. *J Clin Endocrinol Metab* 26:527, 1966.
14. Fray JCS, Park CS: Influence of potassium, sodium, perfusion pressure, and isoprenaline on renin release induced by acute calcium deprivation. *J Physiol* (Lond) 292:363, 1979.
15. Kotchen TA, Maull KI, Luke R, et al: Effect of acute and chronic calcium administration on plasma renin. *J Clin Invest* 54:1279, 1974.
16. Beierwaltes WH, Schryver S, Sanders E, et al: Renin release selectively stimulated by prostaglandin I_2 in isolated rat glomeruli. *Am J Physiol* 243:F276, 1982.
17. Romero JC, Knox FG: Mechanisms underlying pressure-related natriuresis: The role of the renin-angiotensin and prostaglandin systems. *Hypertension* 11:724, 1988.
18. Defforrest JM, Davis JO, Freeman RH, et al: Effects of indomethacin and meclofenamate on renin release and renal hemodynamic function during chronic sodium depletion in conscious dogs. *Circ Res* 47:99, 1980.
19. Tuck ML, Dluhy RG, Williams GH: A specific role for saline or the sodium ion in the regulation of renin and aldosterone secretion. *J Clin Invest* 53:988, 1974.
20. Kirchner KA, Kotchen TA, Galla JH, Luke RG: Importance of chloride for acute inhibition of renin by sodium chloride. *Am J Physiol* 235:F444, 1978.
21. Vander AJ: Effect of catecholamines and the renal nerves on renin secretion in anesthetized dogs. *Am J Physiol* 209:659, 1965.
22. Gordon MB, Moore TJ, Dluhy RG, Williams GH: Dopaminergic blockade of the renin-

angiotensin-aldosterone system: Effect of high and low sodium intakes. *Clin Endocrinol* 19: 415, 1983.

23. Dzau VJ, Hermann HC: Hormonal regulation of angiotensinogen synthesis. *Life Sci* 30:577, 1982.

24. Campbell DJ, Habener J: Angiotensinogen gene is expressed and differentially regulated in multiple tissues in the rat. *J Clin Invest* 78:31, 1986.

25. Dzau VJ, Burt DW, Pratt RE: Molecular biology of the renin-angiotensin system. *Am J Physiol* 255:F563, 1988.

26. Ng KKF, Vane JR: Conversion of angiotensin I to angiotensin II. *Nature* 216:762, 1967.

27. Weare J, Gafford JT, Lu HS, Erdos EG: Purification of human angiotensin converting enzyme using reverse immunoadsorption chromatography. *Anal Biochem* 123:310, 1982.

28. Erdos EG, Johnson AR, Boyden NT: Hydrolysis of enkephalin by cultured endothelial cells and purified dipeptidyl peptidase. *Biochem Pharmacol* 27:843, 1978.

29. Yotsumoto H, Imai Y, Kuzuya N, et al: Increased levels of serum angiotensin converting enzyme activity in hyperthyroidism. *Ann Intern Med* 96:326, 1982.

30. Lieberman J, Sastre A: Serum angiotensin converting enzyme: elevation in diabetes mellitus. *Ann Intern Med* 93:825, 1980.

31. DeRemee RA, Rohrbach J: Serum angiotensin converting enzyme activity in evaluating the clinical course of sarcoidosis. *Ann Intern Med* 92:361, 1980.

32. Zimmerman BG: Adrenergic facilitation by angiotensin: Does it serve a physiologic function? *Clin Sci* 60:343, 1981.

33. Goodfriend TL, Peach MJ: Angiotensin III: Evidence and speculation for its role as an important agonist in the renin-angiotensin system. *Circ Res* 36/37(Suppl 1):38, 1975.

34. Hollenberg NK, Chenitz WR, Adams DF, Williams GH: Reciprocal influence of salt intake on adrenal glomerulosa and renal vascular response to angiotensin II in normal man. *J Clin Invest* 54:34, 1974.

35. Dawson-Hughes BF, Moore TJ, Dluhy RG, et al: Plasma angiotensin concentration regulates vascular but not adrenal responsiveness to restriction of sodium intake in normal man. *Clin Sci* 61:527, 1981.

36. Caldwell PR, Seegal BC, Hsu KC: Angiotensin converting enzyme: Vascular endothelial localization. *Science* 191:1050, 1976.

37. Arriza JL, Weinberger C, Cerelli G, et al: Cloning of human mineralocorticoid receptor complementary DNA: Structural and functional kinship with the glucocorticoid receptor. *Science* 237:268, 1987.

38. August JT, Nelson D, Thorn G: Response of normal subjects to large amounts of aldosterone. *J Clin Invest* 37:1549, 1958.

39. Gonzalez-Campoy JM, Romero JC, Knox FG: Escape from the sodium-retaining effects of mineralocorticoids: Role of ANF and intrarenal hormone systems. *Kidney Int* 35:767, 1989.

40. Young MJ, Fullerton M, Dilley R, Funder JW: Mineralocorticoids, hypertension and cardiac fibrosis. *J Clin Invest* 93:2578, 1994.

41. Douglas JG, Catt KJ: Regulation of angiotensin II receptors in the rat adrenal cortex by dietary electrolytes. *J Clin Invest* 58:834, 1976.

42. Capponi AM, Lew PD, Jornot L, Vallontton MB: Correlation between cytosolic free Ca and aldosterone production in bovine adrenal glomerulosa cells. *J Biol Chem* 259:8863, 1984.

43. Enyedi P, Buki B, Mucsi I, Spat A: Polyphosphoinositide metabolism in adrenal glomerulosa cells. *Mol Cell Endocrinol* 41:105, 1985.

44. Braley LM, Menachery AI, Underwood RH, Williams GH: Is the adrenal angiotensin receptor angiotensin II or angiotensin III-like? *Acta Endocrinol* 102:116, 1983.

45. Braley LM, Menachery AI, Brown EM, Williams GH: Comparative effect of angiotensin II, potassium, adrenocorticotropin, and cyclic adenosine 3',5' monophosphate on cytosolic calcium in rat adrenal cells. *Endocrinology* 119:1010, 1986.

46. Dluhy RG, Axelrod L, Underwood RH, Williams GH: Studies of the control of plasma aldosterone concentration in normal man: II. Effect of dietary potassium and acute potassium infusion. *J Clin Invest* 51:1950, 1972.

47. Kojima I, Kojima K, Rasmussen H: Role of calcium and cAMP in the action of adrenocorticotropin on aldosterone secretion. *J Biol Chem* 260:4248, 1985.

48. Seely ES, Conlin PR, Brent GA, Dluhy RG: Adrenocorticotropin stimulation of aldosterone: Prolonged continuous versus pulsatile infusion. *J Clin Endocrinol Metab* 69:1028, 1989.
49. Oelkers W, Schoneshofer M, Schultze G, et al: Effect of prolonged low-dose angiotensin II infusions on the sensitivity of the adrenal cortex in man. *Circ Res* 36(Suppl 1):I-49, 1975.
50. McDougall JG, Butkus A, Coghlan JP, et al: Biochemical and morphological evidence for inhibition of aldosterone secretion by ACTH in the sheep. *Acta Endocrinol* (Copenh) 94: 559, 1980.
51. Williams GH, Rose LI, Dluhy RG, et al: Aldosterone response to sodium restriction and ACTH stimulation in panhypopituitarism. *J Clin Endocrinol Metab* 32:27, 1971.
52. Krozowski Z, Funder JW: Mineralocorticoid receptors in rat anterior pituitary: Toward a redefinition of "mineralocorticoid hormone." *Endocrinology* 109:1221, 1981.
53. Ganguly A, Hampton T: Calcium-dependence of serotonin-mediated aldosterone secretion and differential effects of calcium-antagonists. *Life Sci* 36:1459, 1985.
54. Lefebvre H, Contesse V, Delarue C, et al: The serotonin-4 receptor agonist cisapride and angiotensin II exert additive effects on aldosterone secretion in normal man. *J Clin Endocrinol Metab* 80:504, 1995.
55. Weidmann P, Beretta-Piccoli C, Ziegler WH, et al: Age versus urinary sodium for judging renin, aldosterone and catecholamine levels: Studies in normal subjects and patients with essential hypertension. *Kidney Int* 14:619, 1978.
56. Creditor MC, Loschky UK: Incidence of suppressed renin activity and of normokalemic primary aldosteronism in hypertensive Negro patients. *Circulation* 37:1027, 1968.
57. Brown JJ: Apparently isolated excess deoxycorticosterone in hypertension. *Lancet* 2:243, 1972.
58. Millar JA, McLean K, Reid JL: Calcium antagonists decrease adrenal and vascular responsiveness to angiotensin II in normal man. *Clin Sci* 61:65s, 1981.
59. Laragh JH: Aldosterone excretion and primary and malignant hypertension. *J Clin Invest* 39: 1091, 1960.
60. Jeunemaitre X, Soubrier F, Kotelevtsev YV, et al: Molecular basis of human hypertension: Role of angiotensinogen. *Cell* 71:169, 1992.
61. Melby JC, Wilson TE, Dale SL: Secretion of 18-hydroxydeoxycorticosterone (18-OH DOC) in human hypertensive disease. *J Clin Invest* 49:64A, 1970.
62. Williams GH, Braley LM, Underwood RH: The regulation of plasma 18-hydroxy-11-deoxycorticosterone in man. *J Clin Invest* 58:221, 1976.
63. Wisgerhof M, Brown RD: Increased adrenal sensitivity to angiotensin II in low renin essential hypertension. *J Clin Invest* 61:1456, 1978.
64. Streeten DHP, Schletter FE, Clift GV, et al: Studies of the renin-angiotensin-aldosterone system in patients with hypertension and in normal subjects. *Am J Med* 46:844, 1969.
65. Shoback DM, Williams GH, Moore TJ, et al: Defect in sodium-modulated tissue responsiveness to angiotensin II in essential hypertension. *J Clin Invest* 72:2115, 1983.
66. Williams GH, Hollenberg NK: Are non-modulating patients with essential hypertension a distinct subgroup? Implications for therapy. *Am J Med* 79(Suppl 3C):3, 1985.
67. Taylor TT, Moore TJ, Hollenberg NK, Williams GH: Converting enzyme inhibition corrects the altered adrenal response to angiotensin II in essential hypertension. *Hypertension* 6:92, 1984.
68. Redgrave JE, Rabinowe SL, Williams GH, Hollenberg NK: Converting enzyme inhibition corrects the altered renovascular responsiveness to angiotensin II in essential hypertension. *J Clin Invest* 75:1285, 1985.
69. Goldblatt H, Lynch J, Hanzal RF, Summerville WW: Studies on experimental hypertension: I. The production of persistent elevation of systolic blood pressure by means of renal ischemia. *J Exp Med* 59:347, 1934.
70. Dzau VJ, Siwek LG, Rosen S, et al: Sequential renal hemodynamics in experimental benign and malignant hypertension. *Hypertension* 3:63, 1981.
71. Fommei E, Ghione S, Palla L, et al: Renal scintigraphic captopril test in the diagnosis of renovascular hypertension. *Hypertension* 10:212, 1987.
72. Clark RA, Alexander ES: Digital subtraction angiography of the renal arteries: Prospective comparison with conventional arteriography. *Invest Radiol* 18:6, 1983.

73. Case DB, Laragh JH: Reactive hyperreninemia in renovascular hypertension after angiotensin blockade with saralasin or converting enzyme inhibitor. *Ann Intern Med* 91:153, 1979.
74. Lyons DF, Stock WF, Kem DC, et al: Captopril stimulation of differential renins in renovascular hypertension. *Hypertension* 5:615, 1983.
75. Martin LG, Price RB, Casarella WJ, et al: Percutaneous angioplasty in clinical management of renovascular hypertension: Initial and long-term results. *Radiology* 155:629, 1985.
76. Salahudeen AK, Pingle A: Reversibility of captopril-induced renal insufficiency after prolonged use in an unusual case of renovascular hypertension. *J Human Hypertens* 2:57, 1988.
77. Corvol P, Pinet F, Plouin P-F, et al: Renin-secreting tumors. *Endocrinol Metab Clin North Am* 23:255, 1994.
78. Squires JP, Ulbright TM, DeSchryver-Kecskemeti K, Engleman W: Juxtaglomerular cell tumor of the kidney. *Cancer* 53:516, 1984.
79. Conn JW: Presidential address: II. Primary aldosteronism: A new clinical syndrome. *J Lab Clin Med* 45:3, 1955.
80. Carey RM, Sen S, Dolan LM, et al: Idiopathic hyperaldosteronism: Defining a possible role for aldosterone-stimulating factor. *N Engl J Med* 311:94, 1984.
81. Kuchel O, Buu NT, Vecsei P, et al: Are plasma aldosterone surges in primary aldosteronism due to a loss of an inhibitory dopaminergic control? *J Clin Endocrinol Metab* 51:337, 1980.
82. Weinberger MH, Grim CE, Hollifield JW, et al: Primary aldosteronism: Diagnosis, localization, and treatment. *Ann Intern Med* 90:386, 1979.
83. Kem DC, Weinberger MH, Mayes DM, Nugent CA: Saline suppression of plasma aldosterone in hypertension. *Arch Intern Med* 128:380, 1971.
84. Blumenfeld JD, Sealey JE, Schlussel Y, et al: Diagnosis and treatment of primary hyperaldosteronism. *Ann Intern Med* 121:877, 1994.
85. Griffing GT, Komanicky P, Aurecchia SA, et al: Amiloride in primary aldosteronism. *Clin Pharmacol Ther* 31:713, 1982.
86. Lifton RP, Dluhy RG, Powers M: The molecular basis of a hypertensive disease: Chimaeric gene duplications result in ectopic expression of aldosterone synthase and glucocorticoid-remediable hyperaldosteronism. *Nature Genet* 2:66, 1992.
87. Stewart PM, Wallace AM, Valentino R, et al: Mineralocorticoid activity of licorice: 11β-hydroxysteroid dehydrogenase deficiency comes of age. *Lancet* 2:821, 1987.
88. Ulick S, Levine LS, Gunczler P, et al: A syndrome of apparent mineralocorticoid excess associated with defects in the peripheral metabolism of cortisol. *J Clin Endocrinol Metab* 49: 757, 1979.
89. Stewart PM, Corrie JET, Shackleton CHL, Edwards CRW: Syndrome of apparent mineralocorticoid excess: A defect in the cortisol-cortisone shuttle. *J Clin Invest* 82:340, 1988.
90. Shimkets RA, Warnock DG, Bositis CM, et al: Liddle's syndrome: Heritable human hypertension caused by mutations in the β subunit of the epithelial sodium channel. *Cell* 79:407, 1994.
91. Schrier RW: Pathogenesis of sodium and water retention in high-output and low-output cardiac failure, nephrotic syndrome, cirrhosis, and pregnancy. *N Engl J Med* 319:10625, 1988.
92. Szatalowicz VL, Arnold PE, Chaimovitz C, et al: Radioimmunoassay of plasma arginine vasopressin in hyponatremic patients with congestive heart failure. *N Engl J Med* 305:265, 1981.
93. Thomas JA, Marks BH: Plasma norepinephrine in congestive heart failure. *Am J Cardiol* 41: 233, 1978.
94. Dzau VJ, Colucci WS, Hollenberg NK, Williams GH: Relation of the renin-angiotensin-aldosterone system to clinical state in congestive heart failure. *Circulation* 63:645, 1981.
95. Dzau VJ, Colucci WS, Williams GH, et al: Sustained effectiveness of converting-enzyme inhibition in patients with severe congestive heart failure. *N Engl J Med* 302:1373, 1980.
96. Dorhout-Mees EJ, Roos JC, Boer P, et al: Observations on edema formation in the nephrotic syndrome in adults with minimal lesions. *Am J Med* 67:378, 1979.
97. Brown EA, Markandu ND, Sagnella GA, et al: Lack of effect of captopril on the sodium retention of nephrotic syndrome. *Nephron* 37:43, 1984.
98. Anderson RJ, Cronin RE, McDonald KM, Schrier RW: Mechanisms of portal hypertension-induced alterations in renal hemodynamics, renal water excretion, and renin secretion. *J Clin Invest* 58:964, 1976.

99. Schrier RW, Arroyo V, Bernardi M, et al: Peripheral arterial vasodilation hypothesis: A proposal for the initiation of renal sodium and water retention. *J Hepatol* 6:239, 1987.

100. Schroeder ET, Anderson GH, Goldman SH, Streeten DHP: Effect of blockade of angiotensin II on blood pressure, renin, and aldosterone in cirrhosis. *Kidney Int* 9:511, 1976.

101. Gregory PB, Broekelschen PH, Hill MD, et al: Complications of diuresis in the alcoholic patients with ascites: A controlled trial. *Gastroenterology* 73:534, 1977.

102. Streeten DHP, Speller PJ: The role of aldosterone and vasopressin in the postural changes in renal excretion in normal subjects and patients with idiopathic edema. *Metabolism* 15:53, 1966.

103. Kuchel O, Cuche JL, Buu NT, et al: Catecholamine excretion in "idiopathic" edema: Decreased dopamine excretion, a pathogenetic factor? *J Clin Endocrinol Metab* 44:639, 1977.

104. Gill JR Jr, Waldmann TA, Bartter FC: Idiopathic edema. *Am J Med* 52:444, 1972.

105. Anderson GH, Streeten DHP: Effect of posture on plasma atrial natriuretic hormone and renal function during salt loading in patients with and without postural (idiopathic) edema. *J Clin Endocrinol Metab* 71:243, 1990.

106. Bartter FC, Pronove P, Gill JR Jr, et al: Hyperplasia of the juxtaglomerular complex with hyperaldosteronism and hypokalemic alkalosis. *Am J Med* 33:811, 1962.

107. Ogihara T, Maruyama A, Nugent CA, et al: Familial Bartter's syndrome. *Arch Intern Med* 145:906, 1982.

108. Gill JR Jr: The role of chloride transport in the thick ascending limb in the pathogenesis of Bartter's syndrome. *Klin Wochenschr* 60:1212, 1982.

109. Delaney VB, Oliver JF, Simms M, et al: Bartter's syndrome: Physiological and pharmacological studies. *Q J Med* 50:213, 1981.

110. Gill JR, Frohlich JC, Bowden RE, et al: Bartter's syndrome: A disorder characterized by high urinary prostaglandins and a dependence of hyperreninemia on prostaglandin synthesis. *Am J Med* 61:43, 1976.

111. Greene LW, Cole W, Greene JB, et al: Adrenal insufficiency as a complication of the acquired immunodeficiency syndrome. *Ann Intern Med* 101:497, 1984.

112. Williams GH, Dluhy RG: Diseases of the Adrenal Cortex. In JD Wilson et al (eds): *Harrison's Principles of Internal Medicine* (13th ed). New York, McGraw-Hill, 1994, p 1711.

113. Oelkers W: Hyponatremia and inappropriate secretion of vasopressin (antidiuretic hormone) in patients with hypopituitarism. *N Engl J Med* 321:492, 1989.

114. Visser HKA, Cost WS: A new hereditary defect in the biosynthesis of aldosterone: Urinary C_{21}-corticosteroid pattern in the three related patients with salt-losing syndrome suggesting an 18-hydroxylation defect. *Acta Endocrinol* 47:589, 1964.

115. Veldhuis JD, Kulin HE, Santen RJ, et al: Inborn error in the terminal step of aldosterone biosynthesis: Corticosterone methyl oxidase type II deficiency in a North American pedigree. *N Engl J Med* 303:118, 1980.

116. Veldhuis J, Melby JC: Isolated aldosterone deficiency in man: Acquired and inborn errors in the biosynthesis or action of aldosterone. *Endocr Rev* 2:495, 1981.

117. Lauber M, Muller J: Purification and characterization of two distinct forms of rat adrenal cytochrome P450 11β: Functional and structural aspects. *Arch Biochem Biophys* 274:109, 1989.

118. White PC: Disorders of aldosterone biosynthesis and action. *N Engl J Med* 331:250, 1994.

119. Lebel M, Grose JH: Angiotensin II effect on plasma steroids in selective hypoaldosteronism. *Horm Metab Res* 14:432, 1982.

120. Battle DC, Arruda JAL, Kurtzman NA: Hyperkalemic distal renal tubular acidosis associated with obstructive uropathy. *N Engl J Med* 304:373, 1981.

121. Tan SY, Shapiro R, Franco R, et al: Indomethacin-induced prostaglandin inhibition with hyperkalemia. *Ann Intern Med* 90:783, 1979.

122. Bravo EL, Dustan HP, Tarazi RC: Selective hypoaldosteronism despite prolonged pre- and postoperative hyperreninemia in primary aldosteronism. *J Clin Endocrinol Metab* 41:611, 1975.

123. Kalin MF, Poretsky L, Seres DS, Zumoff B: Hyporeninemic hypoaldosteronism associated with acquired immune deficiency syndrome. *Am J Med* 82:1035, 1987.

124. Valazquez H, Perazella MA, Wright FS, Ellison DH: Renal mechanism of trimethoprim-induced hyperkalemia. *Ann Intern Med* 119:296, 1993.

125. Zipser RD, Davenport MW, Martin KL, et al: Hyperreninemic hypoaldosteronism in the critically ill: A new entity. *J Clin Endocrinol Metab* 53:867, 1981.
126. Raff H, Findling JW, Diaz SJ, et al: Aldosterone control in critically ill patients: ACTH, metoclopramide, and atrial natriuretic peptide. *Crit Care Med* 18:915, 1990.
127. Kraiem Z, Rosenthal T, Rotzak R, Lunenfeld B: Angiotensin II and K challenge following prolonged ACTH administration in normal subjects. *Acta Endocrinol* (Copenh) 91:657, 1979.
128. Findling JW, Waters VO, Raff H: The dissociation of renin and aldosterone during critical illness. *J Clin Endocrinol Metab* 64:592, 1987.
129. Oster JR, Singer I, Fishman LM: Heparin-induced aldosterone suppression and hyperkalemia. *Am J Med* 98:575, 1995.
130. Cheek DB, Perry IW: A salt wasting syndrome in infancy. *Arch Dis Child* 33:252, 1958.
131. Kuhnle U, Nielson MD, Tietze HU, et al: Pseudohypoaldosteronism in eight families: Different forms of inheritance are evidence for various genetic defects. *J Clin Endocrinol Metab* 70: 638, 1990.
132. Armanini D, Kuhnle U, Strasser T, et al: Aldosterone-receptor deficiency in pseudohypoaldosteronism. *N Engl J Med* 319:1178, 1985.
133. Schambelan M, Sebastian A, Rector FC: Mineralocorticoid-resistant renal hyperkalemia without salt wasting (type II pseudohypoaldosteronism): Role of increased renal chloride reabsorption. *Kidney Int* 19:716, 1981.

The Kidney in Hypertension

Charles R. Nolan and Robert W. Schrier

Historical Perspective: The Link Between Hypertension and Renal Dysfunction

The occurrence of hypertension in the setting of renal disease and its impact on the progression of renal insufficiency have long been of interest to the clinician. The concept that hypertension is in some way related to renal dysfunction was first proposed by Bright in 1863 [1]. He recognized the association between hypertrophy of the heart and contraction of the kidney and postulated that the cause was increased cardiac work required to force blood through a vascular tree constricted by irritating humoral substances that accumulate in renal failure. The role of fluid retention in the genesis of renal hypertension was first outlined by Traube in 1871 [2], who proposed that with shrinkage of the renal parenchyma, a decreasing amount of fluid is removed from the arterial system by urinary secretion, resulting in hypertension.

Mahomed in 1879 [3] was the first to clearly describe hypertension of unknown cause, without evidence of underlying renal disease (now called essential or primary hypertension). He emphasized that in individuals with this type of hypertension, the most frequent complications were cardiovascular and most often occurred in the absence of significant renal dysfunction. However, in 1914, Volhard and Fahr [4] recognized a subgroup of patients with essential hypertension who did eventually develop severe renal involvement. They distinguished two types of hypertensive nephrosclerosis, benign and malignant. The benign type, characterized by hyaline arteriolosclerosis, was accompanied by a slowly progressive course with long-standing cardiac hypertrophy and eventual complications due to heart failure or stroke, with renal function remaining unimpaired. In contrast, the arteriolar necrosis and endarteritis found in malignant nephrosclerosis resulted in rapidly progressive renal failure. Volhard [5] subsequently introduced the concept of the vicious circle in which renal disease causes hypertension, which in turn exacerbates renal injury.

In recent years, it has been reemphasized that the kidney is both "villain and victim" in hypertension [6]. The kidney, even when histologically normal, is felt to play a central role in the pathogenesis of essential hypertension. Clearly, underlying primary renal parenchymal disease or abnormalities of the renal vasculature can cause secondary hypertension. On the other hand, the kidney may also suffer the brunt of hypertension. Essential hypertension that enters a malignant phase can rapidly destroy the kidney. Furthermore, recent evidence suggests that hypertension is a major factor in the progression of chronic renal insufficiency in the setting of underlying primary renal disease.

This chapter will address three major questions with regard to the interaction between the kidney and hypertension: What role does the kidney play in the genesis of essential hypertension? Why does hypertension develop in the setting of primary renal disease? And finally, what is the role of treatment of hypertension in slowing the progression of underlying primary renal disease?

Circulatory Hemodynamics: Complexity in a Simple Relationship

The mean arterial pressure is defined by the product of the cardiac output times the total peripheral resistance. Thus, hypertension can only result from an increase in either of these two variables. The kidney has a major influence on blood pressure, given its central role in the regulation of extracellular fluid (ECF) volume (see Chaps. 1 and 2). An increase in ECF volume due to renal sodium and water retention should cause increased blood volume, venous return, and filling pressure, which in turn should increase stroke volume and cardiac output via the Frank-Starling mechanism and result in hypertension. Volume expansion, resulting from excess sodium intake or an underlying abnormality in renal sodium excretory mechanisms, has been considered to be an important mechanism for the development of hypertension in animal models as well as in humans with essential hypertension or primary renal disease.

The paradox that must be explained is that in human hypertension and in animal models, at least in the chronic phase, an increase in ECF volume or cardiac output is difficult to demonstrate [7]. Hypertension seems to be maintained by an increase in total peripheral resistance arising primarily at the level of precapillary arterioles throughout the circulatory system [8]. This observation forms the basis for the concept that a primary increase in total peripheral resistance is the cause of hypertension, and many theories exist regarding the roles of various vasoconstrictor mechanisms [9] or the absence of vasodilator substances [10, 11].

However, there are complexities in the seemingly simple formula that relates blood pressure to cardiac output and total peripheral resistance. The circulatory system is dynamic, and a perturbation, such as ECF volume expansion, that initially leads to hypertension via an increase in cardiac output may result in compensatory hemodynamic responses that ultimately restore sodium balance and thus normalize ECF volume and cardiac output. However, this restoration of sodium balance may result from a "pressure natriuresis" that occurs in the setting of systemic hypertension, which is maintained by an increase in total peripheral resistance [8, 12–16].

The various theories proposed to account for the phenomenon whereby initially volume-dependent hypertension is transformed into high vascular resistance hypertension are described in detail in the following discussion.

Dietary Salt and Hypertension

Archeologic studies of Paleolithic man suggest that the diet of these hunter-gatherers was very low in sodium and relatively high in potassium. Sodium intake averaged 30 mmol/day, with a ratio of dietary potassium to sodium of 16 : 1 [17]. Since total body sodium is the major determinant of ECF volume, in the face of this limited availability of sodium, a very efficient renal sodium conservation mechanism evolved. In contrast, the modern urban diet contains 120 to 300 mmol of sodium per day [17] and only 65 mmol of potassium per day [18]. Therefore, the human species today is faced with a much higher daily sodium load than that to which it adapted over roughly 2 million years [17]. Since virtually all ingested sodium is absorbed, sodium intake in excess of insensible losses must be excreted by the kidney. Under normal circumstances, even in the face of tremendous dietary sodium excess, humoral and other mechanisms cause an increase in urinary sodium excretion with little increase in ECF volume [19]. However, in a segment of the population, this natriuretic mechanism is aberrant such that an excessive dietary salt intake results in the development of hypertension [12–16, 20].

Epidemiologic Studies

Studies throughout the world have suggested a correlation between the mean dietary sodium intake and the prevalence of hypertension in the population. In parts of Japan where the mean sodium intake is over 400 mmol/day, the prevalence of hypertension approaches 50 percent [21]. In contrast, in certain inland populations where the sodium intake is very low (0.2–51.0 mmol/day), hypertension is virtually nonexistent, and there is no tendency for the blood pressure to rise with age [22]. The INTERSALT Study investigated the relation between dietary sodium intake (defined by 24-hour urinary sodium excretion) and blood pressure in 10,000 subjects in 32 countries [23]. A significant positive correlation was found between sodium intake and blood pressure even when the data were adjusted for age, sex, body weight, and alcohol consumption. The data suggest that habitual high sodium intake (>150 mmol of sodium per day) is a critical environmental factor that contributes to the high prevalence of hypertension in most urban populations, whereas lifelong ingestion of a diet extremely low in sodium (<50 mmol/day) prevents the development of hypertension [22, 23]. Extremely high sodium intake (>800 mmol of sodium per day) has been shown to raise the blood pressure of healthy normotensive individuals [24]. On the other hand, diets with less than 10 mmol of sodium per day have been shown to lower the blood pressure of most hypertensive patients [25]. Additional support for the importance of dietary sodium in the genesis of hypertension is the finding that, in an adult population, long-term lowering of the sodium intake was associated with a fall in the prevalence of hypertension and a concomitant reduction in cerebrovascular mortality [26].

However, the importance of dietary sodium intake as a risk factor for the development of hypertension has recently been questioned. Recent studies fail to demonstrate a consistent relationship between sodium intake and blood pressure among individuals in the same population [27]. Furthermore, the effects on blood pressure of short-term sodium loading or deprivation have been unimpressive [28]. Clinical studies have demonstrated that long-term sodium intake must be lowered to less than 80 mmol/day to obtain a significant decrease in blood pressure [29]. This translates into a daily intake of 2 g of sodium, which is less than 50 percent of the usual intake in the United States. Given compliance issues and the lack of a significant blood pressure response to more modest sodium restriction, the wisdom of recommending sodium restriction to the general public or to patients with mild to moderate hypertension has been questioned [29].

On balance, it is clear that sodium intake must play a permissive role in the development of hypertension, since a lifelong diet very low in sodium prevents hypertension [22]. On the other hand, excessive sodium intake alone is not sufficient to cause hypertension, since the majority of individuals on such a diet fail to develop hypertension. These observations imply that there must be additional predisposing factors that lead to the development of hypertension in certain individuals when the intake of sodium is greater than 60 to 70 mmol/day.

Dietary Salt and Animal Models of Genetic Hypertension

When groups of rats were maintained on a wide range of a dietary sodium, the mean blood pressure in each group was directly related to the sodium intake. Dahl and Schackow [30] noted that at each level of dietary sodium intake, only some rats became hypertensive. By selective inbreeding, they were able to show that the predisposition to develop hypertension was genetically determined, and they produced a salt-sensitive strain that develops hypertension on a high-sodium diet and a salt-resistant strain that remains normotensive.

The Role of the Kidney in Essential Hypertension

Cross-Transplantation Experiments

In renal cross-transplantation experiments between four different strains of genetically hypertensive rats (Dahl salt-sensitive hypertensive rats, Milan hypertensive rats, spontaneously hypertensive rats [SHR], and stroke-prone spontaneously hypertensive rats [SHRSP]), and their respective normotensive control strains, it was found that blood pressure determinants were carried within the kidney [31]. Thus, transplantation of a kidney from a hypertensive strain rat into a bilaterally nephrectomized rat from the normotensive strain results in hypertension in the recipient.

Conversely, transplantation from normotensive strain rat into a nephrectomized hypertensive strain rat prevents the development of hypertension. Thus, the blood pressure of the recipient rat is dependent on the source of the donated kidney.

Alternatively, it could be argued that the post-transplant hypertension in recipients of kidneys from hypertensive strains is not due to a primary defect in the donor kidney but instead results from hypertension-induced changes in the donor kidney and that these acquired secondary structural defects in kidney lead to hypertension in the recipient. To address this question, the development of hypertension in the SHRSP kidney donors was prevented by chronic antihypertensive drug treatment [31]. Despite sustained normalization of blood pressure in the donor rats, the recipients developed post-transplant hypertension. This finding indicates that SHRSP kidneys carry a primary defect that can elicit hypertension.

These experiments suggest that the predisposition to genetic hypertension resides in the kidney and is not determined directly by systemic humoral abnormalities or changes in vascular reactivity that have been described in these models. The latter abnormalities must represent either epiphenomena or secondary changes in response to a primary renal abnormality.

These animal models of hypertension bear a remarkable resemblance to human essential hypertension. Indeed, studies of renal transplant patients also support a primary role for the kidney in the development of essential hypertension. In patients with essential hypertension and renal failure due to malignant nephrosclerosis, bilateral native nephrectomy in conjunction with a well-functioning renal allograft from a normotensive cadaver donor cures essential hypertension [32]. In a study of six such patients, before renal transplantation, mean arterial pressure was 168 ± 9 mm Hg despite treatment with a minimum of a four-drug antihypertensive regimen. However, following bilateral native nephrectomy and successful renal transplantation, at a mean follow-up of 4.5 years, mean arterial pressure without antihypertensive treatment was 92 ± 1.9 mm Hg. In contrast, the incidence of hypertension in recipients of cadaver kidneys seems to correlate with the incidence of essential hypertension in the family of the donor [33]. These intriguing reports support the notion that the defect that causes human essential hypertension resides within the kidney.

Underlying Defect in Natriuretic Capacity

If the relationship between sodium intake and hypertension represents cause and effect, then it is important to explain why a high sodium intake leads to hypertension in only some individuals. In this regard, it has been postulated that in the setting of essential hypertension in humans or in salt-sensitive animal models, there is a genetically predetermined impairment in the ability to excrete sodium [12–16]. This postulated renal abnormality has been termed an "unwillingness to excrete sodium." In studies of isolated, perfused kidneys from Dahl salt-sensitive strains, at age 8 weeks, even before the onset of hypertension, there is a defect in natriuresis such that at any given perfusion pressure, less sodium is excreted than with kidneys from salt-resistant strains [34].

The heritability of essential hypertension has been well established in epidemiologic surveys. The prevalence of hypertension among offspring has been reported to be 46 percent if both parents are hypertensive, 28 percent if one parent is hypertensive, and only 3 percent if neither parent is hypertensive [35]. Analysis of the natriuretic response to slow infusion of saline has revealed that normotensive first-degree relatives of patients with essential hypertension excrete a sodium load less well than control subjects without a family history of hypertension [36]. Among blacks [37] and individuals over 40 years old [38], two groups with an increased incidence of hypertension, studies of normotensive individuals have also demonstrated a slower natriuretic response to saline infusion than in controls, suggesting that a diminished natriuretic capacity may underlie the predisposition to essential hypertension in these groups.

Lithium Clearance Studies

The genetic defect that underlies the development of essential hypertension may be a diminished natriuretic capacity due to a primary increase in proximal tubule sodium reabsorption [39]. Lithium clearance is often used as a measure of proximal sodium reabsorption, since lithium reabsorption occurs in parallel to sodium resorption and is limited to the proximal tubule. A decreased fractional lithium clearance (ratio of lithium clearance to creatinine clearance) therefore implies increased proximal sodium reabsorption. Studies in patients with essential hypertension have revealed a decreased fractional lithium clearance [39]. Furthermore, normotensive subjects with a hypertensive first-degree relative had a lower fractional lithium clearance than subjects with no hypertensive relative [39]. Though most likely an epiphenomenon, increased erythrocyte lithium-sodium countertransport has been shown to correlate with decreased fractional lithium clearance and may serve as a useful marker for the increased proximal sodium reabsorption that possibly underlies the development of essential hypertension [39].

Mechanism of Impaired Natriuresis

Reduced Nephron Mass

It has been postulated that the underlying cause of impaired natriuretic capacity in essential (genetic) hypertension may be a congenitally acquired deficit of effective nephron mass [20]. In the SHR, the fenestrae of the glomerular capillary endothelium are smaller than in normotensive control rats. In the Milan SHR, there is a decreased glomerular ultrafiltration coefficient and increased proximal sodium reabsorption. Salt-sensitive hypertension in rats is associated with a 15 percent reduction in nephron number. In humans, major inborn deficits of nephron number such as oligomeganephronia and congenital unilateral renal agenesis are associated with the development of hypertension. Brenner et al. [20] have postulated that the abnormality that predisposes a minority of the population to essential hypertension in the setting of excessive sodium intake is an inherited deficit of nephrons or glomerular filtration surface area, leading to a diminished capacity to excrete a sodium load, resulting in salt-sensitive hypertension.

Neurohormonal Mechanisms

Several neurohormonal mechanisms act through the kidney in response to perceived changes in blood pressure or intravascular volume to modulate renal sodium excretion. These include the renin-angiotensin system and the sympathetic nervous system. Proximal tubular sodium reabsorption is enhanced by the actions of angiotensin II and α-adrenergic receptor–mediated sympathetic activation [40]. It has been postulated that abnormal response of the renal vasculature to angiotensin II or catecholamines causes the defect in natriuresis found in essential hypertension.

Angiotensin II has been shown to increase renal sodium and water retention independent of its effect to increase aldosterone production [41]. In this regard, angiotensin II–mediated renal hemodynamic changes lead indirectly to increases in tubular sodium reabsorption. Infusion of angiotensin II causes a reduction of renal blood flow with maintenance of near normal glomerular filtration rate due to an increase in filtration fraction consistent with an increase in efferent arteriolar resistance. The increase in efferent arteriolar resistance caused by angiotensin II results in a fall in hydrostatic pressure and an increase in oncotic pressure in the peritubular capillaries of the proximal and distal tubules and collecting ducts, which results in enhanced tubular sodium reabsorption [41]. Angiotensin II has also been shown to directly stimulate sodium reabsorption in the proximal tubule [42].

Recent evidence suggests that renal abnormalities involving disordered regulation of the renin-angiotensin system may be important in the pathogenesis of essential hypertension [43]. These fundamental abnormalities, which are present in 45 percent of patients with essential hypertension, cause an impairment in renal sodium handling that results in sodium-sensitive hypertension. These patients have normal to high plasma renin activity and have been termed nonmodulators because of their inability to adjust renal responsiveness to angiotensin II during changes in sodium intake. In normal individuals or patients with essential hypertension who are "modulators," renal blood flow changes in parallel to sodium intake. With an increase in sodium intake, renal blood flow rises, while with a decrease in sodium intake, renal blood flow declines. In contrast, in nonmodulators, the renal blood flow remains fixed despite changes in sodium intake. This abnormal renal vascular response to changes in sodium intake may account for the limited capacity of the kidney to handle a sodium load. Nonmodulators also demonstrate less suppression of renin in response to sodium loading or angiotensin II infusion compared to normals or modulators with essential hypertension. Treatment of these nonmodulators with an angiotensin-converting enzyme (ACE) inhibitor restores the normal natriuretic response to a sodium load and also normalizes renin suppression in response to a sodium load or angiotensin II infusion. Furthermore, ACE inhibition also results in a decrease in renal vascular resistance, an increase in renal blood flow, and natriuresis [43]. These findings suggest that, in nonmodulators, enhanced renal vascular responsiveness to angiotensin II is present, even in the absence of increased systemic renin and angiotensin II levels, perhaps secondary to in situ angiotensin II production by renal converting enzyme. The resulting decrease in peritubular Starling force and increase in proximal and distal sodium reabsorption may underlie the defect in natriuresis in essential hypertension [41–43]. Moreover, restoration of the ability of the kidney to handle a sodium load may be a major mechanism by which ACE inhibitors reduce blood pressure in patients with low-renin essential hypertension.

A recent study suggests that increased vasoconstrictor responsiveness of the efferent arteriole to α-adrenergic stimuli may cause the intrarenal hemodynamic abnormalities seen in essential hypertension, namely decreased renal blood flow, increased renal vascular resistance, and increased filtration fraction [44]. Akin to the effect of angiotensin II, this primary increase in efferent resistance may cause the defective natriuresis in essential hypertension by decreasing peritubular capillary Starling forces. It should also be noted that increased α-adrenergic activity has been shown to directly stimulate sodium reabsorption in the proximal tubule [45]. Calcium channel blockers decrease renal afferent arteriolar vasoconstriction and improve renal blood flow [44]. The natriuretic response to calcium channel blockers may be secondary to this phenomenon, in addition to their direct effect on tubular sodium transport [46].

Abnormalities in Renal Nitric Oxide

There is increasing evidence that endothelium-derived nitric oxide is tonically synthesized within the kidney and that nitric oxide plays a crucial role in the regulation of renal hemodynamics and sodium excretion [47]. These effects are mediated in part by interactions between nitric oxide and the renin-angiotensin system. Nitric oxide is an important mediator of renal blood flow and the renal microcirculation. Bradykinin and acetylcholine induce renal vasodilation by increasing nitric oxide synthesis, which in turn leads to enhancement of diuresis and natriuresis. Blockade of basal nitric oxide synthesis, with specific inhibitors of the L-arginine nitric oxide pathway (L-NAME or L-NMMA), has been shown to result in an increase in renal vascular resistance with decreases in renal blood flow, urine flow, and sodium excretion. Intrarenal inhibition of nitric oxide synthesis leads to reduction of sodium excretory responses to changes in renal perfusion pressure without an effect on renal autoregulation, suggesting that nitric oxide exerts a permissive or mediatory role in the tubular responses that regulate the pressure natriuresis mechanism [48]. Nitric oxide released from the macula densa may modulate tubulo-glomerular feedback response by affecting afferent arteriolar constriction. In the collecting duct, a nitric oxide–dependent inhibition of solute transport has been suggested. While most studies indicate that nitric oxide synthesis blockade causes reduction in sodium excretion, the exact mechanism is unclear. Reduction in the filtered load of sodium, increased tubular sodium reabsorption, altered medullary blood flow, and decreased renal interstitial hydrostatic pressure may mediate sodium retention during nitric oxide blockade. Taken together, these observations suggest that nitric oxide–dependent mechanisms have a major impact on renal control of body fluid volume.

Abnormalities in renal nitric oxide have been postulated to explain the disordered renal physiology in essential hypertension [47–49]. It has been suggested that a deficiency in the renal synthesis of nitric oxide may constitute an important factor in the development of systemic hypertension, since it interferes with the ability of the kidney to excrete sodium. Moreover, nitric oxide is thought to mediate the natriuretic response to volume expansion.

Impaired Natriuresis: A Prerequisite in Hypertension

Experiments with isolated, perfused kidneys demonstrate that the magnitude of urinary sodium excretion is a direct function of the perfusion pressure [50, 51]. The level of perfusion pressure may alter sodium excretion by changing the peritubular hydrostatic pressure. Thus, an increase in perfusion pressure should increase peritubular hydrostatic pressure with a resultant decrease in sodium reabsorption. Micropuncture studies in the rat have shown an inverse relationship between renal perfusion pressure and proximal sodium reabsorption [52].

It has been argued that if this pressure natriuresis mechanism was operating in a normal fashion, in the presence of hypertension, profound volume depletion would result. The fact that this does not occur suggests that in every hypertensive state, there must be a shift in the pressure natriuresis curve such that a higher perfusion pressure is required to achieve any given level of natriuresis. In this regard, it has been postulated that this shift in the pressure natriuresis curve is actually a reflection of the underlying renal abnormality present in essential hypertension as well as in hypertension caused by underlying renal disease [13, 15, 16]. If a primary defect in natriuresis does exist in hypertension, then to avert disaster due to persistent positive sodium balance with inexorable fluid accumulation, compensatory hormonal responses or other mechanisms must be invoked that restore sodium balance. The theories regarding the pathogenesis of hypertension that follow explain how these compensatory processes restore sodium balance but in the process cause systemic hypertension.

The Na,K-ATPase Inhibitor Hypothesis

In both essential hypertension and secondary hypertension due to renal disease, there must be an underlying abnormality in the kidney's ability to excrete sodium. In individuals with this impairment of natriuretic capacity, if the intake of dietary sodium is greater than 60 mmol/day, there will be a tendency toward sodium and water retention, resulting in ECF volume expansion. Some authors have proposed that in response to this expansion of ECF volume, there is an increase in the plasma concentration of two or more substances that are collectively referred to as "natriuretic hormone" [12, 13, 53, 54]. The responses induced by this natriuretic hormone include an increase in the natriuretic capacity of the plasma, an increase in the ability of the plasma to inhibit Na,K-ATPase, and an increase in vascular responsiveness to vasoconstrictors such as norepinephrine, angiotensin II, and vasopressin. Atrial natriuretic peptide (ANP), which is released from the atria in response to acute volume expansion, causes a brisk increase in renal sodium and water excretion of rapid onset and short duration. However, ANP does not inhibit Na,K-

ATPase or increase vascular reactivity; in fact, ANP decreases systemic vascular resistance. It is proposed that another response to the underlying renal impairment in the ability to excrete sodium is an increase in the plasma concentration of a substance, probably of hypothalamic origin, that inhibits Na,K-ATPase [55, 56]. As a result of inhibition of Na,K-ATPase, renal tubular sodium reabsorption is reduced, and urinary sodium excretion increases, thereby returning sodium balance toward normal. However, this circulating inhibitor also inhibits the sodium pump in other cells such as erythrocytes and leukocytes and, more importantly, in vascular smooth muscle cells. The increase in cellular sodium is associated with increased sodium-calcium exchange and increased cellular calcium concentration. Thus, at the arteriolar level, inhibition of Na,K-ATPase could theoretically cause vasoconstriction secondary to increased intracellular calcium, with a resultant increase in systemic vascular resistance and a rise in blood pressure [53]. This Na,K-ATPase inhibitor might also increase vascular reactivity to pressors [57].

As a result of the compensatory release of these natriuretic substances, sodium balance and ECF volume are restored to normal, but at the expense of systemic hypertension caused by the increase in vascular resistance (Fig. 9-1). Thus, although the underlying cause of this type of salt-sensitive (volume-dependent) hypertension is a defect in renal natriuretic capacity, in the steady-state phase, this does not result in a detectable increase in ECF volume or cardiac output. Instead, the hypertension is maintained by the resulting increase in systemic vascular resistance [12, 13, 53, 54].

Support for this concept of a chronic state of "controlled volume expansion" includes the finding of increased plasma levels of ANP in some patients with essential hypertension [58] and in hypertensive patients with autosomal dominant polycystic kidney disease [59]. Furthermore, cytochemical assays demonstrate increased ability of the plasma to inhibit Na,K-ATPase in patients with essential hypertension [56] and is spontaneously hypertensive rats [60]. It has been postulated that a circulating Na,K-ATPase inhibitor may also be important in the pathogenesis of secondary causes of hypertension in both humans (primary renal parenchymal disease, primary hyperaldosteronism, renal artery stenosis) and animal models of hypertension (reduced renal mass, one-kidney/one-clip Goldblatt hypertension, mineralocorticoid hypertension) [54]. Each of these conditions causes secondary hypertension in conjunction with an underlying tendency for sodium retention that must be overcome and that, via the mechanism illustrated in Figure 9-1, would produce hypertension. For example, in the DOCA/salt model of experimental hypertension, injection of deoxycorticosterone acetate (DOCA) in animals on a high-salt diet initially produces sodium retention, weight gain, and hypertension. However, within a few days, there is an increase in urinary sodium excretion such that, in the chronic phase, there is no detectable increase in ECF or blood volume. Despite this "escape" from the sodium-retaining effects of mineralocorticoid, hypertension is maintained by an increase in systemic vascular resistance. Mineralocorticoid escape in animal models or patients with primary hyperaldosteronism may be due to an increase in ANP and inhibitors of Na,K-ATPase, which act to restore normal sodium balance, but the latter may lead to an increase in systemic vascular resistance [51].

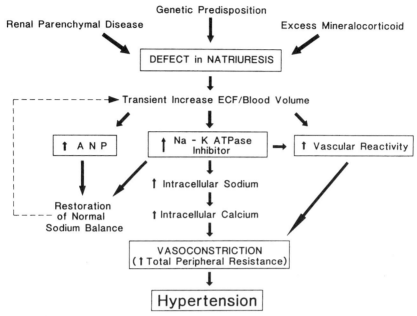

Fig. 9-1. The Na,K-ATPase inhibitor hypothesis. A defect in the natriuretic capacity of the kidney is thought to be the fundamental abnormality that predisposes to the development of hypertension. The resulting tendency toward extracellular fluid (ECF) volume expansion leads to increased circulating levels of two or more substances, collectively called natriuretic hormones. Atrial natriuretic peptide (ANP) and a circulating inhibitor of Na,K-ATPase result in reduced renal tubular sodium reabsorption, thereby compensating for the underlying natriuretic defect and restoring sodium balance and ECF volume to normal. However, Na,K-ATPase inhibition in vascular smooth muscle also causes vasoconstriction, resulting in systemic hypertension. ANP causes vasodilation, thus attenuating the rise in blood pressure.

Cellular Sodium Transport in Essential Hypertension

There is evidence of an increase in intracellular sodium in leukocytes, and probably erythrocytes, in patients with essential hypertension [61]. These abnormalities are not thought to represent hereditary defects intrinsic to the cells. Rather, they appear to result from a diminished activity of the cellular sodium pump, an acquired defect possibly caused by a circulating inhibitor of Na,K-ATPase [62]. Serum from patients with essential hypertension has been shown to increase the sodium content of normal human leukocytes [62]. This ability of plasma to inhibit Na,K-ATPase seems to be proportional to the level of blood pressure and inversely proportional to the plasma renin activity [56], findings that provide evidence of underlying volume expansion (see Fig. 9-1). Systemic resistance vessels may be subject to a similar disorder of sodium transport induced by a circulating Na,K-ATPase inhibitor. A positive correlation between leukocyte sodium content and forearm vascular resistance has been reported [63]. It has been postulated that the circulating Na,K-ATPase inhibitor found in essential hypertension causes an increase in systemic vascular resistance [53]. Inhibition of the vascular smooth muscle sodium pump would lead to an increase in the intracellular sodium content, which in turn would increase intracellular calcium by one of two mechanisms. Inhibition of the sodium pump would result in a small reduction in membrane potential, thereby allowing an increase in calcium influx through voltage-dependent calcium channels. Alternatively, a raised level of sodium in the cell would increase intracellular calcium through an effect on the sodium-calcium exchange mechanism. Increased vascular smooth muscle calcium would, in turn, lead to contraction of vascular smooth muscle and increased responsiveness to vasoconstrictors [53].

Recent evidence suggests that low dietary potassium intake may be an important factor in the genesis of hypertension, especially in blacks [64]. Furthermore, dietary potassium supplementation lowers blood pressure in patients with essential hypertension and in the setting of diuretic-induced hypokalemia [64]. With regard to the Na,K-ATPase inhibitor hypothesis, it is interesting to note that increases in serum potassium within the physiologic range stimulate the activity of Na,K-ATPase [65]. Theoretically, potassium supplementation could lower blood pressure by counteracting the effect of the circulating Na,K-ATPase inhibitor in hypertension.

A major criticism of the hypothesis outlined in Figure 9-1 has been the inability to isolate the circulating substance that inhibits Na,K-ATPase [66]. Recently, however, a highly potent, selective inhibitor of the ion transport functions of the sodium pump has been purified from human plasma. The properties of this substance suggest that it may be a mammalian endogenous digitalis-like factor and that it may be similar to the sodium transport inhibitor detected in the plasma of volume-sensitive forms of experimental and human hypertension [55]. Nonetheless, acceptance of this hypothesis will require proof that a circulating Na,K-ATPase inhibitor can lead to the long-standing increase in systemic vascular resistance that is observed in essential hypertension.

The Guyton Hypothesis

Guyton's hypothesis states that the most important and fundamental mechanism determining the long-term control of blood pressure is the renal fluid–volume feedback mechanism. In simple terms, this is the basic mechanism through which the kidneys regulate arterial pressure by altering renal excretion of sodium and water, thereby controlling circulatory volume and cardiac output. Changes in blood pressure, in turn, directly influence renal excretion of sodium and water, thereby providing a negative feedback mechanism for control of ECF volume, cardiac output, and blood pressure. The hypothesis is that derangements in this renal fluid–volume pressure control mechanism are the fundamental cause of virtually all hypertensive states [14–16, 67].

Renal Function Curves

Interactions of the renal perfusion pressure–sodium excretion mechanism and modulating neurohormonal factors normally operate very precisely to maintain sodium

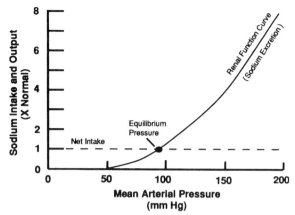

Fig. 9-2. Renal function curve showing the effect of perfusion pressure on urinary sodium excretion in the isolated, perfused kidney. With computer modeling, when the corresponding sodium intake curve is superimposed, an equilibrium pressure point is defined, which represents the unique level at which the arterial pressure will be regulated regardless of primary changes in the cardiac output or systemic vascular resistance. (From A. C. Guyton, Renal function curve: A key to understanding the pathogenesis of hypertension. *Hypertension* 10:1, 1987. By permission of the American Heart Association, Inc.)

balance at a set point of normal arterial pressure [67]. The physiologic basis of the renal-body fluid feedback mechanism for the regulation of arterial pressure is the direct effect of arterial pressure on output of water and sodium from the kidneys. Studies of the isolated, perfused kidney show that an increase in perfusion pressure directly causes the renal output of sodium and water to increase, the so-called pressure natriuresis and diuresis [68, 69]. Figure 9-2 depicts a *renal function curve* showing the effect of perfusion pressure on urinary sodium excretion in the isolated perfused kidney. When the arterial pressure falls to approximately 50 mm Hg, urinary sodium output falls to zero. On the other hand, when the arterial pressure rises from the normal value of 100 mm Hg up to 200 mm Hg, the output of sodium rises six- to eightfold [67]. This effect of arterial pressure on sodium excretion has been demonstrated in isolated, perfused kidneys and in intact animals. However, for the reasons discussed later, the upward slope of the renal function curve in the intact animal is much steeper. The horizontal line in Figure 9-2 represents the level of sodium intake at equilibrium when sodium intake and output are matched. When net intake and output of sodium are matched, the arterial pressure is determined by the point where the two plots intersect, which is known as the *equilibrium pressure point*. Computer model analysis of hypothetical renal function curves in the intact animal suggests that, if the renal function curve and the sodium intake remain unchanged, this is the unique perfusion pressure at which external sodium balance will be maintained [70]. If the pressure rises above this level, the output becomes greater than input, and negative sodium balance occurs, with eventual reduction of ECF volume and cardiac output to a level that returns the blood pressure to the equilibrium point. In contrast, if the blood pressure falls below the equilibrium point, the intake of sodium will be greater than output, and a positive sodium balance will occur until the increases in ECF volume, blood volume, and cardiac output are sufficient to return the pressure to the equilibrium point. Only at the 100 mm Hg pressure set point can sodium balance be maintained.

If this model is correct, it is apparent that a primary increase in cardiac output or systemic vascular resistance cannot result in a sustained increase in blood pressure, since a normally functioning feedback mechanism would result in natriuresis and diuresis, thereby returning the blood pressure to normal. Thus, a primary increase in systemic vascular resistance would be accompanied by an equal and opposite decrease in cardiac output, with return of the blood pressure to normal. This return of the pressure to the equilibrium point illustrates the infinite gain characteristic of the renal fluid–volume feedback mechanism. In this system, a change in the arterial pressure is the critical feedback stimulus that modifies the natriuretic response. In theory, if an initial decrease in blood pressure results from a decrease in cardiac output—for instance, in the setting of congestive heart failure—the compensatory salt and water retention would increase ECF volume but fail to normalize cardiac output and perfusion pressure. Thus, renal sodium and water retention would continue unopposed, resulting in massive fluid overload. This mechanism is consistent with the unifying hypothesis recently proposed to explain body fluid volume regulation in disorders characterized by low effective arterial blood volume [19, 71].

The implication of this renal fluid–volume feedback mechanism, if correct, is that the finding of sustained hypertension must be a reflection of an underlying abnormality that caused a shift of the renal function curve to the right such that a higher blood pressure is required to maintain sodium balance at any given level of sodium intake [70, 72].

Role of the Renin-Angiotensin System in Regulation of Blood Pressure

Unlike the isolated perfused kidney or computer models, in vivo the position of the renal function curve can be shifted by various neural and endocrine factors. For example, changes in the activity of the renin-angiotensin system can result in a shift of the curve and thus either magnify or blunt the basic relation between sodium and water excretion and blood pressure [72, 73]. Different renal function curves can be produced in animals by varying sodium intake in stepwise increments while maintaining angiotensin II levels constant at various levels using combinations of ACE inhibitor and angiotensin II infusion [73] (Fig. 9-3). With the angiotensin II level maintained above normal, there is a shift in the renal function curve to the right consistent with a blunting of the pressure-induced natriuretic response. In contrast, when angiotensin II is totally suppressed with ACE inhibitor, the curve is shifted to the left consistent with an exaggerated pressure natriuresis. The vertical line in Figure 9-3 represents a different type of renal function curve called a *salt-loading renal function curve*. It is obtained when sodium intake is varied in a stepwise fashion in animals with an intact renin-angiotensin system (angiotensin II level

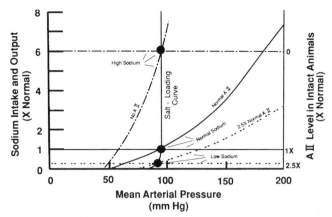

Fig. 9-3. Salt-loading renal function curve obtained when the sodium intake is varied in stepwise increments in animals with an intact renin-angiotensin system. The curve is very steep such that over a wide range of dietary sodium intake, the blood pressure at equilibrium changes very little. Three separate renal function curves were produced by varying the sodium intake in a stepwise fashion in animals, with angiotensin II (A II) levels maintained constant in either the normal range, 2.5 times normal, or with angiotensin II absent. The curve obtained when angiotensin II production is suppressed by converting enzyme inhibitor is shifted to the left, consistent with an enhanced natriuretic response to any given perfusion pressure. In contrast, with an angiotensin II level 2.5 times normal, the curve is shifted to the right, reflecting a blunted natriuretic response to pressure. Superimposition of these individual renal function curves reveals that the steepness of the salt-loading curve in the intact animal is due to changes in the natriuretic response to pressure, which are mediated by changes in the activity of the renin-angiotensin system as a function of the dietary sodium intake. (Adapted from A. C. Guyton, Renal function curve: A key to understanding hypertension. *Hypertension* 10:1, 1987. By permission of the American Heart Association, Inc.)

allowed to vary in response to the sodium intake), which will modulate the intrinsic renal-body fluid feedback mechanism. Thus, the renal function curve in the intact animal is much steeper than that seen in the isolated perfused kidney. In this salt-loading curve, blood pressure at equilibrium for each level of sodium intake changes very little. Analysis of the superimposed renal function curves, with angiotensin II held constant at different levels, illustrates that the steepness of the curve in the intact animal may be due to changes in the activity of the renin-angiotensin system. A high sodium intake suppresses the renin-angiotensin system and shifts the renal function curve to the left, whereas a low sodium intake activates the renin-angiotensin system and shifts the curve to the right. This modulation of the renal function curve by the renin-angiotensin system is thought to be due to the effect of angiotensin II on renal sodium and water reabsorption. Angiotensin II directly enhances proximal tubular sodium reabsorption [42]. In addition, angiotensin II has important renal hemodynamic effects that cause increased tubular sodium reabsorption independent of aldosterone [41]. The predominant efferent vasoconstriction produced by angiotensin II causes a drop in peritubular capillary hydrostatic pressure, leading to enhanced tubular resorption of sodium and water [41, 74].

This dynamic interaction between the renin-angiotensin system and the renal fluid–volume feedback mechanism accounts for the observation that tremendous extremes of dietary sodium intake in normal individuals result in relatively little change in the systemic arterial pressure.

Autoregulation Leads to Increased Systemic Vascular Resistance

The ability to maintain normal blood pressure over a wide range of dietary sodium intake is present only if both the renin-angiotensin system and the kidney function normally. Aberrations in either the renin-angiotensin system or the renal fluid–volume mechanism can lead to a significant increase in blood pressure when the sodium intake is increased. Guyton's hypothesis holds that there are two basic ways in which the pressure equilibrium set point can be increased, with resulting hypertension. A shift of the renal function curve to the right along the pressure axis due to either intrinsic renal abnormalities or overactivity of the renin-angiotensin system can cause hypertension. Alternatively, an increase in the sodium intake without a compensatory leftward shift of the renal function curve can also cause hypertension.

In the setting of an underlying decrease in the inherent natriuretic capacity, the renal fluid–volume feedback mechanism should cause progressive sodium and water retention until the increases in ECF volume, blood volume, and cardiac output are sufficient to raise the blood pressure to the equilibrium pressure point. At the equilibrium point, sodium and water balance is restored; however, this is accomplished at the expense of systemic hypertension (Fig. 9-4). Thus, when the inherent natriuretic capacity is reduced, Guyton's concept holds that an increase in arterial pressure is an essential protective mechanism to restore sodium balance and avert disaster [14–16, 67].

Hypertension caused by a rightward shift of the renal function curve should theoretically be mediated by an increased cardiac output in response to sodium and water retention. However, in animal models and humans with essential hypertension, even though the initiating mechanism for hypertension is sodium retention with increased ECF volume and cardiac output, ultimately an increase in the peripheral vascular resistance perpetuates the hypertension, and the cardiac output and ECF volume return to normal. According to Guyton's hypothesis, this transition from hypertension associated with high cardiac output to the high systemic vascular resistance type of hypertension is explained by the process of autoregulation of blood flow in the systemic circulation [14–16]. Autoregulation is a local tissue phenomenon that adjusts local blood flow when it becomes too high or low. Acutely, autoregulation may be due to local changes in vascular muscle tone; however, in the chronic phase, structural changes in the resistance vessels develop [8]. In theory, when the cardiac output increases as a result of ECF volume expansion, autoregulatory vasoconstriction in all vascular beds eventually returns the cardiac output to normal. Hypertension persists, however, because the fall in cardiac output is accompanied by an equal and opposite increase in systemic vascular resistance. Given the persistent hypertension, sodium balance can still be maintained by the renal fluid–volume mechanism. Figure 9-4 summarizes the pathophysiologic sequence

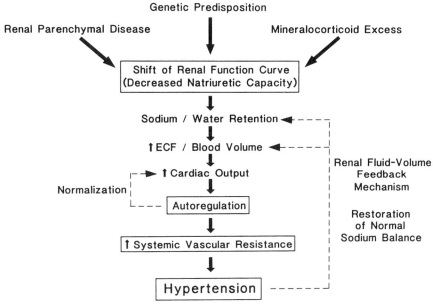

Fig. 9-4. The Guyton hypothesis. In the setting of essential hypertension, primary renal disease, or mineralocorticoid excess, a defect in the intrinsic natriuretic capacity of the kidney, reflected by a rightward shift of the renal function curve, is thought to be the fundamental abnormality that leads to the development of hypertension. Initially, sodium and water retention leads to increases in extracellular fluid (ECF) volume and cardiac output. However, in the long term, circulatory autoregulation restores cardiac output to normal. Via pressure-induced natriuresis, the renal fluid–volume feedback mechanism returns sodium balance and ECF volume to near normal but at the expense of persistent hypertension, which is maintained by increased systemic vascular resistance resulting from autoregulation.

whereby an initial defect in natriuretic capacity (shift of renal function curve to the right) leads to sustained hypertension due to increased systemic vascular resistance in the absence of clinically evident increases in ECF volume, blood volume, or cardiac output.

Renal Function Curves in Essential Hypertension

An impairment of the intrinsic natriuretic capacity of the kidney is easy to conceptualize in the setting of renal artery stenosis, primary renal parenchymal disease, or mineralocorticoid hypertension. However, in the early stages of human essential hypertension, no specific renal histologic abnormality can be identified. At face value, this observation suggests that renal function is entirely normal until damage (nephrosclerosis) secondary to hypertension supervenes. However, if either the Guyton hypothesis or the Na,K-ATPase inhibitor hypothesis is correct, it is clear that with sustained hypertension, regardless of etiology, there must be a rightward shift of the renal function curve such that sodium balance is maintained at a hypertensive level.

Salt-Sensitive and Salt-Resistant Essential Hypertension

In the normal individual, salt balance is maintained at a normal blood pressure. Moreover, the slope of the renal function curve is very steep such that, even with dietary salt loading, the blood pressure remains near normal (Fig. 9-5). Two subsets of patients with essential hypertension have been identified based on their sensitivity to increases in dietary sodium intake: salt-sensitive and salt-resistant patients [75]. Approximately 60 percent of subjects with essential hypertension have greater than a 10 percent increase in blood pressure when given a high-sodium diet (>200 mmol/day) and are defined as salt sensitive, whereas 40 percent are salt resistant. Plasma renin activity is usually normal or high in salt-resistant patients and usually low in salt-sensitive patients. These hypertensive subtypes probably represent differ-

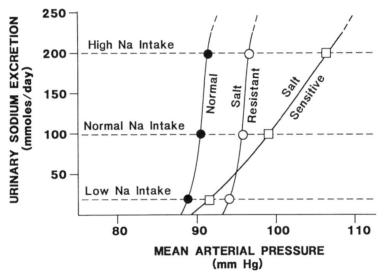

Fig. 9-5. Schematic renal function curves in human essential hypertension. In the normal individual, salt balance is maintained at a normal blood pressure. Moreover, the slope of the renal function curve is very steep such that with dietary salt loading the blood pressure remains near normal. The salt-loading renal function curve in *salt-resistant hypertension* is shifted to the right, but it remains parallel to the curve for normotensive individuals. Thus on a normal sodium intake, salt balance is maintained, but at a higher blood pressure set point. However, since the renal function curve is steep, the blood pressure does not increase with dietary salt loading. In contrast, in *salt-sensitive hypertension*, the rightward shift of the curve is accompanied by a depression of the slope. Thus, not only is the blood pressure set point on a normal sodium diet elevated, but also the blood pressure increases in response to dietary salt loading. Response to strict dietary sodium restriction also differs in the two subtypes. Hypertension responds to lowered sodium intake in salt-sensitive hypertension but not in salt-resistant hypertension.

ences in the adaptation to a sodium load. The salt-loading renal function curve in *salt-resistant hypertension* is shifted to the right, but it remains parallel to the curve for normotensive individuals (see Fig. 9-5). Thus on a normal sodium intake, salt balance is maintained, but at a higher blood pressure set point. However, since the renal function curve is steep, the blood pressure does not increase with dietary salt loading. In contrast, in *salt-sensitive hypertension*, the rightward shift of the curve is accompanied by a depression of the slope. Thus, not only is the blood pressure set point on a normal sodium diet elevated, but also the blood pressure increases in response to dietary salt loading (see Fig. 9-5). Response to strict dietary sodium restriction also differs in the two subtypes. Hypertension responds to reduced sodium intake in salt-sensitive hypertension but not in salt-resistant hypertension.

Experimental evidence suggests that disorders associated with increased renal vascular resistance, such as one-kidney Goldblatt hypertension, tend to induce salt-resistant hypertension. In contrast, salt sensitivity with rightward shift of the curve accompanied by a depression in slope occurs in conditions characterized by increased sodium reabsorption by the renal tubules. This phenomenon occurs in DOCA/salt hypertension in the rat, in patients with primary hyperaldosteronism, in the setting of reduced renal mass, and in conditions characterized by inhibition of the negative feedback of the renin-angiotensin system. In these instances, as sodium intake increases, an incremental rise in blood pressure is required to overcome excessive sodium reabsorption and maintain normal sodium balance [75].

The precise nature of the defect responsible for the altered pressure natriuresis mechanism in human essential hypertension is unknown. Theoretically, any abnormality that increases renal vascular resistance, reduces renal mass, decreases glomerular basement membrane filtration coefficient, or increases tubular sodium reabsorption (angiotensin, α-adrenergic stimulation, deficient renal nitric oxide, aldosterone, alterations in net peritubular Starling forces) could impair renal natriuretic capacity and lead to hypertension [14]. Changes in renal vascular resistance have been clearly documented in human essential hypertension, especially with advanced nephrosclerosis. On the other hand, the mechanism of increased tubular sodium reabsorption in salt-sensitive patients may relate to abnormalities of the sympathetic nervous system [75]. Salt-sensitive patients display an abnormal relation between sodium intake and plasma norepinephrine levels. Although plasma norepinephrine levels are suppressed by salt loading in normal individuals and salt-resistant patients, they tend to increase in salt-sensitive patients. It has been postulated that increased sympathetic activity and reduced renal sodium excretion in salt-sensitive patients may be related to a defect in sodium-coupled cellular calcium transport. In this regard, calcium channel blockers have been shown to have a natriuretic effect and to normalize the derangements in the renal function curve in salt-sensitive essential hypertension in blacks [46, 75].

The Dominant Role of Perfusion Pressure in Aldosterone Escape Phenomenon

To substantiate the role of direct pressure-induced natriuresis in the regulation of sodium balance in mineralocorticoid hypertension, Hall et al. [76] compared the systemic blood pressure and natriuretic effect of aldosterone infusion in a dog model in which the renal perfusion pressure was either allowed to increase or mechanically servocontrolled to maintain pressure at normal levels. In the intact animal, continuous aldosterone infusion caused a transient period of sodium and water retention with a mild increase in blood pressure. However, the sodium retention lasted only a few days and was followed by an escape from the sodium-retaining effects of aldosterone and restoration of normal sodium balance. In contrast, when the renal perfusion pressure was servocontrolled during aldosterone infusion, there was no escape from aldosterone, and there was a relentless increase in sodium and water retention accompanied by severe hypertension, edema, ascites, and congestive heart failure. When the servocontrol device was removed and the perfusion pressure was allowed to rise to the systemic level, a prompt natriuresis and diuresis ensued, with restoration of sodium balance and a fall in blood pressure. The observations highlight the pivotal role of blood pressure in the regulation of renal sodium and water excretion. Similar observations have been made in studies of hypertension produced by angiotensin II [77] or vasopressin infusion [78]. Thus, the natriuretic factors proposed by de Wardener [51] to account for the phenomenon of mineralocorticoid escape are apparently not sufficient to offset the antinatriuretic action of mineralocorticoid in the absence of an accompanying increase in renal perfusion pressure.

Essential Hypertension and Benign Nephrosclerosis

The kidney is usually histologically normal in the early stages of essential hypertension. However, with time there is a gradual loss of nephron mass such that with long-standing benign hypertension, a contracted, granular kidney is found. This progressive reduction in renal size is caused by diffuse cortical atrophy and fibrosis due to hyaline arteriosclerosis, the severity of which is proportional to the duration of the hypertension [79]. In benign nephrosclerosis, the afferent arterioles demonstrate hyaline arteriosclerosis with subintimal deposition of a homogenous eosinophilic material. The interlobular arteries exhibit fibroelastic hyperplasia, which consists of reduplication of the internal elastic lamina. There is patchy ischemic atrophy of glomeruli; while some glomeruli are normal, others are globally sclerotic. Atrophic tubules filled with eosinophilic material are seen in the areas of glomerular ischemia.

Benign Nephrosclerosis and End-Stage Renal Disease

Despite the presence of these renal histologic abnormalities, even with long-standing benign hypertension, the majority of patients never develop clinically significant renal insufficiency. Benign essential hypertension tends to cause much less damage to the kidney than to other target organs such as the heart and brain. Indeed, the relationship between essential hypertension and end-stage renal disease (ESRD) remains circumstantial despite the fact that these syndromes have long been associated in the medical literature. Even though nephrologists credit essential hypertension as the cause of ESRD in 25 percent of patients initiating Medicare-supported renal replacement therapy [80], the widely held notion that benign hypertension with benign nephrosclerosis is a common cause of ESRD is difficult to support. Recent reviews have suggested that the number of patients reaching ESRD attributable to benign nephrosclerosis may have been significantly overestimated [80–82]. Overall, significant renal dysfunction is very rare in uncomplicated essential hypertension. Estimates in white populations have suggested that the relative risk of developing renal failure in essential hypertension is on the order of 1 in 6000 cases [83]. Moreover, serum creatinine levels infrequently increase in patients with long-standing mild to moderate hypertension. An analysis of the data from three recent large clinical trials in patients with essential hypertension revealed that less than 1 percent of 10,000 patients developed advanced renal failure during the 4 to 6 years of follow-up [84, 85]. A very low incidence of clinically significant deterioration of renal function was also noted in the Hypertension Detection and Follow-up Program [86].

Autopsy studies conducted in the pre-antihypertensive era have documented that benign nephrosclerosis is an uncommon cause of ESRD. Among 150 hypertensive patients with ESRD, only one was found to have benign nephrosclerosis as the sole underlying etiology [87]. Moreover, in a study of renal anatomy and histology of 146 patients with bilateral nephrectomy prior to initiation of dialysis, approximately half had glomerulonephritis, and 20 percent had reflux nephropathy [88]. Only three subjects had hypertension as the primary cause of renal failure; two of these had malignant hypertension and one renal artery stenosis. Kincaid-Smith and Whitworth [89] maintain that patients with hypertension and renal impairment in whom renal artery stenosis (ischemic nephropathy) and malignant hypertension have been excluded, most likely have underlying primary renal parenchymal disease rather than benign nephrosclerosis.

Patients classified as having hypertensive ESRD typically present with advanced disease, making the processes that initiated the renal disease difficult to discern. It has been proposed that many patients classified with ESRD secondary to benign nephrosclerosis actually have primary renal parenchymal disease, unrecognized renal artery stenosis with ischemic nephropathy, unrecognized episodes of malignant hypertension, occult renal cholesterol embolic disease, or primary renal microvascular disease [81–83].

Hemodynamic studies in essential hypertension demonstrate a near normal glomerular filtration rate (GFR) despite a significant reduction of renal blood flow, consistent with an increased filtration fraction. Genetic models of essential hypertension in the rat have shown that these alterations in renal hemodynamics arise through an increase in resistance of both the afferent and efferent arterioles, so that glomerular capillary hydraulic pressure is maintained at a normal level [90]. Thus in these models of spontaneous hypertension, the kidney is protected from elevated systemic pressure, and glomerular capillary hypertension does not develop. In contrast, in animal models of diabetic nephropathy [91] and renal ablation [92], afferent arteriolar vasodilation occurs such that an increase in arterial pressure is transmitted to the glomerulus, resulting in glomerular capillary hypertension, which is thought to be a critical factor in the progression of renal insufficiency.

The rarity of significant renal impairment in patients with essential hypertension (nonmalignant) is consistent with these hemodynamic observations. In benign essential hypertension, there appears to be a balanced increase in afferent and efferent resistances, thereby shielding the kidney from the high systemic pressure, while simultaneously enabling the maintenance of near normal GFR.

Hypertension and Renal Disease in Blacks

The critical issue that has yet to be resolved is why blacks constitute a disproportionate percentage of patients with ESRD in the United States. The overall rate of ESRD is four times higher in blacks than in whites [93]. It has been suggested that the higher incidence of ESRD in blacks compared to whites may be the consequence of a higher risk of progressive hypertensive nephrosclerosis among blacks [93]. Epidemiologic studies suggest that essential hypertension occurs more frequently in blacks and is associated with more severe cardiovascular end-organ damage for any given level of blood pressure [94]. In angiographic studies of patients with mild to moderate essential hypertension and normal renal function, blacks tended to have more severe angiographic evidence of nephrosclerosis than whites [95].

There are several plausible explanations for the high frequency with which hypertensive nephrosclerosis is reported as a cause of ESRD in the black population. Since most of the available data are based on clinical diagnoses rather than renal histology, there may be a tendency on the part of physicians to identify hypertension as the cause of ESRD given the known high prevalence of hypertension in blacks [80]. In this regard, there appears to be a racial bias with regard to the diagnosis of hypertensive nephrosclerosis. In a recent survey, nephrologists were asked to review identical case histories of patients with ESRD in which only the race of the patient was randomly assigned as either black or white. It was found that black patients were twice as likely as white patients to be labeled as having ESRD secondary to hypertensive nephrosclerosis [96]. Therefore, in the absence of renal biopsy, it is possible that in many cases ESRD that appears to have resulted from hypertension is in reality due to an undiagnosed primary renal parenchymal disease [82, 88, 89].

Another possibility is that recurrent bouts of unrecognized or inadequately treated malignant hypertension are the actual cause of the increase in ESRD due to hypertension among blacks. The incidence of malignant hypertension is higher in blacks than in whites. Furthermore, in the epidemiologic studies, it is not clear whether the term *hypertensive nephrosclerosis* refers to benign or malignant nephrosclerosis. In the few available studies detailing the pathologic findings in blacks with ESRD due to hypertension, the characteristic findings have been those of malignant nephrosclerosis, namely, musculomucoid intimal hyperplasia of the interlobular arteries and accelerated glomerular obsolescence, rather than benign arteriolar nephrosclerosis [82, 97]. In this regard, a recent study of 100 patients admitted to an inner-city hospital with a diagnosis of hypertensive emergency showed that two-thirds had malignant hypertension based on funduscopic findings [98]. These patients were predominantly young, male, black or Hispanic individuals of lower socioeconomic status. Over 93 percent of these patients had been previously diagnosed as hypertensive, and most reported having received prior pharmacologic treatment for hypertension. However, no source of regular health care could be documented in 60 percent of cases. More than 50 percent were noted to have stopped their antihypertensive medications more than 30 days prior to admission, and only 24 percent had taken any medication on the day of admission. If the overrepresentation of young blacks with ESRD is at least in part due to undiagnosed or inadequately treated malignant hypertension, this would have tremendous public health implications, since malignant hypertension is clearly preventable, and even significant renal dysfunction is potentially reversible with early and aggressive antihypertensive therapy.

Finally, it may be that blacks with essential hypertension tend to develop more severe benign nephrosclerosis that, unlike benign hypertension in whites, results in progressive renal insufficiency and ESRD. This could occur because the hypertension in blacks is more severe or because their renal vasculature is more susceptible to hypertensive damage [99]. Tobian [18] has postulated that the low-potassium diet characteristically consumed by blacks in the United States (30 mmol/day versus 65 mmol/day in the general population) accelerates the intimal thickening of the renal vasculature that occurs due to hypertensive damage. He has proposed that this may account for the increased risk of progressive renal insufficiency due to hypertension among blacks. Dustan [100] has suggested that increased risk of renal injury in essential hypertension in blacks may in part be due to the increased expression of growth factors leading to vascular smooth muscle hypertrophy in renal arterioles.

Link Between Salt Sensitivity and Progressive Renal Disease in Blacks with Essential Hypertension

There is some evidence that essential hypertension may be fundamentally different in blacks and whites. Compared to whites, blacks tend to have a more expanded intravascular volume, lower plasma renin activity, reduced natriuretic response to a sodium load, and better antihypertensive responses to diuretics and calcium channel blockers than to ACE inhibitors or β-blockers. Substantial renal hemodynamic differences between black and white patients with essential hypertension have been described [46, 75]. For instance, black hypertensive patients have a greater reduction in renal blood flow and higher renal vascular resistance than white patients [99]. In addition, black hypertensive patients are more likely to be salt sensitive than white hypertensive patients such that an increase in sodium intake leads to an increase in blood pressure [46].

In a recent study of 17 black patients and 9 white patients with essential hypertension, 11 blacks were found to be salt sensitive, whereas all the whites were salt resistant [46]. Renal hemodynamics were measured during a low-sodium diet (20 mmol/day for 9 days) and during a high-salt diet (200 mmol/day for 14 days). During the low-sodium diet period, salt-sensitive and salt-resistant patients had similar mean arterial pressure, GFR, effective renal plasma flow (ERPF), and filtration fraction. During the high-salt diet period, GFR did not change in either group; ERPF increased in salt-resistant patients but decreased in salt-sensitive patients; filtration fraction decreased in salt-resistant patients but increased in salt-sensitive patients; and glomerular pressure decreased in salt-resistant patients but increased in salt-sensitive patients. Given the high prevalence of salt-sensitive hypertension in black Americans, the documented rise in filtration fraction and in intraglomerular pressure during high sodium intake suggests that these renal hemodynamic derangements might be partially responsible for the greater propensity to hypertension-induced renal failure in this ethnic group [46]. Thus it is possible that in black patients, essential hypertension may lead to progressive renal injury in the absence of malignant hypertension or underlying primary renal disease.

Experimental evidence in genetic models of hypertension supports this possibility. Renal function deteriorates faster in some strains of rats than others with genetic hypertension. In the spontaneously hypertensive rat, hypertension is accompanied by an increase in renal afferent arteriolar resistance, thus protecting the glomerulus from the adverse effects of hypertension so that progressive renal insufficiency does not occur. In contrast, all salt-sensitive rat models of hypertension share the peculiarity of responding to a rise in blood pressure with a decrease in afferent arteriolar resistance, which leads to an increase in glomerular capillary pressure with progressive renal injury [46].

Malignant Hypertension

Malignant hypertension is a distinct clinical and pathologic entity characterized by a marked elevation of the blood pressure (diastolic pressure is often >120–130 mm Hg) and evidence of widespread acute arteriolar injury [101]. The clinical sine qua non of malignant hypertension is the funduscopic finding of *hypertensive neuroretinopathy*, which consists of striate (flame-shaped) hemorrhages, cotton-wool (soft) exudates, and often papilledema. The development of hypertensive neuroretinopathy heralds the onset of a hypertensive vasculopathy that may cause necrotizing arteriolitis in the central nervous system, kidneys, and other vital organs. If the hypertension is untreated, there is rapid and relentless progression to renal failure in less than 1 year, often with associated hypertensive encephalopathy, intracerebral hemorrhage, or congestive heart failure. Regardless of the degree of blood pressure elevation, malignant hypertension cannot be diagnosed in the absence of hypertensive neuroretinopathy [101]. There has been an unfortunate tendency in recent years to diagnose "malignant hypertension" in any patient with markedly elevated blood pressure. However, given the prognostic and therapeutic implications of true malignant hypertension, it is extremely important to make a clear distinction between benign and malignant hypertension. This is not to say that benign hypertension cannot cause a hypertensive crisis. Benign hypertension that is accompanied by acute end-organ dysfunction such as acute pulmonary edema, dissecting aortic aneurysm, or intracerebral bleeding clearly represents a hypertensive crisis requiring immediate reduction of the blood pressure to avert disaster [101]. On the other hand, marked elevation of diastolic blood pressure (>120 mm Hg) frequently occurs in the absence of hypertensive neuroretinopathy or evidence of acute end-organ dysfunction. This entity, which is called *severe asymptomatic hypertension*, does not represent a true hypertensive crisis, and urgent treatment is often not required [101].

Headache and blurred vision are the most common presenting complaints in malignant hypertension. A striking "asymptomatic" presentation is not uncommon, especially in young black males who deny any prior symptoms when they present in the end stage of malignant hypertension with florid failure of the heart, brain, and kidney. In most patients, the diastolic pressure at presentation is over 120 to 130 mm Hg. However, there is no absolute level of pressure above which malignant hypertension develops, and there is considerable overlap of blood pressure readings in patients with benign and malignant hypertension [101].

The patient with malignant hypertension (hypertensive neuroretinopathy) may or may not have clinically apparent end-organ involvement at the time of presentation. However, in the absence of adequate treatment, a variety of organ systems will eventually be damaged by the evolving hypertensive vasculopathy. Nervous system manifestations include hypertensive encephalopathy or intracerebral hemorrhage. Congestive heart failure with recurrent bouts of acute pulmonary edema is the most common cardiac complication. Gastrointestinal involvement may cause acute pancreatitis or an acute abdomen due to necrotizing mesenteric vasculitis. Patients with malignant hypertension may present with a spectrum of renal involvement ranging from minimal albuminuria with normal renal function to ESRD. In the untreated or inadequately treated patient, even if the renal function is initially normal, it is common to observe progressive deterioration to end-stage renal failure over several weeks to months [101].

Pathology of Malignant Nephrosclerosis

Even when terminal renal failure occurs in malignant hypertension, the kidneys may be normal in size. Small, pinpoint petechial hemorrhages on the cortical surface give rise to a peculiar, flea-bitten appearance. Fibrinoid necrosis of the afferent arterioles has traditionally been regarded as the hallmark of malignant nephrosclerosis. There is deposition in the media of a granular material that is pink with hematoxylin-eosin stain and a deep red color with trichrome stain [79]. The characteristic finding in the interlobular arteries is severe luminal narrowing due to intimal thickening [79]. This lesion is known as proliferative endarteritis, endarteritis fibrosa, or the onionskin lesion. The arteriolar lumens are severely narrowed due to thickening of the walls or superimposed fibrin thrombi. In large autopsy series in the pretreatment era, focal and segmental fibrinoid necrosis was the predominant glomerular lesion. However, accelerated glomerular obsolescence due to ischemia is currently the most common finding at renal biopsy. In blacks with malignant hypertension, fibrinoid necrosis of the afferent arterioles is a rare finding. Instead, the afferent arterioles show a marked degree of hyalinization. The most prominent and characteristic finding is musculomucoid intimal hyperplasia of the interlobular arteries and larger arterioles [97] (Fig. 9-6). The intima of interlobular arteries is thickened by hyperplastic smooth muscle cells with variable degrees of fibrosis. The glomeruli show evidence of accelerated glomerular obsolescence with ischemic wrinkling of the glomerular basement membrane on electron microscopy [101].

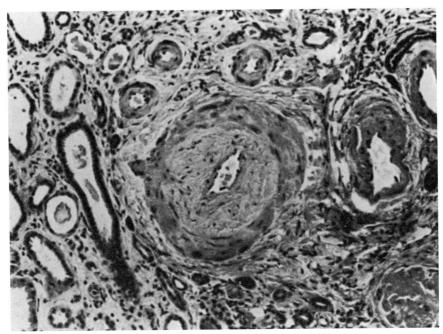

Fig. 9-6. Musculomucoid intimal hyperplasia of an interlobular artery in malignant hypertension. The arterial wall is thickened by hyperplastic smooth muscle cells. A small amount of myxoid material is seen between the smooth muscle cells. (Hematoxylin-eosin stain.) (From J. A. Pitcock, J. G. Johnson, F. E. Hatch, et al., Malignant hypertension in blacks: Malignant arterial disease as observed by light and electron microscopy. *Hum. Pathol.* 7:333, 1976. With permission.)

Pathophysiology of Malignant Hypertension

The mechanism that initiates a transition from benign to malignant hypertension is unknown. Several pathophysiologic mechanisms have been postulated [101]. According to the *pressure hypothesis*, the microvascular damage is a direct consequence of the mechanical stress placed on the vessel wall by hypertension. In contrast, the *vasculotoxic theory* holds that angiotensin II, vasopressin, and catecholamines not only raise blood pressure but also induce direct vascular injury. Pressure-induced natriuresis with volume depletion and reflex activation of the renin-angiotensin system may also result in an unrelenting vicious cycle of hypertension and ischemic renal injury. The development of localized intravascular coagulation or altered metabolism of glucocorticoids, prostaglandins, or kininogens has also been postulated to play a role in acceleration of the vascular injury. Recent evidence suggests that the vascular endothelium plays a crucial role in the regulation of vascular tone through the release of mediators such as endothelium-derived relaxing factor (EDRF) and endothelin-1, which influence the contractile activity of the underlying vascular smooth muscle. Endothelium-derived nitric oxide–mediated vasodilation is impaired in patients with essential hypertension [47]. In contrast, endothelin-1, which is also produced by the vascular endothelium, is a vasoconstrictor with a potency 10 times that of angiotensin II. Additional studies are required to define the potential roles of impaired EDRF-mediated vasodilation or endothelin-1–mediated vasoconstriction in the pathogenesis of malignant hypertension.

The vicious cycle of malignant hypertension is depicted in Figure 9-7. In the setting of severe essential or secondary hypertension, the pressure increases to a critical level or at a rate that overwhelms normal autoregulatory mechanisms and

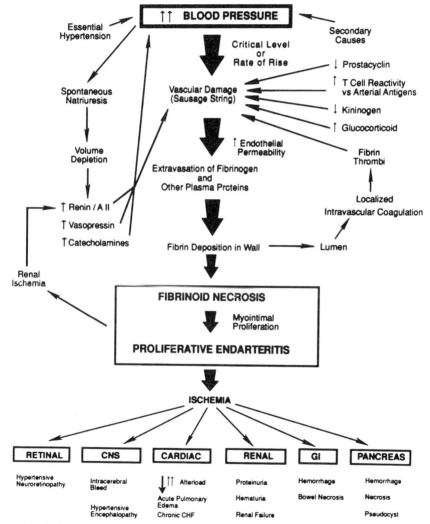

Fig. 9-7. Pathophysiology of malignant hypertension. A II = angiotensin II; CHF = congestive heart failure. (From C. R. Nolan and S. L. Linas, Malignant Hypertension and Other Hypertensive Crises. In R. W. Schrier and C. W. Gottschalk [eds.], *Diseases of the Kidney* [6th ed.]. Boston: Little, Brown, 1997.)

leads to focal areas of overstretched arterioles. The resulting endothelial damage allows extravasation of fibrinogen and other plasma proteins. The deposition of fibrin causes fibrinoid necrosis. Myointimal proliferation occurs, resulting in proliferative endarteritis. In the kidney, there is progressive glomerular injury due to ischemia. Activation of the renin-angiotensin system further increases the blood pressure and leads to amplification of the cycle of hypertension and renal ischemia. The end result is renal failure. This widespread hypertensive vasculopathy also results in ischemic damage to other vascular beds. In the retina, ischemia of nerve fiber bundles leads to cotton-wool spots and papilledema. Hypertensive neuroretinopathy occurs very early in the course and is the clinical hallmark of malignant hypertension.

Response to Treatment in Malignant Hypertension

In the absence of adequate blood pressure control, malignant hypertension has a grave prognosis. In the pre-antihypertensive era, the 1-year mortality rate approached 90 percent, and uremia was the most common cause of death. However, it is now clear that adequate treatment of essential hypertension prevents malignant hypertension. Furthermore, early and aggressive treatment of an established malignant phase prevents progressive renal damage. More severe renal dysfunction at presentation correlates with an increased risk of progression to ESRD. However, there are numerous reports of dramatic recovery of renal function in patients with malignant hypertension, even after months of dialysis requiring renal failure [101]. This recovery of renal function has been attributed to strict blood pressure control with the potent peripheral vasodilator minoxidil used in conjunction with a loop diuretic and a β-blocker. Presumably, the renal vasculopathy heals and the ischemic glomeruli recover when the inciting stimulus (severe hypertension) is removed.

Renovascular Hypertension

The landmark experimental models of hypertension developed by Goldblatt and colleagues demonstrated that persistent hypertension could be produced in dogs either by constricting both renal arteries or by removing one kidney and constricting the artery of the remaining kidney [102]. Another variant of Goldblatt hypertension is produced by clipping the artery of one kidney and leaving the other kidney untouched. This two-kidney/one-clip (2K/1C) hypertension may be analogous to unilateral renal artery stenosis in humans. In this model, constriction of one artery leads to an immediate rise in blood pressure due to increased renin production by the ischemic kidney. The activation of the renin-angiotensin system leads to angiotensin II–mediated vasoconstriction and hypertension. Curiously, after a few days, even though blood pressure continues to rise, the plasma renin activity returns to normal. In the early stages of 2K/1C hypertension, removal of the clipped kidney restores blood pressure to normal. In contrast, later in the course, when the plasma renin activity is no longer elevated, the blood pressure fails to normalize with angiotensin antagonists, removal of the clipped kidney, or unclipping. Of note, however, is the observation that removal of the contralateral "normal kidney" and unclipping normalize blood pressure. These findings imply that vascular changes that develop in the normal kidney when it is chronically exposed to elevated pressure may serve to perpetuate hypertension even after the original cause of the renovascular hypertension has been removed. Guyton's hypothesis would imply that from the very beginning the contralateral kidney must have an abnormal renal function curve with a blunted natriuretic response to the elevated blood pressure. Early in the course, this shift of the renal function curve may be mediated by functional changes induced by local intrarenal formation of angiotensin II [103]. The direct and indirect effects of angiotensin II on renal sodium excretion have been previously discussed in detail. It now seems clear that the angiotensin II–dependent mechanisms that contribute to the development and maintenance of hypertension in the 2K/1C model probably act primarily by attenuating the ability of the animal to exhibit the expected hypertension-induced natriuresis by the nonclipped kidney [103]. In later stages of renovascular hypertension, hypertension-induced structural damage may underlie the reduced natriuretic response to any given level of pressure. These secondary changes in the contralateral kidney may explain the well-known clinical observation that nephrectomy or revascularization for unilateral renal artery stenosis often fails to normalize blood pressure. Preexisting essential hypertension is also a likely explanation in many cases.

Causes of Renal Artery Stenosis

The principal cause of renal artery stenosis is *atheromatous* narrowing of one or both main renal arteries (Fig. 9-8). Atheromatous renal artery stenosis occurs in older individuals, with a peak incidence in the sixth decade. Men are affected twice as often as women. It is most often found in association with diffuse atherosclerotic disease of the aorta, coronary arteries, cerebral arteries, and peripheral vasculature. However, in 15 to 20 percent of cases, renal involvement occurs in the absence of atherosclerotic disease elsewhere [104]. The obstructing atheromatous lesion is usually within the proximal 2 cm of the artery. Not uncommonly, the lesion is actually in the aorta at the origin of the renal artery, the so-called ostial lesion.

A second type of arterial lesion, of obscure etiology, that affects the main renal artery is *fibromuscular dysplasia* (hyperplasia) [104]. The lesion appears as a multifocal "string-of-beads" beginning in the mid–renal artery and often extending into peripheral branches (Fig. 9-9). This variant is typically seen in young to middle-aged females. The risk of progression to total arterial occlusion is small.

Screening for Renovascular Hypertension

Although renovascular hypertension due to renal artery stenosis is the most common cause of potentially remediable secondary hypertension, available estimates suggest that less than 0.5 percent of the hypertensive population has renovascular hypertension [105]. Thus, an aggressive approach to screening for this disorder is often not

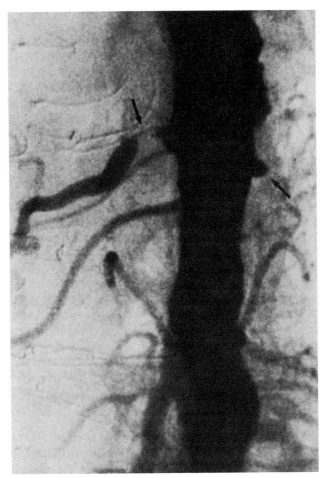

Fig. 9-8. Aortogram demonstrating generalized atherosclerosis with bilateral atherosclerotic renal artery stenosis. The left renal artery is totally occluded at its origin. The right renal artery has a high-grade lesion near its origin (ostial lesion). (Courtesy of Steven D. Brantley, M.D., Department of Radiology, Wilford Hall Medical Center, Lackland Air Force Base, Texas.)

warranted. Several lines of evidence now suggest that an aggressive work-up to exclude renovascular hypertension may not be cost-effective because the yield of curable hypertension is low, and the majority of patients can be successfully managed with medical therapy [106]. The dilemma for the clinician lies in the fact that even the ideal screening test, with high sensitivity and specificity, has a low predictive value when applied indiscriminately to the general hypertensive population, where the prevalence of renovascular hypertension is low [107]. In this regard, aggressive screening leads to the generation of many more false-positive results (essential hypertension) than true-positive results (occult renovascular hypertension). This statistical phenomenon undoubtedly accounts for the numerous highly touted screening tests that have come and gone over the years. The rapid sequence intravenous pyelogram (hypertensive IVP) is no longer routinely used as a screening tool, since it not only is insensitive but also has a false-positive rate of up to 12 percent among patients with essential hypertension [105]. Isotope renography (renal scan) has proved even less accurate than the hypertensive IVP because of an unacceptable frequency of false-positive results in patients with essential hypertension [105]. Casual measurements of plasma renin activity are of little value [105]. The highly touted "captopril test," which measures the increase in venous plasma renin activity in response to captopril, has proved to have low specificity [108].

Thus, it is apparent that sound clinical judgment is essential in the selection of patients in whom an aggressive evaluation for renovascular hypertension is indicated. Certain clinical clues suggest the possibility of underlying renovascular hypertension [105]. The onset of hypertension before age 30 years should suggest secondary hypertension. A truly abrupt onset of hypertension at any age suggests renal vascular disease. However, more often than not, this finding represents newly diagnosed essential hypertension rather than recently developed secondary hypertension. A definite worsening of previously well-controlled hypertension should suggest renovascular hypertension. Clues on physical examination include the finding on

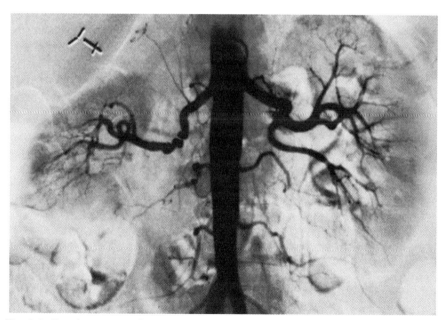

Fig. 9-9. Renal angiogram demonstrating right renal artery stenosis due to medial fibroplasia, the most common variant of the fibromuscular dysplasias. The small right kidney has a mid–renal artery lesion with a "string of beads" appearance due to mural aneurysms, caused by thinning of the internal elastica alternating with areas of narrowing due to fibrovascular ridges. (Courtesy of Steven D. Brantley, M.D., Department of Radiology, Wilford Hall Medical Center, Lackland Air Force Base, Texas.)

funduscopy of striate hemorrhages, cotton-wool spots or papilledema (malignant hypertension) [101], or a continuous systolic and diastolic epigastric bruit [109].

Even in the presence of diffuse atherosclerotic disease, aggressive evaluation for renovascular hypertension is only indicated if the blood pressure is truly resistant (>150/100 mm Hg) to a rational triple-drug regimen that includes a diuretic [105]. Unexplained deterioration of renal function despite adequate blood pressure control suggests the possibility of ischemic nephropathy and should prompt a search for bilateral renal artery stenosis with ischemic nephropathy [109, 110]. Deterioration of renal function upon the addition of an ACE inhibitor suggests the possibility of bilateral renal artery stenosis or stenosis of a solitary kidney. This phenomenon probably reflects maintenance of GFR in the ischemic kidneys by angiotensin II–mediated vasoconstriction of the efferent arteriole to increase filtration fraction [109].

In the patient in whom the probability of renovascular hypertension is high, the conventional screening tests are of little value, since the predictive value of a negative test is low [107]. In this setting, many clinicians proceed immediately to renal angiography, which allows for a definitive diagnosis of renal artery stenosis [105]. Unfortunately, selective renal angiography carries definite risks, including contrast media–associated nephrotoxicity and renal atheroembolic disease [111]. Furthermore, anatomic renal artery stenosis does not always imply functional renovascular hypertension. Incidental renal artery stenosis can clearly occur in essential hypertension. Selective renal vein renin determinations have been used to predict the functional significance of anatomic lesions. A renal vein renin ratio greater than 2 : 1 (involved-uninvolved) is highly predictive of a beneficial response to intervention. However, a significant number of patients with nonlateralizing ratios ultimately prove to benefit from intervention [112]. Preliminary data suggest that a change in the ^{99m}Tc-labeled DTPA or MAG$_3$ renogram after treatment with captopril may help to define the functional significance of a renal artery lesion prior to intervention with surgery or angioplasty [113].

Medical Therapy Versus Angioplasty Versus Surgical Revascularization

The major objectives in the management of renovascular hypertension are adequate control of the blood pressure and preservation of renal function. To date, no prospective, randomized study has been published that addresses the risk-benefit ratio of medical therapy compared to angioplasty or surgical revascularization [114]. In the patient with diffuse atherosclerotic disease, even in the presence of suspected or known renal artery stenosis, medical management may be prudent and entirely appropriate as long as the blood pressure is controlled and the renal function remains stable.

Percutaneous transluminal renal angioplasty provides a nonsurgical method of treating renal artery stenosis. With fibromuscular dysplasia, the technical success rate is 90 percent, and cure of hypertension is obtained in 60 percent [115]. Although hypertension secondary to medial fibroplasia can often be managed medically, angioplasty is usually attempted given the chance of cure, which would obviate the need for lifelong antihypertensive therapy in these young patients.

Patients with atherosclerotic renal artery stenosis and either poor blood pressure control on triple-drug therapy or deteriorating renal function should be considered for surgical revascularization or angioplasty. With angioplasty, the technical success rate with unilateral, nonostial lesions is only 57 percent [116]. Restenosis occurs in 30 percent. Angioplasty in patients with bilateral atherosclerotic disease with occluded renal arteries or ostial lesions has an even lower technical success rate, and complications such as dissection or occlusion are more frequent. Surgical revascularization is now the preferred method of treatment in these patients [114]. Surgical options include aortorenal bypass with saphenous vein grafts, endarterectomy, splenorenal bypass, and hepatorenal saphenous vein bypass [117]. Extracorporeal (bench) microvascular surgery with autotransplantation can now be performed to salvage renal function in selected cases [117].

Ischemic Nephropathy

Although it is appropriate to elect medical therapy in the patient with atherosclerotic renal artery stenosis, the patient should be followed closely for evidence of progressive loss of renal function despite adequate blood pressure control. The threat of ischemic nephropathy secondary to atherosclerotic disease is now recognized as an important clinical concern that is separate and distinct from the issue of renovascular hypertension [109, 110, 114]. Even in the absence of severe or resistant hypertension, angiography should be considered to screen for treatable ischemic nephropathy in patients with generalized atherosclerosis accompanied by a unilaterally small kidney. Ischemic nephropathy should also be considered in the hypertensive patient with mild to moderate renal insufficiency (creatinine >1.5 mg/dl), especially if there is no evidence of primary renal parenchymal disease (normal urine sediment, normal protein excretion), or ultrasound evidence of urinary tract obstruction [118]. Progressive loss of renal function culminating in ESRD can occur with bilateral renal artery stenosis, and studies now suggest that this entity is preventable and treatable [109, 114, 118]. Patients with high-grade atherosclerotic stenosis (>75 percent) affecting the entire renal mass, by virtue of bilateral renal artery stenosis or stenosis of a solitary kidney, should be considered candidates for surgical revascularization [114]. Interestingly, even complete occlusion does not preclude successful return of significant renal function if the lesion developed gradually, allowing for the development of collateral flow [114]. However, revascularization to preserve renal function is generally not worthwhile if the creatinine is over 4.0 mg/dl [114].

Hypertension in Primary Renal Disease

Virtually all forms of primary renal parenchymal disease can lead to secondary hypertension, especially if renal insufficiency is present [83, 89]. Glomerulonephritis and vasculitis are more likely to cause hypertension than chronic interstitial nephritis. Hypertension is present in over 75 percent of cases of acute post-streptococcal glomerulonephritis. In a series of patients with biopsy-proven glomerulonephritis, the overall prevalence of hypertension was 60 percent. Hypertension was found more commonly with IgA nephropathy, membranoproliferative glomerulonephritis and focal segmental glomerulosclerosis, whereas it was less frequent with membranous nephropathy or minimal change disease. In the setting of lupus nephritis, the frequency of hypertension approaches 50 percent. In idiopathic rapidly progressive (crescentic) glomerulonephritis, hypertension is uncommon unless overt fluid overload is present. Hypertension is extremely common in diabetic glomerulosclerosis. Autosomal-dominant polycystic kidney disease (ADPKD) is associated with a greater than 50 percent incidence of hypertension even before the onset of renal insufficiency [59]. Recent studies have found that the incidence of hypertension in ADPKD may be related to the degree of renal cyst enlargement [119].

A variety of disorders of the renal vasculature other than stenosis of the main renal arteries may also produce hypertension. Systemic vasculitis due to classic polyarteritis nodosa is frequently accompanied by hypertension, which may enter a malignant phase. In patients with progressive systemic sclerosis, hypertension plays a central role in the precipitous loss of renal function that occurs with scleroderma renal crisis [120]. Thrombotic microangiopathy due to hemolytic-uremic syndrome or thrombotic thrombocytopenic purpura can also cause severe hypertension. Renal cholesterol embolization syndrome following an angiographic procedure in patients with severe aortic atherosclerosis can cause sudden onset of severe hypertension, which may enter a malignant phase [121].

The prevalence of hypertension increases with progressive chronic renal insufficiency, regardless of cause, such that at end stage, virtually all patients are hypertensive. Among patients with ESRD and hypertension, roughly 70 percent have volume overload, and hemodialysis alone normalizes blood pressure. Approximately 30 percent of patients have dialysis-resistant hypertension, which may be due to hyperactivity of the renin-angiotensin system or sympathetic nervous system and thus require long-term antihypertensive therapy [122]. Hypertension is also extremely common in the renal transplant recipient and may result from a variety of factors including acute or chronic rejection, stenosis of the transplant renal artery, cyclosporine, high-dose glucocorticoids, or increased renin production by diseased native kidneys [123, 124].

Mechanism of Hypertension in Primary Renal Disease

In acute nephritic syndrome due to post-streptococcal glomerulonephritis, the hypertension is clearly due to sodium and water retention with increased ECF volume, plasma volume, and cardiac output with either normal or increased systemic vascular resistance [83, 89]. In contrast, the cause of hypertension in the setting of chronic renal insufficiency due to primary renal disease is more controversial. It has been postulated that the hypertension is caused by volume expansion with inappropriately increased renin release. However, in both humans and animal models with hypertension due to primary renal disease, the ECF volume, plasma volume, and cardiac output are usually normal, and hypertension is maintained by an increased total peripheral resistance. Nonetheless, sodium intake clearly plays an important role in the genesis of hypertension, since blood pressure is much more sodium sensitive in patients with chronic renal insufficiency than in normal subjects [125].

The genesis of hypertension in the setting of primary renal disease can be readily conceptualized on the framework of either the Na,K-ATPase inhibitor or Guyton's hypotheses. Declining nephron mass is associated with a diminished capacity to excrete a sodium load. A compensatory increase in Na,K-ATPase inhibitor may cause an increase in systemic vascular resistance and thus hypertension [13, 53, 54] (see Fig. 9-1). On the other hand, Guyton suggests that in the face of this type of primary natriuretic defect, the renal fluid–volume feedback mechanism restores external sodium balance but does so at the expense of systemic hypertension, which is maintained by an increase in peripheral vascular resistance secondary to the autoregulatory response [15, 16, 67] (see Fig. 9-4).

Hypertension due to intrinsic renal disease may also be related to the activation of renal pressor mechanisms such as the renin-angiotensin system in ADPKD [59, 119] or diminished production of vasodilator substances (bradykinins, prostaglandins, nitric oxide) [89]. The recent demonstration that ninefold increases in circulating inhibitors of nitric oxide synthesis may occur in uremic patients implies that deficiencies of vasodilatory substances may indeed be an important contributor to the elevated systemic vascular resistance in hypertensive patients with renal failure [126].

Role of Hypertension in the Progression of Primary Renal Disease

In the setting of primary renal parenchymal disease, hypertension clearly has its origin in the kidney. There is now substantial clinical and experimental evidence to support the concept that this secondary hypertension in turn aggravates the underlying disorder and is a major factor in the progression of chronic renal insufficiency [127]. Coexistence of hypertension and primary renal disease creates a vicious circle, hastening the progression of renal failure.

Systemic hypertension had traditionally been assumed to accelerate primary renal disease by inducing structural damage in the renal microvasculature (hyaline arteriosclerosis) with resultant glomerular hypoperfusion and ischemia (Fig. 9-10). However, it is now widely accepted that the converse may be true, namely that systemic hypertension induces progressive injury in the already diseased kidneys via hydraulic stress on the glomeruli caused by increased transmission of the elevated systemic pressure to the glomerular capillaries (hyperperfusion theory) [92, 128] (see Fig. 9-10). The differences in the pathophysiologic mechanism of renal injury between essential hypertension (hypoperfusion/ischemia) and secondary hypertension due to primary renal disease (hyperperfusion/glomerular hypertension) may be explained by differences in afferent arteriolar resistance in these disorders. Afferent arteriolar resistance determines the fraction of the systemic pressure that is transmitted to

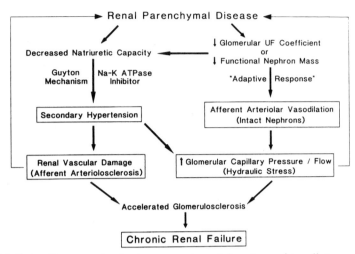

Fig. 9-10. Role of hypertension in the progression of chronic renal insufficiency. Secondary hypertension may contribute to the inexorable progression of renal insufficiency by either of two mechanisms. Hypertensive damage to the renal microvasculature may lead to hyaline arteriolosclerosis of the afferent arteriole with further renal injury via an ischemic mechanism. Alternatively, with nephron loss due to renal disease, compensatory responses in the remaining nephrons could cause afferent arteriolar vasodilation. Though this hemodynamic response helps to maintain whole-kidney GFR, in the long term it may be maladaptive. The decrease in afferent arteriolar resistance allows for transmission of the elevated systemic pressure to the glomerulus. The resulting hemodynamic stress caused by the elevated glomerular capillary flow and pressure may lead to accelerated glomerulosclerosis and progression of chronic renal insufficiency. UF = ultrafiltration.

the glomerular capillaries. In benign essential hypertension, the structural changes in the afferent arterioles increase resistance and presumably serve to prevent transmission of the elevated systemic pressure to the glomeruli. In contrast, the glomerular hemodynamic changes in the setting of primary renal disease may be entirely different.

The most extensively studied model of hypertension in the setting of a reduced number of normally functioning nephrons is the *remnant kidney* model produced by surgical ablation of renal mass in the rat. Reduction of renal mass below a critical level is associated with the development of proteinuria, systemic hypertension, and progressive renal failure due to glomerulosclerosis in the remnant kidney [128]. The reduction of functioning nephrons leads to a compensatory increase in single-nephron GFR in the remaining nephrons. Vasodilation of both the afferent and efferent arterioles leads to a decrease in renal vascular resistance, with a resulting increase in glomerular capillary plasma flow. Because the decrease in efferent resistance is less pronounced than the decrease in afferent resistance, the glomerular capillary pressure increases. Together the increases in glomerular capillary pressure and perfusion account for the observed compensatory single-nephron hyperfiltration. Similar glomerular hemodynamic changes are also observed in the DOCA/salt hypertension model and in the salt-sensitive model of nephrotoxic serum nephritis [129]. Brenner and colleagues [92, 128] have suggested that these compensatory increases in glomerular capillary flow and pressure, though sufficient to maintain whole-kidney GFR in the short term, are in the long term maladaptive and that the resulting hydraulic stress is somehow responsible for the eventual development of glomerulosclerosis in the remaining nephrons.

In animal models, when secondary hypertension due to DOCA/salt administration or renal artery clipping is superimposed on immune complex or nephrotoxic serum nephritis, deterioration of renal function accelerates dramatically [129]. Micropuncture studies have confirmed that in the diseased kidneys autoregulation is lost and afferent arterioles are dilated so that the elevated systemic pressure is transmitted to the glomerulus, resulting in glomerular capillary hypertension, which is thought to induce progressive renal injury (see Fig. 9-10).

In the aforementioned models, treatment of hypertension is associated with a slowing of the progression of renal injury [130]. However, in the renal ablation model, although both ACE inhibitor (enalapril) and triple therapy (reserpine, hydralazine, hydrochlorothiazide) reduce blood pressure equally, only ACE inhibitor treatment ameliorates proteinuria and glomerular scarring [131]. ACE inhibitors also seem to be superior agents for slowing the progression of renal injury in models of diabetic nephropathy [91]. The superiority of ACE inhibitor therapy in these models has been attributed to the fact that it leads to a reduction in intrarenal angiotensin II–mediated efferent arteriolar tone, thereby directly reducing glomerular capillary pressure in addition to lowering systemic blood pressure [91, 131].

A large body of experimental evidence suggests that glomerular capillary hypertension is an important mechanism underlying the adverse impact of systemic hypertension on renal survival. However, glomerular capillary hypertension cannot provide a single unifying hypothesis to explain the progression of all forms of chronic renal disease. The evidence that glomerular hypertension is causally related to glomerular injury does not exclude the possibility that additional factors may also induce progressive glomerular injury [132]. Many nonhemodynamic mechanisms, which are beyond the scope of this discussion, have also been shown to cause progressive glomerulosclerosis, including coagulation abnormalities and metabolic abnormalities such as nephron hypermetabolism, hyperphosphatemia, or hyperlipidemia.

Furthermore, systemic hypertension and glomerular hypertension do not always coexist. A maladaptive increase in glomerular capillary flow and pressure may be a phenomenon that occurs principally in the setting of reduced functioning renal mass due either to ablation or intrinsic renal disease. In the spontaneously hypertensive rat (SHR), systemic hypertension occurs without the development of glomerular capillary hypertension [133]. The glomeruli are protected from the high systemic pressure by afferent arteriolar vasoconstriction, which may explain the absence of progressive renal dysfunction in this model. The critical role that afferent arteriolar tone plays in the protection against hypertensive glomerular injury is illustrated by the fact that reduction of nephron mass by unilateral nephrectomy in the SHR results in a reduction of afferent arteriolar resistance in the remaining kidney. This allows for transmission of the systemic pressure to the glomeruli, and in this model, progressive glomerular injury with glomerulosclerosis does occur [134].

In this regard, most of the available data indicate that ESRD is a rare phenomenon in human benign essential hypertension in the absence of malignant hypertension. In human essential hypertension, there is also a relative intrarenal vasoconstriction. It is tempting to speculate that, at least in patients with salt-resistant essential hypertension, there may be an increase in afferent arteriolar resistance that protects the glomeruli from the deleterious effects of systemic hypertension and thus accounts for the infrequent occurrence of progressive renal insufficiency.

Role of Hypertension in Diabetic Nephropathy

In the diabetic patient, hypertension is a major risk factor for large-vessel atherosclerotic disease affecting the coronary, cerebral, and peripheral vascular beds. The incidence of large-vessel disease is dramatically increased in both type I and type II diabetics and is a major cause of morbidity and premature death. Diabetics have a twofold increased risk of coronary artery disease, a two- to sixfold increased risk of atheroembolic stroke, and a significantly increased risk of peripheral vascular disease [135]. Hypertension also hastens the progression of diabetic microangiopathic complications such as nephropathy and retinopathy [135]. In non–insulin-dependent (type II) diabetes mellitus (NIDDM), hypertension is twice as common as in the nondiabetic population. This increased prevalence of hypertension may relate to underlying insulin resistance. Moreover, control of hypertension, especially in conjunction with the use of ACE inhibitors, has been shown in clinical trials to slow the progression of diabetic nephropathy.

Natural History of Diabetic Nephropathy

Diabetic nephropathy is the most common cause of end-stage renal failure in the United States. The natural history of diabetic nephropathy in insulin-dependent (type I) diabetes mellitus (IDDM) has been well characterized (Fig. 9-11). The cumulative risk of developing nephropathy in IDDM is approximately 30 to 40 percent. The earliest clinical evidence of nephropathy is the development of microalbuminuria (incipient diabetic nephropathy). A radioimmunoassay technique is required to detect this low-level albumin excretion, since standard 24-hour urine protein assays are not sufficiently sensitive. Microalbuminuria is defined by the presence of urinary albumin between 30 and 300 mg in a 24-hour collection. Since there is marked day-to-day variability and severe hyperglycemia, exercise, and urinary tract infections can cause transient elevations in urinary albumin excretion, at least two out of three 24-hour collections should show elevated levels above 30 mg before the patient is diagnosed with microalbuminuria. Roughly 80 percent of patients with IDDM who develop sustained microalbuminuria will progress over the ensuing 5 to 15 years to develop overt nephropathy, which is defined by the presence of clinical albuminuria (>300 mg/24 hr), which can be detected with standard 24-hour urine protein assays (>500 mg/24 hr). In these patients, the magnitude of proteinuria continues to increase, eventually reaching the nephrotic range,

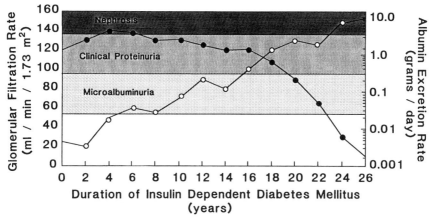

Fig. 9-11. Natural history of nephropathy in insulin-dependent (type I) diabetes mellitus. In the 35 percent of patients who develop diabetic nephropathy, the onset of microalbuminuria (albumin excretion rate 30–300 mg/day) occurs after diabetes has been present for 5 to 15 years. Over the next 10 years, the vast majority of these patients develop clinical proteinuria (albumin excretion rate 300–3000 mg/day). Eventually, the magnitude of the proteinuria exceeds 3 g/day, and nephrotic syndrome ensues. Once clinical proteinuria develops, the glomerular filtration rate begins to fall such that greater than 90 percent of these patients reach end-stage renal disease within the ensuing 20 years. ○—○ = Albumin excretion rate; ●—● = glomerular filtration rate.

and frank nephrotic syndrome often develops. Among type I diabetics, although the GFR may initially be elevated due to hyperfiltration in the early stages of diabetes, once clinical proteinuria develops, the GFR begins to fall such that ESRD develops in 50 percent within 10 years, 75 percent within 15 years, and 90 percent within 20 years [136] (see Fig. 9-11).

Much less is known about the natural history of diabetic nephropathy in type II diabetic patients. Unlike IDDM, NIDDM is often accompanied very early in the course of disease, even at onset, by microalbuminuria or sometimes overt clinical proteinuria [137]. In contrast to IDDM, the presence of microalbuminuria has been reported to be a predictor of clinical proteinuria in only 22 percent of patients with NIDDM. However, in NIDDM patients, proteinuria even at the microalbuminuric stage is a strong predictor of mortality [138]. The 10-year survival rate was 22 percent versus 57 percent for NIDDM patients with and without microalbuminuria. Most of the deaths were related to cardiovascular disease rather than renal disease.

ESRD due to type II diabetes is much more common in the United States than in Europe. The greater prevalence in the United States may reflect the greater frequency of NIDDM and higher risk of significant diabetic renal disease in certain racial groups such as blacks, Mexican-Americans, and Native Americans [137]. The high prevalence of ESRD due to diabetic nephropathy in these groups could possibly relate to earlier age of onset of diabetes, genetic predisposition to hypertension, or differences in diet and level of glycemic control.

Epidemiology of Hypertension in Diabetes

The evolution of hypertension in IDDM (type I diabetes) has been well characterized [139]. In the early years of type I diabetes, hypertension is no more common than in healthy controls. Incipient nephropathy (microalbuminuria) is accompanied by a small but consistent increase in blood pressure compared to controls. With the development of overt diabetic nephropathy (clinically apparent proteinuria), hypertension is the rule, and the severity of the hypertension correlates inversely with the level of renal function. Once the serum creatinine begins to increase, the prevalence of hypertension is over 90 percent.

In the older patient with NIDDM (type II diabetes), the natural history of hypertension is less predictable. Essential hypertension is likely to coexist in a substantial proportion of patients even before the development of nephropathy. Atherosclerotic renal artery stenosis may also cause hypertension in some patients.

Pathogenesis of Hypertension in Patients with Insulin Resistance

Various hypotheses have been proposed to explain the high prevalence of hypertension in type II diabetics compared to nondiabetics. It could be related to obesity and increased sympathetic nervous system stimulation observed in diabetics [135]. Overt diabetic nephropathy with renal insufficiency may also cause hypertension, although this does not explain the vast excess of hypertension seen in the general diabetic population without nephropathy.

It has been observed that glucose intolerance, hyperlipidemia, and essential hypertension tend to cluster in the same patient. In 1988, Reaven [140] proposed that *insulin resistance* is the primary feature that underlies these cardiovascular risk factors, the so-called Syndrome X hypothesis. Insulin resistance, which may be inherited or acquired (due to obesity, dietary factors, or sedentary lifestyle), results in compensatory *hyperinsulinemia*. Eventually the beta-cell output of insulin may become inadequate to compensate for insulin resistance, resulting in glucose intolerance or frank type II diabetes. The hyperinsulinemia induces abnormalities of lipid metabolism with increased low-density lipoprotein and reduced high-density lipoprotein levels. Hyperinsulinemia may also be causally related to the development of hypertension. For instance, increased insulin levels may stimulate the sympathetic nervous system, resulting in an increase in systemic vascular resistance [135]. Moreover, insulin has been shown to play an important role in sodium metabolism. In human studies in which euglycemic hyperinsulinemia was generated using an insulin clamp technique, urinary sodium excretion declined significantly within 60 minutes [141]. This antinatriuretic effect of insulin was observed in the absence of changes in GFR, renal plasma flow, the filtered load of glucose, or plasma aldosterone concentration. The predominant effect of insulin on tubular sodium reabsorption is in more distal parts of the nephron (thick ascending limb of Henle or distal convoluted tubule). Thus, the net effect of insulin resistance and resulting hyperinsulinemia is to induce an impairment of intrinsic renal natriuretic capacity, which would be predicted to lead to the development of compensatory hypertension to maintain sodium balance based on a Guyton's hypothesis or Na,K-ATPase inhibitor type of mechanism.

Role of Systemic and Glomerular Hypertension in the Progression of Diabetic Nephropathy

There are a number of experimental and clinical observations that suggest an important role for hypertension in the pathogenesis of diabetic nephropathy. Hypertension is thought to accelerate diabetic renal injury by exacerbating the underlying abnormalities in renal hemodynamics and further elevating glomerular capillary flow and pressure. Poor glycemic control may magnify these hemodynamic disturbances, in particular afferent arteriole vasodilation, thereby allowing enhanced transmission of the elevated systemic blood pressure to the glomerulus.

Diabetic patients destined to develop nephropathy have a higher prevalence of hypertension and a higher mean blood pressure than diabetics not destined to develop nephropathy. Moreover, there is a threefold increase in risk of nephropathy among type I diabetics with a parental history of hypertension, suggesting that an inherited predisposition to essential hypertension may increase the risk of nephropathy [142].

In a multivariate analysis of patients with overt diabetic nephropathy, more rapid loss of GFR correlated most strongly with higher diastolic blood pressure [143]. In contrast, blood sugar control, assessed by hemoglobin A_{1C}, did not correlate with change in GFR, at least in these patients with overt nephropathy.

In a study of the effect of two-kidney/one-clip Goldblatt hypertension in the streptozotocin-induced diabetic model in the rat, severe diabetic nephropathy was observed in the unclipped kidney exposed to the high systemic pressure, whereas in the clipped kidney, protected from the high systemic pressure, nephropathy did not develop [144]. This experimental demonstration of the central role of hypertension in the pathogenesis of diabetic nephropathy is further supported by reports of autopsy findings in patients with diabetes and unilateral renal artery stenosis. Glomerular basement membrane thickening and nodular Kimmelstiel-Wilson lesions were found only in the kidney with the patent renal artery [145].

In rat models, diabetic nephropathy is produced by injection of streptozocin with maintenance of moderate hyperglycemia with low-dose insulin. Initially, there is a substantial increase in whole-kidney GFR akin to the hyperfiltration observed in young juvenile diabetics. There is also an increase in single-nephron GFR due to intrarenal vasodilation of both afferent and efferent arterioles that results in an increase in glomerular capillary pressure and flow. However, after several weeks, progressive proteinuria, hypertension, and glomerulosclerosis develop [91]. As in the remnant kidney model, it has been proposed that this increase in glomerular hydraulic pressure is maladaptive and eventually leads to progressive renal injury and nephron loss. In this model, normalization of glomerular capillary pressure with chronic ACE inhibitor therapy prevents the development of proteinuria and glomerulosclerosis, supporting the important pathophysiologic role of glomerular capillary hypertension. In these models of diabetic nephropathy, ACE inhibitors appear to be superior to conventional triple-antihypertensive therapy with thiazide diuretic, reserpine, and hydralazine. It has been proposed that this is due to a selective decrease in efferent arteriolar tone with ACE inhibitors, which leads to a direct reduction of glomerular capillary pressure independent of a reduction in systemic pressure [91].

Treatment of Hypertension in the Diabetic Patient

Clinically, it has been shown that effective antihypertensive therapy with a diuretic and a β-blocker can reduce proteinuria and slow the progression of renal disease in patients with established diabetic nephropathy [146]. At least in retrospective studies, the correlation between diastolic blood pressure and rate of progression of diabetic nephropathy is valid even at pressures less than 90 mm Hg [143]. Although not yet confirmed in prospective studies, this observation suggests that the usual therapeutic target for diastolic blood pressure may be too high and that patients may benefit from reductions of blood pressure into the low-normal range.

There is now convincing evidence from clinical trials that ACE inhibitors are beneficial in the treatment of diabetic nephropathy through a mechanism that is independent of their effect on systemic blood pressure. The Collaborative Study Group investigated the effect of ACE inhibitors in type I diabetics, aged 18 to 49 years old, with overt diabetic nephropathy (proteinuria $\geq$ 500 mg/day) [147]. All subjects had serum creatinine levels of 2.5 mg/dl or less. For the 75 percent of patients who were hypertensive on entering the study, treatment was instituted as required with antihypertensive medications other than ACE inhibitors or calcium channel blockers. Subjects (200 in each group) were then randomized to receive either captopril (25 mg) or placebo tablets given three times a day for a median of 3 years. The blood pressure goal during the study was 140/90 mm Hg or below. Over the course of the study, mean arterial pressures were generally slightly (<4 mm Hg) lower in the ACE inhibitor treated group. The primary end point of the study was a doubling of the baseline serum creatinine, which was reached in 25 subjects in the captopril group and 43 in the placebo group (p = 0.007). Captopril treatment reduced the relative risk of doubling serum creatinine by 48 percent. Captopril treatment was also associated with a 50 percent reduction in the relative risk of ESRD or death. Overall, in the captopril group, the mean rate of increase in serum creatinine was 0.2 $\pm$ 0.8 mg/dl/yr versus 0.5 $\pm$ 0.8 mg/dl/yr in the placebo group. Since the inclusion of mean arterial pressure as a time-dependent covariate in the statistical analysis did not alter the risk reduction estimates, it was concluded that there was a specific beneficial effect of ACE inhibitors independent of systemic blood pressure reduction.

Recent studies also suggest that ACE inhibitors are useful in normotensive type I diabetic patients with incipient diabetic nephropathy (microalbuminuria), in that they slow the increase in microalbuminuria and reduce the probability of progression to clinical proteinuria [148, 149]. These studies suggest that ACE inhibitors postpone the development of clinically overt nephropathy in normotensive type I diabetic patients with microalbuminuria. Likewise, ACE inhibitors have been reported to have a stabilizing effect on plasma creatinine and proteinuria in normotensive type II diabetics with microalbuminuria [150].

Given the diverse effects of the renin-angiotensin system in the kidney, ACE inhibitors may have protective effects in diabetic nephropathy in addition to glomerular hemodynamic effects. Postulated protective mechanisms include improvement in glomerular permselectivity with decreased proteinuria, decreased mesangial matrix expansion, inhibition of glomerular hypertrophy, amelioration of insulin resistance, improvement in serum lipid profiles, changes in angiotensin II–mediated renal sodium handling, inhibition of renal procollagen formation, and inhibition of atherogenesis [91].

A few words of caution are in order regarding the use of ACE inhibitors for the treatment of diabetic nephropathy. Although, the beneficial effect of ACE inhibitors has been shown to be independent of the antihypertensive effect of the drug, in the ACE inhibitor trials that have been discussed, the patients were either normotensive or blood pressure was reduced to less than 140/90 mm Hg with concomitant antihypertensive therapy. Thus, ACE inhibitors have not been shown to be a benefit in diabetic nephropathy in the absence of adequate blood pressure control. This is a crucial point, since ACE inhibitor therapy alone may be inadequate to control blood pressure. For instance, in the Collaborative Study Group trial at various time points during follow-up, 74 to 87 percent of hypertensive patients in the captopril-treated group required concomitant therapy with diuretic versus 79 to 93 percent in the placebo-treated group [147]. Likewise, there were no significant differences between the two groups with regard to the use of other classes of antihypertensive agents. This finding can be interpreted to mean that captopril was essentially no more effective than placebo at controlling blood pressure. Thus, the majority of hypertensive diabetic patients with overt nephropathy will require other antihypertensive agents in addition to ACE inhibitors to achieve adequate blood pressure control.

Furthermore, diabetic patients with renal insufficiency are predisposed to the development of hyperkalemia (due to an underlying hyporenin-hypoaldosterone state), which may be exacerbated by the use of ACE inhibitors. Although few patients in the clinical trials have developed significant hyperkalemia, most of the participants in these trials had either normal renal function or mild to moderate renal insufficiency (creatinine $\leq$ 2.5 mg/dl). In clinical practice, diabetic patients with more advanced renal insufficiency are at substantially increased risk of serious hyperkalemia.

Treatment of Hypertension in Nondiabetic Renal Disease

The potential benefits of ACE inhibitor therapy in slowing the progression of nondiabetic renal parenchymal disease remain rather speculative at present. However, a trial in patients with nondiabetic chronic renal failure has shown that ACE inhibitor (enlapril) was more effective in slowing progression than conventional therapy with β-blocker [151]. Moreover, a recent meta-analysis suggests that the beneficial effects of antihypertensive agents on proteinuria and GFR are similar in diabetic and nondiabetic patients with renal disease and that ACE inhibitors and possibly nondihydropyridine calcium antagonists have additional beneficial effects on proteinuria that are independent of blood pressure reductions [152].

Current recommendations are that hypertension should be controlled in patients with chronic renal failure to a target level of 130/80 to 130/85 mm Hg. In patients with proteinuria greater than 1 g/24 hours, the mean blood pressure should be reduced to 92 mm Hg (equivalent to 125/75 mm Hg) if no contraindication such as cerebrovascular disease is present [153].

Treatment of Essential Hypertension

Efficacy and Safety of Diuretics in Treating Hypertension

Since impaired renal handling of sodium plays a central role in the pathogenesis of both essential and secondary forms of hypertension, the use of diuretics has become a cornerstone in the treatment of hypertension. Diuretics have been employed for the treatment of hypertension since the discovery of chlorothiazide in 1957. Over the last 40 years, the efficacy of thiazides and related diuretics in preventing complications of hypertension has been conclusively demonstrated in long-term controlled clinical trials [154–158]. Mild to moderate hypertension often responds to treatment with low-dose thiazide diuretics alone [159]. In the setting of severe hypertension, or with concomitant renal insufficiency, diuretics are often an essential element of a stepped-care, multidrug regimen [159]. Moreover, the failure to include a diuretic in the antihypertensive regimen is a common cause of "resistant" hypertension, which fails to respond to treatment with ACE inhibitors, calcium channel blockers, α-adrenergic blockers, β-blockers, or vasodilators used singly or in combination [160].

The mechanism of the antihypertensive action of diuretics is incompletely understood. The acute effect of diuretic administration is a decrease in ECF and plasma volume with a reduction in cardiac output. However, over a period of weeks to months of chronic thiazide diuretic administration, the negative sodium balance is attenuated such that plasma volume and cardiac output are normalized. Nevertheless, the antihypertensive effect persists, implying a concomitant decrease in peripheral vascular resistance. This secondary *decrease in peripheral vascular resistance* appears to be the long-term mechanism of the antihypertensive action of thiazides and related diuretics [161–164]. The precise mechanism of this reduction in peripheral vascular resistance is unknown. However, in the framework of either the Na,K-ATPase inhibitor or Guyton's hypotheses, a reduction in peripheral resistance and blood pressure as an indirect result of the natriuretic action of the diuretics is easy to conceptualize. As previously discussed, an underlying defect in natriuretic capacity must be present in hypertension, regardless of etiology. Diuretic treatment, by ameliorating this defect in natriuresis, could result in a decrease in the circulating level of the Na,K-ATPase inhibitor, which has been proposed as the cause of the increase in vascular reactivity and systemic vascular resistance in hypertension (see Fig. 9-1). In the context of Guyton's hypothesis, restoration of natriuretic capacity toward normal with diuretics would mean that the renal fluid–volume feedback mechanism would no longer necessitate the presence of systemic hypertension to maintain sodium balance (see Fig. 9-4). Alternatively, diuretics may directly lower vascular resistance independent of their natriuretic action. A direct vasodilatory action of diuretics has been observed in studies of isolated aortic strips. Diuretics also stimulate the kallikrein-kinin and prostaglandin systems, leading to vasodilatory responses [161].

Effects of Thiazide Diuretics on Coronary Heart Disease

During the past decade, there has been a shift away from diuretics as first-line antihypertensive agents toward the preferential use of newer agents such as converting enzyme inhibitors, calcium channel blockers, and selective α-adrenergic blockers because of concern over potentially deleterious metabolic effects of diuretics. Thiazide diuretics have been accused of aggravating cardiac arrhythmias and increasing the complications of coronary heart disease, including myocardial infarction and sudden death.

In all of the long-term randomized clinical trials on morbidity and mortality in essential hypertension, thiazides and related diuretics have been used as primary treatment. Newer agents such as ACE inhibitors and calcium channel blockers have not been tested in this regard. A recent meta-analysis of 14 randomized trials utilizing diuretics as first-line therapy demonstrated a 42 percent reduction in strokes and a 14 percent decrease in coronary heart disease events [158]. The Hypertension Detection and Follow-up Program study revealed a significant reduction at 8-year follow-up in all-cause mortality in its intensively (high-dose diuretic) treated stepped-care group relative to the referred-care control group [155]. For fatal ischemic heart disease, there was a 16 percent risk reduction. This difference was noted primarily in the fatal myocardial infarction classification, in which there was a 23 percent risk reduction. In the European Working Party on High Blood Pressure in the Elderly Trial, a double-blind placebo-controlled trial of low-dose hydrochlorothiazide plus triamterene in patients over the age of 60, total cardiovascular mortality was reduced 38 percent, and deaths from myocardial infarction were reduced by 60 percent [156]. In the Systolic Hypertension in the Elderly Program trial, a double-blind placebo-controlled trial of low-dose chlorthalidone in patients over age 60 with isolated systolic hypertension, the relative risks of stoke, left ventricular failure, nonfatal myocardial infarction or fatal coronary heart disease, and requirement for coronary artery bypass grafting were all significantly reduced in the active treatment group [157].

Despite overall reductions in cardiovascular mortality with the use of thiazide diuretics for the treatment of essential hypertension, controversy persists regarding the risk of ventricular arrhythmias and sudden death in hypertensive patients with diuretic-induced hypokalemia [154]. Short-term studies have failed to show any increase in cardiac arrhythmias on 24- to 48-hour electrocardiographic monitoring during thiazide treatment, even in patients with left ventricular hypertrophy [165]. In the Multiple Risk Factor Intervention Trial, a much publicized increase in risk of sudden death in the special intervention (high-dose diuretic) group was found in a subgroup analysis of those participants with baseline nonspecific electrocardiogram changes. Little known, however, is the 57 percent lower rate of coronary artery disease mortality in the special intervention group compared to the usual care group in the subgroup analysis of men with abnormal exercise electrocardiograms prior to randomization [166]. These findings suggest that men with underlying coronary artery disease may benefit substantially from risk factor reduction even if antihypertensive treatment includes relatively higher doses of thiazide diuretics.

On the other hand, in more recent hypertension trials that have used smaller daily doses of diuretic (hydrochlorothiazide, 12.5–25.0 mg, or chlorthalidone, 12.5 mg), sometimes with a potassium sparing diuretic, the number of sudden deaths was reduced by 30 to 66 percent [154]. These reductions were considerably greater than those in trials that used high-dose thiazide therapy. Moreover, in a recent case-control study, the risk for sudden death was greater in patients who received high doses of diuretics, considerably lower in those receiving small doses, and lowest in those treated with low-dose thiazides combined with potassium sparing diuretics [167].

Side Effects of Diuretic Therapy

Why diuretics reduce coronary heart disease mortality less than they reduce stroke mortality has been the subject of speculation. A number of hypotheses have been suggested. The duration of the clinical trials may have been too short to significantly impact the slowly progressive atherosclerosis of coronary heart disease. Furthermore, hypertension is only one of several risk factors for atherosclerotic disease, and blood pressure reduction alone may have been insufficient to retard progression. Alternatively, various drug-related side effects have been postulated as causal factors, including elevated serum cholesterol levels, glucose intolerance, and various electrolyte abnormalities.

Diuretics and Cholesterol. In short-term studies of 1 year or less, thiazide diuretics increase cholesterol levels by an average of less than 0.3 mmol/L [154]. However, long-term clinical trials demonstrate that this modest increase in cholesterol persists for only the first 6 to 12 months of diuretic therapy, and thereafter cholesterol decreases to pretreatment levels or lower [157, 168, 169]. The data from long-term antihypertensive trials indicate that clinically significant increases in cholesterol levels do not occur with diuretic-based treatment programs.

Diuretics and the Risk of New-Onset Diabetes. Despite evidence that treatment with thiazide diuretics may decrease insulin sensitivity [170], most of the long-term clinical trials show no increase in the risk of diabetes in diuretic-treated patients. In a 10-year controlled trial, no evidence was found that low-dose thiazides increased the incidence of diabetes [171]. A recent case-control study of the New Jersey Medicaid program was designed to quantify the risk for occurrence of hyperglycemia requiring initiation of oral hypoglycemics or insulin among patients taking various antihypertensive agents [172]. The frequency of initiation of hypoglycemic therapy was increased for users of virtually all antihypertensive agents relative to nonusers consistent with the fact that hypertensive individuals are at increased risk of diabetes independent of blood pressure treatment. However, the relative risk for initiation of hypoglycemic therapy was actually lowest for patients receiving thiazide diuretics at 1.40 and ranged from 1.56 to 1.77 for patients receiving other antihypertensive agents such as converting enzyme inhibitors, calcium channel blocker, and adrenergic blocking agents.

Risk of Thiazide-Induced Hypokalemia and Hypomagnesemia. It is widely held that thiazide-induced reduction of the serum potassium levels represents a significant depletion of total-body potassium, which might predispose patients to cardiac arrhythmias. However, since the intracellular potassium is much greater than the extracellular potassium concentration and the former is maintained by a Na,K-ATPase pump, reduction of extracellular potassium does not necessarily influence intracellular levels [154]. Several studies have shown that the reduction of intracellular potassium concentration after administration of thiazide diuretics is usually not biologically significant, since it constitutes only 5 percent of total-body potassium [173]. Moreover, with thiazide diuretic therapy, urinary losses of potassium occur only with the first 2 to 3 days of treatment, after which external potassium balance is restored such that total-body potassium is not continuously drained [174].

Likewise, intracellular magnesium stores are not significantly reduced during thiazide treatment for uncomplicated hypertension [175]. In contrast to loop diuretics, thiazides only modestly effect magnesium excretion because they do not act at the loop of Henle, which is the major nephron site of magnesium reabsorption.

Thiazide Diuretics and Regression of Left Ventricular Hypertrophy. Left ventricular hypertrophy is an independent risk factor for cardiovascular mortality that predisposes to myocardial infarction, sudden death, left ventricular failure, and stroke. Ideally, the goal for treatment of hypertension should be not only blood pressure control but also regression of left ventricular hypertrophy. It has been suggested that diuretic therapy for hypertension may be inadequate in this regard because chronic volume depletion would lead to reflex activation of the sympathetic nervous system and the renin-angiotensin axis, both of which could serve as persistent stimuli for left ventricular hypertrophy.

This argument is based on the misconception that thiazide diuretics lower blood pressure by inducing a chronic negative salt balance with persistent volume depletion. As outlined previously, the mechanism of blood pressure reduction with thiazides is a decrease in systemic vascular resistance without detectable long-term changes in ECF volume. Moreover, in the Treatment of Mild Hypertension Study, patients with diastolic blood pressure less than 100 mm Hg were randomized to one of six treatment groups: placebo, diuretic (chlorthalidone), β-blocker (acebutolol), selective α-blocker (doxazosin), calcium channel blocker (amlodipine), or converting enzyme inhibitor (enalapril) [176]. Echocardiographic left ventricular mass declined in all treatment groups. However, for chlorthalidone, but not the other drug classes, left ventricular mass declined more than for participants given placebo. Thus, the data fail to support the hypothesis that use of thiazide diuretics leads to persistence of left vesticular hypertrophy despite adequate blood pressure control.

Treatment Recommendations for Essential Hypertension

Concern over the adverse effects of low-dose thiazide diuretics has been greatly exaggerated [154, 177, 178]. There is a widespread impression, fostered to a large extent by the pharmaceutical industry, that the use of antihypertensive drugs without metabolic side effects will inevitably have a more favorable impact on coronary artery disease–related morbidity and mortality than thiazide diuretics and β-blockers [179]. Although this may prove correct, none of these agents, including the ACE inhibitors and calcium channel blockers, has been subjected to the rigorous clinical trials that will be required to prove this assumption [179]. It is currently advisable in clinical practice to follow the latest recommendations of the Joint National Committee on Detection, Evaluation, and Treatment of High Blood Pressure [159], which recommends beginning treatment in essential hypertension with low-dose thiazides or related diuretics. Analysis of the wholesale costs of various antihypertensives demonstrates that thiazide diuretics are clearly the least expensive, with the price for generic hydrochlorothiazide ranging from $1 to $5 for 100 tablets [180]. Thus, it appears that the vast majority of patients with essential hypertension can be treated at low cost without compromising quality of care. The fact that drug costs are often a major impediment to patient compliance provides additional sound rationale for first-line use of diuretics [181]. Given existing controversy, a potassium sparing diuretic may also be added for patients who require larger doses of diuretic or in patients with evidence of ischemic heart disease [154, 159]. Serum potassium levels should be determined prior to and at periodic intervals after initiation of treatment.

Although thiazide diuretics provide a safe, effective, and inexpensive form of treatment in the vast majority of hypertensive patients, treatment should be individualized. In some patient groups, drugs other than diuretics may be considered as first-line therapy [159]. For instance, given the evidence that ACE inhibitors have a beneficial effect in slowing the progression of diabetic nephropathy, they should be considered as initial antihypertensive therapy in the treatment of diabetic patients with hypertension. Nonetheless, ACE inhibitors alone may not adequately control blood pressure, and the addition of other classes of antihypertensives may be required. In diabetic patients with resistant hypertension or overt diabetic nephropathy with nephrotic syndrome, the use of thiazide or loop diuretics may be imperative. Converting enzyme inhibitors should also be considered as initial therapy for hypertensive patients with congestive heart failure due to systolic dysfunction. There may also be some benefit of converting enzyme inhibitors in nondiabetic renal disease for slowing the progression of renal disease [151, 152], although further study is required. Since the risk of progressive renal disease in benign essential hypertension is low, there is currently little rationale for the routine use of ACE inhibitors in patients with benign nephrosclerosis.

A number of clinical and demographic factors affect patient response to different agents. As a group, blacks tend to have lower cardiac output, lower plasma renin activity, higher peripheral resistance, and higher blood volume and are more likely to have salt-sensitive hypertension. Thus, blacks tend to respond better to diuretics or calcium channel blockers than to either β-blockers or converting enzyme inhibitors. Moreover, calcium channel blockers may improve renal salt handling and thereby ameliorate the rightward shift of the renal function curve in black patients with salt-sensitive hypertension [46, 75]. In elderly hypertensives, low-dose thiazide diuretics are particularly efficacious even though pretreatment plasma volumes seem to be decreased [157, 164]. Converting enzyme inhibitors are also effective in the elderly even though plasma renin activity is usually low. In the elderly, drugs that cause sedation (centrally acting α-agonists) or orthostatic hypotension (selective α-blockers) should be avoided. In patients with underlying atherosclerotic coronary vascular disease, β-blockers or calcium channel blockers represent logical alternatives for the treatment of hypertension. In hypertensive patients with prior myocardial infarction, β-blockers should be considered first-line therapy because they reduce the risk of reinfarction and sudden death [159]. In the setting of hypertension with coexistent renal insufficiency, diuretics represent very logical first-line therapy. Substitution of the more potent loop diuretics may be required in patients failing to respond to thiazide diuretics [162]. In patients with severe benign hypertension or malignant hypertension, a triple-drug regimen, employing a diuretic and a β-blocker in conjunction with the use of a potent peripheral vasodilator such as hydralazine or minoxidil is often required to achieve adequate blood pressure control [159].

Conclusions

It is apparent that the kidney is both villain and victim in hypertension [6]. The kidney has a central role in the pathogenesis of both essential hypertension and secondary hypertension due to primary renal parenchymal disease, renal artery stenosis, and mineralocorticoid excess. On the other hand, the critical role of hypertension in accelerating the progression of renal parenchymal disease is well established.

Nonetheless, even though it has been more than 150 years since Bright's original description of the relationship between hypertrophy of the heart (hypertension) and contraction of the kidney (renal dysfunction), many questions remain. At present, there is little hard evidence to support the widely held notion that benign essential hypertension is a common cause of ESRD. What then, accounts for the tremendous overrepresentation of blacks in the ESRD population? Is the impact of benign essential hypertension in blacks more pronounced, such that benign nephrosclerosis leads to more rapidly progressive nephron loss? Does low dietary potassium intake play a role in the increased risk of severe hypertensive nephrosclerosis in blacks? Or alternatively, does inadequate treatment of hypertension in the black population allow for the development of recurrent episodes of malignant hypertension, which culminate in ESRD? The ongoing African-American Study of Kidney Disease and Hypertension may help to resolve some of these important issues.

References

1. Bright R: Tabular view of the morbid appearances in 100 cases connected with albuminous urine: With observations. *Guy's Hosp Rep* I:380–402, 1836.
2. Traube L: *Ueber den Zusammenhang von Herz-und Nieren Krankheiten. Gesammelte Beitrage zur Pathologie und Physiologie.* Berlin, Hischwald, 1871, pp 290–350.
3. Mahomed FA: Some of the clinical aspects of chronic Bright's disease. *Guy's Hosp Rep* 24 (Series III):363–436, 1879.

4. Volhard F, Fahr T: *Die Brightische Neirenkrankhert, Klinik Pathologie und Atlas*. Berlin, Julius Springer, 1914.
5. Volhard F: Der arterielle Hochdruck. *Verh Dt Ges Inn Med* 35:134–175, 1923.
6. Klahr S: The kidney in hypertension: Villain and victim. *N Engl J Med* 320:731–733, 1989.
7. Birkenhäger WH, Schalekamp MADH: Body Fluids in Essential Hypertension. In *Control Mechanisms in Essential Hypertension*. New York, Elsevier, 1976, pp 63–77.
8. Folkow B: Cardiovascular structural adaptation: Its role in the initiation and maintenance of primary hypertension. *Clin Sci Mol Med* 55:3s–22s, 1978.
9. Folkow B: Sympathetic nervous control of blood pressure: Role in primary hypertension. *Am J Hypertens* 2:103S–111S, 1989.
10. Muirhead EE, Pitcock JA, Brooks B: The renomedullary system of blood pressure control. *J Hypertens* 4(Suppl 4):S27–S32, 1986.
11. Panza JA, Quyyumi AA, Brush JE Jr, et al: Abnormal endothelium-dependent vascular relaxation in patients with essential hypertension. *N Engl J Med* 323:22–27, 1990.
12. De Wardener HE, MacGregor GA: Dahl's hypothesis that a saluretic substance may be responsible for a sustained rise in arterial pressure: Its possible role in essential hypertension. *Kidney Int* 18:1–9, 1980.
13. De Wardener HE, MacGregor GA: The relation of a circulating sodium transport inhibitor (the natriuretic hormone?) to hypertension. *Medicine* 62:310–326, 1983.
14. Guyton AC: Renal function curve: A key to understanding the pathogenesis of hypertension. *Hypertension* 10:1–6, 1987.
15. Guyton AC, Cowley AW, Coleman TG, et al: Hypertension: A disease of abnormal circulatory control. *Chest* 65:328–338, 1974.
16. Guyton AC, Manning RD, Norman RA, et al: Current concepts and perspectives of renal volume regulation in relationship to hypertension. *J Hypertens* 4(Suppl 4):S49–S56, 1986.
17. Eaton SB, Konner M: Paleolithic nutrition: A consideration of its nature and current implications. *N Engl J Med* 312:283–289, 1985.
18. Tobian L: Potassium and sodium in hypertension. *J Hypertens* 6(Suppl 4):S12–S24, 1988.
19. Schrier RW: Body fluid volume regulation in health and disease: A unifying hypothesis. *Ann Intern Med* 113:155–159, 1990.
20. Brenner BM, Garcia DL, Anderson S: Glomeruli and blood pressure: Less of one, more of the other? *Am J Hypertens* 1:335–347, 1988.
21. Sasaki N: The relationship of salt intake to hypertension in the Japanese. *Geriatrics* 19:735–744, 1964.
22. Carvalho JJM, Baruzzi RG, Howard PF, et al: Blood pressure in four remote populations in the INTERSALT study. *Hypertension* 14:238–246, 1989.
23. Intersalt Cooperative Research Group: Intersalt: An international study of electrolyte excretion and blood pressure. Results for 24 hour urinary sodium and potassium excretion. *Br Med J* 297:319–330, 1988.
24. Murray RH, Luft FC, Bloch R, et al: Blood pressure responses to extremes of sodium intake in normal man. *Proc Soc Exp Biol Med* 159:432–436, 1978.
25. Watkin DM, Froeb HF, Hatch FT, et al: Effects of diet in essential hypertension: II. Results with unmodified Kempner rice diet in fifty hospitalized patients. *Am J Med* 9:441–493, 1950.
26. Joossens JV, Geboers J: Salt and hypertension. *Prev Med* 12:53–59, 1983.
27. Simpson FO: Salt and hypertension: A skeptical review of the evidence. *Clin Sci Mol Med* 57:463s, 1979.
28. Dustan HP, Kirk KA: Corcoran Lecture: The case for or against salt in hypertension. *Hypertension* 13:696, 1989.
29. Luft FC: Salt and hypertension: Recent advances and perspectives. *J Lab Clin Med* 114:215, 1989.
30. Dahl LK, Schackow E: Effects of chronic excess salt ingestion: Experimental hypertension in the rat. *Can Med Assoc J* 90:155–160, 1964.
31. Rettig R: Does the kidney play a role in the aetiology of primary hypertension? Evidence from renal transplantation studies in rats and humans (review). *J Human Hypertens* 7:177–180, 1993.

32. Curtis JJ, Luke RG, Dustan HP, et al: Remission of essential hypertension after renal transplantation. *N Engl J Med* 309:1009–1015, 1983.
33. Guidi E, Bianchi G, Rivolta E, et al: Hypertension in man with kidney transplant: Role of familial versus other factors. *Nephron* 41:14–21, 1985.
34. Tobian L, Lange J, Azar S, et al: Reduction of natriuretic capacity and renin release in isolated, blood perfused kidneys of Dahl hypertension-prone rats. *Circ Res* 43(Suppl I):I92–I98, 1978.
35. Ayman D: Heredity in arteriolar (essential) hypertension: A clinical study of the blood pressure of 1,524 members of 277 families. *Arch Intern Med* 53:792–802, 1934.
36. Grim CE, Luft FC, Miller JZ, et al: Effects of sodium loading and depletion in normotensive first-degree relatives of essential hypertensives. *J Lab Clin Med* 94:764–771, 1979.
37. Luft FC, Grim CE, Higgins JT, et al: Differences in response to sodium administration in normotensive white and black subjects. *J Lab Clin Med* 90:555–562, 1977.
38. Luft FC, Grim CE, Fineberg N, et al: Effects of volume expansion and contraction in normotensive whites, blacks, and subjects of different ages. *Circulation* 59:643–650, 1979.
39. Weder AB: Red-cell lithium-sodium countertransport and renal lithium clearance in hypertension. *N Engl J Med* 314:198–201, 1986.
40. DiBona GF: Neural control of renal tubular solute and water transport. *Miner Electrolyte Metab* 15:66–73, 1989.
41. Hall JE: Intrarenal actions of converting enzyme inhibitors. *Am J Hypertens* 2:875–884, 1989.
42. Cogan MG: Angiotensin II: A powerful controller of sodium transport in the early proximal tubule. *Hypertension* 15:451–458, 1990.
43. Hollenberg NK, Williams GH: Sodium-sensitive hypertension: Implications of pathogenesis for therapy. *Am J Hypertens* 2:809–815, 1989.
44. Frolich ED: Efferent glomerular arteriolar constriction: A possible intrarenal hemodynamic effect in hypertension. *Am J Med Sci* 295:409–413, 1988.
45. Bello-Reuss E, Trevino DL, Gottschalk CW: Effect of renal sympathetic nerve stimulation on proximal water and sodium reabsorption. *J Clin Invest* 57:1104–1107, 1976.
46. Campese VM, Parise M, Karubian F, et al: Abnormal renal hemodynamics in black salt-sensitive patients with hypertension. *Hypertension* 18:805–812, 1991.
47. Bachmann S, Mundel P: Nitric oxide in the kidney: Synthesis, localization, and function. *Am J Kidney Dis* 24:112–129, 1994.
48. Majid DSA, Williams A, Navar LG: Inhibition of nitric oxide synthesis attenuated pressure-induced natriuretic responses in anaesthetized dogs. *Am J Physiol* 264:F79–F87, 1993.
49. Ikenaga H, Suzuki H, Ishii N, et al: Role of NO on pressure natriuresis in Wistar-Kyoto and spontaneously hypertensive rats. *Kidney Int* 43:205–211, 1993.
50. Aperia AC, Broberger CGO, Söderlund S: Relationship between renal artery perfusion pressure and tubular sodium reabsorption. *Am J Physiol* 220:1205–1212, 1971.
51. De Wardener HE: The control of sodium excretion. *Am J Physiol* 235:F163–F173, 1978.
52. Stumpe KO, Lowitz HD, Ochwadt B: Fluid reabsorption in Henle's loop and urinary excretion of sodium and water in normal rats and rats with chronic hypertension. *J Clin Invest* 49:1200–1212, 1970.
53. Blaustein MP: Sodium transport and hypertension. *Hypertension* 6:445–453, 1984.
54. Haddy FJ, Overbeck HW: The role of humoral agents in volume expanded hypertension. *Life Sci* 19:935–948, 1976.
55. Hamlyn JM, Harris DW, Clark MA, et al: Isolation and characterization of sodium pump inhibitor from human plasma. *Hypertension* 13:681–689, 1989.
56. MacGregor GA, Fenton S, Alaghband-Zadeh J, et al: Evidence for a raised concentration of a circulating sodium transport inhibitor in essential hypertension. *Br Med J* 283:1355–1357, 1981.
57. Okada K, Caramelo C, Tsai P, et al: Effect of inhibition of Na^+/K^+-adenosine triphosphatase on vascular action of vasopressin. *J Clin Invest* 86:1241–1248, 1990.
58. Musca A, Cammarella I, Ferri C, et al: Plasma atrial natriuretic peptide in young essential hypertensive patients. *Curr Ther Res* 46:126–133, 1989.
59. Bell PE, Hossack KF, Gabow PA, et al: Hypertension in autosomal dominant polycystic kidney disease. *Kidney Int* 34:683–690, 1988.

60. Millett JA, Holland SM, Alaghband-Zadeh J, et al: Na-K-ATPase-inhibiting and glucose-6-phosphate dehydrogenase stimulating activity of plasma and hypothalamus of the Okamoto spontaneously hypertensive rat. *J Endocrinol* 108:69–73, 1986.
61. Hilton PJ: Cellular sodium transport in essential hypertension. *N Engl J Med* 314:222–229, 1986.
62. Poston L, Sewell RB, Wilkinson SP, et al: Evidence for a circulating sodium transport inhibitor in essential hypertension. *Br Med J* 282:847–849, 1981.
63. Poston L, Gray HH, Crowther A, et al: Cellular sodium concentration and vasoconstrictive state in hypertension. *J Cardiovasc Pharmacol* 6:S16–20, 1984.
64. Krishna GG: Effect of potassium intake on blood pressure. *J Am Soc Nephrol* 1:43–52, 1990.
65. Dunham ET, Glynn IM: Adenosinetriphosphatase activity and the active movements of alkali metal ions. *J Physiol* 156:274–293, 1961.
66. Ives HE: Ion transport defects and hypertension: Where is the link? *Hypertension* 14:590–597, 1989.
67. Guyton AC, Coleman TG, Cowley AW Jr, et al: Arterial pressure regulation: Overriding dominance of the kidneys in long-term regulation and in hypertension. *Am J Med* 52:584–594, 1972.
68. Norman RA, Enobakhare JA, DeClue JW, et al: Arterial pressure–urinary output relationship in hypertensive rats. *Am J Physiol* 234:R98–R103, 1978.
69. Selkurt EE: Effect of pulse pressure and mean arterial pressure modification on renal hemodynamics and electrolyte and water excretion. *Circulation* 4:541, 1951.
70. Guyton AC, Montani JP, Hall JE, et al: Computer models for designing hypertension experiments and studying concepts. *Am J Med Sci* 295:320–326, 1988.
71. Schrier RW: Pathogenesis of sodium and water retention in high-output and low-output cardiac failure, nephrotic syndrome, cirrhosis, and pregnancy (in two parts). *N Engl J Med* 319:1065–1072, 1127–1134, 1988.
72. Hall JE, Granger JP, Hester RL, et al: Mechanisms of sodium balance in hypertension: Role of pressure natriuresis. *J Hypertens* 4(Suppl 4):S57–S65, 1986.
73. Hall JE, Guyton AC, Smith MJ, et al: Blood pressure and renal function during chronic changes in sodium intake: Role of angiotensin. *Am J Physiol* 239:F271–F280, 1980.
74. Ichikawa I, Brenner BM: Importance of efferent arteriolar vascular tone in regulation of proximal tubular fluid reabsorption and glomerulotubular balance in the rat. *J Clin Invest* 65:1192–1201, 1980.
75. Campese VM: Effects of calcium antagonists on deranged modulation of the renal function curve in salt-sensitive patients with essential hypertension. *Am J Cardiol* 62:85G–91G, 1988.
76. Hall JE, Granger JP, Smith MJ, et al: Role of renal hemodynamics and arterial pressure in aldosterone "escape." *Hypertension* 6(Suppl I):I183–I192, 1984.
77. Hall JE, Granger JP, Hester RL, et al: Mechanisms of escape from sodium retention during angiotensin II hypertension. *Am J Physiol* 246:F627–F634, 1984.
78. Hall JE, Montani JP, Woods LL, et al: Renal escape from vasopressin: Role of pressure diuresis. *Am J Physiol* 250:F907–F916, 1986.
79. Heptinstall RH: *Pathology of the Kidney* (4th ed). Boston, Little, Brown, 1992.
80. Whelton PK, Klag MG: Hypertension as a risk factor for renal disease: Review of clinical and epidemiological evidence. *Hypertension* 13(Suppl I):I-19–I-27, 1989.
81. Freedman BI, Iskandar SS, Appel RG: The link between hypertension and nephrosclerosis. *Am J Kidney Dis* 25:207–221, 1995.
82. Schlessinger SD, Tankersley MR, Curtis JJ: Clinical documentation of end-stage renal disease due to hypertension. *Am J Kidney Dis* 23:655–660, 1994.
83. Brown MA, Whitworth JA. Hypertension in human renal disease. *J Hypertens* 10:701–712, 1992.
84. Bulpitt CJ: Prognosis of treated hypertension 1951–1981. *Br J Clin Pharmacol* 13:73, 1982.
85. Labeeuw M, Zech P, Pozet N, et al: Renal failure in essential hypertension. *Contrib Nephrol* 71:90, 1989.
86. Shulman NB, Ford CE, Hall WD, et al: Prognostic value of serum creatinine and effect of treatment of hypertension on renal function: Results from the Hypertension Detection and Follow-up Program. *Hypertension* 13(Suppl I):I-80, 1989.

87. Goldring W, Chasis H: *Hypertension and Hypertensive Disease*. New York, Commonwealth Fund, 1944, pp 53–95.
88. Kincaid-Smith P: *The Kidney: A Clinicopathological Study*. Oxford, Blackwell, 1975, p 212.
89. Kincaid-Smith P, Whitworth JA. Pathogenesis of hypertension in chronic renal failure. *Semin Nephrol* 8:155–162, 1988.
90. Azar S, Johnson MA, Scheinman J, et al: Regulation of glomerular capillary pressure and filtration in young Kyoto hypertensive rats. *Clin Sci* 56:203, 1979.
91. Anderson S: Antihypertensive therapy in experimental diabetes. *J Am Soc Nephrol* 3:S86–S90, 1992.
92. Brenner BM, Meyer TW, Hostetter TH: Dietary protein intake and the progression of kidney disease: The role of hemodynamically mediated glomerular injury in the pathogenesis of progressive glomerulosclerosis in aging, renal ablation, and intrinsic renal disease. *N Engl J Med* 307:652–659, 1982.
93. Rostrand SG, Kirk KA, Rutsky EA, et al: Racial differences in the incidence of treatment for end-stage renal disease. *N Engl J Med* 306:1276–1279, 1982.
94. Entwisle G, Apostolides AY, Hebel JR, et al: Target organ damage in black hypertensives. *Circulation* 55:792–796, 1977.
95. Levy SB, Talner LB, Coel MN, et al: Renal vasculature in essential hypertension: Racial differences. *Ann Intern Med* 88:12–16, 1978.
96. Perneger TV, Whelton PK, Klag MJ, et al: Diagnosis of hypertensive end-stage renal disease: Effect of patient's race. *Am J Epidemiol* 141(1):10–15, 1995.
97. Pitcock JA, Johnson JG, Hatch FE, et al: Malignant hypertension in blacks: Malignant intrarenal arterial disease as observed by light and electron microscopy. *Hum Pathol* 7:333–346, 1976.
98. Bennett NM, Shea S: Hypertensive emergency: Case criteria, sociodemographic profile, and previous care of 100 cases. *Am J Public Health* 78:636, 1988.
99. Frolich ED, Messerli FH, Dunn FG, et al: Greater renal vascular involvement in the black patient with essential hypertension: A comparison of systemic and renal hemodynamics in black and white patients. *Miner Electrolyte Metab* 10:173–177, 1984.
100. Dustan HP: Growth factors and racial differences in severity of hypertension and renal diseases. *Lancet* 339:1339–1340, 1992.
101. Nolan CR, Linas SL. Malignant Hypertension and Other Hypertensive Crises. In RW Schrier and CW Gottschalk (eds), *Diseases of the Kidney* (6th ed). Boston, Little, Brown, 1997, pp 1475–1554.
102. Barger AC: The Goldblatt memorial lecture. Part I: Experimental renovascular hypertension. *Hypertension* 1:447–455, 1979.
103. Ploth DW, Fitzgibbon W: Pathophysiology of altered renal function in renal vascular hypertension. *Am J Kidney Dis* 24:652–659, 1994.
104. Treadway KK, Slater EE: Renovascular hypertension. *Annu Rev Med* 35:665–692, 1984.
105. Working Group on Renovascular Hypertension: Detection, evaluation and treatment of renovascular hypertension: Final report. *Arch Intern Med* 147:820–829, 1987.
106. McNeil BJ, Varady PD, Burrows BA, et al: Measures of clinical efficacy: Cost effectiveness calculations in the diagnosis and treatment of hypertensive renovascular disease. *N Engl J Med* 293:216–221, 1975.
107. Griner PF, Mayewski RJ, Mushlin AI, et al: Selection and interpretation of diagnostic tests and procedures. *Ann Intern Med* 94(Part 2):553–593, 1981.
108. Davidson RA, Barri YM, Wilcox CS: The simplified captopril test: An effective tool to diagnose renovascular hypertension. *Am J Kidney Dis* 24:660–664, 1994.
109. Albers FJ: Clinical characteristics of atherosclerotic renovascular disease. *Am J Kidney Dis* 24:636–641, 1994.
110. Mailloux LU, Napolitano B, Bellucci AG, et al: Renal vascular disease causing end-stage renal disease, incidence, clinical correlates, and outcomes: A 20-year experience. *Am J Kidney Dis* 24:622–629, 1994.
111. Rudnick MR, Berns JS, Cohen RM, et al: Nephrotoxic risks of renal angiography: Contrast media-associated nephrotoxicity and atheroembolism—a critical review. *Am J Kidney Dis* 24: 713–727, 1994.

112. Marks LS, Maxwell MH: Renal vein renin: Value and limitations in the prediction of operative results. *Urol Clin North Am* 2:311–325, 1975.

113. Bourgoignie JJ, Rubbert K, Sfakianakis BN: Angiotensin-converting enzyme–inhibited renography for the diagnosis of ischemic kidneys. *Am J Kidney Dis* 24:665–673, 1994.

114. Novick AC: Current concepts in the management of renovascular hypertension and ischemic renal failure. *Am J Kidney Dis* 13(Suppl 1):33–37, 1989.

115. Tegtmeyer CJ, Elson J, Glass TA, et al: Percutaneous transluminal angioplasty: The treatment of choice for renovascular hypertension due to fibromuscular dysplasia. *Radiology* 143:631–637, 1982.

116. Sos TA, Pickering TG, Sniderman K, et al: Percutaneous transluminal renal angioplasty in renovascular hypertension due to atheroma or fibromuscular dysplasia. *N Engl J Med* 309:274–279, 1983.

117. Novick AC, Khauli RB, Vidt DG: Diminished operative risk and improved results following revascularization for atherosclerotic renovascular disease. *Urol Clin North Am* 11:435–449, 1984.

118. Jacobson HR: Ischemic renal disease: An overlooked clinical entity? *Kidney Int* 34:729–743, 1988.

119. Chapman AB, Johnson A, Gabow PA, et al: The renin-angiotensin-aldosterone system and autosomal dominant polycystic kidney disease. *N Engl J Med* 323:1091–1096, 1990.

120. Cannon PJ, Hassar M, Case DB, et al: The relationship of hypertension and renal failure in scleroderma (progressive systemic sclerosis) to structural and functional abnormalities of the renal cortical circulation. *Medicine* 53:1, 1974.

121. Smith MC, Ghose MK, Henry AR: The clinical spectrum of renal cholesterol embolization. *Am J Med* 71:174, 1981.

122. Zuchhelli P, Santoro A, Zuccala A: Genesis and control of hypertension in hemodialysis patients. *Semin Nephrol* 8:163–168, 1988.

123. Curtis JJ: Hypertension after renal transplantation: Cyclosporine increases the diagnostic and therapeutic considerations. *Am J Kidney Dis* 13(Suppl 1):28–32, 1989.

124. Linas SL, Miller PD, McDonald KM, et al: Role of the renin-angiotensin system in post-transplantation hypertension in patients with multiple kidneys. *N Engl J Med* 298:1440–1444, 1978.

125. Koomans HA, Ross JC, Dorhout Mees EJ, et al: Sodium balance in renal failure: A comparison of patients with normal subjects under extremes of sodium intake. *Hypertension* 7:714–721, 1985.

126. Vallance P, Leone A, Calver A, et al: Accumulation of an endogenous inhibitor of nitric oxide synthetase in chronic renal failure. *Lancet* 339:572–575, 1992.

127. Dworkin LD, Benstein JA. Impact of antihypertensive therapy on progressive kidney damage. *Am J Hypertens* 2:162S–172S, 1989.

128. Hostetter TM, Oslon JL, Rennke HG, et al: Hyperfiltration in remnant nephrons: A potentially adverse response to renal ablation. *Am J Physiol* 241:F85–F93, 1981.

129. Neugarten J, Kaminetsky B, Feiner H, et al: Nephrotoxic serum nephritis with hypertension: Amelioration by antihypertensive therapy. *Kidney Int* 28:135–139, 1985.

130. Baldwin DS, Neugarten J: Treatment of hypertension in renal disease. *Am J Kidney Dis* 5:A57–A70, 1985.

131. Anderson S, Meyer TW, Rennke HG, et al: Control of glomerular hypertension limits glomerular injury in rats with reduced nephron mass. *J Clin Invest* 76:612, 1985.

132. Klahr S, Schreiner G, Ichikawa I: The progression of renal disease. *N Engl J Med* 318:1657–1666, 1988.

133. Arendshorst WJ, Beierwaltes WH: Renal and nephron hemodynamics in spontaneously hypertensive rats. *Am J Physiol* 236:F246–F251, 1979.

134. Dworkin LD, Feiner HD: Glomerular injury in uninephrectomized spontaneously hypertensive rats: A consequence of glomerular capillary hypertension. *J Clin Invest* 77:797–809, 1986.

135. Barnett AH: Diabetes and hypertension. *Br Med Bull* 50(2):397–407, 1994.

136. Krowleski AS, Warram JH, Christlieb AR, et al: The changing natural history of nephropathy in type I diabetes. *Am J Med* 78:785–794, 1985.

137. Tuttle KR, Stein JH, DeFronzo RA: The natural history of diabetic nephropathy. *Semin Nephrol* 10:184–193, 1990.
138. Mogensen CE: Microalbuminuria predicts clinical proteinuria and early mortality in maturity-onset diabetes. *N Engl J Med* 310:356–360, 1984.
139. Mogensen CE, Christensen CK: Blood pressure changes and renal function in incipient and overt diabetic nephropathy. *Hypertension* 7(Suppl II):II64–II73, 1985.
140. Reaven GM: Role of insulin resistance in human disease: Banting Lecture. *Diabetes* 37:1595–1607, 1987.
141. DeFronzo RA: The effect of insulin on renal sodium metabolism: A review of clinical implications. *Diabetologica* 21:165–171, 1981.
142. Viberti GC, Earle K: Predisposition to essential hypertension and the development of diabetic nephropathy. *J Am Soc Nephrol* 3:S27–33, 1992.
143. Dillon JJ: The quantitative relationship between treated blood pressure and progression of diabetic renal disease. *Am J Kidney Dis* 22:798–802, 1993.
144. Mauer SM, Steffes MW, Azar S, et al: The effects of Goldblatt hypertension on the development of the glomerular lesion of diabetes mellitus in the rat. *Diabetes* 27:738–744, 1978.
145. Béroniade VC, Lefebvre R, Falardeau P: Unilateral nodular diabetic glomerulosclerosis: Recurrence of an experiment of nature. *Am J Nephrol* 7:55–59, 1987.
146. Parving H-H, Andersen AR, Smidt UM, et al: Effects of antihypertensive treatment on kidney function in diabetic nephropathy. *Br Med J* 294:1443–1447, 1987.
147. Lewis EJ, Hunsicher LG, Bain RP, et al: The effect of angiotensin-converting-enzyme inhibition on diabetic nephropathy. *N Engl J Med* 329:1456–1462, 1993.
148. Viberti G, Mogensen CE, Groop LC, et al: Effect of captopril on progression to clinical proteinuria in patients with insulin-dependent diabetes mellitus and microalbuminuria. *JAMA* 271:275–279, 1994.
149. Mathiesen ER, Hommel E, Giese J, et al: Efficacy of captopril in postponing nephropathy in normotensive insulin dependent diabetic patients with microalbuminuria. *BMJ* 303:81–87, 1991.
150. Ravid M, Savin H, Jutrin I, et al: Long-term stabilizing effect of angiotensin-converting-enzyme inhibition on plasma creatinine and on proteinuria in normotensive type II diabetic patients. *Ann Intern Med* 118:577–581, 1993.
151. Hannedouche R, Landais P, Boldfarb B, et al: Randomized controlled trial of enalapril and β blockers in non-diabetic chronic renal failure. *BMJ* 309:833–837, 1994.
152. Maki DD, Ma JZ, Louis TA, et al: Long-term effects of antihypertensive agents on proteinuria and renal function. *Arch Intern Med* 155:1073–1080, 1995.
153. Jackobson HR, Striker GE: Report on a workshop to develop management recommendations for the prevention of progression in chronic renal disease. *Am J Kidney Dis* 25:103–106, 1995.
154. Freis ED: The efficacy and safety of diuretics in treating hypertension. *Ann Intern Med* 122:223–226, 1995.
155. Hypertension Detection and Follow-up Program Cooperative Group: Persistence of reduction in blood pressure and mortality of participants in the hypertension detection and follow-up program. *JAMA* 259:2113–2122, 1988.
156. Amery A, Birkenhäger W, Brixko P, et al: Mortality and morbidity from the European Working Party on High Blood Pressure in the Elderly Trial. *Lancet* 1:1349–1354, 1985.
157. SHEP Cooperative Research Group: Prevention of stroke by antihypertensive treatment in older persons with isolated systolic hypertension: Final results of the Systolic Hypertension in the Elderly Program (SHEP). *JAMA* 265:3255–3264, 1991.
158. Collins R, Peto R, MacMahon S, et al: Blood pressure, stroke, and coronary heart disease: Part 2. Short-term reductions in blood pressure: Overview of randomized drug trials in their epidemiological context. *Lancet* 335:827–838, 1990.
159. Joint National Committee on Detection, Evaluation, and Treatment of High Blood Pressure: The fifth report of the Joint National Committee on Detection, Evaluation, and Treatment of High Blood Pressure (JNC V). *Arch Intern Med* 153:154–183, 1993.
160. Gifford RW Jr: An algorithm for the management of resistant hypertension. *Hypertension* 11(Suppl II):II-101, 1988.

161. Bock HA, Stein JH: Diuretics and the control of extracellular fluid volume: Role of counter-regulation. *Semin Nephrol* 8:264–272, 1988.
162. Guédon J, Chaignon M, Lucsko M: Diuretics as antihypertensive drugs. *Kidney Int* 34(Suppl 25):S177–S180, 1988.
163. Shah S, Khatri I, Fries ED: Mechanism of antihypertensive effect of thiazide diuretics. *Am Heart J* 95:611–618, 1978.
164. Vardan S, Mookherjee S, Warner R, et al: Systolic hypertension in the elderly: Hemodynamic response to long-term thiazide diuretic therapy and its side effects. *JAMA* 250:2807–2813, 1983.
165. Papademetriou V, Burris JF, Notargiacoma A, et al: Effect of diuretic therapy on ventricular arrhythmias in patients with or without left ventricular hypertrophy. *Am Heart J* 110:596–599, 1985.
166. Multiple Risk Factor Intervention Trial Research Group. Exercise electrocardiogram and coronary heart disease mortality in the Multiple Risk Factor Intervention Trial. *Am J Cardiol* 55:16–24, 1985.
167. Siscovick DS, Raghunathanan TE, Psary BM, et al: Diuretic therapy for hypertension and the risk of primary cardiac arrest. *N Engl J Med* 330:1852–1857, 1994.
168. Williams WR, Schneider KA, Borhani NO, et al: The relationship between diuretics and serum cholesterol in Hypertension Detection and Follow-up Program participants. *Am J Prev Med* 2:248–255, 1986.
169. Amery A, Birkenhäger W, Bulpitt C, et al: Influence of antihypertensive therapy on serum cholesterol in elderly hypertensive patients: Results of trial by the European Working Party on high blood pressure in the elderly (EWPHE). *Acta Cardiol* 37:235–244, 1982.
170. Pollare T, Lithell H, Berne C: A comparison of the effects of hydrochlorothiazide and captopril on glucose and lipid metabolism in patients with hypertension. *N Engl J Med* 321:868–873, 1989.
171. Berglund G, Andersson O, Widgren B: A low-dose antihypertensive treatment with a thiazide diuretic is not diabetogenic: A 10-year controlled trial with bendroflumethiazide. *J Hypertens* 4(Suppl 5):S525–527, 1986.
172. Gurwitz JH, Bohn RL, Glynn RJ, et al: Antihypertensive drug therapy and the initiation of treatment for diabetes mellitus. *Ann Intern Med* 118:273–278, 1992.
173. Kassirer JP, Harrington JT: Diuretics and potassium metabolism: A reassessment of the need, effectiveness and safety of potassium therapy. *Kidney Int* 11:505–515, 1977.
174. Papademetriou V, Price M, Johnson E, et al: Early changes in plasma and urinary potassium in diuretic-treated patients with systemic hypertension. *Am J Cardiol* 54:1015–1019, 1984.
175. Siegel D, Hulley SB, Black DM, et al: Diuretics, serum and intracellular electrolyte levels and ventricular arrhythmias in hypertensive men. *JAMA* 267:1683–1688, 1992.
176. Neaton JD, Grimm RH Jr, Prineas RJ, et al: Treatment of Mild Hypertension Study: Final results. *JAMA* 270:713–724, 1993.
177. Gifford RW Jr, Borazanian RA: Traditional first-line therapy: Overview of medical benefits and side effects. *Hypertension* 13(Suppl I):I-119, 1989.
178. Moser M: In defense of traditional antihypertensive therapy. *Hypertension* 12:324, 1988.
179. Moser M, Blaufox MD, Freis E, et al: Who really determines your patients' prescriptions? *JAMA* 265:498–500, 1991.
180. Drug Topics Red Book. *Wholesale Prices of Pharmaceuticals* (90th ed). Montvale, NJ, Medical Economics, 1995.
181. Shulman NB, Martinez B, Brogan D, et al: Financial cost as an obstacle to hypertension therapy. *Am J Public Health* 76:1105–1108, 1986.

Acute Renal Failure: Pathogenesis, Diagnosis, and Management

Muhammad M. Yaqoob, Ahmed M. Alkhunaizi,
Charles L. Edelstein, John D. Conger,
and Robert W. Schrier

Approximately 5 percent of all general hospital patients develop acute renal failure [1]. While the incidence of acute renal failure in association with obstetrics and elective surgery has decreased, that occurring in older and more complex patients—often with multiorgan failure and septicemia—has actually increased. Even though the introduction of dialysis has had a significant positive impact, the mortality from acute renal failure continues to be excessive [2, 3]. From 50 to 70 percent of patients with trauma-related acute renal failure [3–6] and 25 percent of patients with acute renal failure unassociated with surgery or trauma still die in the dialysis era [7, 8].

Acute renal failure is defined as a rapid deterioration of renal function associated with the accumulation of nitrogenous wastes in the body (azotemia) that is not due to extrarenal factors. When acute renal failure is not the result of primary vascular, glomerular, or interstitial disorders, it has been referred to as acute tubular necrosis. In fact, in the clinical setting, the terms *acute renal failure* and *acute tubular necrosis* have become synonymous. However, since acute tubular necrosis is a renal histologic finding and may not be consistently detectable in patients with acute renal failure [9, 10], in the strictest sense the terms should not be used interchangeably.

Causes of Acute Renal Failure

A number of factors are etiologically related to acute renal failure. These fall into the general categories of ischemic disorders, nephrotoxic disorders, diseases of small blood vessels and glomeruli, major blood vessel disease, and acute interstitial nephritis (Table 10-1). The diseases of vessels and glomeruli will be dealt with in Chapter 15. This chapter therefore will focus primarily on the ischemic and nephrotoxic causes of acute renal failure and acute interstitial nephritis.

While the majority of ischemic and nephrotoxic causes of acute renal failure are well known, recent evidence has shown the increasingly important roles played by three nephrotoxins—aminoglycoside antibiotics, x-ray contrast media, and nonsteroidal anti-inflammatory drugs (NSAIDs)—in inducing acute deterioration of renal function [11–16].

Table 10-1. Specific disorders that cause acute renal failure

Ischemic disorders
  Major trauma
  Massive hemorrhage
  Crush syndrome
  Septic shock
  Burns, exudative dermatitis
  Transfusion reactions
  Myoglobinuria
  Pregnancy: postpartum hemorrhage
  Postoperative, particularly cardiac, aortic,
    and biliary surgery
  Medical: pancreatitis, gastroenteritis
Nephrotoxins, including hypersensitivity
    reactions
  Heavy metals: mercury, arsenic, lead,
    bismuth, uranium, cadmium, gold
  Carbon tetrachloride
  Ethylene glycol
  Other organic solvents
  X-ray contrast media (particularly in
    patients with diabetes mellitus)
  Pesticides
  Fungicides
  Antibiotics: aminoglycosides, penicillins,
    tetracyclines, amphotericin
  Chemotherapeutic agents: cisplatin,
    methotrexate
  Immunosuppressive agents: cyclosporine
  Other drugs and chemical agents:
    phenytoin, phenylbutazone, uric acid,
    calcium, nonsteroidal anti-
    inflammatory drugs
Diseases of glomeruli and small blood vessels
  Acute poststreptococcal
    glomerulonephritis
  Systemic lupus erythematosus
  Polyarteritis nodosa
  Schönlein-Henoch purpura
  Subacute bacterial endocarditis
  Serum sickness
  Goodpasture's syndrome
  Malignant hypertension
  Wegener's granulomatosis
  Mixed essential cryoglobulinemia
  Hemolytic-uremic syndrome
  Drug-related vasculitis
  Pregnancy: preeclampsia, eclampsia,
    abruptio placentae, abortion with and
    without gram-negative sepsis,
    postpartum renal failure
  Rapidly progressive glomerulonephritis,
    unknown etiology

Major blood vessel disease
  Dissecting aortic aneurysm
  Renal artery thrombosis, embolism, or
    stenosis
  Bilateral renal vein thrombosis
Interstitial nephritis associated with
    infection, granulomas, crystals
  Streptococcal
  Staphylococcal
  Diphtheria
  Leptospirosis
  Brucellosis
  Legionnaires' disease
  Toxoplasmosis
  Infectious mononucleosis
  Salmonella typhi
  Tuberculosis
  Sarcoidosis
  Hyperuricemia
  Hypercalcemia
Interstitial nephritis associated with
    drugs
  Penicillin semisynthetic analogues
  Sulfonamides
  Tetracyclines
  Cephalosporin
  Co-trimoxazole
  Rifampin
  Phenindione
  Warfarin
  Furosemide
  Thiazides
  Azathioprine
  Allopurinol
  Phenytoin
  Cimetidine
  Acyclovir

The aminoglycosides continue to be the major antibiotics in the treatment of serious gram-negative infections. Their increased use and potential nephrotoxic risk have made them one of the most frequent causes of acute renal failure. Gentamicin, kanamycin, tobramycin, amikacin, netilmicin, and sisomicin are all aminoglycosides capable of impairing renal function [17]. The nephrotoxicity of the aminoglycosides probably is related to their binding to the renal cortical tissue [18]. The tissue half-life of the aminoglycosides is much longer than that in serum; specifically, in the rat the half-life in serum of gentamicin has been shown to be 30 minutes, while in renal tissue it is 109 hours [19]. The long tissue half-life explains why renal failure secondary to aminoglycosides can occur even after cessation of the antibiotics. While additional confirmatory studies will be necessary, it appears that aminoglycosides decrease renal function by damaging proximal tubules [13] and decreasing glomerular capillary permeability for filtration [20]. Although the mechanism is not understood fully, recent evidence suggests that amikacin, tobramycin, and netilmicin are less toxic than other aminoglycosides [21].

Several factors may predispose to aminoglycoside nephrotoxicity. These include advancing age, underlying renal disease, volume depletion, hypertension, and recent exposure to aminoglycosides or other nephrotoxic drugs [22–25]. The clinical course of aminoglycoside nephrotoxicity is usually gradual in onset and is related to the dose and duration of drug exposure [15]. Frequently, mild proteinuria, lysozymuria, a defect in concentrating ability, and polyuria precede a decline in glomerular filtration. The acute renal failure of aminoglycoside toxicity is characteristically nonoliguric and reversible, with a low mortality. Dialysis may or may not be required in its management.

Radiocontrast media-induced acute renal failure is clinically similar to that caused by aminoglycosides. It has been recognized to be a cause of renal failure with increasing frequency in the past few years. Predisposing factors include age (>55 years), prior renal insufficiency, diabetes mellitus with neurovascular complications, proteinuria, volume depletion, acute liver failure, and recent nephrotoxic drug exposure [16, 26]. Renal failure has been reported following a variety of arteriographic procedures as well as intravenous urography, computed tomography (CT) scan with contrast medium, cholangiography, and oral cholecystography [11]. The onset of renal failure usually is abrupt—within 24 hours after exposure to contrast media—and is characterized by oliguria, but it may be nonoliguric [27]. While recovery of renal function generally occurs, several patients have experienced irreversible deterioration of renal function and either have required chronic dialysis or have died [16, 28]. The mechanism of renal injury with contrast media is not understood, but recent studies suggest that it involves a posthyperemic vasoconstriction that is accentuated in high-risk individuals and leads to ischemic injury [29]. The contrast-related vasoconstriction involves a calcium-dependent mechanism [29].

NSAIDs, which are commonly used in the management of pain and rheumatic disorders, are increasingly recognized as etiologic factors in acute renal failure. These substances, which include a large group of newer nonsteroidal agents, as well as aspirin and its derivatives, have in common the inhibition of prostaglandin synthesis [14]. They have been incriminated in several renal abnormalities including ischemic acute renal failure [30, 31], acute interstitial nephritis [32–34], hyporeninemic hypo-aldosteronism [14, 35], edema [14], papillary necrosis [36, 37], and nephrotic syndrome [38, 39]. The first two of these disorders will be discussed in this chapter. The results of the studies indicate that NSAID-induced acute renal failure is due to the diminished renal vasodilatory effect of prostaglandins. In individuals receiving a 50-mEq sodium diet daily, indomethacin doses of 150 mg caused decrements in glomerular filtration rate (GFR) of less than 10 percent but no change in renal blood flow [40]. However, chronic renal failure patients treated with the same indomethacin dose and diet regimen had more profound decrements in both GFR and renal blood flow. Similar effects of diminished renal function and blood flow associated with the use of indomethacin and other NSAIDs have been reported in patients with lupus nephritis [41], nephrotic syndrome [42], cirrhosis with ascites [43], and severe congestive heart failure [44]. Common to all of the edematous disorders is reduced effective arterial circulating volume and renal vasoconstriction mediated by stimulation of sympathetic tone and the renin-angiotensin system. This renal vasoconstriction is normally attenuated by the vasodilatory effect of prostaglandins [14]. Blocking prostaglandin synthesis with NSAIDs disrupts this balance, thus causing severe renal vasoconstriction and reduced GFR. In addition to the aforementioned conditions causing arterial underfilling, other predisposing factors to NSAID-induced ischemic renal dysfunction include diuretic use, elderly age group, atherosclerotic cardiovascular disease, renovascular disease, diabetes, and acute gouty arthritis [14, 44]. In most instances, acute renal failure is rapidly reversed when the offending NSAID drug is discontinued [33, 35]. The use of the antiplatelet agent sulfinpyrazone (Anturane) following myocardial infarction and cardiopulmonary bypass has been associated with acute renal deterioration that is thought to be secondary to prostaglandin synthesis inhibition; however, an additional effect of the associated uricosuria cannot be excluded. NSAIDs have also been reported to cause acute renal failure in patients with dysproteinurias and hypercalciuria with or without hypercalcemia. Several of the NSAIDs have been associated with a more chronic variety of renal failure that is highlighted by heavy proteinuria and interstitial nephritis on renal biopsy. This renal failure with NSAIDs is also generally reversible, but in a slower fashion.

An acute deterioration of renal function has also been described with inhibition of angiotensin-converting enzyme in association with bilateral renal artery stenosis, renal artery stenosis in a solitary kidney, congestive heart failure, cirrhosis, and diuretic-induced volume depletion.

Pathogenesis of Acute Renal Failure

Role of Calcium in the Pathogenesis of Ischemic Acute Renal Failure

In 1981 it was proposed that Ca^{2+} ions were important participants in the functional, biochemical, and morphologic disturbances that characterize ischemic acute renal failure [45]. The subtitle of that manuscript, "From MAN-To-MITOCHONDRIA-

To-MAN," described how careful observations of patients by physicians could lead to hypotheses that were testable in the laboratory. Much of the laboratory work in the early 1980s involved the study of normal and deranged bioenergetics. From the results of these cell biology/animal studies, it was hoped that new clinical interventions would soon be forthcoming that would ameliorate the devastating effects of ischemic acute renal failure.

Specifically, building on the hypothesis that homeostatic mechanisms controlling cellular Ca^{2+} were disturbed in acute renal failure, it has been shown that radiocontrast-induced acute renal failure [46, 47] and cadaveric kidney transplant dysfunction [48, 49], for example, can be attenuated by administration of chemically dissimilar calcium channel blockers. These are two clinical conditions in which intense renal vasoconstriction is demonstrable, a situation where delivery of oxygen and nutrients to renal tubules is compromised. The administration of calcium channel blockers reduces the intensity of renal vasoconstriction and provides better delivery of nutrients to renal tissues. With ischemia, the poor nutrient flow to renal tubules also results in tubule Ca^{2+} overload, which can be lessened by the calcium channel blockers. Although calcium channel blockers have been shown to be efficacious in these two aforementioned clinical conditions, a full understanding of the mechanisms by which cytosolic or tissue Ca^{2+} increases in underperfused situations and how this increase may contribute to organ injury is the focus of much recent research. It is important, therefore, to understand the normal cellular calcium regulation before discussing the newer insights that have been gained using experimental approaches to further improve our understanding of the pathogenesis of acute renal failure.

Normal Regulation of Cell Calcium

Three major cellular calcium pools exist: (1) a pool bound to plasma membranes, (2) a pool bound to or sequestered within intracellular organelles, and (3) a pool both free and bound within the cytoplasm [50].

Although 60 to 70 percent of all calcium in renal epithelial cells is located in the mitochondria, cytosolic free ionized calcium is the most critical with regard to regulation of intracellular events. Cytosolic free calcium is normally kept at about 100 nM, which is 1/10,000 of the extracellular level [51]. Calcium efflux is mediated on basolateral membranes by both calcium ATPase, which is adenosine triphosphate (ATP) dependent, and by a Na^+/Ca^{2+} exchanger on the basolateral membrane, which is-ATP independent [52]. Normally, the cell membrane is impermeable to calcium and maintains a steep calcium gradient between the cytosol and the extracellular space. However, when cytosolic calcium increases in response to either increased cellular membrane permeability or decreased calcium efflux or both, the mitochondria and endoplasmic reticulum actively increase their calcium uptake. Mitochondrial uptake and retention of calcium become substantial only when cytosolic levels exceed 400 to 500 nM, as occurs with cell injury [51]. Mitochondrial uptake is regulated by a calcium uniporter in the mitochondrial inner membrane. During cell injury, active mitochondrial sequestration appears to be quantitatively the most important process for buffering elevations in cytosolic calcium.

Calcium Accumulation and Cell Injury

Calcium overload is characteristic of tissues with lethally injured cells, since the breakdown of the plasma membrane barrier to calcium causes a large increase in cytosolic calcium, which is sequestered by the mitochondria. There is accelerated calcium influx into renal cells from the extracellular compartment during ischemic injury [53]. Anoxic rabbit proximal tubules, however, do not show this increase in total tissue calcium, whereas hypoxic rabbit tubules do show a time-dependent increase in calcium [54]. Reasons for this difference may be that in hypoxic tissues, mitochondrial membrane potential is not totally dissipated (as it is with anoxia) so that increased calcium influx is accompanied by mitochondrial calcium sequestration, thus leading to tissue calcium overload [55]. Weinberg's [51] explanation for anoxic tubules not showing an increase in total tissue calcium is that the more substantial acidosis of anoxia inhibits calcium uptake.

Vascular Effects

It was at first thought that calcium channel blockers might be exerting their protective effects entirely at the vascular level by promoting the enhancement of renal blood flow. There are unquestioned renal vascular effects of calcium channel blockers, with renal blood flow improving more rapidly after ischemia with calcium channel blocker treatment [56]. Renal blood flow and glomerular filtration will not decrease as severely during radiocontrast administration in dogs when calcium channel blockers are coadministered [57]. Ischemic acute renal failure is characterized by a loss of autoregulatory ability, an enhanced sensitivity of renal blood flow to renal nerve stimulation, and injury to the endothelial lining of renal vessels [56] (Fig. 10-1). Much of this injury may be related to Ca^{2+} overload in vascular smooth muscle and/or endothelial cells, since verapamil and diltiazem partially obviate the loss of autoregulatory capacity and hypersensitivity to renal nerve stimulation [56]. Warm and cold ischemia during transplantation surgery may also contribute to

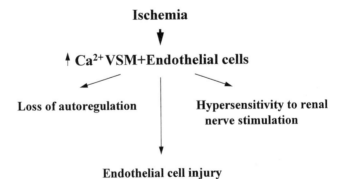

Fig. 10-1. Role of calcium on ischemia-induced perturbation of the renal vasculature. Ischemia increases the cytosolic calcium concentration in the endothelial and vascular smooth muscle cells (VSM), which results in (1) loss of renal autoregulation, (2) enhanced sensitivity of renal blood flow to renal nerve stimulation, and (3) injury to endothelial cells.

vascular injury, and calcium channel blockers are protective in experimental models of these clinical entities [58, 59]. However, other renal vasodilators such as prostacyclin do not restore autoregulatory integrity or reverse the increased sensitivity to renal nerve stimulation [56]. Thus, it also seems that a unique effect of calcium channel blockers is exerted at the vascular level. In vivo studies of intact kidney, however, cannot discriminate between protective effects at the vascular as compared to tubular sites, or a combination thereof. Since the renal proximal tubule is probably the site of the worst cell injury in both toxic nephropathy and ischemic acute renal failure, several laboratories have turned to the study of isolated proximal tubules during conditions of oxygen deprivation either in suspension or in primary culture [60–63].

Tubular Effects

Using microdissection techniques, isolated segments of the proximal nephron (S_1, S_2, S_3) and the distal tubule from rabbit kidneys have been grown in primary culture [61]. When exposed to anoxia in vitro, the proximal and distal nephrons rapidly exhibit cell death after reoxygenation [61]. However, if Ca^{2+} is removed from the bathing medium during the first 2 hours of reoxygenation and then replaced, cell viability is greatly enhanced [61]. Thus, at least a portion of anoxia-induced cell damage that occurred during reoxygenation in vitro was Ca^{2+} dependent. The increased cellular Ca^{2+} could activate calmodulin or other second messenger–mediated events, thereby leading to cell damage. This seems quite plausible because drugs that are calmodulin antagonists, even in the presence of Ca^{2+} ions during the first 2 hours of reoxygenation, also delay cell death and preserve cell viability [62]. Calcium channel blockers have also been shown to delay the onset of anoxic cell death in primary cultures of rabbit proximal tubules and cortical collecting tubules, suggesting that Ca^{2+}-mediated hypoxic cell death is not limited to the proximal tubules [62].

Calcium Influx

Calcium channel blockers have no effects on the rate of Ca^{2+} influx into normoxic proximal tubules. However, during hypoxia or anoxia in vitro, Ca^{2+} influx rate into tubules is increased above normal levels, and calcium channel blockers reduce this rate to or toward normal [60]. This is an important observation because cytosolic-free Ca^{2+} could increase as the result of normal influx rates in the presence of reduced efflux rates secondary to decreased ATP-dependent Ca^{2+}-ATPase or decreased Na^+/Ca^{2+} antiporter activity. The efficacy of calcium channel blockers to prevent the increased Ca^{2+} influx rate during hypoxia and not during normoxia suggests a hypoxia-induced alteration in membrane permeability to Ca^{2+} that is sensitive to calcium channel blockers. This permeability pathway appears to be sensitive, in part, to the decrease in ATP that occurs during hypoxia. For example, reduced ATP levels in rat proximal tubules with a phosphate-free incubation medium results in increased Ca^{2+} influx rate [64]. This ATP-dependent change in Ca^{2+} permeability has not been examined in detail, however, acidosis prevents the increased Ca^{2+} influx rate in tubules and delays the onset of cell injury as assessed by lactate dehydrogenase (LDH) release even though ATP remains at low levels

[65]. Cellular protection is also observed with an acidotic perfusate in the isolated perfused kidney [66]. Intracellular acidosis is more likely to develop in complete anoxia than in hypoxia, and this may explain the only very short-lived increase in Ca^{2+} influx rate [60] as well as the absence of appreciable tissue Ca^{2+} overload during anoxia as assessed by atomic absorption spectroscopy [67].

Based on these observations, the role of Ca^{2+} influx rate in mediating proximal tubule hypoxic injury was examined. By employing a combination of EGTA and various Ca^{2+} concentrations in the tubule bathing medium (Ca^{2+} modified Krebs buffer), a delay in the onset of cell injury during hypoxia was seen when extracellular Ca^{2+} concentration was below 10^{-5} M [68].

Thus, Ca^{2+} ions enter renal proximal tubules at a faster rate than normal during oxygen deprivation. The removal of extracellular Ca^{2+} ions or administration of calcium channel buffers reduces the injury associated with this increased influx rate of Ca^{2+}. Acidosis also reduces Ca^{2+} influx rate [65] and exerts cytoprotective effects [64–67]. Finally, if Ca^{2+} ions do enter hypoxic or anoxic cells, their deleterious effects can be mitigated by calmodulin inhibitors [62]. Together, these data strongly suggest that it is the increased cytosolic or intracellular burden of Ca^{2+} that initiates the development of cell injury.

Cytosolic Free Calcium $(Ca^{2+})_i$

Cytosolic free Ca^{2+} in freshly isolated proximal tubules, as assessed with fura-2, increases significantly after 2 minutes of hypoxia and continues to increase progressively with continued hypoxia [69]. This increase in $(Ca^{2+})_i$ precedes the release of LDH or the uptake by nuclei of the membrane-impermeable dye propidium iodide (PI) [69, 70]. The reduction in PI staining and the reduced LDH release observed when hypoxic rat proximal tubules are incubated either in a Ca^{2+}-free medium [68] or with the intracellular Ca^{2+} chelator BAPTA [71] strongly support the hypothesis that a cause and effect relationship exists between the elevation in $(Ca^{2+})_i$ and the development of hypoxic membrane damage. Furthermore, this early rise in $(Ca^{2+})_i$ after 5 to 10 minutes of hypoxia is reversible, since return to a well-oxygenated medium results in a prompt (1 minute) return of $(Ca^{2+})_i$ to baseline level. If membrane injury had been the cause of the increase in $(Ca^{2+})_i$, a return to basal levels would not have occurred with reoxygenation. Membrane injury with irreversible rise in $(Ca^{2+})_i$ occurs after more prolonged periods of hypoxia [69]. These studies suggest that $(Ca^{2+})_i$ rather than total intracellular burden is more important.

Mechanisms of Calcium-Induced Cell Injury

There is now compelling evidence that hypoxia-induced rise in cytosolic free calcium activates calcium-dependent intracellular events that mediate membrane injury [72] (Fig. 10-2).

Role of Nitric Oxide in Hypoxia-Induced Proximal Tubule Injury. Nitric oxide (NO) is a recently recognized messenger molecule, mediating diverse functions including vasodilatation, neurotransmission, and antimicrobial and antitumor ac-

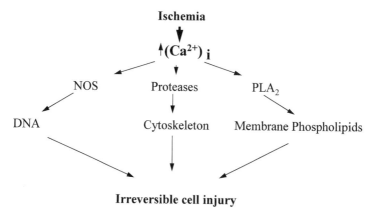

Fig. 10-2. Role of calcium on ischemia-induced renal tubular cell injury. Ischemia promotes an increase of cytosolic free calcium (Ca^{2+})$_i$ concentration, which activates (1) nitric oxide synthase (NOS), with resulting DNA damage, (2) cysteine proteases such as calpain, which attacks cytoskeletal elements, and (3) phospholipases such as phospholipase A_2 (PLA_2), which attacks the phospholipid component of the cell membrane. All these changes ultimately may result in irreversible cell injury.

tivities [73]. A variety of cells produce NO via oxidation of L-arginine by the enzyme nitric oxide synthase (NOS) [74]. Thus far, four distinct NOS isoforms have been isolated, purified, and cloned: neuronal, endothelial, macrophage, and vascular smooth muscle cell/hepatocyte isoform [75, 76]. Identification of the specific isoform of NOS is important because the four isoforms vary in subcellular location, amino acid sequence, regulation and hence functional roles. Neuronal and endothelial NOS are continuously present and thus are termed constitutive NOS (cNOS) [76]. NO is produced by these enzymes when Ca^{2+}/calmodulin interaction permits electron transfer from NADPH via flavin groups within the enzyme to a heme-containing active site [77]. This activation is very short-lived. In contrast, VSMC/hepatocyte and macrophage isoforms are only expressed when the cells have been induced by certain cytokines, microbes, and microbial products and are therefore called inducible NOS (iNOS) [78]. iNOS expression results in sustained production of NO. Unlike cNOS, iNOS activity is believed to be insensitive to changes in intracellular Ca^{2+}, since calmodulin is tightly bound to the molecule. Once synthesized, iNOS remains tonically activated, producing NO continuously for the life of the enzyme [79].

Both cNOS and iNOS isoforms have been identified in the kidney, specifically in macula densa cells (cNOS), inner medullary collecting ducts (cNOS and iNOS), and proximal tubules (cNOS and iNOS) [76, 80]. In the kidney, physiologic amounts of NO play an important role in hemodynamic regulation and salt and water excretion [81].

Recently, it was demonstrated that NOS activity is increased during hypoxia in freshly isolated rat proximal tubules. In this study, membrane damage, as assessed by LDH release into the medium, was prevented by both a nonselective NOS inhibitor (L-NAME) and a NO scavenger (hemoglobin) [82]. A further increase in hypoxic injury was observed when the NOS substrate L-arginine was added to the hypoxic tubule suspension [82]. Hypoxia stimulated prompt and sustained NO release in the proximal tubule suspension as assessed by a NO-selective sensing electrode [83]. NO concentration remained unmeasurable during normoxia. L-NAME completely inhibited hypoxia-induced NO release in parallel to marked cytoprotection. Immunoblotting of tubular extracts with three specific antibodies against nNOS, eNOS, and macrophage NOS (macNOS) confirmed the presence of nNOS, eNOS, and inducible macNOS. The results of this study suggest that all three nNOS isoforms, eNOS, and iNOS are present in proximal tubules. A recent study has demonstrated that in vivo targeting of iNOS with oligodeoxynucleotides protects the rat kidney against ischemia [84]. This study provided direct evidence for the cytotoxic effects of NO produced via iNOS in the course of ischemic acute renal failure. The nonselective NOS inhibitor L-NAME resulted in a deterioration of renal function reinforcing the recent findings of endothelial NOS (eNOS) stimulation early in the course of ARF and profound vasoconstriction accompanying L-NAME infusion.

All isoforms of NOS require tetrahydrobiopterin (BH_4) as a cofactor for NO generation. Depletion of BH_4 or inhibition of enzymes involved in its production is associated with the attenuation of NO production. In a recent preliminary study, the impact of BH_4 availability in rat proximal tubules on NO kinetics and markers of membrane injury was assessed. The results of this study suggest that inhibition of BH_4 synthesis is associated with marked attenuation of NO production and subsequent hypoxia-induced cell injury. These effects are reversible by exogenous BH_4 [85].

Moreover, it has been shown that cNOS (neuronal) can be phosphorylated at specific sites by protein kinase A (PKA), protein kinase C (PKC), and Ca^{2+}/calmodulin protein kinase II. Furthermore, phosphorylation by PKC has been shown to be associated with reduced NOS activity [86]. Phosphorylation of cNOS has also been demonstrated in endothelial cells in response to various drugs and hormones; based on the time course of NOS activation and phosphorylation, these investigators suggested that this NOS phosphorylation deactivates the enzyme [87]. In other studies, inhibition of the activity of phosphatase calcineurin was associated with enhanced phosphorylation of neuronal cNOS and inhibition of nitrite release, thus supporting a role for calcineurin in the activation of cNOS [88].

NO has a very short half-life in oxygenated solutions; however, the half-life of NO generated under low oxygen tension during hypoxia may be greatly prolonged. The resultant accumulation of NO may have a number of consequences during hypoxia. For example, NO has been shown to cause nuclear DNA fragmentation, which in turn activates nuclear poly(ADP-ribose) synthase (PARS) [89]. Enhanced activation of PARS promotes ribosylation of nuclear and cytoskeletal proteins such as filamentous actin (F-actin) utilizing NAD as substrate. Cellular ATP is then shunted to regenerate NAD, an event that may contribute to cell injury because of further decrement in already depleted energy stores during hypoxia [89]. Furthermore, it is possible that NO directly inhibits mitochondrial respiration because of its high affinity for heme-containing compounds (i.e., respiratory chain enzymes). Moreover, hypoxia-induced depletion of ATP would likely result in accelerated protein dephosphorylation due to the dual effect of kinase inhibition and unopposed phosphatase activity. In this regard, the Ca^{2+}-dependent protease calpain has been reported to activate calcineurin [90], and, as discussed in the next section, calpain activity is increased during hypoxia. The dephosphorylation of NOS due to ATP depletion and increased calcineurin activity should favor continued NO generation, potentially exacerbating cell injury. In a preliminary report, Kobryn and Mandel [91] demonstrated a cytoprotective effect of phosphatase inhibition in the anoxic rabbit tubules. In addition, NO may cause membrane damage either by direct attack or by combining with superoxide to form the highly toxic radical peroxynitrite, which can attack cellular membranes by lipid peroxidation [92].

Finally, the mechanism of cytoprotection by low pH during hypoxia remains unclear. It is well recognized that NOS is pH dependent and less active at acidic pH [93]. A pH of 6.8 or lower results in complete inhibition of NOS. Furthermore, low pH promotes the conversion of NO to its noninjurious metabolites nitrite and nitrate [94]. Recent observations suggest that acidosis provides cytoprotection against hypoxia-induced cell injury by inhibiting NOS and NO production [83].

Role of Cysteine Proteases in Hypoxia-Induced Proximal Tubule Injury. The cysteine proteases are intracellular proteases that include cathepsins B, H, L, and S and calpain. The cathepsins are non–calcium-dependent lysosomal proteases. Calpain is the major cytosolic protease and the only Ca^{2+}-dependent cytosolic protease so far described [95]. Renal brush-border membranes are rich in proteases [97], and calpain has been demonstrated in proximal tubules in culture [98] and in both distal and collecting tubules in the rabbit [99, 100]. Calpain exists in the cytosol as the inactive proenzyme procalpain, which translocates from the cytosol to the cell membrane in the presence of μM Ca^{2+}. Autocatalytic activation of procalpain to active calpain occurs at the membrane in the presence of Ca^{2+} and phosphatidyl-inositol [96]. Calpain occurs in two forms: Calpain I is activated by μM and calpain II by mM Ca^{2+} [100]. As well as being Ca^{2+} dependent, the activity of calpain is highly pH dependent. Calpain is active at neutral pH and is inactivated at an acidic pH. In contrast, the lysosomal cathepsins are not Ca^{2+} dependent, are active at an acidic pH, and are inactivated at a pH above 6.5.

In certain circumstances, proteases have been shown to play a role in cellular injury. For example, studies using cultured fibroblasts and the specific lysosomotropic detergent C12-imidazole demonstrated that cell death can be caused by activation and/or release of lysosomal cysteine proteases into the cytoplasm [101]. Studies of cysteine proteases and renal proximal tubule damage, however, have been confined to cyclosporine-induced toxicity. In cultured tubules exposed acutely to cyclosporine, calpain but not cathepsin activity was increased; in addition, lysosomes were intact, suggesting that calpain (but not cathepsins) is involved in acute cyclosporine-induced renal tubular injury [98]. These results are in agreement with previous observations that the non–Ca^{2+}-dependent lysosomal cathepsins do not play a role in lethal injury. These observations are (1) lysosomes are highly resistant to disruption during lethal injury [102], (2) lysosomal proteolysis is inhibited in lethal anoxic injury of rat hepatocytes [103], and lysosomal proteolysis is suppressed by ATP depletion [104]. However, in chronic cyclosporine toxicity, cathepsin activity was found to be increased [105]. Thus, the role of cathepsins in toxic tubular damage may depend on the duration of exposure.

On the other hand, calpain-mediated degradative proteolysis has been implicated as an important mechanism contributing to lethal anoxic cell injury. Specifically, ischemia of hippocampal neurons triggers proteolysis of cytoskeletal spectrin, a preferred substrate of calpain, and inhibition of this proteolysis protects hippocampal neurons from ischemia [106, 107]. Moreover, pH-dependent nonlysosomal proteolysis contributes to lethal anoxic injury of rat hepatocytes [103]. Ca^{2+}-dependent nonlysosomal proteases may also contribute to cell injury during anoxia in myocardium [108, 109]. Additionally, in the past, studies using specific cysteine protease inhibitor were difficult to interpret because these compounds were charged and did not penetrate the cells. However, synthetic uncharged cell-permeable inhibitors of cysteine proteases have recently been developed and are proving useful in the examination of the role of calpain in many cellular processes [110]. Recently, the role of the lysosomal proteases cathepsins B and L and the calcium-dependent cytosolic protease calpain in hypoxia-induced renal proximal tubular injury was investigated [96]. There was no increase in cathepsin activity during hypoxia. However, calpain activity in isolated proximal tubules significantly increased during hypoxia. This increase in calpain activity occurred prior to cell membrane damage, suggestive of a cause and effect relationship. The cysteine protease inhibitor N-Cbz-Val-Phe methyl ester markedly decreased membrane injury and completely prevented the rise in calpain activity during hypoxia. The increase in calpain activity during hypoxia and the inhibitor studies with N-Cbz-Val-Phe methyl ester therefore suggested a role for calpain as a mediator of proximal tubular injury [96].

Cytoskeletal and cell-membrane organizational proteins that anchor cytoskeletal elements to the plasma membrane are excellent substrates for calpain [111]. For example, calpain cleaves actin-binding proteins such as spectrin, talin, filamin, α-actinin, and ankyrin [112]. Spectrin has been extensively studied during forebrain ischemia and has been found to be the major calpain substrate undergoing proteolysis in the hippocampus after forebrain ischemia-reperfusion [106]. Irreversible modification of spectrin, a major lining anchor protein beneath the plasma membrane in the brain, may contribute to this neuronal membrane damage [106, 107]. Molitoris and co-workers [113–115] have shown that ATP depletion during ischemia causes profound alterations in proximal tubular cell polarity by inducing major changes in the actin cytoskeletal architecture. Also, the proximal tubule brush-border structure undergoes pronounced changes during ischemia-reperfusion, and disruption of microvillar cytoskeletal proteins may accompany some of these changes [116, 117]. Specifically, actin binding proteins that link actin to the plasma membrane may dissociate during hypoxia and play a role in microvillar and ultimately plasma membrane damage [118]. Indeed, degradation of the calpain substrates spectrin and ankyrin have been shown in the ischemic rat kidney [119]. Thus, cytoskeletal damage induced by Ca^{2+} activation of calpain during hypoxia may contribute to lethal cellular injury.

Finally, the cytoprotective effects of low intracellular Ca^{2+} and pH have been shown to be in part due to inhibition of calpain activity. Both low intracellular

Ca^{2+} and pH attenuated the hypoxia-induced rise in LDH and calpain activity [120].

Activation of Phospholipase A_2

Phospholipase A_2 (PLA_2) hydrolyzes the acyl bond at the sn-2 position of phospholipids to generate free fatty acids and lysophospholipids. Free fatty acid release has been well documented in rat proximal tubules [63]. This release is thought to be mediated to a large extent by activation of intracellular PLA_2 during hypoxia [121]. It has been shown that both the messenger RNA for PLA_2 and the PLA_2 enzyme activity are increased in hypoxic rabbit tubules [122].

The mechanism of PLA2-induced cell membrane damage is controversial. In proximal tubules hypoxia has been shown to cause an increase in free fatty acids, which was initially believed to contribute to cell injury [63]. However, a recent study has shown that unsaturated free fatty acids protect against hypoxic injury in proximal tubules and that this protection may be mediated by negative feedback inhibition of PLA2 activity [123].

There are various isoforms of PLA_2, and most isoforms of PLA_2 require calcium for catalytic activity [124, 125]. An 85-kDa isoform present in proximal tubules has been identified using amino acid sequence methods [126]. This isoform has two defining characteristics: (1) a 5- to 10-fold preference for the sn-2 arachidonyl-containing phospholipid substrates, and (2) translocation of the activity in either whole-cell or broken-cell preparations from the cytosolic to the particulate membrane fraction at buffered Ca^{2+} concentrations between 300 and 700 nM. This isoform has a 45-amino-acid domain homologous with the calcium binding domain of PKC and partial homology to a lung surfactant protein but no other sequence homology with any of the other isoforms of PLA_2. An expressed fragment of the PKC homologous region has been shown to translocate to the membrane in a calcium-dependent fashion. It has also been shown using ^{45}Ca that there is a single binding site for calcium in a tertiary complex with 85-kDa PLA_2 and phospholipid. However, hydrolytic activity could be obtained in the absence of calcium using high concentrations of NaCl or other salts, implying that calcium is required for interfacial association with the lipid membrane but not for catalysis. Thus this isoform translocates to the membrane in response to changes in intracellular Ca^{2+}. It is unknown whether other proteins are involved in this translocation phenomenon. Activity of this isoform is found in the cytosol when cells are broken in calcium-free buffers, but largely in the microsomal fraction when cells are broken in the presence of calcium concentrations approaching those found in activated cells. Nakamara et al. [127] have shown that the activity of this isoform, which has a molecular mass of 110 kDa using gel electrophoresis, increases after renal ischemia and reperfusion in rat kidney and that cytosolic PLA_2 activity was enhanced when calcium was increased over the range of 10^{-7} to 10^{-6} M, whereas mitochondrial PLA_2 required higher calcium for activation ($>10^{-6}$ M).

The role of PLA_2 activation in hypoxia-induced proximal tubular injury has been evaluated using phospholipase inhibitors. After 10 minutes of hypoxia, dibucaine, a phospholipase inhibitor, reduced LDH release as well as the increase in calcium uptake rate in rat proximal tubules [128]. The membrane-protective effect and effect on calcium uptake rate are not demonstrable after 20 minutes of hypoxia, however, thus suggesting that other events such as oxygen free radicals or proteases may predominate at this time.

A significant fraction of the PLA_2 activity in rabbit proximal tubules has been found to be calcium independent and selective for plasmalogen substrates. The activity of this calcium-independent PLA_2 enzyme was found to play an important role in the pathogenesis of membrane injury during hypoxia in proximal tubules [129].

Mitochondria are important sites of PLA_2 action. It has been proposed that the mechanism responsible for the enhanced mitochondrial swelling and respiratory inhibition induced by calcium loading may involve activation of mitochondrial PLA_2 [130, 131]. This is based on the protective effects demonstrated with local anesthetics and PLA_2 inhibitors. Attenuation of ischemic mitochondrial damage by verapamil has been demonstrated [132, 133], which provides further support for an important role for calcium-activated intracellular phospholipases.

Recent studies have shown the disappearance of a high-molecular-weight (~100 kDa) Ca^{2+}-dependent form of PLA_2 during hypoxia that coincides with the appearance of a low-molecular-weight form (~15 kDa) with the same Ca^{2+} and substrate specificity [121]. These data suggest the possibility that the high-molecular-weight form is converted to the low-molecular-weight form by a protease such as calpain that is activated during hypoxia. This provides further support that calcium-mediated cellular events either alone or in combination mediate hypoxic cellular injury.

Role of Abnormal Vascular Function in Acute Renal Failure

Organ ischemia presents a dilemma in which the restoration of perfusion may add to the problem of organ injury. Extensive current investigation clearly indicates the development of organ dysfunction ascribable to reperfusion in the laboratory, and the breadth of the phenomenon is indicated by its demonstration in heart, lung, brain, intestine, liver, and other organs. The importance of these findings is in their probable contribution to clinical features of myocardial infarction, acute renal failure, and cerebrovascular accident and their implications concerning effects of flow diversion in surgical bypass and for function of transplanted heart, lung, kidney, and other organs.

It is now clear that injury induced by ischemia-reperfusion leads to organ dysfunction in part by direct injury of parenchymal cells. However, abundant evidence indicates a major role for intravascular neutrophil sequestration early in reperfusion with release of oxidants and other injurious substances. Thus, it is not surprising that vascular dysfunction is an early and prominent aspect of ischemia-reperfusion injury, with consequent impairment of blood flow and its regulation. For instance, there may be a progressive loss of regional organ blood flow following ischemia-reperfusion. There also may be exaggerated constriction to neurohumoral agonists, failure to respond to physiologic and pharmacologic vasodilators, and paradoxical vasoconstrictor responses to changes in arterial pressure and blood flow following a period of transient organ ischemia and reperfusion. A growing body of evidence suggests that disordered vascular function subsequent to ischemia-reperfusion injury may itself have a substantial impact on organ recovery, since normalization of blood flow influences the rate of parenchymal cell restoration.

Normal Vascular Tone and Reactivity

Basal Vascular Tone. Basal vascular tone is that level of vessel contraction present in the resting state without the imposition of physiologic or pathologic stress. The level of tone within the small arteries and arterioles of the systemic and pulmonary vasculature is the major component of resistance to blood flow within the general circulation, which in turn maintains appropriate arterial pressures at physiologic levels of cardiac output. The systemic vessels have relatively high basal tone (compared to the lungs). This affords the presumed advantage for maintaining high systemic pressure, which offsets the effects of gravity in upright animals and perhaps provides vasodilator reserve for increased perfusion demand. Without normal tone in the small arterial resistance vessels, there would be vascular collapse and an inability of the cardiac output to adequately support the circulation. The principal factor determining resistance in the small arterial vasculature is vessel lumen diameter, which in large part is determined by active intramural smooth muscle contraction. The level of contraction, or tone, is determined by the local and circulating neurohumoral modulating factors and by the vessel responses to transmural pressure (stretch) and blood flow (shear stress). Of primary importance in determining local neurohumoral activity is metabolic demand of individual organs.

The mechanisms of transduction of stretch and shear stress to basal vascular tone have been examined in a variety of in vivo and in vitro experimental preparations. The constrictor response to stretch is dependent on the presence of extracellular Ca^{2+} [134]. Distention of the vascular smooth muscle cell membrane is associated with Ca^{2+} entry. At least in part, Ca^{2+} entry in response to stretch involves a unique pathway separate from voltage-gated and receptor-operated Ca^{2+} channels. Voltage-gated and stretch-operated Ca^{2+} channels have been shown to be inhibited by inorganic blockers (Mn^{2+} and Mg^{2+}) and the phenylalkylamine Ca^{2+} entry antagonist verapamil [135]. However, the sensitivity is greater for stretch-operated Ca^{2+} channels. In contrast, dihydropyridines, potent inhibitors of voltage-gated Ca^{2+} channels, are much less effective in attenuating myogenic (stretch) vasoconstriction. These results indicated that voltage-gated and stretch-operated mechanisms of vascular tone generation are not identical. It also has been shown in small facial vessels that stretch-induced tone is resistant to concentrations of phenylalkylamine, dihydropyridine, and benzothiazipine Ca^{2+} channel antagonists that block K^+-induced tone [136–139]. Several other experiments carried out in arterioles of hamster cheek pouch [140] and the cerebral circulation [141–143] suggest that Ca^{2+} entry mechanisms are at least partially separate in response to membrane depolarization, receptor activation, and stretch.

Recently, a number of studies have suggested that K^+ channels of vascular smooth muscle cell membranes also contribute to basal vascular tonal balance. Glibenclamide, a predominant K_{ATP} channel blocker, increased baseline vascular resistance in dog diaphragm [144]. Imamura et al. [145] and Samaha et al. [146] found that glibenclamide increased resistance in the coronary circulation of dogs. How K^+ channel activity is related specifically to the myogenic response is unknown.

The role of the endothelium in the stretch-induced component of basal vascular tone is controversial. Some evidence suggests that vessel wall pressure stimulates an endothelium-derived constricting factor [147] or reduced NOS activity [148]. Harder et al. [147] showed that the myogenic response was reduced when the endothelium was removed from cerebral arteries. Similar results were found by Katusic et al. [149]. These studies suggested that the stretch of vessel walls induced release of an endothelial constrictor or inhibited an endothelial dilator. While it is possible that the endothelium plays a modulating role in the pressure-related vasoconstrictor response, there is ample evidence that myogenic activity is present in the absence of the endothelium. Endothelium-independent, stretch-activated tone has been shown in skin [150], lung [151], coronary [152], and brain preparations [153–155] in several mammalian species. Therefore, it is likely that both sensing and transducing mechanisms of myogenic activity are present within the smooth muscle layer of arterial vessel walls.

The influence of blood flow, as opposed to transmural pressure, on the tone of the arterial vasculature is of two types: flow-induced vasoconstriction and flow-induced vasodilation. Flow-related vasoconstriction has been described only in vitro in small artery segments and is of uncertain significance. Several minutes were required to reach a steady-state response, but the recovery was nearly instantaneous with stopping flow [156–157]. Flow-induced contraction was most readily detected in the presence of modest transmural pressure. Unlike myogenic vascular tone, flow constriction was inhibited by dihydropyridines, low extracellular fluid Ca^{2+}, and inorganic Ca^{2+} entry blockers [158]. Sodium dependence of flow constriction has also been noted. The magnitude of tonal response to flow was sensitive to relatively small changes in extracellular sodium [159]. Flow-induced vasoconstriction was unaffected by de-endothelialization in cerebral or skeletal muscle arterial segments [156–160].

Flow-induced vasodilation represents the primary shear stress response of the arterial vasculature. It has been described in arterial vessels of all sizes both in vivo and in vitro. In studies where it specifically has been examined, flow can overcome and inhibit stretch-related vasoconstriction [156–161]. Bevan [162] showed that flow-induced vasodilation was sensitive to extracellular Na^+ concentration. Cationic substitution for Na^+ with a variety of agents significantly attenuated flow vasodilation. Maneuvers that increase intracellular Na^+ have a similar effect. The effect of altering Na^+ concentrations was unaffected by removal of the endothelium. However, de-endothelialization itself has been shown to have a major effect on flow-related vasodilation. In large arteries studied in vivo, removal of the endothelium resulted in disappearance of flow vasodilation [160]. Endothelial dependence of flow vasodilation has also been shown in the microcirculation of skeletal muscle [163] and heart [164]. However, as the arterial vasculature investigated became progressively smaller, it was difficult to be certain that the endothelium was selectively injured.

The finding that the endothelium contributes to flow-related vasodilation suggests that a humoral substance is involved in the transduction of shear stress to a reduction in vascular smooth muscle cell constriction. Some evidence indicates that NO may be a critical humoral factor [165]. Other evidence suggests that an endothelial cyclooxygenase product may contribute to flow-induced vasodilation [163]. The role of large conductance K_{Ca} channels in flow-induced vasodilation, both directly and as a mediator of the effect of endothelial humoral agents, is currently being examined [144, 166].

One humoral factor that should be considered as a constitutive factor in establishing basal arterial tone is NO. Exposure to NOS inhibitors, which are primarily L-arginine analogues, has shown increases in resistance in essentially all vascular beds in normal animals and humans [167–169]. This finding would indicate that endothelial cNOS and NO activity continuously modulate vascular tone under normal physiologic conditions in a paracrine manner. The effect of interrupting NOS activity on physiologic vascular tone is substantially greater than the effect of inhibiting other endogenous constrictor or dilator agonists such as the α-adrenergic nervous system, angiotensin II, endothelins, or prostaglandins, suggesting that the effects of the latter on basal tone are of lesser significance. The role of endothelial NOS/NO activity in setting vascular tone is not solely the result of shear stress (flow) stimulation. In isolated arterial preparations from normal rats in which there is physiologic pressure but no flow, vasoconstrictor responses to NOS inhibitors can be demonstrated [170]. Thus, endothelial NOS/NO activity arguably can be considered an integral part of basal vascular tone along with the direct effects of physical forces. Other neurohumoral agents that participate in adjustments in arterial tone to satisfy metabolic demand in individual organs are adenosine, oxygen, and carbon dioxide tension [171].

In summary, basal vascular tone is essential for perfusion of complex and distinct vascular beds and is dictated in large part by metabolic requirements of individual organs. It is clear that both transmural pressure and shear stress from blood flow contribute to basal arterial vascular tone. The predominant effect of vessel wall pressure is to increase tone; that of flow is to reduce tone. The mechanisms mediating the tonal response to these physical forces are only partially understood. Ca^{2+} entry, at least in part, through unique stretch-operated channels is important in pressure-induced vasoconstriction. Vascular smooth muscle cell transmembrane Na^+ concentrations are a factor in flow-related vasodilation. In addition, endothelial factors (NO, prostaglandins) are involved in flow-related vasodilation. Apart from its role in mediating shear-induced vasodilation, evidence indicates that endothelial-generated NO independently contributes to normal vascular tone. Other neurohumoral factors that contribute to changes in arterial tone dictated by metabolic demand are adenosine, oxygen, and carbon dioxide.

Vascular Reactivity. Vascular reactivity implies a vasomotor response to any neurohumoral stimulus or alteration in basal physical forces brought about by organism stress or metabolic need. For nearly all circulatory beds, concentration or dose responses have been determined to the vast majority of endogenous and exogenous vasoactive substances and to nerve stimulation. Similarly, the nature and magnitude of vascular responses to changes in perfusion pressure and flow have been characterized for most organs. These data not only have pharmacologic and therapeutic implications but also allow projection of an estimated magnitude of vascular response when neurohumoral and physical factors are altered by pathophysiologic conditions. A variety of stress states are associated with increases in vasoactive factors and autonomic nervous system activity. While some of these factors may circulate and have generalized effects such as catecholamines, angiotensin II, and atrial natriuretic peptides, others like thromboxane A_2, prostaglandin H_2 (PGH_2), endothelin-1, adenosine, platelet activating factor, neuropeptide V kinins, histamine, serotonin, NO, and PGI_2 have predominantly localized paracrine or autocrine effects. Sensitivities to these vasoactive agents vary among individual organs based on receptor density and affinity, postreceptor signaling events, and interactions with other vasoactive factors. For example, the kidney has greater vasoconstrictor sensitivity to endothelin-1 than other organs [172, 173], and adenosine, which is a vasodilator in the coronary circulation, has both dilator and constrictor effects in the renal arterial bed [174].

Another form of vasoreactivity besides neurohumoral responses is the adjustment in vascular tone to changes in perfusion pressure and flow. The most familiar type of vascular response to a change in organ perfusion pressure is autoregulation. Descriptively, autoregulation is the phenomenon of maintaining relative constancy of blood flow over a physiologic range of organ perfusion pressures. Autoregulation is a protective mechanism both in terms of preserving organ function and metabolic requirements in states of variable perfusion pressure and in preventing ischemic or hypertensive injury when perfusion pressure varies dramatically. To achieve constancy of blood flow when perfusion pressure is varied, adjustments in arterial vascular resistance are required according to the relationship flow = pressure/resistance. The renal, coronary, and cerebral circulations demonstrate autoregulatory capacity. The mechanisms underlying the autoregulatory response, that is, increase in tone of resistance arterial vessels when perfusion pressure increases and decrease in tone of these same vessels when pressure decreases, are complex and only partially understood. A fundamental component in all organs demonstrating autoregulation is the myogenic stretch response. As previously alluded, there are data supporting the role of several mechanisms in myogenic reactivity including alterations in vascular smooth muscle cell membrane properties leading to activation of ion channels, modulation of cell signaling pathways within vascular smooth mucle cells, length-dependent changes in contractile protein function, and endothelial modulation of vascular smooth muscle cell tone [175]. In addition to the myogenic response, other factors may participate in autoregulation in different organs. In the kidney, for instance, characteristics of tubular fluid flow in the distal nephron modulate arteriolar tone and autoregulation of glomerular filtration to maintain fluid and electrolyte balance (tubuloglomerular feedback). In the coronary circulation and, to a lesser extent, the cerebral circulation, metabolic demand is a major factor in autoregulation. Potential mediators of metabolic demand for stable blood flow include oxygen, carbon dioxide, and adenosine [176]. Carbon dioxide is a potent modulator of cerebral autoregulation [177].

In summary, vascular reactivity is the inherent capability of the resistance arterial vasculature of an organ to respond to circulating and locally generated neuronal and humoral stimuli, as well as to changes in the physical forces and humoral factors that establish basal vascular tone. Under some conditions of stress and metabolic demand, vascular reactivity may be essential to preserving organ function and viability. In certain pathophysiologic circumstances, altered vasoreactive capacity may actually induce or aggravate organ injury.

Mechanisms of Ischemia-Reperfusion Vascular Injury

Among the stresses that can alter basal vascular tone and reactivity is ischemia-reperfusion injury. In the following paragraphs, the ischemia-reperfusion process will be reviewed as it pertains to the arterial microvasculature.

The early effects of ischemia on the vasculature involve platelets, endothelial cells, and vascular smooth muscle cells [178]. Platelets undergo aggregations, adhesion, and release of agonists and procoagulant mediators, resulting in vasoconstriction and thrombosis. In endothelial cells and vascular smooth muscle cells, there is progressive depletion of ATP. There is increased cellular lactate, increased cytosolic Ca^{2+}, and decreased membrane Na^+,K^+-ATPase activity. Membrane and cytosolic phospholipase activity is increased with return of oxygenated blood flow through the vasculature, and the ischemic insult is terminated. However, a secondary series of noxious events ensue that are the consequence of reperfusion.

Oxidizing radicals, O_2^-, and —OH may be generated during the respiratory burst of activated polymorphonuclear neutrophil leukocytes (PMN) and from the endothelial cells subjected to ischemia-reperfusion. In endothelial cells, Ca^{2+}-dependent conversion of xanthine dehydrogenase to xanthine oxidase occurs, which generated O_2^- and H_2O_2 from hypoxanthine and available oxygen. Oxygen radicals attack lipid membranes, nucleic acid, proteins, and carbohydrates. A host of other proteases, vasoactive agonists, and proinflammatory cytokines are also released following reperfusion, both from neutrophils attached to vessel walls and from endothelial cells.

Endothelium. Because of its strategic anatomic position, the vascular endothelium is particularly vulnerable to toxin and ischemic-reperfusion injury. Following ischemia-reperfusion, the endothelium itself produces proinflammatory substances including endothelin-1, platelet activating factor, leukotriene B_4, and reactive oxygen metabolites (—O_2^-) [179] while down-regulating production of protective substances including adenosine, NO, and PGI_2 [180–182]. There is early increased expression of leukocyte components (CD11/CD18, L-selectin) and endothelial components (intracellular adhesion molecule 1 [ICAM-1], P-selectin) of the adhesion molecule system, resulting in leukocyte (primarily neutrophil) adherence and subsequent release of additional proinflammatory mediators from both endothelial cells and neutrophils, including tumor necrosis factor-α, proteinases, oxygen metabolites, platelet activating factor, and other cytokines [179]. These mediators cause endothelial detachment, basal lamina disruption, and promote diapedesis of PMN through the endothelium, where they cause injury of the underlying vessel wall cells.

The endothelial cells undergo morphologic changes as a consequence of ischemia and ischemia-reperfusion. In the cerebral vasculature, for example, ultrastructural abnormalities have ranged from thick fingerlike projections, dark osmophilic cytoplasm, clustering of ribosomal structures, and dilation of tight junctions to frank necrosis and endothelial blebbing, depending on the severity of the ischemia [183]. In the coronary arteries, total ischemia and reperfusion result in partial detachment and blebbing of the endothelial cells and both thickening and thinning of the basal lamina [184]. Comparing the cerebral and coronary vessels to the renal vasculature, there are both similarities and differences. After similar duration of ischemia, the predominant renal endothelial cell abnormality in the early reperfusion period is partial detachment from basal lamina and loss of endothelial cell-to-cell attachment [185, 186]. Unlike cerebral and coronary arterial vessels [187, 188], there are negligible ultrastructural changes of nuclei and cytoplasm of endothelial cells. However, the common abnormality in all three vascular beds is potential exposure of denuded areas of basal lamina and underlying vessel wall cells to cytokines and proteinases. Another difference between postischemic coronary/cerebral and renal endothelial injury is in the rate of restructuring of the endothelium. The intima morphology approaches normal in the kidney by 48 hours, while the ultrastructure of the endothelium remains abnormal for several days in the former vascular beds [184, 187]. The reason for the differences in endothelial recovery rates is unknown but may simply be related to the relative severity and duration of ischemia and rates of reperfusion in the different models.

Basal Lamina. The basal lamina of the arterial resistance vasculature, consisting predominantly of collagen type IV, laminin, entactin, heparan sulfate, and fibronectin [189], provides the attachment ligands for endothelial cell integrins and a supplemental barrier to diffusion of endothelial cell–generated and circulating substances into the vessel wall. While there is evidence indicating increased permeability of capillaries following ischemia and ischemia-reperfusion [190], there are no studies specifically examining disruption of endothelial cell-to-cell attachment or of the basal lamina in the resistance arterial vasculature. In the coronary microvessels following ischemia and reperfusion, increased elastase production has been demonstrated to cause degradation of the basal lamina [179]. While not exclusively related to ischemia, several studies have demonstrated glomerular basement membrane lysis in the kidney by proteinases (elastase; cathepsin G, B, and L; and serine proteinases) produced by inflammatory leukocytes [191]. The matrix proteins degraded were identical to those found in normal arterial vascular basal lamina [189].

Thus, while the evidence is indirect, there are studies that support the possibility that postischemic disruption of the basal lamina occurs during reperfusion. This disruption, due primarily to matrix component degradation by proteinases from leukocytes or endothelial cells, potentially promotes diapedesis and cytokine entry into the vessel wall and contributes to the detachment of endothelial cells by modifying expression of integrin receptors.

Smooth Muscle Cells. In the renal artery clamp model of acute renal failure in rats, Terry et al. [192] found segmental arterial and arteriolar necrosis in up to 40 percent of vessels between 4 and 96 hours after ischemia. Matthys et al. [185] and Conger and Robinette [186] reported arcuate and interlobular artery and afferent arteriolar segmental vascular smooth muscle cell necrosis 48 hours following 40 to

70 minutes of renal ischemia in rats. At 1 week, these groups also described marked thickening and fibrosis of the tunica adventitia of the interlobular arteries and afferent arterioles. The sequence of arterial morphologic changes was defined in greater detail by Conger and Robinette [186] in the norepinephrine acute renal failure model. Vacuoles appear within and between vascular smooth muscle cells 6 hours after ischemia. At 48 hours after ischemia, endothelial reattachment had largely occurred, with less than 20 percent of arterial vessels showing endothelial cell detachment. There were scattered areas of vessel wall necrosis primarily involving vascular smooth muscle cells; however, the fraction of vessels showing frank necrosis was just under 10 percent, significantly less than that reported in the more severe renal artery clamp model [185, 192]. Except for continuing evidence of intercellular vacuoles and occasional PMN or red blood cell within the vessel wall, the vast majority of vascular smooth muscle cells did not show notable ultrastructural changes. The other feature present at 48 hours postischemic insult was an increased number of "fibroblast-like" cells adjacent to the outer vascular smooth muscle cells and outside the lamina externa. By 1 week after the ischemic insult, the endothelium appeared normal. The vascular smooth muscle cells were increased in number, and intercellular vacuoles were less frequent. As was noted in the renal artery clamp model, the perivascular fibrosis was striking. There were both increased numbers of large fibroblast-like cells and extracellular matrix surrounding the arterial vessels. This process of vessel wall injury is not understood, but some evidence would support the following ischemia-reperfusion process. Loss of the endothelial protective barrier, the first event after reperfusion, exposes vessel wall cells to a variety of proinflammatory agents that can produce cytotoxicity. In addition, there is a second consequence of loss of the paracrine "cross talk" function between the intima and vessel wall cells. As a general function, the normal endothelium has a suppressive role regarding vessel wall cell mitogenesis and dedifferentiation [179]. Local production of PGI_2, NO, cyclic nucleotides, and proteoglycans (heparan sulfates) is critical to the maintenance of normal vascular smooth muscle cell and fibroblast growth and behavior in the arterial vessel wall. Recent evidence indicates that disruption of the endothelial barrier, loss of stabilizing endothelial and basal lamina factors, and activation of proinflammatory cytokines may lead to phenotypic changes in vessel wall vascular smooth muscle cells from the mature contractile form to the less differentiated proliferative form [193]. The loss of α-actin in the proliferative vascular smooth muscle cells in addition to the loss of both contraction and relaxation capacity might explain the lack of normal vasoreactivity in renal and coronary resistance vessels after ischemia-reperfusion injury [194].

Vascular Dysfunction Due to Ischemia-Reperfusion Injury

Having considered ischemia-reperfusion as an injury process to the vasculature, attention in this section is directed at the actual changes in blood vessel function in the postischemic phase, when there is variable recovery of organ blood flow. The vascular element of interest in this review is the small arterial resistance component of the circulation.

The Kidney. The kidney model that exemplifies ischemia-reperfusion injury is ischemia-induced acute renal failure. A severe form of this disorder in which the renal artery is clamped for 40 to 70 minutes followed by immediate reflow [186, 195] and a less severe form in which high-dose norepinephrine is infused into the renal artery for 90 minutes with slow spontaneous return of blood flow [186, 196] have been studied extensively in rats. In the former model, there is a brief postocclusion hyperemia, then a sustained small reduction in renal blood flow and attenuated response to endothelium-dependent dilators [196]. In the first few hours after reflow, in the latter model there is a modest reduction in renal blood flow compared to the preischemia level without hyperemia, a decreased response to endothelium-dependent vasodilators, and a small but significant reduction in the constrictor response to the NOS inhibitor L-NAME [197]. There is partial endothelial cell detachment without ultrastructural changes in individual endothelial cells at 6 hours in both the renal artery clamp and norepinephrine acute renal failure models. By 48 hours of reperfusion, the basal renal blood flow remains 20 percent reduced in the renal artery clamp model, and there is a reduced vasoreactive response to changes in renal perfusion pressure to constrictor agonists and to endothelium-dependent and endothelium-independent dilators [170]. The predominant histologic finding at this time in the small resistance arteries and arterioles is vascular smooth muscle cell necrosis, present in 55 to 60 percent of the vessels [185, 193]. It is assumed that the lack of response to vasoactive stimuli is due to the diffuse vascular smooth muscle cell injury related to both the relative severity of ischemia and the rapidity of reperfusion. In the norepinephrine acute renal failure model at 48 hours, the basal renal blood flow also is approximately 20 percent less than normal [170, 186]. However, vascular reactivity is strikingly different from that in the renal artery clamp acute renal failure model. The difference likely is due to less severe ischemia and a slower rate of reperfusion. There is an exaggerated renal vasoconstrictor response to angiotensin II and endothelin-1 both in vivo and in arterioles isolated from these kidneys [170, 198]. Response to endothelium-dependent vasodilators is reduced, but the constrictor response to L-NAME is actually increased [170]. cNOS can be identified as at least as strongly reactive or more reactive than normal, as determined with cNOS monoclonal antibody in the resistance arterial vessels [199]. While there is a dilator response to cyclic adenosine monophosphate–dependent PGI_2 in the 48-hour postischemic renal vasculature, there is no increase in renal blood flow to the NO donor sodium nitroprusside. Taken together, these data indicate that at 48 hours after ischemia in norepinephrine acute renal failure in the rat kidney, vascular cNOS activity is not diminished, but rather is maximal such that it cannot be stimulated further by endothelium-dependent vasodilators. The available NO under basal conditions has fully activated vascular smooth muscle cell soluble cyclic guanosine monophosphate such that there is no additional response to an exogenous NO donor. It is suggested, but not demonstrated, that the increase in NOS activity may be a "protective" response to an underlying vasoconstrictor stimulus that is the direct consequence of the ischemia-reperfusion injury. The nature of the constrictor stimulus is unknown but is not likely to be endothelin-1, thromboxane A_2, or angiotensin II, based on unpublished pharmacologic inhibition studies [200]. However, the exaggerated constrictor response observed both in vivo and in vitro in 48-hour postischemic renal arterial vessels to NOS inhibition indicates that the constrictor stimulus is potent.

In examining the mechanism for the constrictor hypersensitivity in the 48-hour postischemic vasculature in norepinephrine acute renal failure, measurements of vascular smooth muscle cell cytosolic calcium Ca^{2+} have been made in the isolated arterioles from these kidneys perfused at physiologic pressures [198]. Compared to similar vessels from sham acute renal failure kidneys, there is a significantly higher baseline and an earlier and greater increase in vascular smooth muscle cell Ca^{2+} in response to a normal half-maximal constricting concentration (EC_{50}) of angiotensin II, which correlates with the initially lower and more intense reduction in lumen diameter in the postischemic acute renal failure vessels. The mechanism of the basal increase in vascular smooth muscle cell Ca^{2+} and the exaggerated increase in response to a constrictor agonist are as yet undetermined, but the increase in baseline vascular smooth muscle cell Ca^{2+} also suggests that possibility of an ischemia-reperfusion induction of a primary vasoconstrictor stimulus. Another novel observation regarding vascular smooth muscle cell Ca^{2+} in 48-hour postischemic renal arterioles in vitro is a paradoxical change in vascular smooth muscle cell Ca^{2+} in response to changes in lumen pressure. In normal afferent and efferent arterioles, increasing lumen pressure (stretch) within an autoregulatory range for these vessels results in an increase in vascular smooth muscle cell Ca^{2+}. Conversely, decreasing lumen pressure is associated with a decrease in vascular smooth muscle cell Ca^{2+}. In the norepinephrine acute renal failure vessels, the reverse relationships are observed. There are also corresponding paradoxical changes in lumen diameter representing, at least, a loss of the myogenic response and, at most, a "reverse" myogenic response. This abnormal vascular smooth muscle cell Ca^{2+} and myogenic response to pressure is suggested to be the basis of the markedly abnormal in vivo autoregulatory response between 48 hours and 1 week after acute renal failure induction that is likely the most significant and clinically relevant ischemia-reperfusion disorder of vasoreactivity in the kidney.

At 1 week after ischemic injury, the endothelium appears normal, smooth muscle necrosis is less evident, but perivascular fibrosis is marked in the mid- to small-sized arterial vessels [186]. Functionally, the response to endothelium-dependent dilators is reduced, L-NAME constrictor response is increased, and immunologically-detectable NOS is present [199]. There is a decreased dilator response to sodium nitroprusside, but a measurable, albeit slightly reduced dilator response to PGI_2 [199]. These findings suggest maximal endothelial cNOS activity similar to that at 48 hours. Unlike 48-hour vessels, the vasoconstrictor response to angiotensin II was markedly attenuated both in vivo and in vitro at 1 week [170, 200]. On the other hand, as previously alluded, a paradoxical vasoconstriction to a reduction in perfusion pressure in the autoregulatory range could be demonstrated in vivo. It is difficult to suggest a single mechanism that explains this series of functional aberrations at 1 week. It is likely that more than one pathophysiologic process is operating to produce these complex responses.

By 30 days after the ischemia-reperfusion insult in norepinephrine acute renal failure, there is minimal residual fibrosis of the tunica adventitia; the remainder of the vascular morphology appears normal. The functional responses to constrictor and dilator agonists and to changes in pressure and flow have returned to near normal [200].

In summary, ischemia-reperfusion injury is accompanied by dramatic changes in basal and reactive vascular function of the organ involved. There are similarities in altered organ vascular function, particularly in the early reperfusion period of 24 to 48 hours, including changes in permeability, decreased basal organ blood flow, hypersensitivity to vasoconstrictor stimuli, and attenuated response to vasodilators. The reduced responsiveness to endothelium-dependent vasodilators may be due to an actual reduction in endothelial NOS activity or to an actual spontaneous maximal NOS/NO activity that cannot be stimulated further by endothelium-dependent agents. Correlating the actual ischemia-reperfusion injury process with the morphologic changes in the vasculature and specific mechanisms of dysfunction will require considerable additional investigative effort.

Clinical Relevance of Ischemia-Reperfusion Vascular Injury

Are there important clinical implications of these postischemic abnormalities of vascular function? In discussing potential patient-related consequences of ischemia-reperfusion vascular injury, there is a distinction between direct parenchymal cell injury, such as the initial severity of tubular degeneration in acute renal failure, and the abnormalities that occur as the result of subsequent reduced basal blood flow and aberrant vasoreactivity of resistance vessels. The latter, which has been the focus of this review, may have more subtle, but unique clinical consequences.

The course of human ischemia-induced acute renal failure is highly variable. An important and relevant observation regarding the variable duration and, in particular, the prolonged course in acute renal failure patients was made by Solez et al. [201]. In individuals with acute renal failure duration of longer than 3 weeks, a prominent finding in biopsy or autopsy specimens was fresh tubular renal ischemic lesions that could not be related to the remote initial ischemic insult. A possible explanation for the fresh ischemic lesions was altered reactivity of the renal vasculature. Abnormal vascular reactivity in established ischemic acute renal failure animal models includes loss of renal blood flow autoregulation. A number of investigators [185, 200, 202] have found an attenuated autoregulatory response from 2 to 7 days after acute renal failure induction in the renal artery clamp model in rats. In the norepinephrine acute renal failure model in rats, there was an actual paradoxical vasoconstriction with renal perfusion pressure reduction in the autoregulatory range [185]. Kelleher et al. [203] and Conger et al. [204], using this norepinephrine acute renal failure model, have shown that transient reduction in mean renal perfusion pressure to only 90 mm Hg for 4 hours in 1 week after inducing acute renal failure resulted in worsening azotemia and recurrent focal ischemic injury, which prolonged recovery from acute renal failure. This minimal renal perfusion pressure reduction had no effects on sham acute renal failure rats. These data have important clinical implications, as a modest arterial pressure reduction during the course of this disease, such as frequently occurs with hemodialysis treatment, can actually result in recurrent ischemic injury and prolongation of acute renal failure [205].

Role of Vasodilatory Substances

Endogenous vasodilators are involved in the hemodynamic changes that both initiate and maintain acute renal failure. Exogenously administered vasodilators, with or without diuretics, are the principal agents that have been used in the pharmacologic therapy of this disease. Not only are vasodilators of historic interest in pathogenesis and treatment, they continue to represent a major area of focus in investigative efforts in acute renal failure. In this section, the roles of endogenously generated vasodilators in the pathophysiology of ischemic and nephrotoxic acute renal failure will be considered, as well as the therapeutic use of vasorelaxing substances in animal models and in clinical acute renal failure. Emphasis will be placed on findings and observations that have been made in the past decade.

Prostaglandins

Robertson et al. [206] demonstrated in a rat micropuncture study what had been suspected from filtration fraction measurements in whole-kidney experiments, that is, the primary hemodynamic function of the kidney is the autoregulation and maintenance of GFR. When renal perfusion pressure was reduced, as occurs in the initial phase of renal ischemia, preglomerular arterial resistance decreased and efferent arteriolar resistance increased to maintain glomerular capillary hydraulic pressure (P_{GC}) and single-nephron GFR relatively constant. The efferent arteriolar constriction is mediated, in large part, through the local renin-angiotensin system [207]. Activation of the renin-angiotensin system, however, stimulated synthesis of cyclooxygenase products, including the vasodilator prostaglandins PGI_2 and PGE_2 [208]. PGI_2 and PGE_2 oppose the constrictor effects of angiotensin II, thereby attenuating the reduction in renal blood flow as renal perfusion pressure declines. The modulating vasodilator effect of prostaglandins in the setting of impending ischemia appeared to be greater in afferent than efferent arterioles. When PGI_2 and PGE_2 were administered exogenously during reduced renal perfusion, filtration fraction increased, with better preservation of GFR than renal blood flow [209, 210], suggesting that vasodilator prostaglandins preferentially caused preglomerular vasorelaxation under these conditions.

Prostaglandin synthesis was found to be increased in animal models of ischemic acute renal failure [209, 211], aminoglycoside nephrotoxicity [212], sepsis, and endotoxic shock [213, 214]. The indication that an increase in prostaglandin activity was renoprotective (by maintaining glomerular hemodynamics) was the observation that cyclooxygenase inhibitors in these disorders augmented the reduction in renal blood flow and GFR [215, 216].

Other evidence of protection in acute renal failure was the finding that infusion of biologic prostaglandins and their analogues in ischemic [209, 210], mercuric chloride [217], and glycerol-induced acute renal failure [218] improved GFR and attenuated tubular necrosis. In all but one of the studies [219], the protective effect was observed only when prostaglandins were given before or during acute renal failure induction.

A predisposing role of reduced intrinsic prostaglandin activity to the development of acute renal failure has been considered by several investigators. For example, low plasma or urinary prostaglandin metabolites have been found during cyclosporine administration [220], thrombotic thrombocytopenic purpura [221], Henoch-Schönlein purpura [222], hemolytic-uremic syndrome [223], and the hepatorenal syndrome [224].

It has been recognized that treatment with NSAID, an induced state of reduced cyclooxygenase activity, can precipitate acute renal failure in settings of prerenal azotemia such as hepatic cirrhosis [43] and congestive heart failure [44]. There are other data, however, that bring into question the predisposing importance of prostaglandins. Infusion of PGI_2 to thrombotic thrombocytopenic patients did not prevent acute renal failure [225], and a more recent study by Tonshoff et al. [226] suggested that prostaglandin synthesis may actually be increased in the hemolytic-uremic syndrome.

Finally, it should be noted that the protective effects of prostaglandins in disorders of acute renal dysfunction may not be entirely through a hemodynamic mechanism. Prostaglandins have other effects, particularly on immunologic and thrombotic processes [227]. Thus, interpretation of the role of prostaglandins in acute renal failure requires consideration of the potential for complex effects.

Natriuretic Peptides

In 1981 de Bold et al. [228] reported the natriuretic effects of an extract of mammalian atrial myocytes. Subsequently, this substance has been characterized as a polypeptide. There are small species variations in peptide chain length and amino acid sequence. However, the basic structure of the precursor molecule contains approximately 150 amino acids (152 amino acids in humans and rats) [229]. The active portion of the polypeptide is the —COOH terminus, which contains approximately 25 amino acids (28 amino acids in humans) and a cys-cys disulfide bond [230]. There are several natural and synthetic variations of the active peptide component.

The primary stimulus to atrial natriuretic peptide (ANP) synthesis and release is distention of the atria, where storage granules have been identified. Infusion of normal saline into human volunteers increased plasma ANP twofold from basal levels of less than 25 pg/ml [231]. Shenker et al. [232] found that plasma ANP levels were elevated in edematous states that involved increased intravascular volume and atrial enlargement such as congestive heart failure. However, plasma ANP in edematous states not involving atrial stretch (cirrhosis, nephrotic syndrome) has not been found consistently to be increased. In addition to atrial enlargement, endothelins have been found to be potent direct stimuli of cardiac ANP release [233].

ANP has a relatively short plasma half-life of approximately 5 minutes. Clearance receptors are located primarily in the lung, liver, and kidney [234]. Neutral endopeptidase is the principal ANP degradative enzyme in these tissues [235].

Natural and synthetic ANPs cause dose-dependent reductions in systemic arterial pressure. The mechanism involves both peripheral vasorelaxation and a reduction in cardiac output [236, 237]. The magnitude of arterial pressure reduction is dependent on the state of basal vascular tone. The vasorelaxing effect of ANP is greater when there is an increase in peripheral vascular resistance [238, 239]. ANP has been shown to inhibit both secretion and activity of the renin-angiotensin-aldosterone [240] and adrenergic nervous systems [241], as well as that of vasopressin [242] and endothelin-1 [243].

The most notable effects of ANP are on the kidney. The natriuresis induced by ANP is associated with an increase in GFR. In addition, there are direct inhibitory effects of ANP on sodium and water reabsorption that appear to be confined to the distal nephron [244, 245]. Most, but not all investigators have found that in vivo infusion of ANPs, both synthetic and naturally occurring from a variety of species, markedly increased GFR while having a proportionately smaller effect on renal blood flow [238, 246]. Studies by Aalkjaer et al. [247] and Veldkamp and associates [248] suggested that ANP-induced renal vasorelaxation was specific for the preglomerular arterioles. Other studies examining the rat renal microvasculature in vitro by Loutzenhiser et al. [249] and Lanese and associates [250] indicated that ANP not only directly vasodilated the afferent arteriole but also constricted the efferent arteriole. The magnitude of afferent arteriolar relaxation was dependent on the initial vascular tone. The mechanism for the apparent paradoxical effects of ANP on the pre- and postglomerular resistance vessels is unknown, but it does not appear to involve selective mediation by a known second vasoactive agent [250]. Consistent with these in vitro findings was the in vivo micropuncture observation that ANP substantially increased glomerular capillary hydraulic pressure. The tubular natriuretic effects of ANP involve inhibition of sodium and water transport in the loop of Henle, connecting tubules, and collecting duct. Among other possible mechanisms, ANP has been shown to interfere with vasopressin effect and to alter adenylate cyclase activity.

Recently, other natriuretic peptides have been discovered. One such 32 amino acid substance, urodilatin, is four amino acids longer at the NH_2 terminus than human ANP. It is not detectable in the plasma but has been isolated from human urine [251, 252]. It is likely produced by the kidney. Urodilatin has equal or greater natriuretic potency when compared to ANP and is resistant to renal cortical endopeptidase activity. Another class of natriuretic peptides is referred to as brain natriuretic peptide (BNP). It has been isolated from both brain and heart [253, 254]. BNP, which contains 32 amino acids, has diuretic and natriuretic effects similar to ANP, while the hypotensive effect is not as potent. Finally, another newly described natriuretic peptide is termed C-type natriuretic peptide (CNP). It contains 22 amino acids and like ANP has a 17 amino acid ring formed by a disulfide bond [255]. CNP has been isolated from brain and heart endothelium [256]. The vasorelaxing effects of CNP, which predominate over a sodium excretory effect, are mediated through a separate particulate guanylate cyclase smooth muscle receptor probably in a paracrine manner [255]. The effects of BNP and CNP on acute renal failure are presently unknown.

In the late 1980s, a series of reports began to appear that demonstrated a positive effect of ANPs on ischemic and nephrotoxic animal models of acute renal failure. Schafferans et al. [257] found that ANP improved renal function in norepinephrine-induced acute renal failure. Similarly, Nakamoto et al. [258] and Shaw and associates [259] were able to shorten the course of renal artery clamp acute renal failure in rats with ANP and atriopeptin III, respectively. The latter is a 24 amino acid COOH-terminus ANP derivative. Neumayer et al. [260] gave an ANP bolus of 100 μg/kg for 180 minutes intra-arterially after 120 minutes of renal ischemia in dogs. Boluses of ANP were repeated on two subsequent days. Renal blood flow was not changed appreciably, but GFR was twice that of vehicle-treated dogs. Lieberthal et al. [261] have shown that neither ANP nor mannitol alone, but the combination of both agents improved GFR following ischemia in an isolated perfused rat kidney. A13 amino acid ANP analogue (A68828) given after clamp ischemia in rats improved GFR [262]. Dopamine was given to prevent hypotension, which was associated with infusion of the ANP analogue. Conger et al. [263] found a marked improvement in GFR in a rat renal artery clamp model when atriopeptin III (0.2 μg/kg/min) was given intravenously immediately after clamp release in combination with dopamine sufficient to maintain mean arterial pressure above 100 mm Hg. In that study, it was found that the primary effects of atriopeptin III were to increase glomerular capillary hydraulic pressure and plasma flow. In a subsequent study by the same group, atriopeptin III and dopamine were infused intravenously for 4 hours in awake rats 2 days after inducing acute renal failure with norepinephrine [264]. Renal function was examined 2 days thereafter. Renal blood flow and GFR were twofold higher in the atriopeptin III plus dopamine–treated group compared to a saline-treated control group. Tubular necrosis and cast formation were also less in the atriopeptin III plus dopamine–treated group. Intravenous ANP was found to be effective in improving GFR in gentamicin-induced acute renal failure [265]. However, ANP increased GFR only transiently in uranyl nitrate–induced acute renal failure [266]. After the ANP infusion was discontinued, GFR fell to the same reduced level found in saline-treated rats. Capasso et al. [267] gave ANP (12 μg/kg bolus, 1 μg/kg/min maintenance infusion intravenously) to rats 3 days after inducing acute renal failure with cisplatin. There was a prompt doubling of GFR during maintenance ANP infusion. Finally, Shaw et al. [268] showed that urodilatin combined with dopamine reversed ischemic acute renal failure in the rat.

What was most intriguing about the use of ANP in acute renal failure models was that it was effective when given after the initiating insult. In fact, it attenuated the course of acute renal failure when given as late as 2 days after the initiating ischemic event. Except for a rare report with verapamil [269] and prostaglandins [219], this effect was unique. It also made ANP a clinically promising agent in managing acute renal failure patients. In addition, ANP directly increased GFR in pathophysiologic states by altering pre- and postglomerular vascular resistances to increase P_{GC}. ANP also had direct diuretic and natriuretic effects on the distal nephron. These pharmacologic properties made ANP an ideally suited substance to counteract two proposed pathophysiologic mechanism of GFR reduction in acute renal failure: reduced glomerular perfusion and tubular obstruction.

Based on the encouraging animal experimental results and the unique combination of pharmacologic properties, Rahman and associates [270] entered 53 patients meeting clinical and laboratory criteria of established intrinsic acute renal failure to one of two treatment groups. The first group of patients were treated with ANP with or without diuretics. Group II patients were treated with or without diuretics but no ANP. Age, sex, etiology of acute renal failure, entry serum creatinine (group I, 5.3 ± 1.8 mg/dl; group II, 5.1 ± 2.1 mg/dl), and creatinine clearances (C_{cr}) (group I, 9.9 ± 2.1 ml/min; group II, 9.2 ± 2.1 ml/min) were similar in both groups. Thirty group I patients received ANP (0.20 μg/kg/min IV × 24 hours [N = 20] or 0.08 μg/kg/min intra-arterially × 8 hours [N = 10]) and furosemide (0.5 mg/kg/hr × 24 hours), or mannitol (12.5 g every 6 hours × 4), or no diuretic; 23 group II patients received either diuretics as for group I or no diuretic in a similar distribution to group I. C_{cr} (verified with simultaneous inulin clearances $\times$ 12, r = 0.93, $p < 0.001$) increased significantly by 8 hours of ANP treatment to 17.1 $\pm$ 3.2 ml/min and by 24 hours after discontinuing ANP to 21.0 $\pm$ 4.4 ml/min (both $p < 0.05$). There was no corresponding increase in C_{cr} in group II. Dialysis was required in 23 percent of group I and 52 percent of group II patients (different at $p < 0.05$). Mortality rates of 17 percent for group I and 35 percent for group II were not significantly different ($p = 0.11$). Significant hypotension occurred in only one patient. A large study consisting of 504 patients was conducted at more than 60 centers in the United States and Canada to further examine the utility of ANP in the setting of acute renal failure. The preliminary results of the phase III clinical study indicate that ANP did not reduce the need for dialysis in the broad patient population, nor did the drug reduce mortality. The study did, however, demonstrate that ANP significantly reduced the need for dialysis in the oliguric subgroup of patients with acute renal failure [271].

Calcium Channel Blockers

Calcium channel blockers, which inhibit voltage-gated calcium entry, have been used in a number of acute renal failure models. Malis et al. [272] infused verapamil (5 μg/kg/min) before and after ischemic acute renal failure induction with norepinephrine or renal artery clamping in rats. There was no improvement on GFR in the treated groups except when verapamil was given prior to norepinephrine infusion, which in fact attenuated the magnitude of induced ischemia. In contrast to the findings of Malis et al. [272] in rats, Burke et al. [269] found a protective effect of both verapamil (5 μg/kg/min) and nifedipine (2 μg/kg/min) when given before and a reversal effect when given after norepinephrine-induced ischemia in dogs. The preinduction protective effect, as indicated by improved renal blood flow and GFR, was greater than the postinduction reversal effect at 24 hours. Morphology and mitochondrial calcium were also normalized by the calcium channel blockers. Wagner et al. [273] infused diltiazem (5 μg/kg/min) continuously into the aorta for 7 days after ischemic acute renal failure induction or from 3 days before until seven days after ischemia in dogs. There was a smaller postischemic decrease in GFR in the latter, but not the former group compared to saline-infused dogs. In a similar study in rats, Garthoff et al. [274] found that the dihydropyridine nisoldipine added to the diet from 4 days before until 3 days after ischemia improved renal function, decreased renal tissue calcium, and increased ATP content. In a rat model of cisplatin acute renal failure [275], it was found that nifedipine given from 2 days before until 5 days after beginning cisplatin improved renal function if given in a low dose (0.1 μg/kg/day) but actually aggravated acute renal failure when given in higher doses (0.3 and 0.6 μg/kg/day). It was suggested the lower dose may have been cytoprotective, while the larger doses increased GFR, augmenting cisplatin delivery to the renal tubules. In a gentamicin nephrotoxic model, nitrendipine (25 μg/kg/day) during gentamicin exposure improved GFR despite similar tissue aminoglycoside content [276]. Verapamil (10 mg/100 ml drinking water), on the other hand, was not protective in the same aminoglycoside rat model [277]. Dobyan and Bulger [278] found that pretreatment with the nonselective calcium channel blocker chlorpromazine improved GFR and renal morphology 2 to 4 days after acute renal failure induction with mercuric chloride.

While calcium channel blockers have been examined extensively in experimental acute renal failure, few clinical studies have been carried out. Lumlertgul et al. [279] gave gallopamil (40–80 μg/min) for 4 hours intrarenally combined with furosemide (0.8 mg/kg/hr) for 24 hours to five patients with malaria- or leptospirosis-related acute renal failure. Five similar patients were treated with intravenous furosemide only and served as controls. Recovery of GFR was more rapid in the gallopamil-treated group. Other human experience with calcium channel blockers has largely been in the setting of renal transplantation. Duggan et al. [280] found that verapamil improved early graft function when administered to donors prior to harvesting the kidneys. Wagner et al. [281] gave diltiazem to transplant patients immediately after graft placement. The level of graft function was better and the incidence of post-transplant acute renal failure was less in diltiazem-treated patients. While Bakris and Burnett [282] found calcium channel blockers to be protective against radiocontrast-induced reduction in renal blood flow and GFR in rabbits, Caboub et al. [283] did not find a difference in postcontrast serum creatinine elevations in patients with mild chronic renal failure who were and were not being treated with nifedipine for hypertension. Diltiazem also was not found to protect renal function in patients given methotrexate [284].

Tubular Obstruction in Renal Cell Injury

Tubular obstruction is an important pathophysiological event in acute renal failure [285]. Early studies showed that one hour of ischemia causes a dramatic increase in proximal tubular pressure [285]. The potential mechanism of tubular obstruction and increased proximal tubular pressure in acute renal failure has been investigated. It was originally thought that necrotic tubular cells were the major components of casts obstructing the tubular lumen. However, recent studies have found the presence of viable tubular cells in the urine of patients with acute renal failure [286]. This raises the alternative possibility that exfoliation of viable tubular cells is the cause of tubular obstruction. It has been demonstrated in tubular cells exposed to oxidative stress that detachment of viable tubular cells is caused by reorientation of integrins from a predominantly basolateral location to the apical membrane where they can mediate cell–cell adhesion via an arginine-glycine-aspartic acid (RGD) inhibitable mechanism [287]. The RGD sequence is the most common domain contained in a variety of matrix proteins and serves as the recognition site for various integrin receptors. A subsequent in vivo study demonstrated that infusions of a synthetic RGD peptide into the renal artery during the reperfusion period abolished the characteristic elevation of proximal tubular pressure which served as an index of tubular obstruction [288]. The most recent study demonstrated that systemic administration of two highly potent cyclic RGD peptides infused after the release of renal artery clamp ameliorated ischemic acute renal failure in rats [289]. This study also suggested that cyclic RGD peptides inhibited tubular obstruction by predominantly preventing cell-to-cell adhesion, rather than cell-to-matrix adhesion. Another potential mechanism of tubular obstruction is the binding of tubular cells to Tamm Horsfall protein (THP) or uromodulin. THP is the most abundant protein in the urine and is made exclusively in the epithelial cells of the thick ascending limb of the loop of Henle and the early part of the distal convoluted tubule. THP binds to cellular debris in the urine from the proximal tubule, forms a cast in the tubule lumen, and obstructs further flow of urine. Whether tubular cells seen in THP casts are merely physically trapped or whether there are specific receptor-ligand interactions between THP and exfoliated tubular cells is not known. THP released in the tubule tends to gel, potentially aided by a rise in concentration of sodium and other ions in the tubular fluid. Thus, increased distal delivery of sodium in the nephron in acute renal failure would also promote THP to a gel form. The protein sequence of THP is known and there is an RGD sequence at position 143-145. The functional significance of the RGD peptide on THP was suggested by a study which found that neutrophil adhesion to THP was inhibited by synthetic RGD peptides [290]. It is possible that the detached tubular cells adhere to THP in the distal tubule via the RGD sequence. This adhesion of viable tubular cells to the large THP may promote tubule cast formation, distal tubular obstruction and decreased GFR.

Therapeutic Role of Growth Factors

The growth factors, insulin like growth factor (IGF-I), epidermal growth factor (EGF), and hepatocyte growth factor (HGF) are known to bind specific receptors in the proximal tubule and regulate metabolic, transport, and proliferative responses in these cells. Both HGF and IGF-I accelerate the recovery of renal function and regeneration of damaged proximal tubular epithelium and improve the mortality in postischemic rat tubular injury [291, 292]. Clinical studies of IGF-I in ARF are under way.

Diagnosis of Acute Renal Failure

The diagnosis of acute renal failure must be a diagnosis of exclusion, since both prerenal and postrenal factors may lead to an acute deterioration of renal function and cause azotemia. In contrast to acute renal failure, however, the states of prerenal and postrenal azotemia are immediately reversible.

Prerenal Azotemia

Events leading to a decrease in renal perfusion pressure or an increase in renal vascular resistance, or both, may diminish GFR to such a degree that the daily endogenous load of nitrogenous wastes cannot be excreted. The resultant accumulation of wastes may be referred to as prerenal azotemia. Table 10-2 lists some of the clinical circumstances in which this reversible variety of azotemia may occur. The azotemic state can be corrected immediately if the extrarenal circumstance causing the renal ischemia is reversed. Such an improvement in renal function may involve increasing ECF volume, enhancing cardiac output, or correcting the cause of systemic vasodilation, such as bacteremia or excessive use of antihypertensive drugs. Correction or improvement of an insult, such as anesthesia, surgical trauma, liver disease, or bilateral renal vascular occlusion, may also reverse a state of prerenal

Table 10-2. Conditions causing prerenal azotemia

Hypovolemia
   Hemorrhage
   Gastrointestinal losses
   Third space
      Burns
      Peritonitis
      Traumatized tissue
      Diuretic abuse
   Diuretic abuser
Impaired cardiac function
   Congestive heart failure
   Myocardial infarction
   Pericardial tamponade
   Acute pulmonary embolism
Peripheral vasodilatation
   Bacteremia
   Antihypertensive medications
Increased renal vascular resistance
   Anesthesia
   Surgical operation
   Hepatorenal syndrome
Renal vascular obstruction, bilateral
   Embolism
   Thrombosis

azotemia. A careful search by history and physical examination for causes of prerenal azotemia, therefore, must constitute the initial undertaking in the evaluation of patients with the potential diagnosis of acute renal failure.

Postrenal Azotemia

Events occurring subsequent to urine formation and obstructing its elimination from the urinary tract also must be sought in the process of diagnosing acute renal failure. The retention of nitrogenous waste as a result of obstruction of urine may be referred to as postrenal azotemia. Urinary tract obstruction is discussed in detail in Chapter 12. A general list of causes of urinary tract obstruction that may lead to postrenal azotemia is given in Table 10-3. The presence of urethral and bladder-neck obstruction can be evaluated by estimating the volume of residual urine in the bladder after an attempt at complete voiding. Profound obstruction at these sites may lead to a degree of bladder distention that can be detected by suprapubic percussion or palpation. In addition to anatomic causes, functional disturbances of bladder emptying also must be considered. Autonomic insufficiency, spinal cord lesions, and anticholinergic agents may cause functional bladder-neck obstruction and thus postrenal azotemia. Other obstructive sites in the genitourinary tract that may lead to postrenal failure are the ureterovesical, ureteral, and ureteropelvic areas. In the absence of a single kidney or previously impaired renal function, postrenal azotemia occurs

Table 10-3. Conditions causing postrenal azotemia

Urethral obstruction
Bladder neck obstruction
  Prostatic hypertrophy
  Bladder carcinoma
  Bladder infection
  Functional: neuropathy or ganglionic blocking agents
Obstruction of ureters, bilateral
  Intraureteral
    Sulfonamide and uric acid crystals
    Blood clots
    Pyogenic debris
    Stones
    Edema
    Necrotizing papillitis
  Extraureteral
    Tumor: cervix, prostate, endometriosis
    Periureteral fibrosis
    Accidental ureteral ligation during pelvic operation
    Pelvic abscess
    Pelvic hematoma
    Ascites
    Pregnancy

only with bilateral obstruction of the urinary tract at these sites. Since 90 percent of renal calculi are radiopaque, a flat-plate roentgenogram of the abdomen (kidney, ureter, bladder [KUB]) should always be obtained during the evaluation of an azotemic patient. In the absence of knowledge as to the natural history of the renal failure, the KUB roentgenogram may also be helpful in differentiating acute from chronic renal failure, since bilaterally small kidneys suggest an advanced form of chronic renal disease. It should be remembered, however, that patients afflicted with chronic renal disease secondary to diabetes mellitus, amyloidosis, renal vein thrombosis, polycystic disease, and scleroderma may have normal-sized or enlarged kidneys.

Hemorrhage from polycystic or traumatized kidneys or the use of chemotherapy for neoplasms may incriminate blood clots and uric acid crystals, respectively, as causes of bilateral ureteral obstruction. A history of analgesic nephropathy, sickle cell anemia, diabetes mellitus, or acute pyelonephritis may suggest obstruction secondary to papillary necrosis [293]. Acute pyelonephritis also may be associated with unilateral or bilateral ureteral obstruction secondary to accumulation of pyogenic debris. A pelvic examination is mandatory in the evaluation of postrenal azotemia, because patients with cervical or endometrial carcinoma or endometriosis may present with azotemia secondary to bilateral ureteral obstruction. Vague back pain and a history of migraine headaches with chronic ingestion of methysergide suggest the diagnosis of retroperitoneal fibrosis [294]. As with prerenal azotemia and in contrast to acute renal failure, postrenal azotemia is immediately reversible when the obstructive lesion is corrected. The rapidity of the recovery of renal function, however, depends on the duration and completeness of the obstruction. With the recognition and increased evidence of radiocontrast-induced acute renal failure, it is most appropriate to use ultrasonography to exclude urinary tract obstruction. In some cases, retrograde pyelography may be necessary to exclude urinary tract obstruction definitively. Renal ultrasonography will detect pelvicalyceal dilatation secondary to obstruction in more than 90 percent of patients. Staghorn calculi and small shrunken kidneys, however, decrease this sensitivity, and extrarenal pelvices may produce a false-positive diagnosis. Pelvicalyceal dilatation may not occur in some cases of retroperitoneal fibrosis.

Evaluation of Urine Volume, Sediment, and Composition

After prerenal and postrenal failure have been excluded, the diagnosis of acute renal failure can be entertained and supported by evaluation of the urine. In acute renal failure, the urine volume may vary over a wide range. As classically defined, a 24-hour urine volume of less than 400 ml is compatible with the diagnosis of oliguric acute renal failure. However, in as many as half the cases of acute renal failure, the daily urine volume may exceed this amount and actually be as high as 1.5 to 2.0 L/day [295]. This form of acute renal failure has been termed *nonoliguric* acute renal failure. It is frequently associated with nephrotoxin-induced disease and tends to carry a lower morbidity and mortality than oliguric failure. In nonoliguric renal failure, urinary sodium concentration, fractional excretion of sodium, and urine to plasma creatinine ratio are lower at the time of diagnosis than in oliguric acute renal failure [296]. The exact mechanism for the higher urine flow in this variety of acute renal failure is not known. However, the finding of a higher creatinine clearance in nonoliguric patients suggests that the GFR may be better preserved [297]. Despite liberal daily urine volumes, progressive azotemia with nonoliguric acute renal failure may occur in the following manner. Since the abolition of the renal concentration capacity is a characteristic of acute renal failure, approximately 300 mOsm of solute can be excreted in each liter of isotonic urine. The catabolic rate of patients with acute renal failure is often markedly increased. In these individuals, there may be an exogenous plus endogenous solute load as great as 900 mOsm/day. The daily excretion of 2 liters of isotonic urine thus will eliminate only 600 mOsm of the 900-mOsm solute load. Therefore, despite a daily urine output of 2 liters, progressive azotemia will result because of the 300-mOsm daily positive solute balance. Such is the sequence of events that occurs in nonoliguric renal failure.

The renal concentrating capacity is not abolished in prerenal failure, and urine volumes thus are generally in the range of 500 ml/day. In patients with impaired renal concentration, however, polyuria may be present in association with prerenal azotemia [298]. However, since partial urinary tract obstruction may be associated with the abolition of renal concentrating capacity, daily urine volumes in patients with postrenal azotemia may vary over a wide range (500 ml/day to 2–4 L/day). In contrast to patients with acute renal failure, the urine volume in patients with postrenal azotemia may be variable, depending on the constancy of the obstruction. For example, with passage of renal calculi or necrotic papillae, periods of severe oliguria may alternate with periods of polyuria. During the recovery phase of acute renal failure, the urine volumes should gradually increase rather than exhibit marked increases or decreases from day to day. If a progressive rise in urine flow during the recovery phase of acute renal failure reaches what appears to be a premature plateau, or actually decreases, a complicating event such as ECF volume depletion or nephrotoxic drugs should be suspected.

Anuria has been defined in the past as a 24-hour urine volume of less than 75 ml and has been suggested to be more compatible with urinary tract obstruction or renal vascular occlusion than with acute renal failure. Such a definition of anuria, however, is probably not appropriate. During the first few days of oliguric acute renal failure, urine volumes may frequently be less than 75 ml/day when assessed by bladder catheterization. It has been documented that such severe oliguria can occur with acute renal failure in the absence of renal vascular or urinary tract obstruction [299]. Anuria, therefore, is best defined as the excretion of no urine as documented by bladder catheterization. Anuria by this definition may suggest bilateral renal artery occlusion and thus the need for emergency renal arteriography, particularly in the appropriate clinical setting, such as atrial fibrillation with arterial emboli, abdominal trauma, or a dissecting aortic aneurysm. Because of the slower progression of irreversible functional loss with urinary tract obstruction, some minimal delay (a few days) in establishing this diagnosis may be acceptable, depending on the clinical status of the patient.

Assessment of the urinary sediment also is helpful in the diagnosis of acute renal failure. An active sediment with renal tubular epithelial cells, cellular debris, and tubular cell casts supports the diagnosis of acute renal failure. Frequently, however, the urine contains only granular casts without renal tubule cells or tubular cell casts. A few red and white blood cells per high-power field and $1+$ to $2+$ proteinuria by dipstick are compatible with the diagnosis of acute renal failure. Although it is extraordinarily uncommon, some observers have reported the transient occurrence of a few red blood cell casts in the urine of patients with acute renal failure. Large amounts of urinary protein (>3.0 g/24 hr) and numerous red blood cell casts are indicative of acute renal failure secondary to renal parenchymal disease, such as acute oliguric glomerulonephritis or vasculitis. The absence of cellular elements and protein in the urine is most compatible with prerenal and postrenal azotemia. Prerenal azotemia with a urinary protein excretion greater than 3.0 g/24 hr, however, may occur with severe congestive heart failure. Most of these cases were reported, however, in an era when mercurial diuretics were being used. An abundance of crystals in the urine such as uric acid or oxalate crystals secondary to ethylene glycol [300] or methoxyflurane toxicity [301] also may provide a clue to the specific cause of the acute renal failure. Stones, gravel-like material, or tissue (necrotic papillae) passed in the urine should be analyzed in search for a specific cause of the acute renal failure. Straining the urine in suspected cases can be of value.

Considerable information may be obtained from the assessment of the urinary composition [296, 302]. A study by Miller and associates [296] evaluated the differences in urinary composition between prerenal azotemia and both oliguric and nonoliguric acute renal failure. Those differences are summarized in Table 10-4. Since tubular function is preserved in prerenal azotemia, the urinary sodium concen-

Table 10-4. Urine findings in prerenal azotemia and acute renal failure

Laboratory test	Prerenal azotemia	Acute renal failure
Urine osmolality (mOsm/kg)	>500	<400
Urinary sodium (mEq/L)	<20	>40
Urine-plasma creatinine	>40	<20
Renal failure index	<1	>2
Fractional excretion of filtered sodium	<1	>2
Urinary sediment	Normal or occasional granular casts	Brown granular casts, cellular debris

tration decreases in response to the renal ischemia. The renal concentrating mechanism also is activated, so that the urine osmolality exceeds plasma osmolality. With the intact tubular function in prerenal azotemia, tubular fluid resorption causes the concentration of urinary nitrogenous wastes. The urine to plasma (U/P) creatinine ratio therefore should exceed 40 : 1 with prerenal azotemia. This ratio is generally less than 20 : 1 in acute renal failure. Calculation of the "renal failure index," which is the urinary sodium concentration divided by the urine to plasma creatinine ratio and the fractional excretion of filtered sodium (U/P Na ÷ U/P creatinine × 100), may differentiate prerenal azotemia from acute renal failure when other parameters are overlapping [296]. A value of less than 1 for either of these measurements is characteristic of prerenal azotemia, whereas values greater than 2 are characteristic of acute renal failure. If mannitol or a diuretic has been administered within a few hours of obtaining the urine for examination, the interpretation of the urinary composition is difficult, because with prerenal azotemia the administration of either of these substances may raise the urinary sodium concentration and impair renal concentrating capacity. Thus, the urinary composition of such a patient with prerenal azotemia who has received a diuretic may mimic that of a patient with acute renal failure. There are a few other limitations to interpreting the urinary composition in differentiating acute renal failure from prerenal azotemia. The urine of older patients and patients with chronic renal disease may not be concentrated, despite the presence of prerenal azotemia. Also, urine from patients with nonoliguric renal failure occasionally may have a urinary sodium concentration of less than 20 mEq/L [303]. Such a low urinary sodium concentration in nonoliguric acute renal failure, however, is unusual and generally occurs after hypotonic volume expansion.

Evaluation of urinary composition may thus be helpful in differentiating prerenal azotemia and acute renal failure but must be made with caution; it is less helpful in differentiating postrenal azotemia from acute renal failure. Acute urinary tract obstruction for a few hours may be associated primarily with renal hypoperfusion and thus with a urinary composition similar to that in prerenal azotemia. In contrast, chronic urinary tract obstruction is associated with tubular dysfunction, and the urinary composition may be similar to that present in acute renal failure.

Finally, since urea clearances are flow dependent, the decreased urine flow and intact tubular function with prerenal azotemia or acute urinary tract obstruction are associated with reduced urea clearances. The rise in blood urea nitrogen (BUN), therefore, may be more rapid than the increase in serum creatinine concentration, since creatinine clearances are not flow dependent. In this regard, a ratio of BUN to serum creatinine concentration considerably in excess of 10 : 1 suggests prerenal azotemia or acute postrenal failure; with uncomplicated acute renal failure, this ratio usually does not exceed 10 : 1. However, increased protein intake, blood in the gastrointestinal tract, or enhanced endogenous catabolic rate (e.g., fever or trauma) may also increase the ratio of BUN to plasma creatinine. Alternatively, a low-protein diet or liver disease could lower the ratio of BUN to serum creatinine with prerenal or postrenal azotemia, or an increased catabolic rate could increase the ratio to greater than 10 : 1 with acute renal failure. Thus, as with evaluation of the composition of the urine, the interpretation of the ratio of BUN to plasma creatinine must be made with caution.

Acute Interstitial Nephritis

Acute interstitial nephritis is a disorder characterized by acute renal insufficiency usually due to infection, drug exposure, or immunologic processes that have the pathologic changes of an acute interstitial inflammatory exudate and edema. In addition to the morphologic alterations, acute interstitial nephritis is typified by a number of clinical features. These include low-grade fever, rash, blood eosinophilia, and eosinophils in the urinary sediment; it may, however, occur in the absence of any of these findings. Acute interstitial nephritis is increasingly recognized as a cause of abrupt deterioration in renal function, particularly in association with drug substances. In contrast to chronic interstitial nephritis, gross or microscopic hematuria may occur with acute interstitial nephritis.

Etiology

The causes of acute interstitial nephritis are outlined in Tables 10-1 and 10-5. Infectious processes, drug exposure, and immunologic disorders are known to cause acute interstitial nephritis. The earliest cases of this disease were detected in association with diphtheria, syphilis, and streptococcal and other bacterial infections [304]. More recently, acute interstitial nephritis has been diagnosed in leptospirosis [305], legionnaires' disease [306], infectious mononucleosis [307], and falciparum malaria

Table 10-5. NSAID drugs that cause acute interstitial nephritis

Tolmetin	Indomethacin
Zomepirac	Naproxen
Fenoprofen	Diflunisal
Mefenamic acid	Phenylbutazone

[308]. Other protozoan, fungal, and rickettsial agents have also been causally incriminated in acute interstitial nephritis.

In the past, most drug-related reports of acute interstitial nephritis have been with the use of penicillin and, in particular, its synthetic analogues such as methicillin. Less often, other antimicrobial, diuretic, and anticoagulant agents listed in Table 10-1 have been incriminated. Recently, there has been considerable interest in the role of NSAIDs in acute interstitial nephritis. The interstitial disorder associated with NSAIDs can occur separately from the ischemic injury discussed earlier. Table 10-5 lists the specific NSAIDs that have been reported to cause acute interstitial nephritis. Drug-related interstitial nephritis frequently has the clinical findings of a hypersensitivity reaction, with fever, rash, and eosinophilia. However, acute deterioration of renal function may be the only manifestation.

Immunologic types of acute interstitial nephritis are less clearly defined than infection- and drug-related forms of the disease, despite a sizeable body of evidence supporting immunologic mechanisms [309]. In a rat model, antisera to Tamm-Horsfall protein caused in situ granular immune complexes in the ascending limb of the loop of Henle [310]. In another animal model, Brown-Norway rats have been found to develop anti–tubular basement membrane antibodies and tubulointerstitial nephritis when injected with homologous tubular basement membrane [311]. Renal mononuclear cell infiltration has also been shown in rats injected with homologous or heterologous kidney preparations, suggesting a cell-mediated inflammatory response to autologous antigens [312]. Other studies in rats [313] identified activated and immunologically suppressible T cells in inflammatory kidney infiltrates, which also suggests a cell-mediated immunologic response in interstitial nephritis. Human counterparts of these animal studies have been suggested by a number of investigators. Tubular immune complexes have been demonstrated in 50 percent of lupus nephritis patients [309]. Interstitial inflammatory infiltrates are frequently found in association with tubular deposits. Anti–tubular basement membrane antibodies have been detected in patients with anti–glomerular basement membrane–mediated disorders such as Goodpasture's syndrome [309]. Anti–tubular basement membrane antibodies have also been found in renal allografts and poststreptococcal glomerulonephritis [309]. In anti–glomerular basement membrane disease [309], evidence exists that cell-mediated immunity develops against renal antigens. Interstitial lymphocyte infiltrates are frequently seen in this disorder. An understanding of the relationship of immune complex, anti–tubular basement membrane antibody, and cell-mediated immunologic observations to clinical acute interstitial nephritis will require further investigation. As additional information on tubulointerstitial immunologic mechanisms is acquired, many of the drug-related causes of acute interstitial nephritis, such as methicillin, may be found to have an immunologic basis [309]. It should be added that a cause of acute interstitial nephritis cannot always be found. Acute deterioration in renal function secondary to idiopathic acute interstitial nephritis has been reported in as many as 25 percent of cases.

The clinical manifestations of acute interstitial nephritis can vary from an asymptomatic deterioration in renal function to a full-blown hypersensitivity syndrome. Infection-related acute interstitial nephritis usually presents as renal failure complicating the underlying disease. The urinary sediment is not diagnostic, showing mild proteinuria (<1.5 g/24 hr), pyuria, hematuria, and granular casts. Occasionally heavy proteinuria may be present, particularly in association with NSAIDs. Urine protein electrophoresis reveals a "tubular" pattern. Urine cultures are usually negative. Other urinary findings include impaired concentrating ability, sodium conservation, urinary acidification, and potassium excretion. Renal failure is variable. Drug-related acute interstitial nephritis also may have a paucity of clinical findings. However, a presentation suggestive of a systemic drug reaction, with fever, rash, joint pain, and blood eosinophilia, is frequently found. Urinary eosinophilia in addition to pyuria is often present. Other urinary findings are similar to those reported in infection-related acute interstitial nephritis. Raised IgE levels have been reported in the serum of patients with drug-induced interstitial nephritis [314]. Since immune-type interstitial nephritis has been demonstrated only in diseases with simultaneous glomerulopathy, the clinical picture is dominated by the latter disease so that no specific clinical picture has been found.

The pathology as seen on renal biopsy is similar regardless of the etiology. There is interstitial edema with variable numbers of polymorphonuclear leukocytes, eosinophils, mononuclear cells, and plasma cells. The glomeruli appear normal, and the tubules show abnormalities that include necrosis, degeneration, or atrophy. The distribution of the tubular changes is patchy.

Except for idiopathic acute interstitial nephritis where patient history does not suggest the disorder, the clinical setting may suggest the diagnosis. The presence of an etiologically related infection, drug substance, or immunologic disease such as lupus or Goodpasture's syndrome provides an important clue. Fever, skin rash, joint pain, or eosinophilia are frequently found when there is an underlying drug etiology. The urinary sediment and composition are as outlined previously and are not specific except for urinary eosinophilia. Since the Wright stain is pH-dependent, eosinophils in the urine may be detected by the bilobed nature of the nucleus rather than the presence of eosinophilic granules in the cytoplasm. Alkalinization of the urine will also be helpful in detecting the eosinophilic granules. A technique using Hansel's stain has also been described to identify urine eosinophils [315]. A number of studies have shown that radioactive gallium citrate (^{67}Ga) scanning is positive in interstitial nephritis due to the inflammatory cell infiltrate [316]. The test appears to be relatively specific, and there is poor ^{67}Ga uptake with acute tubular necrosis. Pyelonephritis may also show a positive scan; however, the pattern tends to be focal and patchy as opposed to the diffuse pattern seen with interstitial nephritis. In general, recovery occurs with treatment of the underlying disease or removal of the offending drug. However, there have been reports of permanent impairment of renal function or death [308]. There is some indication that heavy proteinuria in the nephrotic range and renal granulomas on biopsy are associated with a poor outcome. The use of steroid therapy is controversial, since there is a paucity of controlled studies that have addressed this issue. A single study in methicillin-related acute interstitial nephritis that approximated a controlled design suggested that recovery rate was more rapid and residual renal functional defects less if short-term prednisone therapy was used [317].

Management of Acute Renal Failure

Fluid and Electrolyte Intake in Acute Renal Failure

With the recognition of the entity of nonoliguric acute renal failure, the management of fluid and electrolyte balance becomes considerably more complex than that of oliguric acute renal failure. Restriction of fluid intake to less than 1 L/day is reasonable if, as in oliguric acute renal failure, daily urine volumes are 500 ml or less and daily insensible losses are estimated to be 500 to 750 ml. However, with nonoliguric renal failure, daily urine losses plus insensible losses may be in excess of 2 L/day. Obviously a severe negative fluid balance could occur if fluid intake is restricted to 1 L/day in these patients. Similarly, electrolyte losses may be considerably more in the nonoliguric form of acute renal failure than in the oliguric form. Thus, severe restriction of sodium and potassium intake may lead to total body deficits of these cations. These comments are not meant to diminish the importance of avoiding positive fluid and electrolyte balances in the patient with acute renal failure, because such complications as hypertension, cardiac failure, hyperkalemia, and hyponatremia may be the life-threatening consequences of such indiscretions. It must be emphasized, however, that careful balance of intake and output of fluid and electrolytes is extremely important in patients with acute renal failure, both oliguric and nonoliguric.

Protein and Calorie Intake in Acute Renal Failure

In addition to maintenance of fluid and electrolyte balance, regulation of protein and calorie intake is important for patients with acute renal failure. Dietary protein restriction may be used to slow the development of azotemia. An intake of adequate nonprotein calories in the form of carbohydrates should be imposed to minimize the rate of endogenous catabolism, that is, the so-called protein-sparing effect of carbohydrates [318, 319]. However, protein restriction may not always be appropriate in acute renal failure. Some patients with a prolonged course of acute renal failure may develop profound negative nitrogen balances on protein-restricted diets. In such cases, the effect of the resulting negative nitrogen balance on wound healing, and thus on predisposition to infections, theoretically may affect ultimate morbidity and mortality. As with chronic renal failure, if liberalization of protein intake seems advisable, more frequent dialysis may be necessary to control the azotemic state and avoid uremic symptoms.

While the theoretic basis for nutritional therapy in acute stress states including acute renal failure is clear, the actual management techniques and their efficacies are highly controversial. Some studies report the beneficial use of parenteral hyperalimentation using various amino acid formulae, while others do not. Usually, consideration of parenteral hyperalimentation is limited to patients with acute renal failure associated with serious underlying catabolic disorders such as trauma, burns, sepsis, peritonitis, rhabdomyolysis, and surgery. The rationale for hyperalimentation treatment, at least in principle, is fairly obvious. Glucose provides an energy source and blunts the gluconeogenesis of stress states. Amino acids also attenuate gluconeogenesis and provide substrate for protein synthesis. Lipids serve as a two-carbon energy source with a high caloric equivalent. Insulin decreases proteolysis and lipid mobilization and increases cellular glucose uptake. Experimental results in rats using glucose plus either essential or a combination of essential and nonessential amino acids in rat models of acute renal failure have been conflicting. Toback [320] showed more rapid recovery of renal function in amino acid–treated rats compared to animals receiving glucose only. On the other hand, Oken [321] found no differences in recovery rates in glucose plus amino acid–treated rats and glucose only–treated rats. Human study results are unclear as well. Several case reports [322, 323] described improved survival and recovery from acute renal failure in hypercatabolic patients who received parenteral glucose and essential amino acid regimens. Abel [324] carried out a double-blind study of 53 acute renal failure patients using glucose and vitamins in one group and added essential amino acids to the treatment in the other group. This author found that recovery of renal function, as well as patient survival, was significantly better in the latter group. Baek and associates [325] found similar mortality results using nearly identical treatment formulas to those of Abel [324] in 129 acute renal failure patients. Other studies by Leonard and colleagues [326] and Feinstein and coworkers [327] have not supported the earlier favorable results. Leonard and colleagues [326] divided 20 acute renal failure patients into essential amino acid plus glucose and glucose only treatment groups. They found mortality to be identical; however, the daily rate of rise of BUN was significantly less in the amino acid–treated group. Feinstein and coworkers [327] examined survival and daily urea nitrogen appearance (UNA) rates as an index of catabolism in 30 acute renal failure patients who were treated according to three protocols. One group received glucose only; a second, glucose and essential amino acids; and a third, glucose and essential plus nonessential amino acids. There was no difference in recovery from renal function or survival in the three groups even though there was a trend toward a better outcome in the glucose and essential amino acid group. The UNA rate was not different between the glucose only and the glucose plus essential amino acid groups; however, the glucose and essential plus nonessential amino acid group had UNA rates significantly higher than those of the group that received only essential amino acids. The UNA rate did not correlate with patient survival. Thus, on balance, the available data do not indicate clearly that hyperalimentation programs using combinations of glucose and amino acids are of benefit in the management of the stress-related acute renal failure patient. However, adequate energy intake, predominantly given as glucose, or glucose plus soluble lipids if volume overload is of concern, at the rate of 20 to 30 kcal/kg/day has been a nearly universal element of previous studies and likely should continue to be a basic nutritional regimen. Additional, large, controlled studies that measure nitrogen balance as well as survival should aid in answering many of the present questions. Ultimately, the increased catabolism associated with acute renal failure may be best treated with agents such as protease inhibitors.

Use of Dialysis in Acute Renal Failure

While proper attention to fluid and electrolyte balance and to calorie and protein intake is important in the treatment of acute renal failure, intermittent dialysis is frequently needed to avoid the symptoms of uremia. The use of dialysis to prevent rather than to treat uremic symptoms after their occurrence has been termed *prophylactic dialysis* [328–330]. In some circumstances, such as traumatic or postsurgical renal failure, this may entail the daily use of hemodialysis.

The various complications of acute renal failure are listed in Table 10-6. The presence of severe hyponatremia may mimic or accentuate symptoms of uremia, and hyperkalemia may lead to severe cardiac disturbances (see Chap. 5). In contrast, hypocalcemia and hyperphosphatemia are generally not associated with symptoms. Hypocalcemia may persist despite normalization of serum phosphate concentration and the presence of secondary hyperparathyroidism [331]. It has been shown that patients with acute renal failure are resistant to the action of parathyroid hormone, but the nature of this resistance remains to be defined [331]. In patients with acute renal failure associated with muscle damage, severe hypocalcemia may develop early, when calcium deposition occurs in necrotic muscles [331, 332]. Later, however, as calcium is mobilized from the damaged muscles, hypercalcemia may develop and be associated with life-threatening metastatic calcification. Hemodialysis with a calcium-free dialysate should be used to treat this cause of hypercalcemia in acute renal failure.

Symptomatic hypermagnesemia probably occurs only when patients with acute renal failure are treated with magnesium-containing antacids [333]. Hyperuricemia of moderate degree (10–14 mg/dl) is a frequent accompaniment of acute renal failure, but the occurrence of gouty arthritis is very rare. In severely catabolic states associated with muscle breakdown, the level of hyperuricemia may be substantially greater (20–30 mg/dl) [334] and thus necessitate treatment with a xanthine oxidase

Table 10-6. Complications of acute renal failure

Metabolic	Hematologic
Hyponatremia	Anemia
Hyperkalemia	Coagulopathies
Hypocalcemia, hyperphosphatemia	Hemorrhagic diathesis
Hypermagnesemia	Gastrointestinal
Hyperuricemia	Nausea
Cardiovascular	Vomiting
Pulmonary edema	Infectious
Arrhythmias	Pneumonia
Hypertension	Urinary tract infection
Pericarditis	Wound infection
Neurologic	Septicemia
Asterixis	
Neuromuscular irritability	
Somnolence	
Coma	
Seizures	

inhibitor such as allopurinol. Both dialysis and allopurinol therapy are needed if the acute renal failure is secondary to hyperuricemia, as may be the situation during the treatment of various malignancies with chemotherapy. Prior to institution of dialysis, however, treatment with potent diuretics and alkalinization of the urine should be tried in cases of uric acid–induced acute renal failure. Recent results indicate that a urinary uric acid to creatinine ratio greater than 1 suggests that the hyperuricemia is the cause rather than the result of the acute renal failure [335].

Fluid overload is generally primarily responsible for the occurrence of hypertension and cardiac failure in acute renal failure, and removal of fluid by dialysis is the most appropriate treatment. Since digoxin is excreted largely by the kidneys, and rapid changes in plasma potassium concentration may occur during dialysis or in catabolic states associated with acute renal failure, the use of digoxin should be reserved for patients who do not respond to removal of excess fluid. Not only dosage of digoxin, but also the dose of all drugs metabolized or excreted by the kidney should be adjusted to the level of renal dysfunction. It is not known whether the increased plasma renin activity in acute renal failure [336–340] contributes to the hypertension that may be present in 50 percent of these patients [8, 341]. In some patients, however, it is clear that the use of antihypertensive medications may be necessary, in addition to fluid removal, to control the hypertension.

Gastrointestinal and neurologic symptoms and hemorrhagic disorders of the uremic patient with acute renal failure should be immediately treated with dialysis. Some care must be taken, however, to carry out the treatment gradually enough to avoid the symptoms of the "disequilibrium syndrome." Initial short periods of hemodialysis (3–4 hours), sometimes with urea or mannitol added to the dialysate, or the use of peritoneal dialysis may prevent the occurrence of the disequilibrium syndrome, which may feature muscle cramps, headaches, mental obtundation, and convulsions. Intravenous infusion of mannitol and slow rates of blood flow through the dialyzer also have been used to prevent this syndrome. The anemia of acute renal failure may occur more rapidly than expected from bone marrow suppression of erythropoiesis, and thus, in contrast to chronic renal failure, hemolysis may have a predominant role [342]. However, the anemia generally does not necessitate treatment with transfusions unless simultaneous blood loss occurs.

Infections remain the main cause of death in patients with acute renal failure despite the vigorous use of dialysis [4, 8]. Thus meticulous aseptic care of intravenous catheters and wounds and avoidance of the use of an indwelling urinary catheter are important in the management of such patients.

The choice of peritoneal dialysis versus hemodialysis in the treatment of acute renal failure should depend primarily on the capacity to prevent the uremic symptoms of the disorder. In some catabolic states, even the continuous use of peritoneal dialysis is inadequate to prevent uremic symptoms [299, 343]. Moreover, in general, the continuous use of peritoneal dialysis should be avoided, since its complications increase in parallel with its duration [344]. After 36 to 48 hours of continuous peritoneal dialysis, the incidence of peritonitis increases. Even with intermittent use, peritonitis is the main complication of this form of dialysis. The persistent elevation of the diaphragm and the immobilization associated with continuous peritoneal dialysis also predispose to respiratory complications, including atelectasis and pneumonia.

Hemodialysis also is not without consequences. The need for heparinization with hemodialysis may exacerbate any bleeding tendency or bleeding already present. The cardiovascular consequences are generally more pronounced with hemodialysis, but peritoneal dialysis also may impair cardiac output. The use of hemodialysis also may not be possible if arterial perfusion pressure is inadequate, and peritoneal dialysis thus may be the only alternative. With connective tissue disorders, diabetes mellitus, malignant hypertension, and heat stroke, peritoneal clearances may be impaired [343]. Thus, if optimal clearances are needed to prevent uremic symptoms, treatment with hemodialysis is indicated.

Continuous arteriovenous hemofiltration (CAVH) and continuous arteriovenous (CAVHD) or venovenous (CVVHD) hemodialysis are alternatives to intermittent hemodialysis that are gaining popularity in the management of acute renal failure. These technologies rely primarily on slow, continuous ultrafiltration. A specifically designed ultrafiltration cell or high-flux dialyzer is connected by blood lines to a large-flow artery and vein. No blood pump is in the circuit. Ultrafiltration is driven by the patient's arterial pressure. Fluid removal rate varies depending on hemodynamic factors and the magnitude of negative pressure (usually gravitational) applied to the filtrate collection side of the system. Generally, fluid removal rates vary between 5 and 15 ml/min. Since this therapy is continuous, fluid removal can be as high 20 L/day. With CAVH, solutes are removed solely by bulk solution transport. With CAVHD and CVVHD, solutes are removed by a diffusional gradient imposed by a continuous, low rate of flow of the dialysis solution. While neither CAVH nor CAVHD or CVVHD has the solute removal efficiency of standard hemodialysis, daily clearances are sufficient to prevent net accumulation of nitrogen wastes and to correct electrolyte imbalances. The advantages of CAVH or CAVHD and CVVHD over intermittent hemodialysis are continuous, slow fluid removal, which reduces the likelihood of dialysis hypotension and osmolar-shift symptoms, and less technical demand for both equipment and personnel. These approaches are ideal for states of fluid volume overload and for hyperalimentation therapy in oliguric patients. Disadvantages of CAVH, CAVHD, and CVVHD include the need for continuous heparinization, arterial access, and strict, long-term monitoring of volume status. Direct comparisons of hemodialysis and CAVH, CAVHD, and CVVHD are limited [345]. Therefore, actual advantages or disadvantages of intermittent or continuous therapy in acute renal failure are uncertain at the present time. Several reviews describing the application and techniques of CAVH, CAVHD, and CVVHD are available [346–348].

The decision with respect to the mode of dialysis must be an individual one. In general, however, a severely catabolic patient with trauma, fever, or rhabdomyolysis, or following an operation, will present initially with a high BUN and have a predicted high mortality. Aggressive and even daily treatment with hemodialysis therefore is indicated for this group of patients. Finally, it should be emphasized that early institution of dialysis may be necessary in patients with uremic symptoms even before prerenal and postrenal causes of azotemia are excluded.

The duration of dialysis necessary prior to the recovery phase is extremely variable, and dialysis may be needed from a few days to 8 to 12 weeks. Dialysis is a replacement therapy and has no beneficial effect on recovery from acute renal failure. In fact, there is some evidence that hemodialysis may prolong recovery from acute renal failure. There is some evidence from animal studies that the recovery may be accelerated by the administration of growth factors. DNA synthesis and mitogenesis were stimulated in rats treated with one dose of epithelial growth factor, compared to controls [349, 350]. Humes et al. [349] have shown that exogenous administration of epidermal growth factor into animals that have sustained ischemic insults to their kidneys has resulted in an earlier recovery of renal function and enhanced renal tubular epithelial proliferation. Similar effects have been suggested using transforming growth factor-α [351]. Miller et al. [352] have shown that rats with ischemic acute tubular necrosis treated with IGF-I recovered renal function more rapidly and sustained less weight loss as compared to controls. The same investigators have also shown that hepatocyte growth factor (HGF) administered following ischemia enhanced recovery of renal function but had no effect on weight loss, indicating that HGF has no anabolic effect [353]. While these findings are interesting, it is not known whether they are of any potential clinical value in shortening the duration of acute renal failure.

References

1. Hou SH, Bushinsky DA, Wish JB, et al: Hospital acquired renal insufficiency: A prospective study. *Am J Med* 74:243, 1983.
2. Board for the Study of the Severely Wounded. Clinical, Physiologic, and Biochemical Correlation in Lower Nephron Nephrosis. In *Surgery in World War II: Physiologic Effects of Wounds.* Washington, DC, Office of the Surgeon General, Department of the Army, 1952.
3. Smith LH, et al: Posttraumatic renal insufficiency in military casualties: II. Management, use of an artificial kidney, prognosis. *Am J Med* 18:187, 1955.
4. Conger JD, Schrier RW: Renal hemodynamics in acute renal failure. *Annu Rev Physiol* 42: 603, 1980.
5. Lordon RE, Burton JR: Posttraumatic renal failure in military personnel in Southeast Asia. *Am J Med* 53:137, 1978.
6. Whelton A, Donadio JV Jr: Post-traumatic acute renal failure in Vietnam. *Johns Hopkins Med J* 124:95, 1969.
7. Granger P, Dalheim H, Thurau K: Enzyme activities of the single juxtaglomerular apparatus of the rat kidney. *Kidney Int* 1:78, 1972.
8. Swann RC, Merrill JP: The clinical course of acute renal failure. *Medicine* (Baltimore) 32: 215, 1953.
9. Finckh ES, Jeremy D, Whyte HM: Structural renal damage and its relation to clinical features in acute oliguric renal failure. *Q J Med* 31:429, 1962.
10. Olsen TS, Skjoldborg H: The fine structure of the renal glomerulus in acute anuria. *Acta Pathol Microbiol Scand* 70:205, 1967.
11. Ansari Z, Baldwin DS: Acute renal failure due to radiocontrast agents. *Nephron* 17:28, 1976.
12. Appel GB, Neu HC: Nephrotoxicity of antimicrobial agents: I, II, and III. *N Engl J Med* 296: 663, 722, and 783, 1977.
13. Bennett WM, Plamp C, Porter GA: Drug-related syndromes in clinical nephrology. *Ann Intern Med* 151:736, 1976.
14. Dunn MJ, Zambraski EJ: Renal effects of drugs that inhibit prostaglandin synthesis. *Kidney Int* 18:609, 1980.
15. Hewitt WL: Gentamicin: Toxicity in perspective. *Postgrad Med J* 50(Suppl 7):55, 1974.

16. Swartz RD, Rubin JE, Leeming BW, et al: Renal failure following major angiography. *Am J Med* 65:31, 1978.
17. Fabre J, et al: Persistence of sisomicin and gentamicin in renal cortex and medulla compared with other organs and serum of rats. *Kidney Int* 10:444, 1976.
18. Luft FC, et al: Experimental aminoglycoside nephrotoxicity. *J Lab Clin Med* 86:213, 1975.
19. Luft FC, Kleit SA: Renal parenchymal accumulation of aminoglycoside antibiotics in rats. *J Infect Dis* 130:656, 1974.
20. Baylis C, Rennke HR, Brenner BM: Mechanisms of gentamicin-induced defect in glomerular filtration. *Clin Res* 25:426A, 1977.
21. Luft FC, et al: Comparative nephrotoxicity of aminoglycoside antibiotics in rats. *J Infect Dis* 138:541, 1978.
22. Bennett WM, et al: Effect of sodium intake on gentamicin nephrotoxicity in the rat. *Proc Soc Exp Biol Med* 151:736, 1976.
23. Butkus EE, de Torrente A, Terman DS: Renal failure following gentamycin in combination with clindamycin. *Nephron* 17:307, 1976.
24. Lane AZ, Wright GE, Blair DC: Ototoxicity and nephrotoxicity of amikacin. *Am J Med* 62:911, 1977.
25. Lawson DH, et al: Effect of furosemide on antibiotic-induced renal damage in rats. *J Infect Dis* 126:593, 1972.
26. VanZee BE, et al: Renal injury associated with intravenous pyelography in nondiabetic and diabetic patients. *Ann Intern Med* 89:51, 1978.
27. Harkonen S, Kjellstrand CM: Exacerbation of diabetic renal failure following intravenous pyelography. *Am J Med* 63:939, 1977.
28. Carvallo A, et al: Acute renal failure following drip infusion pyelography. *Am J Med* 65:38, 1978.
29. Berns AS: Nephrotoxicity of contrast media. *Kidney Int* 36:730, 1989.
30. Fong HJ, Cohen AH: Ibuprofen-induced acute renal failure with acute tubular necrosis. *Am J Nephrol* 2:28, 1982.
31. Tan SY, Shapiro R, Kish MA: Reversible acute renal failure induced by indomethacin. *JAMA* 241:2732, 1979.
32. Finkelstein A, et al: Fenoprofen nephropathy: Lipoid nephrosis and interstitial nephritis. *Am J Med* 72:81, 1982.
33. Katz SM, et al: Tolmetin: Association with reversible renal failure and acute interstitial nephritis. *JAMA* 246:243, 1981.
34. Russell GI, et al: Interstitial nephritis in a case of phenylbutazone hypersensitivity. *Br Med J* 1:1322, 1978.
35. Goller M, Folkert VW, Schlondorff D: Reversible acute renal failure insufficiency and hyperkalemia following indomethacin therapy. *JAMA* 246:154, 1981.
36. Husserl FE, Lange RK, Kantrow CM Jr: Renal papillary necrosis and pyelonephritis accompanying fenoprofen therapy. *JAMA* 242:1896, 1979.
37. Morales A, Steyn J: Papillary necrosis following phenylbutazone ingestion. *Arch Surg* 103:420, 1971.
38. Brezin JH, et al: Reversible renal failure and nephrotic syndrome associated with nonsteroidal anti-inflammatory drugs. *N Engl J Med* 301:1271, 1979.
39. Chatterjee GP: Nephrotic syndrome induced by tolmetin. *JAMA* 246:1589, 1981.
40. Donker AJM, et al: The effect of indomethacin on kidney function and plasma renin activity in man. *Nephron* 17:228, 1976.
41. Kimberly RP, et al: Reduction of renal function by newer nonsteroidal anti-inflammatory drugs. *Am J Med* 64:804, 1978.
42. Arisz L, et al: The effect of indomethacin on proteinuria and kidney function in the nephrotic syndrome. *Acta Med Scand* 199:121, 1976.
43. Zipser RD, et al: Prostaglandins: Modulators of renal function and pressor resistance in chronic liver disease. *J Clin Endocrinol Metab* 48:895, 1979.
44. Riley DJ, Weir M, Bakris GL: Renal adaptation to the failing heart: Avoiding a "therapeutic misadventure." *Postgraduate Med* 98:153–156, 1994.

45. Schrier RW, Burke TJ, Conger JD, et al: New Aspects of Acute Renal Failure. In: *Proceedings of the 8th International Congress of Nephrology, Athens*. New York, S Karger, 1981, pp 63–69.
46. Neumayer HH, Junge W, Kufner A, et al: Prevention of radiocontrast-media–induced nephrotoxicity by the calcium channel blocker nitrendipine: A prospective randomised clinical trial. *Nephrol Dial Transplant* 4:1030–1036, 1989.
47. Russo D, Testa A, Della Volpe L, et al: Randomised prospective study on renal effects of two different contrast media in humans: Protective role of a calcium channel blocker. *Nephron* 55:254–257, 1990.
48. Duggan KA, MacDonald GJ, Charlesworth JA: Verapamil prevents post-transplant oliguric renal failure. *Clin Nephrol* 24:289–291, 1985.
49. Neumayer HH, Wagner K: Prevention of delayed graft function in cadaver kidney transplants by diltiazem: Outcome of two prospective, randomized clinical trials. *J Cardiovasc Pharmacol* 10(S10):S170–S177, 1987.
50. Humes DH: Role of calcium in the pathogenesis of acute renal failure. *Am J Physiol* 250:F579, 1986.
51. Weinberg JM: The cell biology of ischemic renal injury. *Kidney Int* 39:476, 1991.
52. Schrier RW, Arnold PE, Van Putten VJ, et al: Cellular calcium in ischemic acute renal failure: Role of calcium entry blockers (editorial review). *Kidney Int* 32:313, 1987.
53. Burke TJ, Schrier RW: Pathophysiology of Cell Ischemia. In Schrier RW, Gottschalk CW (eds): *Diseases of the Kidney* (5th ed). Boston, Little, Brown, 1992, p 1257.
54. Takano T, Soltoff SP, Murdaugh S, et al: Intracellular respiratory dysfunction and cell injury in short-term anoxia of rabbit renal proximal tubules. *J Clin Invest* 76:2377, 1985.
55. Burke TJ, Sing H, Schrier RW: Calcium handling by renal tubules during oxygen deprivation injury to the kidney prior to reoxygenation. *Cardiovasc Drugs Ther* 4:1319, 1990.
56. Conger JD, Robinette JB, Schrier RW: Smooth muscle calcium and endothelium-derived relaxing factor in the abnormal vascular responses of acute renal failure. *J Clin Invest* 82:532–537, 1988.
57. Bakris GL, Burnette JC Jr: A role for calcium in radiocontrast-induced reduction in renal hemodynamics. *Kidney Int* 27:465–468, 1985.
58. Shapiro JI, Cheung C, Itabashi A, et al: The protective effect of verapamil on renal function after warm and cold ischemia in the isolated perfused rat kidney. *Transplantation* 40:596–600, 1985.
59. Mills S, Chan L, Schwertschlag U, et al: The protective effect of (−) Emopomil on renal function following warm and cold ischemia. *Transplantation* 43:928–930, 1987.
60. Almeida ARP, Bunnachak D, Burnier M, et al: Time dependent protective effect of Ca^{2+} channel blockers on anoxia- and hypoxia-induced proximal tubule injury. *J Pharmacol Exp Ther* 262:526–532, 1992.
61. Wilson PD, Schrier RW: Nephron segment and calcium as determinants of anoxic cell death in primary renal cell cultures. *Kidney Int* 29:1172–1179, 1986.
62. Schwertschlag U, Schrier RW, Wilson PD: Beneficial effects of calcium channel blockers and calmodulin binding drugs on in vitro renal cell anoxia. *J Pharmacol Exp Ther* 238:119–124, 1986.
63. Wetzels JFM, Wang X, Gengaro PE, et al: Glycine protection against hypoxic but not phospholipase A_2 induced injury in rat proximal tubules. *Am J Physiol* 264:94–99, 1993.
64. Almeida ARP, Wetzels JFM, Bunnachak D, et al: Acute phosphate depletion and in vitro proximal tubule injury: Protection by glycine and acidosis. *Kidney Int* 41:1494–1501, 1992.
65. Burnier M, van Putten VJ, Schieppati A, et al: Effect of extracellular acidosis on ^{45}Ca uptake in isolated hypoxic proximal tubules. *Am J Physiol* 254:C839–C846, 1988.
66. Shanley PF, Johnson GC: Calcium and acidosis in renal hypoxia. *Lab Invest* 65:298–305, 1991.
67. Weinberg JM: Oxygen deprivation–induced injury to isolated rabbit kidney tubules. *J Clin Invest* 76:1193–1208, 1985.
68. Wetzels JFM, Yu L, Wang X, et al: Calcium modulation and cell injury in isolated rat proximal tubules. *J Pharmacol Exp Ther* 267:176–180, 1993.
69. Kribben A, Wetzels JFM, Wieder ED, et al: Evidence for role of cytosolic free calcium in hypoxia-induced proximal tubule injury. *J Clin Invest* 93:1922–1929, 1994.

70. Kribben A, Wetzels JFM, Wieder ED, et al: New technique to assess hypoxia-induced cell injury in individual isolated renal tubules. *Kidney Int* 43:464–469, 1993.

71. Kribben A, Wieder ED, Wetzels JFM, et al: Protection of the cytosolic calcium chelator BAPTA against hypoxic injury in rat proximal tubules. International Satellite Symposium on Acute Renal Failure, Halkidiki, Greece, June 20–23, 1993.

72. Schrier RW, Burke TJ: New aspects in pathogenesis of acute renal failure. *Nephrol Dial Transplant* 9(Suppl 4):9–14, 1994.

73. Moncada S, Palmer RMJ, Higgs EA: Nitric oxide: Physiology, pathophysiology, and pharmacology. *Pharmacol Rev* 43:109–142, 1991.

74. Ignarro LJ: Biosynthesis and metabolism of endothelium derived relaxing factor. *Ann Rev Pharmacol Toxicol* 30:535–560, 1990.

75. Knowles RG, Moncada S: Nitric oxide synthases in mammals. *Biochem J* 298:249–258, 1994.

76. Mohaupt MG, Elzie JL, Ahn KY, et al: Differential expression and induction of mRNAs encoding two inducible nitric oxide synthases in rat kidney. *Kidney Int* 46:653–665, 1994.

77. Abu-Soud HM, Stuehr DJ: Nitric oxide synthases reveal a role for calmodulin in controlling electron transfer. *Proc Natl Acad Sci USA* 90:10769–10772, 1993.

78. Nussler AK, Biliar TR: Inflammation, immunoregulation, and inducible nitric oxide synthase. *J Leukocyte Biol* 54:171–178, 1993.

79. Morris SM, Billiar TR: New insights into the regulation of inducible nitric oxide synthesis. *Am J Physiol* 266:E829–E839, 1994.

80. Terada Y, Tomito K, Nonoguchi H, Marumo F: Polymerase chain reaction localization of constitutive nitric oxide synthase and soluble guanylate cyclase messenger RNAs in microdissected rat nephron segments. *J Clin Invest* 90:659–665, 1992.

81. Romero JC, Lahera V, Salom MG, et al: Role of endothelium dependent relaxing factor nitric oxide on renal function. *J Am Soc Nephrol* 2:1371–1387, 1992.

82. Yu L, Gengaro PE, Niederberger M, et al: Nitric oxide: A mediator in rat tubular hypoxia/reoxygenation injury. *Proc Natl Acad Sci USA* 91:1691–1695, 1994.

83. Yaqoob M, Edelstein C, Wieder E, et al: Nitric oxide kinetics during hypoxia in proximal tubules: Effects of acidosis and glycine. *Kidney Int* 49:1314–1319, 1996.

84. Noiri E, Peresleni T, Miller F, et al: In vivo targeting of inducible NO synthase with oligodeoxynucleotides protects rat kidney against ischemia. *J Clin Invest* 97:2377–2383, 1996.

85. Yaqoob M, Edelstein C, Alkhunaizi A, et al: Inhibition of tetrahydrobiopterin synthesis attenuates nitric oxide release and hypoxia-induced proximal tubular injury (abstract). *J Am Soc Nephrol* 6:992, 1995.

86. Bredt DS, Ferris CD, Snyder SH: Nitric oxide synthase regulatory sites. *J Biol Chem* 267:10976–10981, 1992.

87. Michel T, Li GK, Busconi L: Phosphorylation and subcellular translocation of endothelial nitric oxide synthase. *Proc Natl Acad Sci USA* 90:6252–6256, 1993.

88. Dawson TM, Steiner JP, Dawson VL, et al: Immunosuppressant FK506 enhances phosphorylation of nitric oxide synthase and protects against glutamate neurotoxicity. *Proc Natl Acad Sci USA* 90:9808–9812, 1993.

89. Zhang J, Dawson VL, Dawson TW, et al: Nitric oxide activation of poly (ADP-ribose) synthetase in neurotoxicity. *Science* 263:687–689, 1994.

90. Tallant EA, Brumley LM, Wallace RW: Activation of calmodulin-dependent phosphatase by a Ca^{2+}-dependent protease. *Biochemistry* 27:2205, 1988.

91. Kobryn C, Mandel LJ: Decreased protein phosphorylation induced by anoxia in proximal renal tubules. *Am J Physiol* 267:C1073–C1079, 1994.

92. Beckman JS, Beckman TW, Chen J, et al: Apparent hydroxyl radical production by peroxynitrite: Implications for endothelial injury from nitric oxide and superoxide. *Proc Natl Acad Sci* 87:1620–1624, 1990.

93. Fleming I, Hecker M, Busse R: Intracellular alkalinization induced by bradykinin sustains activation of the constitutive nitric oxide synthase in endothelial cells. *Circ Res* 74:1220–1226, 1994.

94. Ujiie K, Star RA: Enzymatic destruction of nitric oxide by carbonic anhydrase. *J Am Soc Nephrol* 5(3):595, 1994.

95. Suzuki K, Saido TC, Hirai S: Modulation of cellular signals by calpain. *Ann NY Acad Sci* 674:218–227, 1992.
96. Edelstein CL, Wieder ED, Yaqoob MM, et al: The role of cysteine proteases in hypoxia-induced rat renal proximal tubular injury. *Proc Natl Acad Sci USA* 92:7662–7666, 1995.
97. Scherberich JE, Wolf G, Stuckhardt C, et al: Characterization and clinical role of glomerular and tubular proteases from human kidney. *Adv Exp Med Biol* 240:275–282, 1988.
98. Wilson PD, Hartz PA: Mechanisms of cyclosporin A toxicity in defined cultures of renal tubule epithelia: A role for cysteine proteases. *Cell Biol Int Rep* 15:1243–1258, 1991.
99. Hayashi M, Kasau Y, Kawashima S: Preferential localization of calcium activated neutral proteases in epithelial tissues. *Biochem Biophys Res Comm* 148:567–574, 1987.
100. Yoshimura N, Hatanaka M, Kitahara A, et al: Intracellular localization of two distinct Ca^{2+}-proteases (calpain I and II) as demonstrated using discriminative antibodies. *J Biol Chem* 259:9847–9852, 1984.
101. Wilson PD, Firestone RE, Lenard J: The role of lysosomal enzymes in killing of mammalian cells by the lysosomotropic detergent n-dodecylimidazole. *J Cell Biol* 104:1223–1229, 1987.
102. Hawkins HK, Ericsson JLE, Biberfeld P, et al: Lysosomal and phagosome stability in lethal cell injury. *Am J Pathol* 68:255–288, 1972.
103. Bronk SF, Gores GJ: pH dependent non lysosomal proteolysis contributes to lethal anoxic injury of rat hepatocytes. *Am J Physiol* 264:G744–G751, 1993.
104. Plomp PJAM, Gordon PD, Meijen AJ, et al: Energy dependence of different steps in the autophagic-lysosomal pathway. *J Biol Chem* 264:6699–6704, 1989.
105. Olbricht CJ, Grone HJ, Gutjahr E, et al: Potential contribution of lysosomal proteases to cyclosporin A induced nephrotoxicity. *Toxic Lett* 53:251–252, 1990.
106. Seubert P, Lee K, Lynch G: Ischemia triggers NMDA receptor linked cytoskeletal proteolysis in hippocampus. *Brain Res* 492:366–370, 1989.
107. Lee KS, Frank S, Vanderklish P, et al: Inhibition of proteolysis protects hippocampal neurons from ischemia. *Proc Natl Acad Sci USA* 88:7233–7237, 1991.
108. Lizuka K, Kawaguchi H, Yasuda H: Calpain is activated during hypoxic myocardial cell injury. *Biochem Med Metab Biol* 46:427–431, 1991.
109. Tolnadi S, Korecky B: Calcium dependent proteolysis and its inhibition in ischemic rat myocardium. *Can J Cardiol* 2:442–447, 1986.
110. Mehdi S: Cell-penetrating inhibitors of calpain. *TIBS* 16:150–153, 1991.
111. Mellgren RL: Calcium dependent proteases: An enzyme system active at cellular membranes? *FASEB J* 1:110–115, 1987.
112. Saido TC, Sorimachi H, Suzuki K: Calpain: New perspectives in molecular diversity and physiological-pathological involvement. *FASEB J* 8:814–822, 1994.
113. Molitoris BA, Geerdes A, McIntosh JR: Dissociation and redistribution of Na^+,K^+-ATPase from its surface membrane cytoskeletal complex during cellular ATP depletion. *J Clin Invest* 88:462–469, 1991.
114. Molitoris BA: Ischemia-induced loss of epithelial polarity: Potential role of the cytoskeleton. *Am J Physiol* 260:F769–778, 1991.
115. Molitoris BA: New insights into the cell biology of ischemic acute renal failure. *J Am Soc Nephrol* 1:1263–1270, 1991.
116. Kellerman PS, Bogusky RT: Microfilament disruption occurs very early in ischemic proximal tubular injury. *Kidney Int* 42:896–902, 1992.
117. Kellerman PS, Clark RAF, Hoilien CA, et al: Role of microfilaments in the maintenance of proximal tubule structural and functional integrity. *Am J Physiol* 259:F279–F285, 1990.
118. Chen J, Doctor B, Mandel MJ: Cytoskeletal dissociation of ezrin during renal anoxia: Role in microvillar injury. *Am J Physiol* 36:C784–C795, 1994.
119. Doctor RB, Bennet V, Mandel LJ: Degradation of spectrin and ankyrin in the ischemic rat kidney. *Am J Physiol* 264:C1003–1013, 1993.
120. Edelstein CL, Yaqoob MM, Alkhunaizi AM, et al: Modulation of hypoxia-induced calpain activity in rat renal proximal tubules. *Kidney Int* 50:1150–1157, 1996.
121. Choi KH, Edelstein CL, Gengaro PE, et al: Hypoxia induces changes in phospholipase A_2 in rat proximal tubules: Evidence for multiple forms. *Am J Physiol* 269:F846–F853, 1995.

122. Portilla D, Mandel LJ, Bar-Sagi D, et al: Anoxia induces phospholipase A₂ activation in rabbit renal proximal tubules. Am J Physiol 262:F354, 1992.
123. Alkhunaizi AM, Yaqoob MM, Edelstein CL, et al: Arachidonic acid protects against hypoxic injury in rat proximal tubules. Kidney Int 49:620–625, 1996.
124. Hazen SL, Stuppy RJ, Gross RW: Purification and characterization of canine myocardial cytosolic phospholipase A₂. J Biol Chem 265:10622, 1990.
125. Bonventre JV, Swidler M: Calcium dependency of prostaglandin E₂ production in rat glomerular mesangial cells: Evidence that protein kinase C modulates the Ca²⁺-dependent activation of phospholipases A₂. J Clin Invest 82:168, 1988.
126. Mayer RJ, Marshall LA: New insights on mammalian phospholipase A₂(s): Comparison of arachidonyl-selective and -nonselective forms. FASEB J 7:339, 1993.
127. Nakamara H, Nemenoff RA, Gronich JH, et al: Subcellular characteristics of phospholipase A₂ activity in rat kidney: Enhanced cytosolic, mitochondrial and microsomal phospholipase A₂ enzymic activity after renal ischemia and reperfusion. J Clin Invest 87:1810, 1991.
128. Bunnachak D, Almeida ARP, Wetzels JFM, et al: Ca²⁺ uptake, fatty acid and LDH release during proximal tubule hypoxia: Effects of mepacrine and dibucaine. Am J Physiol 266:F196, 1994.
129. Portilla D, Shah SV, Lehman PA, et al: Role of cytosolic calcium independent plasmalogen selective phospholipase A₂ in hypoxic injury to rabbit proximal tubules. J Clin Invest 93:1609, 1994.
130. Malis CD, Bonventre JV: Mechanism of calcium potentiation of oxygen free radical injury to renal mitochondria: A model for post-ischemic and toxic mitochondrial damage. J Biol Chem 261:14201, 1986.
131. Scarpa A, Lindsay JG: Maintenance of energy-linked functions in rat liver mitochondria aged in the presence of nupercaine. Eur J Biochem 27:401, 1972.
132. Broekemeier KM, Schmid PC, Schmid HHO, et al: Effect of phospholipase A₂ inhibitors on ruthenium red-induced Ca²⁺ release from mitochondria. J Biol Chem 260:105, 1985.
133. Widener LL, Mela-Riker LM: Verapamil pretreatment preserves mitochondrial function and tissue magnesium in the ischemic kidney. Circ Shock 13:27, 1984.
134. Uchida E, Bohr DF: Myogenic tone in isolated perfused resistance arteries from rats. Am J Physiol 216:1343–1350, 1969.
135. Hwa JJ, Bevan JA: A nimodipine-resistant Ca²⁺ resistant Ca²⁺ pathway is involved in myogenic tone in a resistance artery. Am J Physiol 251:H182–H189, 1986.
136. Cabanac M: Keeping a cool head. News Physiol Sci 1:41–43, 1986.
137. Winquist RJ, Bevan JA: Temperature sensitivity of tone in the rabbit facial vein: Myogenic mechanism for cranial thermoregulation. Science 207:1001–1002, 1980.
138. Laher I, Bevan JA: Stretch of vascular smooth muscle activates tone and ⁴⁵Ca²⁺ influx. J Hypertens 7:S17–S20, 1989.
139. Laher I, van Breemen C, Bevan JA: Stretch-dependent calcium uptake associated with myogenic tone in rabbit facial vein. Circ Res 63:669–772, 1988.
140. Jackson PA, Duling BR: Myogenic response and wall mechanics of arterioles. Am J Physiol 257:H1147–H1155, 1989.
141. McCalden TA, Nath RG: Cerebrovascular autoregulation is resistant to calcium channel blockage with nimodipine. Experientia 45:305–306, 1989.
142. Harris RJ, Banston NM, Symon L, et al: The effects of a calcium antagonist, nimodipine, upon physiologic responses of the cerebral vasculature and its possible influence upon focal cerebral ischaemia. Stroke 13:759–766, 1982.
143. Pearce WJ, Bevan JA: Diltiazem and autoregulation of canine cerebral blood flow. J Pharmacol Exp Ther 242:812–817, 1987.
144. Vanelli G, Hussain SNA: Effects of potassium channel blockers on basal vascular tone and reactive hyperemia of canine diaphragm. Am J Physiol 266(35):H43–H51, 1994.
145. Imamura Y, Tomoike H, Narishige T, et al: Glibenclamide decreases basal coronary blood flow in anesthetized dogs. Am J Physiol 263(32):H399–H404, 1992.
146. Samaha FF, Heineman FW, Ince C, et al: ATP-sensitive potassium channel is essential to maintain basal coronary vascular tone in vivo. Am J Physiol 262(31):C1220–C1227, 1992.

147. Harder DR, Sanchez-Ferrer C, Kauser K, et al: Pressure releases a transferable endothelial contractile factor in cat cerebral arteries. *Circ Res* 65:193–198, 1989.
148. Rubanyi GM: Endothelium-dependent pressure-induced contraction of isolated canine carotid arteries. *Am J Physiol* 255:H783–H788, 1988.
149. Katusic A, Shepherd JT, Vanhoutte PM: Endothelium-dependent contraction to stretch in canine basilar arteries. *Am J Physiol* 252:H671–H673, 1987.
150. Hwa JJ, Bevan JA: Stretch-dependent (myogenis) tone in rabbit ear resistance arteries. *Am J Physiol* 250:H87–H95, 1986.
151. Kulik TJ, Evans JN, Gamble WJ: Stretch-induced contraction in pulmonary arteries. *Am J Physiol* 255:H1391–H1398, 1988.
152. Kalsner S, Quillan M: Non-neurogenic relaxation to field stimulation in coronary arteries. *J Pharmacol Exp Ther* 250:461–469, 1989.
153. Nakayama T, Tanaka Y: Calcium Transients and Stretch-Induced Myogenic Tone in Vascular Tissue in Resistance Arteries. In Halpern W, Pegram BL, Mackey K, et al. (eds), *The Resistance Arteries*. Ithaca, NY, Perinatology Press, 1988, pp 212–218.
154. Osol G, Cipolla M, Knutson S: A new method for mechanically denuding the endothelium of small (50–150 μM) arteries with human hair. *Blood Vessels* 26:320–324, 1989.
155. Asano M, Aoki K, Suzuki Y, et al: Effects of Bay K 8644 and nifedipine on isolated dog cerebral, coronary and mesenteric arteries. *J Pharmacol Exp Ther* 647:646–656, 1987.
156. Garica-Roldan JL, Bevan JA: Flow-induced constriction and dilation of cerebral resistance arteries. *Cir Res* 66:1445–1448, 1990.
157. Garcia-Roldan JL, Bevan JA: Intraluminal flow causes contraction of coronary resistance arteries. *Circulation* 82:III-704, 1990.
158. Bevan JA, Laher I: Pressure and flow-dependent vascular tone. *FASEB J* 5:2267–2273, 1991.
159. Joyce EH, Bevan JA: Unique sensitivity of flow-induced changes in tone to extracellular sodium concentrations (abstract). *FASEB J* 5:A1751, 1991.
160. Koller A, Kaley G: Endothelium regulates skeletal muscle microcirculation by a blood flow velocity sensing mechanism. *Am J Physiol* 258:H916–H920, 1988.
161. Bevan JA, Joyce EH: Flow-induced resistance artery tone: A balance between constrictor and dilator mechanism. *Am J Physiol* 258:H663–H668, 1990.
162. Bevan JA: Flow regulation of vascular tone: Its sensitivity to changes in sodium and calcium (review). *Hypertension* 22(3):273–281, 1993.
163. Koller A, Kaley G: Prostaglandins mediate arteriolar dilation to increased blood flow velocity in skeletal muscle microcirculation. *Circ Res* 67:529–534, 1990.
164. Kuo L, Davis MJ, Chilian WM: Endothelium-dependent, flow-induced dilation of isolated coronary arterioles. *Am J Physiol* 259:H1063–H1070, 1990.
165. Ward ME, Magder SA, Hussain SNA: The role of endothelium-derived relaxing factor in reactive hyperemia in canine diaphragm. *J Appl Physiol* 74:1606–1612, 1993.
166. Roy-Contancin L, Garcia ML, Glavez A, et al: Ca^{2+}-activated K^+ channels in bovine aortic smooth muscle and GH_3 cells: Properties and regulation by guanine nucleotides. *Prog Clin Biol Res* 334:145–170, 1990.
167. Cooke JP, Rossitch E, Andon NA, et al: Flow activates an endothelial potassium channel to release an endogenous nitrovasodilator. *J Clin Invest* 88:1663–1671, 1991.
168. Vane JR, Änggård EE, Botting RM: Regulatory functions of the vascular endothelium. *N Engl J Med* 323:27–36, 1990.
169. Vallance P, Collier J, Moncada S: Effects of endothelium-derived nitric oxide on peripheral arteriolar tone in man. *Lancet* 2:997–1000, 1989.
170. Conger JD, Falk SA: Abnormal vasoreactivity of isolated arterioles from rats with ischemic acute renal failure (ARF). *J Am Soc Nephrol* 4:733A, 1993.
171. Olsson RA, Bugni WJ: Coronary Circulation. In Fozzard HA, et al (eds): *The Heart and Cardiovascular System*. New York, Raven Press, 1986, pp 987–1038.
172. Simonson MS: Endothelins: Multifunctional renal peptides. *Physiol Rev* 73:375, 1993.
173. Goetz KL, Wang BC, Madwed JB, et al: Cardiovascular, renal, and endocrine responses to intravenous endothelin in conscious dogs. *Am J Physiol* 255(24):R1064–R1068, 1988.
174. Spielman WS, Arend LJ: Adenosine receptors and signaling in the kidney. *Hypertension* 17:117–130, 1991.

175. Meininger GA, Davis MJ: Cellular mechanisms involved in the vascular myogenic response. *Am J Physiol* 263(32):H647–H659, 1992.

176. Kanatsuka H, Lamping KG, Eastham CL, et al: Comparison of the effects of increased myocardial oxygen consumption and adenosine on the coronary microvascular resistance. *Circ Res* 65:1296–1305, 1989.

177. Madden JA: The effect of carbon dioxide on cerebral arteries. *Pharmacol Ther* 59:229–250, 1993.

178. Lefer AM: Physiologic and Pathophysiologic Role of Cyclo-oxygenase Metabolites of Arachidonic Acid in Circulating Disease States. In Mehta JI (ed), *Cardiovascular Clinics: Thrombosis and Platelets in Myocardial Ischemia*. Philadelphia, Davis, 1987, pp 85–99.

179. Lefer AM, Lefer DJ: Pharmacology of the endothelium in ischemia-reperfusion and circulatory shock. *Annu Rev Pharmacol Toxicol* 33:71–90, 1993.

180. Engler RL, Gruber HE: Adenosine: An autacoid. In Fozzard HA (ed), *The Heart and Cardiovascular System* (2nd ed). New York, Raven Press, 1991, pp 1745–1764.

181. Johnson G, Tsao PS, Lefer AM: Cardioprotective effects of authentic nitric oxide in myocardial ischemia and reperfusion. *Crit Care Med* 19:244–252, 1991.

182. Ogletree ML, Lefer AM, Smith JB, et al: Studies on the protective effect of prostacyclin in acute myocardial ischemia. *Eur J Pharmacol* 56:95–103, 1979.

183. Del Zoppo GJ: Microvascular changes during cerebral ischemia and reperfusion. *Cerebrovasc Brain Metab Rev* 6:47–96, 1994.

184. Kloner RA, Przyklenk K: Consequences of Ischemia-Reperfusion on the Coronary Microvasculature. In Yellon DM, Jennings RB (eds), *Myocardial Protection: The Pathophysiology of Reperfusion Injury*. New York, Raven Press, 1992, pp 85–103.

185. Matthys E, Patton M, Osgood R, et al: Alterations in vascular function and morphology in ischemic ARF. *Kidney Int* 23:717–724, 1983.

186. Conger JD, Robinette JB: Differences in vascular reactivity in models of ischemic acute renal failure. *Kidney Int* 39:1087–1097, 1993.

187. Pomfy M, Huska J: The state of the microcirculatory bed after total ischaemia of the brain. *Funct Dev Morphol* 2(4):253–258, 1992.

188. VanBenthuysen KM, McMurtry IF: Reperfusion after acute coronary occlusion in dogs impairs endothelium-dependent relaxation to acetylcholine and augments contractile reactivity in vitro. *J Clin Invest* 76:265–274, 1987.

189. Defilippi P, van Hinsbergh V, Bertolotto A, et al: Differential distribution and modulation of expression of alpha1/beta1 integrin on human endothelial cells. *J Cell Biol* 114:855–863, 1991.

190. Öjteg G, Nygren K, Wolgast M: Permeability of renal capillaries: II. Transport of neutral and charged protein molecular probes. *Acta Physiol Scand* 129:287–294, 1986.

191. Humes HD, Nakamura T, Cieslinski DA, et al: Role of proteoglycans and cytoskeleton in the effects of TGF-β1 on renal proximal tubule cells. *Kidney Int* 43:575–584, 1993.

192. Terry BE, Jones DB, Mueller CB: Experimental ischemic renal arterial necrosis with resolution. *Am J Pathol* 58:69–83, 1970.

193. Ueda M, Becker AE, Tsukada T, et al: Fibrocellular tissue response after percutaneous transluminal coronary angioplasty: An immunocytochemical analysis of the cellular composition. *Circulation* 83:1327–1332, 1991.

194. Newcomb PM, Herman IM: Pericyte growth and contractile phenotype: Modulation by endothelial-synthesized matrix and comparison with aortic smooth muscle. *J Cell Physiol* 155:385–393, 1993.

195. Conger JD, Schultz MF, Miller F, et al: Responses to hemorrhagic arterial pressure reduction in different ischemic renal failure models. *Kidney Int* 46:318–326, 1994.

196. Lieberthal W, Wolf EF, Rennke HG: Renal ischemia and reperfusion impair endothelium-dependent vascular relaxation. *Am J Physiol* 256:F894–F900, 1989.

197. Conger JD, Weil JU: Abnormal vascular function following ischemia-reperfusion injury (review). *J Investig Med* 43:431–442, 1995.

198. Conger JD, Falk SA, Robinette JB: Angiotensin II–induced changes in smooth muscle calcium in rat renal arterioles. *J Am Soc Nephrol* 3:1792–1803, 1993.

199. Conger JD, Robinette JB, Villar A: Increased NOS activity despite lack of response to endothelium-dependent vasodilators in post-ischemic acute renal failure in rats. *J Clin Invest* 96: 631–638, 1995.
200. Kelleher SP, Robinette JB, Conger JD: Sympathetic nervous system in the loss of autoregulation in acute renal failure. *Am J Physiol (Renal Fluid Electrolyte Physiol)* 15:F379–F386, 1984.
201. Solez L, Marel-Maroger L, Sraer J: The morphology of acute tubular necrosis in man: Analysis of 57 renal biopsies and comparison with glycerol model. *Medicine* (Baltimore) 58:362–376, 1979.
202. Williams RH, Tomas CE, Navar LG, et al: Hemodynamic and single nephron function during the maintenance phase of ischemic acute renal failure in the dog. *Kidney Int* 19:503–515, 1981.
203. Kelleher SP, Robinette JB, Miller F, et al: Effect of hemorrhagic reduction in blood pressure on recovery from acute renal failure. *Kidney Int* 31:725–730, 1987.
204. Conger JD, Schultz MF, Miller F, et al: Responses to hemorrhagic arterial pressure reduction in different ischemic renal failure models. *Kidney Int* 46:318–326, 1994.
205. Conger JD: Does hemodialysis delay recovery from acute renal failure? *Semin Dial* 3:146–148, 1990.
206. Robertson CR, Deen WM, Troy JL, et al: Dynamics of glomerular ultrafiltration in the rat: III. Hemodynamics and autoregulation. *Am J Physiol* 223:1193, 1972.
207. Meyers BD, Deen WM, Brenner BM: Effects of norepinephrine and angiotensin II on the determinants of glomerular ultrafiltration and proximal tubular fluid reabsorption in the rat. *Circ Res* 37:101, 1975.
208. Stahl RAK, Paravicini M, Schollmeter P: Angiotensin II stimulation of prostaglandin E_2 and 6-keto F1α formation by isolated human glomeruli. *Kidney Int* 26:30, 1984.
209. Torsello G, Schror K, Szabo A, et al: Effects of prostaglandin E_1 (PGE_1) on experimental renal ischemia. *Eur J Vasc Surg* 3:5, 1989.
210. Klausner JM, Paterson IS, Kobzik L, et al: Vasodilating prostaglandins attenuate ischemic renal injury only if thromboxane is inhibited. *Ann Surg* 209:219, 1989.
211. Oliver JA, Sciacca RR, Pinto J, et al: Participation of the prostaglandins in the control of renal blood flow during acute reduction of cardiac output in the dog. *J Clin Invest* 67:229, 1981.
212. Assael BM, Chiabrando C, Gagliardi L, et al: Prostaglandins and aminoglycoside nephrotoxicity. *Toxicol Appl Pharmacol* 78:386, 1985.
213. Badr KF, Kelley VE, Rennke HG, et al: Roles for thromboxane A_2 and leukotrienes in endotoxin-induced acute renal failure. *Kidney Int* 30:474, 1986.
214. Freund HR, Barcellu UO, Muggia-Sullam M, et al: Renal prostaglandin production is increased during abdominal sepsis in the rat and unaffected by infusion of different amino acid formulations. *J Surg Res* 44:99, 1988.
215. Walshe JJ, Venuto RC: Acute oliguric renal failure induced by indomethacin: Possible mechanism. *Ann Intern Med* 91:47, 1979.
216. Fink MP, Mac Vittie TJ, Casey LC: Effects of nonsteroidal anti-inflammatory drugs on renal function in septic dog. *J Surg Res* 36:516, 1984.
217. Papanicolaou N, Darlametsos J, Hatziantonion, et al: Partial protection against acute renal failure by efamol. *Prog Clin Biol Res* 301:271, 1989.
218. Werb R, Clark WF, Lindsay RM, et al: Protective effect of prostaglandins (PGE_2) in glycerol induced acute renal failure in rats. *Clin Sci Mol Med* 55:505, 1978.
219. Casey KF, Machiedo GW, Lyons MJ, et al: Alteration of postischemic renal pathology by prostaglandin infusion. *J Surg Res* 29:1, 1980.
220. Stahl RAK, Kanz L, Kudelka S: Cyclosporine and renal prostaglandin E_2 production. *Ann Intern Med* 103:474, 1985.
221. Hensby CN, Lewis PJ, Hilgard PJ, et al: Prostacyclin deficiency in thrombotic thrombocytopenic purpura. *Lancet* 2:728, 1979.
222. Turi S, Belch JJF, Beattie TJ, et al: Abnormalities of vascular prostaglandins in Henoch-Schonlein purpura. *Arch Dis Child* 61:773, 1986.
223. Turi S, Beattie TJ, Belch JJF, et al: Disturbances of prostacyclin metabolism in children with hemolytic uremic syndrome and in first degree relatives. *Clin Nephrol* 25:193, 1986.

224. Zipser RD, Radvan GH, Kronborg IT, et al: Urinary thromboxane B_2 and prostaglandin E_2 in the hepatorenal syndrome: Evidence for increased vasoconstrictor and decreased vasodilator factor. *Gastroenterology* 84:697, 1983.
225. Budd GT, Bukowski RM, Lucas FU, et al: Prostacyclin therapy of thrombotic thrombocytopenic purpura. *Lancet* 2:915, 1980.
226. Tonshoff B, Momper R, Kuhl PG, et al: Increased thromboxane biosynthesis in childhood uremic syndrome. *Kidney Int* 37:1134, 1990.
227. Pollack R, Dumble LJ, Wiederkehr JC, et al: The immunosuppressive properties of new oral prostaglandin E_1 analogues. *Transplantation* 50:834, 1990.
228. DeBold AJ, Borenstein HB, Veress AT, et al: A rapid and potent natriuretic response to intravenous injection of atrial myocardial extract in rats. *Life Sci* 28:89, 1981.
229. Nakayama K, Ohkubo H, Hirose T, et al: mRNA sequence of human cardiodilatin–atrial natriuretic factor precursor and regulation of precursor in RNA in rat atria. *Nature* 310:699, 1984.
230. Kangawa K, Matsuo H: Purification and complete amino acid sequence of α-human atrial natriuretic polypeptide (α-hANP). *Biochem Biophys Res Commun* 118:131, 1984.
231. Yamaji T, Ishibashi M, Takaku F: Atrial natriuretic factor in human blood. *J Clin Invest* 76:1705, 1985.
232. Shenker Y, Sider RS, Ostafin EA, et al: Plasma levels of immunoreactive atrial natriuretic factor in healthy subjects and in patients with edema. *J Clin Invest* 76:1684, 1985.
233. Goetz KL, Wang BC, Madwed JB, et al: Cardiovascular, renal, and endocrine responses to intravenous endothelin in conscious dogs. *Am J Physiol* 255:R1064, 1988.
234. Perrella MA, Margulies KB, Wei CM, et al: Pulmonary and urinary clearance of atrial natriuretic factor in acute congestive heart failure in dogs. *J Clin Invest* 87:1649, 1991.
235. Sonnenberg JL, Skane Y, Jeng AY, et al: Identification of protease 3.4.24.11 as the major atrial natriuretic factor degrading enzyme in the rat kidney. *Peptides* 9:173, 1988.
236. Bussien JP, Biollaz J, Waeber B, et al: Dose-dependent effect of atrial natriuretic peptide on blood pressure, heart rate, and skin blood flow of normal volunteers. *J Cardiovasc Pharmacol* 8:216, 1986.
237. Lappe RW, Smits JFM, Todt JA, et al: Failure of atriopeptin II to cause arterial vasodilation on the conscious rat. *Circ Res* 56:606, 1985.
238. Camargo MJF, Kleinert HD, Atlas SA, et al: Ca-dependent hemodynamic and natriuretic effects of atrial extract in isolated rat kidney. *Am J Physiol* 254:F447, 1984.
239. Maack T, Camargo MJF, Kleinert HD: Atrial natriuretic factor: Structure and functional properties. *Kidney Int* 27:607, 1985.
240. Lappe RW, Todt JA, Wendt RL: Effects of atrial natriuretic factor on the vasoconstrictor actions of the renin-angiotensin system in conscious rats. *Circ Res* 61:134, 1987.
241. Haass M, Kopin IJ, Goldstein DS, et al: Differential inhibition of alpha adrenoceptor–mediated pressor responses by rat atrial natriuretic peptide in the pithed rat. *J Pharmacol Exp Ther* 235:122, 1985.
242. Dillingham MA, Anderson RJ: Inhibition of vasopressin action by atrial natriuretic factor. *Science* 231:1572, 1986.
243. Kohno M, Yasunari K, Yokokawa K, et al: Inhibition by atrial and brain natriuretic peptides of endothelin-1 secretion after stimulation with angiotensin II and thrombin of cultured human endothelial cells. *J Clin Invest* 87:1999, 1991.
244. Roy DR: Effect of synthetic ANP on renal and loop of Henle functions in the young rat. *Am J Physiol* 251:F220, 1986.
245. Anand-Srivastava MB, Vinay P, Genest J, et al: Effect of atrial natriuretic factor on adenylate cyclase in various nephron segments. *Am J Physiol* 251:F417, 1986.
246. Huang CL, Lewicki J, Johnson LK, et al: Renal mechanism of action of rat atrial natriuretic factor. *J Clin Invest* 75:769, 1985.
247. Aalkjaer C, Mulvany MJ, Nyborg NCB: Atrial natriuretic factors causes specific relaxation of rat arcuate arteries. *Br J Pharmacol* 86:447, 1985.
248. Veldkamp PJ, Carmines PK, Inscho EW, et al: Direct evaluation of the microvascular actions of ANP in juxtamedullary nephrons. *Am J Physiol* 254:F440, 1988.

249. Loutzenhiser R, Hayashi K, Epstein M: Atrial natriuretic peptide reverses afferent arteriolar vasoconstriction and potentiates efferent arteriolar vasoconstriction in the isolated perfused rat kidney. *J Pharmacol Exp Ther* 246:522, 1988.
250. Lanese DM, Yuan BH, Falk SA, et al: Effects of atriopeptin III on isolated rat afferent and efferent arterioles. *Am J Physiol* 261:F1102, 1991.
251. Saxenhofer H, Fitzgibbon WR, Paul RV: Urodilatin: Binding properties and stimulation of cGMP generation in rat glomeruli cells. *Am J Physiol* 264:FS67, 1993.
252. Abassi ZA, Powell JR, Golomb E, et al: Renal and systemic effects of urodilatin in rats with high-output heart failure. *Am J Physiol* 262:F615, 1992.
253. Sudoh T, Kangawa K, Minamino N, et al: A new natriuretic peptide in porcine brain. *Nature* 332:78, 1988.
254. Minamino N, Aburaya N, Ueda S, et al: The presence of brain natriuretic peptide of 12,000 daltons in porcine heart. *Biochem Biophys Res Commun* 155:740, 1988.
255. Wei CM, Kim CH, Khraibi AA, et al: Atrial natriuretic peptide and c-type natriuretic peptide in spontaneously hypertensive rats and their vasorelaxing actions in vitro. *Hypertension* 23:903, 1994.
256. Stingo AJ, Clavell AL, Aarhus LL, et al: Cardiovascular and renal actions of c-type natriuretic peptide. *Am J Physiol* 262:H308, 1992.
257. Schafferhans K, Heidbreder E, Grimm D, et al: Norepinephrine-induced acute renal failure: Beneficial effects of atrial natriuretic factor. *Nephron* 44:240, 1986.
258. Nakamota M, Shapiro JI, Shanley PF, et al: In vitro and in vivo protective effect of atriopeptin III on ischemic acute renal failure. *J Clin Invest* 80:698, 1987.
259. Shaw SG, Weideman P, Hodler J, et al: Atrial natriuretic peptide protects against acute ischemic renal failure in the rat. *J Clin Invest* 80:1232, 1987.
260. Neumayer HH, Blossei N, Scherr-Thots U, et al: Amelioration of postischemic acute renal failure in conscious dogs by human atrial natriuretic peptide. *Nephrol Dial Transplant* 5:32, 1990.
261. Lieberthal W, Sheridan AM, Valeri CR: Protective effect of atrial natriuretic factor and mannitol following renal ischemia. *Am J Physiol* 258:F1266, 1990.
262. Pollock DM, Opgenorth TJ: Beneficial effect of the atrial natriuretic factor analog A68828 in postischemic acute renal failure. *J Pharmacol Exp Ther* 255:1166, 1990.
263. Conger JD, Falk SA, Yuan BH, et al: Atrial natriuretic peptide and dopamine in a rat model of ischemic acute renal failure. *Kidney Int* 35:1126, 1989.
264. Conger JD, Falk SA, Hammond WS: Atrial natriuretic peptide and dopamine in established acute renal failure in the rat. *Kidney Int* 40:21–28, 1991.
265. Schafferhans K, Heidbreder E, Sperber S, et al: Atrial natriuretic peptide in gentamicin-induced acute renal failure. *Kidney Int* 25:S101, 1988.
266. Heidbreder E, Schafferhans K, Heyd A, et al: Uranyl nitrate–induced acute renal failure in rats: Effect of atrial natriuretic peptide on renal function. *Kidney Int* [Suppl] 3:S79, 1988.
267. Capasso G, Anastasio P, Giordani D, et al: Beneficial effects of atrial natriuretic factor on cisplatin-induced acute renal failure in the rat. *Am J Nephrol* 7:228, 1987.
268. Shaw S, Weidmann P, Zimmermann A: Urodilatin, not nitroprusside, combined with dopamine reverses ischemic acute renal failure. *Kidney Int* 42:1153, 1992.
269. Burke TJ, Arnold PE, Gordon JA, et al: Protective effect of intrarenal calcium membrane blockers before or after renal ischemia. *J Clin Invest* 74:1830, 1984.
270. Rahman SN, Kim GE, Mathew AS, et al: Effects of atrial natriuretic peptide in clinical acute renal failure. *Kidney Int* 45:1731–1738, 1994.
271. Allgren RL: Randomized, double-blind, placebo-controlled multicenter clinical trial of anaritide atrial natriuretic peptide in the treatment of acute renal failure. Presented at the International Society of Nephrology Meeting, Madrid, Spain, July 1995.
272. Malis CD, Cheung JY, Leaf A, Bonventre, JV: Effects of verapamil in models of ischemic acute renal failure in the rat. *Am J Physiol* 245:F735, 1983.
273. Wagner K, Schultze G, Molzahn M, et al: The influence of long-term infusion of the calcium antagonist diltiazem on postischemic acute renal failure in conscious dogs. *Klin Wochenschr* 64:P135, 1986.

274. Garthoff B, Hirth C, Federmann A, et al: Renal effects of 1,4-dihydropyridines in animal models of hypertension and renal failure. *J Cardiovasc Pharmacol* 9:S8, 1987.

275. Deray G, Dubois M, Beaufils H, et al: Effects of nifedipine on cisplatinum-induced nephrotoxicity in rats. *Clin Nephrol* 30:146, 1988.

276. Lee SM, Michael UF: The protective effect of nitrendipine on gentamicin acute renal failure in rats. *Exp Mol Pathol* 43:107, 1985.

277. Watson AJ, Gimenez LF, Klassen DK, et al: Calcium channel blockade in experimental aminoglycoside nephrotoxicity. *J Clin Pharmacol* 27:625, 1987.

278. Dobyan DC, Bulger RE: Partial protection by chlorpromazine in mercuric chloride–induced acute renal failure in rats. *Lab Invest* 50:578, 1984.

279. Lumlertgul D, Hutdagoon P, Sirivanichai C, et al: Intrarenal infusion of gallopamil in acute renal failure: A preliminary report. *Drugs* 42(Suppl 1):44–50, 1991.

280. Duggan KA, MacDonald GJ, Charlesworth JA: Verapamil prevents post-transplant oliguric renal failure. *Clin Nephrol* 24:289, 1985.

281. Wagner K, Albrecht S, Neumayer HH: Prevention of posttransplant acute tubular necrosis by the calcium antagonist diltiazem: A prospective randomized study. *Am J Nephrol* 7:287, 1987.

282. Bakris GL, Burnett JC Jr: A role for calcium in radiocontrast-induced reductions in renal hemodynamics. *Kidney Int* 27:465, 1985.

283. Cacoub P, Baumelou A, Jacobs C: No evidence for protective effects of nifedipine against radiocontrast-induced acute renal failure. *Clin Nephrol* 29:215, 1988.

284. Deray G, Khayat D, Cacoub P, et al: The effects of diltiazem on methotrexate-induced nephrotoxicity. *Eur J Clin Pharmacol* 37:337, 1989.

285. Tanner GA, Steinhausen M: Kidney pressure after temporary artery occlusion in the rat. *Am J Physiol* 230:1173–1181, 1976.

286. Racusen LC, Fivush BA, Li YL, et al: Dissociation of tubular cell detachment and tubular cell death in clinical and experimental "acute renal failure." *Lab Invest* 64:546–556, 1991.

287. Gailit J, Colflesh D, Rabiner I, et al: Redistribution and dysfunction of integrins in cultured renal epithelial cells exposed to oxidative stress. *Am J Physiol* 33:F149–F157, 1993.

288. Goligorsky MS, Dibona GF: Pathogenic role of Arg-Gly-Asp recognizing integrins in acute renal failure. *Proc Natl Acad Sci USA* 90:5700–5704, 1993.

289. Noiri E, Gailit J, Sheth D, et al: Cyclic RGD peptides ameliorate ischemic acute renal failure in rats. *Kidney Int* 46:1050–1058, 1994.

290. Toma G, Bates JM, Kumar S: Uromodulin (Tamm-Horsfall Protein) is a leucocyte adhesion molecule. *Biochem Biophys Res Comm* 200:275–282, 1994.

291. Miller SB, Martin DR, Kissane J, et al: Hepatocyte growth factor accelerates recovery from acute ischemic renal injury in rats. *Am J Physiol* 266:F129–F134, 1994.

292. Miller SB, Martin DR, Kissane J, et al: Insulin like growth factor 1 accelerates recovery from ischemic acute tubular necrosis in the rat. *Proc Natl Acad Sci USA* 89:11876–11881, 1992.

293. Harvald B: Renal papillary necrosis. *Am J Med* 35:481, 1963.

294. Graham JR, et al: Fibrotic disorders associated with methysergide therapy for headache. *N Engl J Med* 274:359, 1966.

295. Anderson RJ, et al: Nonoliguric acute renal failure. *N Engl J Med* 296:1134, 1977.

296. Miller TR, et al: Urinary diagnostic indices in acute renal failure: A prospective study. *Ann Intern Med* 89:47, 1978.

297. Meyers C, Roxe DM, Hano JE: The clinical course of nonoliguric acute renal failure. *Cardiovasc Med* 2:669, 1977.

298. Miller PD, et al: Polyuric prerenal failure. *Arch Intern Med* 40:907, 1980.

299. Schrier RW, et al: Nephropathy associated with heat stress and exercise. *Ann Intern Med* 67:356, 1967.

300. Friedman EA, et al: Consequences of ethylene glycol poisoning. *Am J Med* 32:891, 1962.

301. Churchill D, et al: Persisting renal insufficiency after methoxyflurane anesthesia. *Am J Med* 56:575, 1974.

302. Handa SP, Morrin PA: Diagnostic indices in acute renal failure. *Can Med Assoc J* 96:78, 1967.

303. Vertel RM, Knochel JP: Non-oliguric acute renal failure. *JAMA* 200:598, 1967.
304. McCluskey RT, Klassen J: Immunologically mediated glomerular, tubular and interstitial renal disease. *N Engl J Med* 288:564, 1973.
305. Sitprija V, Evans H: The kidney in human leptospirosis. *Am J Med* 49:780, 1970.
306. Poulter N, et al: Acute interstitial nephritis complicating Legionnaires' disease. *Clin Nephrol* 15:216, 1981.
307. Lee S, Kjellstrand CM: Renal disease in infectious mononucleosis. *Clin Nephrol* 9:236, 1978.
308. Baldwin DS, et al: Renal failure and interstitial nephritis due to penicillin and methicillin. *N Engl J Med* 279:1245, 1968.
309. Andres GA, McCluskey RT: Tubular and interstitial renal disease due to immunologic mechanisms. *Kidney Int* 7:271, 1975.
310. Friedman J, Hoyer JR, Seiler MW: Formation and clearance of tubulointerstitial immune complexes in kidneys of rats immunized with heterologous antisera to Tamm-Horsfall protein. *Kidney Int* 21:571, 1982.
311. Lehman DH, Wilson CB, Dixon FJ: Interstitial nephritis in rats immunized with heterologous tubular basement membrane. *Kidney Int* 5:187, 1974.
312. Sugisaki T, Kano K, Andres G, Milgrom F: Antibodies to tubular basement membrane elicited by stimulation with allogenic kidney. *Kidney Int* 21:557, 1982.
313. Husby G, Tung KSK, Williams RC Jr: Characterization of renal tissue lymphocytes in patients with interstitial nephritis. *Am J Med* 70:31, 1981.
314. Oor BS, et al: IgE levels in interstitial nephritis. *Lancet* 1:1254, 1974.
315. Nolan CR, Anger MS, Kelleher SP: Eosinophiluria: A new method of detection and definition of the clinical spectrum. *N Engl J Med* 315:1516, 1986.
316. Wood BC, et al: Gallium citrate Ga67 imaging in noninfectious interstitial nephritis. *Arch Intern Med* 138:1665, 1978.
317. Galpin JE, et al: Acute interstitial nephritis due to methicillin. *Am J Med* 65:756, 1978.
318. Gamble JL: Physiological information gained from studies on the life raft ration. *Harvey Lect* 42:247, 1974.
319. Merril JP: *Fifth Conference on Renal Function.* New York, Josiah Macy, Jr, Foundation, 1953, p 136.
320. Toback FG: Amino acid enhancement of renal regeneration after acute tubular necrosis. *Kidney Int* 12:193, 1977.
321. Oken DE: Amino acid therapy in the treatment of experimental acute renal failure in the rat. *Kidney Int* 17:14, 1980.
322. Abel RM, Abbott WM, Fischer JE: Acute renal failure: Treatment without dialysis by total parenteral nutrition. *Arch Surg* 103:513, 1971.
323. Wilmore DW, Dudrick SJ: Treatment of acute renal failure with intravenous essential L-amino acids. *Arch Surg* 99:669, 1969.
324. Abel RM: Improved survival from acute renal failure after treatment with intravenous L amino acids and glucose. *N Engl J Med* 288:675, 1973.
325. Baek SM, et al: The influence of parenteral nutrition on the course of acute renal failure. *Surg Gynecol Obstet* 141:405, 1975.
326. Leonard CD, Luke RG, Spiegel RR: Parenteral essential amino acids in acute renal failure. *Urology* 6:145, 1975.
327. Feinstein EI, et al: Clinical and metabolic responses to parenteral nutrition in acute renal failure. *Medicine* (Baltimore) 60:124, 1981.
328. Easterling RE, Forland M: A five year experience with prophylactic dialysis for acute renal failure. *Trans Am Soc Artif Organs* 10:200, 1964.
329. Kleinknecht D, et al: Uremic and non-uremic complications in acute renal failure: Evaluation of early and frequent dialysis on prognosis. *Kidney Int* 1:190, 1972.
330. Teschan PE, Baxter CR, O'Brien TF, et al: Prophylactic hemodialysis in the treatment of acute renal failure. *Ann Intern Med* 53:992, 1960.
331. Massry SG, et al: Divalent ion metabolism in patients with acute renal failure: Studies on the mechanism of hypocalcemia. *Kidney Int* 5:437, 1974.
332. Akmal M, et al: Resolution of muscle calcification in rhabdomyolysis and acute renal failure. *Ann Intern Med* 89:928, 1978.

333. Randall RE Jr, et al: Hypermagnesemia in renal failure: Etiology and toxic manifestations. *Ann Intern Med* 61:73, 1974.
334. Schrier RW, et al: Acute Renal Failure Associated with Heat Stress and Exercise. In Gessler U, Schroder K, Weidinger H (eds): *Pathogenesis and Clinical Findings with Renal Failure*. Stuttgart, Thieme, 1971, p 211.
335. Kelton J, Kelley WN, Holmes EW: A rapid method for the diagnosis of acute uric acid nephropathy. *Arch Intern Med* 138:612, 1978.
336. Brown JJ, et al: Renin and acute renal failure: Studies in man. *Br Med J* 1:253, 1970.
337. Kokot F, Kuska J: Plasma renin activity in acute renal insufficiency. *Nephron* 6:115, 1969.
338. Massani ZM, et al: Angiotensin blood levels in hypertensive and non-hypertensive diabetes. *Clin Sci* 30:473, 1966.
339. Ochoa E, Finkielman S, Agrest A: Angiotensin blood levels during the evolution of acute renal failure. *Clin Sci* 38:225, 1970.
340. Tu WH: Plasma renin activity in acute tubular necrosis and other renal diseases associated with hypertension. *Circulation* 31:686, 1965.
341. Teschan PE, Post RS, Smith LH, et al: Post-traumatic renal insufficiency in military casualties: I. Clinical characteristics. *Am J Med* 18:172, 1955.
342. Mathew A, Schrier RW: Pharmacological therapy of acute renal failure: Current practices and future horizons. *IM for the Specialist* 10:101, 1989.
343. Nolph KD, Whitcomb ME, Schrier RW: Mechanisms for inefficient peritoneal dialysis in acute renal failure associated with heat stress and exercise. *Ann Intern Med* 71:317, 1969.
344. Barry KG, et al: Peritoneal dialysis: Current applications and recent developments. *Proc Third Int Cong Nephrol* 3:288, 1966.
345. Kohen JA, Whitley KY, Kjellstrand CM: Continuous arteriovenous hemofiltration: A comparison with hemodialysis in acute renal failure. *Trans Am Soc Artif Intern Organs* 31:169, 1985.
346. Kaplan AA, Longnecker RE, Folbert VW: Continuous arteriovenous hemofiltration: A report of six months' experience. *Ann Intern Med* 100:358, 1984.
347. Kramer P, Kaufhold G, Grone HJ, et al: Management of anuric intensive-care patients with arteriovenous hemofiltration. *Int J Artif Organs* 3:225, 1980.
348. Lauer A, Saccaggi A, Ronco C, et al: Continuous arteriovenous hemofiltration in the critically ill patient. *Ann Intern Med* 99:455, 1983.
349. Humes HD, Cieslinski DA, Coimbra TM, et al: Epidermal growth factor enhances renal tubular cell regeneration and repair and accelerates the recovery of renal function in postischemic acute renal failure. *J Clin Invest* 84:1757, 1989.
350. Norman J, Badie-Dezfooly B, Nord EP, et al: EGF-induced mitogenesis in proximal tubular cells: Potentiation by angiontensin II. *Am J Physiol* 253:F299, 1987.
351. Humes HD, Shigang L: Cellular and molecular basis of renal repair in acute renal failure. *J Lab Clin Med* 124(6):749–754, 1994.
352. Miller SB, Martin DR, Kissane J, Hammerman MR: Insulin like growth factor I accelerates recovery from ischemic acute tubular necrosis in the rat. *Proc Natl Acad Sci USA* 89: 11876–11880, 1992.
353. Miller SB, Martin DR, Kissane J, Hammerman MR: Hepatocyte growth factor accelerates recovery from acute ischemic renal injury in rat. *Am J Physiol* 266:F129–134, 1994.

Chronic Renal Failure: Manifestations and Pathogenesis

Laurence Chan and Allen C. Alfrey

Chronic renal failure is characterized by a decrease in glomerular filtration rate (GFR) and histologic evidence of a reduction in nephron population. The clinical course is typically one of a progressive and unrelenting loss of nephron function ultimately leading to end-stage renal disease (ESRD). However, the time between the initial onset of disease and ultimate development of terminal renal failure may vary considerably not only between different diseases but also in different patients with similar disease processes. The incidence of ESRD shows marked geographic variation as determined by the population base in regard to age, race, and sex. The reported incidence of ESRD in the United states in 1991 was 198 per million population [1]. In 1993, there were 171,479 patients being treated for end-stage renal failure with dialysis. An additional 10,934 patients received a renal transplant. In addition, approximately 50,000 patients were added to the ESRD program in this country in 1993 [1]. The incidence of ESRD in the United States is increasing by approximately 8.7 percent annually. A similar increase in incidence is occurring in most other industrialized countries as well; the reason for this increase in frequency of ESRD is unclear. The distribution of patients by race most recently reported shows that 67.9 percent were white, 28.8 percent were black, with the remaining 3.3 percent being Asian/Pacific islanders and Native Americans. In the U.S. population, it is clear that chronic renal failure is more prevalent in the black population and Native Americans than in the white population.

Although life for chronic renal failure patients can be sustained by chronic dialysis and kidney transplantation, neither form of therapy is totally satisfactory. The current yearly mortality rate in the U.S. dialysis population is 23.6 percent. With the advent of improved immunosuppressive therapy with cyclosporine, results with renal transplantation have improved considerably [1]. The adjusted and averaged 1-year graft survival was approximately 90 percent for living related donors and 77 percent for cadaveric donor transplants in 1991 [1]. With improved transplant outcomes, growth in the number of patients wanting or needing a transplant has outpaced the supply of available organs. Although kidney transplant has become the preferred method of treatment for many ESRD patients, fewer than 25 percent of patients entering ESRD programs receive renal transplantation because of age, associated disease, anatomic abnormalities of the urinary tract, the presence of preformed cytotoxic antibodies, or lack of availability of a suitable donor.

The rehabilitation rate of patients on chronic dialysis has been disappointing, and the cost of this treatment has been of increasing concern [1]. In 1991, the total charges from public and private sources for the treatment of ESRD was $8.59 billion [1]. As the number of patients being treated for ESRD continues to increase, so does the cost of care. Because of both the cost as well as the morbidity and mortality associated with ESRD, every attempt should be made to preserve renal function as long as possible and ideally preventing any further progression of the underlying renal disease.

Causes of Chronic Renal Failure

The cause of renal failure should be established, if possible, since some conditions if corrected may result in partial or full functional recovery. The major causes of chronic renal failure found in patients entering the ESRD program in 1991 are listed in Table 11-1.

Glomerular Diseases

Diabetes mellitus has become the most common cause of chronic renal failure. It is estimated that 40 percent of patients who have had type I diabetes mellitus for over 20 years will have renal disease. Although the incidence of renal failure in patients with type II diabetes is only about 10 percent of that found in type I diabetes, because of the larger number of patients with type II diabetes it is a more frequent cause of ESRD than type I diabetes [2].

Glomerulonephritis represents the third most common cause of ESRD. The most common glomerular diseases are focal glomerulosclerosis and membranoproliferative and lupus glomerulonephritis. However, it should be noted that the majority of glomerular diseases are unclassified. Since IgA nephropathy is the most common glomerular disease responsible for ESRD in most other developed countries, it is possible that this disease accounts for a relatively large fraction of the unclassified glomerular diseases.

Table 11-1. Major causes of chronic renal failure

Cause	Incidence
Diabetes mellitus	30.6%
Hypertension	26.5%
Glomerulonephritis	13.6%
Cystic disease	3.4%
Other urologic	5.4%
Other or unknown	20.5%

Vascular Disease

Hypertension is the second leading reported cause of ESRD. A 15-year follow-up study of 361,659 men with hypertension found that 924 developed ESRD [3]. This represented an incidence of 17.12 per 100,000 person-years. The relative risk for development of ESRD for diastolic blood pressure above 120 mm Hg versus below 70 mm Hg was 30.9. For systolic blood pressure above 200 mm Hg versus below 120 mm Hg, the relative risk was 48.2. Across the entire range, blood pressure represented an independent risk factor. The relative risk for blacks was 1.99 [4]. This increased risk could not be explained by difference in levels of systolic or diastolic pressures or other known risk factors. In general, ESRD from hypertension occurs in black patients with a long history of uncontrolled hypertension or almost any patient with a history of malignant or accelerated hypertension [5–7]. Although the incidence of renal failure from hypertension can be markedly attenuated by treatment of accelerated or malignant hypertension [5, 8], adequate chronic treatment of milder hypertensive states, especially in the black population, may not prevent progression of renal failure [4, 6].

Other less common vascular causes of chronic renal failure are atheroembolic disease and bilateral renal artery stenosis. Atheroembolic disease should be suspected in any individual who develops progressive renal failure following a vascular diagnostic procedure or surgery. In contrast to other vascular renal disease, atheroembolic disease may include high-grade proteinuria, eosinophiluria, and decreased serum complement. Diagnosis of atheroembolic disease largely depends on renal biopsy in which the cholesterol clefts are observed. There is no specific treatment for atheroembolic disease. Bilateral renal artery stenosis, as a cause of renal failure, is suggested by a further reversible reduction in renal function produced by converting enzyme inhibitors.

Arteriography is usually required for the diagnosis of renal artery stenosis. As of this time, there is no good evidence that renal function can predictably be improved in patients with bilateral renal artery stenosis by either angioplasty or surgical correction of the lesions. Uncontrolled studies have, however, suggested that these procedures can improve renal function in some rare instances.

Interstitial Nephritis

Interstitial nephritis is a descriptive term implying fibrosis and an inflammatory response in the interstitium of the kidney. The glomeruli are involved only secondarily as a result of the fibrosis and vascular changes. Because of the potential reversibility or prevention of this group of renal diseases, it is important to differentiate interstitial nephritis from glomerulonephritis.

A number of clinical and biochemical features, listed in Table 11-2, tend to separate these two forms of renal disease. Characteristically, patients with interstitial nephritis complain of polyuria and nocturia. Their urine volume is unusually large (3–5 L/day) because the kidneys' ability to concentrate urine is lost early in the course of renal failure. The diluting capability in interstitial nephritis is maintained even late in the course of renal failure; thus, the urine osmolality and specific gravity may be low when determined on a random collection of urine.

Table 11-2. Features differentiating glomerulonephritis and interstitial nephritis

Feature	Glomerulonephritis	Interstitial nephritis
Proteinuria	>3 g	<1.5 g
Sediment	Numerous cells and red blood cell casts	Few cells and casts
Sodium handling	Normal until late	Sodium wasting
Anemia	Moderate severity until late	Disproportionately severe for degree of renal failure
Hypertension	Common	Less common
Acidosis	Normochloremic	Hyperchloremic
Uric acid	Slightly elevated	Markedly elevated
Urine volume	Normal	Increased

A feature of advanced glomerular diseases is high-grade proteinuria, which usually is in excess of 2.5 g/day. Even with advanced interstitial nephritis, the 24-hour urinary protein excretion is usually less than 1 to 2 g. Furthermore, the urinary protein may be predominantly an α_2- or β-globulin instead of albumin. This finding is characteristic of the so-called tubular type of proteinuria. In the majority of chronic renal diseases, serum uric acid increases only slightly, and clinical gout is uncommon [9]. However, in interstitial nephritis, serum uric acid is commonly elevated, and in one type of interstitial nephritis, lead nephropathy, clinical gout has been recognized in approximately 50 percent of the patients [10]. The urinary sediment in interstitial nephritis may be totally unremarkable, or there may be a few white blood cells and hyaline casts. Renal salt wasting appears to be more common in patients with interstitial nephritis than in other forms of renal disease, and salt supplementation must sometimes be given to maintain extracellular fluid (ECF) volume.

Finally, hypertension is less common in interstitial nephritis than in chronic glomerulonephritis, and anemia may be disproportionately more severe for the degree of compromised renal function.

As is apparent in Table 11-3, a variety of drugs and toxins can be the etiologic agent responsible for causing interstitial nephritis. In general, with the exception of analgesics, drugs cause an acute interstitial nephritis that is reversible when the drugs are discontinued. The severity and chronicity of other forms of interstitial nephritis are largely related to the amount and duration of exposure to the various nephrotoxins. Interstitial nephritis accounts for 3 percent of the patients in this country being treated for ESRD. In this group, currently analgesic nephropathy accounts for 0.8 percent of patients being treated for ESRD. Analgesic nephropathy used to account for up to 20 percent of ESRD in a number of countries [11]. However, following the removal of analgesics containing the combination of aspirin and phenacetin, the incidence of this disease has markedly decreased worldwide. The typical patient with this disease is a depressed, middle-aged woman who gives a history of years of daily ingestion of analgesics containing caffeine, aspirin, and phenacetin. Usually, the total consumption of analgesics amounts to several kilograms. Patients frequently complain of headaches, backache, or other types of chronic pain and state that the analgesics are consumed to relieve this pain. There is evidence that sometimes the headaches may be due to the caffeine or phenacetin ingestion, or both. If the patient can be persuaded to discontinue the analgesics, the headaches may disappear. The patient commonly presents with recurrent urinary tract infections, gross hematuria, or symptoms of uremia. However, since papillary necrosis is common, acute renal failure and ureteral colic may develop as a result of the passing of necrotic papillae down one or both ureters. In this disease, the kidney has a remarkable capacity to recover even after what would appear to be a terminal state of renal failure [11]. With conservative treatment and discontinuation of the analgesics, the patient can achieve significant improvement in renal function and have a relatively good long-term survival. Many times, however, it is very difficult to convince the patient to break a long habit of drug abuse.

Uric acid and oxalate nephropathy and cystinosis represent less than 0.1 percent each of the ESRD population [1]. Renal failure is uncommon in patients with primary gout, and when it does occur, it is slowly progressive and only becomes clinically important late in life [12]. However, in some hematologic disorders, particularly in association with the use of chemotherapeutic agents, there may be marked overproduction of uric acid, which may cause acute renal failure due to deposition of urate crystals in the tubules.

Another compound capable of inducing a severe interstitial nephritis is oxalate. Besides ethylene glycol intoxication [13], increased urinary excretion of oxalate can occur in association with genetic disorders as well as with a number of acquired conditions. Two enzymatic defects have been described that can result in the accumulation of glyoxylic acid and hyperoxaluria. In the first type, urinary excretion of oxalic acid, glyoxylic acid, and glycolic acid is increased as a result of deficiency of 2-oxoglutarate-glyoxylate carboligase [14]. In the second defect, urinary excretion of glycolic acid is normal, but the excretion of L-glyceric acid and oxalate is in-

Table 11-3. Various etiologies of interstitial nephritis

Analgesics	Uric acid
Other drugs	Gouty nephropathy
Sulfonamide	Hematologic disorders
Penicillin and homologues	Oxalate deposition
Furosemide, thiazides	Associated with small-bowel disease
Phenindione	Hereditary
Phenytoin	Anesthetic agents: methoxyflurane
Cimetidine	Ethylene glycol
Nonsteroidal anti-inflammatory agents	Heavy metals
Calcium disorders	Lead
Hyperparathyroidism	Cadmium
Milk-alkali syndrome	Uranium
Sarcoid	Copper
Neoplasms	Miscellaneous
Multiple myeloma	Infection
	Idiopathic

creased. This condition is due to a deficiency of D-glyceric dehydrogenase [14]. Both diseases are characterized by nephrolithiasis, nephrocalcinosis, and renal failure, with few patients living beyond the age of 40 years.

Recently, a number of acquired forms of hyperoxaluria and renal failure have been described. Methoxyflurane anesthesia can cause hyperoxaluria and renal failure [15]. In addition, it has been recognized that patients with distal small-bowel disease may have hyperoxaluria [16]. In this group of patients, calcium oxalate stones are common; however, marked oxalate deposition occasionally may occur in the kidney, resulting in interstitial nephritis and loss of renal function. The mechanism responsible for the hyperoxaluria has been shown to be a consequence of increased absorption of dietary oxalate [16]. It is felt that this results from calcium and possibly magnesium (which normally binds oxalate in the gut, rendering it insoluble and nonabsorbable) being bound to fatty acids in steatorrheic states, allowing the oxalate to be absorbed. Similarly, this condition has been successfully treated by giving supplemental calcium. Furthermore, cholestyramine has also been shown to be effective in decreasing oxalate absorption from the bowel and thus in decreasing urinary excretion of this compound [16].

All other causes of interstitial nephritis are even less prevalent. Conditions that cause hypercalcemia, hypercalciuria, or both can lead to the deposition of calcium in the kidney, with a resulting interstitial nephritis. Radiographic evidence of nephrocalcinosis is frequently a late finding and even then may be observed only by using the technique of nephrotomography. Thus, radiographic evidence of nephrocalcinosis cannot be relied on to establish the diagnosis even when renal function is severely impaired. In this condition, too, if the underlying cause responsible for the disturbance of calcium metabolism such as primary hyperparathyroidism, sarcoid, or milk-alkali syndrome is corrected or treated, further progression of renal failure can be either slowed or prevented [17, 18].

A final group of agents that can produce a chronic interstitial nephritis are some of the heavy metals, including copper, lead, cadmium, and uranium. Lead nephropathy is common in Queensland, Australia [10] and has been reported in some areas of the United States in patients who have consumed moonshine whiskey [19]. Lead nephropathy may occur more commonly than previously suspected in this country. Batuman and associates patients [20] have suggested that patients having the combination of interstitial nephritis and gout should be suspected of having lead nephropathy. This supposition was supported by the finding that ethylenediaminetetraacetic acid (EDTA) mobilized significantly greater amounts of lead in patients with renal failure and gout than in patients with either gout alone or renal failure alone. Cadmium intoxication can also lead to an interstitial nephritis and renal tubular dysfunction. Characteristically, the patients present with aminoaciduria, glycosuria, phosphaturia, and severe osteomalacia [21]. As a result of industrial contamination with the element, chronic cadmium intoxication is especially prevalent in the people living along the Jinzu River in Japan [21]. In Wilson's disease, copper is deposited in the proximal tubule cells and may cause a variety of renal functional abnormalities, including Fanconi's syndrome, proteinuria, and hematuria. However, it would not appear to progress to renal failure.

Evidence so far accumulated suggests that, in the adult, chronic urinary tract

Table 11-4. Normal values used in screening patients with interstitial nephritis

Substance measured	Plasma	Urine
Calcium	9.5–10.5 mg/dl	<300 mg/day
Oxalate	30 ng/dl	<40 mg/day
Uric acid	5–7 mg/dl	<800 mg/day
Lead	<40 ng/dl	<0.5 mg/day*
Cadmium, mercury, and uranium	Normally nondetectable	Normally nondetectable

* Following 1 g of EDTA.

infection without obstruction rarely, if ever, leads to terminal renal failure. However, there are some exceptions in which renal bacterial infections if untreated can lead to chronic renal insufficiency; among them are tuberculosis, multiple renal abscesses, and bacterial infections associated with papillary necrosis.

Since a number of patients with interstitial nephritis have a potentially preventable or reversible form of renal failure, a careful history should be obtained relating to medications, small-bowel disease, and possible environmental exposure to some toxin. In addition, serum and urinary uric acid and calcium should be determined. In selected cases, urinary oxalate excretion should be measured and heavy-metal screens performed. The normal values to be used for these screening procedures are given in Table 11-4.

Reflux Nephropathy

Reflux nephropathy is the second most common renal disease in children [22]. According to the European Dialysis and Transplantation Association, it accounts for 30 percent of advanced renal failure in children under 16 years and 15 to 20 percent of severe renal disease in adults below 50 years of age. The infant kidney is especially susceptible to intrarenal reflux. Most evidence would suggest that scarring usually occurs by 2 years of age [23] and that new scarring is unusual after age 5 [23–25]. Increasing evidence suggests that severe congenital renal damage may already be present at birth [24]. This may represent a disorder in kidney embryogenesis as a result of an abnormal development of the ureteral bud. Prognosis is largely determined by the extent to which the kidney is scarred and contracted when the patient is initially seen. It has also been shown that the severity of the reflux can be correlated with the degree of renal damage and that surgical correction of reflux is associated with eradication of upper urinary tract infection and improvement of renal growth and function. However, a recent study in children would suggest that surgical correction of reflux offers no advantage over good medical management [25]. Although there are no control trials in adults regarding surgical correction of reflux, most studies would suggest that it does not influence the course of renal failure.

Hereditary Renal Disease

Approximately 5 to 8 percent of patients with chronic renal failure have a hereditary form of renal disease such as polycystic kidney disease, Alport's syndrome, Fabry's disease, congenital nephrotic syndrome, medullary cystic disease, cystinosis, or familial amyloidosis. This is another group of renal diseases for which no specific treatment is available [26]. Through genetic counseling, however, a number of these diseases are potentially preventable. The physician therefore has an obligation to advise potential parents of the risk of having children with renal disease and to determine when possible which family members are at risk or have diagnosable renal disease. In adult polycystic kidney disease, which is inherited as an autosomal dominant disorder with complete penetrance, a DNA probe has localized the majority of the cases (>90%) to a mutation to the short arm of human chromosome 16. This technique has been used to diagnose the disease in utero in a 9-week fetus [27]. The potential success of genetic counseling is demonstrated by a study carried out at the genetic clinic at the Hospital for Sick Children in London. Approximately two-thirds of the families who were informed that the chances were greater than 10 percent that their children would develop hereditary disease decided to have no more children, whereas three-fourths of the families informed that the chances were 10 percent or less elected to have more children [28].

Risk Factors for Development of End-Stage Renal Disease

The four major risk factors for the development of ESRD are race, age, sex, and family history.

Race

The incidence of renal failure adjusted for sex in the black population is 550 per million as compared to 140 per million in the white population, or over three times as great [1]. Black men aged 25 to 44 years are 20 times more likely to develop renal disease secondary to hypertension than white men [7, 28]. Black men also have a very high incidence of idiopathic focal and segmental glomerulosclerosis (FSGS) as well as that associated with intravenous drug use and acquired immune deficiency syndrome (AIDS) [1, 29]. The attack rate of FSGS in black men with AIDS is approximately 10 times as great as in white men. In fact, FSGS is the most common cause of renal failure in young adult black men. Blacks also have a fourfold greater risk of developing ESRD from type II diabetes as compared to whites [2]. In contrast, two diseases, cystic kidney disease and especially IgA nephropathy, occur with considerably less frequency in the black population than the white population. In the Native American, diabetes accounts for almost twice as much ESRD (63.9%) as found in the white or black population. The incidence of diabetic ESRD in Native Americans in 1992 in ESRD Network 15 was 80.1 percent. Hispanics also have a high frequency of diabetic ESRD, with a reported incidence of 65 percent, as compared to other ethnic groups in ESRD Network 15, in whom the incidence of diabetic ESRD was 42.6 percent in 1992.

Age

The incidence of ESRD in 1991, adjusted for race, was 95 per million population in adults 20 to 44 years, as compared to 760 per million population in ages 65 to 74 years [1]. The incidence of diabetic renal failure also increases dramatically with age. However, in contrast to the total causes of renal failure, which continue to increase with advanced age, over 66 percent of diabetic ESRD occurs prior to 64 years of age. Excluding diabetes and hypertension, the occurrence of a number of selected causes of renal failure, accounting for approximately 13 percent of all end-stage renal failure, are largely age dependent [1]. Prior to age 40 years, focal glomerulosclerosis, lupus erythematosus, Henoch-Schönlein purpura, AIDS-related nephropathy, and congenital and hereditary disease (e.g., renal agenesis, obstructive nephropathy, Alport's syndrome, and reflux nephropathy) are most commonly seen. In the age group 40 to 55 years, autosomal dominant polycystic kidney disease, membranous glomerulonephritis, membranoproliferative glomerulonephritis, and hemolytic-uremic syndrome are seen with increasing frequency. Over age 55 years, Goodpasture's syndrome, interstitial nephritis, analgesic nephropathy, amyloidosis, multiple myeloma, and Wegener's granulomatosis are the most common diseases in this group.

Sex

Sex is an additional risk factor for the development and progression of certain types of renal disease. Overall, the incidence of ESRD is greater in males than in females (56.3% versus 43.7%) [1]. However, there are certain causes of ESRD such as type II diabetes, interstitial nephritis, lupus erythematosus, scleroderma, and hemolytic-uremic syndrome/thrombotic thrombocytopenia purpura that occur more frequently in females.

Family History

Genetic factors are also important in predisposing individuals to developing ESRD. Patients with diabetes who have a family history of essential hypertension and abnormal lithium-sodium countertransport are at greater risk of developing renal failure [30].

Similarly, there are numerous types of hereditary renal disease such as Alport's syndrome and, autosomal dominant polycystic kidney disease plus a variety of less common and largely recessive or sex-linked hereditary diseases such as Fabry's disease, tuberous sclerosis, medullary cystic disease, sickle cell disease, familial Mediterranean fever, type I glycogen storage disease, cystinosis, oxalate nephropathy, and infantile polycystic kidney disease.

Evaluation of Renal Function

Progression to ESRD occurs at a variable rate. When a patient is first seen with chronic renal failure, it is therefore most important to document the degree of renal impairment and to attempt to determine if potentially reversible factors have contributed to the severity of the renal failure.

For clinical purposes, the creatinine clearance is a simple and reliable method of estimating GFR and thus the degree of impairment of renal function. Approximately 1 mg of creatinine is produced daily by the metabolism of 20 g of muscle [31]. In addition, about 20 percent of urinary creatinine is derived from the ingestion of meat. Small quantities of creatinine are secreted by the renal tubules so that the creatinine clearance slightly overestimates true glomerular filtration. As a result, the 24-hour endogenous creatinine clearance generally exceeds inulin clearance, and this difference increases in patients with advanced chronic renal failure and proteinuria. If lean body mass does not appreciably change, daily urinary creatinine excretion remains relatively constant. Therefore, the serial measurements of serum creatinine can be used to estimate renal function. Alternatively creatinine clearance (C_{cr}) can be estimated from serum creatinine (SrCr) determinations alone using the Crockcroft and Gault equation [32]:

$$C_{cr} \text{ (males)} = \frac{(140 - \text{age}) \text{ (weight kg)}}{(72) \text{ (SrCr mg/dl)}}$$

$$C_{cr} \text{ (females)} = (0.85) \frac{(140 - \text{age}) \text{ (weight kg)}}{(72) \text{ (SrCr mg/dl)}}$$

This equation corrects for the major factors that effect GFR, that is, sex, weight, and age. The normal creatinine clearance established by this method is 140 ± 27 ml/min for men and 112 ± 20 ml/min for women.

For every 50 percent reduction in GFR, the serum creatinine concentration doubles. For example, if a patient has a GFR of 100 ml/min with a serum creatinine of 1 mg/dl, when the GFR falls to 50 ml/min serum creatinine will increase to 2 mg/dl. With a further fall in function to 25 ml/min, serum creatinine again doubles and is 4 mg/dl. As can be appreciated in Figure 11-1, changes in serum creatinine become a very sensitive method of estimating further impairment in renal function when there is already extensive kidney damage, that is, GFR less than 25 ml/min. In most patients with chronic renal failure, a plot of the reciprocal of the serum creatinine against time yields a straight line. The linear decline in the reciprocal serum creatinine value with time is consistent with a linear loss of glomerular filtration. A change in the slope may indicate the superimposition of some additional factor that accelerates renal functional loss such as volume depletion or a nephrotoxic agent if the slope is increased. Conversely, a decrease in the slope represents slowing of the rate of decline in function.

The blood urea nitrogen (BUN) is a less reliable indicator of renal function, since factors other than the GFR including protein intake, state of hydration, antianabolic agents (tetracycline and corticosteroids), blood in the bowel, fever, and infection all can cause changes in BUN in the absence of changes in renal function.

Symptomatology of Chronic Uremia

Early in chronic renal failure, when the GFR is greater than 25 ml/min, that is, approximately 25 percent of normal, the majority of patients have few symptoms,

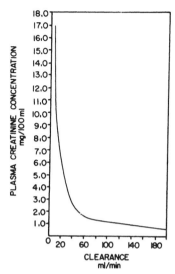

Fig. 11-1. Relationship between serum creatinine concentration and creatinine clearance. (Adapted from P. D. Doolan, E. L. Alpen, and G. B. Thiel, A clinical appraisal of the plasma concentration and endogenous clearance of creatinine. *Am. J. Med.* 32:65, 1962.)

and the biochemical abnormalities are equally unremarkable. Although a rise in serum uric acid has been reported to occur early in renal failure, the increment is usually less than 1 mg/dl [9]. Therefore, with the exception of some patients with interstitial nephritis, secondary gout is uncommon in renal failure. Proteinuria is common at this stage, and in some glomerular diseases the nephrotic syndrome may be present. In association with high-grade proteinuria, the patient may also lose antithrombin III, with resulting antithrombin III deficiency, a hypercoagulable state, and a predisposition to thromboembolic complications [33]. The third major finding in the early stage of renal failure is hypertension. If the hypertension is not treated, arteriolar nephrosclerosis as well as focal glomerulosclerosis may develop and accelerate the loss of renal function. Since it is extremely difficult to determine whether the progressive loss of renal function is a consequence of the underlying renal disease or the hypertensive state, it is imperative that blood pressure be well controlled.

Fluid and Electrolyte Disturbances

As the GFR falls below 25 ml/min, disturbances of fluid and electrolytes may occur. The interesting aspect is that on a normal diet, even with a GFR of 3 to 5 ml/min, there may be only minimal disturbances of plasma electrolytes and the body water content. This is a result of the fact that as GFR falls there is increased fractional clearance of electrolytes, as well as water. This has been termed the magnification phenomenon [34]. This implies that the diseased kidney continues to be under the control of a variety of biologic systems that regulate the excretion of the various electrolytes, and the excretory response per nephron evoked by these systems varies inversely with the number of surviving nephrons. Because of this, the individual with advanced renal failure is able to excrete the elements and waste products obtained from a normal dietary intake, maintaining reasonable water and electrolyte balance.

However, the range over which the individual can maintain balance is limited. Because of the inability to dilute or concentrate urine, if water intake is restricted, the patient will develop increasing dehydration and hypernatremia, and the degree of azotemia may increase secondary to further impaired excretion of nitrogenous waste products. Conversely, if water intake is excessive, hyponatremia may occur.

When placed on a low-sodium diet, the majority of patients with advanced chronic renal failure are either unable to reduce urinary sodium excretion to the level of their sodium intake or else it takes three to four times longer to do so than in a normal person. In a few patients, usually with medullary cystic disease, autosomal dominant polycystic kidney disease, or interstitial nephritis, an excess sodium intake may be necesary to maintain sodium balance [35]. A rare patient may require as much as 10 to 20 g of salt supplementation daily to maintain ECF volume and maximum renal function. In general, such severe renal salt wasting is very infrequent and occurs in the presence of far-advanced renal failure.

In the absence of an endogenous or exogenous potassium load, hyperkalemia rarely occurs in patients who have a GFR above 5 ml/min. Potassium balance is maintained in the majority of patients by a combination of increased tubular secretion of potassium, which is mediated in part by aldosterone [36, 37] and the increased fecal potassium loss [37]. Since these mechanisms must work to the maximum in advanced renal failure, there are several circumstances in which hyperkalemia may develop. Competitive inhibition of aldosterone with spironolactone, or inhibitors of distal potassium secretion, such as amiloride or triamterene, may induce severe hyperkalemia. A second cause of hyperkalemia is an increased intake of potassium, and third is acute acidosis that caused intracellular potassium to be released into the extracellular pool. A rough clinical estimate of the effect of acidosis on serum potassium concentration is as follows: For every decrease of 0.1 pH unit, serum potassium will increase by approximately 0.6 mEq/L.

An additional cause for the spontaneous occurrence of hyperkalemia in patients with renal failure was described by Schambelan and associates [38]. Although all their patients had hyperkalemia in association with chronic renal failure, the degree of renal impairment often was not severe. The majority of their patients had either diabetes mellitus or interstitial nephritis [38]. The highlight of the findings in these patients was diminished plasma levels of renin and aldosterone. It has been suggested that the hyperkalemia is a result of hypoaldosteronism, which is attributable to hyporeninemia. The diminished plasma renin activity may in turn be due to an autonomic neuropathy or sclerosis of the juxtaglomerular apparatus in the diabetic patients. Sickle cell disease, renal transplantation, and lupus nephritis have also been associated with hyperkalemia, probably secondary to diminished tubular secretory capacity. Another cause of hyperkalemia occurs in some patients with chronic obstructive uropathy [39]. In contrast to the hyporeninemic-hypoaldosterone patients, these individuals appear to have a tubular resistance to aldosterone. Thus, when hyperkalemia is noted in patients with chronic renal failure, and other causes have been excluded, these conditions should be considered.

Hypokalemia may also occur in patients with chronic renal insufficiency. A number of factors may be responsible for this finding, including poor dietary intake of potassium, diuretic therapy, hyperaldosteronism secondary to volume depletion or malignant hypertension, or specific renal tubular defects such as those found in association with the Fanconi's syndrome.

Total body burdens of other elements, although not totally corrected by the diseased kidney, are corrected to the extent that the remaining alterations are associated with few, if any, clinical symptomatology until end-stage renal failure has occurred. The fractional clearance of phosphorus, magnesium, and calcium all increase as GFR progressively falls. As a result, plasma magnesium and phosphorus are not elevated until GFR falls below 25 ml/min [40]. Even then, plasma values rarely increase more than 1 to 2 mg/dl until GFR falls below 5 ml/min. The serum magnesium concentration may be slightly elevated when the patient is ingesting a normal magnesium intake. Since such patients have difficulty in excreting large magnesium loads, magnesium-containing antacids and laxatives should be avoided [41].

Although fractional clearance of calcium is increased in renal failure, absolute excretion is actually decreased. In contrast to other elemental disturbances, there may be major consequences as a result of the altered calcium metabolism associated with the uremic state. Parathyroid hormone levels are found to increase when GFR falls to 70 to 80 percent of normal, and 1,25-dihydroxy vitamin D_3 ($1,25[OH]_2D_3$) levels fall when GFR is 40 percent or less than normal. Hypocalcemia is also a common finding in patients with advanced renal failure. Hypocalcemia probably results from a combination of factors including low $1,25(OH)_2D_3$ with decreased gastrointestinal absorption of calcium, hyperphosphatemia, and bone resistance to the calcemic effect of parathyroid hormone.

Acidosis is a common disturbance at a more advanced stage of chronic renal failure. Normally, the kidneys are responsible for excreting 60 to 70 mEq of hydrogen ions daily. Although in a majority of patients with chronic renal failure the urine can be acidified normally [42], these patients have a reduced ability to produce ammonia. With advanced renal failure, total daily acid excretion is usually reduced to 30 to 40 mEq; thus, throughout the remainder of their course of chronic renal failure, many patients may be in a positive hydrogen ion balance of 20 to 40 mEq/day. The retained hydrogen ions probably are buffered by bone salts, although this has not yet been unequivocally proven. On occasion, in the early stage of renal failure, hyperchloremic renal tubular acidosis with a normal anion gap may occur. With more advanced renal failure, the plasma chloride concentration becomes normal, and a fairly large anion gap may develop. In most patients with renal failure, the metabolic acidosis is mild, and the pH is rarely less than 7.35. As with other abnormalities in chronic renal failure, the primary symptomatic manifestations of the acid-base disturbances occur when the patient receives an excessive endogenous or exogenous acid load or loses excessive alkali (e.g., with diarrhea).

The final stage of chronic renal failure occurs when the GFR falls below 5 ml/min.

The deranged metabolic functions present at this stage of renal failure are responsible for the striking clinical features of uremia.

Anemia

Anemia is extremely common at the advanced stage of renal failure and is of the normocytic, normochromic type. The hematocrit is usually first noted to be reduced when the BUN increases to 60 to 80 mg/dl [43]. The hematocrit progressively falls with further deterioration of renal function but only rarely is lower than 18 to 20 percent. The anemia of uremia has been felt to result from a combination of factors, including reduced erythropoietin activity, circulating factors that appear to inhibit the bone marrow response to erythropoietin, and shortened erythrocyte life span. With the recent availability of recombinant erythropoietin, it would appear that the major cause of anemia has been a failure of erythropoietin production by the diseased kidney, since uremic patients typically respond so well to exogenously administered erythropoietin [44].

Bleeding Diathesis

Disturbances in the coagulation system also occur with an advanced stage of chronic renal failure. Approximately 20 percent of uremic patients have a modest degree of thrombocytopenia, but it is rare to find a platelet count of less than 50,000. Severe thrombocytopenia may occur in patients with the hemolytic-uremic syndrome as a consequence of disseminated intravascular coagulation. However, this is not a common cause of chronic renal failure in adults. Platelet factor 3 is reduced and platelet aggregation is decreased [45] in advanced renal failure. This results in prolongation of the Ivy bleeding time and poor clot retraction. Treatment of the uremic state with dialysis improves platelet function in the majority of patients, suggesting some dialyzable factor is responsible for this abnormality. It is of interest that D-deaminoarginine vasopressin (DDAVP) improves the bleeding time without affecting the platelet abnormalities [46]. This suggests that an abnormality in factor VIII or von Willebrand's factor may play a role in the pathogenesis of the bleeding abnormality in the uremic state, since DDAVP has been shown to improve factor VIII levels and the bleeding tendency in von Willebrand's disease [46]. Anemia also contributes to the abnormal bleeding time present in uremic patients. A higher hematocrit causes the platelets to skim at the endothelial surface, which is optimal for platelet endothelium interaction. Such skimming does not occur with hematocrits below 25 to 30 percent.

Serositis

Another complication noted with some frequency in patients with far-advanced renal failure is involvement of the serous membranes as manifested by pericarditis and pleuritis. The involved membrane is markedly thickened, extremely vascular, and infiltrated with plasma cells and histiocytes [47]. Both pleural and pericardial friction rubs may be heard. When pleural and pericardial effusions are present, they are uniformly hemorrhagic and usually contain fewer than 10,000 white blood cells per cubic millimeter. Pericardiocentesis, as well as thoracentesis, is occasionally necessary to relieve clinical symptoms. However, if the uremic state is not improved with treatment of reversible factors or hemodialysis, recurrent effusions are common. Rarely, constrictive pericarditis may follow healing of acute uremic pericarditis.

Chronic ascites also may be a manifestation of uremic serositis and advanced renal failure. This complication arises primarily in patients who have had previous abdominal surgery or peritoneal dialysis. The ascitic fluid is an exudate with the ascitic fluid albumin–plasma albumin concentration ratio of more than 0.5. While fluid overload may worsen uremic ascites, fluid removal frequently is not a successful mode of treatment. Renal transplantation or several consecutive days of intensive dialysis has been useful in treating uremic ascites.

Gastrointestinal Disorders

Most patients with far-advanced renal failure have gastrointestinal symptoms that are a major part of their clinical picture [48]. Specifically, nausea, vomiting, and anorexia are extremely common. Uremic stomatitis, characterized by dry mucous membranes and multiple, bright-red, small, ulcerative lesions, may occur with advanced uremia. Poor dental hygiene appears to contribute to the development of uremic stomatitis. Since saliva in uremic patients has an increased urea content, it has been suggested that the stomatitis results from high levels of ammonium, which is formed by bacteria ureases from the high levels of salivary urea. Inflammation of salivary glands (e.g., parotitis) also may occur in uremic patients and is usually associated with stomatitis. The salivary glands may become markedly swollen in chronic renal failure, but characteristically they are not tender or indurated, as might be seen in inflammatory parotitis.

Pancreatic involvement has also been found on postmortem examination in patients who have died from uremia. Typically, on histologic examination of the pancreas, there is dilatation of the acini, flattening of the epithelial cells, and inspissation of the intra-acinar secretions. Clinical symptoms of pancreatitis also may occur. It was felt previously that uremia alone, as a result of chronic loss of renal function and thus the inability to excrete amylase, could significantly elevate the serum amylase concentration, but this has been shown not to be the case [49]. Rather, when a high elevation of serum amylase concentration is found in patients with chronic renal failure, pancreatitis should be strongly considered. In acute renal failure, however, serum amylase elevations are common but are rarely over twice normal in the absence of clinical evidence of pancreatitis [49]. Other findings in the gastrointestinal tract in advanced uremia include erosive gastritis and uremic colitis characterized by submucosal hemorrhages and small mucosal ulcerations. With the exception of anorexia, nausea, and vomiting, the majority of other gastrointestinal complications of uremia are rarely seen in patients with renal failure now that treatment with dialysis and renal transplantation is possible and initiated relatively early.

Neuromuscular Disturbances

The neuromuscular disturbances occurring in patients with advanced renal failure were some of the earliest clinical symptoms described in uremia [50]. The initial symptoms are mild and consist of emotional lability, insomnia, and a lack of facility in abstract thinking. If the uremic state is allowed to progress, more striking changes are noted, consisting of increased deep tendon reflexes, clonus, asterixis, and stupor, which progress to coma, convulsions, and death.

Uremic neuropathy is another major and potentially disabling complication of chronic renal failure. The earliest feature is the restless legs syndrome, in which the patient has a tendency to avoid inactivity of the lower extremities because of a sensation of numbness. This syndrome is followed by a sensory neuropathy that is characterized by paresthesia and hypalgesia, especially of the feet. In the most severe cases, a motor neuropathy also may occur. Typically, there is symmetric involvement of the lower extremities, which is more severe distally and usually is manifested initially by bilateral footdrop [50]. Uremic neuropathy occasionally can progress rapidly to a state of total quadriplegia. Histologically, the damage in the peripheral nerve occurs in the distal portion of the medullated fibers and involves a loss of myelin. For unknown reasons, the motor neuropathy is much more common in males than in females.

Skeletal Abnormalities (Renal Osteodystrophy)

Other major causes of disability in chronic renal failure, especially in children, are the abnormalities in the skeletal system. Growth is markedly retarded in children with chronic renal failure. The reasons are not well understood, but there is evidence that dialysis, especially chronic cyclic peritoneal dialysis, will improve the growth rate. A high caloric and protein intake may also be helpful. Even with these measures, however, children on dialysis rarely grow normally. The use of corticosteroids after kidney transplantation is also associated with growth retardation. More recently, recombinant human growth hormone has been used with considerable success to increase height velocity in uremic children and in children who have received transplants [51].

Severe rickets with resulting deformities and disability can develop in children with advanced chronic renal failure. The typical radiographic feature of rickets is an irregular and fragmented line that separates the metaphysis from the growth cartilage (Fig. 11-2). The space separating the metaphyseal line and the epiphyseal nucleus is widened, and the epiphyseal center appears late. Although this radiographic finding is classic of vitamin D–deficient rickets, uremic children with this finding characteristically show histologic changes of hyperparathyroidism rather than osteomalacia. Vitamin D and calcium therapy may be effective in correcting this abnormality.

The most common skeletal disturbance found in adults with advanced chronic renal failure is hyperparathyroid bone disease, which is characterized by increased osteoclastic bone resorption. Bone histomorphometry performed in 60 nondialyzed uremic patients revealed that over 80 percent showed evidence of hyperparathyroid

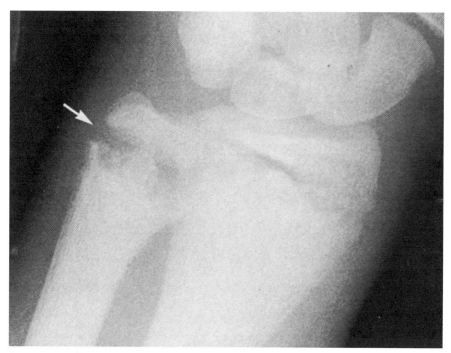

Fig. 11-2. Radiographic features of rickets. The metaphysis of the ulna is fragmented and irregular, and the space separating the metaphysis from the epiphyseal nucleus is widened (*arrow*).

bone disease [52]. Only one patient in this series had histologic evidence of osteomalacia, and this patient was an alcoholic with chronic pancreatitis, suggesting an etiology other than uremia. The parathyroid glands may be markedly hyperplastic, and parathyroid hormone levels are increased. Characteristically, there are few symptoms, and the diagnosis is made by finding the typical radiographic features of subperiosteal resorption. Figure 11-3 shows the subperiosteal resorption in the phalanges and the "salt-and-pepper" pattern in the skull of a patient with severe secondary hyperparathyroidism associated with advanced renal failure. Such patients occasionally develop large osteoclastic tumors (brown cysts) in the skeleton around weight-bearing areas, as shown in Figure 11-4. Under these conditions, parathyroidectomy is indicated, following which there is usually dramatic healing of the cyst (see Fig. 11-4). The hyperparathyroid state usually resolves following renal transplantation [53]. On occasion, however, persistent hypercalcemia that is endangering the integrity of the kidney graft may necessitate parathyroidectomy.

With the advent of chronic hemodialysis, osteomalacia has been noted with increased frequency in uremic patients. This appears to result largely from aluminum intoxication rather than uremia per se (see Inorganic Substances, p. 532, this volume). This disease is characterized by bone pain, fracturing bone disease, and proximal myopathy. Unlike other types of bone disease, osteomalacia is unresponsive to any vitamin D analogues.

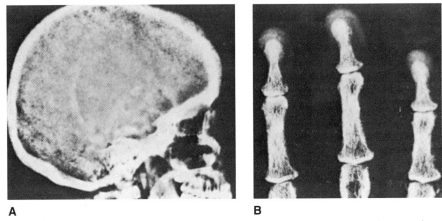

A   **B**

Fig. 11-3. Typical radiographic features of severe secondary hyperparathyroidism involving the skull (note "salt-and-pepper" pattern) (A) and phalanges with lacy subperiosteal reabsorption (B).

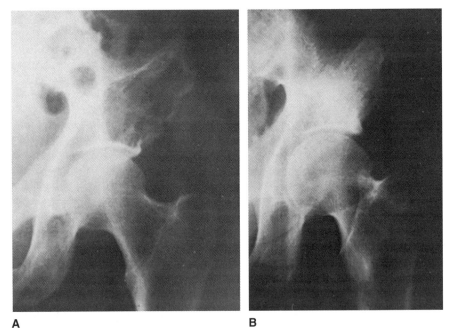

A   **B**

Fig. 11-4. (A) Biopsy-proven osteoclastic tumor (brown cyst) in the left ileum. (B) Appearance 1 year following parathyroid surgery. Healing of the cyst is essentially complete, as judged radiologically.

Recently a third type of bone disease, adynamic bone disease, has been described [54]. This is a histologic diagnosis showing lack of bone formation and resorption. There are usually no clinical findings, and there is a real question as to whether it requires any type of therapy.

Metastatic Calcification

A serious complication associated with chronic renal failure is metastatic calcification. Three distinct types of metastatic calcium phosphate deposits have been described in uremic patients. The specific mechanisms responsible for the development of these deposits have not been well delineated, and it is possible all three have different pathogenic mechanisms.

One of the most potentially devastating forms of metastatic calcification is vascular calcification. An example of diffuse calcification in the arterial vessels of the hand of a patient with advanced renal failure appears in Figure 11-5. This vascular calcification can affect virtually any medium-sized artery in the body and rarely can cause severe vascular insufficiency with the production of gangrene of the extremi-

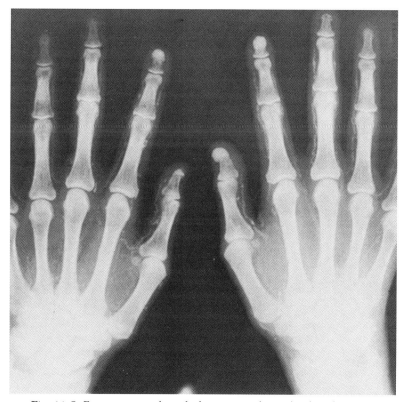

Fig. 11-5. Extensive vascular calcification involving the digital arteries.

ties [55] and ischemic ulcerations of the skin and gastrointestinal tract. Although improvement is occasionally observed following renal transplantation, in general, this vascular calcification persists after renal transplantation or parathyroidectomy. Histologic evidence of vascular calcification occurs even in young individuals with uremia, and by age 50 years, radiographic evidence of vascular calcification is present in almost 100 percent of uremic patients [56]. It is felt that vascular calcification results from an accelerated aging process of the vessels in the uremic state.

The second variety of calcium phosphate deposit is felt to result from hyperphosphatemia. This is based on the fact that these deposits can be rapidly mobilized by reducing the serum phosphorus and thus the calcium phosphate product by dialysis, the use of phosphate-binding antacids, or transplantation [53]. These deposits occur in three forms. Conjunctival calcification causes a redness and gritty feeling in the eyes. Periarticular calcification occurs over pressure points and around joints (Fig. 11-6). The major symptoms associated with these deposits is a limitation of joint movement because of the size of the deposits. The third type of deposit resulting from hyperphosphatemia is acute arthritic episodes secondary to hydroxyapatite crystal deposition in the synovium and joint fluid.

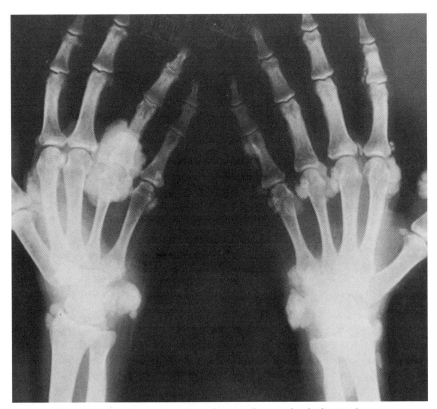

Fig. 11-6. Periarticular calcium phosphate deposits (tumoral calcification) in a patient with advanced renal failure.

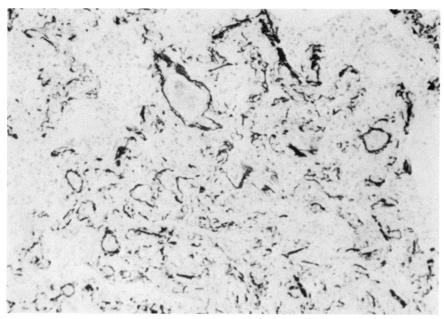

Fig. 11-7. Extensive calcification of the lung. The dark-staining material (von Kossa's stain) present in the alveolar septa and walls of the small arteries is the calcium phosphate deposit.

The final type of calcification found in uremic patients is visceral calcification, which occurs in the lung, skeletal muscle, and myocardium. This is an amorphous calcium phosphate deposit that has markedly different chemical and thermochemical properties from the other two types of calcium phosphate deposits. The vascular and hyperphosphatemic-induced calcifications appear to consist of hydroxyapatite, while visceral calcifications have the thermochemical properties of whitlockite. In cardiac calcification, the deposits occur initially in the conducting system and may cause severe arrhythmias. With far-advanced cardiac calcification, however, there is extensive involvement of the entire myocardium, and death may result from a low cardiac output state. When calcification occurs in the lung, it characteristically causes a fibrous response in the small arteries and alveolar septa (Fig. 11-7). This results in restrictive and diffusion abnormalities and can lead to hypoxemia. The pathogenic mechanism responsible for the development of these visceral calcium phosphate deposits is not well understood. Furthermore, it is unknown whether once present they can be mobilized by either transplantation or reduction of the plasma calcium-phosphate product.

Generalized pruritus is an extremely bothersome complication of chronic renal failure. Some authors have suggested that high skin calcium content may be responsible for it. However, it is possible that skin calcium content also may be secondarily increased as a result of the scratching. Parathyroidectomy has been used in a few cases as a method of treatment of pruritus. However, the majority of patients can be adequately controlled with less radical forms of treatment such as local lubrication, cyproheptadine (Periactin), and reduction of the serum phosphorus with phosphate-binding gels or intensified dialysis.

Immunologic Alterations

The immune response is also blunted in the majority of patients with advanced renal failure, as manifested by depressed delayed hypersensitivity, prolonged survival of skin allografts, and reduced lymphocyte response to phytohemagglutinin [57]. The uremic patient also appears to have a poorer immune response to some infections than nonuremic subjects. This is perhaps best exemplified by the frequent occurrence of positivity for hepatitis B surface antigen (HBsAG) in patients with advanced chronic renal failure [58]. Although these patients usually do not manifest clinical symptoms of hepatitis, they become chronic carriers of the hepatitis-associated antigen. This continuing positivity for HBsAG has recently been related to low interferon levels in uremic patients [59].

Most studies show that otherwise humoral immunity is normal. It has recently been shown that $1,25(OH)_2D_3$ modulates the proliferation, differentiation, and immune function of lymphocytes and monocytes. Based on this finding, it has been suggested that part of the compromised immune function in uremia may be a consequence of the low $1,25(OH)_2D_3$ present in this state [60].

Other Metabolic Disturbances

Finally, a variety of generalized metabolic disturbances are present in the uremic patient. As a result of anorexia, nausea, poor dietary intake, and occasional vomiting, many patients with advanced renal failure present in a chronic state of negative nitrogen balance and protein-calorie malnutrition.

Approximately 70 percent of uremic patients present with glucose intolerance. In contrast to patients with diabetes mellitus, the fasting blood sugar of uremic patients is normal, but postprandial glucose levels are increased [61]. Plasma insulin levels in response to intravenously administered glucose are normal or even accentuated, thus suggesting that the glucose intolerance is a result of peripheral resistance to insulin. There is evidence that this abnormality in glucose metabolism may be improved by hemodialysis. Although glucagon levels are known to be increased in patients with advanced renal failure, dialysis may improve glucose intolerance without altering glucagon levels.

A number of patients with renal failure have type IV hyperlipidemia with increased levels of serum triglycerides and reduced HDL cholesterol. Bagdade and associates [62] have suggested that the hypertriglyceridemia is a result of increased hepatic synthesis of triglyceride-rich lipoprotein and reduced clearing activity of lipoprotein lipase. Whether this disturbance has any clinical importance has not yet been established, but there is some evidence of acceleration of atherosclerosis in patients treated by chronic intermittent hemodialysis. In addition, experimental evidence suggests that abnormal lipid metabolism may contribute to the progression of renal disease.

Pathogenesis of the Uremic Syndrome

Although the metabolic consequences of uremia have been reasonably well defined, the specific uremia toxins responsible for most of these metabolic alterations have not been identified. It is apparent, however, that certain organic compounds, hormonal alterations, and inorganic substances that are affected by the uremic state may cause a number of defects (Table 11-5).

Organic Compounds

Most studies of organic compounds have been directed at determining the toxicity of the various nitrogenous waste products, which consist of urea, ammonia, guanidine, guanidinosuccinic acid, and methylguanidine. Since urea is characteristically elevated and can be correlated with the severity of impairment of renal function, a large number of studies have been directed at determining the role of urea in producing the uremic symptomatology. However, the results of most studies have been disappointing, and at present the only abnormalities that have been suggested as resulting at least in part from urea retention are nausea, anorexia, uremic stomatitis, and possibly uremic colitis.

Guanidine has been found to be increased in the blood of uremic patients. When injected into laboratory animals, guanidine produces muscle twitching, hyperexcitability, paresis, and convulsions. However, recent studies in uremic patients have failed to show a correlation between high guanidine levels and central nervous system symptoms [63].

Another potentially toxic organic compound is myoinositol, a natural constituent of food that is also synthesized in vivo. The concentration of this compound in plasma and cerebrospinal fluid is increased in uremia. Experimentally, myoinositol has been shown to be a neurotoxin, and therefore it has been suggested that this compound might be involved in the pathogenesis of uremic neuropathy [64]. Plasma cyclic adenosine 3',5'-monophosphate (cyclic AMP) levels have also been found to be increased in uremic patients [65]. Plasma cyclic AMP levels have been found to correlate inversely with platelet aggregation, and in vitro, cyclic AMP has been shown to inhibit platelet aggregation [65]. Thus cyclic AMP may be in part responsible for the altered platelet function in uremia.

Possibly the strongest evidence that some of the nitrogenous waste products may be toxic in uremic patients are the studies of Walser and co-workers [66]. In their studies, a number of patients were placed on diets extremely low in nitrogen to

Table 11-5. Partial list of compounds incriminated as "uremic toxins"

Urea	Parathyroid hormone
Polyamines	Myoinositol
Guanidines	β_2-Microglobulin
Middle molecules	

reduce the production of nitrogenous waste products. The diets were supplemented with the ketoanalogues of the essential amino acids. These ketoanalogues were used to supply the carbon skeletons for the essential amino acids and thus to prevent the breakdown of tissue protein. There was marked improvement in the patients' sense of well-being and possibly in some other abnormalities associated with the uremic syndrome. Although these results are not conclusive in demonstrating that nitrogenous waste products have a role in producing some uremic symptoms, they are deserving of further study.

Another organic toxin recently identified in dialyzed uremic patients is the protein β_2-microglobulin. Normally the kidney is responsible for the elimination of this protein, which has a molecular weight of 11,800 dalton. The 150 to 200 mg produced each day is filtered by the glomerulus and catabolized in the proximal tubule. With renal failure, elimination of this protein is prevented, and it is retained, increasing plasma levels by up to 50-fold and causing it to be deposited in tissues. The protein is deposited in tissues as amyloid, with its deposition being present largely in joint capsules, synovial membranes, the carpal tunnel, subchondral bone, tendons, intervertebral disks, and bone marrow [67]. Clinical symptomatology from β_2-microglobulin deposition includes carpal tunnel syndrome, bone cysts, destructive spondylarthropathy, effusive arthritis, scapulohumeral periarthritis, and camptodactyly. This complication has usually been seen in dialyzed uremic patients probably because it requires a minimum of 6 years of almost total loss of renal function for enough β_2-microglobulin to be deposited to cause any clinical disturbances. Once deposited, it would appear that even following reinstitution of renal function with a successful renal transplant, this amyloid is not mobilized.

Hormonal Alterations

Hormonal alterations occur in uremia as a result of four mechanisms. First, the diseased kidney may be unable to produce certain hormones normally, such as erythropoietin and $1,25(OH)_2D_3$ [68]. Second, the kidney normally excretes or degrades a variety of hormones: growth hormone, prolactin, luteinizing hormone, gastrin, insulin, glucagon, and parathyroid hormone. Levels of these hormones may be increased in patients with chronic renal failure because of lack of ability of the diseased kidney to metabolize or excrete these substances. Third, the diseased kidney as a result of ischemia may cause increased renin secretion, which in turn increases angiotensin and aldosterone production. The final mechanism for hormone alteration in uremia is the "trade-off" hypothesis [69].

The various hormonal alterations present in the uremic state may result in a variety of clinical disturbances (Table 11-6). However, the mere finding of increased levels of immunoreactive hormones does not necessarily mean that they are biologically active. That some of these hormones lack biologic activity is suggested by the fact that gastrin levels are not correlated with basal acid secretion in uremic patients. It has also been suggested that the measured growth hormone and possibly glucagon are not biologically active. Furthermore, it has been shown that the largest fraction of the elevated levels of immunoreactive parathyroid hormone is the inactive C-terminal, which is normally disposed of by the kidney.

Table 11-6. Hormonal alterations in uremia

Hormone	Potential metabolic consequences
Increased	
Prolactin	Lactation
Luteinizing hormone	Gynecomastia
Gastrin	Gastritis
Renin-aldosterone	Hypertension
Glucagon	Glucose intolerance
Growth hormone	
Parathyroid hormone	Osteitis fibrosis
Decreased	
1,25-Dihydroxyvitamin D_3	Osteitis fibrosa
Erythropoietin	Anemia
Somatomedin	Decreased linear growth
Testosterone	Impotence
Follicle-stimulating hormone	Impotence

Elevated parathyroid hormone levels have been incriminated in the pathogenesis of numerous abnormalities found in the uremic state, including neuropathy, encephalopathy, anemia, pruritus, impotence, and carbohydrate and lipid alterations [70]. Although parathyroid hormone has been shown in vitro to increase red cell osmotic fragility, decrease erythropoiesis, and decrease myocardial function and in vivo to be associated with increased brain calcium content and electroencephalographic (EEG) alterations, it is still unclear what role parathyroid hormone plays in the uremic symptomatology found in humans.

Bricker [69] has proposed another conceptual approach to the pathogenesis of uremia, the so-called trade-off hypothesis. This theory suggests that with the progressive destruction of nephrons, a number of adaptive mechanisms are brought into play to allow the remaining nephrons to maintain normal body homeostasis. The adaptive changes that occur to maintain sodium balance in the patient with advanced renal failure have been used as an illustrative example of the trade-off hypothesis. With a normal sodium intake of 120 mEq/day and a normal GFR, approximately 0.5 percent of the filtered load of sodium is excreted. However, on a similar sodium intake, when GFR has fallen to 2 ml/min, approximately 30 percent of the filtered load of sodium must be excreted to maintain sodium balance. The assumption is made that there is a substance that inhibits the tubular reabsorption of sodium, possibly a natriuretic hormone. It is further suggested that this inhibitor is present in high concentrations in the uremic patient's serum and that it may affect a variety of cellular transport systems and in turn lead to functional changes in other organs and organ systems. The trade-off is that the effects of such a hormone would be beneficial for the kidney and sodium balance but might cause some of the symptoms of uremia by inhibiting transport systems in other organs.

The increased parathyroid hormone levels found in patients with chronic renal failure have been suggested to be another example of a trade-off phenomenon. In this instance, it is proposed that as nephrons are lost, even early in the course of renal failure, phosphate excretion is reduced, and serum phosphorus rises. The elevated serum phosphorus then causes serum calcium concentration to fall, an effect that leads to increased parathyroid hormone release. The increased parathyroid activity is then associated with a decrease in tubular reabsorption of phosphorus, which results in increased phosphorus excretion and returns the serum phosphorus to near-normal levels. As more nephrons are lost and the amount of filtered phosphate further decreases, higher serum concentrations of parathyroid hormone are required to maintain phosphorus balance. The trade-off for the maintenance of phosphorus would be the clinical consequences of secondary hyperparathyroidism on the bony skeleton. More recently, it has been suggested that hyperphosphatemia per se can stimulate parathyroid hormone secretion. However, other factors as well are also probably important in the pathogenesis of the hyperparathyroid state. It has been shown that there is a reduced number of calcitriol receptors on the parathyroid gland in the uremic state [71]. Since calcitriol suppresses the synthesis of parathyroid hormone, the combination of decreased calcitriol receptor number and impaired renal production of $1,25(OH)_2D_3$ would markedly decrease this hormone's inhibitor effect on parathyroid hormone synthesis [72]. Bone resistance to parathyroid hormone in patients with renal failure may be an additional cause of the secondary hyperparathyroidism.

Inorganic Substances

The role of inorganic substances in producing some of the uremic symptomatology has received increasing interest. Brain and peripheral nerve calcium levels have been found to be increased in uremic patients. The elevated calcium levels have been associated with impairment of neurologic function, EEG disturbances [73], and reduced motor nerve conduction velocities [73]. The finding that the elevated calcium levels and altered neurologic function can be prevented by parathyroidectomy suggests that parathyroid hormone is involved in the pathogenesis of these disturbances. The observation of increased calcium levels in peripheral nerves, however, awaits confirmation.

Phosphorus represents another inorganic toxin. As already stated, phosphorus retention is probably quite important in the pathogenesis of the secondary hyperparathyroidism state in uremic subjects [69]. Phosphorus retention is also involved in the pathogenesis of metastatic calcification.

Based on strong biochemical and epidemiologic studies, it is now firmly established that aluminum intoxication is responsible for major neurologic and skeletal toxicity in uremic patients [74, 75]. Although aluminum intoxication was initially felt to result only from aluminum-contaminated dialysate, it is now apparent that toxicity can also result from the orally administered, aluminum-containing phosphate-binding gels commonly given to uremic patients. Aluminum-induced neurologic toxicity is characterized by a distinctive speech disturbance, myoclonus, seizures, and dementia. It is progressive, with death usually occurring 6 to 8 months after the onset of the first symptoms [74]. The bone disease associated with aluminum intoxication is fracturing osteomalacia, which is resistant to treatment with vitamin

D analogues [75]. Recent studies suggest that both the encephalopathy and osteomalacia can be cured by chelation of the aluminum with desferrioxamine. A microcytic hypochromic anemia also attributed to aluminum intoxication has been found to improve following desferrioxamine treatment.

Although zinc deficiency has been implicated as the cause of impotence and anorexia in uremic patients, zinc replacement has given conflicting results, with some investigators finding improvement in potency, smell, taste, and appetite, while others find no effect at all. There is little evidence that other trace element alterations are responsible for any additional symptomatology found in uremic patients.

It would thus appear that a variety of toxins are responsible for the array of clinical signs and symptoms of the uremic state and that a number of different pathogenetic mechanisms are involved. However, only a relatively small number of toxins and mechanisms have been identified or defined to explain the wide spectrum of uremic symptomatology.

Progression of Renal Failure

It has been well documented that when a critical loss of nephron population occurs from a variety of different causes, the remaining renal tissue will ultimately be lost, resulting in ESRD. The most classic example of this phenomenon in humans is oligomeganephronia [76]. This is a congenital disease in which the child is born with a markedly reduced number of nephrons. The nephrons that are present are greatly hypertrophied. However, these hyperfunctioning nephrons undergo spontaneous destruction over the first few years of life, and the child usually dies of uremia by 3 or 4 years of age. Other examples supporting the concept that secondary or compensatory changes resulting from loss of renal mass may promote further injury are unilateral renal agenesis [77] and severe reflux nephropathy, both of which may develop glomerulosclerosis and progress to ESRD.

The compensatory mechanisms resulting from loss of renal function that mediate this injury have not been totally defined, although altered intrarenal hemodynamics [78] and systemic hypertension [79] are currently felt to be of major importance. It has been shown that when renal mass is surgically reduced, glomerular plasma flow, intraglomerular hydraulic pressure, and GFR of the remaining nephrons are markedly increased. These altered intrarenal hemodynamic events may lead to glomerular injury, resulting in glomerular sclerosis and functional deterioration. Any injury or disease that reduces nephron population appears to cause a compensatory afferent arteriolar dilatation, which allows the glomerular capillary bed to be exposed to increased hydraulic pressure with resulting injury. This is supported by the fact that hypertension is especially injurious to the glomeruli of a diseased kidney and that treatment of hypertension markedly reduces the rate and severity of glomerular injury in renal diseases such as diabetic glomerulosclerosis and experimental glomerulonephritis. The evidence for the harmful effects of altered intrarenal hemodynamics on the diseased kidney is strong. However, other secondary or compensatory changes such as compensatory glomerular hypertrophy may result in glomerular injury. Similarly, increased intrarenal energy requirement, renal parenchymal calcification, or tubule fluid iron may also be of importance in promoting tubulointerstitial injury in a diseased kidney.

Reversible Factors Compromising Renal Function

Renal function in chronically diseased kidneys can be further compromised by a number of potentially reversible factors (Table 11-7).

Volume Depletion

The most common reversible factor that can cause rapid deterioration of renal function is depletion of the ECF volume. If ECF volume depletion develops in a patient who already has compromised renal function, a vicious cycle of events may ensue. The diminished renal function that accompanies ECF volume depletion may cause worsening of the azotemic state. With the increased azotemia, nausea and vomiting may occur, leading to more volume depletion, further compromising GFR, and intensifying the uremia state, thus repeating the cycle. The diagnosis of severe volume depletion is easy, since the patient will demonstrate tachycardia, postural hypotension, a dry furrowed tongue, and loss of skin elasticity. At an earlier stage of volume depletion, however, physical findings may be minimal. A history of over-zealous treatment with potent diuretic agents or stringent salt restriction may suggest the diagnosis of modest volume depletion in patients with chronic renal failure who have had recent deterioration of renal function. It is frequently necessary to treat the patient with salt supplementation to determine whether renal function will improve. A weight gain of 1 to 3 kg generally constitutes a reasonable indication of ECF volume expansion.

Infection and Obstruction

Since many urinary tract infections are asymptomatic, a urine culture should be obtained on the initial evaluation of patients with chronic renal failure. To prevent the introduction of a bacterial infection, instrumentation and indwelling catheterization of the urinary tract also are best avoided in such patients. Another potentially reversible cause of renal failure is urinary tract obstruction. Obstruction can be excluded with about 95 percent confidence by performing ultrasound studies; retro-

Table 11-7. Reversible factors responsible for renal function deterioration

Infection	Hypertension
Urinary tract obstruction	Pericardial tamponade
Extracellular fluid volume depletion	Hypercalcemia
Nephrotoxic agents	Hyperuricemia > 15–20 mg/dl
Congestive heart failure	Hypokalemia

grade pyelograms, therefore, are seldom necessary, even when the patient has severely compromised renal function. Ultrasound will also give valuable information in regard to the presence of two kidneys as well as kidney size. A postvoid residual urine as assessed by a straight catheterization will allow exclusion of important bladder-neck obstruction (>50 ml of residual urine). A flat-plate radiograph of the abdomen with nephrotomograms can also help establish renal size and exclude the presence of radiopaque calculi.

Nephrotoxic Agents

Another potential cause of reversible renal failure are nephrotoxic agents. The most common are the antimicrobials and antitumor agents, including aminoglycosides, colistin, amphotericin, gallium, and cisplatin. An additional group of agents that can further compromise renal function in patients with chronic renal failure is radiocontrast media. Predisposing factors to contrast media–induced renal failure include diabetes mellitus, advanced age, volume depletion, other nephrotoxic agents such as aminoglycosides, and preexisting renal failure. While the use of these agents in patients with chronic renal failure is not contraindicated, they should be used with the consideration that they can cause permanent as well as reversible changes in renal function. Since toxicity is somewhat dose dependent, the smallest dose consistent with obtaining an adequate study should be administered. In addition, the patient's volume status should be optimized prior to their administration. Mannitol (20 g IV) at the time of the contrast media administration may also be protective; however, the results of a recent study favored the protective effect of saline [90].

Pharmacologic Reduction in Function

Recently, two other drug classes, converting enzyme inhibitors and cyclooxygenase inhibitors [80, 81], have been shown to decrease renal function acutely and reversibly in patients with underlying renal disease. The nonsteroidal anti-inflammatory agents cause this effect by inhibiting renal prostaglandins and their vasodilatory effect, which causes a reduction in renal blood flow and GFR. The converting enzyme inhibitors exert their effect by inhibiting angiotensin II constriction of the glomerular efferent arteriole. This causes a reduction in filtration pressure and, in turn, GFR. The effects of these agents on GFR are most commonly seen when renal arterial flow is reduced as a consequence of volume depletion, congestive heart failure, or bilateral renal artery stenosis, where filtration pressure is largely being maintained by angiotensin II–induced efferent arteriolar constriction. The effects of both the cyclooxygenase inhibitors and converting enzyme inhibitors on reducing GFR are rapidly reversed by discontinuing their administration. When indicated, therefore, the use of these drugs in patients with chronic renal failure is not universally contraindicated.

Cardiovascular Effects

Congestive heart failure in the uremic patient can result from a variety of causes, such as atherosclerosis, hypertension, and fluid overload. Treatment of congestive heart failure may improve kidney function. Blood pressure should be normalized by fluid removal, antihypertensive agents, or both. A diuresis can usually be accomplished with large doses of furosemide; however, when renal failure is severe, dialysis may be indicated to remove the excess body fluid. Since digoxin is largely excreted by the kidney, the dosage has to be modified in patients with compromised renal function.

In patients with far-advanced renal failure, the possibility of uremic pericarditis with associated pericardial effusion and tamponade should be considered. The clinical features of this diagnosis consist of increased jugular venous pulsations with a paradoxical inspiratory accentuation (Kussmaul's sign), pulsus paradoxus, and a reduction in systemic blood pressure and pulse pressure. A pericardial friction rub may or may not be present. With an extremely severe cardiac tamponade, the paradoxical pulse may not be present, and the only finding may be a reduction in blood and pulse pressures. The diagnosis is easily confirmed by ultrasound or blood-pool scanning. Pericardiocentesis may be lifesaving; in addition, by relieving the tamponade, it may improve cardiac output and renal function. Finally, treatment of severe hypercalcemia, hypokalemia, and hyperuricemia also may lead to improvement in renal function.

Decreasing Rate of Functional Deterioration

Diabetic Renal Disease

Several factors have been identified that might either prevent the development of diabetic renal disease or slow its progression to ESRD. Both animal and human studies have shown that, with strict control of the blood glucose levels, renal functional as well as anatomic alterations may be prevented or actually reversed. Further support for the beneficial effect of tight glucose control is that transplantation of a kidney in conjunction with a pancreas in patients with ESRD from diabetes has been found to prevent mesangial expansion and thickening of the basement membrane in the transplanted kidney [82]. These glomerular changes are commonly observed when the kidney alone is transplanted into diabetic patients. Finally, a recent multicenter study involving 1441 patients with type I diabetes showed that intensive insulin therapy delayed the onset and slowed the progression of diabetic retinopathy, nephropathy, and neuropathy [83].

A recent multicenter study involving over 400 patients with type I diabetes clearly showed that the converting enzyme inhibitor captopril protected against deterioration of renal function significantly more than blood pressure control alone [84]. This protective effect was especially noted in type I diabetics with serum creatinine greater than 1.5 mg/dl. These studies clearly show that converting enzyme inhibitors are protective not only as a consequence of blood pressure control but probably more importantly because of their intrarenal effects on decreasing efferent arteriolar constriction and a reducing proteinuria. Based on this study, the Food and Drug Administration approved the use of captopril in diabetic patients to protect against renal functional deterioration. Angiotensin-converting enzyme (ACE) inhibitors probably should be given to all patients with type I and probably type II diabetic renal disease, hypertensive or not, even when there is only early renal involvement manifested by microalbuminuria, unless their use is specially contraindicated.

Hypertension

Increasing evidence suggests that the control of hypertension can have a major effect on reducing the progression of chronic renal failure in patients with essential hypertension as well as patients with primary renal disease. Blacks are especially at risk of renal failure from hypertension [4, 6]. Therefore, hypertension should be aggressively controlled in most patients by virtually any agent(s) shown to be effective. The possible exception is patients with proteinuric renal disease, for whom ACE inhibitors may be the drug of choice for management of hypertension.

Proteinuric Renal Disease

In proteinuric renal disease (glomerular disease), evidence is accumulating strongly suggesting that any means of reducing urinary protein excretion exerts a protective effect on renal function. The means that have been applied for this purpose are dietary protein restriction and ACE inhibitors. However, a large multicenter trial carried out in 840 patients with chronic renal disease showed that a very low–protein diet had minimal effect on slowing the progression of renal functional deterioration [85]. In view of this study, as well as poor patient acceptance, the potential for inducing protein malnutrition, and expense of dietary management and amino acid supplementation, dietary protein restriction does not appear to be a feasible or effective means of treating patients with chronic renal failure. However, there is increasing evidence that ACE inhibitors are effective not only in diabetic renal disease but also in any proteinuric renal disease [86, 87]. There are studies, however, in which these ACE inhibitors have decreased proteinuria and yet worsened renal function. While calcium channel blockers in general do not decrease proteinuria to the degree of ACE inhibitors, some studies using animals have shown protective and additive effects on proteinuria with ACE inhibitors and non-dihydropyridine calcium channel blockers. ACE inhibitors have only been shown to have a protective effect in proteinuric renal disease. Otherwise, any protection exerted in nonproteinuric renal disease is probably only a result of blood pressure control. It has been estimated that 10 to 15 percent of patients may not tolerate these drugs because of their causing chronic coughing or hyperkalemia.

Management of the Uremic State

Fluid and Electrolytes

Because of the accompanying decrease in tubule processing of the filtrate associated with progressive functional loss, a greater fraction of the filtrate is excreted as urine. As a result, the patient with chronic renal failure is able to maintain fluid and major elemental balance throughout the course of renal functional deterioration until GFR has fallen to a critical value of less than 5 percent of normal. By maintaining a urine volume of approximately 2 L/day, the patient with advanced renal failure is able to excrete the normal fluid (2 liters), sodium (140 mEq), potassium (70 mEq), osmotic load (600 mOsm), and nitrogen (12 g, equivalent to 72 g of protein) present in the average American diet without excreting a concentrated or dilute urine. Therefore, dietary restrictions, which may cause protein-calorie malnutrition, are not required in the majority of uremic patients throughout the entire course of renal failure up to, and even including, end-stage disease. Similarly, dietary sodium and potassium restriction is not required in the majority of patients with chronic renal failure and can actually be harmful, as described previously. A high-potassium diet, potassium sparing diuretics, and a high-sodium diet are contraindicated in advanced renal failure because of hyperkalemia, hypertension, and fluid overload, respectively.

The mild acidosis present in the majority of patients with chronic renal failure can readily be treated by the administration of 12 mEq (1 g) of sodium bicarbonate given three times daily. This amount of bicarbonate has minimal effect on blood pressure and ECF volume [88]. However, not all nephrologists believe that there is a need to treat the mild acidosis of chronic renal failure.

Chronic renal failure causes edema by two distinct mechanisms: (1) hypoalbuminemia (serum albumin < 2.5 g/dl) secondary to urinary protein loss and (2) when the ingestion of sodium and water exceeds the ability of the diseased kidney to eliminate the ingested loads. Management of the first cause is discussed in Chapter 14. In general, development of edema from the latter cause is a consequence of advanced renal failure and marked reduction in GFR. This frequently necessitates institution of treatment for ESRD, that is, dialysis or transplantation of sodium and water restriction with loop diuretics is ineffective.

Calcium and Phosphate

Patients with advanced renal failure have decreased $1,25(OH)_2D_3$ levels, are commonly mildly hypocalcemic, have hyperphosphatemia, and usually have histologic evidence of mild hyperparathyroid bone disease. However, these conditions are usually mild and asymptomatic and do not require the routine administration of $1,25(OH)_2D_3$. Severe hyperparathyroid bone disease is rarely seen in nondialyzed uremic patients. There is increasing evidence suggesting that pulse therapy with up 1 to 3 μg of calcitriol administered intravenously is more effective in treating hyperparathyroid bone disease than usual daily oral doses of 0.5 to 1.0 μg of calcitriol. These large intravenous doses of calcitriol result in much higher plasma levels, which more effectively occupy receptors on the parathyroid gland and suppress parathyroid hormone synthesis. In addition, intravenously administered calcitriol has less effect on gastrointestinal absorption of calcium than orally administered calcitriol, resulting in less hypercalcemia. However, intravenous calcitriol therapy has only been reportedly used in dialyzed uremic patients.

Prevention of progressive hyperphosphatemia at this stage of renal failure can be accomplished by administering compounds that bind dietary phosphate in the gut, thus preventing its absorption. Aluminum salts were initially used, but because of the occurrence of aluminum loading and toxicity from their ingestion, they are no longer recommended. Currently, calcium carbonate and calcium acetate are the most widely used phosphate binders. To improve their effectiveness and decrease the chance of causing hypercalcemia, these drugs (1–2 g) should be given with meals.

Anemia

Anemia is common in patients with chronic renal failure. However, it is usually not severe until late in the course of renal failure, when the hematocrit may fall to around 20 percent. The hematocrit rarely needs treatment with erythropoietin in patients with chronic renal disease prior to ESRD. However, if treatment is required prior to ESRD because of associated conditions such as cardiac or pulmonary disease, erythropoietin, although quite expensive, is effective [89]. Prior to erythropoietin administration, iron stores should be documented to be adequate by the measurement of serum ferritin, iron, and total iron binding capacity. The initial dosage of erythropoietin should be 50 units/kg subcutaneously twice weekly. An adequate response to erythropoietin therapy will result in an increased reticulocyte count within 1 week and rise in hematocrit after 2 to 4 weeks. A potential complication of increasing the hematocrit with erythropoietin is hypertension, which can have an adverse effect on renal function.

Bleeding Diathesis

The bleeding diathesis present in uremia usually requires no treatment unless the patient requires surgery or experiences a traumatic event. Correction of anemia with either transfusion of packed cells or administration of recombinant human erythropoietin may improve hemostasis. The minimum target hematocrit should be approximately 26 percent. Fifty to seventy-five percent of uremic patients have improvement or correction of the bleeding time with DDAVP. The usual dosage is 0.3 μg/kg given intravenously, subcutaneously, or intranasally. It is effective within 1 to 2 hours, with its effect persisting for approximately 4 hours. Tachyphylaxis can occur within 24 to 48 hours. Conjugated estrogens improve bleeding time in approximately 80 percent of the patients. The usual dosage is 0.6 mg/kg daily for five consecutive days. The initial effect on bleeding time occurs within 6 hours with peak response in 5 to 7 days, which persists for up to 14 days. Cryoprecipitate is also effective in controlling the uremic bleeding diathesis. The usual infusion of cryoprecipitate is 10 bags. It affects the bleeding time within 1 hour and persists for 18 hours. Platelet infusions are also effective but are recommended only for life-threatening emergencies.

Miscellaneous Disturbances

In general, other disturbances that occur with chronic renal failure such as mild glucose intolerance, hypertriglyceridemia, and mild elevation of uric acid require no treatment. However, because of the inability of renal excretion of large loads of magnesium, magnesium-containing antacids and laxatives should be largely avoided. Similarly, as stated previously, potassium supplementation, even with diuretic administration, potassium sparing diuretics, and salt substitutes, should be avoided unless hypokalemia is present.

Indications for Initiation of ESRD Therapy

Symptomatic uremia usually develops when serum creatinine reaches 8 to 10 mg/dl and BUN is greater than 100 mg/dl. Classically, the first manifestations are gastrointestinal symptoms of nausea, anorexia, and possibly vomiting. However, other symptoms and findings of advanced uremia such as intractable itching, malnutrition, volume overload, protracted hyperkalemia, and impairment of cognitive function represent additional indications for the consideration of initiating ESRD treatment. Serositis (pericarditis and pleuritis) does not respond to conservative measures but usually resolves following initiation of dialysis or transplantation. In addition, uremic motor neuropathy is a progressive and debilitating condition in the uremic state. However, progression can be prevented by adequate dialysis or transplantation. Therefore, both serositis and motor neuropathy represent specific indications for the immediate initiation of ESRD therapy. As stated previously, both anemia and the bleeding disorder can be improved by ESRD therapy. However, neither represents an absolute indication for commencement of ESRD therapy, since other treatment modalities are available.

References

1. U.S. Renal Data System: *USRDS 1994 Annual Report, National Institute of Arthritis, Metabolism and Digestive and Kidney Disease.* Bethesda, MD, National Institutes of Health, 1994.
2. Cowie CC, Port FK, Wolfe RA, et al: Disparities in incidence of diabetic end-stage renal disease according to race and type of diabetes. *N Engl J Med* 321:1074–1079, 1989.
3. Klag MJ, Whelton PK, Neaton JD, et al: Blood pressure and incidence of ESRD in men in the MRFIT screened cohort. *JASN* 5:334, 1994 (Abst.).
4. Klag MJ, Whelton PK, Neaton JE, et al: Higher incidence of ESRD in African-American men in the MRFIT screened cohort. *JASN* 5:334, 1994 (Abst.).
5. Woods JW, Blythe WB, Huffines WD: Malignant hypertension and renal insufficiency. *N Engl J Med* 291:10–14, 1974.
6. Rostand SG, Brown G, Kirk KA, et al: Renal insufficiency in treated essential hypertension. *N Engl J Med* 320:684–688, 1989.
7. Rostand SG, Kirk KA, Rutsky EA, et al: Racial differences in the incidence of treatment for end-stage renal disease. *N Engl J Med* 306:1276–1279, 1982.
8. Mroczek WJ, Davidson M, Gavrilavich L, et al: The value of aggressive therapy in the hypertensive patient with azotemia. *Circulation* 40:893–904, 1969.
9. McPhaul JJ Jr: Hyperuricemia and urate excretion in chronic renal disease. *Metabolism* 17:430–438, 1968.
10. Emmerson BT: Chronic lead nephropathy. *Kidney Int* 4:1–5, 1973.
11. Kincaid-Smith P: Analgesic nephropathy. *Kidney Int* 13:1–8, 1978.
12. Talbott JH, Terplan KL: The kidney in gout. *Medicine* (Baltimore) 39:405–462, 1960.
13. Berman LB, Schreiner GE, Feys J: The nephrotoxic lesion of ethylene glycol. *Ann Intern Med* 46:611–619, 1957.

14. Williams HE, Smith LH Jr: Disorders of oxalate metabolism. *Am J Med* 45:715–735, 1968.
15. Frascino JA, Vanamee P, Rosen PP: Renal oxalosis and azotemia after methoxyflurane anesthesia. *N Engl J Med* 283:676–679, 1970.
16. Stauffer JQ, Humphreys MH, Weir GJ: Acquired hyperoxaluria with regional enteritis after ileal resection. *Ann Intern Med* 79:383–391, 1973.
17. Britton DC, Thompson MH, Johnston ID, et al: Renal function following parathyroid surgery in primary hyperparathyroidism. *Lancet* 2:74–75, 1971.
18. Burnett CH, Commons RR, Albright F, et al: Hypercalcemia without hypercalciuria or hyperphosphatemia, calcinosis and renal insufficiency: Syndrome following prolonged intake of milk and alkali. *N Engl J Med* 240:787–798, 1949.
19. Crutcher JC: Clinical manifestations and therapy of acute lead intoxication due to ingestion of illicitly distilled alcohol. *Ann Intern Med* 59:707–715, 1963.
20. Batuman V, Maesaka JK, Haddad B, et al: The role of lead in gout nephropathy. *N Engl J Med* 304:520–523, 1981.
21. Ui J: Pollution disasters in Japan. *Lakartidningen* 69:2789–2795, 1972.
22. Aperia A, Broberger O, Ericson NO, et al: Effect of vesicoureteric reflux on renal function in children with recurrent urinary infections. *Kidney Int* 9:418–423, 1976.
23. Smellie M, Edwards D, Hunter N, et al: Vesico-ureteric reflux and renal scarring. *Kidney Int* 8(Suppl 4):S65–72, 1975.
24. Assael BM, Claris-Appiani A, Acerbi L, et al: Congenital renal damage in males with vesicoureteric reflux. *JASN* 5:387, 1994.
25. Smellie JM, Tamminen-Mobius T, Olbing C, et al: Five-year study of medical or surgical treatment in children with severe reflux: Radiological renal findings. *Pediatr Nephrol* 6:223–230, 1992.
26. Perkoff GT: The hereditary renal diseases. *N Engl J Med* 277:79–85, 1967.
27. Reeders ST, Zerres K, Gal A, et al: First prenatal diagnosis of autosomal dominant polycystic kidney disease using a DNA probe. *Lancet* 2:6–7, 1986.
28. Horton R: Trials and technology in nephrology. *Lancet* 344:1287, 1994.
29. Pontier PJ, Patel TG: Racial differences in the prevalence and presentation of glomerular disease in adults. *Clin Nephrol* 42:79–84, 1994.
30. Krolewski AS, Canessa M, Warram JH, et al: Predisposition to hypertension and susceptibility to renal disease in insulin-dependent diabetes mellitus. *N Engl J Med* 318:140–145, 1988.
31. Alleyne GAO, Millward DJ, Scullard GH: Total body potassium, muscle electrolytes, and glycogen in malnourished children. *J Pediatr* 76:75–81, 1970.
32. Cockcroft DW, Gault MH: Prediction of creatinine clearance from serum creatinine. *Nephron* 16:31–35, 1976.
33. Kaufman RH, Veltkamp JJ, Van Tilburg NH, et al: Acquired antithrombin III deficiency and thrombosis in the nephrotic syndrome. *Am J Med* 65:607–613, 1978.
34. Bricker NS, Fine LG, Kaplan M, et al: "Magnification" phenomenon in chronic renal disease. *N Engl J Med* 299:1287–1293, 1978.
35. Stanbury SW, Mailer RF: Salt-wasting renal disease: Metabolic observations on a patient with "salt-losing nephritis." *Q J Med* 28:425–447, 1959.
36. Schrier RW, Regal EM: Influence of aldosterone on sodium, water and potassium metabolism in chronic renal disease. *Kidney Int* 1:156–168, 1972.
37. Hayes CP, McLeod MF, Robinson RR: An extrarenal mechanism for the maintenance of potassium balance in severe chronic renal failure. *Trans Assoc Am Physicians* 80:207–216, 1967.
38. Schambelan M, Stockist JR, Biglieri EG: Isolated hypoaldosteronism in adults: A renin-deficiency syndrome. *N Engl J Med* 287:573–578, 1972.
39. Battle DC, Arruda JAL, Kurtzman NA: Hyperkalemic distal renal tubular acidosis associated with obstruction. *N Engl J Med* 304:373–379, 1981.
40. Bricker NS, Slatopolsky E, Reiss E, et al: Calcium, phosphorus, and bone in renal disease and transplantation. *Arch Intern Med* 123:543–553, 1969.
41. Randall RE Jr, Chen MD, Spray CC, et al: Hypermagnesemia in renal failure: Etiology and toxic manifestation. *Ann Intern Med* 61:73–88, 1964.

42. Seldin DW, Coleman AJ, Carter NW, et al: The effect of Na2SO4 on urinary acidification in chronic renal disease. *J Lab Clin Med* 69:893–903, 1967.
43. Verel D, Turnbull A, Tudhope GR, et al: Anemia in Bright's disease. *Q J Med* 28:491–504, 1959.
44. Eschbach JW, Abdulhad MH, Browne JK, et al: Recombinant human erythropoietin in anemic patients with end-stage renal disease. *Ann Intern Med* 111:992–1000, 1989.
45. Castaidi PA, Rozenberg MC, Stewart JH: The bleeding disorder of uremia: A qualitative platelet defect. *Lancet* 2:66–69, 1966.
46. Eberst ME, Berkowitz LR: Hemostasis in renal disease: Pathophysiology and management. *Am J Med* 96:168–179, 1994.
47. Alfrey AC, Goss JE, Ogden DA, et al: Uremic hemopericardium. *Am J Med* 45:391–400, 1968.
48. Schreiner GE, Maher JF: *Uremia: Biochemistry, Pathogenesis and Treatment.* Springfield, IL, Thomas, 1961.
49. Levitt MD, Rapoport M, Cooperband SR: The renal clearance of amylase in renal insufficiency, acute pancreatitis and macroamylasemia. *Ann Intern Med* 71:919–925, 1969.
50. Tyler HR: Neurologic disorders in renal failure. *Am J Med* 44:734–748, 1968.
51. Rees L, Rigden SPA, Ward GM, et al: Treatment of short stature by recombinant human growth hormone in children with renal disease. *Arch Dis Child* 65:856–862, 1990.
52. Dahl E, Nordal KP, Attramadal A, et al: Renal osteodystrophy in predialysis patients without stainable bone aluminum. *Acta Med Scand* 224:157–164, 1988.
53. Alfrey AC, Jenkins D, Groth CG, et al: Resolution of hyperparathyroidism, renal osteodystrophy and metastatic calcification after renal homotransplantation. *N Engl J Med* 279:1349–1356, 1968.
54. Sherrard DJ, Herez G, Pei Y, et al: The spectrum of bone disease in end-stage renal failure: An evolving disorder. *Kidney Int* 43:436–442, 1993.
55. Massrey SG, Coburn JW, Popovtzer MM, et al: Secondary hyperparathyroidism in chronic renal failure: The clinical spectrum in uremia, during hemodialysis and after renal transplantation. *Arch Intern Med* 124:431–441, 1969.
56. Meema HE, Oreopoulus DG: Morphology, progression and regression of arterial and periarterial calcification in patients with end-stage renal disease. *Radiology* 158:671–677, 1986.
57. Wilson WEC, Kirkpatrick CH, Talmadge DW: Suppression of immunologic responsiveness in uremia. *Ann Intern Med* 62:1–14, 1965.
58. London WT, Di Figlia M, Sutnick A, et al: An epidemic of hepatitis in a chronic hemodialysis unit: Australian antigens and differences in host response. *N Engl J Med* 281:571–578, 1969.
59. Sanders CV Jr, Luby JP, Sanford JP, et al: Suppression of interferon responses in lymphocytes from patients with uremia. *J Lab Clin Med* 77:768–776, 1971.
60. Manolagas SC, Hustmyer FG, Yu XP: Immunomodulating properties of 1,25-dihydroxyvitamin D_3. *Kidney Int* 38(Suppl 29):S-9–16, 1990.
61. Cerletty JM, Engoring NH: Azotemia and glucose intolerance. *Ann Intern Med* 66:1097–1108, 1967.
62. Bagdade JD, Porte D Jr, Bierman EL: Hypertriglyceridemia: A metabolic consequence of chronic renal failure. *N Engl J Med* 279:181–185, 1968.
63. Olsen NS, Bassett JW: Blood levels of urea nitrogen, phenol, guanidine and creatinine in uremia. *Am J Med* 10:52–59, 1951.
64. Liveson JA, Gardner J, Bernstein MB: Tissue culture studies of possible uremic neurotoxins: Myoinositol. *Kidney Int* 12:131–136, 1977.
65. Wathem R, Smith M, Keshaviah P, et al: Depressed in vitro aggregation of platelets of chronic hemodialysis patients (CHDP): A role for cyclic AMP. *Trans Am Soc Artif Intern Organs* 21:320–328, 1975.
66. Walser M, Coulter AW, Dighe S, et al: The effect of keto-analogues of essential amino acids in severe chronic uremia. *J Clin Invest* 52:678–690, 1973.
67. Alfrey AC: Beta$_2$-microglobulin amyloidosis. *AKF Nephrol Letter* 6:27–33, 1989.
68. Fraser DR, Kodicek E: Unique biosynthesis by kidney of a biologically active vitamin D metabolite. *Nature* 228:764–766, 1970.
69. Bricker NS: On the pathogenesis of the uremic state: An exposition of the "trade-off" hypothesis. *N Engl J Med* 286:1093–1099, 1972.

70. Massrey SG: Parathyroid Hormone as a Uremic Toxin. In Masrey SG, Glassock RS (eds): *Textbook of Nephrology*. Baltimore, Williams & Wilkins, 1983.
71. Korkor AB: Reduced binding of [3H] 1,25 dihydroxyvitamin D_3 in patients with renal failure. *N Engl J Med* 316:1573–1577, 1987.
72. Silver J, Naveh-Many T, Mayer H, et al: Regulation by vitamin D metabolites of parathyroid gene transcription in vivo in the rat. *J Clin Invest* 78:1296–1301, 1986.
73. Goldstein DA, Chui LA, Massey SG: Effect of parathyroid hormone and uremia on peripheral nerve calcium and motor nerve conduction velocity. *J Clin Invest* 62:88–93, 1978.
74. Alfrey AC, LeGendre GR, Kaehny WD: The dialysis encephalopathy syndrome: Possible aluminum intoxication. *N Engl J Med* 294:184–188, 1976.
75. Ott SM, Maloney NA, Coburn JW, et al: Bone aluminum in renal osteodystrophy: Prevalence and relationship to response to 1,25-dihydroxy vitamin D. *N Engl J Med* 307:709–713, 1982.
76. Scheinman JL, Abelson HJ: Bilateral renal hypoplasia with oligonephroma. *J Pediatr* 76:389–397, 1970.
77. Kiprov DD, Colvin RB, McCluskey RT: Focal and segmental glomerulosclerosis and proteinuria associated with unilateral renal agenesis. *Lab Invest* 46:275–281, 1982.
78. Brenner BM, Meyer TW, Hostetter TH: Dietary protein intake and the progressive nature of kidney disease: The role of hemodynamically mediated glomerular injury in the pathogenesis of progressive glomerular sclerosis in aging, renal ablation, and intrinsic renal disease. *N Engl J Med* 307:652–659, 1982.
79. Meyer TW, Rennke HG: Progressive glomerular injury after limited renal infarction in the rat. *Am J Physiol* 254:F856–862, 1988.
80. Hricik DE, Browning PJ, Kopelman R, et al: Captopril-induced functional renal insufficiency in patients with bilateral renal-artery stenosis or renal artery stenosis in a solitary kidney. *N Engl J Med* 308:373–376, 1983.
81. Kimberly RP, Gill JR Jr, Bowden RE, et al: Elevated urinary prostaglandins and the effect of aspirin on renal function in lupus erythematosus. *Ann Intern Med* 89:336–341, 1978.
82. Bilous RW, Mauer SM, Sutherland DER: The effect of pancrease transplantation on the glomerular structure of renal allografts in patients with insulin dependent diabetes. *N Engl J Med* 321:80–85, 1989.
83. The Diabetes Control and Complications Trial Research Group: The effect of intensive treatment of diabetes on the development and progression of long-term complications in insulin-dependent diabetes mellitus. *N Engl J Med* 329:977–986, 1993.
84. Lewis EJ, Hunsicker LG, Bain RP, et al: The effect of angiotensin-converting-enzyme inhibition on diabetic nephropathy. *N Engl J Med* 329:1456–1462, 1993.
85. Klahr S, Levey AS, Beck GJ, et al: The effects of dietary protein restriction and blood pressure control on the progression of chronic renal disease. *N Engl J Med* 330:877–884, 1994.
86. Elving LD, Wetzels JF, de Nobel E, et al: Captopril acutely lowers albuminuria in normotensive patients with diabetic nephropathy. *Am J Kidney Dis* 20:559–563, 1992.
87. Praga M, Hernandez E, Montoyo C, et al: Long-term effects of angiotensin-converting enzyme inhibitors beneficial in patient with nephrotic syndrome. *Am J Kidney Dis* 20:240–248, 1992.
88. Husted FC, Nolph KD, Maher JF: NAHCO$_3$ and NaCl tolerance in chronic renal failure. *J Clin Invest* 56:414–419, 1975.
89. Lim VS, Kirchner PT, Fangman J, et al: The safety and the efficacy of maintenance therapy of recombinant human erythropoietin in patients with renal insufficiency. *Am J Kidney Dis* 14:496–506, 1989.
90. Solomon R, Werner C, Mann D, et al: Effects of saline mannitol and furosemide to prevent decreases in renal function induced by radiocontrast agents. *N Engl J Med* 331:1416–1420, 1994.

12

Obstructive Nephropathy: Pathophysiology and Management

Saulo Klahr

Obstructive uropathy, hydronephrosis, and *obstructive nephropathy* are terms commonly used to describe urinary tract obstruction or its consequences. Obstructive uropathy refers to the structural changes of the urinary tract that impair urine outflow and necessitate a rise in proximal pressure to transmit the usual flow through the point of narrowing. Proximal to the site of obstruction, dilatation occurs. Hydronephrosis describes this dilatation. However, a widened ureteral and caliceal system does not necessarily indicate the presence of obstructive uropathy. Vesicoureteric reflux, primary megaureter, and diabetes insipidus are examples of nonobstructive causes of ureteral dilatation. Nevertheless, in each of these cases renal parenchymal damage may occur. Obstructive nephropathy refers to the renal disease that results from impaired flow of urine. Such impedance to flow causes initially high back pressure, which has direct and indirect effects on the renal parenchyma.

Obstructive nephropathy may be manifested clinically either as an abrupt or as a gradual and insidious decline in renal function. Such a decrease in renal function may be halted and even reversed if the obstruction is relieved. Thus, obstructive nephropathy is different from most of the diseases affecting the kidney in that it is potentially curable.

Causes, Incidence, and Impact

Obstructive uropathy may be due to functional or anatomic abnormalities of the urethra, bladder, ureters, or renal pelvis. These abnormalities may be congenital or acquired. Obstructive uropathy may also occur during the course of diseases extrinsic to the urinary tract. The major causes of obstructive uropathy are summarized in Table 12-1.

The exact incidence and cost of obstructive uropathy are difficult to ascertain because obstruction occurs in a variety of diseases that may warrant hospitalization and surgical intervention. Obstructive uropathy has a bimodal distribution in humans. It is common in childhood mainly due to congenital anomalies of the urinary tract. It declines with age until late adulthood. At age 60 the incidence begins to

544

Table 12-1. Causes of urinary tract obstruction

I. Upper urinary tract
  A. Intrinsic causes
    1. Intraluminal
      (a) Intratubular deposition of crystals (uric acid)
      (b) Ureter: urolithiasis, blood clots, renal papillae, fungus ball
    2. Intramural
      (a) Ureteropelvic junction or ureterovesical junction dysfunction
      (b) Ureteral valve, ureteral polyp, ureteral stricture
  B. Extrinsic causes
    1. Vascular lesions
      (a) Aneurysm: abdominal aorta, iliac vessels
      (b) Aberrant vessels: ureteropelvic junction
      (c) Venous: retrocaval ureter, puerperal ovarian vein thrombophlebitis
      (d) Fibrosis following vascular reconstructive surgery
    2. Originating in the reproductive system
      (a) Uterus: pregnancy, prolapse, tumors, endometriosis
      (b) Ovary: abscess, tumors, ovarian remnants
      (c) Gartner's duct cyst, tubo-ovarian abscess
    3. Lesions of the gastrointestinal tract: Crohn's disease, diverticulitis, appendiceal abscess, tumors, pancreatic tumors, abscess, cysts
    4. Diseases of the retroperitoneum
      (a) Retroperitoneal fibrosis (idiopathic, radiation)
      (b) Inflammatory: tuberculosis, sarcoidosis
      (c) Hematomas
      (d) Primary retroperitoneal tumors (lymphoma, sarcoid, etc.)
      (e) Tumor metastatic to the retroperitoneum (cervix, bladder, colon, prostate, etc.)
      (f) Lymphocele
      (g) Pelvic lipomatosis
II. Lower urinary tract
  1. Phimosis, meatal stenosis, paraphimosis
  2. Urethra: strictures, stones, diverticulum, posterior or anterior urethral valves, periurethral abscess, urethral surgery
  3. Prostate: benign prostatic hyperplasia, prostatic calculi, abscess, prostatic carcinoma
  4. Bladder
    (a) Neurogenic bladder: spinal cord defect or trauma, diabetes, multiple sclerosis, cerebrovascular accidents, Parkinson's disease
    (b) Bladder neck dysfunction
    (c) Bladder calculus
    (d) Bladder cancer
  5. Trauma
    (a) Straddle injury
    (b) Pelvic fracture

Source: S. Klahr, Obstructive Uropathy. In H. R. Jacobson, G. E. Striker, and S. Klahr (eds.): *The Principles and Practice of Nephrology.* Philadelphia: B.C. Decker, 1991. Pp. 432–441.

rise, particularly in men, predominantly due to the increase in the occurrence of prostatic disease. In 1985 in the United States, 397,000 hospital discharges were coded as obstructive uropathy. In addition, there were 482,348 discharges for benign prostatic hyperplasia, and it is probable that most of these admissions were due to obstruction secondary to the prostatic disease. Taken together, this number of discharges coded as urinary tract obstruction is second only to urinary tract infections for hospital discharges due to kidney and urologic diseases in the United States.

Classification

Obstructive uropathy is classified according to (1) the duration, (2) the degree, and (3) the site of the obstruction. When the obstruction is of short duration, less than a few days, it is said to be acute and is usually due to calculus, blood clot, or sloughed papilla. Obstruction that develops slowly and is long lasting is said to be chronic, as in congenital ureteropelvic or ureterovesical abnormalities and retroperitoneal fibrosis. The obstruction is said to be high grade when it is complete or low grade when it is partial or incomplete. Upper tract obstruction is that located above the ureterovesical junction; this type of obstruction is usually unilateral in nature. Lower tract obstruction refers to lesions located below the ureterovesical junction and by definition is bilateral in nature.

Consequences of Urinary Tract Obstruction

Urine moves from the calices and pelvis into the ureter due to electrical impulses generated by pacemaker sites in the calices [1]. This electrical activity causes pelvoureteral contraction and peristalsis, which propel the urine from the renal pelvis to the bladder [1]. At low or normal urine flows, propagation of the electrical activity is usually blocked at the renal pelvis or at the ureteropelvic junction, resulting in a greater frequency of calyceal contractions than ureteric contractions. When urine flow increases, ureteric and calyceal contractions occur at the same frequency. Intrapelvic pressure rises, as the renal pelvis fills with urine, and urine is extruded into the ureter [1]. Since the ureter is collapsed prior to urine evacuation from the pelvis, a bolus of urine forms in the most proximal portion of the ureter. Contraction of the proximal ureter moves the bolus of urine in a distal direction [1]. For efficient propulsion of the urine bolus, the peristaltic contraction must completely collapse the ureteral walls (coaptation). Basal or resting ureteral pressures are approximately 0 to 5 cm H_2O, and peristaltic contraction waves of 20 to 60 cm H_2O are superimposed on this baseline pressure at intervals of approximately 10 to 30 seconds. The urine enters the bladder across the ureterovesical junction, which under normal conditions permits only unidirectional urine transport [2]. Intraureteral pressure at the ureterovesical junction must exceed intravesical pressure for urine to move unimpeded from the ureter to the bladder.

When the movement of urine in the ureter becomes inadequate, urine stasis develops, leading to ureteral dilatation and ultimately to cessation of peristaltic activity. In this setting, urine may flow from the pelvis to the bladder as a continuous column of fluid. As in other systems, the ureter can efficiently transport a maximum amount of fluid per unit of time [3]. Inadequate transport of fluid may result from either too much fluid entering the system or too little fluid exiting the ureter per unit of time. Thus, ureteral dilatation and impaired peristaltic activity may result from obstruction to outflow or excessive urine flow into the system [3].

It has been postulated that the major damage to renal tissue, which is the direct consequence of increased pressure, occurs soon after the onset of ureteral obstruction. The clinical observations that support this conclusion are as follows: (1) The highest measured ureteral pressures (40–50 mm Hg) occur during acute obstruction as seen during the passage of stones [1]. (2) In patients with incomplete obstruction there is an inverse correlation between intrapelvic pressures and time. (3) Patients with obstructive uropathy due to congenital anomalies, which tend to be static, may have relatively well-preserved renal function in the fourth and fifth decades of life [4]. Thus, damage in the obstructed kidney will be potentiated by those conditions that acutely increase ureteral pressure, such as increases in urine flow (i.e., an increase in fluid intake or after administration of diuretics) or augmentation of the degree of obstruction, or both.

The effects of obstructive uropathy on the kidney are due to a variety of factors with complex interactions that alter both glomerular hemodynamics and tubular function [5]. Studies in experimental animals have been used to examine the pathophysiology of obstruction, since it is usually impossible both to define the exact time of onset of obstruction in humans and to obtain repetitive functional measurements. Most studies in experimental animals have examined the effects of complete acute ureteral obstruction (<48 hours) on renal function. Animal models with either unilateral or bilateral ureteral obstruction have been studied. It is apparent that significant differences exist between these two models. The effects of long-standing urinary tract obstruction or partial urinary tract obstruction have been less well studied. For the convenience of the reader, the alterations in renal function that occur during obstruction have been divided into those affecting glomerular function and those affecting tubular function. Despite this artificial division, it is important to realize that such alterations in function are interdependent.

Pathophysiology of Obstructive Nephropathy

The Effects of Acute Ureteral Obstruction on Glomerular Function

Glomerular filtration rate (GFR) falls following the onset of complete ureteral obstruction [6]. The maintenance of residual GFR after ureteral ligation is due to (1) continuous reabsorption of salt and water along the nephron, (2) the ability of the renal tract to dilate, and (3) alterations in renal hemodynamics. Glomerular filtration has four major determinants: (1) the mean difference in hydrostatic pressure between the glomerular capillary lumen and Bowman's space (ΔP); (2) renal plasma flow (Q_A); (3) the ultrafiltration coefficient of the glomerular capillary wall (K_f), which reflects both the total surface area available for filtration and the intrinsic permeability characteristics of the filtering apparatus; and (4) the mean oncotic pressure difference across the glomerular capillary wall ($\Delta \pi$). The manner in which these parameters are affected by ureteral obstruction depends on the duration of the obstruction, the volume status of the animal, and whether or not a contralateral functioning kidney is present.

Changes in Hydrostatic Pressure Gradients

Ligation of the ureter increases ureteral pressure. These changes are instantaneously reflected in changes in proximal tubular pressure, the latter being higher than that in the ureter. The rise in intratubular pressure depends on the degree of hydration of the animal, mean urine flow rate, and whether one or both kidneys are obstructed. Nevertheless, independent of the volume status, within an hour of ureteral obstruction, intratubular pressure rises (Fig. 12-1). Concomitantly there is an increase in glomerular capillary hydrostatic pressure [7]. But this increase in intraglomerular pressure is not proportional to the rise in intratubular pressure [7]. Therefore, the net hydrostatic pressure difference across glomerular capillaries decreases. This results in a decline in GFR. After approximately 5 to 6 hours of ureteral obstruction, proximal intratubular pressure begins to decline [8]. After 24 hours, intratubular pressures are lower than [8, 9] or equal to [10] values prior to obstruction in animals with unilateral ureteral obstruction, but this does not restore an effective filtration pres-

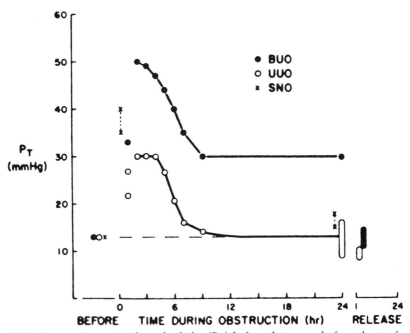

Fig. 12-1. Pressure in proximal renal tubules (P_T) before, during, and after release of complete obstruction of one ureter (UUO), both ureters (BUO), or single nephrons (SNO).

sure, since intraglomerular capillary hydrostatic pressure declines at an even faster rate [8, 10] and falls below the levels seen prior to obstruction. In animals with bilateral ureteral obstruction, proximal intratubular pressures are initially twofold higher [8, 11] than those seen in rats with unilateral ureteral obstruction (see Fig. 12-1). By 24 hours, the levels of intratubular pressure have fallen but not back to baseline [11, 12]. At this time glomerular capillary pressure is no different from preobstruction values. Thus, in this setting, high intratubular pressures contribute significantly to the decrease in GFR.

Changes in Renal Blood Flow

Ureteral obstruction causes a transient increase in renal blood flow [13]. Decreased resistance of the afferent arteriole accounts for the increase in blood flow to the unilaterally obstructed kidney [13, 14]. This phenomenon is observed in both the denervated and the isolated perfused kidney, suggesting that this hyperemic phase is mediated through an intrarenal mechanism. Measurements of the distribution of blood flow during this phase indicate that inner cortical blood flow is increased [15–17]. There is a progressive decrease in blood flow to the inner medulla during ureteral obstruction [18]. This increase in renal blood flow may represent a hemodynamic response intended to maintain GFR. The increase in renal blood flow and afferent arteriolar dilatation leads to an increase in glomerular capillary pressure (Fig. 12-2). This response maintains GFR at approximately 80 percent of preobstruction values despite the substantial increase in proximal tubular pressure. The mechanism underlying this response involves a signal generated at the single-nephron level, since a wax plug placed in the proximal tubule generates an identical hemodynamic response in a single glomerulus. Tanner [19] suggested that the fall in afferent

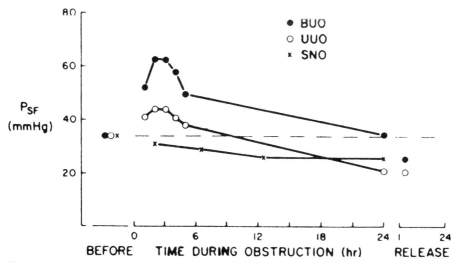

Fig. 12-2. Proximal tubule stop-flow pressure (P_{SF}), a reflection of glomerular capillary pressure before, during, and after release of complete ureteral obstruction of one ureter (UUO), both ureters (BUO), or single nephrons (SNO).

arteriolar resistance was due to tubular glomerular feedback related to interrupting acutely distal delivery of tubular fluid to the macula densa. Ichikawa [20], however, demonstrated that glomerular blood flow does not rise if proximal tubular pressure is maintained in the normal range in the face of tubule blockade, suggesting that the altered glomerular hemodynamics are a result of intratubular dynamics rather than cessation of distal delivery of tubule fluid. The transient increase in renal blood flow after ureteral obstruction can be prevented by the administration of inhibitors of prostaglandin synthesis such as indomethacin [21]. Thus, vasodilatory prostaglandins, such as prostaglandin E_2 and prostacyclin, may account for this initial vasodilatory effect. At this time interval, the renal vascular bed is particularly resistant to vasoconstriction induced either by electrical stimulation of renal nerves or by an infusion of catecholamines. In addition, autoregulation of renal blood flow is impaired, suggesting a prominent vasodilating influence following the onset of ureteral obstruction. Usually the increase in blood flow following obstruction peaks at about 2 to 3 hours.

In a second phase, approximately 3 to 5 hours after the onset of obstruction, renal blood flow starts to decline while ureteral pressure continues to increase. This may be in part a consequence of augmented renal resistance due to increased interstitial pressure. In this phase, ureteral pressure starts to fall toward control values, and renal plasma flow continues to decline, reaching about 30 to 50 percent of control values by 24 hours [22, 23]. This vasoconstrictive response of the kidney to unilateral ureteral obstruction results predominantly from an increased resistance of afferent arterioles.

In animals with bilateral ureteral obstruction, the changes in renal hemodynamics are similar to those seen following unilateral ureteral obstruction. There is also an initial hyperemic phase [11, 14], which is blocked by cyclooxygenase inhibitors [21], and the decline in GFR is thus secondary to a rise in intratubular pressure. Renal plasma flow falls progressively and is similar at 24 hours to that seen after unilateral ureteral obstruction, although afferent arteriole resistance may not increase as much. As a result of the persistently high proximal tubular pressure and the decline in renal plasma flow, it would be expected that the decline in GFR would be greater after bilateral ureteral obstruction than after unilateral ureteral obstruction. However, this is not the case and may reflect the effect of a higher intraglomerular capillary pressure and a greater number of filtering nephrons prior to and after release of an obstruction of 24 hours' duration in rats with bilateral ureteral obstruction than in those with unilateral ureteral obstruction [24].

Changes in the Ultrafiltration Coefficient

After ureteral obstruction, GFR falls to a greater extent than renal plasma flow [6]. Thus, filtration fraction decreases. This may reflect preferential constriction of the preglomerular blocked vessels, as this would lower both blood flow and glomerular capillary pressure, thus resulting in a greater decrement in GFR than in blood flow. Alternatively, it is suggested that there is either diversion of blood to nonfiltering areas of the kidney or that there is a reduced area available for filtration per glomerulus. That the latter occurs is suggested by the finding that K_f values in rats with ureteral obstruction are lower than those typically obtained in normal rats [25].

Alterations in Net Oncotic Pressure

There is no information on whether changes in the oncotic pressure difference across the glomerular wall can modify glomerular hemodynamics after ureteral obstruction.

In summary, the fall in single-nephron GFR in obstruction is due to a decrease in net hydrostatic pressure across the glomerular capillary wall. The fall in net hydrostatic filtration pressure is due initially to an increase in intratubular pressure. After 24 hours of obstruction, the main mechanism responsible for the decrement in the net hydrostatic pressure across the glomerular capillary wall is a fall in intraglomerular pressure. In animals with bilateral ureteral obstruction, both a persistent increase in intratubular pressure and a decrease in intraglomerular pressure contribute to the decrease in net hydrostatic pressure across glomerular capillaries. There is also evidence that the ultrafiltration coefficient is decreased. The greater decrease in total kidney GFR than in single-nephron GFR after 24 hours of obstruction is due to the fact that some nephrons cease to function during the period of obstruction.

Renal Hemodynamics in Animals with Unilateral or Bilateral Ureteral Obstruction

As indicated previously, the renal hemodynamics of animals with unilateral or bilateral ureteral obstruction differ [5, 8]. Whereas 24 hours after ureteral ligation the decrease in single-nephron GFR in animals with unilateral obstruction is due almost exclusively to a decrease in intraglomerular capillary pressure, in rats with bilateral ureteral obstruction both a decrease in intraglomerular capillary pressure and a persistent elevation of intratubular pressure account for the decrease in net filtration pressure. Furthermore, the number of filtering nephrons after 24 hours of ureteral ligation is greater in animals with bilateral obstruction than in those with unilateral obstruction [24]. The causes for these hemodynamic differences between unilateral and bilateral ureteral obstruction have not been elucidated. The levels of circulating atrial natriuretic peptide (ANP), a potent vasodilator, are higher in rats with bilateral ureteral obstruction than in rats with unilateral ureteral obstruction [26]. ANP causes preglomerular vasodilatation and postglomerular vasoconstriction and has been demonstrated to increase K_f in the isolated perfused glomerular preparation. In addition, the administration of exogenous ANP increases GFR following release of unilateral or bilateral ureteral obstruction [26, 27]. Since ANP antagonizes the vasoconstrictive effects of angiotensin II, it is probable that in vivo the elevated levels of endogenous ANP in animals with bilateral ureteral obstruction minimize the renal vasoconstriction that occurs, as compared to animals with unilateral ureteral obstruction.

Effects of Prolonged Complete or Partial Ureteral Obstruction on Glomerular Filtration Rate and Renal Plasma Flow. After ureteral obstruction in the rat, GFR reaches 2 percent of control values by 48 hours and remains at this low level. Renal plasma flow also declines but to a lesser extent [22]. Identical observations have been obtained in the dog [28]. Although the changes in the dog are less severe than those in the rat, GFR of the obstructed kidney, 2 weeks after the onset of obstruction, was 10 percent of the values obtained in the contralateral unobstructed kidney. After 4 weeks, the GFR of the obstructed dog kidney was less than 1 percent of normal. Changes in renal blood flow were also less severe in the dog. Three weeks after ureteral ligation, renal blood flow was 50 percent of the original value and by the fourth week averaged 30 percent of that in the contralateral nonobstructed kidney [28]. The effects of partial chronic obstruction of the ureter depend on both the degree and the duration of the obstruction. Whole-kidney GFR may be reduced to one-third of control values 2 to 4 weeks following partial ureteral obstruction in the rat [29]. Single-nephron GFR, however, was only reduced by 20 percent of control levels, suggesting that the decline in whole-kidney function was a result of a loss in the number of functioning nephrons not accessible to micropuncture, that is, juxtamedullary nephrons [29].

Rats with partial obstruction of 2 to 4 weeks' duration had a 30 percent decrease in the ultrafiltration coefficient. GFR and single-nephron plasma flow were maintained near normal due to an increase in glomerular capillary pressure secondary to a greater decrease in afferent than efferent arteriolar resistance. This vasodilatation was prostaglandin mediated, since indomethacin administration increased both afferent and efferent arteriolar resistance and caused a decline in single-nephron GFR [30].

Role of Vasoactive Compounds

Two major vasoconstrictors, angiotensin II and thromboxane A_2 [31], and several other vasoactive compounds [31] play a role in the changes in plasma flow per nephron and single-nephron GFR seen in obstruction. Inhibition of thromboxane A_2 synthesis in rats with ureteral obstruction increases plasma flow per nephron, due to decreased vasoconstriction of both afferent and efferent arterioles [32]. Thromboxane may also decrease K_f through mesangial cell contraction and a decrease in the surface area available for filtration. Although infusion of angiotensin II into normal animals increases net filtration pressure, presumably due to greater vasoconstriction of the efferent than the afferent arteriole, blockade of angiotensin II formation after relief of obstruction increases GFR [32]. This increase in GFR may be due to a greater filtering surface area, since angiotensin II causes mesangial cell contraction [5] and therefore can reduce the total glomerular capillary area available for filtration. In addition, angiotensin II decreases plasma flow per nephron, which also contributes to the fall in single-nephron GFR. The central and critical role of these two vasoconstrictors in modulating postobstructive renal hemodynamics is illustrated (Fig. 12-3) by the fact that rats pretreated with both angiotensin-converting enzyme and thromboxane synthase inhibitors, prior to obstruction, demonstrate almost normal renal function after release of the obstruction [27].

Vasodilatory prostaglandins, produced in increased amounts by the obstructed kidney, may prevent further decrements in GFR by antagonizing the vasoconstrictive effects of thromboxane A_2 and angiotensin II. Indeed, it has been demonstrated that after release of obstruction in rats, in the setting of prior inhibition of the thromboxane synthase, administration of inhibitors of the cyclooxygenase causes a marked decrease in whole-kidney GFR and in renal plasma flow [32].

Role of Infiltrating White Blood Cells in the Decrement in Glomerular Filtration Rate and Renal Plasma Flow.

An infiltration of mononuclear cells and a proliferation of interstitial fibroblasts were found in the renal parenchyma of rabbits

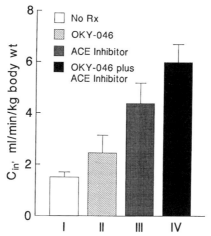

Fig. 12-3. Baseline levels of inulin clearance (C_m) in four groups of rats measured 3 to 4 hours after unilateral release of bilateral ureteral obstruction of 24 hours' duration. Values for inulin clearance were significantly greater in rats of group II (pretreated with an inhibitor of thromboxane synthesis [OKY-046]), in rats of group III (pretreated with an inhibitor of angiotensin-converting enzyme [ACE]), and in rats of group IV (treated with a combination of both a thromboxane synthase inhibitor and an inhibitor of angiotensin-coverting enzyme) as compared to rats of group I, which were untreated (No Rx). Notice that the values for inulin clearance in group III rats are significantly higher than those in group II ($p < 0.01$) and that the combination of enalapril and OKY-046 resulted in the highest values of GFR observed after release of obstruction (group IV). (From M. L. Purkerson and S. Klahr, Prior inhibition of vasoconstrictors normalizes GFR in postobstructed kidneys. *Kidney Int.* 35:1310–1314, 1989.)

with chronic ureteral obstruction [33]. Schreiner and co-workers [34] found that a leukocyte influx is one of the earliest responses of the kidney to ureteral obstruction. The infiltrate was observed within 4 hours of obstruction, but its peak response occurred at 24 hours, after which a plateau was observed (Fig. 12-4).

Normal kidneys have a small number of resident leukocytes, predominantly macrophages, in the renal cortex, mainly in the glomeruli. The normal medulla, however, is completely devoid of resident leukocytes. In obstruction, however, the medulla is also invaded by mononuclear cells to an extent comparable to that of the cortex. The mononuclear cell infiltrate present in the obstructed kidney consists mainly of macrophages. The second most abundant leukocytes are T lymphocytes of the cytotoxic suppressor cell subclass (Fig. 12-5).

The infiltrate is slowly reversible, requiring several days after release of obstruction to revert to near-normal levels [34]. Two days after release of obstruction, the macrophage content of the cortical interstitium appeared to increase modestly and then to fall to near-normal levels by 6 days after release of the obstruction. In contrast, the T lymphocytes in the cortex diminish rapidly to less than 20 percent of their values during obstruction 2 days after release of the ureteral ligation, with a further decrement noted 4 days later. Even 1 week after release of the obstruction, a small increase in both cell populations was noted when compared to normal kidneys.

The functional significance of this leukocyte infiltration has been examined [35]. The kinetics of arrival of the macrophages and T lymphocytes correlate temporally with the decline in GFR. As mentioned previously, following the onset of obstruction there is an initial increase in renal blood flow, which is mediated by prostaglandins. Four hours after obstruction, renal blood flow decreases, and by 24 hours values for renal plasma flow are between 40 and 70 percent of those observed prior to obstruction. This progressive vasoconstriction is in part due to augmented production of thromboxane A_2. The chronically obstructed kidney displays an enhanced ability to metabolize arachidonic-acid [5, 31], and thromboxane synthase activity is increased. Inhibition of thromboxane synthase dramatically improves postobstructive renal hemodynamics and reverses partially the renal vasoconstriction of acute ureteral obstruction [27, 32].

To examine the potential role of the infiltrating cells in the decrease in GFR and renal plasma flow seen with ureteral obstruction, Harris and associates [35]

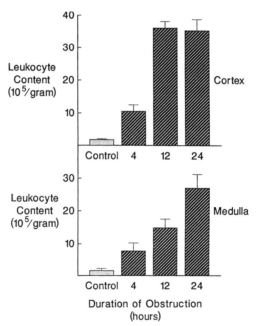

Fig. 12-4. The effect of bilateral ureteral obstruction on the number of cells expressing the leukocyte common antigen in kidneys at timed intervals after obstruction. The results represent the mean ± standard error of single kidneys of three rats. Representative portions of cortex and medulla were dissected out, weighed, subjected to enzymatic digestion, and labeled. The control kidneys were taken from littermates that did not undergo any procedure. (From G. F. Schreiner, K. P. G. Harris, M. L. Purkerson, and S. Klahr, Immunological aspects of acute ureteral obstruction: Immune cell infiltrate in the kidney. *Kidney Int.* 34:487–493, 1988.)

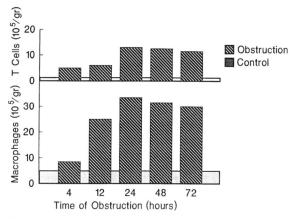

Fig. 12-5. The T lymphocyte (*upper panel*) and macrophage (*lower panel*) content, expressed as 10^5 cells per gram of tissue, of the obstructed kidneys of rats at different time intervals after the initiation of unilateral obstruction. Control values represent normal kidneys from nonobstructed littermates. Results are expressed as mean ± standard error. (From G. F. Schreiner, K. P. G. Harris, M. L. Purkerson, and S. Klahr, Immunological aspects of acute ureteral obstruction: Immune cell infiltrate in the kidney. *Kidney Int.* 34: 487–493, 1988.)

studied rats that underwent total body radiation prior to the onset of obstruction. Irradiation abolished the leukocyte infiltration observed in the kidney after 24 hours of obstruction. Irradiation had no effect on renal morphology or function in normal rats. By contrast, elimination of the infiltrate by prior irradiation of the rats with bilateral ureteral obstruction decreased thromboxane B_2 excretion in the urine and significantly improved renal hemodynamics in the postobstructed kidney [35]. This implies that the infiltrating leukocytes contribute to the hemodynamic changes observed in the postobstructed kidney. The leukocytic infiltrate may contribute to the decline in GFR and renal plasma flow seen after obstruction, possibly via the production of vasoactive prostanoids such as thromboxane A_2. Indeed, it is of note that renal plasma flow, which increases for the first few hours after obstruction, only begins to decline 4 hours after the onset of obstruction at a time when the leukocyte infiltrate is becoming evident.

Eliminating the leukocyte infiltrate from the renal parenchyma does not, however, return the function of the postobstructed kidney to normal. Furthermore, the elimination of the infiltrating macrophages by prior irradiation does not reduce the excretion of thromboxane B_2 in the urine to baseline levels. This is consistent with obstruction causing enhanced production of this vasoactive prostanoid by structures intrinsic to the kidney such as glomerular epithelial or mesangial cells [36]. Such leukocyte-independent sources of thromboxane A_2 may also modulate renal hemodynamics [5, 31].

Yanagisawa et al. [36] reported that glomeruli isolated from animals with bilateral ureteral obstruction produce greater quantities of prostaglandin E_2, 6-keto-prostaglandin $F_{1\alpha}$ (the stable metabolite of prostacyclin), and thromboxane B_2 (the stable metabolite of thromboxane A_2) than glomeruli isolated from kidneys of normal animals. Since there is a depletion of endogenous macrophages from the glomeruli of the obstructed kidney, the increased synthesis of thromboxane B_2 in isolated glomeruli is related to its production by an intrinsic glomerular cell. Most likely this reflects increased production of thromboxane A_2 by mesangial cells; however, this has not been established in the obstructed model. The increased synthesis of prostanoids by isolated glomeruli was restored to levels comparable to those seen in glomeruli of normal kidneys when the animals were pretreated with an angiotensin-converting enzyme inhibitor prior to the onset of ureteral obstruction [36]. This suggests that endogenous angiotensin II has an important role in the increased synthesis of prostanoids found in isolated glomeruli from rats with ureteral obstruction. The most likely explanation may be a marked stimulation of phospholipase A_2 or cyclooxygenase, or both, by angiotensin II in glomeruli from rats with bilateral ureteral obstruction. Thus, the increased thromboxane excretion in the urine of animals with bilateral ureteral obstruction may have two origins: increased release by intrinsic glomerular cells and production by macrophages that invade the renal parenchyma during obstruction.

Whether or not other substances or factors released by infiltrating macrophages modulate epithelial cell function in obstruction has not been established. What contribution, if any, the infiltrating suppressor T lymphocytes make to the renal response to obstruction requires further characterization. Finally, the nature of the stimulus coupling urinary tract obstruction to the appearance of a leukocyte infiltrate in the renal parenchyma has not been completely defined. Initial evidence indicates that there is release of macrophage-chemoattractant substances by the obstructed kidney. The nature of these chemoattractant agents has not been completely elucidated [37, 38].

Polymorphonuclear leukocytes and monocytes are present in the renal interstitium of rabbits subjected to ureteral obstruction for 3 days. The obstructed kidney, when perfused ex vivo, exhibits an exaggerated increase in the elaboration of eicosanoids in response to bradykinin and the chemotactic peptide, N-formilmethionil-leucil-phenylalanine. Essential fatty acid deficiency (i.e., deprivation of N-6-fatty acids) attenuated the elaboration of eicosanoids by the obstructed kidney perfused ex vivo. It also prevented the increase in the activities of microsomal cyclooxygenase and thromboxane synthase seen after 3 days of ureteral occlusion. Fatty acid deficiency also attenuated the renal influx of macrophages; this effect was attributed to inhibition of leukotriene B_4 synthesis, a known chemoattractant for monocytes [39].

The long-term effects of this immunologic infiltrate on renal function and structure in obstructive nephropathy are not well defined. Focal segmental glomerulosclerosis is a common histologic finding in patients with ureteropelvic obstruction [40]. This focal segmental glomerulosclerosis was present in areas closely associated with intense interstitial and periglomerular inflammation. It could be envisioned that growth factors released by invading leukocytes have a role in the development and progression of fibrotic and sclerotic changes that occur in the chronically obstructed kidney. It is therefore likely that the cellular infiltrate may contribute to the renal damage and to the progressive decrease in renal function observed with chronic urinary tract obstruction.

Role of Reactive Oxygen Metabolites in the Pathophysiology of Obstructive Uropathy. Reactive oxygen metabolites, including free radicals (i.e., superoxide anion and hydroxy radical) and other toxic oxygen metabolites (i.e., hydrogen peroxide and hypochlorous acid), appear to be important mediators in several models of immune-mediated toxic and ischemic tissue injury. Specifically, recent studies suggested that reactive oxygen metabolites may have an important role in the pathophysiology of renal disease [41]. The possibility that in obstructive nephropathy, oxidants generated by infiltrating leukocytes and intrinsic renal cells may account for some of the functional and morphologic changes observed should be considered. Modi and colleagues [42] examined the effects of probucol, an antioxidant and lipid-lowering agent, on renal function in normal rats and rats with unilateral release of bilateral ureteral obstruction of 24 hours' duration. Rats were fed either a standard diet or a standard diet containing 1% probucol for 2 weeks prior to study. Probucol lowered serum cholesterol in both normal rats and rats with bilateral ureteral obstruction. The drug did not affect renal function in normal rats. By contrast, rats with bilateral obstruction given probucol had greater values for GFR and renal plasma flow both at 4 hours and 3 days after release of the obstruction that did similar rats that did not receive the lipid-lowering drug. Another lipid-lowering drug, lovastatin, did not modify renal function in rats with bilateral ureteral obstruction. This suggests that the decrease in cholesterol was not responsible for the effects observed.

The kidneys from rats with bilateral ureteral obstruction had higher levels of malondialdehyde, an index of lipid peroxidation; a greater number of infiltrating leukocytes in the cortex; decreased levels of reduced glutathione; and increased levels of oxidized glutathione [42]. In contrast, the kidneys of rats with ureteral obstruction given probucol had significantly higher levels of reduced glutathione and a lesser number of infiltrating leukocytes. These observations suggest a potential role for reactive oxygen species in the pathophysiology of obstructive nephropathy. The improved renal function seen in rats with bilateral ureteral obstruction given probucol may be due to an effect of this drug on the accumulation of reactive oxygen metabolites or to a decrease in the number of leukocytes infiltrating the renal cortex, or to both.

Recovery of Glomerular Filtration Rate After Release of Ureteral Obstruction. The degree of recovery of GFR after release of ureteral obstruction depends on the severity and duration of the obstruction. Recovery of renal function has been examined in both dogs and rats with ureteral obstruction. Sequential determinations of GFR have been made in dogs after release of complete unilateral ureteral obstruction of 2 weeks' duration [43]. The control GFR for each kidney was assumed to be half of the level of GFR obtained for the whole animal prior to ureteric ligation. It was found that after release of obstruction, GFR in the postobstructed kidney averaged 25 percent of ipsilateral control values and 16 percent of the concurrent values for the contralateral kidney, the latter having undergone a compensatory increase in GFR. Subsequent studies in the same animals revealed an increase in the GFR of the postobstructed kidney and a fall in the GFR of the normal kidney. Such values stabilized at about 2 months after the release of obstruction. In no instance was there a complete restoration of GFR to normal in the obstructed kidney. After 2 years, the GFR of the experimental kidney was approximately 50 percent below the value obtained for the contralateral kidney. The changes in effective renal plasma flow mirrored the changes seen in GFR. Vaughan et al. [28] found that the recovery of GFR was dependent on the duration of the obstruction. A week or less of obstruction was followed by complete recovery of GFR after release of the obstruction.

In rats, a permanent decrease in GFR occurs if ureteral obstruction has been present for more than 72 hours. With periods of obstruction lasting less than 30 hours, recovery of GFR is complete as assessed by whole-kidney clearances. Such data suggest that short-term obstruction is completely reversible and that most of the decrease in GFR is functional. However, there is evidence to indicate that the normalization in GFR may not be a consequence of homogeneous recovery in single-nephron GFR for all nephrons [44]. Values for whole-kidney GFR calculated from measurements of surface single-nephron GFR were greater than those obtained from direct whole-kidney clearance measurements [24]. This may be explained by the fact that 40 percent of superficial nephrons (those accessible to micropuncture) were found not to be filtering immediately after release of the obstruction, whereas only 12 percent of juxtamedullary nephrons were filtering, suggesting a selective loss of juxtamedullary nephrons. Subsequent studies revealed that 3 to 6 hours after release of unilateral ureteral obstruction of 24 hours' duration, GFR values were one-sixth of those observed prior to ligation of the ureter [44]. With time there was an increase in the GFR such that by 14 and 60 days after the release of obstruction, values in the experimental kidney were comparable to those in the contralateral untouched kidney [44]. However, when single-nephron GFR and the number of filtering nephrons were determined using a modification of Hansen's technique, a decrease in the total number of filtering nephrons was found in the postobstructed kidney such that only 85 percent of the nephrons in this kidney were filtering, compared to 100 percent in the contralateral untouched kidney [44]. The normalization of whole-kidney GFR occurred, therefore, at the expense of hyperfiltration (increase in single-nephron GFR) in the remaining functional nephrons (Fig. 12-6). There was, however, a decrement in the total number of functional nephrons. This decrement appears to be permanent. The mechanism responsible for this loss of nephrons after ureteral obstruction remains to be defined, as does its long-term significance in terms of the development of chronic renal failure following obstructive uropathy.

Alterations in Renal Tubule Function

Abnormalities in renal tubule function are common in obstructive uropathy. Major defects appear to be located in distal segments of the nephron. Thus, a common characteristic of obstructive nephropathy is a decreased ability to concentrate the urine. In addition to alterations in sodium reabsorption, the reabsorption or secre-

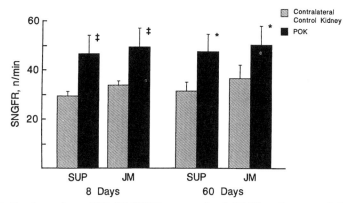

Fig. 12-6. Single-nephron GFR (SNGFR) in superficial (SUP) and juxtamedullary (JM) nephrons of rats 8 days and 60 days after release of unilateral ureteral obstruction of 24 hours' duration. The single-nephron GFR values for the postobstructed kidney (POK) were significantly greater (*asterisk*) than those of the contralateral kidney.

tion of solutes such as potassium, magnesium, calcium, and hydrogen may be altered in obstructive uropathy.

Renal Tubular Reabsorption of Sodium and Water

Effects of Release of Unilateral Ureteral Obstruction. In spite of a decrease in GFR and hence in the filtered load of sodium, the excretion of sodium by the postobstructed kidney of rats with unilateral ureteral obstruction is similar to that of the contralateral kidney [45]. Thus, fractional sodium excretion is greater from the postobstructed than from the contralateral kidney. Similar findings have been reported in the dog and in humans after more prolonged periods of obstruction [4]. These findings indicate significant changes in the tubular reabsorption of sodium and water by the previously obstructed kidney. Changes in intravascular volume may affect the absolute and fractional excretion of salt and water by the postobstructed kidney. Absolute sodium excretion after release of unilateral ureteral obstruction is reduced in rats with volume depletion studied under anesthesia when compared to awake rats. In contrast, expansion of the extracellular fluid (ECF) volume with saline solution increases both absolute and fractional sodium excretion. These increases are greater in the postreleased kidney than in the contralateral untouched kidney.

Effects of Release of Bilateral Ureteral Obstruction. The release of bilateral ureteral obstruction results in a different quantitative excretion of salt and water than what occurs after release of unilateral ureteral obstruction. There is a dramatic increase in the absolute amount of sodium and water excreted in the urine after release of bilateral ureteral obstruction in humans [46, 47] and experimental animals [9, 12, 48–50]. The potential mechanisms responsible for this so-called postobstructive diuresis are discussed elsewhere in this chapter. The differences in salt and

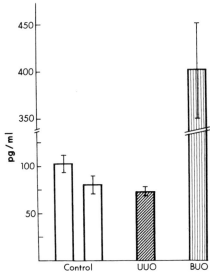

Fig. 12-7. Mean values of atrial peptide in plasma of four groups of rats ($n = 5$ in each group). Open bars show mean values ± standard error in sham-operated rats (controls) that were anesthetized (*1st open bar*) or awake (*2nd open bar*). The other two bars show mean values for atrial peptide in awake rats with either unilateral ureteral obstruction (UUO) or bilateral ureteral obstruction (BUO) of 24 hours' duration. Mean values for atrial peptide in plasma were significantly greater in the rats with bilateral ureteral obstruction than in the other groups ($p < 0.01$).

water excretion after release of bilateral ureteral obstruction and unilateral ureteral obstruction may be due to differences in the levels of urea and potential expansion of the ECF volume during the period of bilateral ureteral obstruction as compared to unilateral ureteral obstruction. In addition, the circulating levels of ANP are significantly greater in rats with bilateral ureteral obstruction than in those with unilateral obstruction [26] (Fig. 12-7).

Segmental Changes in Sodium and Water Reabsorption Along the Nephron. After the release of unilateral ureteral obstruction in rats, the fraction of the filtered sodium and water that is reabsorbed in the proximal tubule of superficial nephrons is increased [45, 51]. In contrast, after release of bilateral ureteral obstruction, where GFR is also reduced to the same extent, the fraction of the glomerular filtrate reabsorbed in the proximal tubule of surface nephrons is either unchanged [9, 48] or decreased. Reabsorption of salt and water by the proximal tubules of deep or juxtamedullary nephrons is decreased after the release of both bilateral and unilateral ureteral obstruction. There is also decreased reabsorption of salt in the thick ascending limb of Henle's loop, as is discussed in the section on the concentrating defect. After release of bilateral obstruction, the fraction of filtered water delivered to the early distal segment is increased [9]. This finding suggests that both unilateral and bilateral ureteral obstruction diminished the ability of the thick ascending limb of

Henle's loop to reabsorb salt. On the other hand, the reabsorption of salt and water is decreased in surface distal nephrons in bilateral ureteral obstruction, but it is increased in unilateral ureteral obstruction. The effects of ureteral obstruction on collecting duct function have been explored by micropuncture and microcatheterization techniques. After release of unilateral obstruction in rats, fractional fluid delivery to the base of the papillae is increased [52]. A large proportion of this fluid is reabsorbed along the terminal collecting duct. This suggests adequate function of this segment of the nephron. It is important to note that the increased fractional delivery of salt and water to this segment of the collecting duct after release of unilateral obstruction occurs even though surface proximal and distal tubules reabsorb an increased fraction of the glomerular filtrate. This suggests that much of the salt that appears in the urine after release of unilateral ureteral obstruction is derived from marked alterations in either the medullary collecting duct function or the function of deep nephrons. Although greater in magnitude, similar increases in the delivery of sodium and water to the collecting duct were found in micropuncture studies after release of bilateral obstruction [48]. Reabsorption of salt and water along the terminal collecting duct also occurred. These results contrast with studies that used the technique of microcatheterization. In these studies, the fraction of filtered water and sodium arriving at the base of the collecting duct was also increased. However, in contradistinction to the micropuncture study results, microcatheterization studies failed to demonstrate reabsorption. Rather there was net addition of water and sodium along the length of the papillary collecting duct [50]. The explanation for these differences is not clear, although the animals studied using the two methods were of different ages. Although these various studies examined the changes in salt and water reabsorption in several segments of the nephron after release of bilateral or unilateral ureteral obstruction, they did not permit determination as to whether the changes observed were due to intrinsic alterations in the nephron, whether they represent a response to extrinsic factors, or whether they are due to a combination of both intrinsic and extrinsic factors. Studies of isolated segments of rabbit nephrons have helped to clarify these different possibilities [53]. When isolated nephron segments from rabbits subjected to either bilateral or unilateral obstruction were compared in vitro, the results were nearly indistinguishable. The in vitro behavior of nephrons from both types of obstruction, however, differed from the behavior of nephrons obtained from normal kidneys. In the in vitro studies, reabsorption of salt and water by surface proximal tubules was unchanged. Reabsorption was decreased in ascending thick limbs of Henle's loop and in juxtamedullary proximal tubules obtained from rabbits with ureteral obstruction [53]. The decreased reabsorption in these two nephron segments was comparable in animals with unilateral and those with bilateral ureteral obstruction. These studies suggest that 24-hour obstruction, either by increasing intratubular pressure, by changes in renal blood flow, or by some other factor, affects the intrinsic reabsorptive capacity of these nephron segments. The in vitro data also suggest that the marked differences in reabsorption by surface nephrons in vivo after release of unilateral versus bilateral ureteral obstruction are not due to alterations intrinsic to the nephron but must result from extrinsic changes.

Impaired Ability to Concentrate the Urine

Patients with partial obstruction of the urinary tract or patients after relief of partial or complete urinary obstruction have impaired renal concentrating capacity [4, 54, 55]. Some patients have persistently hypotonic urine and polyuria, both of which are unresponsive to the administration of vasopressin [56, 57]. If fluid intake is inadequate, severe dehydration and hypernatremia can develop in such patients. This inability to concentrate the urine may disappear after a long period following relief of obstruction. Several mechanisms may contribute to this defect in renal concentrating ability.

Decreased Hypertonicity of the Medullary Interstitium. After relief of unilateral obstruction of 24 hours' duration in rats, the urine osmolality from the postobstructed kidney seldom exceeds 400 mOsm/kg H_2O, as compared to approximately 2000 mOsm/kg H_2O in the contralateral untouched rat kidney. This decrease in urine osmolality is accompanied by a marked decrease in medullary hypertonicity [58, 59]. There is a decrease in the concentrations of both sodium and urea in the interstitium of the renal medulla. This decrease in the hypertonicity of the renal medullary interstitium may be due to a decrease in the reabsorption of sodium chloride in the ascending limb of Henle's loop. Such a decrease in reabsorption would result in a fall in solute present in the medulla and would lower the tonicity of the medullary interstitium, and thus the osmotic driving force for the movement of water from the lumen of the collecting duct into the interstitium. Hanley and Davidson [53] showed that sodium chloride transport was markedly decreased in in vitro perfused thick ascending limb of Henle's loop, microdissected from obstructed kidneys. Decreased Na, K-ATPase activity in the outer medulla of obstructed kidneys may contribute to this defect in sodium reabsorption [60]. Increased prostaglandin synthesis may contribute to this defect [61].

Another cause for the decreased medullary hypertonicity may be an increase in medullary blood flow during the period of obstruction. Increases in blood flow through the medullary region may remove excessive amounts of both sodium and urea present in the medulla and hence would result in decreased medullary hypertonicity. Although medullary blood flow is decreased during obstruction, a marked overshoot in medullary blood flow is observed following relief of obstruction. The concentrating defect may persist in the postobstructed kidney of experimental animals even 2 months after relief of the obstruction [44]. This may be due to the loss of juxtamedullary nephrons and hence destruction of the longest loops of Henle, which are responsible for the reabsorption of solutes and the creation of a hypertonic medulla. A decrease in the number of juxtamedullary nephrons may decrease the generation of a maximally concentrated medullary interstitium and may cause a permanent defect in the concentrating ability of the postobstructed kidney. However, this concentrating defect is not as marked as that seen in the acute stages of obstruction but is still evident when compared to the concentrating ability of the contralateral nonobstructed kidney of the same animals [44].

Insensitivity of the Cortical Collecting Duct to the Action of Vasopressin. The movement of water from the collecting duct into the interstitium is due to an increase in the hydraulic permeability of collecting duct cells in response to vasopressin. Administration of vasopressin in the setting of partial urinary obstruction, however, does not decrease urine flow and usually does not increase urine osmolality [57]. Vasopressin-resistant isotonic urine can be attributed to impaired generation of a hypertonic medullary interstitium. However, since the medullary interstitium is not hypotonic in obstructed kidneys, the presence of hypotonic urine suggests an inability to achieve complete osmotic equilibration between the fluid in the collecting duct and the fluid in the interstitium due to a failure of vasopressin to appropriately increase water permeability across the collecting duct. Campbell and associates [62] demonstrated that vasopressin-dependent water reabsorption was reduced in isolated perfused cortical collecting ducts obtained from kidneys of rabbits whose ureter had been obstructed for 4 hours. A decreased hydro-osmotic response of the cortical collecting duct obtained from rabbits with ureteral ligation of 4 hours' duration was also elicited when adenosine 3',5'-cyclic monophosphate (cyclic AMP) was utilized. Inhibition of prostaglandin synthesis only partially reversed the defect.

In patients or animals with bilateral ureteral obstruction, release of the obstruction results in a mild postobstructive diuresis and an inability to concentrate the urine very much above isotonicity. In addition to the mechanisms described previously, the osmotic effect of solutes retained during the period of obstruction contributes to the generation of an isotonic urine after relief of bilateral ureteral obstruction. Thus, an osmotic diuresis per nephron may contribute to the impaired renal concentrating capacity associated with obstructive uropathy, particularly in the setting of bilateral ureteral obstruction, which leads to the accumulation of urea and other osmotically active solutes in blood during the period of obstruction.

Defective Urinary Acidification

In humans and experimental animals, acid excretion is impaired following the release of bilateral or unilateral ureteral obstruction [54, 63–65]. Most studies suggest that a form of distal renal tubular acidosis with an inability to lower the urine pH to normal minimum values in response to acidemia is common in patients with urinary tract obstruction. Berlyne [54] found that six of seven patients with chronic hydronephrosis were unable to acidify their urine below a pH of 5.3 after a short ammonium chloride load. However, in two patients, following relief of obstruction, the acidification defect was corrected after several weeks. Better and associates [66] described urine pH values of 6.5 to 7.5 in the postobstructed kidney of a patient with complete unilateral ureteral obstruction of 3 months' duration. After ammonium chloride loading, the urine pH from the postobstructed kidney fell from 6.7 to 5.7, while the normal kidney had a normal response.

A defect similar to that seen in humans is observed in both the rat [65] and the dog [64] after release of ureteral obstruction. In this setting, urine pH from the postobstructed kidney is approximately 7.0 and is not significantly affected by an acid load. Bicarbonate titration studies revealed no decrease in proximal reabsorption of bicarbonate after release of unilateral ureteral obstruction, as compared to sham-operated rats [65]. Micropuncture experiments also failed to demonstrate decreased bicarbonate reabsorption in proximal or distal segments of surface nephrons. Urine carbon dioxide pressure (P_{CO_2}) values remained low after bicarbonate loading. These data suggest that the acidifying defect after release of unilateral ureteral obstruction is due either to decreased hydrogen ion secretion in the distal tubule of surface nephrons and the collecting duct or to marked alterations in the reabsorption of bicarbonate in juxtamedullary nephrons. Laski and Kurtzman [67], using perfused tubules from rabbits with obstructive uropathy found that a decrease in bicarbonate transport (JT_{CO_2}) occurs first in perfused medullary collecting duct segments. Only later was there a slight fall in JT_{CO_2} in cortical segments. These data suggest that the initial defect in acidification appears in medullary segments. Sabattini and Kurtzman [68], using an indirect N-ethyl-malcimide (NEM) method, examined the activity of H^+-ATPase in microdissected segments of rat nephrons after 24 hours of obstructive uropathy. NEM-sensitive ATPase activity was markedly reduced in animals with acute ureteral obstruction. In the cortical collecting duct, activity fell significantly but to a lesser degree than in the medullary collecting duct. If indeed NEM-sensitive ATPase is an adequate measure of H^+-ATPase activity, this finding suggests that there is an abnormality in the cortical collecting duct but that the major defect in acidification in obstruction is located at the level of the medullary collecting duct. Using monoclonal antibodies to the 31-kDa subunit of the H^+-ATPase, Purcell and associates [69] reported a decrease in the apical staining for H^+-ATPase in collecting duct intercalated cells of rats with ureteral obstruction. This decrease in apical staining implies a removal of H^+-ATPase from the apical border of intercalated cells during the period of obstruction. Three to five days after release of obstruction, the staining for H^+-ATPase in the apical border was normal, and this was accompanied by a urine pH in the postobstructed kidney similar to that in the contralateral kidney. These data suggest that a decrease in the number of H^+-ATPase pumps in the apical surface of intercalated cells may account for the acidifying defect that occurs with ureteral obstruction. The mechanisms underlying the removal of pumps from the apical membrane of intercalated cells remain to be determined.

The acidifying defect seems to be reversible in the majority of patients. In certain patients, however, the acidifying defect may persist.

Abnormal Potassium Excretion

Hyperkalemic hyperchloremic acidosis has been described in patients with chronic obstructive uropathy [63]. At any given level of GFR, the fractional excretion of potassium was found to be less in patients with obstructive uropathy than in a comparable group of patients with renal insufficiency due to a variety of renal diseases (Fig. 12-8). Three major mechanisms may explain, at least in part, the development of hyperkalemic hyperchloremic acidosis in individuals with obstructive uropathy: (1) a selective deficiency of aldosterone secretion probably secondary to diminished production of renin by the kidney (hyporeninemic-hypoaldosteronism); (2) a defect in renal hydrogen ion secretion with an inability to lower pH of the urine maximally in the presence of systemic acidosis and decreased urinary excretion of both ammonium and titratable acid (type 4 distal renal tubular acidosis); and (3) a combination of these two defects. It is also possible that part of the defect may relate to a decreased sensitivity of the distal tubule to the action of aldosterone on potassium secretion. Batlle and co-workers [63] suggested that a

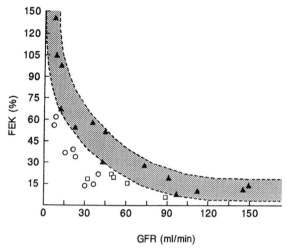

Fig. 12-8. Relation of fractional excretion of potassium (FEK) to GFR under baseline conditions. The area inside the broken lines depicts the normal adaptive increase in fractional potassium excretion observed with a chronic reduction in GFR. These data were obtained from 14 normokalemic controls (*solid triangles*) with different GFRs. Each patient (*open symbols*) had a baseline fractional potassium excretion lower than that expected for the corresponding GFR. Open circles denote patients with distal renal tubular acidosis (group I); open squares represent patients with hyperkalemic metabolic acidosis due to selective aldosterone deficiencies (group II). (Reprinted by permission from D. C. Batlle, J. A. L. Arruda, and N. A. Kurtzman, Hyperkalemic distal renal tubular acidosis associated with obstructive uropathy. *N. Engl. J. Med.* 304:373–380, 1981.)

defect in sodium reabsorption in the distal nephron results in a decrease in the intraluminal negative potential difference. This could be the primary cause of diminished hydrogen ion and potassium secretion, that is, a voltage-dependent defect. This defect may be in part due to an altered response of this segment of the nephron to the action of aldosterone during obstruction.

Kimura and Mujais [70] found a progressive decrease in in situ turnover of the Na-K pump in intact cortical collecting ducts in rats with unilateral ureteral obstruction. This was associated with impaired ability of the obstructed kidney to excrete an acute potassium load. The authors suggested that the impaired in situ turnover of the Na-K pump contributes significantly to the abnormal potassium excretion that accompanies obstructive uropathy.

Effects of Ureteral Obstruction on Calcium and Magnesium Reabsorption

Calcium Reabsorption. The effects of obstructive uropathy on calcium reabsorption have not been adequately studied. Twelve hours after release of complete obstruction of 3 weeks' duration, calcium excretion was three times greater than the predicted values in one patient. Calcium excretion paralleled sodium excretion and decreased fourfold during the time of observation. Similar results were reported by Better and co-workers [71]. In the rat, calcium excretion was found to be unchanged after release of bilateral ureteral obstruction. After release of obstruction, calcium excretion is increased if the animals have had parathyroidectomy. This may suggest a difference in calcium excretion after release of obstruction in humans and rats.

After release of unilateral obstruction, calcium excretion from the postreleased kidney is reduced out of proportion to the decrement in GFR and the filtered load of calcium. Better and co-workers [72] reported that at any level of GFR, the fractional excretion of calcium was decreased after release of unilateral obstruction. Similar changes in calcium excretion occur in the rat after release of unilateral obstruction of 24 hours' duration [73]. The specific sites and mechanisms of altered calcium reabsorption in the nephron have not been determined.

Magnesium Reabsorption. Magnesium excretion in the urine is increased following release of bilateral or unilateral ureteral obstruction. Urinary losses of magnesium may be considerable following release of bilateral obstruction [71]. Indeed, profound magnesium depletion has been reported in men after release of bilateral ureteral obstruction. Moreover, in contrast to calcium, magnesium excretion is increased following release of unilateral ureteral obstruction. In the patient described by Better and colleagues [72], fractional and absolute magnesium excretion after relief of unilateral ureteral obstruction was significantly greater from the postreleased kidney than from the normally functioning kidney. Magnesium excretion is also markedly increased following release of unilateral ureteral obstruction in rats [73]. This change is not modified by magnesium restriction in the diet. It is likely that the differences in magnesium and calcium excretion seen after release of unilateral ureteral obstruction in the rat relate to the greater reabsorption of calcium than magnesium in the proximal tubule. Since in the rat a major portion of the magnesium filtered is reabsorbed in the thick ascending limb, a defect in reabsorption in this segment may account for the marked increase in magnesium excretion in the urine.

Phosphate Reabsorption After Relief of Ureteral Obstruction

The reabsorption of phosphorus by the postobstructed kidney depends on both the duration of the obstruction and whether the obstruction is bilateral or unilateral [73–75]. After release of bilateral ureteral obstruction of 24 hours' duration, phosphate excretion parallels sodium and water excretion and is increased in absolute terms and when expressed as a fraction of the filtered load [71]. This increased excretion is not affected by parathyroidectomy and cannot be accounted for by an increase in ECF volume [74]. The increase in phosphate excretion, however, can be prevented by phosphate restriction in the diet prior to bilateral ureteral obstruction, to forestall the rise in serum phosphorus that usually occurs. In addition, increasing the phosphorus levels of normal rats to concentrations similar to those seen after bilateral ureteral obstruction results in a similar degree of phosphaturia [74]. These observations suggest that the filtered load of phosphorus is the major determinant of the rate of phosphate excretion after release of bilateral ureteral obstruction. Although no studies have examined the nephron site of impaired phosphate reabsorption, it is assumed that it is in the proximal tubule because of the magnitude of the change involved and the fact that the major site of phosphate reabsorption is in this segment of the nephron.

In contrast, phosphate excretion after release of unilateral ureteral obstruction is decreased in the postobstructed kidney and increased in the contralateral kidney in humans [66], rats [75], and dogs [76]. The increase in phosphate excretion by the contralateral kidney in rats with unilateral ureteral obstruction is abolished by parathyroidectomy. Aortic constriction mimics the effects of unilateral ureteral obstruction inasmuch as it causes phosphate retention. The increase in phosphate retention by the postobstructed kidney may be due to a decrease in single-nephron GFR and an increase in the phosphate reabsorption by proximal segments. In summary, after release of unilateral ureteral obstruction, altered phosphorus excretion results primarily from altered renal hemodynamics, and following release of bilateral ureteral obstruction, phosphate excretion is modulated to a large extent by extrarenal factors, mainly the serum levels of phosphate.

Altered Hormone Responsiveness and Sensitivity of the Postobstructed Kidney

After release of ureteral obstruction, there is a change in the response of the postobstructed kidney to hormones [77]. The consequences of obstructive nephropathy include (1) decreased excretion and altered renal metabolism of hormones produced in extrarenal endocrine organs, (2) altered rates of production of hormones within the kidney, and (3) altered responsiveness and sensitivity of the obstructed kidney to hormones.

Parathyroid Hormone. After release of unilateral ureteral obstruction, the fractional excretion of phosphorus is markedly reduced in the postobstructed kidney [75] and increased in the contralateral kidney. The obstructed kidney responds to exogenous parathyroid hormone administration with an increase in urine phosphate and cyclic AMP excretion. However, the magnitude of the response is less in the postobstructed kidney than in the contralateral kidney [75]. This decrease in response to the hormone is accompanied by decreased generation of cyclic AMP, decreased activation of adenylate cyclase by the hormone in basolateral membranes obtained from the proximal tubule of postobstructed kidneys, and the apparent loss of parathyroid hormone receptors from the same membrane [78].

After relief of bilateral ureteral obstruction, absolute and fractional phosphate excretion is increased and does not increase further following the administration of parathyroid hormone [74]. However, when the filtered load of phosphate is restored to normal by dietary manipulations, which prevent the increase in phosphorus that occurs with bilateral ureteral obstruction, the excretion of phosphorus by the postobstructed kidney is normalized, and so is the response to parathyroid hormone.

Ureteral obstruction blunts the calcemic response of bone to parathyroid hormone, presumably as a result of the decreased production of 1,25-dihydroxyvitamin D_3 by the obstructed kidney or as a consequence of increased levels of circulating parathyroid hormone.

Angiotensin II. The role of the renin-angiotensin system in the pathophysiology of obstructive uropathy has been discussed already. The postobstructed kidney has an increased capacity to release prostaglandins in response to angiotensin II, and those response curves suggest that there is an increase in the number or affinity, or both, of the receptors for the hormone. In addition, the contractile responses of the renal cortex to angiotensin were enhanced in rabbit kidneys that had been obstructed for 8 to 32 days, compared to normal kidneys that showed minimal response, suggesting that the sensitivity of the postobstructed kidney to angiotensin II is increased. On the other hand, in isolated glomeruli from obstructed kidneys, the eicosanoid production in response to the in vitro addition of angiotensin II is blunted [36].

Antidiuretic Hormone (Vasopressin). An unresponsiveness of the collecting duct to the effect of antidiuretic hormone (ADH) on water permeability may contribute to the concentrating defect seen after ureteral obstruction. The cyclic AMP response to exogenous ADH is markedly blunted in rats with bilateral ureteral obstruction, compared to nonobstructed rats. In addition, ADH-induced osmotic water flow is significantly impaired in cortical collecting tubules isolated from obstructed kidneys of rabbits [53, 62]. The mechanisms responsible for the alterations in hormone sensitivity are not immediately apparent. The decreased activation of the adenylate cyclase system may be due to alterations in the guanine nucleotide regulatory proteins, with Ns, the stimulatory component, being decreased after ureteral obstruction. In addition, another signal pathway, the polyphosphoinositide pathway, may be altered by ureteral obstruction. Thus, the generation of both phosphatidylinositol-1,4,5-triphosphate, which mobilizes calcium from intracellular organelles, as well as diglyceride, which can activate protein kinase C and thus effect the phosphorylation of proteins, may be impaired. Indeed, phosphatidylinositol-4,5-biphosphate, the precursor of inositol triphosphate, and diglyceride are decreased in the obstructed kidney of rats with unilateral ureteral obstruction, compared to the contralateral kidney.

Changes in Renal Metabolism in the Obstructed Kidney

A variety of changes of renal metabolism occur following ureteral obstruction. These changes are summarized in Table 12-2.

Changes in the Activity of Renal Enzymes

The activities of brush-border alkaline phosphatase, of basolateral Na,K-ATPase, and glucose-6-phosphatase all decrease acutely (within 2 days of ureteral obstruction) and return to normal following the release of obstruction [77]. In contrast, the activities of the enzymes of the pentose shunt pathway increase after ureteral obstruction. In the normal kidney, there is a characteristic distribution of the isoenzymes of lactate dehydrogenase (LDH) with LDH-1 (the aerobic or H form) found predominantly in the cortex and LDH-5 (the anaerobic or N form) found in the

Table 12-2. Effects of urinary tract obstruction on renal metabolism

I. Changes in enzyme activity
    Decreased:
        Alkaline phosphatase
        Na^+,K^+-ATPase
        Glucose-6-phosphatase
        Succinic dehydrogenase
        NADH & NADPH dehydrogenase
        α-Glycerophosphate dehydrogenase
        LDH 1,2,3 isoenzymes
    Increased:
        Glucose phosphate dehydrogenase
        6-Phosphogluconic dehydrogenase
        LDH 4,5 isoenzymes
II. Energy and substrate metabolism
    Decreased O_2 consumption
    Decreased substrate uptake
    Increased anaerobic glycolysis
    Decreased levels of adenine nucleotides
    Decreased renal gluconeogenesis
    Decreased ammoniagenesis
III. Hormonal changes and responsiveness
    Decreased phosphaturia in response to PTH
    Decreased effect of ADH on water reabsorption
    Decreased effects of aldosterone?
    Increased prostaglandin synthesis in response to angiotensin II and bradykinin
    Increased renin secretion

LDH = lactate dehydrogenase; PTH = parathyroid hormone; ADH = antidiuretic hormone.
Source: K. Kurokawa, L. G. Fine, and S. Klahr, Renal metabolism in obstructive nephropathy. *Semin. Nephrol.* 2:31–39, 1982.

inner medulla, possibly as a result of the progressive decrease in oxygen tension that occurs from the cortex to the medulla. With ureteral obstruction, there is a fall in LDH-1 and a reciprocal rise in LDH-5 in the cortex [79], which are compatible with the kidney's adapting to an anaerobic pattern of metabolism. Following ureteral obstruction, Na,K-ATPase activity is decreased along most segments of the nephron [68]. The mechanism for this decline in enzyme activity is not well understood, but a loss of medullary tonicity, which is known to be a stimulus to Na,K-ATPase activity, in the obstructed kidney may have a causal role. Recent observations indicate that the mass of the Na,K-ATPase is preserved in obstructed kidneys. This suggests that the decrease in activity of the enzyme may be related to either tertiary alterations in the configuration of the enzyme, sequestration of the enzyme, and/or changes in the lipid environment in which the enzyme operates [80]. The loss of activity of the Na,K-ATPase in the distal tubule and thick ascending limb may contribute to the pathogenesis of the postobstructive diuresis that is seen in humans and experimental animals.

Changes in Energy and Substrate Metabolism

After ureteral obstruction, oxygen consumption is markedly decreased with a concomitant decrease in carbon dioxide production [81, 82]. The increase in respiratory quotient suggests a switch to anaerobic glycolysis. Indeed, anaerobic glycolysis may increase by as much as 10-fold over normal levels with prolonged (10–14 days) obstruction [81], and such abnormalities may persist even after release of the obstruction [82]. Although the exact mechanism responsible for the switch to anaerobic metabolism in the kidney in response to ureteral obstruction remains to be defined, electron micrographs have shown that ureteral obstruction results in structural changes of mitochondria after 24 hours of ureteral ligation [83]. Adenosine triphosphate levels fall to 50 to 70 percent of normal values within 24 hours of ureteral obstruction [83, 84] with a proportional increase in adenosine diphosphate and AMP levels. These levels return to normal after the release of short periods of ureteral obstruction even though the functional derangements persist. Thus, the pathophysiologic consequences of these changes remain uncertain.

The pars recta and the convoluted portion of the proximal tubule are normally capable of gluconeogenesis and uniquely possess the enzyme phosphoenol-pyruvate carboxykinase (PEPCK), which is a key enzyme for gluconeogenesis. Twenty-four hours of ureteral obstruction reduces the rate of gluconeogenesis by the obstructed kidney by 20 to 40 percent when the substrate is α-ketoglutarate, malate, or pyruvate but not when it is glycerol [83]. Since the latter enters the metabolic pathway above PEPCK, this would suggest that the activity of PEPCK is depressed by ureteral obstruction [83, 84].

Cortical slices obtained from postobstructed kidneys exhibit a decreased capacity to produce ammonia from glutamine, when compared to slices obtained from the contralateral kidney [83]. These experiments demonstrated a decrease in glutamine uptake and oxidation, a decreased oxygen consumption, and impaired gluconeogenesis and ammoniagenesis, but no changes in enzymes were investigated. The decrease in ammoniagenesis may contribute to the inability to excrete acid following ureteral obstruction.

In addition to changes in enzyme activity, ureteral obstruction also causes changes in gene transcription both in the obstructed kidney and in the contralateral kidney [85].

Changes in Lipid Metabolism

After 24 hours of ureteral obstruction, the triglyceride content of the obstructed kidney is increased compared to the contralateral untouched kidney or to the kidneys of sham-operated rats [86]. Concomitantly, there is a decrease in the total phospholipid content of the obstructed kidney. There is an increase in the net synthetic rate of triglyceride by the obstructed kidney that is related to both a decrease in fatty acid oxidation and an increase in the release of fatty acids from phospholipids, presumably due to an increase in phospholipase activity. Further experiments using basolateral membranes isolated from renal tubular cells have shown that following obstruction there is a decrease in phospholipid content of the membrane [87]. Since the lipid composition, or physical state of the membrane (fluidity), affects the activity of membrane-bound enzymes and water permeability, it is possible that selective changes in the lipid composition of basolateral membranes following obstruction could account for both the altered transport characteristics and the altered response to hormones seen after release of ureteral obstruction.

Histopathologic Consequences of Urinary Tract Obstruction

The morphologic alterations of the kidney caused by obstruction can be predicted from the major causes of parenchymal damage: (1) decreased renal blood flow, (2) increased ureteral pressure, (3) invasion by macrophages and lymphocytes, and (4) bacterial infection. Chronic partial obstruction may result in grossly hydronephrotic kidneys with a widely dilated renal pelvis, with the renal papilla either flattened or hollowed out. The first structures to be affected are the ducts of Bellini. Subsequently, other papillary structures are damaged. Ultimately, there is an encroachment on renal cortical tissue, which in advanced cases may be reduced to a thin rim of renal tissue surrounding a large saccular ureteral pelvis.

Histologically, the initial changes of hydronephrosis comprise dilatation of the tubular system, predominantly the collecting duct and distal tubular segments [88, 89]. Subsequently, cellular flattening and atrophy of the cells lining the proximal tubule occur. In most instances, the glomerular architecture is preserved. Bowman's space may be acutely dilated, and ultimately some periglomerular fibrosis may develop. Sequelae of tubular ischemia are the consequence of the combined effects of decreased renal blood flow and the development of interstitial fibrosis and mononuclear infiltration. Invading cells, particularly macrophages, by releasing inflammatory and growth factors, may contribute to interstitial cell proliferation and scarring and widening of the interstitium space. The increased distance between peritubular capillaries and tubular cells may contribute to the ischemia [90]. Superimposed bacterial infection (pyelonephritis) may play an additive role in the development of parenchymal fibrosis and in the pathologic changes that are observed [91].

Tubulointerstitial Fibrosis in Obstructive Uropathy

The tubulointerstitium occupies approximately 80 percent of total kidney volume. Renal epithelial tubular cells represent the major compartment of the kidney. A number of entities can result in the development of tubulointerstitial pathology. Renal interstitial fibrosis is a common consequence of long-standing obstructive uropathy [92, 93]. Fibrosis very likely develops due to an imbalance between extracellular matrix synthesis, matrix deposition, and matrix degradation. In the 1970s, Nagle and Bulger [92] reported that rabbits with unilateral ureteral ligation had a widened interstitial space 7 days after the onset of obstruction; they found increased collagen fibers and numerous fibroblasts at this time, and by day 16 collagen was greatly increased and was arranged in large bundles. Nagle et al. [94] also described a mononuclear cell infiltrate and proliferation of interstitial cells in the renal paren-chyma of rabbits with chronic unilateral ureteral obstruction. Sharma et al. [93] described increased renal synthesis of several extracellular matrix components (col-lagen types I, III, and IV; fibronectin; heparan sulfate proteoglycans) in the renal interstitium of rabbits with ureteral obstruction of 3 and 7 days' duration.

The relative volume of the cortical interstitium is increased after 3 days of unilat-eral ureteral obstruction in the rat [95]. Increased deposition of collagen types I, III, and IV was evident in the tubulointerstitium by the third day of unilateral ureteral obstruction. In addition, the level of messenger RNA (mRNA) for collagen α_1 (IV) was significantly elevated in the obstructed kidney at this time interval. Thus, events leading to interstitial fibrosis are initiated promptly after the onset of obstruction. The amount of collagens I, III, and IV did not change in the glomeruli of the obstructed kidney at day 5 after unilateral ureteral obstruction. Additionally, transforming growth factor-β_1 (TGF-β_1) mRNA levels did not change in glomeruli of the obstructed kidney but did increase in the tubulointerstitium during ureteral obstruction [96]. These results are consistent with the finding that glomeruli appear normal by light microscopy through 7 days of obstructive nephropathy [94, 95]. Both interstitial collagen (types I and III) and the basement membrane collagen (type IV) are deposited in the interstitial space of the obstructed kidney [95]. Colla-gens I and III were increased in the interstitial space only, while collagen IV was deposited both in the interstitium of the obstructed kidney and in the tubular basement membrane. Furthermore, we found that collagen IV is the major collagen that increases in the renal cortex of the adult rat during unilateral ureteral obstruc-tion. The increase in collagen IV in both the interstitial space and in the basement membrane of renal tubules may contribute to alterations in tubular function in the obstructed kidney.

Renal tubular cells in culture produce collagen types I, III, and IV. There is increased expression of collagen α_1 (IV) mRNA in the tubules of the obstructed kidney. Thus, renal tubule cells may contribute to the increased production of collagen IV in both tubular basement membrane and interstitium. Fibroblasts mi-grate and proliferate in the interstitium of the obstructed kidney during unilateral ureteral obstruction [92]. Several cytokines secreted by infiltrating macrophages and T lymphocytes act as chemoattractants and stimulate fibroblast proliferation [97]. Interstitial fibroblasts produce collagens I, III, and IV. The substantial increase in collagens I and III in the interstitium of the obstructed kidney at 3 or 5 days after unilateral ureteral obstruction is consistent with the increased cellularity due to fibroblast proliferation and infiltrating mononuclear cells. Thus, interstitial fibro-blasts may contribute to an increase in the production of collagens in the obstructed kidney of rats with unilateral ureteral obstruction.

The expression of TGF-β_1 mRNA is increased in the obstructed kidney, and this increase is confined to tubular cells [96]. TGF-β_1 has substantial effects on matrix protein production [98]. It causes (1) an increase in the mRNA of extracellular matrix components, particularly the collagens, (2) a decrease in proteinases degrad-ing these proteins, and (3) an increase in metalloproteinase inhibitors (Fig. 12-9). Thus, an increase in TGF-β_1 in the cortical tubules of the obstructed kidney may

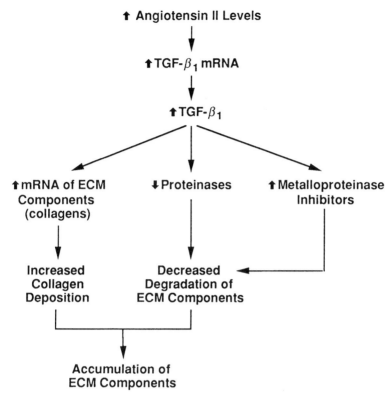

Fig. 12-9. Pathogenesis of interstitial fibrosis in obstructive nephropathy. TGF-β_1 = transforming growth factor-β_1; mRNA = messenger RNA; ECM = extracellular matrix. (From S. Klahr, S. Ishidoya, and J. Morrissey, Role of angiotensin II in the tubulointerstitial fibrosis of obstructive nephropathy. *Am. J. Kidney Dis.* 26:141–146, 1995.)

result in increased collagen α_1 (IV) mRNA. The increase in collagen IV protein is undoubtedly the consequence of the increase in the mRNA.

Both an angiotensin-converting enzyme inhibitor, enalapril, and an angiotensin II receptor antagonist, SC-51316, ameliorate the increased production of extracellular matrix protein in the tubulointerstitium of the obstructed kidney. Blockade of angiotensin II synthesis or inability of angiotensin II to bind to its receptor lessened the increased levels of mRNA for TGF-β and collagen IV found in the obstructed kidney of untreated rats (see Fig. 12-9). A monocyte/macrophage infiltration was present in the obstructed kidney of untreated rats or rats treated with the angiotensin II receptor antagonists. By contrast, this infiltrate was almost completely absent in the obstructed kidney of rats treated with enalapril. The reason for this different effect of enalapril versus the angiotensin II receptor antagonist on the macrophage infiltrate seen in obstructive nephropathy has not been elucidated. Thus, both an angiotensin-converting enzyme inhibitor (enalapril) and a receptor antagonist of angiotensin II ameliorate the tubulointerstitial fibrosis that follows complete unilateral ureteral obstruction in the rat. We suggest that an increased level of angiotensin II has a major role in the development of tubulointerstitial fibrosis following ureteral obstruction.

Clinical Consequences of Urinary Tract Obstruction

Obstruction of the urinary tract is a common cause of renal failure. The symptoms and signs of obstructive uropathy are often nonspecific, and the clinical abnormalities may be dominated by impaired renal function, by manifestations related to urinary tract infection, and sometimes by extrarenal manifestations of the underlying pathologic process responsible for the development of obstructive uropathy, such as tumors or metastases from distal tumors.

Renal Failure Associated with Urinary Tract Obstruction

Bilateral obstruction of the urinary tract is one of the many causes of acute or chronic renal failure. Acute renal failure may also occur when a solitary kidney is obstructed. If acute renal failure presents with complete anuria or if periods of anuria alternate with periods of polyuria, the possibility of obstructive uropathy should be seriously entertained. With partial or intermittent obstruction, polyuria may be present [56, 57], and thirst may be a prominent symptom. A number of patients presenting with the signs and symptoms of chronic uremia may have undetected, long-standing urinary tract obstruction. Urinary tract obstruction may occur in the setting of underlying parenchymal renal disease of another etiology and manifest itself by a change in the rate of progression of renal insufficiency. In some patients, however, obstruction is the only cause of end-stage renal failure. Occasionally, in patients with retroperitoneal fibrosis in whom the onset of obstruction is slow and progressive, far-advanced renal failure may be an initial presenting complaint. Urinary tract obstruction should be considered in patients with uremia and no previous history of renal disease and a relatively benign urinary sediment. It also should be considered in patients with known renal disease who develop an abrupt decrease in renal function that is otherwise unexplained.

Pain and Renal Enlargement

Pain may be the presenting complaint in patients with obstruction. This is usually the case in patients with acute or rapidly developing obstruction. Acute ureteral obstruction may be characterized by steady, crescendo pain radiating downward toward the groin, the testicles, or labia. Pain may be absent, especially in patients with chronic slowly progressive obstruction. Occasionally, such patients may complain of dull flank pain usually related to increased fluid intake or to the use of diuretics. Flank pain occurring during micturition is said to be pathognomic of ureterovesical reflux. Kidney size may increase, sometimes notably in long-standing obstruction. Patients may note increased abdominal girth or a palpable flank mass. Sometimes marked hydronephrosis may present as a flank mass on physical examination. This is often the case in children with hydronephrosis who are younger than 2 years.

Urinary Tract Infection

There is a striking association between urinary tract infection and obstructive uropathy [99]. Infection tends to be more common with obstruction of the lower urinary tract, that is, obstruction that is located below the ureterovesical junction. Several factors may condition the development of infection in the setting of obstruction: (1) the increase of residual urine in the bladder, since urine is an excellent culture medium; and (2) altered properties of the bladder that facilitate bacterial adhesion and growth. Alterations in the glycoprotein composition of epithelial cells of the bladder may explain the greater predisposition to infection in certain patients with urinary tract obstruction than in others. Obstruction of the upper urinary tract is not necessarily accompanied by infection. Obstruction associated with urinary tract infection should be suspected when the infections are repetitive in nature or recurrent or when they are resistant to usual therapeutic agents to which the cultured bacteria have demonstrated susceptibility.

Hypertension

Hypertension may occur in patients with acute or chronic hydronephrosis, either unilateral or bilateral [100–104]. The hypertension could be coincidental or could be related to the hydronephrosis. The mechanisms may relate either to increased ECF volume, owing to decreased sodium excretion, or to an abnormal release of renin and increased generation of angiotensin II. In patients with bilateral hydronephrosis, the increased exchangeable sodium and the usual prompt reversal of the hypertension after catheter drainage and diuresis suggest that the hypertension is due to abnormal retention of salt and water subsequent to the obstructive process. Thus, these patients appear to have a volume-dependent type of hypertension. In addition, the concentrations of renin in renal venous blood and peripheral venous blood are normal in hypertensive patients with bilaterally hydronephrotic kidneys. After corrective surgery, reversal of the hypertension is associated with an osmotic diuresis and a negative salt and water balance, further suggesting that this type of hypertension is volume dependent.

On the other hand, hypertension in patients with unilateral ureteral obstruction may be renin dependent [100, 101, 103]. Elevated values for renal vein renin have been found in unilaterally hydronephrotic kidneys. After appropriate surgery, the hypertension abated, and the renin values returned to normal [100]. Animal studies have demonstrated increased renin release following acute ureteral obstruction [105]. In dogs, acute unilateral ureteral obstruction is associated with an increase in blood pressure and a rise in ipsilateral renal vein renin in spite of a concurrent rise in renal blood flow. The causal relation between renin release and the increase in blood pressure is suggested by the fact that pretreatment with desoxycorticosterone acetate (DOCA) and salt abolished the rise in renin and blood pressure. In contrast, chronic studies in animals have shown that the renin release is not sustained and that the peripheral renin is normal with prolonged unilateral ureteral occlusion. This suggests that chronic, established hypertension in the setting of unilateral obstruction may not be related to increased renin secretion. Since corrective surgery may result in improvement in some of these patients, other abnormalities not related to renin may be operative in obstruction. Whether these abnormalities relate to subtle changes in volume or to the lack of release of vasodepressive substances by the obstructed kidney has not been established.

Polycythemia

Polycythemia has been reported in a few instances of hydronephrosis and is probably related to increased production of erythropoietin by the obstructed kidney. In experimental animals, unilateral hydronephrosis results in elevated plasma levels of erythropoietin that precede the increase in hemoglobin levels.

Hyperkalemic Hyperchloremic Acidosis

In certain patients with obstruction, hyperkalemic hyperchloremic acidosis (renal tubular acidosis type 4) may be a clinical manifestation of partial obstruction of the urinary tract [63, 106]. The pertinent mechanisms have been described in the pathophysiology section of this chapter.

Hypernatremia

Children with partial obstructive uropathy and marked polyuria, due to a greater loss of water than sodium, may develop hypernatremia. Thus, the finding of hypernatremia in children should raise the suspicion of partial urinary tract obstruction.

Diagnosis

Diagnostic Approach to the Patient with Obstructive Uropathy

The approach to the patient with obstructive uropathy varies with the clinical setting and presenting symptoms, the spectrum of which extends from patients presenting with acute pain to patients with acute renal failure and anuria. Thus, the diagnostic approach and the urgency with which the diagnosis must be made are highly variable. When obstructive uropathy is suspected, certain information is essential. A history of similar symptoms, the presence or absence of urinary tract infection, and the kinds of drugs ingested should be noted. Questions directed toward eliciting lower urinary tract symptoms are clearly important. Review of hospital records may reveal abrupt changes in urine output. Physical examination with particular reference to the flank and abdomen is important. Tenderness in the costovertebral angle may or may not be present. A mass in the flank area, especially in children, may be found by palpation or percussion. Muscle rigidity over the kidney may be found, and rebound tenderness may be elicited, particularly if acute infection is present. Analysis of the urine may provide important information. The presence of hematuria alone may lead one to suspect that the obstructive lesion is a calculus, a sloughed papilla, or a tumor. The urine sediment should be examined carefully for the presence of crystals. Sulfonamide, cysteine, or uric acid crystals may be the first indication as to the type of stone causing the ureteral obstruction or the intrarenal obstruction resulting in acute renal failure. Laboratory studies should include determination of serum creatinine and urea nitrogen levels in addition to the usual blood chemistries.

Hydronephrosis and genitourinary abnormalities [107, 108] can be diagnosed prenatally. In neonates and infants, obstructive uropathy may not be suspected until failure to thrive, voiding difficulties, fever, hematuria, or symptoms of renal failure appear. Oligohydramnios at the time of delivery should raise the suspicion of obstructive uropathy. Newborns with third-degree hypospadias and other congenital anomalies should be evaluated for the presence of urinary tract obstruction. Nonurologic anomalies may also suggest obstructive uropathy. Newborns with a single umbilical artery or ear deformities [109] require urologic investigation. The urinary tract should also be examined in infants born with an imperforate anus or a rectourethral or rectovaginal fistula. The existence of a neurogenic bladder with associated obstructive uropathy should be suspected in infants with neurologic abnormalities.

Differential Diagnosis of Obstructive Uropathy

The entities that should be considered in the differential diagnosis of obstruction vary, depending on the clinical presentation of the obstructive lesion. Patients with anuria and acute renal failure should be evaluated for other potential causes of acute renal failure such as ischemia and nephrotoxins (see Chap. 10). The presentation of patients with partial obstruction and polyuria may mimic that of patients with nephrogenic diabetes insipidus. Patients with obstruction presenting with hyperchloremic, hyperkalemic metabolic acidosis should be distinguished from patients who have the same syndrome on the basis of low levels of renin and aldosterone secretion. Renal colic due to stones may mimic flank pain due to a gastrointestinal pathologic condition. In children, the manifestations of obstructive uropathy may include gastrointestinal symptoms such as nausea, vomiting, and abdominal pain.

Diagnosis of Urinary Tract Obstruction

Upper Urinary Tract Obstruction

Upper urinary tract obstruction is relatively easy to diagnose in most instances. Occasionally, however, it may be difficult to make the diagnosis. Not all dilated collecting systems represent obstruction, and this should be considered when evaluating a patient with hydronephrosis. Several radiologic techniques can be used to diagnose suspected upper urinary tract obstruction. These techniques include a plain film of the abdomen, sonography, excretory urography, retrograde pyelography, isotopic renography, pressure-flow studies, and voiding cystography.

Plain Films. A plain film of the abdomen (the kidney, ureter, and bladder [KUB]) should be obtained early in patients with renal failure in whom excretory urography is not contemplated. It provides information on renal and bladder morphology, such as size differences between the two kidneys or a large bladder suggestive of outlet obstruction. Ureteral radiopaque calculi (90%) may be visualized on the KUB film.

Sonography. Sonography (ultrasound) is a noninvasive test used as a screening procedure for obstruction [110, 111]. The main finding detected by sonography is dilatation of the urinary tract. However, in patients with acute obstruction, dilatation of the urinary tract may occasionally not occur, and sonography may be unrevealing. In a few instances, sonography may give false-positive results suggesting obstruction because anatomic variations of the pyelocaliceal system (e.g., extrarenal pelvis) may be interpreted as dilatation of the urinary tract.

Excretory or Intravenous Pyelography. The intravenous pyelogram (IVP) is used frequently to investigate suspected upper urinary tract obstruction [112]. The excretion of contrast medium may be delayed in patients with low GFR, due to a decrease in the filtered load of the dye. In such patients, the procedure should be extended until the collecting system and the site of obstruction are identified [113]. This may require obtaining films as long as 1 day after radiocontrast injection. Intravenous urography may sometimes disclose both the site and the cause of the obstruction. The IVP is not helpful in patients with marked decreases in renal function. Visualization of the urinary tract is usually poor in patients with serum creatinine values greater than 5 mg/dl. Furosemide administration during the performance of an IVP may be helpful. Dilatation of the collecting system may only be seen after furosemide administration, and the concomitant reappearance of renal colic strongly suggests obstruction. However, patients with marked renal insufficiency do not have a diuresis after furosemide administration, making the test less useful. The nephrotoxicity of the contrast material should be considered when ordering an IVP, as compared with other diagnostic procedures, particularly in patients older than 60 years and in patients with diabetes mellitus, renal insufficiency, or dehydration.

Retrograde Pyelography. Retrograde pyelography involves the retrograde injection of radiocontrast material and is used to visualize the ureter and collecting system when the IVP cannot be done or is not justified. Retrograde pyelography can identify both the site and the cause of the obstruction [114]. It is helpful to include a postdrainage film, which is generally obtained 10 minutes after the retrograde injection of the radiocontrast. If the contrast medium does not persist in the collecting system, obstruction is unlikely. In some instances, however, retrograde pyelography cannot differentiate between obstruction and dilatation of the urinary tract. A markedly dilated, but not obstructed ureter will eliminate the contrast medium, mainly by gravity and by constant production of urine. In a patient who is dehydrated, supine, and in the lithotomy position for the performance of the retrograde pyelography, a dilated, but not obstructed ureter will most likely reveal residual contrast material on a postdrainage film. Urinary tract infections may occur as a consequence of retrograde pyelography. If obstruction is present, the risk of introducing overwhelming infection, which is difficult to control with conventional therapy, is great. Hence, if obstruction is diagnosed during retrograde pyelography, it is mandatory to provide adequate drainage of the obstruction to avoid the unfortunate consequences of infection in an obstructed urinary tract.

Isotopic Renography. Isotopic renography can be used to diagnose upper urinary tract obstruction. It requires the intravenous injection of a radionuclide with imaging using a gamma scintillation camera. This can be combined with furosemide, administered intravenously 20 to 30 minutes after injecting the isotope. Theoretically, the diuretic should cause a rapid washout of the isotope in a dilated nonobstructed system. Persistence of the isotope suggests that the system is not only dilated but also obstructed. Several tracings are summarized in Figure 12-10. Tracing I pertains to a patient with a normal urinary tract. Tracing II strongly suggests obstruction because the radioisotope is retained in the pelvis and collecting system. There is no excretion following furosemide administration. Tracing III can be interpreted as showing dilatation without obstruction, since after furosemide administration there is rapid disappearance of the isotope. Although the isotopic renogram is relatively noninvasive [115] and can be performed in most hospitals and clinics, it is seldom the definitive test in making the diagnosis of obstruction. Markedly reduced renal function limits the usefulness of this test because the diuretic response to furosemide may be absent, making interpretation difficult.

Computed Tomography and Magnetic Resonance Imaging. Other diagnostic procedures for obstructive uropathy include computed tomography and magnetic resonance imaging. Computed tomography is particularly useful in the diagnosis of causes of obstruction. The advantages of magnetic resonance imaging include no need to use radiocontrast material with iodine, better tissue contrast, better multiplanar imaging, and no ionizing radiation.

Pressure-Flow Relationships (Whitaker Test). Sometimes upper urinary tract obstruction is difficult to diagnose using the techniques described, and pressure-flow studies may be required [116]. After the collecting system is punctured with a fine-gauge needle and the bladder is catheterized, fluid is perfused at a rate of 10 ml/min. At this perfusion rate, the differential pressure between the bladder and the collecting system should not exceed 15 cm H_2O. A differential pressure greater than 20 cm H_2O indicates obstruction, and a pressure gradient between 15 and 20 cm H_2O is equivocal in diagnosing obstruction. An evaluation of the rise in pelvic pressure during perfusion diuresis also provides useful information. Usually, a steep rise in pelvic pressure is found when high differential pressures and decreased renal function are present. The pressure-flow study should be done both with an empty

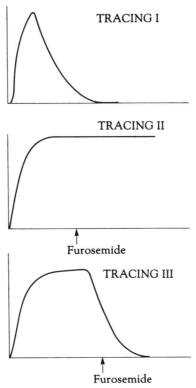

Fig. 12-10. Patterns of isotopic renography. Tracing I = normal excretory pattern; tracing II = obstruction of the urinary tract; tracing III = stasis of urine with obstruction. (From R. Gonzalez and R. K. Chiou. The diagnosis of upper urinary tract obstruction in children: Comparison of diuresis renography and pressure flow studies. J. Urol. 133:646–649, 1985.)

and with a full bladder because sometimes the obstruction is only evident when the bladder is full. During pressure-flow studies, antegrade pyeloureterograms can be obtained and may help define the site of the obstruction and eliminate the need for retrograde pyelography.

Voiding Cystourethrogram. The voiding cystourethrogram is utilized to investigate the presence of vesicoureteral reflux as a cause of the dilatation of the urinary tract.

Diagnosis of Lower Urinary Tract Obstruction

Obstruction of the lower urinary tract may be evaluated by cystoscopy, radiologic tests, and urodynamic tests. *Cystoscopy* allows visual inspection of the entire urethra and the bladder. This procedure, however, requires the use of anesthesia in children and young adults.

The usefulness of the IVP in investigating bladder outlet obstruction due to benign disorders is debatable [117]. Some argue that the IVP does not modify the therapeutic approach for outlet obstruction. Others hold that the test is necessary because lower urinary tract studies should not be performed without a thorough evaluation of the anatomy of the upper urinary tract. When the obstruction is due to malignancy, an IVP should be obtained to evaluate the upper urinary tract and help in cancer staging. Oblique films of the bladder and urethra during voiding (excretory cystogram) and after voiding are useful in evaluating the site of obstruction and the amount of residual urine.

An IVP should generally be obtained in children with congenital anomalies, since marked effects of lower urinary tract obstruction on the upper urinary tract may be detected. Hydronephrosis may be due to increased intravesical pressures or to obstruction of the distal ureter caused by hypertrophy of the detrusor muscle. In general, a retrograde voiding cystourethrogram offers better definition than the excretory cystogram because of greater filling and opacification of the bladder. However, since bladder catheterization is required, this procedure cannot always be done, particularly if the infravesical obstruction is due to urethral stricture or prostatic cancer.

Urodynamic tests measuring urine flow rate per unit of time (debimetry) are useful to evaluate bladder outlet obstruction. This test examines the interplay between the expulsive force of the detrusor muscle and urethral resistance [118]. The patient voids into a container that has a sensor connected to a recorder that plots micturition time and urine flow rate. From this plot, the urine volume, duration of micturition, average urine flow rate, maximum urine flow, and time required to reach the maximum flow rate can be calculated. The maximum flow rate is useful in assessing bladder outlet obstruction, but the pattern (continuous or intermittent) of flow is also useful. Physiologic filling of the bladder makes this test more reliable. Residual urine may be measured after voiding.

Since micturition requires the coordinated effects of expulsive force and urethral resistance, a decrease in bladder tone, for example, or an increase in resistance (i.e., benign prostatic hyperplasia) may produce symptoms of bladder outlet obstruction. *Cystometrography* can be used to assess the force of the detrusor muscle. The procedure quantitates the pressure-volume relationship of the bladder. The resistance of voiding may increase due to an anatomic lesion, such as a urethral stricture, or due to failure of the external sphincter to relax during micturition. Inability of the bladder sphincter to relax (dyssynergia) during contraction of the detrusor muscle is seen in patients with neurologic disorders. This condition is better analyzed by *electromyography* and *urethral pressure profile*.

Treatment

General Considerations

After obstructive uropathy is diagnosed, a decision should be made as to whether surgery or instrumentation is required [119]. Complete bilateral obstruction, with acute renal failure, requires prompt intervention. The site of obstruction will determine the approach in these patients. Introduction of a urethral catheter may suffice if the obstruction is distal to the bladder. In some cases, a suprapubic cystostomy may be necessary. In upper urinary tract obstruction, placement of nephrostomy tubes or retrograde introduction of a ureteral catheter may be required. Tubes should be placed in both obstructed renal calices, since the potential for functional recovery of either kidney is not easily predicted a priori. This may avoid the need for dialysis and allow sufficient time to determine the site and etiology of the obstructing lesion. In addition, the nephrostomy tube can be used for the local infusion of pharmacologic agents to treat infection, calculi, and so on. Patients with urinary tract infection and generalized sepsis require appropriate antibiotics and supportive therapy.

Surgical intervention can be delayed in patients with low-grade acute obstruction or partial chronic obstruction. However, prompt relief of partial obstruction is indicated when (1) the patient has significant symptoms (flank pain, dysuria, voiding dysfunction), (2) there is urinary retention, (3) there are multiple repeated episodes of urinary tract infection, and (4) there is evidence of progressive renal damage.

Management of Upper Urinary Tract Obstruction

Calculi are a common cause of ureteral obstruction. Their treatment includes relief of pain, elimination of obstruction, and treatment of infection [120]. Pain can be relieved by intramuscular injection of a narcotic analgesic. High fluid intake to increase urine volume to at least 1.5 to 2.0 liters daily may help mobilize the stone. The urine must be strained through a gauze sponge to recover the calculi for analysis. If the obstruction is partial and there is no infection or pain, surgical therapy may be delayed. Stones larger than 7 mm usually are not passed spontaneously.

Surgery or instrumentation for caliceal or ureteral calculi is indicated when there is persistent colic, urinary tract infection, or complete obstruction; when the calculus is greater than 7 mm; or if smaller, when the calculus has not moved despite an adequate period of observation and increased fluid intake. Radiologists or urologists can place a percutaneous nephrostomy and dilate the tract to as large as 12 mm. This provides a direct conduit to the kidney for removal of obstructing pelvic and upper ureteral stones. Rigid or flexible endoscopes can be introduced through the nephrostomy tract to remove calculi less than 1.5 cm in diameter. For larger stones, lithotriptor probes that use ultrasonic or electrohydraulic energy to disintegrate calculi have been utilized under direct visualization. Endourologic methods can be used to treat obstructing stones successfully in about 98 percent of patients. In addition, this approach shortens the hospital stay to 3 to 4 days and the convalescence period to only 4 to 7 days.

Extracorporeal shock wave lithotripsy [121] involves the focusing of electrohydraulically or ultrasonically generated shock waves to disintegrate the stone. The treatment is effective for calculi of 7 to 15 mm; in 90 percent of patients, the stone will be disintegrated, and all particulate matter will pass within a 3-month period. Morbidity is low. In selected individuals, the procedure can be done on an outpatient basis. Most patients can resume work 2 to 3 days after shock wave therapy.

Calculi located distal to the pelvic brim can be approached from below and can be removed from the ureter using a variety of loops or baskets. This procedure is successful in about 70 percent of patients. If it fails, dilatation of the ureter or ultrasonic disintegration of the stone can be accomplished using the ureterorenoscope.

Broad-spectrum antibiotics are useful when infections complicate renal calculi. Choice of antibiotic depends on appropriate urine culture results and sensitivities. It should be remembered, however, that relief of obstruction is indispensable for antimicrobial therapy to be effective.

Use of Nephrostomy in Ureteral Obstruction

Nephrostomy is the insertion of a tube through the kidney into the renal pelvis to provide urine drainage [122]. It can be performed with local anesthesia. Indications for placement of a nephrostomy tube include removal of stones through the tube, relief of obstruction due to malignancy or inflammatory disease, or conditions that do not permit the use of other procedures. Refractory infection due to unmanageable obstruction is another indication.

Complications of nephrostomy include perirenal hemorrhage and acute obstruction due to clots. Dislodgment of the nephrostomy tube should be considered an emergency, and the tube should be replaced immediately. Long-term complications such as calculus formation, infection, or pyelonephritis may occur and may lead to renal failure.

Treatment of Lower Urinary Tract Obstruction

Urethral and bladder-neck obstruction requires surgery in patients with recurring infections who are ambulatory, particularly when reflux, renal parenchymal damage, total urinary retention, repeated bleeding, or other severe symptoms are present. Obstruction secondary to benign prostatic hyperplasia does not always progress. Therefore, patients with minimal symptoms, no infection, and a normal upper urinary tract may be followed safely until the patient and the physician agree that surgery is desirable. Urethral strictures in men can be treated by dilation or direct-vision internal urethrotomy. The incidence of bladder-neck and urethral obstruction in women is low. Hence, urethral dilatation, internal urethrotomy, meatotomy, and revision of the bladder neck in women are seldom indicated. Suprapubic cystostomy may be necessary for bladder drainage in patients who cannot void after injury to the urethra or those who have an impassable urethral stricture.

When obstruction is the result of neuropathic bladder function, dynamic studies are essential to determine therapy. The main goals of therapy should be (1) to establish the bladder as a urine storage organ while preventing renal parenchymal injury, and (2) to provide a mechanism for bladder emptying that is acceptable to the patient. Two groups of patients are seen: those with atonic bladders secondary to lower motor neuron injury and those with unstable bladder function due to upper motor neuron disease. In both cases, ureteral reflux and parenchymal damage may develop, although this is more common in patients with a hypertonic bladder. A neurogenic bladder in diabetes mellitus is usually due to lower motor neuron disease.

Voiding at regular intervals will achieve satisfactory emptying of the bladder in these patients. Occasionally these individuals respond to cholinergic agents. Recent reviews on the use of bethanechol chloride (Urecholine), 50 mg orally, have seriously questioned its long-term use. In such patients, overdistention of the bladder may impair emptying. Thus, bladder outlet obstruction may be a major problem. α-Adrenergic blockers relax urethral sphincter tone but have only limited success due to side effects.

The best treatment for patients with significant residual urine and recurrent bouts of urosepsis is the establishment of clean intermittent catheterization at regular intervals. The goal should be to catheterize four to five times per day such that the amount of urine drained from the bladder does not exceed 400 ml. This useful technique requires patient acceptance and adequate training.

In patients with hypertonic bladder function, the major goal is to improve the storage function of the bladder. The use of anticholinergic agents such as oxybutynin (Ditropan), 5 mg every 4 to 6 hours, may be indicated. Occasionally chronic clean intermittent catheterization is necessary.

In all patients with neurogenic bladders, chronic indwelling catheters should be avoided if possible. Indwelling catheters usually lead to the formation of bladder stones, urosepsis, urethral erosion, and squamous cell carcinoma of the bladder. Patients with chronic indwelling catheters for more than 5 years should have yearly cystoscopic examinations.

Treatment of Postobstructive Diuresis

Postobstructive diuresis refers to the marked polyuria that can occur after relief of obstructive uropathy [46]. This polyuria is characterized by the excretion of large amounts of sodium, potassium, magnesium, and other solutes. Although self-limited in duration, the losses of salt and water may result in hypokalemia, hyponatremia or hypernatremia, hypomagnesemia, and/or marked contraction of the ECF volume and peripheral vascular collapse. In many patients, however, a brisk diuresis after relief of obstruction may represent a physiologic response to expansion of the ECF volume occurring during the period of obstruction. This postobstructive diuresis is "appropriate" and does not compromise the volume status of the patient. Postobstructive diuresis in this setting can be perpetuated or prolonged by overzealous administration of salt and water after relief of obstruction. Fluid replacement is justified only when there are excessive losses of sodium and water that are inappropriate for the volume status of the patient and are presumably due to an intrinsic tubular defect for sodium and water reabsorption.

Fluid replacement in patients with postobstructive diuresis should be guided by what is excreted. Intravenous fluid administration may be necessary, but urine losses should be replaced only to the extent necessary to prevent ECF volume contraction or electrolyte imbalance. Orthostatic hypotension and tachycardia are good indicators of when intravenous fluid administration is required. Sometimes to distinguish between inappropriate diuresis and appropriate excretion of fluid retained or excess fluid administered, it may be necessary to decrease fluid replacement to levels below those of urine output plus insensible losses and to observe the patient carefully for signs of volume depletion. Fluid replacement is based on frequent measurements of urine volume and serum and urine electrolytes. With massive diuresis, such measurements may be needed as often as every 6 hours. It is necessary to obtain weights once or twice daily. Fluids administered should be tailored to match excretion of water and electrolytes in the urine.

Urine losses of salt and water are usually replaced with 0.45% sodium chloride to which sodium bicarbonate and potassium chloride are added. Magnesium can be replaced by adding magnesium sulfate (supplied as 2-ml ampules containing 8 mEq of magnesium) to the sodium chloride solution. In some instances, replacement of phosphate losses may be necessary.

Acknowledgments. The author would like to thank Mr. James Havranek for his assistance in the preparation of this chapter.

References

1. Weiss RM: Physiology and Pharmacology of the Renal Pelvis and Ureter. In Walsh PC, Retik AB, Stamey TA, et al (eds): *Campbell's Urology* (6th ed). Philadelphia, Saunders, 1992, pp 111–141.
2. Tanagho EA, Pugh RCB: The anatomy and function of the ureterovesical junction. *Br J Urol* 35:151–165, 1963.
3. Biancani P, Hausman M, Weiss RM: Effect of obstruction on ureteral circumferential force-length relations. *Am J Physiol* 243:F204–F210, 1982.
4. Gillenwater JY, Westervelt FF Jr, Vaughan ED Jr, et al: Renal function after release of chronic unilateral hydronephrosis in man. *Kidney Int* 7:179–186, 1975.
5. Klahr S, Harris KPG, Purkerson ML: Effects of obstruction on renal functions. *Pediatr Nephrol* 2:34–42, 1988.
6. Harris RH, Gill JM: Changes in glomerular filtration rate during complete ureteral obstruction in rats. *Kidney Int* 19:603–608, 1981.
7. Dal Canton A, Stanziale R, Corradi A, et al: Effects of acute ureteral obstruction on glomerular hemodynamics in rat kidney. *Kidney Int* 12:403–411, 1977.
8. Wright FS: Effects of urinary tract obstruction on glomerular filtration rate and renal blood flow. *Semin Nephrol* 2:5–16, 1982.
9. Yarger WE, Aynedjian HS, Bank N: A micropuncture study of postobstructive diuresis in the rat. *J Clin Invest* 51:625–637, 1972.
10. Dal Canton A, Corradi A, Stanziale R, et al: Effects of 24-hour unilateral obstruction on glomerular hemodynamics in rat kidney. *Kidney Int* 15:457–462, 1979.
11. Gaudio KM, Siegel NJ, Hayslett JP, et al: Renal perfusion and intratubular pressure during ureteral occlusion in the rat. *Am J Physiol* 238:F205–F209, 1980.
12. Dal Canton A, Corradi A, Stanziale, R, et al: Glomerular hemodynamics before and after release of 24-hour bilateral ureteral obstruction. *Kidney Int* 17:491–496, 1980.
13. Moody TE, Vaughan ED Jr, Gillenwater JY: Relationship between renal blood flow and ureteral pressure during 18 hours of total unilateral ureteral occlusion: Implications for changing sites of increased renal resistance. *Invest Urol* 13:246–251, 1975.
14. Moody TE, Vaughan ED Jr, Gillenwater JY: Comparison of the renal hemodynamic response to unilateral and bilateral ureteral occlusion. *Invest Urol* 14:455–459, 1977.
15. Abe Y, Kishimoto T, Yamamoto K, et al: Intrarenal distribution of blood flow during ureteral and venous pressure elevation. *Am J Physiol* 224:746–751, 1973.
16. Bay WH, Stein JH, Rector JB, et al: Redistribution of renal cortical blood flow during elevated ureteral pressure. *Am J Physiol* 222:33–37, 1972.

17. Edwards GA, Suki WN: Effect of indomethacin on changes of acute ureteral pressure elevation in the dog. *Renal Physiol* 1:154–165, 1978.
18. Solez K, Ponchak S, Buono RA, et al: Inner medullary plasma flow in the kidney with ureteral obstruction. *Am J Physiol* 231:1315–1321, 1976.
19. Tanner GA: Effects of kidney tubule obstruction on glomerular function in rats. *Am J Physiol* 237:F379–F385, 1979.
20. Ichikawa I: Evidence for altered glomerular hemodynamics during acute nephron obstruction. *Am J Physiol* 242:F580–F585, 1982.
21. Blackshear JL, Edwards BS, Knox FG: Autoregulation of renal blood flow: Effects of indomethacin and ureteral pressure. *Miner Electrolyte Metab* 2:130–136, 1979.
22. Provoost AP, Molenaar JC: Renal function during and after a temporary complete unilateral ureter obstruction in rats. *Invest Urol* 18:242–246, 1981.
23. Siegel NJ, Feldman RA, Lytton B, et al: Renal cortical blood flow distribution in obstructive nephropathy in rats. *Circ Res* 40:379–384, 1977.
24. Buerkert J, Martin D: Relation of nephron recruitment to detectable filtration and recovery of function after release of ureteral obstruction. *Proc Soc Exp Biol Med* 173:533–540, 1983.
25. Ichikawa I, Purkerson ML, Yates J, et al: Dietary protein intake conditions the degree of renal vasoconstriction in acute renal failure caused by ureteral obstruction. *Am J Physiol* 249:F54–F61, 1985.
26. Purkerson ML, Blaine EH, Stokes TJ, et al: Role of atrial peptide in the natriuresis and diuresis that follows relief of obstruction in rats. *Am J Physiol* 256:F583–F589, 1989.
27. Purkerson ML, Klahr S: Prior inhibition of vasoconstrictors normalizes GFR in postobstructed kidneys. *Kidney Int* 35:1306–1314, 1989.
28. Vaughan ED Jr, Sweet RE, Gillenwater JY: Unilateral ureteral occlusion: Pattern of nephron repair and compensatory response. *J Urol* 109:979–982, 1973.
29. Wilson DR: Micropuncture study of chronic obstructive nephropathy before and after release of obstruction. *Kidney Int* 2:119–130, 1972.
30. Ichikawa I, Brenner BM: Local intrarenal vasoconstrictor-vasodilator interactions in mild partial ureteral obstruction. *Am J Physiol* 236:F131–F140, 1979.
31. Klahr S: New insights into the consequences and the mechanisms of renal impairment in obstructive nephropathy. *Am J Kidney Dis* 18:689–699, 1991.
32. Yarger WE, Schocken DD, Harris RH: Obstructive nephropathy in the rat: Possible roles for the renin-angiotensin system, prostaglandins, and thromboxanes in postobstructive renal function. *J Clin Invest* 65:400–412, 1980.
33. Nagle RB, Johnson ME, Jervis HR: Proliferation of renal interstitial cells following injury induced by ureteral obstruction. *Lab Invest* 35:18–22, 1976.
34. Schreiner GF, Harris KPG, Purkerson ML, et al: Immunological aspects of acute ureteral obstruction: Immune cell infiltrate in the kidney. *Kidney Int* 34:487–493, 1988.
35. Harris KPG, Schreiner GF, Klahr S: Effect of leukocyte depletion on the function of the postobstructed kidney in the rat. *Kidney Int* 36:210–215, 1989.
36. Yanagisawa H, Morrissey J, Morrison AR, et al: Role of ANG II in eicosanoid production by isolated glomeruli from rats with bilateral ureteral obstruction. *Am J Physiol* 258:F85–F93, 1990.
37. Rovin BH, Harris KPG, Morrison A, et al: Renal cortical release of a specific macrophage chemoattractant in response to ureteral obstruction. *Lab Invest* 63:213–220, 1990.
38. Diamond JR, Kees-Folts D, Ding G, et al: Macrophages, monocyte chemoattractant peptide-1 and transforming growth factor-β in experimental hydronephrosis. *Am J Physiol* 266:F926–F933, 1994.
39. Spaethe SM, Freed MS, DeSchryver-Kecskemeti K, et al: Essential fatty acid deficiency reduces the inflammatory cell invasion in rabbit hydronephrosis resulting in suppression of the exaggerated eicosanoid production. *J Pharmacol Exp Ther* 245:1088–1094, 1988.
40. Steinhardt GF, Ramon G, Salinas-Madrigal L: Glomerulosclerosis in obstructive uropathy. *J Urol* 140:1316–1318, 1988.
41. Shah SV: Role of reactive oxygen metabolites in experimental glomerular disease. *Kidney Int* 35:1093–1106, 1989.

42. Modi KS, Morrissey J, Shah SV, et al: Effects of probucol on renal function in rats with bilateral ureteral obstruction. *Kidney Int* 38:843–850, 1990.
43. Kerr WS Jr: Effects of complete ureteral obstruction in dogs on kidney function. *Am J Physiol* 184:521–526, 1956.
44. Bander SJ, Buerkert JE, Martin D, et al: Long-term effects of 24 hour unilateral ureteral obstruction on renal function in the rat. *Kidney Int* 28:614–620, 1985.
45. Buerkert J, Martin D, Head M, et al: Deep nephron function after release of acute unilateral ureteral obstruction in the young rat. *J Clin Invest* 62:1228–1239, 1978.
46. Peterson LJ, Yarger WE, Schocken DD, et al: Post-obstructive diuresis: A varied syndrome. *J Urol* 113:190–194, 1975.
47. Vaughan ED Jr, Gillenwater JY: Diagnosis, characterization and management of post-obstructive diuresis. *J Urol* 109:286–292, 1973.
48. Buerkert J, Head M, Klahr S: Effects of acute bilateral ureteral obstruction on deep nephron and terminal collecting duct function in the young rat. *J Clin Invest* 59:1055–1065, 1977.
49. Harris RH, Yarger WE: The pathogenesis of post-obstructive diuresis: The role of circulating natriuretic and diuretic factors, including urea. *J Clin Invest* 56:880–887, 1975.
50. Sonnenberg H, Wilson DR: The role of medullary collecting ducts in postobstructive diuresis. *J Clin Invest* 57:1564–1574, 1976.
51. Harris RH, Yarger WE: Renal function after release of unilateral ureteral obstruction in rats. *Am J Physiol* 227:806–815, 1974.
52. Buerkert J, Martin D, Head M: Effect of acute ureteral obstruction on terminal collecting duct function in the weanling rat. *Am J Physiol* 236:F260–F267, 1979.
53. Hanley MJ, Davidson K: Isolated nephron segments from rabbit models of obstructive nephropathy. *J Clin Invest* 69:165–174, 1982.
54. Berlyne GM: Distal tubular function in chronic hydronephrosis. *Q J Med* 30:339–355, 1961.
55. McDougal WS, Persky L: Renal functional abnormalities in post-unilateral ureteral obstruction in man: A comparison of these defects to post-obstructive diuresis. *J Urol* 113:601–604, 1975.
56. Knowlan D, Corrado M, Schreiner GE, et al: Periureteral fibrosis, with a diabetes insipidus-like syndrome occurring with progressive partial obstruction of a ureter unilaterally. *Am J Med* 28:22–31, 1960.
57. Roussak NJ, Oleesky S: Water-losing nephritis: A syndrome simulating diabetes insipidus. *Q J Med* 23:147–164, 1954.
58. Berlyne GM, Macken A: On the mechanism of renal inability to produce a concentrated urine in chronic hydronephrosis. *Clin Sci* 22:315–324, 1962.
59. Suki WN, Guthrie AG, Martinez-Maldonado M, et al: Effects of ureteral pressure elevation on renal hemodynamics and urine concentration. *Am J Physiol* 220:38–43, 1971.
60. Wilson DR, Knox WH, Sax JA, et al: Postobstructive nephropathy in the rat: Relationship between Na-K-ATPase activity and renal function. *Nephron* 22:55–62, 1978.
61. Stokes JB: Effect of prostaglandin E_2 on chloride transport across the rabbit thick ascending limb of Henle: Selective inhibition of the medullary portion. *J Clin Invest* 64:495–502, 1979.
62. Campbell HT, Bello-Reuss E, Klahr S: Hydraulic water permeability and transepithelial voltage in the isolated perfused rabbit cortical collecting tubule following acute unilateral ureteral obstruction. *J Clin Invest* 75:219–225, 1985.
63. Batlle DC, Arruda JAL, Kurtzman NA: Hyperkalemic distal renal tubular acidosis associated with obstructive uropathy. *N Engl J Med* 304:373–380, 1981.
64. Thirakomen K, Kozlov N, Arruda JAL, et al: Renal hydrogen ion secretion after release of unilateral ureteral obstruction. *Am J Physiol* 231:1233–1239, 1976.
65. Walls J, Buerkert JE, Purkerson ML, et al: Nature of the acidifying defect after the relief of ureteral obstruction. *Kidney Int* 7:304–316, 1975.
66. Better OS, Tuma S, Kedar S, et al: Enhanced tubular reabsorption of phosphate. *Arch Intern Med* 135:245–248, 1975.
67. Laski ME, Kurtzman NA: Site of the acidification defect in the perfused post-obstructed collecting tubule. *Miner Electrolyte Metab* 15:195–200, 1989.
68. Sabatini S, Kurtzman NA: Enzyme activity in obstructive uropathy: Basis for salt wastage and the acidification defect. *Kidney Int* 37:79–84, 1990.

69. Purcell H, Bastani B, Harris KPG, et al: Cellular distribution of H^+-ATPase following acute unilateral ureteral obstruction in the rat. *Am J Physiol* 261:F365–F376, 1991.

70. Kimura H, Mujais SK: Cortical collecting duct Na-K pump in obstructive nephropathy. *Am J Physiol* 258:F1320–F1327, 1990.

71. Better OS, Tuma S, Richter-Levin D, et al: Intrarenal resetting of glomerulotubular balance in a patient with post-obstructive uropathy. *Nephron* 9:131–145, 1973.

72. Better OS, Arieff AI, Massry SG, et al: Studies on renal function after relief of complete unilateral ureteral obstruction of three months' duration in man. *Am J Med* 54:234–240, 1973.

73. Purkerson ML, Slatopolsky E, Klahr S: Urinary excretion of magnesium, calcium and phosphate after release of unilateral ureteral obstruction in the rat. *Miner Electrolyte Metab* 6: 182–189, 1981.

74. Beck N: Phosphaturia after release of bilateral ureteral obstruction in rats. *Am J Physiol* 237: F14–F19, 1979.

75. Purkerson ML, Rolf DB, Chase LR, et al: Tubular reabsorption of phosphate after release of complete ureteral obstruction in the rat. *Kidney Int* 5:326–336, 1974.

76. Weinreb S, Hruska KA, Klahr S, et al: Uptake of Pi in brush border vesicles after release of unilateral ureteral obstruction. *Am J Physiol* 243:F29–F35, 1982.

77. Kurokawa K, Fine LG, Klahr S: Renal metabolism in obstructive nephropathy. *Semin Nephrol* 2:31–39, 1982.

78. Stokes TJ, Martin KJ, Klahr S: Impaired parathyroid hormone receptor–adenylate cyclase system in the postobstructed canine kidney. *Endocrinology* 116:1060–1065, 1985.

79. Cestonaro G, Emanuelli G, Calcamuggi G, et al: Renal lactate dehydrogenase (LDH) isoenzyme pattern in short-term experimental obstructive nephropathy. *Invest Urol* 17:46–49, 1979.

80. Brunskill N, Hayes C, Morrissey J, et al: Changes in lipid environment decrease Na,K-ATPase in obstructive nephropathy. *Kidney Int* 39:843–849, 1991.

81. Middleton GW, Beamon CR, Panko WB, et al: Effect of ureteral obstruction on the renal metabolism of α-ketoglutarate and other substrates in vivo. *Invest Urol* 14:255–262, 1977.

82. Stecker JF Jr, Vaughan ED Jr, Gillenwater JY: Alteration in renal metabolism occurring in ureteral obstruction in vivo. *Surg Gynecol Obstet* 133:846–848, 1971.

83. Blondin J, Purkerson ML, Rolf D, et al: Renal function and metabolism after relief of unilateral ureteral obstruction (38976). *Proc Soc Exp Biol Med* 150:71, 1975.

84. Nito H, Descoeudres C, Kurokawa K, et al: Effect of unilateral ureteral obstruction on renal cell metabolism and function. *J Lab Clin Med* 91:60–71, 1978.

85. Sawczuk IS, Hoke G, Olsson CA, et al: Gene expression in response to acute unilateral ureteral obstruction. *Kidney Int* 13:1315–1319, 1989.

86. Tannenbaum J, Purkerson ML, Klahr S: Effect of unilateral ureteral obstruction on metabolism of renal lipids in the rat. *Am J Physiol* 245:F254–F262, 1983.

87. Morrissey J, Windus D, Schwab S, et al: Ureteral occlusion decreases phospholipid and cholesterol of renal tubular membranes. *Am J Physiol* 250:F136–F143, 1986.

88. Sheehan HL, Davis JC: Experimental hydronephrosis. *Arch Pathol* 68:185–225, 1959.

89. Shimamura T, Kissane JM, Gyorkey F: Experimental hydronephrosis: Nephron dissection and electron microscopy of the kidney following obstruction of the ureter and in recovery from obstruction. *Lab Invest* 15:629–640, 1966.

90. Møller JC, Jørgensen TM, Mortensen J: Proximal tubular atrophy: Qualitative and quantitative structural changes in chronic obstructive nephropathy in the pig. *Cell Tissue Res* 244: 479–491, 1986.

91. Møller JC, Skriver E: Quantitative ultrastructure of human proximal tubules and cortical interstitium in chronic renal disease (hydronephrosis). *Virchows Arch [A]* 406:389–406, 1985.

92. Nagle RB, Bulger RE: Unilateral obstructive nephropathy in the rabbit: II. Late morphologic changes. *Lab Invest* 38:270–278, 1978.

93. Sharma AK, Mauer SM, Kim Y, Michael AF: Interstitial fibrosis in obstructive nephropathy. *Kidney Int* 44:774–788, 1993.

94. Nagle RB, Bulger RE, Cutler RE, et al: Unilateral obstructive nephropathy in the rabbit: I. Early morphologic, physiologic, and histochemical changes. *Lab Invest* 28:456–467, 1973.

95. Kaneto H, Morrissey J, McCracken R, et al: Enalapril reduces collagen type IV synthesis and expansion of the interstitium in the obstructed rat kidney. *Kidney Int* 45:1637–1647, 1994.

96. Kaneto H, Morrissey J, Klahr S: Increased expression of TGF-β1 mRNA in the obstructed kidney of rats with unilateral ureteral ligation. *Kidney Int* 44:313–321, 1993.
97. Kuncio GS, Neilson EG, Haverty T: Mechanisms of tubulointerstitial fibrosis. *Kidney Int* 39: 550–556, 1991.
98. Roberts AB, McCune BK, Sporn MB: TGF-β: Regulation of extracellular matrix. *Kidney Int* 41:557–559, 1992.
99. Santoro J, Kaye D: Recurrent urinary tract infections: Pathogenesis and management. *Med Clin North Am* 62:1005–1020, 1978.
100. Belman AB, Kropp KA, Simon NM: Renal-pressor hypertension secondary to unilateral hydronephrosis. *N Engl J Med* 278:1133–1136, 1968.
101. Nemoy NJ, Fichman MP, Sellers A: Unilateral ureteral obstruction: A cause of reversible high renin content hypertension. *JAMA* 225:512–513, 1973.
102. Palmer JM, Zweiman FG, Assaykeen TA: Renal hypertension due to hydronephrosis with normal plasma renin activity. *N Engl J Med* 283:1032–1033, 1970.
103. Squitieri AP, Ceccarelli FE, Wurster JC: Hypertension with elevated renal vein renins secondary to ureteropelvic junction obstruction. *J Urol* 111:284–287, 1974.
104. Weidmann P, Beretta-Piccoli C, Hirsch D, et al: Curable hypertension with unilateral hydronephrosis: Studies of the role of circulating renin. *Ann Intern Med* 87:437–440, 1977.
105. Kaloyanides GJ, Bastron RD, DiBona GF: Effect of ureteral clamping and increased renal arterial pressure on renin release. *Am J Physiol* 225:95–99, 1973.
106. Pelleya R, Oster JR, Perez GO: Hyporeninemic hypoaldosteronism, sodium wasting and mineralocorticoid-resistant hyperkalemia in two patients with obstructive uropathy. *Am J Nephrol* 3:223–227, 1983.
107. Crombleholme TM, Harrison MR, Longaker MT, et al: Prenatal diagnosis and management of bilateral hydronephrosis. *Pediatr Nephrol* 2:334–342, 1988.
108. Gray DL, Crane JP: Prenatal diagnosis of urinary tract malformation. *Pediatr Nephrol* 2: 326–333, 1988.
109. Taylor WC: Deformity of ears and kidneys. *Can Med Assoc J* 93:107–110, 1965.
110. Coleman BG: Ultrasonography of the upper urinary tract. *Urol Clin North Am* 12:633–644, 1985.
111. Parisky YR, Boswell WD, Raval J, et al: Diagnostic Use of Ultrasound for Kidney and Bladder. In Massry SG, Glassock RJ (eds): *Textbook of Nephrology* (3rd ed). Baltimore, Williams & Wilkins, 1995, pp 1818–1866.
112. Banner MP, Pollack HM: Evaluation of renal function by excretory urography. *J Urol* 124: 437–443, 1980.
113. Kaye AD, Pollack HM: Diagnostic imaging approach to the patient with obstructive uropathy. *Semin Nephrol* 2:55–73, 1982.
114. McGuire EJ: Retrograde Pyelography. In Rosenfield AT, Glickman MG, Hodson J (eds): *Diagnostic Imaging in Renal Disease*. New York, Appleton-Century-Crofts, 1979, pp 103–112.
115. Powers TA, Grove RB, Baureidel JK, et al: Detection of obstructive uropathy using ^{99m}technetium diethylenetriaminepentaacetic acid. *J Urol* 124:588–592, 1980.
116. Whitherow RO, Whitaker RH: The predictive accuracy of antegrade pressure flow studies in equivocal upper tract obstruction. *Br J Urol* 53:496–499, 1981.
117. Andersen JT, Jacobsen O, Stangaard L: The diagnostic value of intravenous pyelography in infravesical obstruction in males. *Scand J Urol Nephrol* 11:225–230, 1977.
118. Drach GW, Binard W: Disposable peak urinary flowmeter estimates lower urinary tract obstruction. *J Urol* 115:175–179, 1976.
119. Klahr S: Obstructive Uropathy. In Glassock RJ (ed): *Current Therapy in Nephrology and Hypertension* (3rd ed). St. Louis, Mosby-YearBook, 1992, pp 81–87.
120. Lemann J Jr, Worcester EM: Nephrolithiasis. In Massry SG, Glassock RJ (eds): *Textbook of Nephrology* (2nd ed). Baltimore, Williams & Wilkins, 1989, pp 920–941.
121. Drach GW, Dretler S, Fair W, et al: Report of the United States cooperative study of extracorporeal shock wave lithotripsy. *J Urol* 135:1127–1133, 1986.
122. Saxton HM: Percutaneous nephrostomy: Technique. *Urol Radiol* 1:131–139, 1981.

13

Renal Function in Pregnancy

Arlene B. Chapman, Verena A. Briner,
and Robert W. Schrier

Anatomic Alterations of the Kidney During Normal Pregnancy

Increased renal size and dilation of the urinary tract occurs in the first trimester of pregnancy and is maintained until term [1]. The increase in renal size is due to an increase in both vascular volume and interstitium [2]. Glomerular size increases during pregnancy without an increase in cell number [3]. Repeated radiographic measurements at term and then 6 months after delivery demonstrate a decrease in renal length by approximately 1 cm [4]. Ureteral dilation and physiologic hydronephrosis are the most dramatic changes that occur during pregnancy, which is usually asymptomatic. Ureteral dilation occurs as early as 8 weeks' gestation, with an abrupt onset often occurring at 20 weeks' gestation [1]. It occurs more often and more severely on the right as compared to the left side owing to an anatomic combination of dilated uterine veins with the enlarging uterus and the iliac artery compressing the right ureter. This results in a striking dilation of calices, renal pelvis, and ureter, which often results in the iliac sign (Fig. 13-1) on pyelography, where the right ureter is abruptly cut off at the pelvic brim where it crosses the iliac artery [5]. Obvious resolution of ureteric dilation occurs in 50 percent of women within 48 hours of delivery, with the remaining 50 percent requiring up to 12 weeks for normalization [6]. Given that ureteral dilation is seen early in pregnancy, other etiologies (most likely hormonal) are also responsible for the changes seen in the urinary tract during pregnancy [7]. Postmenopausal women treated with estrogen have some dilation of the urinary tract. Progesterone and estrogen decrease peristaltic activity and tone of the ureter, and hypertrophy of the ureteral smooth muscle is seen during gestation. The renal structural changes seen during pregnancy and their often slow resolution postpartum make it important to perform renal function studies during pregnancy with the patient well hydrated and in the recumbent position. As well, any interpretation of an excretory urogram, ultrasonogram, or renogram with respect to obstruction must be made with caution during this period.

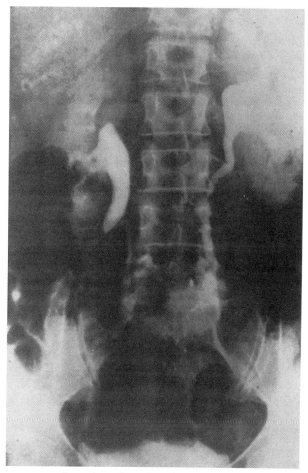

Fig. 13-1. Intravenous pyelograph performed in the second trimester in a woman with normal renal function demonstrating cutoff sign of the right ureter, representing physiologic hydronephrosis.

Systemic and Renal Hemodynamics During Normal Pregnancy

The initial hemodynamic change seen in pregnancy is a decrease in systemic vascular resistance leading to a decrease in mean arterial pressure [8] of approximately 6 mm Hg by the sixth week of gestation (Fig. 13-2) and reaching a 7 to 10 mm Hg decrement by the middle of the second trimester [9]. The decrease in peripheral vascular resistance is accompanied by a 10 to 20 percent increase in cardiac output by the fifth to sixth week of gestation [8–10], increasing as much as 30 to 40 percent throughout the total gestation. Plasma volume increases approximately 10 percent

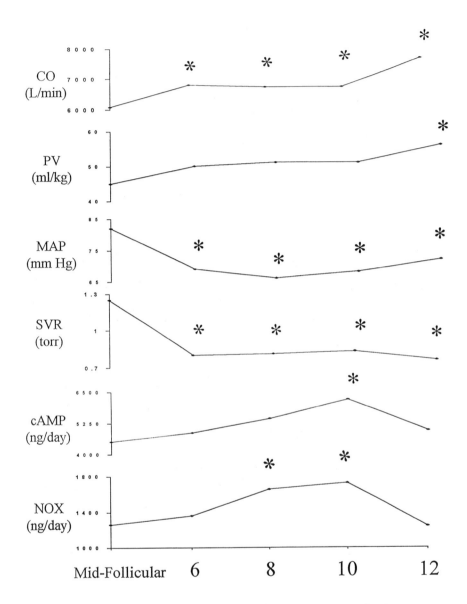

WEEKS GESTATION

Fig. 13-2. Hemodynamic profile for 10 pregnant women in early pregnancy. A significant rise in cardiac output (CO), and decrease in mean arterial pressure and peripheral vascular resistance occurs prior to 6 weeks of gestation. Plasma volume (PV) increases later by 12 weeks' gestation. These changes are accompanied by an increase in cAMP and NO_2/NO_3 excretions (NOX). (From ref. 8.)

by the twelfth week of gestation [8] and continues to maximally increase 40 percent by the middle of the third trimester [11]. The peripheral vasodilation found early in human gestation is also seen in the baboon species prior to volume expansion [12] and in pseudopregnant rats where vaginal stimulation results in alterations in maternal hormonal responses identical to normal pregnancy in the absence of a fetal-placental unit [13]. The etiology of the peripheral vasodilation and change in systemic hemodynamics found in normal human gestation is not completely understood but is important to review given its relevance to both the normal physiology of pregnancy and the pathogenesis of hypertensive disorders of pregnancy, which will be discussed later in this chapter.

Production of vasodilating prostaglandins such as PGE_2 and prostacyclin (PGI_2) and their second messenger cyclic adenosine monophosphate (AMP) is known to increase early in pregnancy [14, 15]. These compounds are produced in large amounts by the endothelium as well as the ovary, uterus, and placenta [16]. Urinary cAMP excretion has been found to increase significantly by the eight week of gestation, prior to placentation in human gestation [8]. The peripheral vasodilation found in normal pregnancy is accompanied by a blunted pressor response to infused angiotensin II [17], vasopressin [18], and norepinephrine [18] as early as the end of the first trimester [19]. While these blunted pressor responses can be reversed by administration of cyclooxygenase inhibitors and converting enzyme inhibitors [20–22], the reversal is not complete [23], suggesting that other potent vasodilators are involved in the peripheral vasodilation found in pregnancy. Moreover, platelet thromboxane A_2, a potent vasoconstrictor, increases markedly at the same time as PGI_2 increases, thus keeping vasoconstrictor and vasodilating prostanoids in relative balance [15].

Endothelium-derived relaxing factor (EDRF), or nitric oxide, is also released by the endothelium and has potent vasorelaxing effects, and the endothelial calcium-dependent nitric oxide synthase is stimulated by estrogen [24]. EDRF production is increased in animal pregnancy [25] and can abolish the pressor effects of angiotensin II, vasopressin, and norepinephrine [26]. Urinary and plasma levels of nitrate, the stable metabolite of nitric oxide (EDRF), as well as cyclic guanosine monophosphate (GMP), the second messenger for nitric oxide–induced dilation, are elevated in human gestation [27] as early as the sixth week of gestation prior to placentation [8]. Importantly, the perfused human placenta and ovary have been shown to generate and respond to nitric oxide [28]. Although these vasodilating compounds have been discussed in detail, others such as estrogen, human chorionic gonadotropin, prolactin, relaxin, and atrial natriuretic peptide (ANP) are presently under investigation with regard to their role in the peripheral vasodilation found in pregnancy.

Because of this vasodilation, blood pressure during normal gestation is less than in the general population, and an increase in blood pressure even to within normal limits should be considered abnormal. Absolute blood pressure levels within the nonpregnant normal range have been shown to correlate positively with pregnancy complications and neonatal mortality [29]. The major change in blood pressure during pregnancy is due to a decrease in diastolic blood pressure, resulting in a widened pulse pressure and decreased mean arterial pressure [30]. There is no universal agreement about the correct measurement of blood pressure during pregnancy.

Controversy remains whether Korotkoff phase 4 (muffling of sounds) or phase 5 (disappearance of sounds) is the preferable estimate of diastolic pressure during pregnancy [31]. In repeated studies, Korotkoff 4 overestimates intra-arterial diastolic measurements by 8 to 15 mm Hg [32], is more variable than Korotkoff 5 mesurements, and is usually 2 to 13 mm Hg greater than simultaneous Korotkoff 5 measurements [33]. However, due to the hyperkinetic circulation of pregnancy, a minority of women (<10%) will demonstrate wider discrepancies between Korotkoff 4 and 5 measurements, and Korotkoff 5 measurements may be 0 mm Hg or undetectable. Therefore, present recommendations are to use the Korotkoff 5 measurement during pregnancy, and when there is a large discrepancy between Korotkoff 4 and 5, both should be recorded.

As with renal hemodynamic measurements (see below), patient position at the time of blood pressure determination is extremely important, particularly as the uterus enlarges and the pregnancy progresses. For example, if a woman is kept in the left lateral recumbent position and her arm is kept at her right side, blood pressure recordings may be reduced by as much as 10 to 14 mm Hg. Regardless of the posture, care must be taken to keep the brachial artery at the level of the heart. Based on practical considerations, it is recommended that blood pressure be measured in the patient after being in a quiet sitting position for at least 10 minutes in the outpatient setting.

Renal hemodynamic changes are dramatic and also develop early in human pregnancy. Renal plasma flow increases 30 percent by the sixth week of gestation [8], reaching 150 to 180 percent of preconception values by the end of the second or early third trimester [34]. Recent studies show a decrease in renal plasma flow toward, but not to, pregestational values in the late third trimester, when the patient is in the correct (left lateral decubitus) position, with good hydration to correct for inaccuracies associated with poor bladder drainage and the increased dead space of the dilated collecting system [34]. Glomerular filtration rate (GFR), as measured by inulin clearance or endogenous creatinine clearance, also increases significantly and early in human gestation, although later than renal plasma flow with significant increases seen by the tenth week of gestation [8, 34, 35]. The GFR increases in parallel with changes in renal plasma flow, although to a lesser extent, thus resulting in a decrease in filtration fraction early in pregnancy (Fig. 13-3). Toward the end of pregnancy, GFR is maintained, resulting in a return of filtration fraction to a level found in the nonpregnant state [34]. The mechanism of the early rise in GFR and renal plasma flow and GFR in pregnancy is not fully understood. However, the increase in renal plasma flow during pregnancy occurs prior to maximal plasma volume expansion [11] and is greater than changes found secondary to experimental plasma volume expansion, high protein intake, or uninephrectomy. Importantly, a direct correlation between maximal increase in renal plasma flow and NO production has been found in rodent species during pregnancy [35a]. The increase in RPF is reversed when inhibitors of NO production are given [35a].

Women who have undergone renal transplantation or who have chronic renal disease with mild renal impairment will demonstrate the same hemodynamic changes during pregnancy as seen in healthy women but to a lesser extent [36]. A number of hemodynamically significant humoral factors have been suggested to

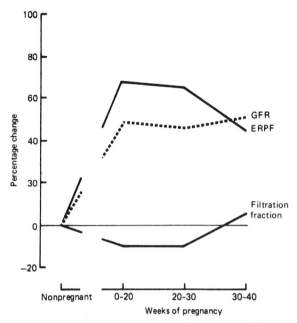

Fig. 13-3. Relative changes in renal hemodynamics during normal human pregnancy. ERPF = effective renal plasma flow; GFR = glomerular filtration rate. (Reprinted from *Kidney International* [Vol. 18:152–161, 1980], with permission.)

play a role in the augmentation of renal plasma flow and GFR including estrogen, cortisol, placental lactogen, chorionic gonadotropin, progesterone, and prostacyclins. The relative importance of each of these factors in the renal hemodynamic changes seen in pregnancy has yet to be determined. Although creatinine clearance increases by 50 percent by the end of the first trimester, there is little change in creatinine production, resulting in a fall in serum creatinine level from 0.67 ± 0.07 mg/dl preconception to 0.45 ± 0.06 mg/dl during gestation. At the same time, blood urea nitrogen (BUN) decreases from 13.0 ± 3.0 mg/dl to 8.7 ± 1.5 mg/dl. Therefore, one must consider that values considered normal in nonpregnant women may reflect decreased renal function during pregnancy. Roughly, serum creatinine concentration values of 0.80 mg/dl or BUN of 16.0 mg/dl or above require further assessment of renal function [37].

Tubular Function During Normal Pregnancy

Structural and functional tubular changes are found during pregnancy. Increased proximal tubular length and increased renal microsomal Na,K-ATPase activity have been documented. Coupled with these observations is the consistent documentation that proximal tubular function remains normal in the setting of increased GFR [38–40], indicating a compensatory increase in fractional reabsorption of most compounds. Functional changes in distal tubular sites have also been suggested, accounting in part for the presence of glucosuria [40] and the absence of kaliuresis in the presence of elevated levels of aldosterone [41].

Glucose

Glucosuria is one of the commonest abnormal urinary findings during normal pregnancy and may contribute to a propensity for urinary tract infections during this time. Importantly, isolated glucosuria does not indicate an increased risk for gestational diabetes mellitus. Urinary glucose excretion increases early in pregnancy. Ninety percent of pregnant women intermittently excrete more than 100 mg/day (upper limit of normal excretion) unrelated to blood glucose levels [42], and urinary glucose returns to normal within 1 week after delivery [43]. The rise in filtration of glucose during pregnancy is accompanied by an increase in tubular reabsorption and urinary excretion of glucose. The pathogenesis of glucosuria found in pregnancy remains controversial. The major factor thought to be involved in glucosuria is the increased filtered load due to the increase in GFR [40]. However, the highest levels of glucosuria have been shown to correlate with the lowest fractional reabsorption rates [42, 44], indicating a lower tubular maximum (T_m) glucose (normal 160–180 mg/dl) in those patients. However, 5 percent of the filtered glucose normally escapes proximal tubular reabsorption and is reabsorbed in the loop of Henle and collecting ducts. Functional changes in these more distal tubular sites thus have been suggested to contribute to the glucosuria of pregnancy [40].

Amino Acids

The urinary excretion of most amino acids is increased in pregnancy [45] with the exception of asparagine, methionine, ornithine, glutamic acid, and isoleucine. Those amino acids that normally have the lowest fractional reabsorption in the proximal tubule are excreted the most during pregnancy. Excretion of glycine, threonine, alanine, histidine, and serine is doubled by 16 weeks and increases four to five times above nonpregnant values at term. The remaining amino acids, lysine, phenylalanine, valine, cystine, tyrosine, and leucine, have a twofold increase in urinary excretion by 16 weeks, which then remains constant. Amino acid losses can be as great as 2 g/day, and with a normal diet this is not clinically relevant, but in situations of poor nutrition these losses can become significant.

Protein

Accurate determination of urinary protein excretion during pregnancy carries important prognostic significance, as will be seen later in the hypertensive disorders of pregnancy. Urinary protein excretion increases during pregnancy and should not be considered abnormal until it is greater than 300 mg/day [2]. The components of urinary protein during normal pregnancy are similar to the nonpregnant state. Normal urinary protein excretion is usually found as trace or 1 + on dipstick. Given that urine volume increases during pregnancy, dipstick analysis for estimates of urinary protein excretion is not accurate enough, and thus a 24-hour urine collection is required for accurate determination.

Uric Acid

In normal pregnancy, the serum uric acid is 25 percent lower than in nonpregnant women in the first two trimesters [46]. The hypouricemia reflects alterations in the fractional clearance of uric acid with a decrease in net tubular reabsorption [46]. The serum uric acid levels return to normal levels in the third trimester. An early increase in serum uric acid concentrations have been considered to be a marker of preeclampsia and intrauterine growth retardation [35, 46]. The significance of the hyperuricemia and alterations in renal clearance of uric acid that occur in patients with preeclampsia of pregnancy will be discussed later.

Water Metabolism and Osmoregulation During Pregnancy

The average weight gain during a normal pregnancy is 12 to 14 kg, of which 6 to 8 liters is accounted for by an increase in total body water. Four to six liters of this fluid is extracellular. Measurements of total body sodium and water have shown that the relative increase in total body water exceeds that of sodium [47–49]. Importantly, serum osmolality decreases approximately 10 mOsm/kg during pregnancy [50] beginning as early as 4 weeks after conception and plateauing by 10 to 12 weeks' gestation [51, 52]. Serum sodium concentration decreases approximately 3 to 5 mEq/L along with its associated anions, accounting for the majority of the change observed in serum osmolality. In fact, changes in serum urea concentration contribute relatively little to the change in serum osmolality seen [53]. Although changes in serum osmolality are complete before the end of the first trimester, most water retention occurs after the thirtieth week of gestation [54]. The decreased extracellular tonicity is maintained throughout pregnancy by decreasing the osmotic threshold for vasopressin release and for thirst [55, 56]. Both human and rat gestational studies have demonstrated that the threshold for vasopressin release is set at a lower level, while the sensitivity of the response is unaffected [55, 57]. The mechanism responsible for the change in extracellular tonicity that occurs during normal pregnancy is not completely understood. Women maintain a normal urinary concentrating ability and diluting capacity, when studied in the appropriate position, in the presence of lower serum tonicity [50, 53], and serum osmolality is maintained over a wide range of sodium intake [58]. The respiratory alkalosis found early in pregnancy may alter the threshold for vasopressin release in the setting of polydipsia often reported [59]. A number of isolated hormones such as human chorionic gonadotropin [50] and prolactin [60] have been shown to alter the osmotic threshold for vasopressin release, whereas progesterone and estrogen [53] administration has not. Also, alterations in intracellular tonicity have been suggested in normal gestation, as increases in erythrocyte sodium-lithium countertransport have been reported

[61]. In addition to these factors, vasodilation, which decreases effective arterial blood volume, may increase vasopressin release in a nonosmotic fashion and account for the "resetting" of the osmotic threshold in pregnancy [62].

In contrast to early pregnancy, diabetes insipidus occurring late in the third trimester or in the peripartum period has been reported [63]. Vasopressinase is produced in increasing quantities by the placenta as pregnancy progresses and inactivates both vasopressin and oxytocin [64]. This may lead to the clinical manifestations of vasopressin-resistant diabetes insipidus; a response to desmopressin acetate (DDAVP), however, should occur in these patients, since vasopressinase does not destroy this antidiuretic agent.

Sodium Metabolism During Normal Pregnancy

One of the most dramatic physiologic changes in pregnancy is the kidneys' ability to respond to an increased filtered load of 5000 to 10,000 mEq of sodium per day, maintaining glomerulotubular balance and providing a positive sodium balance of approximately 950 mEq during gestation [65]. Most of the sodium is present in the extracellular fluid (ECF) volume of the mother and the amniotic fluid. As previously discussed, plasma volume increases approximately 40 percent during normal gestation [11], with half of the increase occurring in the first trimester. Therefore, during a phase of increasing GFR, renal plasma flow, and hormones that are natriuretic in nature (Table 13-1), the pregnant woman is in positive sodium balance. There is thus also a resetting of volume homeostatic mechanisms so that sodium excretion is regulated, "reset," and at an increased ECF volume [66]. This appears to be similar to the phenomenon of mineralocorticoid escape where ECF volume is increased and sodium balance is reestablished at a new steady state. Usually mineralocorticoid escape occurs when positive sodium balance exceeds 400 mEq, which is less than the increase found in normal pregnancy. Importantly, Erhlich [41] demonstrated in an additive manner that pregnant women are extremely sensitive to exogenous mineralocorticoid administration and demonstrated sodium retention, weight gain, and subsequent mineralocorticoid escape when given deoxycorticosterone acetate (DOCA). Conceptually it would seem appropriate to consider that a decrease in effective arterial blood volume is present in spite of an expanded ECF volume, primarily related to the peripheral arterial vasodilation and decrease in systemic vascular resistance seen early in pregnancy. This may be the strongest stimulus for sodium retention in the presence of natriuretic forces.

As with mineralocorticoid administration, the renin-angiotensin-aldosterone system (RAAS) responds appropriately to alterations in sodium intake, aldosterone inhibition, and alterations in posture, although during sodium loading plasma renin activity (PRA) does not decrease to nonpregnant levels. With exogenous angiotensin II administration, urinary sodium excretion and fractional excretion of sodium decreases, although not as much as in the nonpregnant population [67, 68]. Plasma

Table 13-1. Factors that influence renal sodium handling
in pregnancy

Increased sodium excretion
    50% increase in glomerular filtration
    Hormonal factors
        Increased progesterone production
        Prostaglandins, vasopressin, melanocyte-stimulating hormone
        Digoxin-like factors, dopamine
    Physical factors
        Decreased plasma albumin concentration
        Decreased renal vascular resistance
        Decreased postglomerular oncotic pressure
        Decreased filtration fraction
Decreased sodium excretion
    Hormonal factors
        Increased aldosterone secretion
        Increased deoxycorticosterone
        Increased estrogen secretion
        Increased plasma cortisol levels
    Physical factors
        Placental shunts
        Increased uterine pressure
        Exaggerated response to change in posture

Source: Modified from M. D. Lindheimer and A. I. Katz, *Kidney Function and Disease in Pregnancy*. Philadelphia: Lea & Febiger, 1977.

levels of other hormones such as estrogen and nonprotein-bound cortisol are also elevated in pregnancy. Although these hormones have sodium-retaining properties, their relative roles in determining sodium balance during gestation are not fully understood.

Progesterone, which increases in concert with PRA in the first trimester of pregnancy, has been shown to be natriuretic by inhibiting proximal tubular reabsorption of sodium [69] and competitively inhibiting the salt-retaining effects of aldosterone in the distal nephron [70]. ANP has been demonstrated to be increased or unchanged in pregnancy. However, in well-controlled studies of healthy pregnant women, ANP levels initially decrease, most likely in response to decreased venous return secondary to the vasodilatory properties of the hormone [8, 71].

Considerable controversy has occurred regarding optimal sodium intake and use of diuretics in normal pregnancy. On one hand, although between 30 and 90 percent of women will develop edema during some phase of their pregnancy, the positive sodium balance seen during this time appears to be appropriate given the degree of peripheral arterial vasodilation and reduction in systemic vascular resistance. Thus, sodium restriction or diuretic use appears to be contraindicated. However, in those pregnant women with large increases in intravascular volume such as those with chronic renal failure and cardiovascular disease, both sodium restriction and diuretic use should be considered.

The Renin Angiotensin Aldosterone System During Pregnancy

The basic physiology of the RAAS has been discussed in Chapter 8 and will not be repeated here. Given the importance of the role of RAAS in sodium balance as well as in the control of blood pressure, vascular reactivity, and in extrarenal tissues of reproductive origin, this hormonal system has been extensively studied in normal and hypertensive pregnancy.

Prorenin, which acts in the kidney as a biosynthetic precursor to active renin, is one of the first components of the RAAS to change during pregnancy. Prorenin increases in parallel with human chorionic gonadotropin by the fourth week of gestation (Fig. 13-4A). It reaches a peak by week 5 and plateaus at that level until delivery [72]. The 10-fold rise in prorenin that occurs early in pregnancy does not occur in women with ovarian failure, suggesting an ovarian source for prorenin [73].

In the second and third trimesters, prorenin is secreted by uterine and placental tissues [74] and most likely acts locally, as very high levels are found in the chorion laeve and amniotic fluid [75]. Whether prorenin has a role in the control of uteroplacental blood flow, the cardiovascular changes found in gestation, and the early peripheral vasodilation that occurs in pregnancy prior to placentation awaits further study. Angiotensinogen or renin substrate increases gradually during pregnancy, reaching levels five times greater than in the nonpregnant state in the third trimester and corresponding to increases in estrogen levels [76]. A similar rise in renin substrate occurs in nonpregnant women taking estrogen-containing compounds. Increases in renin substrate, however, do not account entirely for the elevation in PRA found during pregnancy [77], and 20 percent of renin found in the peripheral

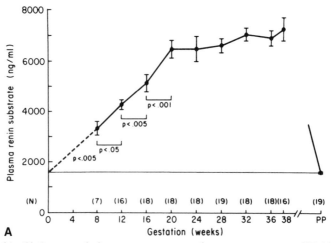

Fig. 13-4. (A–C) Sequential changes in prorenin, plasma renin activity (PRA), and plasma and urinary aldosterone during pregnancy all related to urinary sodium excretion. Dashed line in B represents values normalized to the postpartum substrate levels.

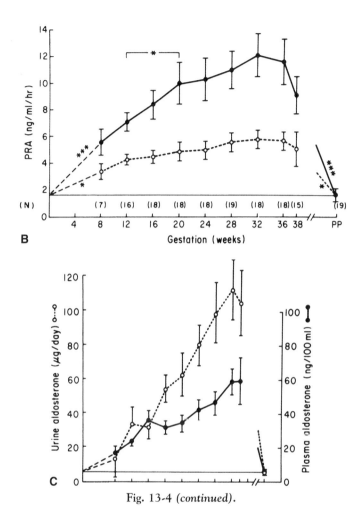

Fig. 13-4 *(continued)*.

circulation originates from the placenta [78]. PRA increases significantly by the sixth week of pregnancy [8], rising to levels four times greater than in the nonpregnant state by the end of the first trimester (Fig. 13-4B). Care and attention must be given to handling samples for PRA in pregnant women, as in vitro cryoactivation of plasma prorenin to renin will occur if samples are not collected at room temperature or immediately frozen [79]. The increases in PRA during late pregnancy follow different patterns in different individuals, increasing less so in older women [80]. PRA increases with sodium restriction and is suppressed by high salt intake, although not to nonpregnant levels [66]. Renin also arises from extrarenal sites including the placenta and uterus, and this source of renin may play a hemodynamic role during pregnancy in some species by controlling uteroplacental blood flow [81, 82]. The role of extrarenal renin in the control of cardiovascular events that occur in human pregnancy is however unclear at this time. Angiotensin II, although technically difficult to measure, has been shown to be elevated in normal pregnancy [83]. Aldosterone increases during pregnancy with significant rises present before the sixth week of gestation [8, 12, 84], continuing throughout pregnancy to levels 10-fold greater than in nonpregnant women in the third trimester [84] (Fig. 13-4C). Changes in urinary aldosterone excretion mirror changes in serum aldosterone levels during pregnancy, and both respond to alterations in PRA [80], as well as sodium balance [84].

The significance of the RAAS in normal pregnancy can be demonstrated when evaluating sodium balance, blood pressure regulation, vascular reactivity, and control of uteroplacental blood flow. Human and primate gestation is marked by primary peripheral vasodilation that occurs extremely early prior to gestation. Both PRA and aldosterone levels have been demonstrated to rise prior to volume expansion in the baboon [12] and out of proportion to volume expansion in humans [8]. This suggests that activation of the RAAS early in pregnancy is due to peripheral arterial vasodilation with a consequent decrease in renal perfusion pressure. In support of this is the marked decrease in blood pressure following administration of converting enzyme inhibitors in experimental animals during pregnancy as well as in humans [20, 21, 85], indicating angiotensin II dependence of blood pressure during pregnancy.

Angiotensin II infusion also demonstrates a decreased pressor response during normal pregnancy as early as the end of the first trimester [17, 67]. The pressor response to the administration of exogenous angiotensin is inversely related to the endogenous levels of the hormone, most likely due to greater occupancy of vascular angiotensin II receptors or a decrease in receptor number or affinity [86]. Importantly, when animals are given converting enzyme inhibitors, a blunted pressor response to angiotensin II still exists [18], indicating that variables other than receptor occupancy affect vascular reactivity to angiotensin II. The possibility that prostaglandins mediate the blunted responsiveness to angiotensin II is supported by the observation that administration of indomethacin or aspirin in doses large enough to block production of prostacyclin significantly increases angiotensin II responsiveness in pregnant women [17]. When low-dose aspirin is given, however, a circumstance in which thromboxane A_2 is selectively inhibited, vascular responsiveness to angiotensin II continues to be blunted [87]. Other vasodilators thought to play a role in the decreased pressor response to angiotensin II include estradiol-17β, prolactin, and nitric oxide [18, 88, 89]. Further studies delineating their relative roles have yet to be undertaken.

In addition to maintaining normal blood pressure and regulating sodium balance as discussed previously, there is evidence that the RAAS plays an important vasodilating role in modulating uteroplacental blood flow. Angiotensin II has demonstrated a paradoxical vasodilation in the uterine circulation of rabbits, dogs, and ewes [76, 90, 91], and converting enzyme inhibitors have been associated with a high incidence of stillbirths in pregnant rabbits [92]. Given that angiotensin II stimulates arachidonic acid release from phospholipids of cell membranes and promotes prostaglandin synthesis and that angiotensin II infusions have been shown to increase concentrations of PGE_2 in uterine veins of pregnant monkeys, it is likely that the vasodilating effects of angiotensin II are mediated by prostaglandins [93].

Importantly, a local RAAS exists in the uteroplacental-fetal unit, where angiotensin-converting enzyme and angiotensin II receptors are present and the placenta has the functional capacity to convert angiotensin I to angiotensin II [94, 95]. In summary, the RAAS is activated and plays a physiologic role in pregnancy with regard to blood pressure regulation, vascular reactivity, sodium balance, and control of the uteroplacental blood flow.

Hypertensive Disorders of Pregnancy

Hypertensive disorders in pregnancy remain common, occurring in up to 10 percent of all pregnancies, with about half due to preeclampsia and the remaining majority due to transient hypertension and chronic essential hypertension. The incidence of eclampsia is approximately 4.9 in 10,000 in Great Britain [96]. Hypertension alone and particularly preeclampsia are associated with increased fetal mortality, maternal morbidity and mortality, and small for gestational age infants. Recently, it has been suggested that the deprived intrauterine environment created by these conditions that leads to small for gestational age infants may later impact on the prevalence of essential hypertension in adulthood in the involved individuals [97]. Therefore, it is important to carry clear diagnostic criteria for the diagnosis of hypertensive disorders during pregnancy, to understand the pathophysiology associated with each disorder, and to apply this knowledge to the correct preventive and interventional therapy for each disorder.

Much confusion has arisen concerning the correct classification of hypertensive disorders of pregnancy for two reasons. Multiple nomenclatures used in the past encumbered more than one hypertensive disorder and included pregnancy-induced hypertension, pregnancy-associated hypertension, toxemia, and gestosis. As well, there is difficulty in accurately diagnosing preeclampsia versus chronic hypertension versus preexisting renal disease based on clinical grounds alone [98, 99]. The simplest, most concise, and practical classification system originated in 1972 by the Committee on Terminology of the American College of Obstetricians and Gynecologists [100] has recently been endorsed by the U.S. National High Blood Pressure Education Program Working Group [101] and separates hypertensive disorders of pregnancy into the following four categories:

1. Preeclampsia-eclampsia
2. Chronic hypertension of whatever cause
3. Chronic hypertension with superimposed preeclampsia-eclampsia
4. Transient or late hypertension

Preeclampsia-Eclampsia

Preeclampsia is a systemic disorder specific to human pregnancy that can be explosive and progressive, as the derivation from the Greek word *eclampsus* (lightning) intimates. Eclampsia is the development of generalized seizures in a patient with preeclampsia and is undoubtedly the most dramatic complication of the disease.

Preeclampsia becomes apparent in the latter half of pregnancy, usually after the twentieth week of gestation, and is clinically manifested by the presence of hypertension, proteinuria, and edema. As many as 75 percent of cases are documented after the thirty-seventh week, and the clinical signs may arise during labor (antepartum) or between 48 hours and 10 days after delivery (postpartum). Hypertension is defined as blood pressure greater than 140/90 mm Hg or an increase in diastolic and systolic level by 15 and 30 mm Hg, respectively [101]. Blood pressure typically is labile, and the usual circadian rhythm is lost [102]. The decrease of change in blood pressure to make the diagnosis of hypertension during pregnancy is necessary given the hemodynamic changes found in normal pregnancy (see Systemic and Renal Hemodynamics During Normal Pregnancy, pp. 591–595). For example, the rise in diastolic blood pressure of approximately 10 mm Hg during the third trimester in normal gestation [84] could lead to the overdiagnosis of hypertension in pregnancy. However, given that preeclampsia is the disorder most often associated with severe maternal and fetal complications, overdiagnosis is preferred to underdiagnosis. Proteinuria needs to be in excess of 300 mg/day, and although diffuse edema can be found in 30 percent and lower-extremity edema in 90 percent of normal pregnancies [103], it is still included in the clinical trial required for the usual diagnosis of preeclampsia [101].

Proteinuria is extremely variable, but nephrotic range proteinuria is not uncommon. In fact, preeclampsia is the most common cause of the nephrotic syndrome during pregnancy [98]. The degree of proteinuria correlates with the severity of the renal histologic lesion in nephrotic patients as well as perinatal mortality and blood pressure level [98, 104]. Classification of preeclampsia based on these criteria alone, particularly high blood pressure, may overemphasize the importance of hypertension. Up to 20 percent of patients with eclampsia have blood pressures below 140/90 mm Hg [96, 105], and up to 40 percent may have little or no edema [106]. Given the systemic nature of preeclampsia, variations in presentation occur, often including coagulation or liver function abnormalities even in the absence of hypertension [107].

Preeclampsia typically presents in the primigravida at the extremes of age and occurs in higher frequency in multigravidas with multiple gestations, a family history of preeclampsia, molar pregnancy, preexisting hypertension or renal disease, or diabetes mellitus. Preeclampsia that occurs prior to 20 weeks' gestation is usually more severe in nature and most commonly occurs in those with underlying renal disorders or hypertension. Antepartum or postpartum eclampsia also appears to have a more fulminant course. Signs and symptoms of the disorder are multiple and can vary in severity from mild blood pressure elevations and subtle laboratory abnormalities to a full-blown explosive disease of severe hypertension, acute renal failure, seizures, liver failure, and disseminated intravascular coagulation. Table 13-2 provides the premonitory signs and symptoms typically associated with severe preeclampsia. It is important to note that there is a deceptive variant of preeclampsia characterized by minimal elevation in blood pressure, modest declines in platelet count, mild liver abnormalities, and little or no renal dysfunction. This benign situation can rapidly progress to a life-threatening syndrome designated the HELLP (hemolysis, elevated liver enzymes, low platelet counts) syndrome, the manifestations of which

Table 13-2. Clinical and laboratory features of severe preeclampsia

Blood pressure greater than 160 mm Hg systolic or greater than 110 mm Hg diastolic or an increase of greater than 60 mm Hg systolic or greater than 30 mm Hg diastolic over baseline levels

Proteinuria of greater than 5 g/24 hr or 3–4+ by dipstick

Oliguria (less than 400 ml/24 hr)

Cerebral or visual disturbances; i.e., lethargy, headache, scotomata, blurred vision

Extreme hyperreflexia or clonus

Epigastric or right upper quadrant pain

Abnormal liver function tests

Hemoconcentration

Pulmonary edema

Thrombocytopenia

Microangiopathic hemolysis; disseminated intravascular coagulation (DIC)

Source: L. E. Feinberg, Hypertension and Preeclampsia. In R. S. Abrams and P. Wexler (eds.), *Medical Care of the Pregnant Patient*. Boston: Little, Brown, 1983. P. 163.

include hemolysis and rapid deterioration of coagulation and liver parameters, requiring prompt termination of the pregnancy [108].

Systemic and Renal Hemodynamic Changes in Preeclampsia

Measurements of cardiac output in women with preeclampsia have given conflicting results. The majority of studies are methodologically flawed, not controlled for intervention with either magnesium sulfate or antihypertensive medications with afterload-reducing potential prior to measurement of cardiac output, and include patients with a questionable diagnosis of preeclampsia [109–111]. Visser and Wallenburg [112] carefully studied nulliparous gravidas who developed third trimester hypertension and proteinuria prior to any therapeutic intervention. Cardiac output was decreased, the hypertension was maintained by increased peripheral vascular resistance, and pulmonary capillary wedge pressure (PCWP) was low or normal. These changes have since been confirmed using noninvasive echocardiography and in women with eclampsia, presumably a more severe form of disease [113, 114].

Plasma volume has consistently been shown to be decreased in preeclamptic women, measured primarily with Evans blue dye techniques [115, 116], presumably due to the primary vasoconstriction resulting in a smaller intravascular compartment. The decrease in intravascular volume, whether primary or secondary, is often associated with hypoalbuminemia and hemoconcentration with evidence of increased capillary permeability [117]. The decrease in the vasoconstricted intravascular compartment suggests that although PCWP, cardiac output, and plasma volume may be decreased in preeclamptic patients, fluid or colloid replacement may be dangerous. Both GFR and renal plasma flow decrease in preeclampsia, with GFR decreasing more so that filtration fraction decreases. The decrease in GFR is of the order of magnitude of 25 to 35 percent, bringing GFR into the "normal" nonpregnant range [118]. Rarely, marked renal insufficiency can be present in the form of acute tubular necrosis or bilateral cortical necrosis and is usually in the setting of disseminated intravascular coagulation or abruptio placentae [119]. Urate excretion is decreased, and the level of hyperuricemia has been shown to correlate better with birth weight and neonatal outcome than blood pressure level in preeclampsia [120]. Urinary sodium excretion following an acute sodium challenge is impaired in preeclampsia as compared to normotensive pregnancy [116], and decreased fractional excretion of calcium, leading to striking hypocalciuria, also occurs [121]. The mechanisms responsible for these abnormalities have yet to be elucidated. Although the RAAS is stimulated in normal pregnancy, PRA, plasma aldosterone concentration, and angiotensin II levels are relatively decreased in women with preeclampsia and in those with essential hypertension who go on to develop preeclampsia [122] as compared to normal pregnant women. This is coupled with a loss of refractoriness to the pressor effects of angiotensin II, which can become even more marked than in the nongravid state. In a classic prospective serial study, Magness et al. [123] demonstrated that the marked pressor resistance to angiotensin II that occurs early in gestation would be lost in those women destined to develop preeclampsia and could be seen as early as the twenty-third week of gestation (Fig. 13-5). As well, increased response to angiotensin II has been described in both resistance and

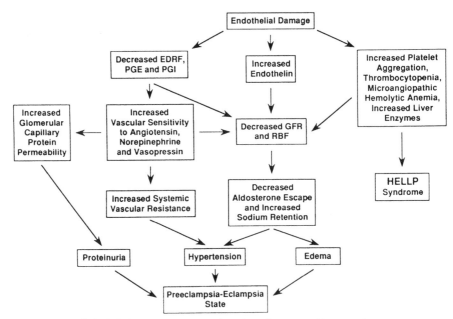

Fig. 13-5. Endothelial damage attenuates the physiologic vasodilation of pregnancy, leading to pathophysiologic events that characterize preeclampsia-eclampsia. EDRF = endothelium-derived relaxing factor; PGE = prostaglandin E; PGI = prostaglandin I; GFR = glomerular filtration rate; RBF = renal blood flow. (From R. W. Schrier and V. A. Briner, Peripheral arterial vasodilatation hypothesis of sodium and water retention in pregnancy: Implications of pathogenesis of preeclampsia-eclampsia [editorial]. *Obstet. Gynecol.* 77:632, 1991.)

conduit-sized vessels obtained from preeclamptic women at cesarean sections and studied in vitro [124, 125]. Although plasma norepinephrine levels are unchanged in preeclampsia and cardiovascular and sympathetic response to cold pressor and isometric hand grip tests are unaltered in preeclampsia, pressor sensitivity to norepinephrine increases, and preeclamptic women demonstrate exaggerated decrements in blood pressure in response to head-up tilt tests [126]. Therefore, increased systemic vascular resistance, rising blood pressure, and loss of vascular refractoriness to pressor agents usually found in normal pregnancy are the hallmarks of preeclampsia.

Pathogenesis of Preeclampsia

Although toxemia has been considered a misnomer for the condition of preeclampsia, recent evidence suggests that a circulating cytotoxin arising from the placenta, particularly toxic to the endothelial cell, may be responsible for the preeclamptic state [126]. As well, antivascular endothelial cell antibodies [127] have been identified in plasma from pregnant women with preeclampsia but not in plasma from normal pregnant women. Plasma from eclamptic patients infused into nonpregnant women has also been shown to cause vasoconstriction [128]. Placental hypoperfusion appears to be the main culprit responsible for the release of cytotoxic material from the placenta. It is possible that lipid peroxides, which are known to be produced in excess in response to ischemia or hypoxic stress, may mediate endothelial damage [129]. Figure 13-5 shows our hypothesis in which endothelial damage may initiate many of the known characteristics of the preeclampsia-eclampsia state.

There is substantial evidence showing that alterations in prostaglandin metabolism occur in preeclampsia. Thorough and careful work has demonstrated that PG_{12} production from the placenta and uterus (measured as 2,3-dinor-6-keto-$PGF_{1\alpha}$) is diminished as early as the first trimester in women destined to become preeclamptic [14] (Fig. 13-6), whereas thromboxane A_2 production is unchanged. The important balance between PG_{12} and thromboxane A_2 production may therefore be lost so that a relative excess of thromboxane A_2 with platelet activation in the placenta occurs, leading to vasoconstriction and platelet aggregation in microcirculation of multiple organ systems. Given that the placenta has a local RAAS that is vasodilatory in the presence of PG_{12}, it is not surprising that diminished PG_{12} production is associated with increased placental vascular resistance in the presence of RAAS, resulting in decreased placental flow [130]. Models of decreased placental perfusion in animals have been the closest at providing clinical features of preeclampsia that is specific to humans [131]. Although decreased placental PG_{12} production was thought to be specific to preeclampsia, it is also found in pregnancies complicated by intrauterine growth retardation or placental insufficiency [132]. Placentas from women with preeclampsia demonstrate failure of the spiral arteries to transform from their usual thick-walled, muscular character to saclike, flaccid vessels to provide greater volumes of blood to the uteroplacental unit. This is usually accomplished by invasion of the spiral artery wall by the endovascular trophoblast and is normally complete by the twentieth week of gestation. This fails to occur in women with preeclampsia [133]. Why this abnormal placental vascularization occurs in preeclampsia is still under investigation, but it is suggested that early in pregnancy,

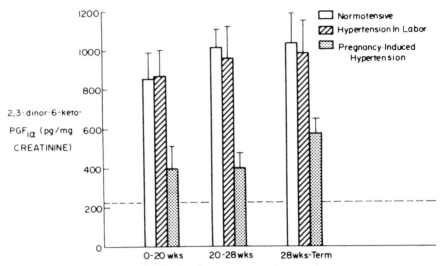

Fig. 13-6. 2-3-Dinor-6-keto-$PGF_{1\alpha}$ levels in women with normal pregnancies, pregnancy-induced hypertension, and patients exhibiting increased blood pressure during labor. The hatched bar represents the upper limits of normal in nonpregnant subjects. (From P. August, M. Lindheimer, Pathophysiology of preeclampsia. In J. H. Laragh and B. M. Brenner [eds], *Hypertension: Pathophysiology, Diagnosis and Management* [Vol. 2]. New York: Raven, 1995. P. 2410.)

cytotrophoblastic cells fail to express adhesion molecules important in the process of vascular invasion and transformation of the spiral arteries [134].

If proper vascularization of the fetal-placental unit cannot occur, it is not surprising that the uterine vessels, normally producing 100-fold greater amounts of PG_{12} than maternal vessels, will produce less of this compound [135]. Other compounds with vasodilatory capacity that are normally produced by the placenta are also shown to be decreased in preeclamptic women. Prospective studies of women with essential hypertension suggest that women with lower estradiol levels are more apt to develop preeclampsia [122]. Although early studies of chronic blockade of nitric oxide did not give rise to blood pressure in pregnant rodents [136], studies since that time using inhibitors of nitric oxide have demonstrated a syndrome with features resembling preeclampsia [136a]. Further support for a decrease in EDRF activity in preeclampsia has been obtained from human studies where EDRF production is impaired in umbilical vessels and subcutaneous fat pads [137, 138] and lower plasma nitrite levels have been reported in preeclamptic as compared to normal women [139].

Alternatively, compounds with vasoconstrictor potential that are produced in the endothelium and the placenta, such as endothelin [140], have been shown to be increased in preeclamptic patients [141]. In a longitudinal study of preeclamptic patients, an increase of a digoxin-like factor that inhibits the NA,K-ATPase as compared to normal pregnancy has been reported [142]. This factor may contribute to the increased vascular sensitivity to vasoconstrictors by increasing intracellular sodium and calcium concentrations [143]. Consistent with this observation are the findings of elevated intracellular calcium levels in platelets from preeclamptic women [144, 145].

Pathologic Consequences of Preeclampsia

Placenta. Consistent with a state of placental hypoperfusion in preeclampsia, there is a greater degree of placental infarction in preeclampsia as compared to uncomplicated pregnancies and evidence of acute atherosis where accumulation of fat-laden macrophages and perinuclear cell infiltrates occur. This is primarily due to focal disruption of the endothelium of the spiral arteries, allowing the infiltration of plasma components into the damaged arterial wall, leading to vasospasm and fibrinoid necrosis. Clearly, cytotoxic components can then be released into the maternal circulation, leading to increased vascular reactivity and diffuse platelet aggregation.

Renal. In 1959, Spargo and colleagues [146, 147] first described in kidneys from preeclamptic women a narrowing of glomerular capillary lumen, which was caused by swelling of endothelial cells (so-called glomerular endotheliosis). The glomerulus is significantly enlarged in this condition without hypercellularity, and the basement membrane and epithelial cells are normal by light microscopy (Fig. 13-7). This endothelial cell swelling has also been found in electron microscopic studies and is accompanied by vacuolization [148]. Of interest, the foot processes are usually well preserved, even when severe proteinuria is present. The occasional existence of electron-dense deposits in the endothelial cells and basement membrane of glomerular capillaries has been described [148]. Immunofluorescence studies revealed that these depositions more likely are fibrin and fibrinogen derivatives than immunoglobulins [149]. In general, however, fibrin deposits and IgG and IgM deposits are rare in biopsy specimens from patients with pathologic changes of preeclampsia. It is therefore possible that immune deposits simply represent nonspecific trapping of plasma proteins in narrowed capillary lumina. Whether glomerular endotheliosis is specific or pathognomonic for preeclampsia is a subject of considerable controversy [150]. The renal histologic changes, however, are clearly different from those that are encountered in essential hypertension, and they appear to regress rapidly after delivery. Pathologic changes in preeclampsia are found in the liver, brain, lungs, and heart, given that it is a systemic disorder [151].

Long-Term Sequelae of Preeclampsia

The difficulty of performing prospective studies in which preeclampsia is histologically and clinically differentiated from other hypertensive and renal disorders has been responsible in part for the conflicting reports about the late sequelae of preeclampsia. Some studies suggest that in previously normal women, renal functional recovery is complete after an episode of preeclampsia. On the other hand, a considerable percentage of patients with previous chronic hypertension and preeclampsia have persistent abnormalities on renal biopsy, and persistent hypertension develops in almost 20 percent of preeclamptic patients [119]. The results of the remarkable studies conducted by Chesley and his collaborators [152] in which as many as 267

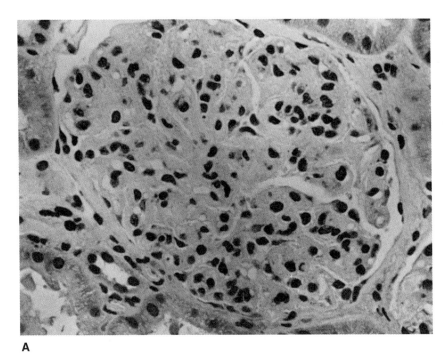

A

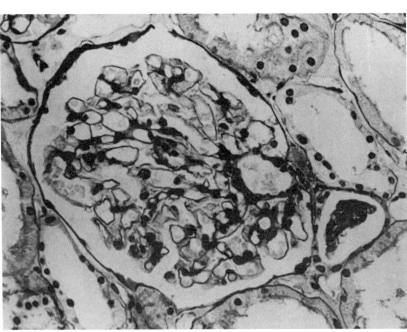

B

women who survived eclampsia were followed for up to 40 years demonstrated that distribution of systolic and diastolic blood pressure in women who had eclampsia in their first pregnancy was not different from that of a comparable matched population. Fischer and colleagues [98], who confirmed the diagnosis of preeclampsia by renal biopsy, showed similar findings. The prevalence of hypertension at follow-up was 10 percent, the expected rate for age-matched women. This does not, however, change the increased risk of preeclampsia (approximately 20%) in subsequent pregnancies [153]. The data obtained by Chesley and associates [152] were primarily applicable to a white population, since the number of blacks in the study was small. In a study of 53 black women with documented preeclampsia followed for a mean of 68 months, the prevalence of hypertension was similar to that of a matched population. However, the incidence of hypertension in the matched population that was normotensive during gestation was severalfold below the expected prevalence in the age- and race-matched population [98].

Prevention and Treatment of Preeclampsia

Preeclampsia is a disease of placental insufficiency, and the curative procedure for the treatment of this disorder is delivery of the fetus. Given that such a decision is not always in favor of the fetus, particularly prior to 36 weeks' gestation, other preventative or therapeutic maneuvers have been considered. In considering any therapy aimed at prevention of or treatment of preeclampsia, three factors need to be kept in mind:

1. The need to obtain or maintain optimal blood flow through the fetal-placental unit.
2. Preeclampsia is a state of high peripheral vascular resistance with low cardiac output and plasma volume.
3. Endothelial damage is present and leads to increases in interstitial fluid with low or normal filling pressures.

With these caveats in mind, specific approaches to the preeclamptic patient or the patient at risk for preeclampsia can be made.

Given that edema is one of the clinical triads commonly found in preeclampsia, diuretics were commonly given in the 1960s to prevent or treat the disorder. Recently, a meta-analysis was performed of nine prospective randomized trials where diuretic therapy was used in pregnant women with edema or extremely fast weight gain [154] showing benefit in the diuretic-treated group. However, no data were available concerning the presence of proteinuria or hypertension specific to preeclampsia, and stillbirth rates were not different between groups. Given the risk of decreasing already compromised fetal-placental blood flow in patients most often

Fig. 13-7. (A) Light microscopy of glomerulus demonstrating changes consistent with glomeruloendotheliosis. (From R. H. Heptinstall, Renal Disease in Pregnancy. In R. H. Heptinstall [ed.], *Pathology of the Kidney* [4th ed.]. Boston: Little, Brown, 1992. P. 1773.) (B) Normal glomerulus. (From M. A. Venkatachalam and W. Kriz, Anatomy. In R. H. Heptinstall [ed.], *Pathology of the Kidney* [4th ed.]. Boston: Little, Brown, 1992. P. 37.)

volume contracted, there is no direct indication for diuretic therapy as a prophylactic or treatment measure in preeclampsia.

Given the large body of evidence that prostacyclin deficiency plays a role in the increased vascular reactivity and peripheral vascular resistance found in preeclampsia, early uncontrolled trials demonstrated improved fetal survival and birth weight in women at risk for preeclampsia as well as decreased incidence of preeclampsia in those treated with low-dose aspirin (100 mg/day) [155, 156]. The thought behind such therapy is that doses of aspirin less than 100 mg/day will preferentially inhibit platelet thromboxane production while maintaining endothelial prostacyclin production, thereby protecting against pathologic vasoconstriction and clotting (Fig. 13-8). However, results from three large prospective trials performed in the United States, Great Britain, and Italy involving over 13,500 healthy pregnant nulliparous

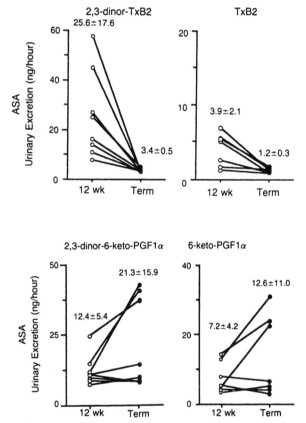

Fig. 13-8. Urinary excretion of 6-keto-PGF$_{1\alpha}$ (*lower right*) and its metabolite 2,3-dinor-6-keto-PGF$_{1\alpha}$ (*lower left*) did not change with administration of 60 mg/day of aspirin (ASA). Urinary excretion of 2,3-dinor-thromboxane B$_2$ decreased by 80 percent (*upper left*) and renal thromboxane B$_2$ excretion decreased by 60 percent (*upper right*) with administration of 60 mg/day of aspirin.

women, although demonstrating a 25 percent reduction in the incidence of pre-eclampsia in those treated with low-dose aspirin, showed no differences in fetal morbidity or mortality [157–159]. Importantly, the frequency of potential side effects to the fetus including cardiovascular complications such as early closure of the patent ductus arteriosus and intraventricular hemorrhage was not increased in the treated patients [157]. As well, no effect on the regional or central circulation of the fetus was found [158]. In the American study, a slightly higher rate of abruptio placentae was found in the aspirin-treated group (0.7% versus 0.1%), although these rates are both similar to that reported in the general obstetric population. These results provide support for the following tentative conclusion. Low-dose aspirin can be safely administered in the asymptomatic pregnant woman prior to the development of hypertension, and there may be a subset of high-risk women with underlying hypertension, renal disease, previous preeclampsia, or diabetes mellitus who may benefit from early prophylactic therapy. However, it is not advisable to treat every nulliparous woman with low-dose aspirin. In addition, therapy with aspirin may mask the clinical features of preeclampsia while the pathologic processes secondary to placental insufficiency continue to develop.

Reports in the 1980s suggested that women with calcium-deficient diets are at increased risk for the development of preeclampsia or pregnancy-induced hypertension [160, 161] and that preeclamptic women are notably hypocalciuric [121]. In support of a role for calcium in blood pressure regulation in pregnancy, calcium supplementation has been shown to increase the pressor resistance to infused angiotensin II [162] as well as reduce the occurrence of gestational hypertension [163]. Urinary calcium excretion increases in normal human pregnancy by the sixth week of gestation. A second rise is seen in the middle of the second trimester. The initial increase in urinary calcium occurs in association with increases in both urinary sodium excretion and GFR [163a]. Further studies are needed to determine if calcium supplementation will reduce the incidence of preeclampsia specifically and/or reduce fetal morbidity and mortality associated with this condition.

When treating established preeclampsia, it is important to note that delivery is always indicated regardless of gestational age if there is evidence of advanced disease or impending eclampsia. Given the explosive nature of preeclampsia and that the clinical course can change quickly, hospitalization is recommended for all patients with preeclampsia. Therefore, the decision to continue the pregnancy with an expectant management approach always increases the risk of eclampsia, acute renal failure, abruptio placentae, disseminated intravascular coagulation, hepatic infarction, and maternal mortality. Some centers have described success in treating women with mild preeclampsia followed at extended care facilities or with home visits; however, this practice requires a trained staff well versed in the treatment of preeclampsia and a patient population that is reliable and transportable.

Although the general wisdom has held that both bed rest in the left lateral decubitus position and sodium restriction are helpful in the treatment of hypertension, edema, and proteinuria in preeclampsia, studies carefully assessing these modalities demonstrate no benefit in fetal or maternal outcome [164]. Given that venous return is maximal in the supine left lateral decubitus position during pregnancy and that central hemodynamic measurements suggest that intravascular volume is decreased in the preeclamptic state, this may be the most hemodynamically correct position for the preeclamptic patient. However, total bed rest need not be enforced and carries the increased risk of thromboembolism. Sodium restriction may actually be detrimental and decrease perfusion to the fetal-placental unit. Antihypertensive medications are recommended to treat the hypertension of preeclampsia when Korotkoff V diastolic pressures exceed 100 mm Hg [101]. Evidence now indicates that early treatment with antihypertensive medication to prevent the occurrence of preeclampsia is of no benefit [165–167] and may be associated with lower birth weight infants [168, 169]. In those women whose midtrimester blood pressures are known to be quite low (diastolic blood pressure <60 mm Hg), antihypertensive medication can be considered if diastolic pressure increases to 85 mm Hg in the preeclamptic state. Given that increased systemic vascular resistance is the hallmark of preeclampsia, medication aimed at reducing vascular resistance that is safe for the fetus should be considered first (Table 13-3). Intravenous hydralazine, which acts directly on the vascular smooth muscle and causes vasorelaxation and a decrease in peripheral vascular resistance, has been used for many years to treat hypertension in preeclamptic women. Maternal side effects include facial flushing, headaches, tachycardia, and a possible increase in ventricular arrhythmias [170]. Importantly, preeclamptic women are extremely sensitive to the blood pressure–lowering effects of antihypertensive medications, with occasional marked decrements in blood pressure and the development of oliguria with small doses of hydralazine [171]. Given that fetal distress has been reported with the use of parenteral hydralazine [172, 173], it is recommended to start with small doses with a minimal time interval of 20 minutes.

Between dosages, α-methyldopa, commonly used in the treatment of chronic

Table 13-3. Therapeutic agents available for the treatment of acute severe hypertension in pregnancy

Drug	Dosage	Onset of action	Adverse effects
Hydralazine	5 mg IV/IM, then 5–10 mg q20–40 min	IV 10 min IM 10–30 min	Headache, flushing, tachycardia, nausea, vomiting, ventricular arrhythmias
Magnesium sulfate	4–6 g IV/IM, then 1 g/hr IV	5–10 min	Maternal and fetal respiratory and cardiac depression
Labetalol	20 mg IV, then 20–80 mg q20–30 min up to 300 mg or infuse 1–2 mg/min until desired blood pressure achieved	5–10 min	Flushing, nausea and vomiting, maternal and fetal bradycardia and fetal hypoglycemia
Nifedipine	5 mg PO, repeat in 30 min if necessary, then 10–20 mg PO q3–6h	10–15 min	Flushing, headache, nausea, tachycardia, inhibition of labor
Diazoxide	30–50 mg IV, q5–15 min	2–5 min	Inhibits labor, hyperglycemia

hypertension in pregnancy (see next section), also has an extremely safe risk profile but is not available parenterally and is not used during the acute management of hypertension of preeclampsia. Recently, experience has accumulated with both labetalol, which has combined β- and α_1-blocking properties, and nifedipine, a calcium channel blocker of the dihydropyridine class. Although data are more limited than with hydralazine, it appears that labetalol is equally efficacious, with the possibility of decreased maternal ventricular arrhythmias [170], although reports of fetal bradycardia exist [174]. Also, animal studies suggest that fetal compensatory responses to stress such as hypoxemia require intact adrenergic mechanisms that may be blocked by labetalol [175]. Nifedipine, which also directly relaxes vascular smooth muscle, has been shown to successfully lower blood pressure in preeclamptic patients [176, 177]. To date, no adverse effects on fetal placental hemodynamics or fetal well-being have been reported; however, experience is limited. In preeclamptic women with severe hypertension that does not respond to these three relatively safe agents, delivery should be considered if possible. However, two other potent agents have been used with some success in transiently controlling blood pressure: diazoxide and sodium nitroprusside. Although both agents take effect immediately, decreases in uterine blood flow have been reported with both [178, 179], and diazoxide has been reported to arrest labor and cause neonatal hyperglycemia [180]. Nitroprusside is known to cause accumulation of cyanide, which will accumulate in fetal tissue and should be used sparingly.

Magnesium sulfate, which is used to prevent the progression from preeclampsia to eclampsia and as an anticonvulsant, acts directly on vascular smooth muscle to increase vasorelaxation by inhibiting calcium uptake, thereby reducing peripheral vascular resistance and lowering blood pressure. Interpreting studies of cardiac output and central hemodynamics during preeclampsia may be hampered by the prior institution of magnesium sulfate therapy. Magnesium sulfate has been shown to increase prostacyclin production, decrease endothelin-1 levels, and increase production of urinary cyclic GMP, as well as improve relaxation of the uteroplacental vasculature [181–184]. Importantly, when magnesium sulfate is given with nifedipine, profound hypotension and neuromuscular blockade have been reported, most likely due to excessive calcium channel blockade [185, 186].

Given the sensitivity of preeclamptic patients to antihypertensive medications and their volume-contracted state, one consideration has been to provide volume expansion prior to medication administration. However, endothelial integrity is markedly abnormal in preeclamptic patients, and pulmonary or cerebral edema therefore can occur easily. Although volume expansion in experimental settings with close central hemodynamic monitoring has demonstrated an increase in cardiac output and a decrease in peripheral vascular resistance [187, 188], no improvement in fetal or maternal mortality or uteroplacental blood flow has been found [185–189]. Therefore, aggressive volume expansion should rarely be performed, as in the presence of oliguria, azotemia, congestive heart failure, or pulmonary edema, and when performed needs central hemodynamic monitoring. Finally, other therapeutic modalities for the treatment of severe preeclampsia have been reported and include plasma exchange [190], prostacyclin infusion [191], prostaglandin A_1 administration [192], and anticoagulation therapy [193]; however, these treatments have serious side effects and risk to both fetus and mother and have been studied in too few patients to be considered for recommendation at this time.

Chronic Hypertension of Whatever Cause

Chronic hypertension in pregnancy is defined as elevated blood pressure (>140/90 mm Hg) prior to pregnancy or that persists more than 6 weeks after delivery [101]. Women with chronic hypertension are at increased risk for preeclampsia, abruptio placentae, acute renal failure, and intrauterine growth retardation. The prevalence of chronic hypertension in pregnancy is not known but is seen in about 1 to 5 percent of pregnancies [152]. Given that some women are not diagnosed prior to pregnancy, those with similar blood pressure elevations to those found in preeclampsia prior to the twentieth week, particularly in the absence of proteinuria, are considered to have chronic hypertension. Importantly, blood pressure in many hypertensive women will decrease more than in their normotensive counterparts throughout pregnancy, making the diagnosis of chronic hypertension during pregnancy difficult [194]. However, there are an equal number of hypertensive women whose blood pressure either increases or does not decrease in the first half of gestation who appear to be at higher risk for complications during pregnancy. Those women with mild essential hypertension (diastolic blood pressure < 105 mm Hg) generally have uncomplicated pregnancies [194]. Approximately 10 percent of hypertensive women develop preeclampsia, which is the group of women at highest risk for fetal and maternal mortality. The reason for the higher frequency of preeclampsia and the greater complication rate in these women is most likely due to the decreased placental reserve and intrauterine growth retardation seen in women with chronic hypertension [195]. Given the diagnostic difficulty in differentiating chronic hypertension from preeclampsia, Table 13-4 provides characteristics that are specific to each disorder. Clearly, those women with moderate to severe hypertension with evidence of end-organ damage such as renal insufficiency or left ventricular hypertrophy due to long and sustained high blood pressure are at extreme risk for complications during pregnancy [105]. It is strongly recommended to follow these women closely with antihypertensive medication started early in pregnancy, and they should be counseled early concerning the risks to themselves and the decreased chances of fetal survival. The majority of patients in the category of chronic hypertension have essential hypertension, but every other cause of secondary hypertension including renal artery stenosis, Cushing's disease, primary aldosteronism, coarctation of the aorta, and pheochromocytoma may occur and should be considered given differences in maternal and fetal outcome as well as different approaches to management.

Management of Chronic Hypertension in Pregnancy

There are several drugs now available for the treatment of chronic hypertension during pregnancy (Table 13-5). As with the treatment of essential hypertension, there are as many opinions about the appropriate approach to medical management of the hypertensive gravida as there are options [196]. Although no complete consensus exists, we recommend the institution of therapy in all women whose Korotkoff V diastolic measurements are greater than 100 mm Hg [101]. Great care must

Table 13-4. Clinical and laboratory characteristics differentiating preeclampsia and chronic hypertension

Characteristics	Preeclampsia	Chronic hypertension
Age	Extremes	Older
Parity	Nulliparous	Multiparous
History	Negative	Positive pregnancy history
Onset	3rd trimester	Early, often <20 wk
Fundi	Retinal edema, arteriolar vasospasm	Arteriolosclerosis
Cardiac status	Normal	Ventricular hypertrophy
Deep tendon reflexes	Hyperactive	Normal
Hematocrit	Possibly increased	Normal
Blood smear	Schistocytes	Normal
Platelet count	Decreased	Normal
Proteinuria	>300 mg/day	Absent or minimal
Uric acid	Often elevated	Usually normal
Liver function	Some elevation with pain and tenderness	Normal
Von Willebrand's factor VIII	Elevated	Normal
Urinary prostacyclin	Decreased	Normal
Plasma endothelin	Increased	Normal
Urinary cyclic guanosine monophosphate	Decreased	Normal
Antithrombin III	Decreased	Normal
Plasma fibronectin	Increased	Normal
Urinary calcium	Decreased	Normal
Angiotensin II sensitivity	Increased	Decreased
Rollover test	Abnormal	Normal

be considered in choosing an antihypertensive agent during pregnancy given that little is known about the long-term effect of most agents on infant and childhood development. Those women who are taking an antihypertensive medication prior to pregnancy that is safe for the fetus are not recommended to stop taking their medication [101]. Some medications, specifically angiotensin converting enzyme inhibitors, although not teratogenic, have been shown to cause acute renal failure in the fetus [197] and fetal demise [198, 199] and are contraindicated past the first trimester of pregnancy [101].

Methyldopa [Aldomet], a central adrenergic inhibitor, has the longest history of effective use in pregnancy and has been studied prospectively for as long as 7 years of the treated offspring [200]. Although some authors have suggested that there is a decrease in second-trimester stillbirths in women with hypertension treated with methyldopa [201], this has not been supported in other studies [194, 202]. The side effect profile of methyldopa indicates that maternal and fetal adverse side effects

Table 13-5. Therapeutic agents available for the treatment of
chronic hypertension in pregnancy

Drug	Daily dose	Adverse effects
First-line agent		
Methyldopa	500–3000 mg/day given q6–12h	
Second-line agent		
Hydralazine	50–300 mg/day q6–12h	Reports of neonatal thrombocytopenia
Other alternatives		
Labetalol	200–1200 mg/day q8–12h	Fetal bradycardia, fetal response to stress impaired, ? intrauterine growth retardation with long-term use
Other β-adrenergic inhibitors		
Nifedipine	30–120 mg/day	Limited data; inhibits uterine contractions, synergistic effect with $MgSO_4$
Clonidine	0.1–0.8 mg/day	Limited data
Prazosin	1–30 mg/day	Limited data; hepatic dysfunction
Thiazide diuretics	Varies	Volume depletion, electrolyte imbalance, pancreatitis, thrombocytopenia
Contraindicated		
Angiotensin-converting enzyme inhibitors		Fetal loss in animals, intrauterine growth retardation, neonatal anuria and renal failure, oligohydramnios

are mild and well tolerated [203]. Other authors have claimed that clonidine, also
an α_2-antagonist, is as effective as methyldopa with no significant differences in
side effects. However, follow-up of treated children suggests that some excess sleep
disturbances may be present [204]. Given the longer-standing record of methyldopa
and the question of long-standing effects with clonidine when both drugs are equally
efficacious, we recommend methyldopa as a first-line therapy for the treatment of
chronic hypertension in pregnancy. Hydralazine has been used successfully in the
chronic setting during pregnancy in combination with methyldopa or a β-blocker.
No studies have been performed on infants who have been exposed to hydralazine
for prolonged periods of time, and there are occasional reports of neonatal thrombocytopenia when mothers were treated with this drug. We consider this a second-line
agent for the treatment of chronic hypertension in pregnancy. β-Adrenoreceptor
blocking agents are the second most widely studied antihypertensive agents in pregnancy after methyldopa. Although early retrospective studies suggested that propranolol was associated with intrauterine growth retardation, neonatal respiratory
depression, bradycardia, and hypoglycemia, recent prospective randomized studies

of atenolol, metoprolol, and pindolol suggest no adverse maternal or fetal effects compared to placebo even at 1 year follow-up [205]. Studies performed in the United Kingdom with oxyprenolol, an agent not available in the United States, suggests equal efficacy to methyldopa in treating chronic hypertension in pregnancy. However, most studies are small, with therapy initiated late in pregnancy (after 29 weeks), and using these agents for extremely long periods during pregnancy is still not advised. Labetalol has also demonstrated equivalent efficacy to methyldopa in the treatment of chronic hypertension in pregnancy but has not been demonstrated to improve fetal outcome or to have a lower side effect profile. No studies to determine the long-term effects of labetalol on exposed children have been performed to date. Calcium channel blockers have been used in the treatment of acute hypertension in pregnancy, but there are only anecdotal case reports of use of these agents for long-term therapy in chronic hypertension in pregnancy [206]. Therefore, these agents are best reserved for those patients who are unresponsive to or do not tolerate the previously mentioned medications.

Chronic Hypertension with Superimposed Preeclampsia

Preeclampsia can occur in women with chronic hypertension. Some authors suggest that 15 to 25 percent will ultimately develop preeclampsia; however, well-performed studies suggest that between 6 and 10 percent will develop preeclampsia [207]. Typically these women develop preeclampsia very early and are at greatest risk for fetal loss. As well, this group is more predisposed to developing abruptio placentae, liver infarction, and acute renal failure. The classic definition is that of preeclampsia, although some authors suggest that high levels of proteinuria should be required so that the disorder is not mistaken for chronic hypertension developing in the third trimester [98].

Transient Hypertension

Late or transient hypertension is a poorly understood entity that refers to transient elevations of blood pressure that develop very late in pregnancy, during labor, or 24 hours postpartum and resolve within 10 days of delivery. It appears that these patients with this condition are at higher risk for development of transient hypertension in subsequent pregnancies and may develop chronic hypertension [208]. The condition usually is benign and resolves spontaneously without intervention.

Renal Diseases Commonly Associated with Pregnancy

Urinary Tract Infections

Infections of the urinary tract are the most frequent infection of pregnancy and represent the most common renal complication of pregnancy. Asymptomatic bacteriuria occurs in 4 to 7 percent of pregnant women, which is similar to the general population [209]. Factors associated with increased risk for bacteriuria in pregnant women include increased maternal age, multiparity, low socioeconomic level, diabetes mellitus, sickle cell trait, previous urinary tract infection, certain glomerular diseases such as analgesic nephropathy, chronic obstruction or reflux nephropathy, and possibly hypertension [210]. Those women with diabetes mellitus and a previous history of urinary tract infection are at greatest risk. Importantly, untreated asymptomatic bacteriuria places gravidas at greater risk for either cystitis (80%) or pyelonephritis (25–30%) sometime during the pregnancy or in the postpartum period as compared to their nonpregnant counterparts [209]. An increased risk for bacteriuria in women during pregnancy is due to alterations in bladder and ureteric tone and peristalsis, leading to incomplete bladder emptying and dilatation of the ureters associated with urinary stasis, and the occurrence of partial ureteric obstruction often associated with reflux during the normal course of pregnancy. Bacteriuria, if present, is usually found in the first trimester. Fifty percent of symptomatic urinary tract infections will demonstrate bacteriuria on routine asymptomatic screening, and if bacteriuria is properly treated, the risk for developing subsequent pyelonephritis decreases by 80 to 90 percent during pregnancy as well as for 1 year following delivery [211]. If no bacteriuria is found in early pregnancy, there is less than a 2 percent chance of having a urinary tract infection in later stages of gestation as compared to 20 to 40 percent of those who have asymptomatic bacteriuria. A screening test for bacteriuria with effective treatment and follow-up is therefore essential at the time of the first prenatal examination.

Significance

Acute cystitis occurs most commonly in the second trimester, and pyelonephritis occurs with equal frequency in the second and third trimesters [212]. Importantly, in those women who develop acute pyelonephritis during pregnancy, there is a 20 to 50 percent increased risk of premature delivery, low birth weight infants, or perinatal death. Two or more episodes of acute pyelonephritis in either pregnant or nonpregnant women warrant a careful postpartum radiographic examination to exclude the possibility of an obstructive lesion. Given that physiologic hydronephrosis occurs during normal pregnancy and may not resolve until 12 weeks postpartum, timing of the evaluation is important. Maternal morbidity associated with acute pyelonephritis includes renal insufficiency, renal abscess, gram-negative bacteremia, and sepsis. Of 130 patients with third-trimester pyelonephritis, the GFR was lower than 80 ml/min in 25 percent of patients and lower than 60 ml/min in 10 percent [213]. Although it is clear that pyelonephritis is associated with premature labor and delivery, an association with bacteriuria is less clear [210, 214]. Kincaid-Smith [210] found a highly significant increase in premature delivery among women with bacteriuria. However, this population may be skewed, with a high incidence of underlying renal disease found in postpartum radiographic studies. The association is potentially confounded by the association between lower socioeconomic status and both asymptomatic bacteriuria and premature delivery. However, a recent meta-analysis of randomized clinical trials indicates a direct adverse effect of untreated asymptomatic bacteriuria on birth weight where a review of randomized clinical trials showed that antibiotic treatment was effective in reducing the rate of low birth weight infants when compared with placebo treatment [215]. In particular, premature delivery seems distinctly more frequent among patients whose urinary tract infections cannot be eradicated. Although a cause-effect relationship appears to exist between asymptomatic bacteriuria and prematurity, it probably accounts for only a small percentage of all premature births [214]. The mechanism by which bacteriuria induces premature delivery is not well understood but may be related to increased production of phospholipase A_2 or an adverse effect of endotoxin on myometrial contractility or an interruption of the placental vasculature. The evidence is less convincing that asymptomatic bacteriuria is associated with an increased risk of maternal hypertension [210, 214], preeclampsia, or anemia [216].

Diagnosis and Treatment

Significant bacteriuria is defined as that level of bacteriuria considered to be a reliable indicator of true infection of the urinary tract. The diagnosis of infection is usually based on bacterial colony counts in voided urine. Recent studies in nonpregnant women have shown that a threshold of 10^2 colony-forming units of a uropathogen per milliliter of voided urine has the best sensitivity and specificity for diagnosing acute urinary tract infections in women, and it seems reasonable to apply this to pregnant women [212]. Asymptomatic bacteriuria is not associated with urinary symptoms, whereas women with acute cystitis have some combination of dysuria, frequency, urgency, suprapubic pain, or suprapubic tenderness. Dysuria is the most suggestive of urinary tract infection or urethritis due to *Neisseria gonorrhoeae* or *Chlamydia trachomatis*. However, dysuria may be caused by genital herpes or vaginal infections. Acute pyelonephritis is suggested by flank pain, nausea/vomiting, fever, and/or costovertebral angle tenderness. The same colony counts used for the diagnosis of asymptomatic bacteriuria can be used for cystitis and pyelonephritis.

Asymptomatic bacteriuria can be treated with antibiotics appropriate to the susceptibility of the organism. Both amoxicillin and nitrofurantoin are inexpensive and safe. If the organism is resistant, broader-range second- or third-generation cephalosporins are reasonable alternatives. Although single-dose regimens appear effective for the treatment of asymptomatic bacteriuria in pregnancy in several studies, none has had sufficient power to provide a definitive answer as to whether single-dose therapy is as effective as longer regimens. Therefore, 7- to 10-day regimens have generally been recommended. Recently, 3-day regimens, believed to be more effective than single-dose regimens, have been advocated for the treatment of asymptomatic bacteriuria as long as follow-up cultures are obtained [217]. In acute cystitis, however, single-dose regimens have been associated with a high rate of failure (31%) in pregnancy [217]. Therefore, longer regimens of 7 to 10 days should be used for the treatment of acute cystitis in pregnancy [217]. The same antibiotic choices apply as with asymptomatic bacteriuria, with the consideration of amoxicillin-clavulanate in patients with more severe symptoms. The fluoroquinolones are contraindicated in pregnancy and should only be used in an unusual situation of antimicrobial resistance with no other therapeutic alternative.

Pregnant women who develop pyelonephritis should be hospitalized for volume replacement and parenteral therapy. After cultures are obtained and no evidence of gram-positive pathogens are evident by Gram's stain, empiric therapy with a second- or third-generation cephalosporin or an aminogycoside (perhaps with ampicillin) can be initiated. Patients can be switched to oral antibiotics after 48 hours if a response is seen. The duration of therapy has not been established, but given the potential consequences of pyelonephritis in pregnancy, a total of 14 days should be considered. Given that recurrence occurs in 25 percent of patients during pregnancy, monthly cultures during the pregnancy should be obtained [218].

Acute Renal Failure Associated with Pregnancy

Obstetric acute renal failure accounted for approximately 40 percent of all cases of acute renal failure prior to legalization of abortion; however, today the estimated frequency is only 1 in 10,000 in developed countries [219]. A list of causes of acute renal failure specific to pregnancy is provided in Table 13-6. Importantly, obstetric acute renal failure still accounts for approximately 20 percent of all acute renal failure in developing countries, secondary to poor access to medical care, poverty, and nontherapeutic abortions [220, 221]. The major cause of acute renal failure in this setting is infection, hemorrhage, and hypovolemia leading to acute tubular necrosis (see Chap. 10) and is usually reversible. Acute renal failure occurring in

Table 13-6. Causes of acute renal failure specific to pregnancy

Sepsis
Abortion
    Intrauterine fetal death
    Puerperal sepsis
Hemorrhage
    Ectopic pregnancy
    Abortion
    Chorionic villus sampling
    Uterine hemorrhage
    Placenta previa
    Abruptio placentae
Obstruction
    Uterine enlargement
        Incarceration
        Polyhydramnios
        Gravid uterus
    Scleroderma
    Solitary kidney with hydronephrosis
      of pregnancy
Preeclampsia/eclampsia
HELLP (hemolysis, elevated liver enzymes, and low platelet count) syndrome
Acute fatty liver of pregnancy
Postpartum acute renal failure

the first half of pregnancy in industrialized nations today have been reported due to hyperemesis gravidarum or complications following chorionic villus sampling [222]. A number of cases of acute renal failure due to urinary tract obstruction during pregnancy have been reported. This appears to occur in women with a solitary kidney, polyhydramnios, multiple gestations, or renal disease or rarely with the occurrence of acute urate nephropathy, scleroderma, or enlarged fetal renal cyst [219]. Fetal mortality is due primarily to prematurity, and resolution can often be obtained with temporary retrograde or percutaneous nephrostomy stints or repeated amniocenteses. With improved obstetric care, the causes of acute renal failure late in pregnancy have become multifactorial usually in the setting of preeclampsia with superimposed abruptio placentae, disseminated intravascular coagulation, the HELLP syndrome, and antepartum hemorrhage. Importantly, the HELLP syndrome is present in over 90 percent of those patients with preeclampsia and acute renal failure. In patients with uncomplicated preeclampsia, the incidence of acute renal failure is low, less than 1 percent [219, 213]. Those preeclamptic patients who develop acute renal failure usually develop preeclampsia superimposed on renal disease or preexisting hypertension [223]. Diagnostic ambiguity is often present in these cases where the gravida is multiparous or the triad of proteinuria, edema, and hypertension is not always present. Those women with pure preeclampsia and superimposed acute renal failure have lower fetal mortality, better maternal outcome, and less requirement of chronic dialysis than those with chronic hypertension or preexisting renal disease [224]. Bilateral cortical necrosis, either confluent or patchy, is common in this group of women and is usually irreversible in more than 50 percent, particularly in those with confluent changes on biopsy. It appears that disturbances in the coagulation mechanism, disseminated intravascular coagulation, and increased response to vasoactive compounds are involved in the development of this disorder. Acute fatty liver of pregnancy occurs rarely in 1 in 13,000 pregnancies and accounts for approximately 5 percent of acute renal failure in pregnancy and may be a preterminal event in up to 60 percent of patients with this disorder.

Postpartum Renal Failure

Idiopathic postpartum acute renal failure is a rare but serious disorder characterized by acute renal failure, mild to moderate hypertension, and evidence of microangiopathic hemolytic anemia after an uneventful pregnancy and delivery. It accounts for 5 to 9 percent of obstetric acute renal failure and was first reported in 1968 [225], with fewer than 200 cases reported to date. The peak incidence is between 2 and 5 weeks postpartum, but it can occur up to 10 weeks after delivery. Renal histologic lesions vary depending on the time of biopsy with respect to the onset of disease [226]. Glomerular and arteriolar lesions are distinct and dominate the pathologic findings and resemble the adult hemolytic-uremic syndrome with fibrin deposition, thickening of glomerular capillary walls, and subendothelial swelling with large granular subendothelial deposits, possibly representing incompletely polymerized fibrin. Arterial lesions predominate later in the course of the disease and include intimal proliferation of the interlobular arteries with fibrin deposition. The severity of arterial involvement corresponds with decreased renal survival. The pathogenesis of this disorder is unknown; however, associations with gastrointestinal symptoms, oral contraceptive pill use, retained placental fragments, and ergotamine compounds or oxytocic agents have been implicated.

Renal recovery occurs in a minority of patients, as late as 1 year after onset of disease. Overall, maternal mortality is 60 percent in this group of patients. Treatment options are sparse, and although improved mortality has been reported with the use of heparin, studies are too small and uncontrolled to be applicable. Other potential, but as yet untested, modalities include prostacyclin infusion, plasma infusion, plasma exchange, and antiplatelet therapy.

Pregnancy in Patients with Renal Disease

Overall fertility is decreased in patients with renal disease, but renal insufficiency by no means precludes conception. The diagnosis of chronic renal disease can be made with reasonable certainty when significant proteinuria, hypertension, abnormal urinary sediment, and a decrease in renal function are noted early in pregnancy. In the second half of gestation, the differentiation is much more difficult to establish on clinical grounds, and renal biopsy may be necessary to make a diagnosis [98].

The major determinants of the successful outcome of pregnancy in women with chronic renal disease are (1) the presence of hypertension, (2) the severity of pregestational renal insufficiency, and (3) the type of primary renal disease. The dissociation of these three factors as independent variables is extremely difficult, but each shall briefly be discussed individually.

Role of Hypertension

Since Mackay [227] originally described the untoward effects of hypertension in patients with renal failure, both for the mother and fetus, the subject has been reexamined by others. Most of the specific risks of hypertension in pregnancy appear to be mediated through superimposed preeclampsia [228]. In women with intact renal function, the presence of hypertension is the prime determinant of fetal morbidity and mortality [228, 229]. Those with hypertension as compared to normotension have an increased incidence of intrauterine growth retardation, preterm delivery, and renal deterioration [230]. Table 13-7 provides a summary of the effect of hypertension on pregnancy outcome from several studies [99, 231]. As is evident

Table 13-7. Pregnancy complications in 1902 women with chronic renal disease

Renal status	Problems (%)	Successful pregnancy (%)	Long-term problems (%)
Mild	26	96	<3
Moderate	47	89	25
Severe	86	46	53

(From J. Davison and C. Baylis, Pregnancy in Patients with Chronic Renal Disease or Renal Transplant. In Jacobsen, Striker, Klahr [eds.], *The Principles and Practice of Nephrology* [2nd ed.]. St. Louis: Mosby, 1996. P. 465)

from Table 13-7, hypertension in gravidas with preexisting renal disease is associated with an incidence of perinatal mortality of 42 percent and preeclampsia in 54 percent as compared to 6 and 11 percent, respectively, in normotensive gravidas with underlying renal disease. The better control of the blood pressure and the later the occurrence of hypertension during pregnancy, the less likely adverse fetal or maternal effects are to be [229]. Therefore, the presence of hypertension is clearly a major determinant of pregnancy outcome for women with chronic renal disease.

Role of Severity of Pregestational Renal Insufficiency

Patients can lose 50 percent of their renal function before serum creatinine concentrations are greater than 1.5 mg/dl. The level of renal impairment prior to pregnancy has the ability to affect both pregnancy outcome and remote renal prognosis, depending on the etiology of the underlying renal disease. Given that pregestational renal function affects both fetal and maternal outcome, it is worthwhile to categorize women prior to conception with regard to their renal status to aid in management and pregestational counseling. Those women with serum creatinine concentrations less than or equal to 1.4 mg/dl are considered to have mild impairment and can fare quite well throughout pregnancy (see Table 13-7). In those with moderate (serum creatinine concentration between 1.4 and 2.8 mg/dl) or severe renal involvement (>2.8 mg/dl), fetal and renal prognosis is more guarded. In a review of 1902 women with 2813 pregnancies between 1973 and 1993, those with severe renal involvement had a less than 50 percent chance of having a successful pregnancy outcome or surviving the pregnancy unharmed. Given the grave fetal and maternal prognosis in those women with severe renal involvement, it may benefit those women to wait if possible to consider pregnancy until after entering end-stage renal disease and renal transplantation, when fetal and maternal outcome are much better [232]. Micropuncture studies have shown no change in mean ultrafiltration pressure or glomerular hydrostatic pressure during pregnancy in rats with and without underlying hypertension [233]. Consistent with this is the lack of untoward effects on long-term renal function in women with underlying renal disease but normal renal function without hypertension who undergo pregnancy [228, 229]. On the other hand, those women with exacerbation of their renal disease or the development of severe preeclampsia during pregnancy with underlying renal insufficiency appear to progress more quickly to renal failure, as compared to their nonpregnant counterparts.

Effect of Specific Renal Disorders on Pregnancy

Primary Glomerular Disease
With all underlying renal diseases, those women with normal renal function, normotension, and mild urinary sediment activity have minimal maternal or fetal complications [230]. In specific conditions such as focal segmental glomerular sclerosis (FSGS), IgA nephropathy, and diffuse, focal, or membranoproliferative glomerulo-

nephritis, a diagnosis prior to pregnancy has been found to be protective, most likely as a result of increased medical surveillance during pregnancy [234, 235]. In contrast, increased histopathologic disease activity has been shown to be associated with poorer fetal and maternal outcome in each of these conditions [236, 237]. For unclear reasons, both FSGS and IgA nephropathy may exacerbate from a quiescent state during pregnancy [234]. Those women with isolated proteinuria as in lipoid nephrosis and membranous nephropathy often develop extremely high levels of proteinuria, which predisposes them to increased thromboembolic risk during a time of predisposition to coagulation; however, unless preexisting hypertension or renal dysfunction is present, the pregnancy is usually uneventful. Preexisting hypertension potentially complicates the course of pregnancy in all women with glomerular disease, resulting in a higher frequency of intrauterine growth retardation and premature delivery [211]. Importantly, treatment of hypertension during pregnancy in these women does improve fetal and maternal outcome [230, 238].

Lupus Nephropathy

Women with lupus nephropathy demonstrate an increased incidence of spontaneous abortion [239]. Circulating autoantibodies, lupus anticoagulant, or anticardiolipin antibodies have been suggested to account for the high frequency of abortion and the development of congenital heart block [239]. Although the influence of pregnancy on the course of lupus nephropathy remains uncertain, retrospective series indicate that clinical disease activity of any type within 6 months prior to conception is associated with a four times higher incidence of fetal wastage (30% versus 8%) than in pregnancies conceived after a 6-month period of clinical remission [240]. As well, development of systemic lupus erythematosus during pregnancy has an unfavorable effect on fetal prognosis. Treatment of stable but clinically active systemic lupus erythematosus with steroids is associated with no adverse effects for the mother but still carries a high fetal risk. In addition, steroid dosages need to be adjusted during labor and delivery. Finally, there is no evidence that the long-term course of lupus nephropathy is affected by pregnancy [241].

Diabetic Nephropathy

Diabetes is one of the most common disorders encountered among high-risk obstetric patients. In succeeding decades where insulin therapy was first introduced, fetal survival improved from 59 percent to 90 percent, close to that found in the general population. Although diabetes is clearly associated with an increased risk (two- to fivefold increase) of preeclampsia, bacteriuria, large for gestational age babies, and some congenital abnormalities, few series are available reporting the outcome of pregnancy in diabetic mothers with overt renal disease. In those women without diabetic renal involvement or preexisting hypertension, little evidence exists for acute loss of renal function during the pregnancy. Risk factors for complications during pregnancy are similar to those for women with other renal disease and include preexisting hypertension and renal insufficiency [242].

Chronic Interstitial Nephritis

The vast majority of patients with "chronic pyelonephritis" have renal disease unrelated to infection. In the majority of childbearing women, the diseases represented by this term include reflux nephropathy and analgesic abuse. One small series of patients with reflux nephropathy who underwent pregnancy had poor fetal (47% perinatal mortality) and maternal outcomes [243]. However, the majority of these patients had pregestational renal insufficiency. Similarly, the outcome of pregnancy in the patients with analgesic abuse is related to the presence of hypertension and the degree of renal insufficiency [99].

Polycystic Kidney Disease

Most women of childbearing potential with polycystic kidney disease have normal renal function and are normotensive. Therefore, the vast majority of pregnancies (>80%) are uncomplicated [228]. There is an increased risk for the development of preeclampsia or pregnancy-induced hypertension, which is a harbinger for the future development of chronic hypertension in autosomal dominant polycystic kidney disease (ADPKD) patients. Hypertensive polycystic women develop preeclampsia often (45%) and are at increased risk for fetal prematurity and mortality. Women with ADPKD who become pregnant have a greater incidence of acute renal failure related to the presence of hypertension and abruption placentae. Complications in pregnancy specifically related to polycystic kidney disease include cyst hemorrhage, cyst infection, and urolithiasis. Long-term renal function appears to suffer as a consequence of pregnancy in those hypertensive polycystic women who complete more than three pregnancies.

Urolithiasis

The prevalence of renal stones varies between 0.03 and 0.35 percent during pregnancy [244]. A study of 78 women with preexisting renal stones who underwent 148 pregnancies revealed that stone disease had no adverse effect on pregnancy; however, the number of urinary tract infections during pregnancy was increased [245]. Endoscopic basket extraction has been performed safely during pregnancy when it was necessary to remove a stone [246].

Effect of Pregnancy on the Course of Renal Disease

There has been much controversy regarding the effect of pregnancy on the natural history of the underlying renal disorder. The difficulty in ascertaining a negative effect on long-term renal function is because study numbers with a particular renal disease are limited and prospective studies with ample population sizes are impossible to obtain. Therefore, much of the information is derived from either retrospective analysis or cross-sectionally designed studies. With these limitations in mind, most studies report no adverse relationship between pregnancy and postpartum renal function [246, 247]. More recent studies have addressed risk factors in women who become pregnant with regard to a more aggressive course of renal disease following their pregnancy. ADPKD women with preexisting hypertension have a more aggressive renal course if they undergo more than three pregnancies. Women with glomerulonephritis or lupus nephropathy have a worse renal outcome if disease activity on biopsy is high close to the time of pregnancy and if the lesion is diffuse [235, 237]. Finally, in patients with preexisting renal disease who become pregnant, the risk for maternal complications increases with the attendant risk for acute irreversible renal deterioration. Therefore, in those women without hypertension, renal insufficiency, or severe disease activity or diffuse lesions on biopsy, there is a high likelihood that pregnancy will be successful, without complications and without adverse effects on long-term renal outcome.

Pregnancy and Dialysis

Hemodialysis has been used in women with chronic renal failure from a variety of causes who either became pregnant while on maintenance hemodialysis or required maintenance hemodialysis because of the development of end-stage renal disease during pregnancy [248]. The largest reported experience of pregnant patients on maintenance hemodialysis comes from Europe [249], where approximately 1 in 200 women become pregnant. This may underestimate the fertility of women on maintenance hemodialysis, as missed periods and menstrual irregularities are common and may represent early spontaneous abortions. Those who conceive have a very poor fetal outcome, with only 7 of 74 pregnancies successful, 32 resulting in therapeutic abortion, and 35 resulting in spontaneous abortion. When excluding spontaneous abortions, the best fetal survival in experienced hands reaches 30 percent [250]. The issues specific to women requiring dialysis who become pregnant include the risk of hypotension to the fetus, the increased risk of hemorrhage with heparin, the lack of flexibility in tolerating large shifts in intravascular volume with regard to the increased cardiovascular risk, and more difficult to control blood pressure in this group of women [251]. Finally, nutritional considerations become paramount, with intrauterine growth combating uremia and volume overload. Women undergoing hemodialysis during pregnancy have a high rate of prematurity, with uterine contractions occurring frequently immediately following dialysis. Given these observations, some modifications in dialytic technique have been proposed for pregnant women [248]. Hypotension on dialysis should be treated or prevented with albumin rather than saline. Ultrafiltration and dialysis should not be performed simultaneously because peripheral vascular resistance is diminished in pregnancy. More aggressive dialysis (increasing by 50%) should be sought, with attempts at keeping predialytic BUN to less than 70 mg/dl [248, 251]. The increase in dialysis time will also improve blood pressure control and minimize intradialytic weight gain [252]. Clearly, multiple health caregivers are required if a successful pregnancy is to occur.

Peritoneal dialysis is a possible alternative to hemodialysis during pregnancy [253]. The advantages of this modality is that nutritional restrictions can be lifted and dialysis is slow and steady, avoiding large shifts in intravascular volume, hypotension, and uterine contractions. Heparin is not used, and therefore one risk for bleeding is minimized. The risks of premature labor, sudden intrauterine death, hypertension, anemia, and abruptio placentae remain, however, and the possibility of peritonitis is always present [249].

Pregnancy Following Renal Transplant

Fertility improves following renal transplantation, with 1 in 50 becoming pregnant. Approximately 40 percent do not pass the first trimester, but over 90 percent of those that continue past early pregnancy end successfully [254]. Approximately half of renal allograft recipients will have a problem in pregnancy, with 12 percent having long-term problems related to gestation. The recommended wait for planning a pregnancy following transplantation varies; however, usually a wait of at least 2 years with stable renal function and without acute rejection within 6 months of conception is recommended. Interestingly, renal function in the transplanted kidney increases during gestation, and transient reductions in the third trimester are not uncommon and do not usually represent a deteriorating situation [255]. Approximately 15 percent will develop acute renal deterioration that will persist past the pregnancy [256]. Proteinuria occurs in the third trimester in approximately 40 percent of patients but in the absence of hypertension is not clinically significant. The proteinuria resolves with delivery. The occurrence rate of acute transplant rejection during pregnancy is no different than the nonpregnant population, but an increased occurrence appears to exist in the peripartum period. Chronic rejection is difficult to diagnose and requires a high level of suspicion to identify correctly. Renal biopsy is always necessary to make the diagnosis. Preeclampsia occurs in approximately 30 percent of patients, and an increased incidence of infection and diabetes occurs in this group of patients. Immunosuppressive agents are given, and the goal of therapy is to maintain levels similar to nonpregnancy. Cyclosporin A has not been well studied in pregnancy but appears to have similar pregnancy outcome rates as other immunosuppressive regimens [252, 257].

References

1. Fried AW: Hydronephrosis of pregnancy: Ultrasonographic study and classification of asymptomatic women. *Am J Obstet Gynecol* 135:1066, 1979.
2. Davison JM: The kidney in pregnancy: A review. *J R Soc Med* 76:485–501, 1983.
3. Sheehan HL, Lynch JP: *Pathology of Toxemia of Pregnancy*. Baltimore, Williams & Wilkins, 1973.
4. Davison JM, Lindheimer MD: Changes in renal hemodynamics and kidney weight during pregnancy in the unanesthetized rat. *J Physiol* 301:129–136, 1980.
5. Dure-Smith P: Pregnancy dilatation of the urinary tract: The iliac sign and its significance. *Radiology* 96:545, 1970.
6. Roberts JA: Hydronephrosis of pregnancy. *Urology* 8:1, 1976.
7. Fried W, Woodring JH, Thompson DS: Hydronephrosis in pregnancy: A prospective sequential study of the course of dilation. *J Ultrasound Med* 2:255, 1982.
8. Chapman AB, Zamudio S, Abraham W, et al: Renal and hemodynamic changes in the first trimester of human pregnancy (P) occur prior to placentation. *XIVth International Society of Nephrol.* Presented in Madrid, Spain, July 2–5, 1995.
9. Page EW, Christianson R: The impact of mean arterial blood pressure in middle trimester upon the outcome of pregnancy. *Am J Obstet Gynecol* 125:740, 1976.
10. Robson SC, Hunter S, Boys RJ, Dunlop W: Serial study of factors influencing changes in cardiac output during human pregnancy. *Am J Physiol* 256:H1060–H1065, 1989.

11. Zamudio S, Palmer SK, Dahms TE, et al: Blood volume expansion, preeclampsia, and infant birth weight at high altitude. *J Appl Physiol* 75(4):1566–1573, 1993.
12. Phippard AF, Horvath JS, Glynn EM, et al: Circulation adaptation to pregnancy: Serial studies of hemodynamics, blood volume, renin and aldosterone in the baboon. *J Hypertens* 4:733, 1986.
13. Baylis C: Glomerular ultrafiltration in the pseudopregnant rat. *Am J Physiol* 242:F300, 1982.
14. Fitzgerald JD, Entmann S, Mulloy K, Fitzgerald GA: Decreased prostacyclin biosynthesis preceding the clinical manifestations of pregnancy-induced hypertension. *Circulation* 75: 956–963, 1987.
15. Fitzgerald JD, Mayo G, Catella F, et al: Increased thromboxane biosynthesis in normal pregnancy is mainly derived from platelets. *Am J Obstet Gynecol* 157:325–330, 1987.
16. Fitzgerald DJ, Fitzgerald A: Eicosanoids in the Pathogenesis of Preeclampsia. In Laragh J, Brenner BM (eds): *Hypertension: Pathophysiology, Diagnosis and Management.* New York, Raven Press, 1990, pp 1789–1807.
17. Gant NF, Whalley PJ, Everett RB, et al: Control of vascular reactivity in pregnancy. *Am J Kidney Dis* 9:303–307, 1987.
18. Paller MS: Mechanisms of decreased pressor responsiveness to ANG II, NE, and vasopressin in pregnant rats. *Am J Physiol* 247:H100, 1984.
19. Brown MA, Boughton Pipkin F, Symonds EM: The effects of intravenous angiotensin II upon blood pressure and sodium and urate excretion in human pregnancy. *J Hypertens* 6:457–464, 1988.
20. August Taufield P, Mueller FB, Edersheim TG, et al: Blood pressure regulation in normal pregnancy: Unmasking the role of the renin angiotensin system with captopril. *Clin Res* 35: 433A, 1988.
21. Olssen K, Fyrquist F, Benlamlih K: Effects of captopril on arterial blood pressure, plasma renin activity and vasopressin concentration in sodium-repleted and sodium-deficient goats: A serial study during pregnancy, lactation and anestrus. *Acta Physiol Scand* 121:73–80, 1984.
22. Everett RB, Warley RJ, MacDonald PC: Effect of prostaglandin synthesis inhibitors in pressin response to angiotensin II in human pregnancy. *J Clin Endocrinol Metab* 46:1007–1010, 1978.
23. Conrad KP, Colpoys MC: Evidence against the hypothesis that prostaglandins are the vasodepressor agents of pregnancy: Serial studies in chronically instrumented, conscious rats. *J Clin Invest* 77:236, 1986.
24. Weiner CP, Lizasoain I, Baylis SA, et al: Induction of calcium-dependent nitric oxide synthase by sex hormones. *Proc Natl Acad Sci USA* 91:5212–5216, 1994.
25. Conrad KP, Joffe GM, Krusayna H, et al: Identification of increased nitric oxide biosynthesis during pregnancy in rats. *FASEB J* 7:566–571, 1993.
26. Molinar M, Hertelendy F: Nw-nitro L-arginine, an inhibitor of nitric oxide synthesis, increases blood pressure in rats and reverses the pregnancy-induced refractoriness to vasopressor agents. *Am J Obstet Gynecol* 166:1560–1567, 1992.
27. Cameron IT, van Papendorp CL, Palmer RMJ, et al: Relationship between nitric oxide synthesis and increase in systolic blood pressure in women with hypertension in pregnancy. *Hypertens Pregnancy* 12:85–92, 1993.
28. Myatt L, Brewer A, Brockman DE: The action of nitric oxide in the perfused human fetal-placental circulation. *Am J Obstet Gynecol* 164:687–692, 1991.
29. Ales KL, Norton ME, Druzin ML: Early prediction of antepartum hypertension. *Obstet Gynecol* 73:928–933, 1989.
30. Villar J, Repke J, Markush L, et al: The measuring of blood pressure during pregnancy. *Am J Obstet Gynecol* 161:1019–1024, 1989.
31. Johenning AR, Barron WM: Indirect blood pressure measurement in pregnancy: Korotkoff phase 4 versus phase 5. *Am J Obstet Gynecol* 167(3):577–580, 1992.
32. Ginsburg J, Duncan S: Direct and indirect blood pressure measurements in pregnancy. *J Obstet Gynecol Br Commonw* 76:705–710, 1969.
33. Perry IJ, Beevers DG, Luesley DM: Recording diastolic blood pressure in pregnancy. *BMJ* 302:179–180, 1991.
34. Davison JM: Renal hemodynamics and volume homeostasis in pregnancy. *Scand J Clin Lab Invest* [Suppl] 169:15–24, 1984.

35. Dunlop W: Serial changes in renal hemodynamics during normal human pregnancy. *Br J Obstet Gynaecol* 88:1–8, 1981.

35a. Deng A, Engels K, Baylis C: Impact of nitric oxide deficiency on blood pressure and glomerular hemodynamic adaptations to pregnancy in the rat. *Kidney Int* 50:1132–1138, 1996.

36. Sturgiss SN, Davison JM: Effect of pregnancy on long-term function of renal allografts. *Am J Kidney Dis* 19:167–172, 1992.

37. Imbasciati E, Ponticelli C: Pregnancy and renal disease. *Am J Nephrol* 11:353–362, 1991.

38. Atherton JC, Bielinska A, Davison JM, et al: Sodium and water reabsorption in the proximal and distal nephron in conscious pregnant rats and third trimester women. *J Physiol* (Lond) 396:457–470, 1988.

39. Alfrey AC, Durr JA, Miller N: The determination of endogenous lithium (li) as a marker of proximal tubular Na and H_2O handling. *Kidney Int* 31:189, 1987.

40. Bishop JHV: Glucose handling by distal portions of the nephron during pregnancy in the rat. *J Physiol* 336:131, 1983.

41. Erhlich EN, Lindheimer MD: Effect of administered mineralocorticoids of ACTH in pregnant women: Attenuation of kaliuretic influence of mineralocorticoids during pregnancy. *J Clin Invest* 51:1301, 1972.

42. Davison JM, Hytten FE: The effect of pregnancy on the renal handling of glucose. *Br J Obstet Gynaecol* 82:374, 1975.

43. Fine J: Glycosuria in pregnancy. *Br Med J* 1:205, 1967.

44. Welsh GW III, Sims EA: The mechanism of renal glucosuria in pregnancy. *Diabetes* 9:363, 1960.

45. Hytten FE, Cheyne GA: The aminoaciduria of pregnancy. *Br J Obstet Gynaecol* 79:242, 1972.

46. Dunlop W, Davison JM: The effect of normal pregnancy upon the renal handling of uric acid. *Br J Obstet Gynaecol* 84:13, 1977.

47. Gray MJ, et al: Regulation of sodium and total body water metabolism in pregnancy. *Am J Obstet Gynaecol* 89:760, 1964.

48. Barron WM, Davison J, Lindheimer MD: Water metabolism in pregnancy. *Semin Nephrol* 4:334, 1984.

49. Pipe NG, Smith T, Halliday D: Changes in fat free mass and body water in normal human pregnancy. *Br J Obstet Gynecol* 86:929–933, 1979.

50. Davison JM, Valloton MB, Lindheimer MD: Plasma osmolality and urinary concentration and dilution during and after pregnancy: Evidence that lateral recumbency inhibits maximal urinary concentrating ability. *Br J Obstet Gynaecol* 88:472, 1981.

51. Davison JM, Shiells EA, Philips PR, et al: Serial evaluation of vasopressin and thirst in human pregnancy. *J Clin Invest* 81:798, 1988.

52. Lindheimer MD, Barron WM, Durr JA, Davison JM: Water homeostasis and vasopressin release during rodent and human gestation. *Am J Kidney Dis* 9:270–275, 1987.

53. Barron WM, Schreiber J, Lindheimer MD: Effect of ovarian sex steroids on osmoregulation and vasopressin secretion in the rat. *Am J Physiol* 250:E352, 1986.

54. Hytten FE: Physiological changes in early pregnancy. *J Obstet Gynec Br Commonw* 75:1193–1197, 1968.

55. Davison JM, Gilmore EA, Durr J, et al: Altered osmotic threshold for vasopressin secretion and thirst in human pregnancies. *Am J Physiol* 246:F105, 1984.

56. Robertson GL: Abnormalities in thirst regulation. *Nephrol Forum Kidney Int* 25:460–469, 1984.

57. Durr JV, Stamoutsos B, Lindheimer MD: Osmoregulation during pregnancy in the rat. *J Clin Invest* 68:337, 1981.

58. Brown MA, Gallery EDM: Sodium excretion in human pregnancy: A role for arginine vasopressin. *Am J Obstet Gynecol* 154:914–919, 1986.

59. Hytten FE, Thompson AM, Taggart N: Total body water in normal pregnancy. *Br J Obstet Gynaecol* 73:553, 1966.

60. Walker J, Garland HO: Single nephron function during prolactin-induced pseudopregnancy in the rat. *J Endocrinol* 107:127–131, 1985.

61. Worley RJ, Hentschel WM, Cormier C, et al: Increased sodium-lithium countertransport in erythrocytes of pregnant women. *N Engl J Med* 307:412–416, 1982.

62. Schrier RW, Briner VA: Peripheral arterial vasodilation hypothesis of sodium and water retention in pregnancy: Implication for pathogenesis of preeclampsia-eclampsia. *Obstet Gynecol* 77:632–639, 1991.

63. Durr JA, Hoggard JG, Hunt JM, et al: Diabetes insipidus in pregnancy associated with abnormally high circulating vasopressin activity. *N Engl J Med* 316:1070, 1987.

64. Davison JM, Shiells EA, Barron WM, et al: Changes in the metabolic clearance of vasopressin and of vasopressinase throughout human pregnancy. *J Clin Invest* 83:1313, 1989.

65. Nolten WE, Ehrlich EM: Sodium and mineralocorticoids in normal pregnancy. *Kidney Int* 18:162, 1980.

66. Brown MA, Nicholson E, Ross MR, et al: Progressive resetting of sodium-renin-aldosterone relationship in human pregnancy. *Clin Exp Hypertens [B]* B5(3):349–375, 1986/1987.

67. Brown MA, Boughton Pipkin F, Symonds EM: The effects of intravenous angiotensin upon blood pressure and sodium and urate excretion in human pregnancy. *J Hypertens* 6:457–464, 1988.

68. Chesley LC: Simultaneous renal clearance of urea and uric acid in the differential diagnosis of late toxemias. *Am J Obstet Gynecol* 59:960, 1950.

69. Oparil S, Ehrlich EN, Lindeheimer M: Effects of progesterone on renal sodium handling in man: Relation to aldosterone excretion and plasma renin activity. *Clin Sci Mol Med* 49:139–147, 1975.

70. Wambach G, Higgens JR: Antimineralocorticoid action of progesterone in the rat: Correlation of the effect on electrolyte excretion and interaction with renal mineralocorticoid receptors. *Endocrinology* 102:1686–1693, 1978.

71. Thomsen JK, Fogh-Anderson N, Jaszczak P, Giese J: Atrial natriuretic peptide (ANP) decreases during normal pregnancy as related to hemodynamic changes and volume regulation. *Acta Obstet Gynecol Scand* 72:103–110, 1993.

72. Sealey JE, McCord D, Taufield PA, et al: Plasma prorenin in first trimester pregnancy: Relationship to changes in human chorionic gonadotropin. *Am J Obstet Gynecol* 153:514–519, 1985.

73. Derkx FH, Alberda AT, DeJong FH, et al: Source of plasma prorenin in early and late pregnancy: Observations in a patient with primary ovarian failure. *J Clin Endocrinol Metab* 65:349–354, 1987.

74. Brar HS, Doy-S, Tam HB, et al: Uteroplacental unit as a source of elevated circulating prorenin levels in normal pregnancy. *Am J Obstet Gynecol* 155(6):1223–1226, 1986.

75. Poisner AM, Words GW, Poisner R, Inagami T: Localization of renin in trophoblast in human chorion laeve at term pregnancy. *Endocrinology* 109:1150–1154, 1981.

76. Rosenfeld CR, Gant NF: The chronically instrumented ewe: A model for studying vascular reactivity to angiotensin II in pregnancy. *J Clin Invest* 67:486, 1981.

77. Tewksbury DA, Dent RA: Elevated high molecular weight angiotensinogen levels in hypertensive pregnant women. *Hypertension* 4:729–734, 1982.

78. Tewksbury DA, Tyler ES, Burrill RE, Dart RA: High molecular weight angiotensinogen: A pregnancy associated problem. *Clin Chem Acta* 158:7–12, 1986.

79. Sealey JE, Atlas SA, Laragh JH: Prorenin and other large molecular weight forms of renin. *Endocr Rev* 1:365–391, 1980.

80. Sealey JE, Wilson M, Morganti AA, et al: Changes in active and inactive renin throughout normal pregnancy. *Clin Exp Hypertens* 4A:2372–2384, 1982.

81. Gorden P, Ferris TF, Mulrow PJ: Rabbit uterus as a possible site of renin synthesis. *Am J Physiol* 212:703–706, 1967.

82. Albertini R, Seino M, Scicli AG, Carretoero OA: Uteroplacental renin in regulation of blood pressure in the pregnant rabbit. *Am J Physiol* 239:H266–H271, 1980.

83. Venuto RC, O'Dorisio T, Stein JH, et al: Uterine prostaglandin E secretion and uterine blood flow in pregnant rabbit. *J Clin Invest* 55:193, 1975.

84. Wilson M, Marganti AA, Zeroudakis I, et al: Blood pressure, the renin-aldosterone system and sex steroids throughout normal pregnancy. *Am J Med* 68:97–102, 1980.

85. Broughton-Pipkin F, Symonds EM, Turner SR: The effect of captopril upon mother and fetus in the chronically cannulated ewe and in the pregnant rabbit. *J Physiol* 323:415, 1982.

86. Baler PN, Broughton Pipkin F, Symonds EM: Platelet angiotensin II binding and plasma renin concentration, plasma renin substrate and plasma angiotensin II in human pregnancy. *Clin Sci* 79:403–408, 1990.

87. Sanchez-Ramos L, O'Sullivan MJ, Garrido Calderon J: Effect of low-dose aspirin on angiotensin II pressor response in human pregnancy. *Am J Obstet Gynecol* 156:193–194, 1987.

88. Rosenfeld CR, Jackson GM: Estrogen-induced refractoriness to the pressor effects of infused angiotensin II. *Am J Obstet Gynecol* 148:429, 1984.

89. Conrad KP: Possible mechanisms for changes in renal hemodynamics during pregnancy: Studies from animal models. *Am J Kidney Dis* 9:253–259, 1987.

90. Ferris TF, Stein JH, Kauffman J: Uterine blood flow and uterine renin secretion. *J Clin Invest* 51:2827, 1972.

91. Terragno NA, Terragno DA, Pacholczyk D, et al: Prostaglandins and the regulation of uterine blood flow in pregnancy. *Nature* 249:57, 1974.

92. Ferris TF, Weir EK: Effect of captopril on uterine blood flow and prostaglandin E synthesis in the pregnant rabbit. *J Clin Invest* 71:809, 1983.

93. Franklin GO, Dowd AJ, Caldwell BV, Speroff L: The effect of angiotensin II intravenous infusion on plasma renin activity and prostaglandin A, E, and F levels in the uterine vein of the pregnant monkey. *Prostaglandins* 6:261–280, 1974.

94. Wilkes BM, Krim E, Mento PF: Evidence for a functional renin-angiotensin system in full term fetoplacental unit. *Am J Physiol* 249:E466–E373, 1985.

95. Alhenc-Gelas F, Tache A, Saint-Andre JP, et al: The renin-angiotensin system in pregnancy and parturition. *Adv Nephrol* 15:25–33, 1986.

96. Douglas KA, Redman CWG: Eclampsia in the United Kingdom. *Br Med J* 309:1395–1400, 1994.

97. Barker DJP, Bull AR, Osmond C, Simmonds SJ: Fetal and placental size and risk of hypertension in adult life. *Br Med J* 301:259–262, 1990.

98. Fisher KA, Luger A, Spargo BH, et al: Hypertension in pregnancy: Clinicopathologic correlation and remote prognosis. *Medicine* 60:267, 1981.

99. Katz AI, Davison JM, Hayslett JP: Pregnancy in women with kidney disease. *Kidney Int* 18:192, 1980.

100. Hughes ED (ed): *Obstetric-Gynecologic Terminology.* Philadelphia, FA Davis, 1972, pp 422–423.

101. The National High Blood Pressure Education Program Working Group: Report on high blood pressure in pregnancy. *Am J Obstet Gynecol* 163:1689–1712, 1990.

102. Miyamoto S, Shimokawa H, Sumioki H, et al: Circadian rhythm of plasma atrial natriuretic peptide, aldosterone and blood pressure during the third trimester in normal and preeclamptic pregnancies. *Am J Obstet Gynecol* 158:393–399, 1988.

103. Saftlas AF, Olson DR, Franks AL, et al: Epidemiology of preeclampsia and eclampsia in the United States, 1979–1986. *Am J Obstet Gynecol* 163:460–465, 1990.

104. Naeye RL, Friedman EA: Causes of perinatal death associated with gestational hypertension and proteinuria. *Am J Obstet Gynecol* 133:8, 1979.

105. Redman CWG: Treatment of hypertension in pregnancy. *Kidney Int* 18:267, 1980.

106. Sibai BM, McCubbin JH, Anderson GD, et al: Eclampsia: I. Observations from 67 recent cases. *Obstet Gynecol* 58:609–613, 1981.

107. Arnoudse JG, Houthoff HJ, Weits J, et al: A syndrome of liver damage and intravascular coagulation in the last trimester of normotensive pregnancy. *Br J Obstet Gynecol* 93:145–155, 1986.

108. Weinstein L: Preeclampsia/eclampsia with hemolysis, elevated liver enzymes and thrombocytopenia. *Obstet Gynecol* 66:657, 1985.

109. Cotton DB, Wesley L, Huhta J, Dorman KF: Hemodynamic profile of severe pregnancy-induced hypertension. *Am J Obstet Gynecol* 158:523–529, 1988.

110. Mabie WC, Ratts TE, Sibai BM: The central hemodynamics of severe preeclampsia. *Am J Obstet Gynecol* 161:1443–1448, 1989.

111. Easterling TR, Benedetti TJ, Schmucker RC, Millard SP: Maternal hemodynamics in normal and preeclamptic pregnancies: A longitudinal study. *Obstet Gynecol* 76:1061–1069, 1990.

112. Visser W, Wallenburg HCS: Central hemodynamic observations in untreated preeclamptic patients. *Hypertension* 17:1072–1077, 1991.

113. Lang RM, Pridjian G, Feldman T, et al: Alterations in left ventricular mechanics in pregnancy induced hypertension (preeclampsia): Increased afterload or cardiomyopathy? *Am Heart J* 121:1768–1775, 1991.

114. Hankins GDV, Wendel DG, Cunningham FG, Leveno KJ: Longitudinal evaluation of hemodynamic changes in eclampsia. *Am J Obstet Gynecol* 150:506–512, 1984.

115. Brown MA, Zammit VC, Mitar DFM: Extracellular fluid volumes in pregnancy-induced hypertension. *J Hypertens* 10:61–68, 1992.

116. Brown MA, Gallery EDM: Volume homeostasis in normal pregnancy and preeclampsia. *Clin Obstet Gynecol* (Bailliere), 1994.

117. Brown MA, Zammit VC, Lowe SA: Capillary permeability and extracellular fluid volumes in pregnancy-induced hypertension. *Clin Sci* 77:599–604, 1989.

118. Chesley LC, Duffus GM: Pre-eclampsia, posture and renal function. *Obstet Gynecol* 38:1, 1971.

119. Sibai BM, Villar MA, Mabie BC: Acute renal failure in hypertensive disorders of pregnancy: Pregnancy outcome and remote prognosis in thirty-one consecutive cases. *Am J Obstet Gynecol* 162:777, 1990.

120. Redman CWG, Berlin LJ, Bonnar J, et al: Plasma-urate measurements in predicting fetal death in hypertensive pregnancy. *Lancet* II:1370–1376, 1976.

121. Taufield PA, Ales K, Resnick L, et al: Hypocalciuria in preeclampsia. *N Engl J Med* 316:715–718, 1986.

122. August P, Lenz T, Ales KL, et al: Longitudinal study of the renin angiotensin system in hypertensive women: Deviations related to the development of superimposed preeclampsia. *Am J Obstet Gynecol* 163:1612–1621, 1990.

123. Magness RR, Cox K, Rosenfeld CR, Gant NF: Angiotensin II metabolic clearance rate and pressor responses in nonpregnant and pregnant women. *Am J Obstet Gynecol* 171:668–679, 1994.

124. Aalkjaer C, Johannesen P, Petersen EB, et al: Characteristics of resistance vessels in preeclampsia and normotensive pregnancy. *J Hypertens* 2(Suppl 3):183–185, 1984.

125. Aalkjaer C, Danielsen H, Johannesen P, et al: Abnormal vascular function and morphology in preeclampsia: A study of isolated resistance vessels. *Clin Sci* 69:483–492, 1985.

126. Nissell H, Hjemdahl P, Linde B, Lunell N-O: Cardiovascular responses to isometric handgrip exercise, an invasive study in pregnancy-induced hypertension. *Obstet Gynecol* 70:339–343, 1987.

127. Rappaport VJ, Hirata G, Yap HK, et al: Antivascular endothelial cell antibodies in severe preeclampsia. *Am J Obstet Gynecol* 162:138, 1990.

128. Piranai BB, MacGillivray I: The effect of plasma retransfusion on the blood pressure in the puerperium. *Am J Obstet Gynecol* 121:221, 1975.

129. Wang Y, Walsh S, Kaig M: Placental lipid peroxides and thromboxane are measured and prostacyclin decreased in women with preeclampsia. *Am J Obstet Gynecol* 167:946–949, 1992.

130. Parisi VM, Rankin JHG: The effect of prostacyclin on angiotensin II induced placental vasoconstriction. *Am J Obstet Gynecol* 151:444–449, 1985.

131. Ferris TF, Venuto RC, Baer WH: Studies of the Uterine Circulation in Pregnant Rabbits. In Lindheimer MD, Katz AI, Zuspan FR (eds): *Hypertension in Pregnancy.* New York, Wiley, 1976.

132. Stuart MJ, Clark D, Sundrys SG: Decreased prostacyclin production: A characteristic of chronic placental insufficiency syndrome. *Lancet* 1:1126, 1981.

133. Arkwright PD, Rademacher TW, Dwek RA, Redman CWG: Preeclampsia is associated with an increase in trophoblast glycogen content and glycogen synthase activity, similar to that found in hydatiform moles. *J Clin Invest* 91:2744–2753, 1993.

134. Zhou Y, Damsky CH, Chiu K, et al: Preeclampsia is associated with abnormal expression of adhesion molecules by invasive cytotrophoblasts. *J Clin Invest* 91:950–960, 1993.

135. Remuzzi G, Marchesi D, Zoja C: Reduced umbilical and placental vascular prostacyclin in severe preeclampsia. *Prostaglandins* 20:105–110, 1980.

136. Umans JG, Lindheimer MD, Barron WM: Pressor effect of endothelium-derived relaxing factor inhibition in conscious virgin and gravid rats. *Am J Physiol* 259:F293, 1990.
136a. Danielson LA, Conrad KP: Acute blockade of nitric oxide synthase inhibits renal vasodilation and hyperfiltration during pregnancy in chronically instrumented conscious rats. *J Clin Invest* 96:482–490, 1995.
137. Pinto A, Sorrentino R, Sorrentino P, et al: Endothelial-derived relaxing factor released by endothelial cells of human umbilical vessels and its impairment in pregnancy induced hypertension. *Am J Obstet Gynecol* 164:507–513, 1991.
138. McCarthy AL, Woolfso RG, Rajui SK, Poston L: Abnormal endothelial cell function of resistance arteries from women with preeclampsia. *Am J Obstet Gynecol* 168:(4):1323–1330, 1993.
139. Seligman SP, Abramson SB, Young BK, Buyon JP: The role of nitric oxide (NO) in the pathogenesis of preeclampsia. *Am J Obstet Gynecol* 170:290, 1994.
140. Gaspari F, Benigni A, Orisio S, et al: Human placenta expresses the endothelin gene and the corresponding protein is excreted in the urine in increasing amounts during the course of normal pregnancy (abstract). *J Am Soc Nephrol* 1:415, 1990.
141. McMahan LP, Redman CWG, Futh JD: Expression of the three endothelin genes and plasma levels of endothelin in preeclamptic and normal gestations. *Clin Sci* 85:417–424, 1993.
142. Kerkes SA, Postin L, Wolf CD: A longitudinal study of maternal digoxin-like immunoreactive substances in normotensive pregnancy and pregnancy induced hypertension. *Am J Obstet Gynecol* 162:783–787, 1990.
143. Strazzullo P, Nunziata V, Cirillo M, et al: Abnormalities of calcium metabolism in essential hypertension. *Clin Sci* 65:137, 1983.
144. Zemel MB, Zemel PC, Berry J, et al: Altered platelet calcium metabolism as an early predictor of increased peripheral vascular resistance and preeclampsia in urban black women. *N Engl J Med* 323:434, 1990.
145. Nardulli G, Proverbio F, Limingi FG, et al: Preeclampsia and calcium adenosine triphosphatase activity of red blood cell ghosts. *Am J Obstet Gynecol* 171(5):1361–1365, 1994.
146. Spargo B, McCartney CP, Winemiller R: Glomerular capillary endotheliosis in toxemia of pregnancy. *AMA Arch Pathol* 68:593, 1959.
147. Gabei LW, Spargo BH, Lindheimer MD: The Nephropathy of Preeclampsia-Eclampsia. In Tisher CC, Brenner BM (eds): *Renal Pathology* (2nd ed). Philadelphia, Lippincott, 1994, pp 419–441.
148. Sheehan HL: Renal morphology in preeclampsia. *Kidney Int* 18:241, 1980.
149. Petrucco, OM: Immunofluorescent studies in renal biopsies in preeclampsia. *Br Med J* 1:473, 1986.
150. Packham DK, Mathews DC, Fairley KF, et al: Morphometric analysis of pre-eclampsia in women biopsied in pregnancy and post-partum. *Kidney Int* 34:704–711, 1988.
151. Sheehan HL, Lynch JB: *Pathology of Toxemia of Pregnancy*. London, Churchill Livingstone, 1973.
152. Chesley LC: *Hypertensive Disorders in Pregnancy*. New York, Appleton-Century-Crofts, 1978.
153. Chesley LC, Cooper DW: Genetics of hypertension in pregnancy: Possible single gene control of pre-eclampsia and eclampsia in the descendants of eclamptic women. *Br J Obstet Gynecol* 93:898, 1986.
154. Collins R, Yusuf S, Peto R: Overview of randomized trials of diuretics in pregnancy. *Br Med J* 290:17, 1985.
155. Beaufils M, Uzan S, Donsimoni R, et al: Prevention of preeclampsia by early antiplatelet therapy. *Lancet* 1:840, 1985.
156. Schiff E, Peleg E, Goldenberg M, et al: The use of aspirin to prevent pregnancy-induced hypertension and lower the ratio of thromboxane A_2 to prostacyclin in relatively high risk pregnancies. *N Engl J Med* 321:351, 1989.
157. CLASP (Collaborative Low-Dose Aspirin in Pregnancy) Collaborative Group. CLASP: A randomized trial of low-dose aspirin for the prevention and treatment of preeclampsia among 9,364 pregnant women. *Lancet* 343:619–629, 1994.
158. Italian Study of Aspirin in Pregnancy. Low-dose aspirin in prevention and treatment of

intrauterine growth retardation and pregnancy-induced hypertension. *Lancet* 341:396–400, 1993.

159. Sibai BM, Caritis SN, Thom E, et al: Low-dose aspirin for the prevention and treatment of preeclampsia in healthy, nulliparous, pregnant women. *N Engl J Med* 329:1213–1218, 1993.

160. Belizan JM, Villar J, Gonzalez L, et al: Calcium supplementation to prevent hypertensive disorders of pregnancy. *N Engl J Med* 325:1399–1405, 1991.

161. Repke JT, Villar J: Pregnancy-induced hypertension and low birth weight: The role of calcium. *Am J Clin Nutr* 54:2375–2415, 1991.

162. Kawasaki N, Matsui K, Ito M, et al: Effect of calcium supplementation on the vascular sensitivity to angiotensin II in pregnant women. *Am J Obstet Gynecol* 153:576–582, 1985.

163. Lopez-Jaramillo P, Narvaez M, Weigel RM, Yepez R: Calcium supplementation reduces the risk of pregnancy-induced hypertension in an Andes population. *Br J Obstet Gynecol* 96: 648–655, 1989.

163a. Osono F, Johnson A, Linas L, Chapman A: Pregnancy-induced hypercalciuria occurs early in pregnancy, prior to fetal placentation. *J Am Soc Nephrol* 12:471.

164. Brown MA: Non-pharmacological management of pregnancy induced hypertension. *J Hypertens* 8:295–301, 1990.

165. Sibai BM, Mabie WC, Shamsa F, et al: A comparison of no medication versus methyldopa or labetalol in chronic hypertension during pregnancy. *Am J Obstet Gynecol* 162:960–967, 1990.

166. Cruickshank DJ, Roberson AA, Campbell DM, MacGllivaray I: Does labetalol influence the development of proteinuria in pregnancy hypertension? A randomized controlled study. *Eur J Obstet Gynecol Reprod Biol* 45:47–51, 1992.

167. Plouin PF, Breart G, Llado J, et al: A randomized comparison of early *???* with conservative use of antihypertensive drugs in the management of pregnancy-induced hypertension. *Br J Obstet Gynecol* 97:134–141, 1990.

168. Blake S, MacDonald D: The prevention of the maternal manifestations of preeclampsia by intensive antihypertensive treatment. *Br J Obstet Gynecol* 98:244–248, 1991.

169. Butters L, Kennedy S, Rubin PC: Atenolol in essential hypertension during pregnancy. *Br Med J* 301:587–589, 1990.

170. Bhorat IE, Naidoo DP, Rout CC, Moodley J: Malignant ventricular arrhythmias in eclampsia, a comparison of labetalol with hydralazine. *Am J Obstet Gynecol* 168:1292–1296, 1993.

171. Belfort M, Uys P, Dommissee J, Davey DA: Hemodynamic changes in gestational proteinuria hypertension: The effects of rapid volume expansion and vasodilator therapy. *Br J Obstet Gynecol* 96:634–641, 1989.

172. Harper A, Hurnaghan GA: Maternal and fetal hemodynamics in hypertensive pregnancies during maternal treatment with intravenous hydralazine or labetalol. *Br J Obstet Gynecol* 98: 453–459, 1991.

173. Vink GJ, Hoodley JM, Philpott RM: Effect of dihydralazine on the fetus in the treatment of maternal hypertension. *Obstet Gynecol* 55:519–522, 1980.

174. Garden A, Davey DA, Dommisse J: Intravenous labetalol and intravenous dihydralazine in severe hypertension in pregnancy. *Clin Exp Hypertens Part B Hypertension Pregnancy* B1(2 & 3):371–383, 1991.

175. Kjellmer I, Dagbjartsson A, Hrbek A, et al: Maternal beta-adrenoreceptor blockade reduces fetal tolerance to asphyxia. *Acta Obstet Gynecol Scand* 118:75–80, 1984.

176. Martins-Costa S, Ramos JG, Barros E, et al: Randomized controlled trial of hydralazine versus nifedipine in preeclamptic women with acute hypertension. *Clin Exp Hypertens Pregnancy* B11(1):25–44, 1992.

177. Fenakel IC, Fenakel G, Appelman Z, et al: Nifedipine in the treatment of severe preeclampsia. *Am J Obstet Gynecol* 77:331–337, 1991.

178. Henrich WL, Cronin R, Miller PD, Anderson RJ: Hypotensive sequelae of diazoxide and hydralazine therapy. *JAMA* 237(3):264–265, 1977.

179. Naulty J, Cefalo RC, Lewis PE: Fetal toxicity of nitroprusside in the pregnant ewe. *Am J Obstet Gynecol* 139:708–711, 1981.

180. Neumann J, Weiss B, Rabello Y, et al: Diazoxide for the acute control of severe hypertension complicating pregnancy: A pilot study. *Am J Obstet Gynecol* 53:550–555, 1979.

181. Nadler JL, Goodson S, Rude RK: Evidence that prostacyclin mediates the vascular action of magnesium in humans. *Hypertension* 9:379–383, 1987.
182. Barton JR, Sibai BM, Ahokas RA, et al: Magnesium sulfate therapy in preeclampsia is associated with increased urinary cyclic guanosine monophosphate excretion. *Am J Obstet Gynecol* 167:931–934, 1992.
183. Mastrogiannis DS, Kalter CS, Õ'Brien WF, et al: Effect of magnesium sulfate on plasma endothelin-1 levels in normal and preeclamptic pregnancies. *Am J Obstet Gynecol* 167:1554–1559, 1992.
184. Nelson SH, Suresh MS: Magnesium sulfate-induced relaxation of uterine arteries from pregnant and nonpregnant patients. *Am J Obstet Gynecol* 164:1344–1350, 1991.
185. Snyder SW, Cardwell MS: Neuromuscular blockade with magnesium sulfate and nifedipine. *Am J Obstet Gynecol* 161:35–36, 1985.
186. Waisman GD, Mayarga LM, Camera MI, et al: Magnesium plus nephedripine: Potentiation of hypotensive effect of preeclampisa? *Am J Obstet Gynecol* 159:308–309, 1988.
187. Lowe SA, Hetmanski DJ, MacDonald I, et al: Intravenous volume expansion therapy in pregnancy-induced hypertension: The role of vasoactive hormones. *Hypertens Pregnancy* 12:139–151, 1993.
188. Gallery EDM: The role of volume expansion in clinical management of hypertensive pregnant women. *Hypertens Pregnancy* 12:9–13, 1993.
189. Jouppila P, Jouppila R, Koivula A: Albumin infusion does not alter the intervillous blood flow in severe pre-eclampsia. *Acta Obstet Gynecol Scand* 62:345–348, 1983.
190. d'Apice AJ, Reet LL, Pepperell RJ: Treatment of severe preeclampsia by plasma exchange. *Aust NZ J Obstet Gynaecol* 20:231, 1980.
191. Lewis PJ, Shepherd GL, Ritter J, et al: Prostacyclin and preeclampsia. *Lancet* 1:559, 1981.
192. Toppozada MK, Ismail AA, Hegab HM, et al: Treatment of preeclampsia with prostaglandin A_1. *Am J Obstet Gynecol* 159:160, 1988.
193. Bonnard J, Redman CWG, Sheppard BL: Treatment of fetal growth retardation in utero with heparin and dipyridamole. *Eur J Obstet Gynecol Reprod Biol* 5:123–134, 1975.
194. Sibai BM, Abdella TN, Anderson GD: Pregnancy outcome in 211 patients with mild chronic hypertension. *Obstet Gynecol* 61:571, 1983.
195. Martikainen AM, Jeomprmem KM, Saarolpsio SV. The effect of hypertension in pregnancy on fetal and neonatal condition. *Int J Gynecol Obstet* 30:213–220, 1989.
196. Dunlop W, Furness C, Hill LM: *Br J Obstet Gynecol* 85:938–940, 1978.
197. Kreft C, Ploudin PF, Tchobioutshy C, et al: Angiotensin converting enzyme inhibitors during pregnancy: A summary of 22 treated patients given captopril and 9 given enalapril. *Br J Obstet Gynecol* 95:420–422, 1988.
198. Schubiger G, Flury G, Nassberger J: Enalapril for pregnancy-induced hypertension: Acute renal failure in a neonate. *Ann Intern Med* 108:215–216, 1988.
199. Knott PD, Thorpe SS, Lamont CAR: Congenital renal dysgenesis possibly due to captopril. *Lancet* 1:451, 1989.
200. Redman CWG, Berlin LJ, Bonner J, et al: Fetal outcome in trial of antihypertensive treatment in pregnancy. *Lancet* 2:753, 1976.
201. Redman CWG: Controlled trials of antihypertensive drugs in pregnancy. *Am J Kidney Dis* 17:149–153, 1991.
202. Sibai MB, Anderson GD: Pregnancy outcome of intensive therapy in severe hypertension in the first trimester. *Obstet Gynecol* 67:517–522, 1986.
203. Olunsted M, Cockburn J, Moar VA, et al: Maternal hypertension with superimposed preeclampsia: Effects on child development at $7\frac{1}{2}$ years. *Br J Obstet Gynecol* 90:644–649, 1983.
204. Huisjes MJ, Haddeus-Algea M, Touwen BCL: Is clonidine a behavioral teratogen in the human? *Early Hum Dev* 14:43–48, 1986.
205. Buffers L, Kennedy S, Rubin P: Atenolol and fetal weight in chronic hypertension (abstract). *Clin Exp Hypertens* 88:468, 1989.
206. Lunell NO, Garoff L, Grunewald C, et al: Isradipine, a new calcium antagonist: Effects on maternal and fetal hemodynamics. *J Cardiovasc Cardiol* 18(Suppl 3):537–540, 1991.
207. Cockburn J, Moar VA, Ounsted M, et al: Final report of study on hypertension during preg-

nancy: The effects of specific treatment in the growth and development of the children. *Lancet* 1:647, 1982.
208. Adams EM, MacGillivray I: Long-term effect of preeclampsia on blood pressure. *Lancet* 2: 1373, 1961.
209. Patterson TF, Andriole VT: Bacteriuria in pregnancy. *Infect Dis Clin North Am* 1:807–822, 1987.
210. Kincaid-Smith P: Bacteriuria and urinary infection in pregnancy. *Clin Obstet Gynecol* 11:533, 1968.
211. Lindheimer MD, Katz AI: Gestation in women with kidney disease. *Clin Obstet Gynaecol* 1: 921, 1987.
212. Martens MG: Pyelonephritis. *Obstet Gynecol Clin North Am* 16:305–315, 1989.
213. Whalley P, Cunningham GF: Short term versus continuous antimicrobial therapy for asymptomatic bacteriuria in pregnancy. *Obstet Gynecol* 49:262, 1977.
214. Mead PB, Guys DW: Asymptomatic Bacteriuria in Pregnancy. In de Alvarez RR (ed): *The Kidney in Pregnancy.* New York, Wiley, 1976.
215. Romero R, Oyarzun E, Mazor M, et al: Metaanalysis-analysis of the relationship between asymptomatic bacteriuria and preterm delivery/low birth weight. *Obstet Gynecol* 73:576–582, 1989.
216. McGregor JA, Well R, LaForce M: Infectious Diseases. In Abrams RS, Wexler P (eds): *Medical Care of the Pregnant Patient.* Boston, Little, Brown, 1983.
217. Zinner SH: Management of urinary tract infections in pregnancy: A review with comments on single dose therapy. *Infection* 20(Suppl):280–285, 1992.
218. Gilstrap LC, Cunningham FG, Whalley PJ: Acute pyelonephritis in pregnancy: A retrospective study. *Obstet Gynecol* 57:409, 1981.
219. Chapman AB, Schrier RW: Acute Renal Failure in Pregnancy. In Jacobsen HR, Striker GE, Klahr S (eds): *Principles and Practice of Nephrology.* St. Louis, Mosby–Year Book, 1994, pp 445–459.
220. Chugh KS, et al: Changing trends in ARF in third-world countries: The Chandigarh study. *Q J Med* 272:1117–1123, 1985.
221. Seedat YK, Nathoo BC: ARF in blacks and Indians in South Africa: Comparison after ten years. *Nephron* 64(2):198–201, 1993.
222. Bareli AI: Septic shock with renal failure after chronic villus sampling. *Am J Obstet Gynecol* 154(5):1100–1102, 1986.
223. Barton JR, Sibai BM: Acute life-threatening emergencies in preeclampsia-ecampsia. *Clin Obstet Gynecol* 35(2):402–413, 1992.
224. Barton JR, Sibai BM: Acute life-threatening emergencies in preeclampsia-eclampsia. *Clin Obstet Gynecol* 35(2):402–413, 1992.
225. Robson JS, et al: Irreversible post-partum renal failure: A new syndrome. *Q J Med* 37:423, 1968.
226. Morel-Maroger I, Kaurfer A, Solez K: Prognostic importance of vascular lesions in acute renal failure with microangiopathic hemolytic-anemia: Clinico-pathologic study in 20 adults. *Kidney Int* 15:548, 1979.
227. Mackay EV: Pregnancy and renal disease: A ten year survey. *NZ J Obstet Gynaecol* 3:21, 1963.
228. Chapman AB, Johnson AM, Gabow PA: Pregnancy outcome and its relationship to progression of renal failure in autosomal dominant polycystic kidney disease. *J Am Soc Nephrol* 5(5): 1178–1185, 1994.
229. Jungers P, Houillier P, Forfget D, Henry-Amar M: Specific controversies concerning the natural history of renal disease in pregnancy. *Am J Kidney Dis* 17:116–122, 1991.
230. Surian M, Imbasciati E, Bonfi G, et al: Glomerular disease and pregnancy: A study of 123 pregnancies in patients with primary and secondary glomerular diseases. *Nephron* 36:101, 1984.
231. Fielding C: The obstetric prognosis in chronic renal disease. *Acta Obstet Gynecol Scand* 47: 168, 1968.
232. Cunningham FG, Cox SM, Harstad TW, et al: Chronic renal disease and pregnancy outcome. *Am J Obstet Gynecol* 163:453–459, 1990.

233. Baylis C: Renal hemodynamics in the pseudopregnant rat. *Am J Physiol* 234:F300–F305, 1982.
234. Packham DK, North RA, Fairley NKF, et al: Pregnancy in women with primary focal and segmental hyalinosis and sclerosis. *Clin Nephrol* 29:185–192, 1988.
235. Packham D, North RA, Fairley KF: Primary glomerulonephritis and pregnancy. *Q J Med* 266: 537–553, 1989.
236. Abe S: The influence of pregnancy on the long-term renal prognosis in women with IgA nephropathy. *Clin Nephrol* 41:61–64, 1994.
237. Packham D, Whitworth JA, Fairley KF, Kincaid-Smith P: Histological features of IgA glomerulonephritis as predictors of pregnancy outcome. *Clin Nephrol* 30:22–26, 1988.
238. Jungers P, Forget D, Houillier P, et al: Pregnancy in IgA nephropathy, reflux nephropathy and focal glomerular sclerosis. *Am J Kidney Dis* 9:334, 1987.
239. McCune AB, Weston WL, Lee LA: Maternal and fetal outcome in neonatal lupus erythromatosus. *Ann Intern Med* 106:518, 1987.
240. Petri M, Howard D, Repke J: Frequency of lupus flare in pregnancy: The Hopkins Lupus Pregnancy Center experience. *Arthritis Rheum* 34:1538–1545, 1991.
241. Hayslett JP: Maternal and fetal complications in women with systemic lupus erythematosus. *Am J Kidney Dis* 17:123–126, 1991.
242. Kitzmiller J, Brown E, Phillipe M, et al: Diabetic nephropathy and perinatal outcome. *Am J Obstet Gynecol* 141:741, 1981.
243. Becker G, Ihle BU, Fairley KF, et al: Effect of pregnancy on moderate renal failure in reflux nephropathy. *BMJ* 292:796–798, 1986.
244. Roopnarinesingh S: Renal calculi in pregnancy. *West Indian Med J* 21:35, 1972.
245. Coe FLC, Parks JH, Lindheimer MD: Nephrolithiasis during pregnancy. *N Engl J Med* 298: 324, 1978.
246. Swanson SK: Personal communication and *Trans Am Urol Assoc*, 1981.
247. Hayslett JP: Pregnancy does not exacerbate primary glomerular disease. *Am J Kidney Dis* VL(4):273–277, 1985.
248. Hou S: Frequency and outcome of pregnancy in women on dialysis. *Am J Kidney Dis* 23: 60–63, 1994.
249. Jacobs R, Brunner FP, Chautler C, et al: Combined report on regular dialysis and transplantation in Europe. *Proc Eur Dial Transplant Assoc* 14:3, 1977.
250. Rizzoni G, Ehrich JHH, Broyer M, et al: Successful pregnancies in women on renal replacement therapy: Report from the EDTA Registry. *Nephrol Dial Transplant* 7:1–9, 1992.
251. Hou S: Peritoneal dialysis and hemodialysis in pregnancy. *Bailliere's Clin Obstet Gynecol*, Vol 8, 1994.
252. Elliot JP, Okeefe DF, Schon DA, Cherem LB: Dialysis in pregnancy: A critical review. *Obstet Gynecol Surv* 46:319–324, 1991.
253. Jacobi P, Ohel G, Szylman P, et al: Continuous ambulatory peritoneal dialysis as the primary approach in the management of severe renal insufficiency in pregnancy. *Obstet Gynecol* 79: 808–810, 1991.
254. Armenti VT, Ahlsede BA, Moritz MJ, Jarrel BE: National Transplantation Registry: Analysis of pregnancy outcomes of female kidney recipients with relation to time interval from transplantation to conception. *Transplant Proc* 25:1036–1037, 1993.
255. Sturgiss SN, Davison JM: Effect of pregnancy on long-term function of renal allografts. *Am J Kidney Dis* 12(2):167–172, 1992.
256. Salmela KT, Kyllonen LEJ, Holmberg C, et al: Impaired renal function after pregnancy in renal transplant recipients. *Transplantation* 56:1372–1375, 1993.
257. Haugen G, Fauchald P, Sodal G, et al: Pregnancy outcome in renal allograft recipients: Influence of cyclosporin A. *Eur J Obstet Gynecol Reprod Biol* 29:25–29, 1991.

14

Proteinuria and the Nephrotic Syndrome

George A. Kaysen

Serum protein concentration is normally about 8 mg/ml. At a normal glomerular filtration rate (GFR), approximately 1.4 kg of plasma protein would be lost into the urine each day if the kidney were not capable of efficiently preventing the transglomerular trafficking of plasma proteins. The ability of the kidney to retain plasma proteins is therefore essential for life. Normal urine contains no more than 150 mg of protein per day, and only a small fraction is of serum origin. Detection of abnormal amounts or types of protein in the urine is frequently the first sign of significant renal or systemic disease. The presence of abnormal amounts of protein in the urine may reflect (1) systemic diseases resulting in the inability of the kidney to normally reabsorb proteins presented to the renal tubules, (2) the overproduction of plasma proteins capable of passing the normal glomerular basement membrane (GBM) so that they enter tubular fluid in quantities that exceed the capacity of the normal proximal tubule to reabsorb them, or (3) a defect in the glomerular barrier that allows abnormal amounts of proteins of intermediate molecular weight to enter Bowman's space.

Renal Handling of Proteins

While urinary protein excretion may be as much as 150 mg/day in normal patients, the major constituent of urinary protein is the Tamm-Horsfall protein, a component of the glycocalix secreted by renal tubular cells and not of serum origin [1]. Since plasma proteins are heterogeneous with respect to size, charge, and shape, different mechanisms have evolved to retain proteins of different classes. Proteins of less than 20 kDa in mass freely pass the glomerular barrier, are reabsorbed, and for the most part are catabolized by proximal tubular cells [2–4] with the amino acids reclaimed. The kidney serves as the primary site for catabolism of low-molecular-weight proteins, peptides, hormones (parathyroid hormone, insulin), fragments of immunoglobulins (light chain, β_2-microglobulin), and enzymes (lysozyme, amylase, cationic trypsinogen). Since these proteins are freely filtered normally, their appearance in the urine may result from a pathologic increase in their generation so that the capacity of the renal tubule to metabolize them is exceeded. This occurs with the increased production of light chains of immunoglobulin in patients with multiple myeloma [5, 6]. Another cause of proteinuria is a consequence of an intrinsic inability of the proximal tubule to reabsorb filtered proteins [6, 7] as a result of proximal tubular damage. Proteins of intermediate size, between 40 and 150 kDa, corresponding to a Stokes-Einstein radius of between 3.5 nM and 6 nM, are nearly completely restricted from glomerular ultrafiltrate in the absence of disease because of their charge and size. These proteins are however lost in greatest quantity when the glomerular barrier is altered [8, 9]. Proteins typical of this class are albumin, IgG, transferrin, ceruloplasmin, α_1-acid glycoprotein (α_1-AG), and high-density lipoprotein (HDL). Very large proteins (IgM, α_1- and α_2-macroglobulins, fibrinogen) are completely restricted by the normal glomerulus. Even when glomerular permselectivity is greatly altered, only small quantities of these large proteins pass into glomerular ultrafiltrate.

Methods of Measuring Proteinuria

The standard method for assessing urinary protein excretion is based on the binding of the pH-sensitive bromcresol green dye by albumin. When bromcresol green is bound to albumin, the dissociation constant of the dye changes so that it is in its ionized form at all physiologic urine pH values and turns to a green color. This method does not detect other urinary proteins well and is relatively insensitive, the lower limit of detection being slightly less than 30 mg/dl. If total urine volume is 1 liter, urinary albumin excretion will reach the threshold of detection with this method at slightly less than 300 mg/day. Since clinically important albuminuria occurs well below this value (>22 mg/day) [10], more sensitive, immunologically based assays must be employed to detect small amounts of albumin in the urine that may reveal the presence of clinically significant renal diseases, such as diabetic nephropathy, in their early stages.

Diseases that alter the glomerular filtration barrier invariably cause albuminuria, but proteinuria can also occur in the absence of an alteration in the glomerular filtration barrier and hence not cause a great increase in urinary albumin excretion. Large amounts of immunoglobulin fragments appear in the urine of patients with multiple myeloma, but this protein may not be detected by the standard colorimetric test used to detect albumin. Measurement of formation of a precipitate by sulfosalicylic acid or trichloroacetic acid will detect any type of protein present in urine, although these methods also detect albumin more readily than other proteins [1]. Both tests have a lower limit of sensitivity of about 20 mg/L.

In some cases, it is important to detect specific proteins that appear in the urine in small amounts as a result of proximal tubular dysfunction. β_2-microglobulin is efficiently reabsorbed by the normal proximal tubule, but subtle damage to the proximal tubule caused by nephrotoxins results in the urinary loss of this and other proteins in quantities detectable by sensitive immunoassays [11]. Electrophoretic methods are also useful in initial evaluation of urinary protein to determine whether the pattern of protein excretion is most compatible with that resulting from a tubular lesion, from overflow of abnormal proteins into the urine, or from glomerular pathology.

Detecting Proteinuria Before the Onset of Overt Renal Disease

Some progressive renal diseases, especially diabetes, declare themselves early in their course by the presence of small amounts of albumin in the urine. Mogensen and Christiansen [10] found that patients with microalbuminuria, albuminuria in the range of 15 to 150 μg/min (between 22 and 220 mg/day), were those who, with the passage of time, developed progressive renal injury. Early treatment of hypertension forestalled the development of renal failure in these patients [12]. More recently it has been established that early treatment of diabetic patients with angiotensin-converting enzyme (ACE) inhibitors prevents the onset of microalbuminuria and the progression of microalbuminuria to clinically overt albuminuria in insulin-dependent diabetic patients [13, 14]. Chronic proteinuria may directly lead to increased interstitial damage [15, 16]. The early detection of albumin in the urine therefore may permit effective treatment of the underlying condition altering glomerular permselectivity [13]. Reduction of proteinuria may also prevent nephrotoxic effects of filtered proteins. Thus, it is possible that aggressive treatment may prevent or delay the eventual development of renal failure [12–14].

Overflow proteinuria may also cause acute or even chronic renal failure [5, 15–17]. Renal failure caused by multiple myeloma may be irreversible and shorten survival of patients with this disease. The early detection and treatment of light-chain proteinuria, myoglobinuria, or hemoglobinuria not only can prevent the development of acute or chronic renal failure but also can provide diagnostic evidence of treatable diseases in time to alter the course of those diseases. The early detection of myoglobinuria may alert the physician to the presence of a crushed extremity or of serious metabolic abnormality in time to intervene with preventive measures. β_2-Microglobulinuria may herald the onset of renal failure caused by nephrotoxic antibiotics, such as aminoglycosides, so that timely discontinuation or dosage adjustment of the drug is possible. β_2-Microglobulinuria may also allow the detection of environmental toxins [18, 19].

Tubular Proteinuria

Tubular proteinuria results from an inability of the proximal tubule to reabsorb proteins filtered by the normal glomerulus in normal amounts. Ideally, urinary protein resulting from tubular abnormalities should consist of a concentrate of proteins present in normal glomerular ultrafiltrate. The total amount of protein in the urine will generally be above 150 mg/day and below 1.5 g/day. Despite its high molecular weight, albumin is still a major constituent of urinary protein, even when the glomerular barrier is normal. Since this protein is present in such great concentrations in blood, appreciable amounts of albumin enter the urine even though the filtration fraction is only 1/10,000 that of inulin. In contrast, both transferrin and IgG are essentially absent from the urine. Many of the proteins found in the urine of patients with pure tubular proteinuria are of low molecular weight, such as β_2-microglobulin (11.8 kDa) and α_2-microglobulin [20].

In its most severe state, proximal tubular dysfunction leads to Fanconi's syndrome [21], a syndrome characterized by the inability of the proximal tubule to reabsorb glucose, amino acids, uric acid, phosphate, bicarbonate, and other normal components of proximal tubular fluid in addition to proteins. As a consequence, Fanconi's syndrome causes a non–anion gap metabolic acidosis, hypouricemia, hypophosphatemia, aminoaciduria, and glycosuria in addition to proteinuria. The syndrome generally results from one of several inherited metabolic disorders [20], although it can also be caused by exposure to cadmium [18, 19], ingestion of outdated tetracycline [20], multiple myeloma, amyloidosis, and other processes detailed in Table 14-1. It is important to recognize the presence of Fanconi's syndrome both to identify and to manage the underlying disease and the metabolic acidosis. Proteinuria, however, is not believed to contribute to the renal disease process associated with Fanconi's syndrome, although as will be discussed subsequently, proteinuria may participate in causing renal injury and not just serve as a marker of renal damage.

Tubular proteinuria may also result from more subtle damage to the proximal tubule. The increased presentation of high-molecular-weight proteins to the proximal tubular cells may even cause an increase in the urinary excretion of low-molecular-weight proteins [22]. β_2-Microglobulin may appear in the urine early in the course of aminoglycoside toxicity [23, 24] prior to any decrease in GFR or the appearance of more overt forms of proximal tubular dysfunction. β_2-Microglobulinuria may also be the first manifestation of cadmium or other heavy-metal intoxication [18, 19, 25], although the level of β_2-microglobulin also increases early in the course of chronic cadmium nephropathy and contributes to the increased appearance of this protein in the urine [26]. Heavy-metal intoxication may also cause an increased renal clearance of albumin and IgG, as well as increased excretion of low-molecular-weight proteins [22], thus leading to a "mixed" form of proteinuria. Urinary β_2-microglobulin excretion is monitored in workers exposed to nephrotoxic metals in an effort to avoid the development of chronic renal disease [18, 19, 25, 26]. As with Fanconi's syndrome, the appearance of β_2-microglobulin and other low-molecular-weight proteins in the urine is not in and of itself injurious. However, detection of these proteins is important in the diagnosis of exposure to nephrotoxic agents.

Overflow Proteinuria

Park and Maack [27] showed in elegant studies, using isolated perfused rabbit proximal tubule, that the absorptive capacity for albumin by the healthy proximal tubule is quite high. Prior to this observation, the low affinity of the renal tubule for albumin predicted that an increase in albuminuria should occur with only a slight increase in its filtered load. An increase in the filtered load of several proteins does result in their appearance in the urine. The most common causes of overflow

Table 14-1. Disorders causing disordered renal reabsorption of filtered proteins at normal filtered loads

Congenital disorders
  Fanconi's syndrome
    Hereditary
      Cystinosis
      Wilson's disease
      Heritable fructose intolerance
      Oxalosis
      Hereditary tyrosinemia [239]
      Glycogen storage diseases
      Galactosemia
    Acquired
      Heavy-metal poisoning
      Outdated tetracycline
      Multiple myeloma
      Amyloidosis
      Vitamin D intoxication
  Bartter's syndrome
  Familial asymptomatic tubular proteinuria
  Oculocerebrorenal dystrophy
  Renal tubular acidosis
  Renal dysplasia
  Renal cystic disorders (polycystic kidney disease)
Systemic disease
  Hereditary
    Galactosemia
    Glycogen storage disease
  Acquired
    Balkan nephropathy
    Sarcoidosis
    Systemic lupus erythematosus
Acute renal disease
  Acute tubular necrosis
  Renal infarction
  Transplant rejection
Infectious disease
  Pyelonephritis
    Viral or bacterial associated interstitial nephritis
    Drugs and toxins
  Acute hypersensitivity interstitial nephritis
    (penicillins, cephalosporins, sulfonamides)
    Aminoglycoside toxicity
    Analgesic nephropathy
    Cyclosporine toxicity
    Cadmium, lead, arsenic, mercury, ethylene glycol,
      carbon tetrachloride
    Vitamin D intoxication

Table 14-2. Causes of overflow proteinuria

Multiple myeloma
Monocytic and myelomonocytic leukemia
Hemoglobinuria
Myoglobinuria
Systemic inflammatory processes
    Trauma
    Sepsis
    HIV infection

proteinuria are listed in Table 14-2. The most significant of these is the appearance of Bence Jones proteins in the urine in multiple myeloma.

Electrophoretic methods used to characterize urinary and serum proteins in clinical laboratories separate them on the basis of charge, not of molecular weight. Those proteins that move the farthest to the left are those with the greatest net negative charge, such as albumin, while those that move farthest to the right bear a net positive charge.

Figure 14-1A shows the result of protein electrophoresis of urine from a patient with this disorder. There is a large quantity of light chain protein in the urine (a so-called spike). Some myeloma light chain proteins are quite nephrotoxic, depending on their isoelectric points (pKi) and other factors. Myeloma light chain proteins with a pKi of around 5 are generally most toxic, in part because of their reduced

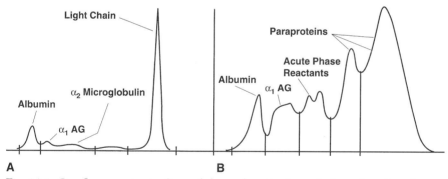

Fig. 14-1. Overflow proteinuria: Scan of electrophoresis of protein from the urine of a patient with multiple myeloma (A) and a patient with acquired immune deficiency syndrome (AIDS) (B). Note the predominance of protein in a single band in the urine of the patient with multiple myeloma. This is caused by the overflow of a homogeneous cationic immunoglobulin fragment (light chains). In the patient with AIDS, urinary protein is composed of a heterogeneous mixture of acute phase reactant proteins and polyclonal immunoglobulin fragments. Protein concentration was 16 mg/dl in the urine in A. Albumin represented 13.4% of total protein, α_1-acid glycoprotein (α_1 AG) 7.6%, α_2-microglobulin 8.1%, β-globulins 5.3%, and gamma globulin 65.6% of total urinary protein. Protein concentration was 220 mg/dl in the urine in B. Albumin represented 7.6% of total protein, α_1 AG 11.7%, α_2-microglobulin 13.3%, β-globulins 18.3%, and gamma globulin 49.2% of total urinary protein.

solubility in the acid milieu of the renal papilla [28]. The continued excretion of these proteins may produce progressive and irreversible renal failure [5]. Early treatment of multiple myeloma may prevent the development or progression of renal failure. Maintenance of an alkaline diuresis may also be therapeutic. For this reason, protein electrophoresis is an important component in the evaluation of any patient with proteinuria, especially in the evaluation of patients over the age of 40.

A modest increase in urinary protein excretion can occur in patients during acute inflammatory conditions, such as in patients with human immunodeficiency virus (HIV) infection, following trauma, or as a consequence of severe infection. This is due to increased excretion of a number of low-molecular-weight proteins produced in response to stress, immunoglobulins, and acute phase reactant proteins. Their filtration is increased beyond the tubular capacity for their reabsorption, and they spill into the urine and should be distinguished from glomerular proteinuria, which can also be caused by HIV infection. Figure 14-1B shows the result of protein electrophoresis of urine from a patient with acquired immune deficiency syndrome (AIDS) with the overflow pattern of urinary protein excretion. Acute phase reactant proteins of relatively low molecular weight appear in the urine as well as immunoglobulin fragments (paraproteins). These represent the filtration of a variety of polyclonal immunoglobulin fragments produced in excess as a result of HIV infection [29, 30] and can clearly be distinguished from the monoclonal gammopathy illustrated in Figure 14-1A.

Myoglobinuria

Damage to striated muscle causes the appearance of myoglobin in the blood. This low-molecular-weight protein is freely filtered by the glomerulus and may appear in the urine in large quantities [31]. The urine may be turbid or clear but generally has a brown color. After centrifugation of the urine, the supernatant will test positive for blood using the benzidine test, even in the absence of red blood cells. It is important to identify this entity for two reasons. Most importantly, myoglobinuria is an important cause of acute renal failure [32, 33]. Prompt treatment with intravenous infusion of mannitol and sodium bicarbonate can prevent the occurrence of acute renal failure [34].

It is also important to identify the cause of rhabdomyolysis. Permanent disability resulting from crush injuries may be avoided by early surgical intervention [32, 33, 35]. Metabolic disorders that predispose to rhabdomyolysis including hypophosphatemia [36], hypothermia, and hypokalemia [22, 37] require therapy, while inherited disorders [38–41] require both management and genetic counseling.

Hemoglobinuria

Hemoglobinuria results from intravascular hemolysis and occurs when the capacity of haptoglobin to bind free hemoglobin is exceeded. The urine may vary from pink to black in color. Spectroscopic methods may be necessary to distinguish hemoglobinuria from myoglobinuria. Since hemoglobinuria can also cause acute renal failure [42], it is important to identify this entity. As with myoglobinuria, renal failure caused by hemoglobinuria [43] may be averted by mannitol infusion, hydration, and urinary alkalinization, although this approach remains controversial. Pure hemoglobin has little or no toxic effect when transfused [44], but red cell stroma alone can cause renal failure [45]. The cause of acute renal failure associated with hemoglobinuria therefore may involve a mechanism other than tubular obstruction by filtered hemoglobin.

Hemoglobinuria may be an initial manifestation of conditions causing acute intravascular hemolysis, which may be life-threatening even in the absence of acute renal failure. These conditions include incompatible blood transfusions [42, 43, 45]; arsine poisoning [46–48]; falciparum malaria; red cell enzyme defects; immune hemolytic anemias; and acute hemolysis due to drugs, chemicals [49], burns, hypophosphatemia [50], infections, eclampsia, or the entrance of hypotonic solutions into the blood, such as hypotonic infusions during prostatectomy. Anemia alone may cause death from many of these entities long before renal failure becomes a clinical problem.

Chronic intravascular hemolysis may also cause hemoglobinuria. Although neither severe acute anemia nor acute renal failure develops as a consequence of chronic intravascular hemolysis, hemoglobinuria or hemosiderinuria may be the first recognizable symptom of one of several chronic disorders. Diseases responsible for chronic intravascular hemolysis include paroxysmal nocturnal hemoglobinuria [51], paroxysmal cold hemoglobinuria, march hemoglobinuria [52] (resulting from mechanical disruption of red cells during exercise, the pigment excreted may also be myoglobin), and mechanical disruption of red blood cells due to prosthetic heart valves [53].

Glomerular Proteinuria

Mechanisms of Altered Glomerular Permselectivity

Since proteins are not only filtered by the glomerulus but also reabsorbed by the renal tubule [54], it is not possible to probe directly the permeability characteristics of the glomerular filtration barrier by measuring urinary protein excretion alone. Neutral and negatively charged dextrans are filtered by the glomerulus, but are neither reabsorbed nor catabolized by the renal tubule and thus serve as probes of glomerular size and charge selectivity [55]. Neutral dextrans and other nonmetabolized organic molecules [56] are restricted from the urine on the basis of size and shape, but not of charge [8, 57]. Negatively charged molecules are more restricted than are neutral molecules [56, 58] because of electrostatic interaction with the glomerular filtration barrier. The normal glomerulus therefore restricts proteins on the basis of both size and charge. The negative charge results from the rich content of heparan sulfate that coats the glomerular filtration barrier [59]. The primary site of impedance for filtration of proteins is the glomerular epithelial cell [60]. Figure 14-2 shows a urine electrophoretic pattern from two patients with glomerular proteinuria. Unlike the previous two patterns, the predominant proteins are of high molecular weight: albumin, transferrin, and to a lesser extent, IgG. Only small amounts of low-molecular-weight proteins are present.

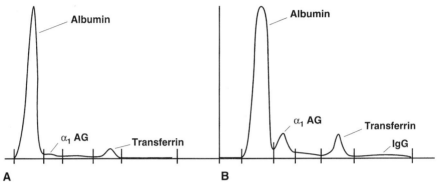

Fig. 14-2. Glomerular proteinuria: Scans of electrophoresis of protein from the urine of patients with the nephrotic syndrome. (A) Selective proteinuria. Protein concentration was 63 mg/dl in the urine. Albumin comprises 84.4% of total protein, α_1-acid glycoprotein (α_1 AG) 3.6%, α_2-microglobulin 3.4%, β-globulins 5.9%, and gamma globulin 2.6% of total urinary protein. (B) Nonselective proteinuria. Protein concentration was 680 mg/dl in the urine. Albumin comprises 71.1% of total protein, α_1 AG 10.1%, α_2-microglobulin 4.1%, β-globulins 9.6%, and gamma globulin 5.2% of total urinary protein. Albumin is still the predominant protein, but filtration of transferrin, which migrates here as β-globulin, is increased compared to A, and IgG is also present in greater amounts. Unlike the immunoglobulin fragments found in the urine of patients with tubular proteinuria, immunoglobulins present in the urine of patients having glomerular proteinuria are full-sized IgG.

Figure 14-3 shows the relative renal clearance of neutral dextrans of increasing molecular radius. The curves bearing open symbols represent the clearance of dextrans by the normal human kidney. As the radius of dextrans increases, their clearance relative to inulin, and therefore to water, decreases. One may depict the normal glomerular filtration barrier as being occupied by a series of pores that allow the unrestricted passage of low-molecular-weight solutes and progressively restrict the passage of molecules of greater molecular radius. Figure 14-4 (left panel) is a hypothetical representation of the surface of such a filtration barrier. The vast majority of the surface is represented as covered by many pores of similar size, small enough to restrict the passage of large- or intermediate-molecular-weight proteins, but freely permeable to water and small-molecular-weight peptides and carbohydrate polymers. These pores are estimated to have a radius of between 5.1 and 5.7 nM [8, 61]. A second, much smaller population of much larger pores is also represented on this hypothetical glomerular filtration barrier. These pores are relatively unselective to molecules of intermediate size and form a shunt pathway that allows proteins to pass into the ultrafiltrate unencumbered [8]. Proteinuria results predominantly from the passage of a fraction of glomerular ultrafiltrate through the large nonselective pores.

When the filtration barrier is altered, the total filtration surface is reduced. Figure 14-5 shows electron micrographs comparing the thickness of the GBM from a normal patient (Fig. 14-5B) with that from a patient with diabetes (Fig. 14-5C) and from a patient with membranous nephropathy (Fig. 14-5A). All three panels are

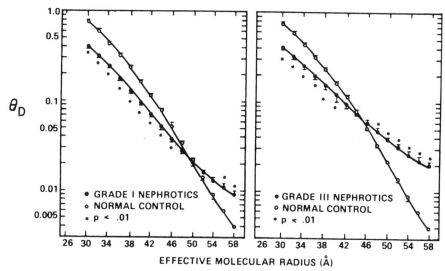

Fig. 14-3. Fractional dextran clearances plotted as a function of effective molecular radius. Data from normal subjects are represented by curves bearing open symbols in both panels. Data from patients with the nephrotic syndrome are represented by curves bearing closed symbols. Dextran sieving curves from patients with mild renal damage are represented in the left panel, and sieving curves from patients with severe glomerular lesions are represented in the right panel. All results are expressed as means ± SE. Statistical differences between control and experimental values are connoted by * and reflect a difference at $p < 0.01$ (From W. M. Deen, C. R. Bridges, B. M. Brenner, and B. D. Meyers, Heteroporous model of glomerular size selectivity: Application to normal and nephrotic humans. *Am. J. Physiol.* 249:F374, 1985.)

of equal magnification, as can be seen by comparing the size of the endothelial cell nuclei. Despite thickening of the GBM in the course of a variety of conditions that cause the nephrotic syndrome, the diseased glomerulus is far more permeable to proteins than normal but is less permeable to water and to molecules of lower molecular weight. The reason for this apparent contradiction is that the GBM itself is not the barrier to protein filtration, but instead the greatest impedance to the filtration of proteins is at the glomerular epithelial cell [60]. Deen and colleagues [8] have mathematically modeled the glomerular filtration barrier using data derived from the filtration of neutral dextrans presented in Figure 14-3. They found a reduction in the filtration of low-molecular-weight dextrans, shown in Figure 14-3 by the curves bearing closed symbols and represented in the right-hand panel in Figure 14-4. The filtration of low-molecular-weight dextrans is reduced relative to normal in the diseased glomerulus. In contrast, the filtration of high-molecular-weight dextrans is increased in patients with the nephrotic syndrome. In the left panel of Figure 14-3 are data derived from patients with less severe renal disease compared to normal subjects. The data in the right panel of Figure 14-3 are derived from patients with more severe renal impairment and less selective proteinuria. The mathematical model proposes that the area of the glomerular filtration barrier cov-

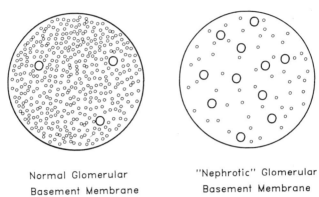

Normal Glomerular   "Nephrotic" Glomerular
Basement Membrane   Basement Membrane

Fig. 14-4. Hypothetical representation of the porous surface of a normal glomerular basement membrane (GBM) (*left panel*) and the GBM from a patient with the nephrotic syndrome (*right panel*). The normal GBM is covered predominantly with small pores that are both size and charge selective. They bear a negative charge and exclude anionic proteins more readily than cationic proteins of similar size. Proteinuria results from the development of a separate population of larger pores that allow proteins of intermediate size to pass the GBM unencumbered.

ered by small charge- and size-selective pores, and thus available for clearance of water and inulin, is greatly reduced in these patients (illustrated in Fig. 14-4, right panel), but the population of larger pores is increased. The larger pores allow proteins such as albumin, transferrin, and IgG to pass the glomerular barrier unrestricted, but contribute very little to the total filtration surface, and therefore do not offset the surface lost by obliteration of the area covered by smaller pores. High-molecular-weight dextrans pass the glomerular filtration barrier more easily in the abnormal kidney, even though the total filtration surface is reduced, leading to a decline in GFR. This phenomenon is responsible for the crossing of the two curves in Figure 14-3. The fractional clearance of low-molecular-weight dextrans is decreased in nephrotic patients, while the fractional clearance of high-molecular-weight dextrans is increased. As renal disease progresses, the fraction of GFR passing through the population of large pores increases, while the total filtering surface occupied by the normal small pores decreases. Figure 14-2A shows the electrophoretic pattern of urinary proteins from a patient with only a mild disruption in glomerular barrier function; the pattern consists predominantly of albumin and 39.5-kDa highly negatively charged α_1-AG and is referred to as a "selective" pattern of glomerular proteinuria. The dextran sieving pattern from such a patient would be expected to be similar to that in the left panel of Figure 14-3. In contrast, Figure 14-2B is from a patient with a greater loss of glomerular size selectivity and consists of transferrin (79.5 kDa) and IgG (150 kDa) in addition to albumin and α_1-AG. The sieving pattern from such a patient would be similar to that in the right panel of Figure 14-3. Most diseases that cause the nephrotic syndrome in humans primarily cause a loss of glomerular size selectivity (an increase in glomerular permeability to large uncharged dextrans) without a loss of charge selectivity [8, 61, 62].

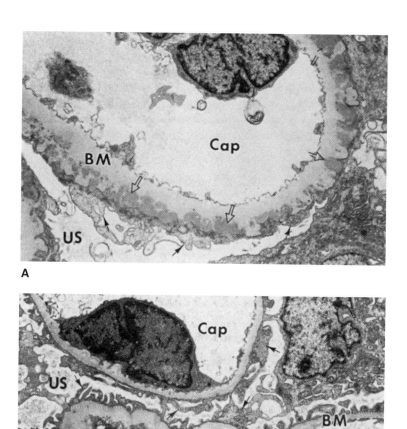

Fig. 14-5. Electron micrographs from glomeruli from a patient with membranous nephropathy (A), a normal patient (B), and a patient with diabetes mellitus (C). All three micrographs are at the same magnification. Note the great thickening of the glomerular basement membrane (GBM) in the specimens obtained from the diabetic patient and the patient with membranous nephropathy. Despite the thickening, the GBMs from the two patients with renal disease are far more permeable to proteins than is the normal GBM. Fusion of the epithelial foot processes results from the loss of heparan sulfate on the cell surface; however, proteinuria in both diabetes and membranous nephropathy results from a loss of size selectivity rather than from a loss of charge selectivity [4, 8, 61, 62]. BM = basement membrane; Cap = capillary lumen; US = urinary space; Mes = mesangium. Small arrows indicate foot processes, and open arrows indicate electron-dense deposits consisting of antigen-antibody complexes.

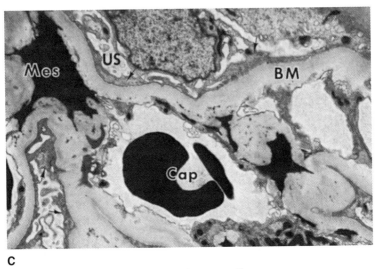

C

Fig. 14-5 (continued).

Hormonal Factors That Alter Glomerular Permselectivity

Although changes in the physical dimensions of the glomerular filtration barrier may be responsible for altered glomerular permselectivity, alterations in permselectivity can occur quickly, may be transient [63], and may be hemodynamically or hormonally mediated [63–65]. Constriction of the renal vein in the rat causes an increase in the filtration of high-molecular-weight dextrans, consistent with an increased fraction of glomerular ultrafiltrate passing through a population of large pores. This occurs in conjunction with a nearly 10-fold increase in proteinuria and can be almost entirely prevented by infusion of saralasin, an angiotensin II antagonist [63]. Angiotensin II may therefore play a role in the development of alterations in size permselectivity [56, 63, 66]. Thromboxane synthesis may also play a role in the development of proteinuria in some forms of renal diseases [64, 65]. Both cyclooxygenase inhibitors and ACE inhibitors reduce proteinuria in patients with the nephrotic syndrome in part by reducing the fraction of glomerular filtrate that passes through the large pores [67]. The fact that the products of ACE and of cyclooxygenase may contribute to the defective filtration barrier in some proteinuric renal disease provides the basis of the pharmacologic means for treating proteinuria in some patients, discussed subsequently.

Nitric oxide is a potent vasodilator released by vascular endothelial cells and macrophages, is derived from the guanidino group on arginine, and plays a role in the regulation of renal blood flow in normal and pathologic states [68, 69]. Baylis et al. [70] recently reported that inhibition of nitric oxide caused both glomerular hypertension and proteinuria in normal rats. It is not known at this time whether nitric oxide modulates proteinuria in the nephrotic syndrome in patients.

Table 14-3. Causes of glomerular proteinuria

Diseases confined to the kidney
    Minimal change nephrotic syndrome
    Membranous nephropathy
    Focal segmental glomerulosclerosis
    Mesangial proliferative glomerulonephritis
    Mesangiocapillary glomerulonephritis
    Acute poststreptococcal glomerulonephritis
Systemic diseases
    Diabetes mellitus
    Henoch-Schönlein purpura
    Systemic lupus erythematosus
    Amyloidosis
    Goodpasture's syndrome
Hereditary disorders
    Congenital nephrotic syndrome
    Hereditary nephritis (Alport's syndrome)
    Partial lipodystrophy

Selectivity of Glomerular Proteinuria

Urinary protein electrophoresis patterns have been used in the past to distinguish between different diseases causing glomerular proteinuria. Minimal change nephrotic syndrome has classically been regarded as causing "selective" proteinuria characterized by a predominance of albumin in comparison to other proteins of intermediate molecular weight. It was believed that minimal change nephrotic syndrome resulted from loss of charge selectivity, so that highly negatively charged albumin was lost in the urine because albumin was restricted on the basis of charge alone, while other larger but more neutrally charged proteins were retained. More recently, it has been determined that minimal change nephrotic syndrome is also characterized by altered size selectivity, similar to other diseases that cause the nephrotic syndrome [62]. Many disease entities that can cause proteinuria may cause selective or nonselective proteinuria. The urinary protein electrophoretic pattern encountered in these diseases is determined by the relative fraction of glomerular ultrafiltrate that passes through these large pores.

Renal biopsy has long replaced measurement of the relative concentrations of different proteins in the urine for determination of glomerular pathology. Urinary protein electrophoresis is useful for distinguishing between tubular proteinuria, overflow proteinuria, and glomerular proteinuria but has little utility for distinguishing between diseases of glomerular origin (Table 14-3).

The Nephrotic Syndrome

The nephrotic syndrome results from alterations in the permselective characteristics of the GBM that allow increased passage of proteins of intermediate size into the urine and consists of the constellation of heavy proteinuria (≥ 3.5 g/day), hypoal-buminemia, hyperlipidema, increased concentration of several high-molecular-weight proteins, and edema formation [71, 72]. Not all components of this syndrome need be present. It is not known why all manifestations of the nephrotic syndrome are expressed in some patients and not in others. Proteinuria in excess of 3.5 g/day, however, is predictive of any of several serious renal diseases listed in Table 14-3 and defines nephrotic proteinuria.

It is somewhat surprising that all of these manifestations may result from the daily urinary loss of the amount of protein in half a hen's egg. The mean value for proteinuria in a number of studies of the nephrotic syndrome is about 8 g/day [73–76], but viewed in the context of normal protein intake, even this external loss is small. Although it is experimentally more difficult to quantitate the losses of tissue protein, continuous massive proteinuria causes marked muscle wasting [77, 78], sometimes obscured by edema. How do these extensive metabolic derange-ment's result from a relatively small amount of protein loss? What are the homeo-static adaptations that result from urinary protein loss? Why are urinary protein losses resistant to replacement by dietary protein augmentation? These are questions that will be approached in the ensuing sections.

Albumin Metabolism in the Nephrotic Syndrome

In the absence of external albumin loss, before the onset of albuminuria, a fixed quantity of albumin is synthesized each day, and an identical quantity is destroyed by catabolism. Three principal adaptive mechanisms may be brought into play to defend the plasma albumin pool when this steady state is disturbed by the develop-ment of albuminuria: The extravascular albumin pool may be mobilized into the intravascular space, the rate of albumin synthesis may be increased, or albumin catabolic rate may be decreased. Of these three adaptive mechanisms, only the last two are capable of reestablishing steady state, such that albumin production is again equal to the sum of external albumin loss plus catabolism.

Albumin Catabolism

The bulk of albumin catabolism occurs in a compartment in rapid equilibrium with the vascular compartment and not in any predominant organ [79–82]. In the ab-sence of renal disease, approximately 10 to 20 percent of albumin catabolism takes place in the kidney [78, 83], and this represents the amount of albumin filtered by the normal glomerulus [9, 84, 85]. When glomerular filtration of albumin is in-creased, more albumin is presented to the proximal tubular cells, and it is possible for the rate of renal albumin catabolism to be increased. However, micropuncture studies in both normal and nephrotic rats suggest that albumin reabsorption by the renal tubules of nephrotic animals might be saturated at near physiologic levels [86–88]. Most of the increased albumin filtered by the abnormal glomerulus may in fact be lost in the urine and not catabolized by the renal tubular epithelium. Urinary albumin excretion is therefore not a gross underestimate of the total albumin lost from the total albumin pool in the nephrotic syndrome.

The absolute rate of albumin catabolism decreases and the rate of albumin synthe-

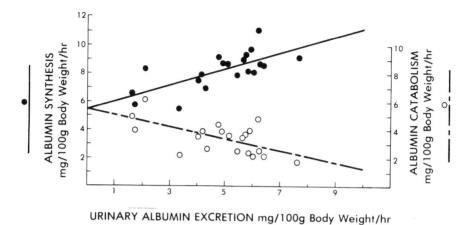

Fig. 14-6. Changes in albumin synthesis (*closed circles, solid line*) and albumin catabolism (*open circles, broken line*) that occur with increasing urinary albumin loss in rats with passive Heymann nephritis. (Data from G. A. Kaysen, W. G. Kirkpatrick, and W. G. Couser, Albumin homeostasis in the nephrotic rat: Nutritional considerations. *Am. J. Physiol.* 247 [*Renal Fluid Electrolyte Physiol.* 16]:F192, 1984.)

sis increases in nephrotic rats almost to an equal extent as albuminuria becomes progressively severe [89] (Fig. 14-6). The fractional rate of albumin catabolism is also increased in nephrotic patients, while the absolute rate of albumin catabolism is reduced [73, 74]. These findings are compatible with a reduced rate of extrarenal albumin catabolism coupled with an increase in intrarenal albumin catabolism. Since total albumin catabolic rate is reduced to about 50 percent of normal in nephrotic rats and patients, and since approximately 20 percent of albumin catabolism occurs in the kidney normally, the maximum increase in intrarenal albumin catabolism that could be sustained in the nephrotic syndrome would be an increase of about 2.5 times that which occurs in the absence of proteinuria, assuming that all extrarenal albumin catabolism ceased. An increased rate of albumin catabolism is therefore not the principal cause of a failure to protect albumin stores in the nephrotic syndrome. Rather a reduced rate of albumin catabolism occurs and is an important homeostatic response to urinary protein losses.

Albumin Synthesis

Albumin synthesis is predominantly regulated by the availability of adequate dietary protein [90–93] and is suppressed during inflammation [94] and during acute metabolic acidosis. The rate of albumin synthesis is increased under conditions when plasma oncotic pressure is reduced, such as during the nephrotic syndrome. Albumin synthesis is increased as a consequence of increased transcription of the cognate gene [95, 96], but the specific mechanisms responsible for altered albumin gene expression are unknown. Conditions that cause an increase in plasma oncotic pressure reduce the rate of albumin synthesis in vivo [97–101]; however, there is no clear relationship between plasma albumin concentration and albumin synthetic rate in nephrotic patients [4, 73, 74] or animals [89]. While albumin synthesis increases in direct proportion to albuminuria in both nephrotic patients [4, 73, 74] and animals [89] (see Fig. 14-6), the response fails to maintain albumin pools or plasma concentration in or near the normal range.

Effect of Dietary Protein on Albumin Synthesis. The rate of albumin synthesis responds rapidly to acute changes in diet [90–92]. When severely malnourished animals or people are refed, the rate of albumin synthesis increases promptly, even while total-body protein stores are still severely depleted [102, 103]. The most important nutritional constituent is dietary protein. The maintenance of a normal plasma albumin concentration and a normal rate of albumin synthesis depends both on total protein availability in the diet and on the relative proportion of protein to nonprotein calories. Diets that provide adequate calories but are poor in protein have a more deleterious effect on albumin synthesis and on albumin stores than do diets that contain the same amount of protein but are deficient in calories [104, 105]. A balanced diet that is inadequate in both protein and calories does not cause hypoalbuminemia. A diet containing adequate calories but insufficient protein results in reduced albumin synthesis, albumin concentration, and total-body albumin mass [106], producing kwashiorkor. One would predict that an ideal diet for patients with the nephrotic syndrome, a disorder that bears much similarity to protein malnutrition, would contain adequate calories, but above all an adequate or preferably high protein content. Diets containing large excesses of protein (3–4 g/kg body weight) have been prescribed in the past [107], although no data are available demonstrating effectiveness of these diets in restoring protein pools. Increased dietary protein intake in fact fails to increase either albumin concentration or body albumin pools in patients with the nephrotic syndrome [74, 77, 78, 108] or in animals with experimentally induced nephrotic syndrome [89, 95, 109]. Instead, much of the ingested protein is catabolized rather than used for net protein synthesis. In addition, dietary protein exerts an effect on the kidney causing a reversible increase in glomerular permeability to large macromolecules [108, 109], so that most of the additional albumin synthesized is lost in the urine [74, 89]. Figure 14-7 shows the effect of diets containing either 2 g/kg or 0.6 g/kg of protein on the renal clearance of neutral dextrans when fed to nephrotic patients [108]. It can be clearly seen that patients clear high-molecular-weight dextrans more easily when fed a high-protein diet. Thus, a change in dietary protein may alter the permselectivity characteristics of the glomerular filtration barrier in these patients.

Virtually every study of the effect of altered dietary protein intake on the nephrotic syndrome noted that urinary albumin or protein excretion varied with dietary protein intake [22, 74, 77, 78, 83, 108, 110–113]. The potential adverse consequences of increased dietary protein intake were largely ignored until recently [74, 89, 110–113]. Continued maintenance of a high-protein diet may have the consequence of causing permanent rather than transient changes in the kidney and accelerate the progression of renal diseases [110–113].

The fractional renal clearance of albumin increases in both the normal rat and in the rat with Heymann nephritis [114, 115] within only 48 hours of institution of a high-protein diet. Similar reversible changes occur in the human kidney after only a short period of eating a diet rich in protein [74, 108]. When dietary protein

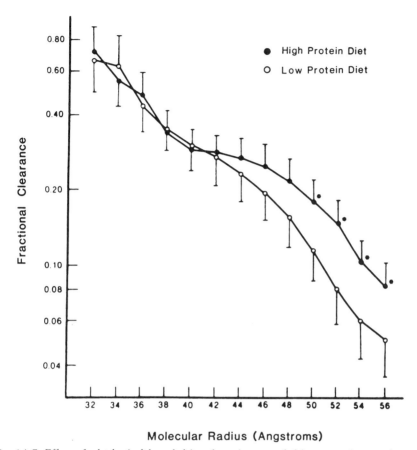

Fig. 14-7. Effect of a high- (*solid symbols*) or low- (*open symbols*) protein diet on the fractional renal clearance of neutral dextrans in nephrotic patients. (From M. E. Rosenberg, J. E. Swanson, B. L. Thomas, and T. H. Hostetter, Glomerular and hormonal responses to dietary protein intake in human renal disease. *Am. J. Physiol.* 253 [*Renal Fluid Electrolyte Physiol.* 22]:F1083, 1987.)

is increased in nephrotic patients, both urinary albumin excretion and the rate of albumin catabolism increase (Fig. 14-8). Although augmentation of dietary protein also causes an increase in the rate of albumin synthesis in both animals and patients with the nephrotic syndrome, neither protein concentration nor albumin concentration increases as a consequence [74, 89, 95]. The reason lies in the fact that these three processes offset one another, so that albumin concentration actually may tend to decrease during consumption of a high-protein diet. If the increase in urinary albumin excretion that follows dietary protein augmentation is prevented by administration of an ACE inhibitor, a high-protein diet will cause an increase in albumin concentration in nephrotic rats [95], although this has yet to be shown in patients. The therapeutic approach to maximizing albumin concentration in nephrotic patients should therefore primarily be aimed at reducing urinary albumin excretion.

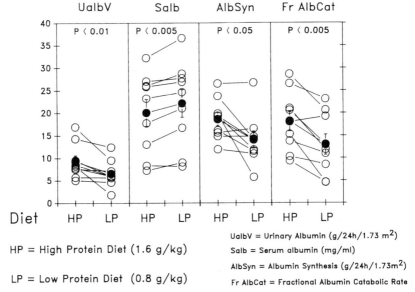

Fig. 14-8. Changes in urinary albumin excretion that occur with isocaloric reduction in dietary protein intake (*first panel*), in serum albumin concentration (*second panel*), in the rate of albumin synthesis (*third panel*), and in the fractional rate of albumin catabolism (*fourth panel*) in patients with the nephrotic syndrome of various etiologies. Fractional albumin catabolic rate is the percent of the vascular albumin pool catabolized in 24 hours. Closed circles represent the mean values for the group. (Data from G. A. Kaysen, J. Gambertoglio, I. Jiminez, et al., Effect of dietary protein intake on albumin homeostasis in nephrotic patients. *Kidney Int.* 29:572–577, 1986.)

Metabolism of Nonalbumin Serum Protein in the Nephrotic Syndrome

Plasma protein composition is greatly altered in the nephrotic syndrome [116]. Albumin and proteins of similar size are lost into the urine, and their concentration in plasma is decreased. In contrast, the plasma concentration of several proteins of high molecular weight is increased [116]. Urinary protein loss is accompanied by increased synthesis of several proteins secreted by the liver [117]. For the most part, the compensatory response to urinary protein loss, if indeed the response can be viewed as compensatory, is an increased synthesis of specific proteins secreted by the liver. The response is confined almost, if not entirely to the liver. For example, the synthesis of both apolipoprotein A-I and transferrin is increased in the liver in the nephrotic syndrome [118], while there is no change in synthesis of apo A-I by the gut [119], the other organ that secretes apo A-I, and there is no change in transferrin gene expression by extrahepatic tissues [120].

Transferrin Metabolism

Transferrin has a molecular weight of 79.5 kDa and is the principal iron carrier protein in plasma. Each mole of this protein lost in the urine carries potentially 2 moles of iron. A microcytic hypochromic anemia has been described in the ne-phrotic syndrome, although this is uncommon [121–124] and has been attributed to iron loss. Transferrin synthesis is increased in the nephrotic syndrome [121], and as in the case of iron deficiency, this response is confined to the liver [120]. Unlike iron deficiency, however, augmentation in transferrin gene expression cannot be suppressed by administration of even large amounts of iron parenterally, and trans-ferrin synthesis is also increased in hereditary analbuminemia [125], a condition not associated with urinary iron loss. These findings suggest that augmentation in transferrin synthesis is not proof of iron deficiency. Iron deposited in the renal tubules from reabsorbed transferrin may also play a role in the putative nephrotoxic effects of proteinuria [126].

Erythropoietin is synthesized by the kidney and regulates red blood cell levels. This protein is also lost in the urine in both nephrotic patients [127] and rats [128], but synthesis of erythropoietin, like that of other nonliver-derived proteins, is not increased in response, and plasma levels are decreased, as is hematocrit in nephrotic rats. Erythropoietin deficiency could potentially play a role in the development of anemia in some nephrotic patients, although this has not been established [127, 128]. While urinary iron excretion also increases in the nephrotic syndrome as a consequence of urinary transferrin loss [124], the loss of erythropoietin may be a critical factor in development of anemia. No controlled studies have been performed to determine whether administration of either iron or erythropoietin corrects ane-mia in nephrotic patients to test the hypothesis that either erythropoietin or iron deficiency is responsible for anemia in some nephrotic patients.

Immunoglobulin Metabolism

Hypogammaglobulinemia has long been recognized as a serious manifestation of the nephrotic syndrome [129] and is an important factor in the reduced defenses against bacterial infections [130] in nephrotic patients. In addition to albumin, IgG is lost in the urine when glomerular permselectivity is severely altered [8]. The urinary loss of this protein undoubtedly plays a significant role in causing hypogam-maglobulinemia in the nephrotic syndrome. As glomerular permselectivity is pro-gressively lost, the renal clearance of IgG approaches that of albumin, despite the much larger effective molecular radius of IgG. Like albumin, the fractional catabolic rate of IgG varies directly with concentration in humans and in rodents, increasing from 2 percent during severe hypogammaglobulinemia to as high as 18 percent when IgG concentration is high [131]. As in the case of albumin metabolism, the increased fractional rate of IgG catabolism is inappropriate because of the presence of hypogammaglobulinemia in nephrotic patients [76, 132]. This phenomenon most likely reflects increased renal catabolism of IgG despite a decrease in IgG catabolism elsewhere in the body.

Although IgG production may be increased in vivo in patients with the nephrotic syndrome [133], the rate of IgG production is depressed [134, 135] in lymphocytes isolated from patients with the nephrotic syndrome of various etiologies when they are exposed to mitogens in culture. This apparent contradiction has not yet been resolved, but it must be remembered that the nephrotic syndrome may be the conse-quence of immunologically mediated disease in some situations, and changes in immunoglobulin may reflect the underlying disease and not the physiologic response to urinary protein loss or changed plasma protein composition.

It has been proposed that the urinary losses of IgG cannot alone be an adequate explanation for the low blood levels, since the various subclasses of IgG are depressed asymmetrically [136], but it is more likely that IgG levels fall because, unlike the case of liver-derived proteins of the same size class, there is no compensatory increase in IgG synthetic rate. When the nephrotic syndrome is induced in experimental animals, there is no increase in IgG synthesis, and both plasma levels and total-body pools are dramatically reduced [137]. Ultimately, at final steady state, very little IgG is found in the urine because plasma levels are so low.

Of the immunoglobulins, IgG is most severely depleted in the nephrotic syndrome [138], most likely because it is smallest and its renal clearance greatest. IgA levels are also reduced, but less so. In contrast to IgG, IgM levels are increased [139]. Although it has been speculated that increased IgM levels might play a role in causing some forms of the nephrotic syndrome, such as minimal change nephrotic syndrome, this is unlikely, since the increase in IgM concentration has been reported almost universally. The increase in concentration of this very large, essentially unfilterable protein is similar to the response of many liver-derived proteins [140–142], the metabolism of which will be reviewed subsequently.

Defects in Hormone Binding Proteins

Thyroxine-binding globulin is found in the urine of nephrotic patients [143–146], but the concentration of this protein is reduced only in patients with extremely high urinary protein output [145]. Nephrotic patients are euthyroid, as serum thyrotropin levels are not increased, and thyroid function tests, as assessed by radioactive iodine uptake, are normal. Similarly, although steroid binding proteins [143] (corticosteroid-binding globulin) are reduced, there is no evidence that this leads to clinically significant reductions in free corticosteroid levels.

Vitamin D Binding Protein and Hypocalcemia in the Nephrotic Syndrome

Hypocalcemia has been long recognized in nephrotic patients [147, 148], but only recently has it been realized that ionized calcium as well as total calcium is reduced. The urinary loss of vitamin D binding protein (65 kDa) in nephrotic syndrome [149] may lead to major derangements in calcium metabolism. Hypocalcemia therefore does not result entirely from a reduction in the fraction of calcium bound to albumin. Vitamin D levels are reduced [150, 151], and the decrease in vitamin D concentration correlates with urinary albumin excretion [148]. Albumin concentration and vitamin D concentration correlate closely. Vitamin D binding protein is also identifiable in the urine of nephrotic patients [152, 153], and vitamin D levels normalize when proteinuria resolves [150, 151]. Labeled vitamin D appears rapidly in the urine of nephrotic subjects [153]. Hypovitaminosis D is not the result of loss of renal mass, since serum vitamin D levels are suppressed in nephrotic patients with normal renal function [148, 149, 151]. While it is possible that proteinuria might in some way inhibit vitamin D_1-hydroxylase, an enzyme located in the renal proximal tubule, such an explanation seems unwarranted. Hypovitaminosis D of the nephrotic syndrome may cause rickets, especially in children [154, 155]. Nephrotic patients malabsorb calcium [150, 151], a defect that can be corrected with exogenously administered vitamin D [150]. It is not known whether synthesis of vitamin D binding protein is altered in response to its urinary loss or is modulated by dietary protein intake. However, unlike many of the other manifestations of the nephrotic syndrome, hypovitaminosis D can be managed with replacement therapy.

Metabolism of High-Molecular-Weight Serum Proteins in the Nephrotic Syndrome

The concentration of several proteins that either are not lost in the urine or are lost in only limited amounts is increased in plasma because of their increased hepatic synthesis [117–119]. It is not known why the liver responds in the way that it does to urinary protein loss (or to reduction in plasma albumin concentration or oncotic pressure), but this seems to be a basic component of the nephrotic syndrome both in patients and in experimental models. The increased plasma concentration of several of these proteins (β-, α_1-, and α_2-macroglobulins) [73, 156] causes no readily identifiable clinical effect. In contrast, the increased concentration of lipids may pose atherogenic risk, as will be discussed subsequently, and the increased concentration of several large proteins involved in hemostasis contribute to the thrombotic tendency that complicates the nephrotic syndrome.

Thrombosis

The nephrotic syndrome is complicated by venous thrombosis [157]. Renal vein thrombosis results from, rather than causes, the nephrotic syndrome [158, 159]. The significant increase in thromboembolic disorders is caused in part by the urinary loss of several proteins that are inhibitors of blood coagulation, specifically antithrombin III [140] and proteins S and C [160, 161], and the increased plasma concentration of several high-molecular-weight proteins, including the binding proteins for proteins C and S.

The plasma concentration and the hepatic synthesis of fibrinogen (340 kDa) [141] are both increased in the nephrotic syndrome. Although total protein C and S may be elevated in the nephrotic syndrome [140, 160], these measurements reflect total concentration of the proteins. Increased total concentration results from an increment in the plasma concentration of their high-molecular-weight carrier protein C4b [161]. The plasma concentration of the biologically active free form of these intermediate-molecular-weight inhibitors of blood coagulation is decreased as a result both of their increased urinary loss [160, 161], and of their increased binding in inactive form to C4b. The combination of the increased concentration of high-molecular-weight procoagulants and the decreased concentration of intermediate-molecular-weight anticoagulants produce the clotting diathesis that complicates the nephrotic syndrome.

Hyperlipidemia

The characteristic disorder in blood lipid composition in nephrotic patients is an increase in the low-density lipoprotein (LDL), very-low-density lipoprotein (VLDL)

[162], and/or intermediate-density lipoprotein (IDL) fractions, but no change [162] or a decrease in HDL [163], resulting in an increase in the LDL/HDL cholesterol ratio. Lipoprotein particles rich in phospholipid and esterified and nonesterified cholesterol resembling VLDL remnants (intermediate-density lipoprotein [LDL]) and chylomicron remnants accumulate. Apolipoproteins B (apo B) and C-III are increased in the serum of nephrotic patients [64], but the concentrations of apo A-I, A-II, and C-II remain unchanged. HDL subtypes found in plasma of nephrotic patients are also abnormally distributed [164]. HDL_3 is modestly elevated, while HDL_2 is markedly reduced. Since it is primarily the latter subclass of HDL that is protective against atherosclerosis, the combination of reduced HDL_2 in conjunction with increased LDL, VLDL, and IDL cholesterol potentially poses significant risk for cardiovascular disease.

Lp(a) lipoprotein has recently been identified as a prominent risk factor in atherogenesis [165, 166]. Generally the quantity of this lipoprotein in plasma is genetically determined [167]. Lp(a) consists of a molecule of LDL to which one molecule of the apolipoprotein apo(a) has been covalently attached to apo B-100. The size of the apo(a) molecule in Lp(a) is genetically determined and distributed in the population in a non-normal fashion [168]. Individuals having the largest apo(a) subtypes are most common and have the lowest plasma concentration of Lp(a) [69]. Lp(a) levels are increased in patients with a variety of renal diseases, including the nephrotic syndrome [169]. Unlike inherited increases in plasma Lp(a) levels, these increases in Lp(a) are acquired and are not associated with increased size of apo(a) [169].

Hyperlipidemia is a consequence both of their increased synthesis [170] and the decreased clearance of the principal triglyceride-bearing lipoproteins, chylomicrons [171] and VLDL [172]. The working hypothesis is that increased lipoprotein synthesis is a consequence of reduced plasma albumin concentration or reduced plasma oncotic pressure [170]. Data supporting this hypothesis are that infusion of albumin or nonprotein macromolecules partially corrects nephrotic hyperlipidemia [173, 174] and that synthesis of apolipoproteins can also be suppressed in tissue culture by increasing oncotic pressure with either albumin [175] or nonprotein solutes [176].

While hepatic apolipoprotein synthesis is increased in the nephrotic syndrome, not all apolipoproteins are affected to the same degree, and the mechanisms causing increased synthesis of the various apolipoproteins are also different. Secretion of apo A is increased approximately sixfold [170], while synthesis of apo B and E is increased only about twofold. Synthesis of the C apolipoproteins is not increased. Apo A-I messenger RNA (mRNA) is increased at the level of transcription in livers of both nephrotic [118, 120] and analbuminemic rats [118], consistent with the hypothesis that reduced plasma albumin concentration or oncotic pressure, but not proteinuria, is responsible for the change in apo A-I gene expression. While plasma apo B and E are both increased in nephrotic and analbuminemic rats, there is little or no change in the amount of these mRNAs in liver and no change in the rate of transcription of their cognate genes [118, 119]. Thus, if increased synthesis of these apolipoproteins plays a role in establishing the increased levels of these apolipoproteins in plasma, the mechanisms involved are most likely post-transcriptional, in contrast to apo A-I. The mechanisms whereby reduction in plasma albumin concentration or oncotic pressure affects hepatic lipoprotein synthesis are not known.

Lipoprotein Catabolism in the Nephrotic Syndrome

Catabolism of both chylomicrons and VLDL is greatly reduced in the nephrotic syndrome [177]. Chylomicrons are secreted by the intestine (Fig. 14-9), and VLDL is secreted by the liver (Fig. 14-10). Both then are transported to the vascular endothelium where their triglycerides are subject to catabolism by lipoprotein lipase (LPL). The free fatty acids are released and taken up by adjacent parenchymal tissue, while the residual remnant particles are released and either are taken up directly by the liver through the remnant receptor or, in the case of VLDL remnants, may be converted to LDL. The first stage of lipolysis of both chylomicrons and VLDL is greatly reduced in the nephrotic syndrome [177–179]. Hepatic uptake of chylomicron remnants is also impaired in nephrotic rats [179], and plasma remnants

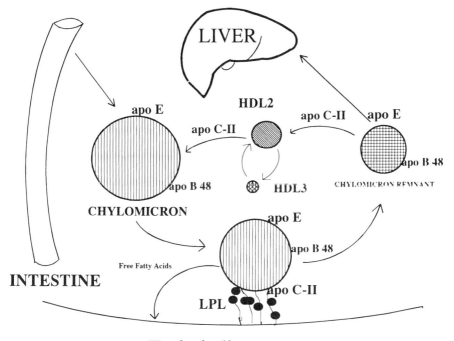

Endothelium

Fig. 14-9. Metabolism of chylomicrons. Chylomicrons are synthesized in the intestine. Apo B is required for their secretion. The isoform secreted by the liver is apo B-48 and is not recognized by the low-density lipoprotein receptor. HDL$_2$ transfers apo C-II to newly secreted chylomicrons. Chylomicrons are then subjected to lipolysis by lipoprotein lipase (LPL). Once they have been depleted of much of their triglycerides, chylomicron remnants are released, their apo C-II transferred back to HDL$_2$, and are then rapidly taken up by the remnant receptor on the liver. This receptor recognizes the apo E moiety, but not apo B-48. HDL = high-density lipoprotein.

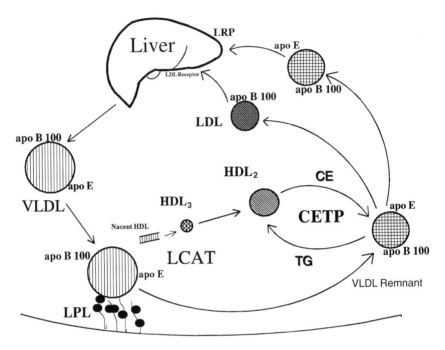

Endothelium

Fig. 14-10. Metabolism of very-low-density lipoprotein (VLDL). VLDL is secreted by the liver and is hydrolyzed on the vascular endothelium by lipoprotein lipase (LPL). LPL (*small filled circles*) is bound electrostatically to heparan sulfate and, in the presence of apo C-II, hydrolyzes triglycerides (TG), releasing free fatty acids, monoglycerides, and diglycerides for cellular uptake. Other surface constituents of VLDL, free cholesterol, and phospholipids participate in the formation of nascent high-density lipoprotein (HDL). The free cholesterol on the surface of nascent HDL is esterified by the action of lecithin–cholesterol acyltransferase (LCAT) to produce cholesterol esters. These sink into the core as nascent HDL is metabolized to the small, dense HDL_3 and finally into the cholesterol ester (CE)–rich HDL_2. The relatively TG-depleted VLDL remnant particle is released from the endothelial surface and then either is taken up by the liver directly via the remnant receptor [low-density lipoprotein receptor-related protein (LRP)], which recognizes apo E, or interacts with CE-rich HDL_2. In that interaction, catalyzed by cholesterol ester transfer protein (CETP), the CE-rich core of HDL_2 is exchanged for the TG-rich core of the VLDL remnant, yielding a TG-rich HDL molecule (*not shown*) and LDL, which is then taken up by the LDL receptor in the liver, which recognizes apo B-100, the isoform secreted by the liver. HDL_2 is processed by lipases to HDL_3 to continue the cycle.

are increased. LDL catabolism has been reported to be either normal or reduced [180] in patients with the nephrotic syndrome and only marginally reduced in nephrotic rats [181].

There are several potential mechanisms that might contribute to delayed lipolysis of chylomicrons and VLDL in the nephrotic syndrome, but none satisfactorily explains all of the data available. Free fatty acids are known to inhibit the action of

LPL, and albumin normally binds free fatty acids in plasma. Thus, one hypothesis for reduced lipolysis is that hypoalbuminemia leads to increased free fatty acid concentration, which in turn inhibits LPL. Rats with hereditary analbuminemia, however, catabolize chylomicrons and VLDL at a normal rate despite the absence of albumin from their plasma [177], disproving that hypothesis. When proteinuria is caused in rats with hereditary analbuminemia, a severe defect in clearance of both chylomicrons and LPL develops (Fig. 14-11) even though there has been no change in plasma albumin concentration. Thus defective chylomicron and VLDL clearance follows urinary protein loss but has little to do with plasma albumin concentration.

When proteinuria is reduced in patients with the nephrotic syndrome, blood lipid levels decrease [182] even if plasma albumin concentration or oncotic pressure is unchanged, suggesting that proteinuria plays a role independently of plasma albumin concentration in the nephrotic syndrome in humans as well as in experimental models of the nephrotic syndrome in animals. It is not yet known how proteinuria causes this defect in lipolysis; however, there are clear abnormalities in lipoprotein metabolism that have been defined in the nephrotic syndrome that might offer insight into the derangements in lipid catabolism.

LPL requires C-II for full activity [183]. This low-molecular-weight apolipoprotein is carried on the surface of VLDL and chylomicrons and is presented to LPL at the site of lipolysis. Following lipolysis, apo C-II is released and transferred to HDL (see Fig. 14-10). Although total plasma apo C-II is normal in nephrotic patients, the amount of this LPL cofactor is reduced by more than 50 percent per unit of VLDL, since the total amount of VLDL is increased while apo C-II is not [184].

One function of HDL is to shuttle apo C-II from remnant particles to nascent VLDL and chylomicrons. Normal catabolism of both lipoproteins therefore requires the presence of normally functioning HDL. HDL is derived from apolipoproteins synthesized either in the liver or gut and cholesterol and phospholipids released by lipolysis of other lipoproteins (see Fig. 14-10). HDL initially appears as discoid nascent HDL containing little or no cholesterol esters [185]. Surface cholesterol is esterified by the enzyme lecithin–cholesterol acyltransferase (LCAT) [185, 186]. Phospholipids are hydrolyzed, the fatty acid, usually arachidonate, is combined to cholesterol to form cholesterol ester, and a mole of lysolecithin is liberated. As in the case of fatty acid transport, albumin serves to bind liberated lysolecithin and accelerates activity of LCAT, thus facilitating the maturation of HDL [187]. The hydrophobic cholesterol esters formed by the LCAT reaction sink into the core of nascent (discoid) HDL and form a spheroid HDL_3 particle with a molecular weight of about 200 kDa. By further action of LCAT, HDL_3 is converted into the 400-kDa HDL_2 particle, a form of HDL more capable of transporting apo C-II. Without recycling of apo C-II by HDL_2, the action of LPL on chylomicrons and VLDL will be greatly reduced. The nephrotic syndrome in humans is characterized by reduced HDL_2.

Changes in the Activities of Liporegulatory Enzymes and of Lipoprotein-Lipoprotein Interactions in the Nephrotic Syndrome

Garber et al. [172] found that LPL activity was reduced in nephrotic rats and suggested that this was responsible for delayed lipolysis. We found that uptake of triglyc-

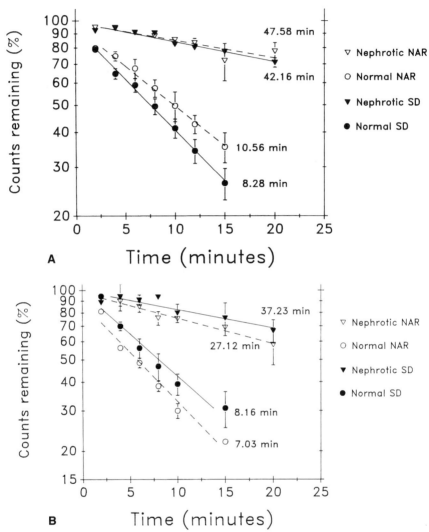

Fig. 14-11. (A) Chylomicron (CM) clearance in normal and nephrotic Sprague-Dawley, (SD) and Nagase analbuminemic rats (NAR). CM clearance was measured by the disappearance of [³H] labeled CMs after intravenous injection. NAR is represented by open symbols and broken lines, SD by solid symbols and lines, nephrotic rats by inverted triangles, and non-nephrotic rats by circles. The half-life of each subgroup is indicated in the figure. Normal SD, N = 6; normal NAR, N = 6; nephrotic SD, N = 8; nephrotic NAR, N = 7. (B) Very-low-density lipoprotein clearance in normal and nephrotic Sprague-Dawley and Nagase analbuminemic rats. (Reproduced from R. W. Davies, I. Staprans, F. N. Hutchison, and G. H. Kaysen, Proteinuria, not altered albumin metabolism, effects hyperlipidemia in the nephrotic rat. *J. Clin. Invest.* 86:600, 1990. By copyright permission of the American Society for Clinical Investigation.)

erides was reduced to about 30 percent of normal in all organs [188], even in heart, which is reported to have normal levels of LPL activity [178]. Chylomicron uptake by hearts isolated from nephrotic rats was decreased in vitro, and the LPL pool bound to the vascular endothelium was reduced by approximately 90 percent. LPL activity not bound to the vascular endothelium, and hence unable to interact with large lipoproteins, was normal [188]. Thus specific reduction of LPL attached to the vascular endothelium may play a role in the reduced catabolism of VLDL and chylomicrons in the nephrotic syndrome [188].

Studies in patients with the nephrotic syndrome have not been as detailed as in the rat; however, when comparable studies are evaluated, both species exhibit similar disturbances in lipid metabolism. The fractional turnover rate of triglycerides is reduced in nephrotic subjects compared to controls, and the half-life of triglycerides is prolonged from 4 to 11 hours in VLDL [189]. Not only is VLDL catabolism decreased, but also the disappearance curve has an unusual shape presumed to result from a delay in the conversion of VLDL to IDL [190]. The delay in lipolysis in humans, as in rats, is proposed to be due to a decrease in LPL activity. Evidence supporting this hypothesis is that LPL activity is reduced in children with the nephrotic syndrome and increases after remission. Furthermore, there is a strong inverse correlation between LPL and the concentration of triglycerides in the VLDL fraction [191].

In addition to changes in LPL activity, the activities of several other enzymes that regulate lipoprotein metabolism are also altered in the nephrotic syndrome. Cholesterol ester transfer protein (CETP) is an enzyme that catalyzes the transfer of the cholesterol ester–rich core of HDL_2 to VLDL remnant particles creating LDL (see Fig. 14-10), increasing LDL cholesterol at the expense of HDL cholesterol. CETP is increased in the plasma of nephrotic patients and correlates positively with VLDL cholesterol and negatively with HDL cholesterol [192]. CETP levels decrease significantly following reduction of proteinuria after treatment with an ACE inhibitor [193], in conjunction with a reduction in VLDL and LDL.

Plasma LCAT activity is increased in plasma of nephrotic patients when measured in assays using excess exogenous substrate [193]. HDL free cholesterol correlates inversely with LCAT activity. Reduction in proteinuria causes a partial normalization of LCAT activity and decreases VLDL and LDL cholesterol. LCAT activity is also increased in nephrotic rats when similar assay conditions are used [194]. These findings are opposite to those of Sestack et al. [195]. Differences may be explained by the different assay conditions used, but the physiologic consequences of these studies depend on the specific reaction catalyzed by LCAT in vivo. The protein LCAT catalyzes two separate reactions: the transfer of an acyl group to free cholesterol, increasing the cholesterol ester content of HDL, and the lysolecitin acyltransferase (LAT) reaction, which takes place on LDL. Sestack et al. [195] found that while esterified cholesterol correlated positively with LCAT activity in normal rats, it correlated negatively in nephrotic animals, suggesting that increases in enzyme activity in vivo may increase the LAT rather than the LCAT reaction.

The observation that HDL_3 is preserved in plasma in nephrotic patients at the apparent expense of HDL_2 is consistent with a reduction in the LCAT reaction; however, increased activity of CETP could also explain this pattern of HDL distribution. This model would also clarify the HDL pattern in rats with the nephrotic syndrome characterized by increased HDL_2. Rats lack CETP, and thus the cycle would be interrupted. Against this explanation is the observation by Warwick et al. [196] that the transition of apo B from VLDL to LDL is impeded in nephrotic humans.

Furukawa et al. [197] report that HDL isolated from normal animals corrects defective lipolysis of VLDL isolated from nephrotic rats by LPL in vitro while HDL isolated from nephrotic rats does not, suggesting that HDL isolated from nephrotic animals may be dysfunctional, and indeed HDL isolated from nephrotic animals is structurally abnormal, even though HDL in the nephrotic rat is predominantly the larger, putatively more functional HDL_2. Thus, multiple separate defects in the peripheral catabolism of triglyceride-rich lipoproteins may be responsible for delayed lipolysis.

Clinical Implications of Hyperlipidemia in Renal Disease

The changes that occur in blood lipoprotein composition in the nephrotic syndrome [163, 198]—reduced HDL_2 cholesterol, a relative increase in HDL_3 cholesterol, and the massive increase in total cholesterol, mostly found in the LDL, IDL, and VLDL fractions—should be expected to cause increased risk of atherosclerotic disease. These abnormalities are further complicated by the increase in plasma Lp(a) levels, increased platelet aggregability [199], increased plasma viscosity, increased concentration of highly atherogenic remnants of VLDL, and chylomicron catabolism in plasma. Indeed, accelerated atherosclerosis has been reported in patients with proteinuria and hyperlipidemia and in some studies has been associated with a sharply increased incidence of cardiovascular disease and stroke [200]. One study reported an 85-fold increase in the incidence of ischemic heart disease in such patients [201]. In another recent retrospective analysis of 142 patients with proteinuria greater than 3.5 g/day, the relative risk of myocardial infarction was found to be 5.5 and the risk of cardiac death 2.8 compared to age-matched, sex-matched controls [202]. For this reason, there is no rationale for leaving pronounced hyperlipidemia untreated for prolonged periods of time in a patient with the nephrotic syndrome.

Disordered lipid metabolism could also play a role in the cycle of progressive renal failure that occurs following the initiation of renal injury [203], although again this link has by no means been established in humans or in animal models of renal disease that are not associated with substantial increases in cholesterol levels. While the association between hyperlipidemia and progression of renal disease has not as yet been confirmed in humans, one disorder that causes hypercholesterolemia in humans, hereditary LCAT deficiency, may be linked to progressive mesangial and glomerular sclerosis [204].

Treatment of Hyperlipidemia

It is not indicated to treat the qualitative abnormalities that characterize the lipid disorders of the nephrotic syndrome or to treat hyperlipidemia if the underlying cause of the nephrotic syndrome is directly treatable, such as in minimal change nephrotic syndrome. If the duration of hyperlipidemia is anticipated to be prolonged, however, it is wise to initiate therapy. The first goal of treatment should be to reduce urinary protein excretion, if possible. Treatment of nephrotic patients with either ACE inhibitors [205] or cyclooxygenase inhibitors [67, 206] results in a decline in both proteinuria and blood lipid levels [182, 193] even if plasma albumin concentration does not increase [182] or increases only slightly [207]. The decline in blood lipid levels includes a decrease in total cholesterol, Lp(a) [169], a decrease in VLDL and LDL cholesterol, and a decrease in the activity of LCAT [193]. The effect of ACE inhibitors is a class effect and appears to be shared by all drugs within this class.

It is probably prudent to restrict dietary cholesterol and saturated lipids in patients with the nephrotic syndrome. If conservative therapy (reduction in proteinuria, dietary fat restriction) does not effectively reduce hyperlipidemia, a variety of lipid-lowering drugs including the 3-hydroxy-3-methylglutaryl coenzyme A reductase (HMG-CoA reductase) inhibitors [208], antioxidants [209], and fibric acid derivatives [210] can be useful, but review of this subject is beyond the scope of this chapter.

Edema Formation: Defenses Against Reduced Plasma Oncotic Pressure

Capillary hydrostatic pressure serves to force fluid from the vascular compartment into the interstitial space. This hydrostatic force is partially balanced by the difference between plasma oncotic pressure and that exerted by interstitial proteins. Interstitial protein concentration is between 25 and 50 percent that of plasma protein [211], and the difference between oncotic pressure exerted by plasma and interstitial proteins ($\Delta\bar{\pi}$) serves to retain salt and water in the vascular space. Fluid not reabsorbed by the time blood has reached the venous end of the capillary bed is returned to the vascular space via the lymphatics.

In steady state:

$$\text{Lymph flow} = Kf\,(\Delta\bar{P} - \Delta\bar{\pi})$$

where Kf = capillary hydraulic conductivity, $\Delta\bar{P}$ = capillary hydrostatic − tissue hydrostatic pressure, and $\Delta\bar{\pi}$ = plasma π − tissue π [212, 213].

When the fall in $\Delta\bar{\pi}$ becomes great enough, the net amount of fluid filtered by the capillaries will exceed maximal lymph flow, and edema will inevitably occur. This increased net transport of fluid into the interstitial space should lead to plasma volume contraction. However, Meltzer et al. [214] subsequently identified a group of patients with the nephrotic syndrome who had a normal or expanded plasma volume and reduced plasma renin activity, despite a profound reduction in oncotic pressure. These patients represented a subset who had nephritic disease as opposed to patients with minimal change nephrotic syndrome. Some patients with minimal

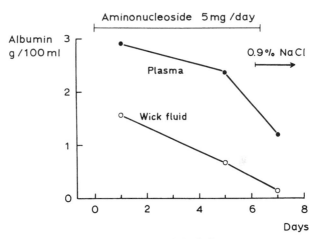

Fig. 14-12. Plasma and subcutaneous interstitial fluid albumin concentration in a rat during development of experimental nephrotic syndrome. Sodium chloride was added to drinking water at day 6. (Adapted from K. Aukland, Autoregulation of interstitial fluid volume: Edema-preventing mechanisms. *Scand. J. Clin. Lab. Invest.* 31:247, 1973.)

change nephrotic syndrome have also been found to have an increased plasma and blood volume [215, 216].

How is it possible to maintain a normal or even expanded plasma volume when oncotic pressure is greatly reduced? If it is indeed possible to maintain a normal plasma volume, why does the kidney retain salt and water in nephrotic patients? The answer to the first question lies in part in the fact that interstitial albumin mass is reduced to an even greater extent than is the plasma albumin mass in the nephrotic syndrome [81]. The mobilization of extravascular albumin is a rapid, hemodynamically mediated response to a decrease in plasma oncotic pressure or to an increase in transcapillary hydrostatic pressure [211, 212, 217–220]. Figure 14-12 illustrates the parallel decrease in interstitial albumin that occurs following the development of proteinuria in a rat with an experimental form of the nephrotic syndrome induced by injection of puromycin aminonucleoside [221]. Although albumin decreases, $\Delta\bar{\pi}$ decreases little or not at all because interstitial protein is swept into the vascular compartment by increased lymphatic flow. In addition, since the capillary endothelium is far more permeable to water than to protein, when transcapillary hydraulic flux increases, the resulting plasma ultrafiltrate is much poorer in protein than when hydraulic flux is reduced. $\Delta\bar{\pi}$ did not decrease in nephrotic rats until saline was administered (see Fig. 14-12).

Edema formation in the nephrotic syndrome may involve two parallel processes (Fig. 14-13). Reduced plasma oncotic pressure leads to augmented net flux of fluid across the systemic capillary bed, but these alterations may be entirely or largely offset by increased lymphatic return from the periphery and reduction in interstitial oncotic pressure so that $\Delta\bar{\pi}$ remains unchanged. Edema formation is not generally obligated to occur until total proteins decrease to around 4 g/dl. The second process results from a reduced ability of the nephrotic kidney to excrete a sodium load,

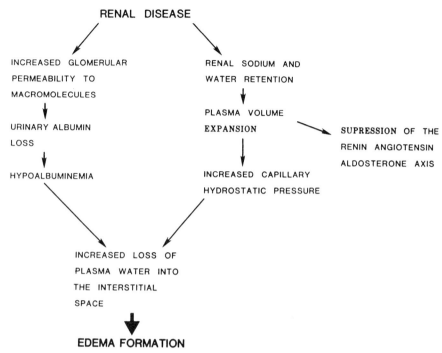

RENAL DISEASE

INCREASED GLOMERULAR PERMEABILITY TO MACROMOLECULES

RENAL SODIUM AND WATER RETENTION

URINARY ALBUMIN LOSS

PLASMA VOLUME EXPANSION

SUPRESSION OF THE RENIN ANGIOTENSIN ALDOSTERONE AXIS

HYPOALBUMINEMIA

INCREASED CAPILLARY HYDROSTATIC PRESSURE

INCREASED LOSS OF PLASMA WATER INTO THE INTERSTITIAL SPACE

EDEMA FORMATION

Fig. 14-13. Primary renal sodium retention with resultant edema formation. Renal salt and water retention occurs as a result of the renal disease itself and causes plasma volume expansion. This produces increased capillary hydrostatic pressure, which in conjunction with the increased transcapillary flux of fluid resulting from hypoalbuminemia causes edema. Edema formation is not a direct consequence of reduced osmotic pressure alone, nor is renal salt and water retention a consequence of increased transudation of fluid into the interstitial space with resultant activation of the renin-angiotensin-aldosterone axis. (From G. A. Kaysen, B. D. Myers, W. G. Couser, et al., Mechanisms and consequences of proteinuria. *Lab. Invest.* 54:479, 1986.)

either in response to plasma volume expansion [222–224] or in response to atrial natriuretic factor (ANF) [225–227]. The inability of the nephrotic kidney to excrete a salt load is intrinsic to the nephrotic kidney itself and is unrelated to systemic volume needs. Studies utilizing unilateral models of proteinuria most clearly demonstrate that impedance to sodium excretion is intrinsic to the nephrotic kidney and not reflective of plasma volume regulation. In one such study, Perico et al. [226] demonstrated an inability of a proteinuric kidney to excrete fluid or sodium in response to infused ANF even though ANF increased GFR in both the proteinuric kidney and the normal contralateral kidney equally. Clearly both the normal contralateral kidney and the proteinuric kidney were exposed to the same oncotic pressure and the same levels of circulating hormones responsible for plasma volume regulation.

Regardless of the mechanism, the proteinuric kidney avidly reabsorbs filtered salt in the distal nephron [228] even in the presence of plasma volume expansion. As a consequence of these combined effects, the systemic capillary bed is faced with increased hydrostatic pressure at the very time that defense mechanisms normally employed to counteract edema formation, increased lymphatic flow and decreased interstitial protein concentration, have already been maximized. Edema results from the combined effect of primary renal salt and water retention coupled with reduced defenses against edema formation resulting from the urinary losses of proteins of intermediate weight, with the resulting decrease in both intravascular and interstitial oncotic pressure. These processes deprive the lymphatic system of the capacity to respond to increased hydrostatic pressure.

Nutritional Recommendations for Patients with Nephrotic Syndrome

Dietary Protein

In patients with nephrotic syndrome, dietary protein augmentation above 1 g/kg/day is not of demonstrated benefit and may cause increased urinary albumin losses. These patients' diets should provide 0.8 to 1.0 g/kg/day of protein and 35 kcal/kg/day of energy. Twenty-four hour urinary protein excretion should be measured every 2 to 3 months and urinary urea excretion monitored to ensure that patients are eating the quantity of protein recommended and that proteinuria decreases and albumin and protein concentration do not decrease when dietary protein intake is restricted to these levels.

Dietary protein intake can be estimated because, in steady state, dietary protein is equal to protein catabolic rate. If total-body urea pools do not change (blood urea nitrogen is neither decreasing or increasing), it is possible to estimate the amount of protein that has been eaten by the following formula:

Protein catabolic rate = (10.7 + 24-hour urinary urea excretion/0.14) g/day

+ urinary protein excretion

If there is variance from the prescribed diet, an accurate nutritional history should be obtained and the diet adjusted accordingly.

In addition to these nutritional recommendations, processes that cause inflammation should be identified and treated if possible, since these directly suppress albumin synthesis [229, 230]. Obvious hormonal deficiency states, such as hypoadrenalism, hypothyroidism, or diabetes, should also be identified and treated.

Dietary Fat

Hyperlipidemia is common in the nephrotic syndrome and is a consequence of both increased synthesis of lipids and apolipoproteins [170] and their decreased catabolism [171, 177, 231]. The characteristic disorder in blood lipid composition in nephrotic patients is an increase in the LDL, VLDL [162], and/or IDL fractions, but no change [162] or a decrease in HDL [163], resulting in an increased LDL/HDL cholesterol ratio. The IDL fractions probably arise as VLDL and chylomicron remnants and are atherogenic [232]. The atherogenic lipoprotein Lp(a) also increases in patients with the nephrotic syndrome [12, 169]. All of these changes are characteristic of those associated with accelerated atherogenesis in other clinical settings.

Soy or Vegan diets have been shown to reduce urinary protein excretion in patients with the nephrotic syndrome [233]. While it is claimed that this effect is a consequence of the reduced lipid content of the diets [233], there is no convincing data presented that changes in dietary lipids are responsible for the salutary effects of these diets. Lipids however represent a wide variety of substances, including steroids, saturated and unsaturated fatty acids, phospholipids, and other compounds, many of which are either directly biologically active or are precursors of important biologically active metabolites. Much attention has been focused on the effect of polyunsaturated fatty acids on renal hemodynamics and on expression of renal injury.

In studies involving human subjects, Gentile et al. [234] added 5 g of fish oil per day to the diet of patients with the nephrotic syndrome who had been maintained on a soy vegetarian diet and found no beneficial effect on either proteinuria or on blood lipids when compared to patients maintained on the soy diet without fish oil supplementation. In contrast, Hall et al. [235] found that 15 g of fish oil per day caused a decrease in total triglycerides and LDL triglycerides and an increase in LDL cholesterol. Donadio et al. [236] treated 55 patients with 12 g of fish oil per day in a recently concluded prospective randomized placebo-controlled study and found a significant reduction in the rate of progression of renal disease using a 50 percent increase in serum creatinine concentration as a study end point. At the end of the treatment period, the fish oil–treated group had a lower prevalence of hypertension, elevated serum creatinine, and nephrotic range proteinuria. These studies suggest that while alterations in dietary polyunsaturated fatty acids may alter some manifestations of the nephrotic state, the effects are dependent on the model being investigated and should still be viewed with caution. These agents may be neither predictable nor salutary for all patients with renal disease.

Pharmacologic Means to Reduce Glomerular Proteinuria

Angiotensin-Converting Enzyme Inhibitors

ACE inhibitors reduce proteinuria in experimental models of the nephrotic syndrome and in some nephrotic patients as well. ACE inhibitors reduce proteinuria by decreasing the fraction of glomerular ultrafiltrate that passes through the nonselective shunt pathway, described previously, and increases the fraction passing through the normal population of small pores. GFR is generally not reduced by ACE inhibitors. Proteinuria is reduced, accompanied by an increase in serum albumin concentration and reduction in blood lipid levels in rats with experimental models of the nephrotic syndrome, but it has not yet been definitely established whether reduced albuminuria is accompanied by correction of reduced albumin and hyperlipidemia in nephrotic patients.

The antiproteinuric effect of ACE inhibitors seems to be shared by all drugs of this class studied to date; however, this property is not shared by all other antihypertensive agents [109]. Results obtained with both α-antagonists and certain classes of calcium channel blockers have been inconsistent and not sufficiently well documented to warrant clinical use of these agents for control of proteinuria at this time.

It is important when prescribing an ACE inhibitor for the purpose of reducing proteinuria to monitor the patient closely for either a reduction in blood pressure or a decrease in GFR. It is also important to discontinue diuretic therapy for several days preceding initiation of therapy with an ACE inhibitor to avoid inhibition of ACE in the presence of a plasma volume contracted state. Therapy should be initiated with a very low dose (2.5 mg of enalapril or 12.5 mg of captopril) and the blood pressure checked within 24 hours, with the aim of ultimately reducing mean arterial pressure by about 10 mm Hg. The dose of the ACE inhibitor should be increased every other week to attain that end point. It is also important to obtain measurements of renal function at 1, 2, and 4 weeks, as well as to monitor potassium concentration, especially in individuals who have significant renal insufficiency (creatinine > 3 mg/dl), diabetes, or underlying hyperkalemia. ACE inhibitors should be discontinued if potassium concentration remains persistently elevated above 5.5 mEq/L. Urinary protein should be monitored once every month or two to evaluate the clinical response. In the still limited experience, decreased urinary protein excretion occurs gradually over several weeks. In some instances, neither the blood pressure nor proteinuria responds to rather large doses of ACE inhibitors, and therapy with these agents should then be discontinued. Some patients, especially those with renal artery stenosis, may exhibit marked reduction in blood pressure and in GFR with even low doses of ACE inhibitors. It is important to identify these patients as well and to discontinue ACE inhibitor therapy if a marked reduction in GFR occurs.

Cyclooxygenase Inhibitors

Cyclooxygenase inhibitors are another class of drugs that may prove helpful in reducing proteinuria in nephrotic patients, although unlike ACE inhibitors, they generally cause a reduction in GFR. Proteinuria is reduced by a combined effect both to reduce total GFR and to reduce the fraction of glomerular ultrafiltrate that passes through the large nonselective pores in the GBM [67]. The antiproteinuric action of these agents may be potentiated by a low-sodium diet and the use of diuretics. Large doses of cyclooxygenase inhibitors, such as 50 mg of indomethacin three times a day, may still be necessary. As with ACE inhibitors, treatment with cyclooxygenase inhibitors may cause hyperkalemia [237], especially in patients with diabetic renal disease and patients with underlying hyperkalemia. The decrease in GFR caused by these agents may also limit their utility. Unlike ACE inhibitors, cyclooxygenase inhibitors are likely to increase renal sodium retention, potentially worsening edema formation or increasing the need for diuretic therapy [238]. Treatment of nephrotic patients with an ACE inhibitor and a cyclooxygenase inhibitor simultaneously may be clinically hazardous, resulting in a marked decrease in GFR and in hyperkalemia. Other potential risks of cyclooxygenase inhibition include acute renal failure and interstitial nephritis, in addition to gastrointestinal disturbances.

Acknowledgment. This work was supported in part by the research service of the United States Department of Veterans Affairs and in part by a grant from the National Institutes of Health RO1 DK 42297.

References

1. Waller KV, Ward KM, Mahan JD, Wismatt DK: Current concepts in proteinuria. *Clin Chem* 35:755–765, 1989.
2. Maack T: Renal handling of low molecular weight proteins. *Am J Med* 58:57–64, 1975.
3. Moglielnicki RP, Waldmann TA, Strober W: Renal handling of low molecular weight proteins: I. L-chain metabolism in experimental renal disease. *J Clin Invest* 50:901–909, 1971.
4. Kaysen GA, Myers BD, Couser WG, et al: Mechanisms and consequences of proteinuria. *Lab Invest* 54:479–498, 1986.
5. Kyle R: Multiple myeloma: Review of 869 cases. *Mayo Clin Proc* 50:29–40, 1975.
6. Hall CL, Hardwicke J: Low molecular weight proteinuria. *Annu Rev Med* 30:199–211, 1979.
7. Harrison JF, Cantab MB: Urinary lysozyme, ribonuclease, and low-molecular-weight protein in renal disease. *Lancet* 1:371–375, 1968.
8. Deen WM, Bridges CR, Brenner BM, Myers BD: Heteroporous model of glomerular size selectivity: Application to normal and nephrotic humans. *Am J Physiol* 249:F374–F389, 1985.
9. Baldamus CA, Galaske R, Eisenbach GM, et al: Glomerular protein filtration in normal and nephrotic rats: A micropuncture study. *Contr Nephrol* 1:37–49, 1975.
10. Mogensen CE, Christiansen CE: Predicting diabetic nephropathy in insulin-dependent patients. *N Engl J Med* 311:89–93, 1984.
11. Woo J, Floyd M, Cannon DC: Albumin and β_2-microglobulin radioimmunoassays applied to monitoring of renal-allograft function and in differentiating glomerular and tubular diseases. *Clin Chem* 27:709–713, 1981.
12. Mogensen CE: Progression of nephropathy in long-term diabetics with proteinuria and effect of initial anti-hypertensive treatment. *Scand J Clin Lab Invest* 36:383–386, 1976.
13. Viberti G, Mogensen CE, Groop LC, Pauls JF: Effect of captopril on progression to clinical proteinuria in patients with insulin-dependent diabetes mellitus and microalbuminuria: European Microalbuminuria Captopril Study Group. *JAMA* 271:275–279, 1994.
14. Lewis EJ, Hunsicker LG, Bain RP, Rohde RD: The effect of angiotensin-converting-enzyme inhibition on diabetic nephropathy: The Collaborative Study Group. *N Engl J Med* 329:1456–1462, 1993.
15. Eddy AA: Interstitial nephritis induced by protein-overload proteinuria. *Am J Pathol* 135:719–733, 1989.
16. Thomas ME, Schreiner GF: Contribution of proteinuria to progressive renal injury: Consequences of tubular uptake of fatty acid bearing albumin. *Am J Nephrol* 13:385–398, 1993.
17. Border WA, Cohen AH: Renal biopsy diagnosis of clinically silent multiple myeloma. *Ann Intern Med* 93:43–46, 1980.
18. Buchet JP, Roels H, Bernard A Jr, Lauwerys R: Assessment of renal function of workers exposed to inorganic lead, cadmium or mercury vapor. *J Occup Med* 22:741–750, 1980.
19. Kjellström T: Exposure and accumulation of cadmium in populations from Japan, the United States, and Sweden. *Environ Health Perspect* 28:169–197, 1979.
20. Butler EA, Flynn FV: The proteinuria of renal tubular disorders. *Lancet* 2:978–982, 1958.
21. DeFronzo RA, Thier SO: Inherited Disorders of Renal Tubule Function. In Brenner BM, Rector FFC Jr (eds): *The Kidney* (3rd ed). Philadelphia, Saunders, 1985, pp 1297–1339.
22. Hutchison FN, Kaysen GA: Albuminuria causes lysozymuria in rats with Heymann nephritis. *Kidney Int* 33:787–791, 1988.

23. Kaye WA, Griffiths WC, Camara PD, et al: The significance of β_2-microglobulinuria associated with gentamicin therapy. *Ann Clin Lab Sci* 11:530–537, 1981.

24. Schentag JJ, Sutfin TA, Plaut ME, Jusko WJ: Early detection of aminoglycoside nephrotoxicity with urinary β_2-microglobulin. *J Med* 9:201–210, 1978.

25. Tsuchiya K, Iwao S, Sugita M, Sakurai H: Increased urinary β_2-microglobulin in cadmium exposure: Dose-effect relationship and biological significance of β_2-microglobulin. *Environ Health Perspect* 28:147–153, 1979.

26. Lauwerys RR, Roels HA, Bucher JP, et al: Investigations on the lung and kidney function in workers exposed to cadmium. *Environ Health Perspect* 28:137–145, 1979.

27. Park CH, Maack T: Albumin absorption and catabolism by isolated perfused proximal convoluted tubules of the rabbit. *J Clin Invest* 73:767–777, 1984.

28. Hill GS, Morei-Maroger L, Mery JP, et al: Renal lesions in multiple myeloma: Their relationship to assorted protein abnormalities. *Am J Kidney Dis* 2:423–438, 1983.

29. Ng VL, Chen KH, Hwang KM, et al: The clinical significance of human immunodeficiency virus type 1-associated paraproteins. *Blood* 74:2471–2475, 1989.

30. Ng VL, Hwang KM, Reyes GR, et al: High titer anti-HIV antibody reactivity associated with a paraprotein spike in a homosexual male with AIDS related complex. *Blood* 71:1397–1401, 1988.

31. Ravnskov U: Low molecular weight proteinuria in association with paroxysmal myoglobinuria. *Clin Nephrol* 3:65–69, 1975.

32. Gabow PA, Kaehny WD, Kelleher SP: The spectrum of rhabdomyolysis. *Medicine* 61:141–152, 1982.

33. Koffler A, Friedler RM, Massry SG: Acute renal failure due to nontraumatic rhabdomyolysis. *Ann Intern Med* 85:23–28, 1976.

34. Eneas JF, Schoenfeld PY, Humphreys MH: The effect of infusion of mannitol–sodium bicarbonate on the clinical course of myoglobinuria. *Arch Intern Med* 139:801–805, 1979.

35. Owen CA, Mubarak SJ, Hargens AR, et al: Intramural pressures with limb compression: Clarification of the pathogenesis of drug-induced muscle-compression syndrome. *N Engl J Med* 300:1169–1172, 1979.

36. Knochel JP: Hypophosphatemia in the alcoholic. *Arch Intern Med* 140:613–615, 1980.

37. Knochel JP, Schlein EM: On the mechanism of rhabdomyolysis in potassium depletion. *J Clin Invest* 51:1750–1758, 1972.

38. Bank WJH, DiMauro S, Bonilla E, et al: A disorder of muscle lipid metabolism and myoglobinuria: Absence of carnitine palmityl transferase. *N Engl J Med* 292:443–449, 1975.

39. Patten BM, Wood JM, Harati Y, Howell RR: Familial recurrent rhabdomyolysis due to carnitine palmityl transferase deficiency. *Am J Med* 67:167–171, 1979.

40. Layzer RB, Rowland LP, Ranney HM. Muscle phosphofructokinase deficiency. *Arch Neurol* 17:512–523, 1967.

41. Paster SB, Adams DF, Hollenberg NK: Acute renal failure in McArdle's disease and myoglobinuric states. *Radiology* 114:567–570, 1979.

42. Todd D: Diagnosis of haemolytic states. *Clin Haematol* 4:63–81, 1975.

43. Goldfinger D: Acute hemolytic transfusion reactions: A fresh look at pathogenesis and considerations regarding therapy. *Transfusion* 17:85–98, 1977.

44. Relihan M, Litwin MS: Effects of stroma free hemoglobin solution on clearance rate and renal function. *Surgery* 71:395–399, 1972.

45. Schmidt PJ, Holland PV: Pathogenesis of the acute renal failure associated with incompatible transfusion. *Lancet* 2:1169–1172, 1967.

46. Fowler BA, Weissberg JB: Arsine poisoning. *N Engl J Med* 291:1171–1174, 1974.

47. Levinsky WJ, Smalley RV, Hillyer PN, Shindler RL: Arsine hemolysis. *Arch Environ Health* 20:436–440, 1970.

48. Pinto SS: Arsine poisoning: Evaluation of the acute phase. *J Occup Med* 18:633–635, 1976.

49. Chan TK, Najm LW, Bg RP: Methemoglobinemia, Heinz bodies and acute massive intravascular hemolysis in lysol poisoning. *Blood* 38:739–744, 1971.

50. Jacob HS, Amsden T: Acute hemolytic anemia with rigid red cells in hypophosphatemia. *N Engl J Med* 285:1446–1450, 1971.

51. Rosse WF: Paroxysmal nocturnal hemoglobinuria: Present status and future prospects. *West J Med* 132:219–228, 1980.
52. Davidson RJL: March or exertional haemoglobinuria. *Semin Hematol* 6:150–161, 1969.
53. Crexells C, Aerucgudem N, Bonny Y, et al: Factors influencing hemolysis in valve prostheses. *Am Heart J* 84:161–170, 1972.
54. Maack T, Johnson V, Kau ST, et al: Renal filtration, transport, and metabolism of low-molecular weight proteins: A review. *Kidney Int* 16:251–270, 1979.
55. Brenner BM, Baylis C, Deen WM: Transport of molecules across renal glomerular capillaries. *Physiol Rev* 56:502–534, 1976.
56. Bohrer MP, Deen WM, Robertson CR, Brenner BM: Mechanism of angiotensin II induced proteinuria in the rat. *Am J Physiol* 233:(*Renal Fluid Electrolyte Physiol* 2):F13–F21, 1977.
57. Deen WM, Bridges CR, Brenner BM: Biophysical basis of glomerular permselectivity. *J Membrane Biol* 71:1–10, 1983.
58. Chang RLS, Deen WM, Robertson CR, Brenner BM: Permselectivity of the glomerular capillary wall: III. Restricted transport of polyanions. *Kidney Int* 8:212–218, 1975.
59. Kanwar YS: Biophysiology of glomerular filtration and proteinuria. *Lab Invest* 51:7–21, 1984.
60. Daniels BS, Deen WM, Mayer G, et al: Glomerular permeability barrier in the rat: Functional assessment by in vitro methods. *J Clin Invest* 92:929–936, 1993.
61. Myers BD, Winetz JA, Chui F, Michaels AS: Mechanisms of proteinuria in diabetic nephropathy: A study of glomerular barrier function. *Kidney Int* 21:633–641, 1982.
62. Hashimoto H, Sibley R, Myers BD: A comparison between the glomerular injuries of minimal change (MCN) and focal/segmental sclerosis (FSGS) in nephrotic humans. *Kidney Int* 37:507A, 1990.
63. Yoshioka T, Mitarai T, Kon V, et al: Role for angiotensin II in an overt functional proteinuria. *Kidney Int* 30:538–545, 1986.
64. Lianos EA, Andres GA, Dunn MJ: Glomerular prostaglandin and thromboxane synthesis in rat nephrotoxic serum nephritis. *J Clin Invest* 72:1439–1448, 1983.
65. Remuzzi G, Imberti L, Rossini M, et al: Increased glomerular thromboxane synthesis as a possible cause of proteinuria in experimental nephrosis. *J Clin Invest* 75:94–101, 1985.
66. Eisenbach GM, Van Liew JB, Boylan JW: Effect of angiotensin on the filtration of protein in the rat kidney. *Kidney Int* 8:80–87, 1975.
67. Goldbetz H, Black V, Shemesh O, Myers BD: Mechanism of the antiproteinuric effect of indomethacin in nephrotic humans. *Am J Physiol* 256:(*Renal Fluid Electrolyte Physiol* 25): F44–F51, 1989.
68. Shultz PJ, Tolins JP: Adaptation to increased dietary salt intake in the rat: Role of endogenous nitric oxide. *J Clin Invest* 91:642–650, 1993.
69. Zatz R, De Nucci G: Effects of acute nitric oxide inhibition on rat glomerular inhibition on rat glomerular microcirculation. *Am J Physiol* 261:(*Renal Fluid Electrolyte Physiol* 30): F360–F363, 1991.
70. Baylis C, Mitruka B, Deng A: Chronic blockade of nitric oxide synthesis in the rat produces systemic hypertension and glomerular damage. *J Clin Invest* 90:278–281, 1992.
71. Earley LE, Farland M: Nephrotic syndrome. In Strauss MB, Welt LG (eds): *Diseases of the Kidney* (3rd ed). Boston, Little, Brown, 1979, pp 765–813.
72. Earley LE, Havel RJ, Hopper J, Graus H: Nephrotic Syndrome. *Calif Med* 115:23–41, 1971.
73. Jensen H, Rossing N, Anderson SB, Jarnum S: Albumin metabolism in the nephrotic syndrome in adults. *Clin Sci* 33:445–457, 1967.
74. Kaysen GA, Gambertoglio J, Jiminez I, et al: Effect of dietary protein intake on albumin homeostasis in nephrotic patients. *Kidney Int* 29:572–577, 1986.
75. Kaitz AL: Albumin metabolism in nephrotic adults. *J Lab Clin Med* 53:186–194, 1959.
76. Gitlin D, Janeway CA, Farr LE: Studies on the metabolism of plasma proteins in nephrotic syndrome: I. Albumin, gamma-globulin and iron-binding globulin. *J Clin Invest* 35:44–55, 1956.
77. Keutmann EH, Bassett SH: Dietary protein in hemorrhagic Bright's disease: II. The effect of diet on serum proteins, proteinuria and tissue proteins. *J Clin Invest* 14:871–888, 1935.
78. Peters JP, Bulger HA: The relation of albuminuria to protein requirement in nephritis. *Arch Intern Med* 37:153–185, 1926.

79. Baynes JW, Thorpe SR: Identification of sites of albumin catabolism in the rat. *Arch Biochem Biophys* 206:372–379, 1981.
80. Waldmann TA: Albumin Catabolism. In Rosemoer M, Oratz M, Rothschild A (eds): *Albumin Structure, Function and Uses.* New York, Permagon, 1977, pp 255–273.
81. Sellers AL, Katz J, Bonorris G, Okyyama S: Determination of extravascular albumin in the rat. *J Lab Clin Med* 68:177–185, 1966.
82. Reeve EB, Chen AY: Regulation of Interstitial Albumin. In Rothschild MA, Waldmann T (eds): *Plasma Protein Metabolism: Regulation of Synthesis, Distribution, and Degradation.* New York, Academic, 1970.
83. Yedgar S, Carew TE, Pittman RC, Beltz WF: Tissue sites of catabolism of albumin in rabbits. *Am J Physiol* 244:(*Endocrinol Metab* 7):E101–E107, 1983.
84. Katz J, Rosenfeld S, Sellers AL: Role of the kidney in plasma albumin catabolism. *Am J Physiol* 198:814–818, 1960.
85. Galaske RG, Baldamus CA, Stolte H: Plasma protein handling in the rat kidney: Micropuncture experiments in the acute heterologous phase of anti-gbm-nephritis. *Pflugers Arch* 375:269–277, 1978.
86. Landwehr DM, Carvalho JS, Oken DE: Micropuncture studies of the filtration and absorption of albumin by nephrotic rats. *Kidney Int* 11:9–17, 1977.
87. Lewy JE, Pesce A: Micropuncture study of albumin transfer in aminonucleoside nephrosis in the rat. *Pediatr Res* 7:553–559, 1973.
88. Oken DE, Cotes SC, Mende CW: Micropuncture study of tubular transport of albumin in rats with aminonucleoside nephrosis. *Kidney Int* 1:3–11, 1972.
89. Kaysen GA, Kirkpatrick WG, Couser WG: Albumin homeostasis in the nephrotic rat: Nutritional considerations. *Am J Physiol* 247:(*Renal Fluid Electrolyte Physiol* 16):F192–F202, 1984.
90. Rothschild MA, Oratz M, Evans CD, Schreiber SS: Albumin Synthesis. In Rosemoer M, Oratz M, Rothschild A (eds): *Albumin Structure, Function and Uses.* New York, Pergamon, 1977, pp 227–255.
91. Rothschild MA, Oratz M, Schreiber SS: Albumin Synthesis. In Javitt NB (ed): *Liver and Biliary Tract Physiology: I. International Review of Physiology.* Baltimore, University Park Press, 1980, vol 21, pp 249–274.
92. Morgan EH, Peters T Jr: The biosynthesis of rat serum albumin. *J Biol Chem* 246:3500–3507, 1971.
93. Kirsch R, Frith L, Black E, Hoffenberg R: Regulation of albumin synthesis and catabolism by alteration of dietary protein. *Nature* 217:578–579, 1968.
94. Moshage HJ, Janssen JAM, Franssen JH, et al: Study of the molecular mechanisms of decreased liver synthesis of albumin in inflammation. *J Clin Invest* 79:1635–1641, 1987.
95. Kaysen GA, Jones H Jr, Martin V, Hutchison FN: A low protein diet restricts albumin synthesis in nephrotic rats. *J Clin Invest* 83:1623–1629, 1989.
96. Yamauchi A, Imai E, Noguchi T, et al: Albumin gene transcription is enhanced in liver of nephrotic rats. *Am J Physiol* 254:(*Endocrinol Metab* 17):E676–E679, 1988.
97. Rothschild MA, Oratz M, Franklin EC, Schreiber SS: The effect of hypergammaglobulinemia on albumin metabolism in hyperimmunized rabbits studied with albumin I-131. *J Clin Invest* 41:1564–1571, 1967.
98. Rothschild MA, Oratz M, Wimer E, Schreiber SS: Studies on albumin synthesis: The effect of dextran and cortisone on albumin metabolism in rabbits studied with albumin I-131. *J Clin Invest* 40:545–554, 1961.
99. Rothschild MA, Oratz M, Mongelli J, Schreiber SS: Albumin metabolism in rabbits during gamma globulin infusions. *J Lab Clin Med* 66:733–740, 1965.
100. Rothschild MA, Oratz M, Mongelli J, Schreiber SS: Effect of albumin concentration on albumin synthesis in the perfused liver. *Am J Physiol* 216:117–1130, 1969.
101. Dich J, Hansen SE, Thieden HID: Effect of albumin concentration and colloid osmotic pressure on albumin synthesis in the perfused rat liver. *Acta Physiol Scand* 89:352–358, 1973.
102. Hoffenberg R, Black E, Brock JF: Albumin and gamma-globulin tracer studies in protein depletion states. *J Clin Invest* 45:143–152, 1966.
103. James WP, Hay AM: Albumin metabolism: Effect of the nutritional state and the dietary protein intake. *J Clin Invest* 47:1958–1972, 1968.

104. Smith JE, Lunn PG: Albumin-synthesizing capacity of hepatocytes isolated from rats fed diets differing in protein and energy content. *Ann Nutr Metab* 28:281–287, 1984.
105. Lunn PG, Austin S: Excess energy intake promotes the development of hypoalbuminemia in rats fed on low-protein diets. *Br J Nutr* 49:9–16, 1983.
106. Coward WA, Sawyer MB: Whole-body albumin mass and distribution in rats fed on low-protein diets. *Br J Nutr* 37:127–134, 1977.
107. Blainey JD: High protein diets in the treatment of the nephrotic syndrome. *Clin Sci* 13:567–581, 1954.
108. Rosenberg ME, Swanson JE, Thomas BL, Hostetter TH: Glomerular and hormonal responses to dietary protein intake in human renal disease. *Am J Physiol* 253(*Renal Fluid Electrolyte Physiol* 22):F1083–F1090, 1987.
109. Hutchison FN, Schambelan M, Kaysen GA: Modulation of albuminuria by dietary protein and converting enzyme inhibition. *Am J Physiol* 253:(*Renal Fluid Electrolyte Physiol* 22):F719–F725, 1987.
110. Zatz R, Meyer TW, Rennke HG, Brenner BM: Predominance of hemodynamic rather than metabolic factors in the pathogenesis of diabetic glomerulopathy. *Proc Natl Acad Sci USA* 82:5963–5967, 1985.
111. Brenner BM, Meyer TW, Hostetter TH: Dietary protein intake and the progressive nature of kidney disease: The role of hemodynamically mediated glomerular injury in the pathogenesis of progressive glomerular sclerosis in aging, renal ablation and intrinsic renal disease. *N Engl J Med* 307:652–659, 1982.
112. Klahr S, Buerhert J, Purkerson ML: Role of dietary factors in the progression of chronic renal disease. *Kidney Int* 24:579–587, 1983.
113. Hostetter TH, Olson JL, Rennke HG, et al: Hyperfiltration in remnant nephrons: A potentially adverse response to renal ablation. *Am J Physiol* 241:(*Renal Fluid Electrolyte Physiol* 10):F85–F93, 1981.
114. Kaysen GA, Rosenthal C, Hutchison FN: GFR increases before renal mass or ODC activity increase in rats fed high protein diets. *Kidney Int* 36:441–446, 1989.
115. Hutchison FN, Martin V, Jones H Jr, Kaysen GA: Differing actions of dietary protein and enalapril on renal function and proteinuria. *Am J Physiol* 258:(*Renal Fluid Electrolyte Physiol* 27):F126–F132, 1990.
116. Kaysen GA. Plasma composition in the nephrotic syndrome. *Am J Nephrol* 13:347–59, 1993.
117. Sun X, Martin V, Weiss RH, Kaysen GA: Selective transcriptional augmentation of hepatic gene expression in the rat with Heymann nephritis. *Am J Physiol* 264:F441–F447, 1993.
118. Sun X, Jones H Jr, Joles JA, et al: Apolipoprotein gene expression in analbuminemic rats and in rats with Heymann nephritis. *Am J Physiol* 262:(*Renal Fluid Electrolyte Physiol* 31):F755–F761, 1992.
119. Marshall JF, Apostolopoulos JJ, Brack CM, Howlett GL: Regulation of apolipoprotein gene expression and plasma high-density lipoprotein composition in experimental nephrosis. *Biochim Biophys Acta* 1042:271–279, 1990.
120. Kaysen GA, Sun X, Jones H Jr, et al: Non-iron mediated alteration in hepatic transferrin gene expression in the nephrotic rat. *Kidney Int* 47:1068–1077, 1995.
121. Jensen H, Bro-Jorgensen K, Jarnum S, et al: Transferrin metabolism in the nephrotic syndrome and in protein-losing gastroenteropathy. *Scand J Clin Lab Invest* 21:293–304, 1968.
122. Rifkind D, Kravetz HM, Knight V, Schade AL: Urinary excretion of iron-binding protein in the nephrotic syndrome. *N Engl J Med* 265:115–118, 1961.
123. Ellis D: Anemia in the course of the nephrotic syndrome secondary to transferrin depletion. *J Pediatr* 90:953–955, 1977.
124. Hancock DE, Onstad JW, Wolf PL: Transferrin loss into the urine with hypochromic, microcytic anemia. *Am J Clin Pathol* 65:72–78, 1976.
125. Esumi H, Sato S, Okui M, et al: Turnover of serum proteins in rats with analbuminemia. *Biochem Biophys Res Commun* 87:1191–1199, 1979.
126. Alfrey AC, Hammond WS: Renal iron handling in the nephrotic syndrome. *Kidney Int* 37:1409–1413, 1990.
127. Vaziri ND, Kaupke CJ, Barton CH, Gonzales E: Plasma concentration and urinary excretion of erythropoietin in adult nephrotic syndrome. *Am J Med* 92:35–40, 1992.

128. Zhou XJ, Vaziri ND: Erythropoietin metabolism and pharmacokinetics in experimental nephrosis. *Am J Physiol* 263:F812–F815, 1992.
129. Longsworth LG, MacInnes DA: An electrophoretic study of nephrotic sera and urine. *J Exp Med* 71:77–82, 1940.
130. Arneil GC: 164 children with nephrosis. *Lancet* 2:1103–1110, 1961.
131. Rothschild MA, Oratz M, Schreiber SS: Albumin Synthesis and Albumin Degradation. In Sgouris JT, Rene A (eds): *Proceedings of the Workshop on Albumin.* Washington, DC: Department of Health, Education, and Welfare, 1975, pp 57–74.
132. Waldmann TA, Strober W, Mogielnicki RP: The renal handling of low molecular weight proteins: II. Disorders of serum protein catabolism in patients with tubular proteinuria, the nephrotic syndrome or uremia. *J Clin Invest* 51:2162–2174, 1972.
133. Perheentupa J: Serum protein turnover in the congenital nephrotic syndrome. *Ann Paediatr Fenn* 12:189–233, 1966.
134. Heslan JM, Lautie JP, Intrator L, et al: Impaired IgG synthesis in patients with the nephrotic syndrome. *Clin Nephrol* 18:144–147, 1982.
135. Ooi BS, Ooi YM, Hsu A, Hurtsubise PE: Diminished synthesis of immunoglobulin by peripheral lymphocytes of patients with idiopathic membranous glomerulonephropathy. *J Clin Invest* 65:789–797, 1980.
136. Bernard DB: Metabolic Abnormalities in Nephrotic Syndrome: Pathophysiology and Complications. In Brenner BM, Stein JH (eds): *Contemporary Issues in Nephrology 9: Nephrotic Syndrome.* New York, Churchill Livingstone, 1982, pp 85–120.
137. Al-Bander H, Martin VI, Kaysen GA: Plasma IgG levels are not defended when urinary protein loss occurs. *Am J Physiol* 262:F333–F337, 1992.
138. Giangiacomo J, Cleary TG, Cole BR, et al: Serum immunoglobulins in the nephrotic syndrome: A possible cause of minimal-change nephrotic syndrome. *N Engl J Med* 293:8–12, 1975.
139. Chan MK, Chan KW, Jones B: Immunoglobulins (IgG, IgA, IgM, IgE) and complement components (C3,C4) in nephrotic syndrome due to minimal change and other forms of glomerulonephritis: A clue for steroid therapy? *Nephron* 47:125–130, 1987.
140. Kauffmann RH, Veltkamp JJ, Van Tilburg NH, Van Es LA: Acquired antithrombin III deficiency and thrombosis in the nephrotic syndrome. *Am J Med* 65:607–613, 1978.
141. Rydzewski A, Myslieiec M, Soszka J: Concentration of three thrombin inhibitors in the nephrotic syndrome in adults. *Nephron* 42:200–203, 1986.
142. Girot R, Jaubert F, Leon M, et al: Albumin, fibrinogen prothrombin, and antithrombin III variations in blood, urines and liver in rat nephrotic syndrome (Heymann nephritis). *Thromb Haemost* 49:13–17, 1983.
143. Robbins J, Rall JE, Petermann ML: Thyroxin-binding by serum and urine proteins in nephrosis: Qualitative aspects. *J Clin Invest* 36:1333–1342, 1957.
144. Musa BU, Seal US, Doe RP: Excretion of corticosteroid-binding globulin, thyroxine-binding globulin and total protein in adult males with nephrosis: Effect of sex hormones. *J Clin Endocr* 27:768–774, 1967.
145. Gavin LA, McMahon FA, Castle JN, Cavalieri RR: Alterations in serum thyroid hormones and thyroxine-binding globulin in patients with nephrosis. *J Clin Endocrinol Metab* 46:125–138, 1978.
146. Afrasiabi AM, Vaziri ND, Gwinup G, et al: Thyroid function studies in the nephrotic syndrome. *Ann Intern Med* 90:335–338, 1979.
147. Salvesen HA, Linder GC: Inorganic bases and phosphates in relation to the protein of blood and other body fluids in Bright's disease and in heart failure. *J Biol Chem* 58:617–634, 1923.
148. Emerson K Jr, Beckman WW: Calcium metabolism in nephrosis: I. A description of an abnormality in calcium metabolism in children with nephrosis. *J Clin Invest* 24:564–572, 1945.
149. Goldstein DA, Haldimann B, Sherman D, et al: Vitamin D metabolites and calcium metabolism in patients with nephrotic syndrome and normal renal function. *J Clin Endocrinol Metab* 53:116–121, 1981.
150. Goldstein DA, Oda Y, Kurokawa K, Massry SG: Blood levels of 25-hydroxyvitamin D in nephrotic syndrome: Studies in 26 patients. *Ann Intern Med* 87:664–667, 1977.

151. Lim P, Jacob E, Chio LF, Pwee HS: Serum ionized calcium in nephrotic syndrome. *Q J Med* 45:421–426, 1976.
152. Haddad JG Jr, Walgate J: Radioimmunoassay of the binding protein for vitamin D and its metabolites in human serum: Concentrations in normal subjects and patients with disorders of mineral homeostasis. *J Clin Invest* 58:1217–1222, 1976.
153. Barragry JM, France MW, Carter ND, et al: Vitamin D metabolism in nephrotic syndrome. *Lancet* 2:629–632, 1977.
154. Stickler GB, Rosevear JW, Ulrich JA: Renal tubular dysfunction complicating the nephrotic syndrome: The disturbance in calcium and phosphorus metabolism. *Proc Mayo Clin* 37:376–387, 1962.
155. Stickler GB, Hayles AB, Power MH, Ulrich JA: Renal tubular dysfunction complicating the nephrotic syndrome. *Pediatrics* 26:75–85, 1960.
156. Yssing M, Jensen H, Jarnum S: Albumin metabolism and gastrointestinal protein loss in children with nephrotic syndrome. *Acta Paediatr Scand* 58:109–115, 1969.
157. Llach F: Nephrotic Syndrome: Hypercoagulability, Renal Vein Thrombosis, and Other Thromboembolic Complications. In Brenner BM, Stein JH (eds): *Contemporary Issues in Nephrology 9: Nephrotic Syndrome*. New York, Churchill Livingstone, 1982, pp 121–144.
158. Llach F, Arieff AI, Massry SG: Renal vein thrombosis and nephrotic syndrome: A prospective study of 36 adult patients. *Ann Intern Med* 83:8–14, 1975.
159. Trew P, Biava C, Jacobs R, Hopper J: Renal vein thrombosis in membranous glomerulonephropathy: Incidence and association. *Medicine* 57:69–82, 1978.
160. D'Angelo S, D'Angelo A, Kaufman CE Jr, et al: Protein S deficiency occurs in the nephrotic syndrome. *Ann Intern Med* 107:42–47, 1987.
161. Cosio FG, Harker C, Batard MA, et al: Plasma concentrations of the natural anticoagulants protein C and protein S in patients with proteinuria. *J Lab Clin Med* 106:218–222, 1985.
162. Joven J, Villabona C, Vilella E, et al: Abnormalities of lipoprotein metabolism in patients with the nephrotic syndrome. *N Engl J Med* 323:579–584, 1990.
163. Gherardi E, Rota E, Calandra S, et al: Relationship among the concentrations of serum lipoproteins and changes in their chemical composition in patients with untreated nephrotic syndrome. *Eur J Clin Invest* 7:563–570, 1977.
164. Muls E, Rosseneu M, Daneels R, et al: Lipoprotein distribution and composition in the human nephrotic syndrome. *Atherosclerosis* 54:225–237, 1985.
165. Kostner GM, Avogaro P, Cazzolato G, et al: Lipoprotein Lp(a) and the risk for myocardial infarction. *Atherosclerosis* 38:51–61, 1981.
166. Utermann G: The mysteries of lipoprotein(a). *Science* 246:904–910, 1989.
167. Boerwinkle E, Menzel HJ, Kraft HG, Utermann G: Genetics of the quantitative Lp(a) lipoprotein trait: III. Contribution of Lp(a) glycoprotein phenotypes to normal lipid variation. *Hum Genet* 82:73–78, 1989.
168. Gavish D, Azrolan N, Breslow J: Plasma Lp(a) concentration is inversely correlated with the ratio of kringle IV/kringle V encoding domains in the apo(a) gene. *J Clin Invest* 84:2021–2027, 1989.
169. Wanner C, Rader D, Bartens W, et al: Elevated plasma lipoprotein(a) in patients with the nephrotic syndrome. *Ann Intern Med* 119:263–269, 1993.
170. Marsh JB: Lipoprotein metabolism in experimental nephrosis. *J Lipid Res* 25:1619–1623, 1984.
171. Staprans I, Felts JM, Couser WG: Glycosaminoglycans and chylomicron metabolism in control and nephrotic rats. *Metabolism* 36:496–501, 1987.
172. Garber DW, Gottlieb BA, Marsh JB, Sparks CE: Catabolism of very low density lipoproteins in experimental nephrosis. *J Clin Invest* 74:1375–1383, 1984.
173. Kaysen GA, Hoye E, Jones H Jr, et al: Effect of oncotic pressure on apolipoprotein A-I metabolism in the rat. *Am J Kidney Dis* 26(1):178–186, 1995.
174. Soothill JA, Kark RM: The effects of infusions of salt-poor human serum albumin on serum cholesterol cholinesterase, and albumin levels in healthy subjects and in patients ill with the nephrotic syndrome. *Clin Res Proc* 4:140–141, 1956.
175. Pullinger CR, North JD, Teng BB, et al: The apolipoprotein B gene is constitutively expressed in HepG2 cells: Regulation of secretion by oleic acid, albumin, and insulin, and measurement of the mRNA half-life. *J Lipid Res* 30:1065–1077, 1989.
176. Yamauchi A, Yamamoto S, Fukuhara Y, et al: Oncotic pressure regulates the levels of albumin

(Alb) mRNA and apolipoprotein B (ApoB) mRNA in cultured rat hepatoma cells (H4IIE). *Kidney Int* 35:441A, 1989.

177. Davies RW, Staprans I, Hutchison FN, Kaysen GA: Proteinuria, not altered albumin metabolism, effects hyperlipidemia in the nephrotic rat. *J Clin Invest* 86:600–605, 1990.
178. Levy E, Ziv E, Bar-On H, Shafrir E: Experimental nephrotic syndrome: Removal and tissue distribution of chylomicrons and very-low-density lipoproteins of normal and nephrotic origin. *Biochim Biophys Acta* 1043:259–266, 1990.
179. Kaysen GA, Mehendru L, Pan XM, Staprans I: Both peripheral chylomicron catabolism and hepatic uptake of remnants are defective in nephrosis. *Am J Physiol* 263:F335–F341, 1992.
180. McKenzie IFC, Nestel PJ: Studies on the turnover of triglyceride and esterified cholesterol in subjects with the nephrotic syndrome. *J Clin Invest* 47:1685–1695, 1968.
181. Joven J, Masana L, Villabona C, et al: Low density lipoprotein metabolism in rats with puromycin aminonucleoside-induced nephrotic syndrome. *Metabolism* 38:491–495, 1989.
182. Kaysen GA, Don B, Schambelan M: Proteinuria, albumin synthesis and hyperlipidemia in the nephrotic syndrome. *Nephrol Dial Transplant* 6:141–149, 1991.
183. Schaefer EJ, Levy RI: Pathogenesis and management of lipoprotein disorders. *N Engl J Med* 312:1300–1310, 1985.
184. Kashyap ML, Srivastava LS, Hynd BA, et al: Apolipoprotein CII and lipoprotein lipase in human nephrotic syndrome. *Atherosclerosis* 35:29–40, 1980.
185. Havel RJ: Lipid transport function of lipoproteins in blood plasma. *Am J Physiol* 253:(*Endocrinol Metab* 16):E1–E5, 1987.
186. Eisenberg S: High density lipoprotein metabolism. *J Lipid Res* 25:1017–1058, 1984.
187. Cohen SL, Cramp DG, Lewis AD, Tickner TR: The mechanism of hyperlipidemia in nephrotic syndrome: Role of low albumin and the LCAT reaction. *Clin Chim Acta* 104:393–400, 1980.
188. Kaysen GA, Pan XM, Couser WG, Staprans I: Defective lipolysis persists in hearts of rats with Heymann nephritis in the absence of nephrotic plasma. *Am J Kidney Dis* 22:128–134, 1993.
189. Kekki M, Nikkilä EA: Plasma triglyceride metabolism in the adult nephrotic syndrome. *Eur J Clin Invest* 1:345–351, 1971.
190. Vega GL, Grundy SM: Lovastatin therapy in nephrotic hyperlipidemia: Effects on lipoprotein metabolism. *Kidney Int* 33:1160–1168, 1988.
191. Yamada M, Matsuda I: Lipoprotein lipase in clinical and experimental nephrosis. *Clin Chim Acta* 30:787–794, 1970.
192. Moulin P, Appel GB, Ginsberg HN, Tall AR: Increased concentration of plasma cholesteryl ester transfer protein in nephrotic syndrome: Role in dyslipidemia. *J Lipid Res* 33:1817–1822, 1992.
193. Dullaart RP, Gansevoort RT, Dikkeschei BD, et al: Role of elevated lecithin:cholesterol acyltransferase and cholesteryl ester transfer protein activities in abnormal lipoproteins from proteinuric patients. *Kidney Int* 44:91–97, 1993.
194. Agbedana ED, Yamamoto T, Moriwaki Y, et al: Studies on abnormal lipid metabolism in experimental nephrotic syndrome. *Nephron* 64:256–261, 1993.
195. Sestak TL, Alavi N, Subbaiah PV: Plasma lipids and acyltransferase activities in experimental nephrotic syndrome. *Kidney Int* 36:240–248, 1989.
196. Warwick GL, Packard CJ, Demant T, et al: Metabolism of apolipoprotein B-containing lipoproteins in subjects with nephrotic-range proteinuria. *Kidney Int* 40:129–138, 1991.
197. Furukawa S, Hirano T, Mamo JCL, et al: Catabolic defect of triglyceride is associated with abnormal very-low-density lipoprotein in experimental nephrosis. *Metabolism* 39:101–107, 1990.
198. Muls E, Rosseneu M, Daneels R, et al: Lipoprotein distribution and composition in the human nephrotic syndrome. *Atherosclerosis* 54:225–237, 1985.
199. Zwaginga JJ, Koomans HA, Sixma JJ, Rabelink TJ: Thrombus formation and platelet-vessel wall interaction in the nephrotic syndrome under flow conditions. *J Clin Invest* 93:204–211, 1994.
200. Mallick NP, Short CD: The nephrotic syndrome and ischaemic heart disease. *Nephron* 27:54–57, 1981.

201. Berlyne GM, Mallick NP: Ischemic heart disease as a complication of nephrotic syndrome. *Lancet* 2:399–400, 1969.
202. Ordonez JD, Hiatt RA, Killebrew EJ, Fireman BH: The increased risk of coronary heart disease associated with nephrotic syndrome. *Kidney Int* 44:638–642, 1993.
203. Schmitz PG, Kasiske BL, O'Donnell MP, Keane WF: Lipids and progressive renal injury. *Semin Nephrol* 9:354–369, 1989.
204. Larger DJ, Rosenberg BF, Shapiro H, Bernstein J: Lecithin cholesterol acyltransferase deficiency: Ultrastructural examination of sequential renal biopsies. *Modern Pathol* 4:331–335, 1991.
205. Don BR, Kaysen GA, Hutchison FN, Schambelan M: The effect of angiotensin-converting enzyme inhibition and dietary protein restriction in the treatment of proteinuria. *Am J Kidney Dis* 17:10–17, 1991.
206. Gansevoort RT, Heeg JE, Vriesendorp R, et al: Antiproteinuric drugs in patients with idiopathic membranous glomerulopathy. *Nephrol Dial Transplant* 7(Suppl 1):91–96, 1992.
207. Keilani T, Schlueter WA, Levin ML, Batlle DC: Improvement of lipid abnormalities associated with proteinuria using fosinopril, an angiotensin-converting enzyme inhibitor. *Ann Intern Med* 118:246–254, 1993.
208. Tokoo M, Oguchi H, Terashima M, et al: Effects of pravastatin on serum lipids and apolipoproteins in hyperlipidemia of the nephrotic syndrome. *Nippon Jinzo Gakkai Shi* 34:397–403, 1992.
209. Modi KS, Schreiner GF, Purkerson ML, Klahr S: Effects of probucol in renal function and structure in rats with subtotal kidney ablation. *J Lab Clin Med* 120:310–317, 1992.
210. Groggel GC, Cheung AK, Ellis-Benigni K, Wilson DE: Treatment of nephrotic hyperlipoproteinemia with gemfibrozil. *Kidney Int* 36:266–271, 1989.
211. Aukland K, Nicolaysen G: Interstitial fluid volume: Local regulatory mechanisms. *Physiol Rev* 61:556–643, 1981.
212. Guyton AC, Taylor AE, Granger HJ (eds): *Circulatory Physiology II: Dynamics and Control of Body Fluids*. Philadelphia, Saunders, 1975, pp 149–165.
213. Taylor AE: Capillary fluid filtration starling forces and lymph flow. *Circ Res* 49:557–575, 1981.
214. Meltzer JI, Keim HJ, Laragh JH, et al: Nephrotic syndrome: Vasoconstriction and hypervolemia types indicated by renin-sodium profiling. *Ann Intern Med* 67:387–384, 1979.
215. Dorhout Mees EJ, Roos JC, Boer P, et al: Observations on edema formation in the nephrotic syndrome in adults with minimal lesions. *Am J Med* 67:378–384, 1979.
216. Geers AB, Koomans HA, Roos JC, et al: Functional relationships in the nephrotic syndrome. *Kidney Int* 26:324–330, 1984.
217. Katz J, Sellers AL, Bonorris G: Plasma albumin metabolism during transient renin proteinuria. *J Lab Clin Med* 64:709–716, 1964.
218. Garlick DG, Renkin EM: Transport of large molecules from plasma to interstitial fluid and lymph in dogs. *Am J Physiol* 219:1595–1605, 1970.
219. Taylor AE. Capillary fluid filtration starling forces and lymph flow. *Circ Res* 49:557–575, 1981.
220. Fadnes HO, Reed RK, Aukland K: Mechanisms regulating interstitial fluid volume. *Lymphology* 11:165–257, 1978.
221. Aukland K: Autoregulation of interstitial fluid volume: Edema-preventing mechanisms. *Scand J Clin Lab Invest* 31:247–254, 1973.
222. Koomans HA, Geers AB, Meiracker AHVD, et al: Effects of plasma volume expansion on renal salt handling in patients with the nephrotic syndrome. *Am J Nephrol* 4:227–234, 1984.
223. Keeler R, Feuchuk D, Wilson N: Atrial peptides and the renal response to hypervolemia in nephrotic rats. *Can J Physiol Pharmacol* 65:2017–2075, 1987.
224. Peterson C, Madsen B, Perlman A, et al: Atrial natriuretic peptide and the renal response to hypervolemia in nephrotic humans. *Kidney Int* 34:825–831, 1988.
225. Rabelink AJ, Koomans HA, Gaillard CA, Dorhout Mees EJ: Renal response to atrial natriuretic peptide in nephrotic syndrome. *Nephrol Dial Transplant* 2(6):510–514, 1987.
226. Perico N, Delaini F, Lupini C, et al: Blunted excretory response to atrial natriuretic peptide in experimental nephrosis. *Kidney Int* 36:57–64, 1989.

227. Hildebrandt DA, Banks RO: Effect of atrial natriuretic factor on renal function in rats with nephrotic syndrome. *Am J Physiol* 254:(*Renal Fluid Electrolyte Physiol* 23):F210–F216, 1988.

228. Ichikawa I, Rennke HG, Hoyer JR, et al: Role for intrarenal mechanisms in the impaired salt excretion of experimental nephrotic syndrome. *J Clin Invest* 71:91–104, 1983.

229. Koj A, Gauldie J, Sweeney GD, et al: A simple bioassay for monocyte-derived hepatocyte stimulating factor: Increased synthesis of α_2-macroglobulin and reduced synthesis of albumin by cultured rat hepatocytes. *J Immunol Methods* 76:317–327, 1985.

230. Bauer J, Weber W, Tran-Thi T, et al: Murine interleukin 1 stimulates α_2-macroglobulin synthesis in rat hepatocyte primary cultures. *FEBS Lett* 190:271–274, 1985.

231. Garber DW, Gottlieb BA, Marsh JB, Sparks CE: Catabolism of very low density lipoproteins in experimental nephrosis. *J Clin Invest* 74:1375–1383, 1984.

232. Chung BH, Segrest JP, Smith K, et al: Lipolytic surface remnants of triglyceride-rich lipoproteins are cytotoxic to macrophages but not in the presence of high density lipoprotein: A possible mechanism of atherogenesis? *J Clin Invest* 83:1363–1374, 1989.

233. D'Amico G, Gentile MG, Manna G, et al: Effect of vegetarian soy diet on hyperlipidaemia in nephrotic syndrome. *Lancet* 339:1131–1134, 1992.

234. Gentile MG, Fellin G, Cofano F, et al: Treatment of proteinuric patients with a vegetarian soy diet and fish oil. *Clin Nephrol* 40:315–320, 1993.

235. Hall AV, Parbtani A, Clark WF, et al: Omega-3 fatty acid supplementation in primary nephrotic syndrome: Effects on plasma lipids and coagulopathy. *J Am Soc Nephrol* 3: 1321–1329, 1992.

236. Donadio JV Jr, Bergstralh EJ, Offord KP, et al: A controlled trial of fish oil in IgA nephropathy. *N Engl J Med* 331:1194–1199, 1994.

237. Tan SY, Shapiro R, Franco R, et al: Indomethacin-induced prostaglandin inhibition with hyperkalemia. *Ann Intern Med* 90:783–785, 1979.

238. Tiggeler RGWL, Koene RAP, Wijdeveld PGAB: Inhibition of furosemide-induced natriuresis by indomethacin in patients with the nephrotic syndrome. *Clin Sci Mol Med* 52:149–152, 1977.

239. Goldsmith LA, Laberge C: Tyrosinemia and Related Disorders. In Scriver C, Beaudet AL, Sly WS, Valle D (eds): *The Metabolic Basis of Inherited Disease* (6th ed). New York, McGraw-Hill, 1989, vol 1, pp 547–562.

15

The Glomerulopathies

Richard J. Glassock

The approach to understanding the multitude of disorders that constitute the glomerulopathies is varied and challenging. Several levels of classification can be simultaneously applied, namely *etiology, pathogenesis, morphology,* and *clinical syndromes* [1, 2]. For some disorders, a more or less complete picture at all levels has been elucidated; for many, complete information is lacking. Unique pathogenetic events give rise to diverse morphologic patterns, and discrete morphologic abnormalities may be associated with a spectrum of clinical syndromes.

Etiology

Glomerular disease can arise from the effects of environmental agents (e.g., microbes or drugs) or from endogenous perturbations (e.g., neoplasia or autoimmunity). In many instances, both the environmental factors and the immune system interact to produce injury when the underlying genetic milieu is conducive to generation of disease.

Pathogenesis

Broadly considered, alterations of glomerular structure and function can occur from immunologic abnormalities, coagulation disturbances, intrinsic biochemical (often heredofamilial) defects, and direct toxic insults. Immunologic mechanisms appear to play a prominent role [3]. A classification of the underlying immunopathogenesis of glomerular disease is given in Table 15-1. Direct examination of renal tissue by immunofluorescence and electron microscopy and other methods provide clues to underlying pathogenesis but do not, in most instances, define the precise mechanism involved. Serologic investigation can also be extremely helpful in uncovering clues to pathogenesis.

Table 15-1. Classification of immunopathogenetic mechanisms of human glomerular disease

Mechanism	Clinical prototype
Antitissue antibody–mediated disease	
Antibody to "native" glomerular basement membrane antigens	
Exogenous	Antilymphocyte serum treatment
Endogenous	Goodpasture's disease and some forms of primary crescentic glomerulonephritis
Antibody to other "native" glomerular antigens (in situ immune-complex disease)	
Exogenous	None known
Endogenous	Membranous glomerulopathy (?)
Antibody to "planted" glomerular antigens	
Exogenous	None known
Endogenous	Systemic lupus erythematosus (?) drugs (?), poststreptococcal glomerulonephritis (?)
Circulating immune complex–mediated disease	
Endogenous antigen	Systemic lupus erythematosus, cryoimmunoglobulinemia, neoplasia-associated glomerular disease
Exogenous antigen	
Nonreplicating	Serum sickness
Replicating	Bacterial, viral, protozoal-associated glomerulonephritis
Cell-mediated disease	Minimal change disease (lipoid nephrosis) (?), allograft glomerulopathy (?), some forms of primary crescentic glomerulonephritis

Antibody-Dependent Mechanisms

With antibody-dependent mechanisms, a circulating antibody reacts in the circulation or in situ with its relevant antigen, which may be either exogenous (replicating or nonreplicating) or endogenous [3]. When antibody (usually of the IgG isotype) reacts with *circulating antigen*, immune complexes are formed [4]. These immune complexes may be removed rapidly by the mononuclear phagocyte system or trapped in the glomerular capillary circulation and give rise to irregular or granular deposits of immunoglobulin by immunofluorescence (Fig. 15-1). The size of the immune complexes, rapidity of formation, nature of the antigen (charge or valence), characteristics of the antibody (affinity, isotype, ability to fix complement), and physiologic attributes of the glomerular capillary circulation all interact to define the phlogistic and tissue deposition of immune complexes. Extensive deposition of large insoluble immune complexes capable of activating complement tends to provoke proliferative and inflammatory glomerular lesions associated with extensive subendothelial elec-

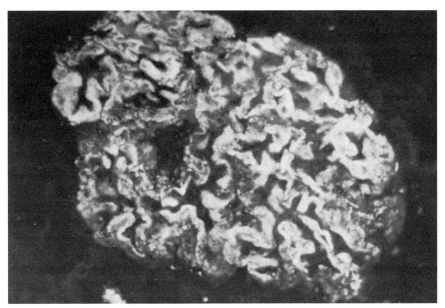

Fig. 15-1. Fluorescent-antibody study of the glomerulus, demonstrating discrete granular deposition of immunoglobulin along the basement membrane, which is characteristic of immune complex–mediated glomerulopathies. The immune complexes contained within the granular deposits may have deposited from the circulation *or* formed locally (in situ) as a consequence of interaction of a circulating antibody with a native glomerular capillary wall antigen or an extrinsic antigen planted in the glomerulus because of an affinity for constituents of the capillary wall.

tron-dense deposits by electron microscopy. Small and more soluble immune complexes may at times permeate the capillary wall and evoke a noninflammatory, nonproliferative lesion characterized by electron-dense deposits in the subepithelial space.

Antibody to *fixed and native antigens* in the glomerular capillary wall lead to a spectrum of glomerular disease, depending on the nature of the antigen and its distribution within the glomerulus [3]. When the antigen is diffusely and uniformly expressed along the capillary wall, a linear pattern of immunoglobulin deposits along the basement membrane may be observed (Fig. 15-2). In experimental animals, the classic example of this form of disease is Masugi nephritis, which is produced by a heterologous antiserum to basement membrane antigens. In humans, the classic example is Goodpasture's disease (see later discussion). Goodpasture's disease is due to the formation of autoantibodies to an epitope on the noncollagenous domain of the $\alpha 3$ chain of type IV collagen present in the lamina densa of the glomerular basement membrane (GBM) (and also in the alveolar basement membrane of the lung) [5, 6]. Antibodies to other native glomerular antigens give rise to different patterns. For example, in experimental animals, an autoantibody to an antigen present on the surface of the glomerular epithelial cell gives rise to electron-dense

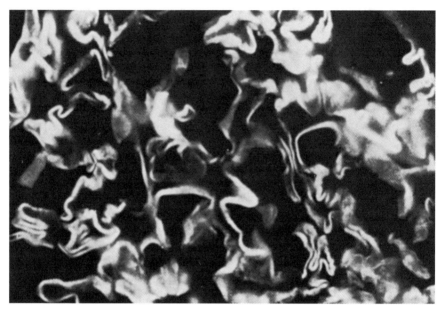

Fig. 15-2. Fluorescent-antibody study of the glomerulus, showing discrete linear deposition of immunoglobulin, which is characteristic of anti–glomerular basement membrane–mediated glomerulopathies and Goodpasture's disease. The immunoglobulin deposits represent autoantibody that has reacted with a native glycoprotein (noncollagen) constituent of the glomerular basement membrane.

deposits in the subepithelial space and "granular" deposits of immunoglobulin [7]. Autoantibodies to other structures, such as the mesangium, may give rise to differing appearances of immunoglobulin deposition by immunofluorescence.

Sometimes *exogenous* substances having an affinity for glomerular structures (e.g., lectins, cationic proteins) may deposit or "plant" in various sites along the capillary wall or mesangium and thereby serve as targets for circulating antibody directed to the newly "planted" antigen that is not normally an intrinsic constituent of the glomerulus [7, 8]. The pattern of immunoglobulin deposition as determined by immunofluorescence microscopy will depend on the sites where the antigen was "planted" in the glomerulus [3, 4]. Among antibody-dependent mechanisms, it is not possible to clearly discriminate the *specific* pathogenesis when a nonlinear pattern of immunoglobulin deposition is observed by immunofluorescence.

Cell-Mediated Immunity

Cell-mediated immune processes may likewise be involved in glomerular disease, although much less is known about the way sensitized T cells cause glomerular injury [3, 4]. Release of putative soluble factors affecting glomerular capillary permeability into the circulation may be one way glomerular structure or function is altered (see Chap. 14). Cell-mediated cytotoxicity directed against the cellular constituents of the glomerulus may be another. The release of cytokines from sensitized T cells may also call forth a variety of additional injurious factors, such as monocytes and promotion of coagulation, and may participate in production of proliferative or sclerosing lesions. It must also be emphasized that cell-mediated immunity and antibody-mediated mechanisms are not mutually exclusive, and both probably occur simultaneously in many diseases.

Mediator Systems

Primary pathogenetic events require participation of mediator systems to bring the disease process to full clinical expression. Indeed, the nature and extent of involvement of these mediator systems have profound effects on the severity, morphology, and clinical expression of disease and may represent potential targets for therapeutic intervention [9–12]. Mediator systems can be characterized as either humoral or cellular or both (Table 15-2). Humoral mediators include the complement system, the coagulation cascade, platelet activating factors, cytokines, growth factors, pro- and anti-inflammatory lipids, and hemodynamically active peptides and amines. Cellular mechanisms include polymorphonuclear leukocytes, monocytes, eosinophils, macrophages, T cells, and platelets. These cellular participants also serve as the source for many of the locally produced soluble factors such as cytokines, growth factors, procoagulant proteins, and lipids. In addition, these mediators may secondarily generate tissue-damaging factors such as toxic oxygen radicals (hydroxyl radical, hydrogen peroxide, superoxide anion) and proteases (cathepsins, elastase, neutral proteases). Growth factors, such as transforming growth factor-β, platelet-derived growth factor, and fibroblast growth factor, are also generated in the course

Table 15-2. Mediator systems involved in glomerulonephritis

Soluble, humoral
  Complement (C3b, C3a, C5a, C5b,6,7,8,9 [membrane attack complex])
  Fibrinogen-fibrin
  Prostaglandins (PGE$_2$, PGI$_2$, thromboxane A$_2$, PGF$_{2\alpha}$)
  Leukotrienes (LTB$_4$, LTC$_4$, LTD$_4$, LTE$_4$)
  Platelet-activating factor (acetylglycerylether phosphocholine)
  Toxic oxygen radicals (H$_2$O$_2$, O$_2^-$, OH$^{\cdot}$)
  Angiotensin II
  Catecholamines
  Histamine
  Serotonin
  Cytokines (e.g., interleukin-2, interleukin-6)
  Growth factors (transforming growth factor-β; fibroblast growth factor, insulin-like growth factor I, platelet-derived growth factor)
Insoluble, cellular
  Polymorphonuclear leukocytes
  Eosinophils
  Monocytes/macrophages
  Lymphocytes (cytotoxic T cells)
  Platelets

of glomerular inflammation and play important roles in the chronic sequelae of acute or ongoing injury, particularly in the development of fibrosis and sclerosis. Specific diseases may be associated with particular patterns of cytokine and growth factor release, but in most glomerular diseases, a wide variety of effector and mediator systems are involved.

Morphology

The glomerular capillary circulation has a rather limited array of morphologic responses to underlying pathogenetic events (Table 15-3). Some lesions are quite specific for certain diseases (e.g., diabetic glomerulosclerosis, amyloidosis, nonamyloid fibrillary glomerulonephritis). Each of the nonspecific lesions can be associated with multisystem diseases or hereditary or biochemical abnormalities, or they may occur in a primary or idiopathic form. Special histologic stains, immunofluorescence microscopy, and electron microscopy are often quite helpful in elucidating possible etiologic or pathogenetic factors.

Table 15-3. Morphologic classification of glomerular disease

Nonspecific lesions
  Minimal change disease (with or without focal or global glomerular obsolescence)
  Focal and segmental glomerulosclerosis and hyalinosis (focal glomerular sclerosis)
  Membranous glomerulonephritis
  Proliferative glomerulonephritis
    Diffuse endocapillary proliferative glomerulonephritis (with or without exudation)
    Diffuse extracapillary proliferative (crescentic) glomerulonephritis (with or without endocapillary proliferation)
    "Pure" mesangial proliferative glomerulonephritis
    Focal and segmental proliferative or necrotizing glomerulonephritis
    Membranoproliferative glomerulonephritis (type I)
    Chronic sclerosing glomerulonephritis
Specific lesions
  Diabetic (nodular) glomerulosclerosis
  Amyloidosis
  Light or heavy chain glomerulopathy
  Macroglobulinemic nephropathy
  Fibrillary/immunotactoid glomerulonephritis
  Fabry's disease
  Nail-patella syndrome
  Thin-basement-membrane nephropathy
  Alport's syndrome
  Quartan malarial glomerulopathy
  Lupus nephritis (with hematoxyphil bodies)
  Berger's disease (IgA nephropathy)
  Collagen (type III) glomerulopathy
  Lipoprotein glomerulopathy
  Membranoproliferative glomerulonephritis type II (dense deposit disease)

Clinical Syndromes

At the clinical level, the expression of glomerular disease constitutes various permutations and combinations of *hematuria, proteinuria*, and *alterations in glomerular filtration rate* (GFR) [1, 2]. The clinical findings aggregate into five common patterns or clinical syndromes: *acute glomerulonephritis, rapidly progressive glomerulonephritis* (RPGN), *chronic glomerulonephritis, nephrotic syndrome*, and *"asymptomatic" hematuria and/or proteinuria*.

Acute glomerulonephritis is characterized by the relatively abrupt onset of hematuria (often with erythrocyte casts), proteinuria, and reduced GFR. These abnormalities are associated with prominent fluid retention, circulatory congestion, edema, and hypertension. Acute glomerulonephritis is often associated with an underlying infectious process, such as group A β-hemolytic streptococcal infection. Spontaneous resolution is the rule. Morphologically, diffuse endocapillary proliferative glomerulonephritis is often observed.

RPGN is characterized by a more insidious onset of hematuria and proteinuria with a rather marked and rapid decline in GFR, often eventuating in oliguria. Recovery, in the absence of therapy, is uncommon. The morphologic lesion most commonly associated with RPGN is diffuse extracapillary (crescentic) proliferative glomerulonephritis. Hypertension is frequently absent or mild.

Chronic glomerulonephritis is characterized by persisting abnormalities in the urinary sediment and proteinuria accompanied by a slow and inexorable decline in GFR. It is a common pathway through which many glomerular diseases progress. No morphologic lesion is characteristic, but extensive global and/or segmental glomerulosclerosis with chronic tubulointerstitial fibrosis and renal parenchymal atrophy is often seen. Hypertension is almost universally present.

Nephrotic syndrome (see also Chap. 14) is characterized by the abrupt or insidious onset of heavy proteinuria (>3.5 g/day/1.73 m^2) with or without changes in the urinary sediment or GFR. Massive proteinuria is often accompanied by a decrease in plasma albumin concentration, increased serum lipids, and edema. No morphologic lesion is characteristic of this syndrome. Hypertension may be present, but is dependent on the nature of the underlying lesion.

"Asymptomatic" hematuria and/or proteinuria is characterized by persistent or recurrent hematuria and/or proteinuria. GFR is normal, and symptoms referable to the urinary tract are absent. When present, proteinuria is less than 3.5 g/day/1.73 m^2. Hypertension may or may not be present. Typically, segmental proliferative glomerulonephritis is a common underlying lesion, but many glomerular abnormalities can evoke this syndrome.

These clinical syndromes can occur as primary (or idiopathic) diseases in which clinical evidence of extrarenal involvement is lacking. Alternatively, they can appear as a secondary manifestation of a wide variety of diseases with or without well defined etiologic events, and often with multisystem involvement.

Hematuria and proteinuria, as indicated previously, are important signs of glomerular disease. Urinary erythrocytes in glomerular disease are often *dysmorphic* [13]. The red cells in the urine are small and distorted and have lost most or all of their hemoglobin content. Such dysmorphic cells can easily be recognized by careful examination of the urinary sediment, particularly the use of special stains or phase-contrast microscopy. *Normo-* or *isomorphic* hematuria is usually a sign of nonglomerular urinary tract disease. The urinary red cells in these circumstances retain their normal biconcave shape and size and in isotonic or hypertonic urine will also retain their hemoglobin content. Proteinuria in glomerular disease consists of albumin and/or globulins depending on the nature of the underlying glomerular permselectivity defect (see also Chap. 14) [14]. The quantity of protein excreted is of little diagnostic help, although proteinuria less than 3.5 g/day/1.73 m^2 may be indicative of a vascular or tubulointerstitial rather than a glomerular lesion, whereas urinary protein excretion greater than 3.5 g/day/1.73 m^2 most often signifies a predominant glomerular lesion. Although a measurement of 24-hour urinary protein excretion rates is commonly performed, the ratio of protein to creatinine concentrations in random urines may also provide reasonable estimates as to the rate of protein excretion. Values above 3.0 mg of protein per milligram of creatinine generally indicate "nephrotic range" proteinuria.

Fluid (sodium chloride and water) retention, edema, and hypertension are common although not universal accompaniments of glomerular disease. Chapters 2, 9, and 14 deal with these abnormalities, and they will only be briefly discussed here. Acute glomerulonephritis is associated with pronounced *primary* renal sodium chloride and water retention probably because of abnormal reabsorption of filtered sodium at more distal sites in the nephron [1]. Although decreased sodium chloride delivery due to a fall in GFR also occurs, it is seldom sufficient to account for the severe sodium chloride and fluid retention, circulatory congestion, and hypertension seen in this clinical syndrome. Hypertension accompanied by mild to moderate volume expansion is commonly seen in chronic glomerulonephritis. The renin-angiotensin system may be incompletely suppressed, perhaps contributing to elevated blood pressure.

In the nephrotic syndrome, the loss of protein in the urine eventually results in hypoproteinemia and hypoalbuminemia. The lowered plasma oncotic pressure secondary to reduced albumin concentration results in a disturbance in Starling forces in the peripheral capillary [15]. These changes favor movement of fluid into the interstitium (edema), but since interstitial oncotic pressure also falls, the transcapillary oncotic pressure gradient remains relatively normal until the plasma oncotic pressure falls by 30 to 50 percent or more. Thus, movement of fluid from the intravascular compartment into the interstitial compartment may not always occur secondary to a reduced plasma albumin concentration and plasma oncotic pressure. Simultaneous with the loss of urinary protein, the renal reabsorption of filtered sodium chloride and water is augmented chiefly at distal tubular sites (e.g., collecting duct). This sodium chloride and water retention is intrinsic to the kidney and not dependent on circulating factors. It may be due to an acquired resistance to atrial natriuretic factor or to an activation of Na,K-ATPase at the tubular level [15, 16]. The combination of *primary* renal sodium chloride retention and altered Starling forces in the peripheral capillary wall leads to a spectrum of abnormalities of intravascular volume. A minority of patients present with intravascular volume depletion [15]. These patients are largely those with *severe* hypoalbuminemia and/or a more generalized defect in capillary permeability. In most patients with nephrotic syndrome, and especially those with abnormally reduced GFR, intravascular volume is normal or elevated, despite hypoalbuminemia and a reduction in plasma oncotic pressure. In combination with incompletely suppressed renin-angiotensin, moderate or even severe hypertension may ensue. Rarely, pulmonary edema in the low-pressure pulmonary vascular circuit may develop, associated with profound hypoalbuminemia.

Primary (Idiopathic) Glomerular Diseases

The primary glomerular diseases are defined by the absence of recognizable multisystem abnormalities, heredofamilial or metabolic disease, or other precipitating factors such as drug exposure or infection. This group is ordinarily further classified into specific clinical pathologic "entities" based on light, electron, and immunofluorescence microscopy of renal tissue.

Minimal Change Disease

Minimal change disease is associated with normal or minimally altered glomeruli by light microscopy, absent or scanty deposits of immunoglobulin by immunofluorescence, and very diffuse epithelial cell foot process effacement (fusion) by electron microscopy [1, 17]. Electron-dense deposits are usually absent, although a few may be seen in the mesangium. Mild degrees of mesangial hypercellularity, focal tubular abnormalities, and occasionally globally sclerotic glomeruli are also compatible with this diagnosis. If the renal tissue sample size is small (<10 glomeruli), areas of focal and segmental glomerulosclerosis can be easily missed. A similar or identical lesion can also be seen in association with Hodgkin's disease, certain carcinomas (renal cell, pancreas, prostate, mesothelioma), pollen or milk allergies, and nonsteroidal anti-inflammatory drugs [1]. The etiology and pathogenesis of minimal change disease are unknown but are suspected to be associated with disturbances in T-cell pathophysiology leading to the secretion of a permeability-promoting lymphokine [18]. The urine contains principally albumin, probably the result of a defect in the anionic charge barrier of the capillary wall [19] (see Chap. 14).

Minimal change disease accounts for 80 to 85 percent of idiopathic nephrotic syndrome seen in children, with a peak prevalence between the ages of 4 and 8 [1, 20]. Approximately 20 percent of adults with idiopathic nephrotic syndrome may also be demonstrated to have this lesion. Males are affected somewhat more commonly than females. The onset is usually abrupt, and nearly all patients will present with nephrotic syndrome and relatively well-preserved GFR. A reversible form of acute renal failure may rarely be seen. The urinary sediment is typically benign, but in about 20 percent of patients, microhematuria may be present. Cholesterol and triglyceride concentrations are strikingly elevated. Serum complement concentrations (C3, C4) are typically normal. There is an increased incidence of atopy, and the HLA antigens B8, B13, and DR7 are increased [21, 22].

Minimal change disease uncomplicated by superimposed focal and segmental glomerulosclerosis or severe mesangial hypercellularity is a relatively benign disease. Spontaneous remissions may occur in 30 to 40 percent of cases. Less than 5 percent of patients will progress to end-stage renal failure. However, because of the distressing manifestations of nephrotic syndrome and enhanced susceptibility to thrombosis and infection (see Chap. 14), most children and young adults are treated. Glucocorticoids clearly will increase the tendency for remission. Over 90 percent of children can be induced to full remission with 60 mg/m^2/day or 1 mg/kg of oral prednisone or prednisolone (maximum 80 mg/day) for 4 to 6 weeks, followed by 35 to 40 mg/m^2 every other day for an additional 4 to 6 weeks. Intravenous methylprednisolone, 7 to 15 mg/kg daily for 3 days, is also effective in inducing remissions, but relapses are common.

Nonresponders often have some other underlying disease process unrecognized in initial renal biopsy, such as focal and segmental glomerulosclerosis. The responder group will commonly relapse when steroids are withdrawn or during the alternate-day phase of therapy, especially when steroids are rapidly withdrawn. Overall, about 60 percent of patients experience at least one relapse. These steroid-dependent and relapsing patients sometimes require more prolonged treatment. Delayed or less frequent relapses can be managed by repeated courses of glucocorticoids, unless severe steroid toxicity supervenes. Adults require more prolonged therapy with prednisone or prednisolone, 1 mg/kg/day (maximum dose 80 mg/day) or 2 mg/kg every other day for 8 to 10 weeks followed by alternate-day therapy for an additional 8 to 12 weeks. Overall remission rates in adults may be somewhat less than in children (about 80–85%) [23].

Steroid-dependent or frequently relapsing children and adults can also be treated successfully with alkylating agents [1, 20, 24, 25]. Oral cyclophosphamide, 2 to 3 mg/kg/day for 10 to 12 weeks, appears to be an effective and relatively safe regimen. Cumulative dose of cyclophosphamide should not exceed 200 mg/kg. A remission should be initially induced with steroids whenever possible. About 50 to 60 percent of patients so treated will enter into a prolonged disease-free remission. If a relapse occurs, one additional course of cyclophosphamide can be tried. Cyclosporine (initially 5–6 mg/kg/day plus low-dose glucocorticoids) may be an alternate to cyclophosphamide therapy or be used for patients who do not respond to or relapse early following cyclophosphamide treatment [26, 27]. Unfortunately, relapses frequently occur when cyclosporine is withdrawn. Overall, about 70 to 75 percent of patients will respond to cyclosporine treatment (85–90% of steroid-sensitive and 60–70% of steroid-resistant patients). If patients can be induced into remission with doses of cyclosporine of 5.5 mg/kg/day or less, they can be maintained on this or a slightly lower dosage for 12 months before attempting to taper and discontinue the agent. Failure to respond to cyclosporine after 3 months usually indicates nonresponsive disease. Rarely, levamisole or azathioprine can be used to induce or maintain a remission in multiple relapsing disease [28, 29]. The long-term course of minimal change disease is quite favorable, and very few patients will develop renal failure. Most deaths are related to infection, thrombosis, or complications of treatment.

Focal and Segmental Glomerulosclerosis (Focal Sclerosis)

Focal sclerosis is associated with the appearance of focal and segmental glomerulosclerosis and hyalinosis on a background of diffuse foot process effacement similar to that seen in minimal change disease [1, 30, 31]. Focal sclerosis may be a variant of minimal change disease with more severe glomerular involvement. Mild to moderate mesangial hypercellularity and chronic tubulointerstitial lesions may also be present. Focal deposition of IgM in the sclerotic areas is observed. The deeper juxtamedullary glomeruli are initially affected, and the glomeruli are consistently hypertrophic (increased cross-sectional diameter) compared to minimal change disease. A variant of focal sclerosis known as "collapsing glomerulopathy" is associated with severe sclerosis rapidly leading to collapse of the glomerular architecture [32]. Heavy proteinuria and progressive renal failure are very common in this lesion.

Lesions morphologically similar to focal sclerosis can also be found in human immunodeficiency virus (HIV)–associated nephropathy, heroin abuse nephropathy, vesicoureteral reflux nephropathy, cystinosis, oligonephronia, underlying neoplasia, and with long-standing hypertension (especially of the volume-dependent variety) [1]. In addition, the segmental scars associated with healed proliferative or necrotizing glomerulonephritis can occasionally resemble the lesions of focal sclerosis. The etiology and pathogenesis of focal sclerosis are unknown but a nonimmunoglobulin circulating permeability-promoting factor is suspected to be involved based on studies of plasma exchange and immunoabsorption and the frequent recurrence of disease following transplantation [18].

Clinically, the majority of patients present with nephrotic-range proteinuria, although persisting non-nephrotic proteinuria is relatively common. Occasionally patients may develop massive proteinuria (>20 g/day) with severe clinical manifestations, hypoalbuminemia, and hyperlipidemia. Such patients tend to rapidly progress to end-stage renal failure.

The focal sclerosis lesion is found in 10 to 15 percent of children and about 20 to 25 percent of adults with idiopathic nephrotic syndrome [1, 30, 31]. Elevated blood pressure, impaired GFR, and abnormal urinary sediment (leukocyturia and erythrocyturia) are common findings at presentation. Urine protein selectivity is poor, and over 85 percent of patients excrete large amounts of IgG in addition to albumin. Serum complement component concentrations are normal. A permeability-promoting nonimmunoglobulin factor is present in the circulation of many patients, which may account for the prominent tendency of this lesion to recur following renal transplantation [18].

Spontaneous remissions of proteinuria are rare. In the absence of treatment, this disorder tends to progress to end-stage renal failure at variable rates. The tendency to progress is associated with high urinary protein excretion rates, impaired GFR at discovery, poorly controlled hypertension, and extensive chronic tubulointerstitial lesions. Forty to sixty percent of patients can be induced into a complete or partial remission of proteinuria with prolonged aggressive glucocorticoid therapy [27, 33–35]. Six to nine months of treatment with daily or alternate-day prednisone may be required [34, 35]. Patients who respond with a diminution of proteinuria to non-nephrotic levels appear to have an improved prognosis with respect to progressive renal failure [35]. Treatment of patients with advanced glomerular lesions, impaired GFR, and/or chronic tubulointerstitial pathology is much less successful, arguing for early aggressive management. Some patients may respond in a fashion similar to those with minimal change disease, with multiple steroid-induced remissions followed by relapse. It is difficult to predict which patients will respond to glucocorticoids based on clinical or morphologic features, although mild glomerular and tubulointerstitial involvement may augur a more favorable outcome with treatment.

Some studies have suggested that a combined intravenous methylprednisolone and oral cytotoxic drug regimen may produce a higher remission rate than prolonged oral glucocorticoids alone [35]. This has not yet been tested in a randomized prospective trial. The addition of an oral alkylating agent (e.g., cyclophosphamide) to a regimen of oral prednisone or prednisolone appears to be of limited value, although occasionally a complete remission ensues or the lesion becomes more steroid responsive. Cyclosporine in doses of about 5 mg/kg/day in adults (up to 7 mg/kg/day in children) combined with low-dose alternate-day prednisone may result in remissions in 50 to 60 percent of patients with focal sclerosis who fail to respond to steroids alone [27, 35]. Unfortunately, relapses are common when cyclosporine is withdrawn, and prolonged therapy is required. An initial renal biopsy showing significant chronic tubulointerstitial lesions increases the risk of cyclosporine-associated nephrotoxicity, and this approach cannot be recommended for those with advanced disease (e.g., serum creatinine >2.0 mg/dl). Responses to cyclosporine, if they are to occur at all, will usually be observed in the first 3 months of treatment.

Other experimental approaches include prolonged treatment with nonsteroidal anti-inflammatory agents and the use of inhibitors of thromboxane action, plasma exchange, or immunoabsorption. Angiotensin-converting enzyme (ACE) inhibitors will decrease the rate of protein excretion by 50 percent in most patients and may thereby slow the rate of progression. Recurrences in renal allografts are common (30–40%), especially in those patients with rapidly progressive disease [1]. Plasma exchange (or immunoabsorption) at the time of transplantation combined with higher-dose cyclosporine induction therapy may lower the risk of recurrence or modify the adverse consequences of recurrence on graft survival [36, 37].

Mesangial Proliferative Glomerulonephritis

Mesangial proliferative glomerulonephritis comprises a heterogeneous group of rather poorly characterized disorders having in common moderate but definite diffuse hypercellularity in the mesangial (axial) zones of glomeruli [1, 38]. The lesion is often but not necessarily accompanied by immunoglobulin and/or complement component deposits in the mesangium. When heavy mesangial IgA deposits are present, the lesion is separately categorized as *IgA nephropathy* or *Berger's disease*. Heavy IgM deposits may also connote a distinct entity known as *IgM nephropathy* [39]. Some patients may have an underlying autoimmune disease such as systemic lupus erythematosus (SLE) or rheumatoid arthritis or be in the resolving phase of postinfectious glomerulonephritis. The pathogenesis of the lesion is largely unknown, but immunopathologic studies have suggested the involvement of immune complexes.

Clinically, most patients present with a combination of hematuria and proteinuria, sometimes with frank nephrotic syndrome. The long-term outcome is not well understood, as some patients may undergo spontaneous recovery, while others progress, most often in association with heavy proteinuria and the development of superimposed lesions of focal and segmental glomerulosclerosis. Heavy deposits of IgM in the mesangium associated with distinct mesangial proliferation may connote a poor prognosis [39]. Treatment of the lesion is controversial, but a trial of glucocorticoids is probably indicated in those patients with nephrotic-range proteinuria. Alkylating agents may also increase the likelihood of remission.

Membranous Glomerulonephritis

Membranous glomerulonephritis is characterized by barely perceptible to advanced thickening of the glomerular capillary wall, usually in the absence of significant cellular proliferation [1, 40, 41] (Fig. 15-3). Immunofluorescence studies reveal typical beadlike and granular deposits of IgG and to a lesser extent C3 outlining the glomerular capillary loops and sparing the mesangium. Electron microscopy reveals multiple subepithelial dense deposits often associated with spikelike projections of basement membrane material between the deposits. In the very advanced stages of the disease and following remission of proteinuria, the electron-dense deposits become more lucent, and the basement membrane may become quite thickened and have a moth-eaten or Swiss cheese appearance. Similar morphologic lesions can be seen in a variety of disorders (Table 15-4), especially chronic viral infection (e.g., hepatitis-B), neoplasia, drug exposure, and autoimmune disease.

The etiology and pathogenesis of the idiopathic disorder are unknown, but studies in experimental animals have suggested that the subepithelial immune deposits are

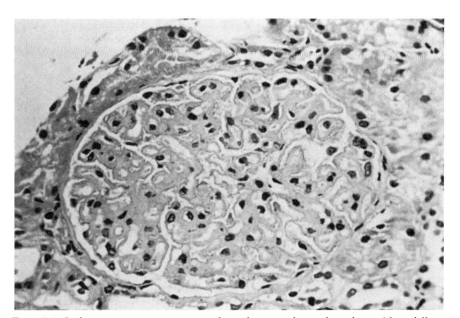

Fig. 15-3. Light-microscopic appearance of membranous glomerulonephritis. Note diffuse thickening of the capillary walls without associated inflammatory response.

Table 15-4. Causes of membranous glomerulonephritis

Idiopathic

Secondary

Systemic lupus erythematosus (and uncommonly mixed connective tissue disease or rheumatoid arthritis)

Drug induced (penicillamine, gold, mercury, probenecid, trimethadione, captopril)

Neoplasia (carcinoma of lung, colon, stomach, breast, etc.)

Infections (syphilis, leprosy, chronic hepatitis B, hepatitis C, malaria, schistosomiasis, filariasis)

Miscellaneous (sickle cell disease, thyroiditis, chronic allograft rejection, sarcoidosis, Sjögren's syndrome)

caused by an interaction of a circulating autoantibody to an antigen present on the surface of glomerular epithelial cells [1, 3, 7]. Thus, immune complexes are formed in situ and grow to form electron-dense deposits in the subepithelial space. Altered glomerular permeability appears to be due to local activation of complement with the subsequent generation of toxic oxygen radicals [42, 43]. Increased urinary excretion of C5b–C9 (the membrane attack complex) or C3dg (a degradation product of C3) and/or glomerular deposition of C3 may signify "active" formation of in situ immune complexes [44]. Unfortunately, the precise nature of the antigen in human disease is unknown, and other mechanisms could also be responsible for the immunoglobulin deposition in glomerular capillary wall.

Clinically, over 80 percent of patients with membranous glomerulonephritis will present with nephrotic-range proteinuria, and the remainder manifest isolated non-nephrotic proteinuria [1, 44]. Overall, membranous glomerulonephritis accounts for about 30 to 40 percent of cases of idiopathic nephrotic syndrome in adults, but it is quite uncommon in children. Most patients will present with normal or near-normal GFR. Complement levels are normal, and the urinary protein selectivity is quite variable.

In the absence of treatment, approximately 30 percent of patients will progress to end-stage renal failure over 10 to 20 years [45, 46]. Patients who maintain normal renal function over the first 5 years of follow-up following initial recognition are not likely to progress to renal failure subsequently. Overall, approximately 40 percent of patients will experience one or more spontaneous complete or partial remissions to proteinuria, and in such patients progressive renal failure is uncommon [46]. A progressive course with renal insufficiency is associated with persisting heavy proteinuria (usually over 8–10 g/day for over 6–8 months), male sex, older age at onset, poorly controlled hypertension, impaired renal function at discovery, and chronic tubulointerstitial lesions on biopsy [45, 46].

The treatment of membranous glomerulonephritis is controversial, since spontaneous full or partial recovery is so common and since the lesion only slowly progresses to end-stage renal failure in about one-third of patients [1, 27, 47, 48]. Glucocorticoids given alone appear to have little overall beneficial effect, except in a very small minority of patients who manifest a steroid-responsive, multiple-relapsing course. The addition of an alkylating cytotoxic agent (either cyclophosphamide or chlorambucil) significantly enhances the likelihood of a complete or partial remission, but protection from progressive renal failure by these regimens remains a controversial area [48–50]. Either cyclical therapy with intravenous methylprednisolone, oral prednisolone, and oral chlorambucil for 6 months or daily oral cyclophosphamide with combined with alternate-day prednisone for 6 to 9 months appears effective [4, 49, 50]. Sixty to eighty percent of patients are likely to exhibit improvement with such regimens, but relapses do occur following discontinuance of treatment. One additional course of therapy may be indicated, but multiple and repeated attempts to reduce remissions with regimens containing cytotoxic drugs should be avoided due to cumulative toxicity, which includes oncogenesis, mutagenesis, azoospermia, amenorrhea, bladder toxicity, and enhanced viral or opportunistic infections [1].

Patients with progressive disease may also be "rescued" from end-stage renal failure by combined cytotoxic and steroid therapy after impaired renal function is noted, providing that therapy is begun before the serum creatinine rises to values greater than about 3.5 mg/dl [1, 51, 52]. Chronic therapy of patients with slowly progressive disease using combinations of azathioprine and prednisone or cyclosporine and prednisone may also prove beneficial [53, 54]. High-dose intravenous immunoglobulins can also induce complete or partial remissions of proteinuria in some patients but are usually ineffective when renal failure is present [55]. Nonsteroidal anti-inflammatory agents may also stabilize renal function, but these regimens are poorly tolerated. Angiotensin converting enzyme therapy will often reduce proteinuria and may delay onset of renal failure. These approaches require further evaluation in large-scale prospective trials.

Patients with mild disease who are at low risk for complications or progressive renal failure should be treated conservatively and followed closely for spontaneous remission or the delayed onset of renal functional impairment. Membranous glomerulonephritis secondary to a defined etiology (e.g., hepatitis B or C virus infection, SLE, neoplasia) require specific management [56] (see later discussion). Patients with membranous glomerulonephritis and severe nephrotic syndrome (serum albumin < 2.0–2.5 g/dl) are at increased risk for thromboembolic phenomena, including renal vein thrombosis (see also Chap. 14). Prophylactic anticoagulation with warfarin may be indicated in such patients [57]. A search for renal vein thrombosis may be indicated in patients with clinically evident pulmonary emboli but is probably not necessary in most cases. Magnetic resonance imaging and duplex Doppler ultrasound studies are good screening approaches for the detection of renal vein thrombosis, but the definitive diagnosis requires renal venous angiography [1]. Acute allergic interstitial nephritis (often due to diuretics) and crescentic glomerulonephritis may occasionally complicate the course of membranous glomerulonephritis and lead to rapid loss of renal function. These complications require renal biopsy for definitive diagnosis.

The overall mortality in membranous glomerulonephritis is rather low and is mostly attributed to cardiovascular events. Hypercholesterolemia associated with the nephrotic syndrome contributes to an increased risk of cardiovascular disease. The pathogenesis and treatment of the lipid disorders associated with the nephrotic syndrome are covered in Chapter 14.

Crescentic Glomerulonephritis

Crescentic glomerulonephritis is characterized by the presence of extracapillary proliferation involving 50 percent or more of the glomeruli [1, 58, 59] (Fig. 15-4).
Crescents are usually circumferential and may be associated with varying degrees
of glomerular capillary proliferation or segmental necrosis. Electron microscopy frequently reveals gaps or discontinuities in the capillary wall or Bowman's capsule.
Immunofluorescence reveals fibrin-related antigens within Bowman's space. Many
disorders can evoke this lesion (Table 15-5); most are secondary to defined disorders
such as systemic necrotizing angiitis, Goodpasture's disease, or chronic or acute
infections [1]. Primary crescentic glomerulonephritis, in which no extrarenal involvement can be detected, is of diverse pathogenesis. In approximately 10 to 25
percent of cases, antibodies to GBM can be detected and linear deposits of IgG are
seen in immunofluorescence. The anti-GBM antibodies are directed to a well-
defined epitope on the noncollagenous domain of the $\alpha3$ chain of type IV collagen
[5, 6]. This lesion can be regarded as a renal-limited form of Goodpasture's disease.
In another 10 to 15 percent of cases, heavy deposits of IgG can be detected in the
glomeruli. If these deposits are predominantly IgA, then the patient can be classified
as IgA nephropathy or Berger's disease. In 50 to 80 percent of cases, immunoglobulin
deposits are quite scanty (pauci-immune crescentic glomerulonephritis) [1, 60]. The
majority of such cases are also associated with circulating antineutrophil cytoplasmic
autoantibodies (ANCA) [61], similar to those found in systemic necrotizing angiitis,

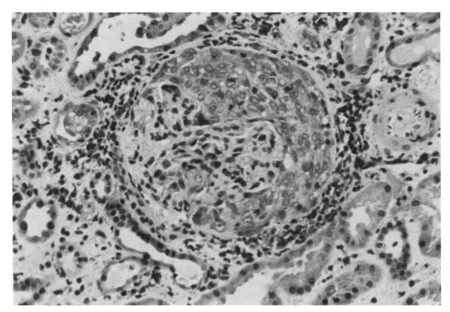

Fig. 15-4. Light-microscopic findings characteristic of crescentic glomerulonephritis. Note
necrotizing glomerulonephritis with marked extracapillary reaction, including crescent
and periglomerular fibrosis.

Table 15-5. Causes of extracapillary (crescentic) glomerulonephritis

Primary
    Anti–glomerular basement membrane antibody mediated
    Immune complex mediated
    "Pauci-immune" (antineutrophil cytoplasmic antibody associated)
    Other
Secondary
    Infectious diseases
        Infective endocarditis, poststreptococcal glomerulonephritis, visceral sepsis, hepatitis B
    Multisystem disease
        Systemic lupus erythematosus, Goodpasture's disease, Henoch-Schönlein purpura, microscopic polyangiitis, Wegener's granulomatosis, cryoglobulinemia, relapsing polychondritis, malignancy
    Drug associated
        Allopurinol, rifampicin, D-penicillamine, hydralazine
Complicating other primary renal diseases
    Membranous glomerulonephritis
    Membranoproliferative glomerulonephritis (especially type II)
    IgA nephropathy

such as microscopic polyangiitis or Wegener's granulomatosis, and thus the lesion may represent a renal-limited form of systemic necrotizing angiitis. In about 10 to 20 percent of cases, both anti-GBM autoantibodies and ANCA coexist or neither autoantibodies are detected [62, 63]. The latter may be regarded as representing truly "idiopathic" crescentic glomerulonephritis.

From the clinical viewpoint, all forms of crescentic glomerulonephritis present in a similar fashion with clinical features of glomerular inflammation (hematuria and proteinuria) accompanied by rapid loss of renal function. The clinical syndrome of RPGN is commonly associated with the crescentic glomerulonephritic lesion. Multisystem complaints are more common in those patients with granular immunoglobulin deposits or with scanty deposits in glomeruli. In the absence of therapy, over 80 percent of patients will require renal replacement therapy within 2 to 6 months from the time of discovery. Spontaneous recovery is unusual, except if the glomerular involvement is less than 50 percent, if the patient has a background of infection, or has developed an exacerbation of IgA nephropathy.

Treatment of the lesion is empiric [1]. Intensive plasma exchange combined with glucocorticoids and cytotoxic agents appears to be beneficial in those patients with anti-GBM antibody–induced disease, providing therapy is begun before dialysis is required. Approximately 60 to 80 percent of patients so treated will respond, and long-term remissions may ensue [64]. Daily or alternate-day plasma exchange (removing approximately 4 liters of plasma and replacing it with 5% albumin) may be required. Anti-GBM antibody levels fall quickly with such treatment. Only 10 percent of those patients treated after the onset of dialysis dependency will respond to this form of treatment. Relapses are rare.

Plasma exchange is usually not needed for the management of other forms of primary crescentic glomerulonephritis, except perhaps as an adjunct to glucocorticoids and cytotoxic drugs in patients who quickly become dialysis dependent and who have biopsy evidence of potentially reversible disease [65]. High doses of intravenous methylprednisolone (1000 mg of methylprednisolone daily for 3 days) combined with oral prednisone (1 mg/kg/day) and oral cyclophosphamide (2–3 mg/kg/day depending on bone marrow tolerance) appear to be the treatment of choice for the non–anti-GBM antibody–mediated forms of crescentic glomerulonephritis, especially in the presence of positive serologic tests for ANCA. Overall, 80 percent of patients with non–anti-GBM antibody–mediated disease treated in this fashion will experience full or partial recovery [65]. Long-term management is usually required. Relapses are common if the therapy is withdrawn when ANCA titers remain positive. Persistent proteinuria, hypertension, and impaired renal function are best managed by chronic administration of ACE inhibitors.

Membranoproliferative Glomerulonephritis (Mesangiocapillary Glomerulonephritis)

Membranoproliferative glomerulonephritis (MPGN) is a very heterogeneous collection of disorders characterized by diffuse proliferation of mesangial cells accompanied by expansion of mesangial matrix, and by the extension of cells and cytoplasm into the capillary wall, leading to a thickened or reduplicated appearance [1, 66, 67]. At *least* four types are recognized on the basis of electron microscopy [1, 66]. Type I demonstrates extensive subendothelial electron-dense deposits containing immunoglobulins, type II manifests an electron-dense alteration of the basement membrane (so-called dense deposit disease), type III is associated with extensive fragmentation and duplication of the basement membrane; and type IV is associated with both subendothelial and subepithelial deposits resembling membranous glomerulonephritis. The pathogenesis of MPGN is unknown, but immune complex deposition or in situ formation is suggested as being involved in type I disease. C3 is extensively deposited in type II in a "railroad track" appearance in the capillary wall and in nodules or "rings" in the mesangium. Several diseases can give rise to type I MPGN including SLE, chronic viral (especially hepatitis C virus) and bacterial infection, and cryoimmunoglobulinemia (Table 15-6).

Table 15-6. Causes of membranoproliferative glomerulonephritis

Idiopathic
    Type I (subendothelial deposits)
    Type II (dense deposit disease)
    Other variants (type III, etc.)
Secondary (usually resembles type I)
    Infections: "shunt nephritis, malaria, chronic viral infections (e.g., hepatitis B, C)
    Neoplasia
    Multisystem disease: systemic lupus erythematosus, mixed connective tissue disease
    Miscellaneous: sickle cell disease, α_1-antitrypsin deficiency, light-chain nephropathy, cryoglobulinemia, malignancies

Clinically, patients present with features of acute nephritis and/or nephrotic syndrome [1, 67]. The urine usually contains dysmorphic erythrocytes and abnormal proteinuria. Serum complement levels tend to be decreased, often with C3 disproportionately lowered compared to C1q or C4, suggesting alternate pathway activation [68]. Some patients also present with decreased C3 and C4, suggesting classic pathway activation. An autoantibody to the classic pathway C3 convertase (C3b,Bb, also known as C3 Nef) may also be found, particularly in type II disease [1, 68]. The blood pressure is commonly elevated and renal function impaired at the time of discovery. MPGN accounts for 5 to 10 percent of cases of nephrotic syndrome in children and a somewhat higher percentage in adults.

The prognosis for MPGN is guarded, since spontaneous remissions are unusual. Untreated, most patients will have persistence of signs of glomerulonephritis, and over 50 percent will progress to end-stage renal failure within 10 years of discovery, often in association with persisting nephrotic-range proteinuria and poorly controlled hypertension [1, 67, 69]. Crescentic involvement as well as advanced chronic tubulointerstitial lesions is associated with a poor prognosis. Treatment is controversial [70–72]. Uncontrolled studies have suggested that long-term alternate-day prednisone therapy may be helpful in children, providing treatment is initiated before progressive renal insufficiency appears [70]. Prospective randomized clinical trials have not conclusively proved that this approach is beneficial. Combinations of aspirin and dipyridamole may also delay the onset of renal insufficiency [72], and some uncontrolled studies have suggested that judicious use of glucocorticoids and cytotoxic agents may also be beneficial [71]. However, overall the effects of therapy are modest, and there is no compelling evidence that over the long term any form of treatment is effective. MPGN may also recur in the renal allograft. Type II disease (dense deposit disease) recurs in virtually all allografts but does not necessarily lead to a loss of renal function. Type I disease recurs much less frequently [73].

IgA Nephropathy (Berger's Disease)

IgA nephropathy is a very common primary glomerular disease that is characterized by diffuse and generalized mesangial deposits of IgA, often accompanied by C3, IgM, and IgG [1, 74–76] (Fig. 15-5). A variety of patterns are seen in light microscopy, most commonly focal and segmental proliferative or diffuse proliferative glomerulonephritis [74, 77].

Superimposed crescents are relatively common, especially following episodes of macroscopic hematuria often consequent to upper respiratory infection. Rarely, crescentic involvement will be extensive (>50% involvement of glomeruli). Membranous and membranoproliferative patterns are very uncommon. By electron microscopy, mesangial electron-dense deposits are seen.

The pathogenesis of IgA nephropathy is unknown but is thought to be related to immune complex formation and deposition or due to an abnormality in the IgA molecule itself [77, 78]. A variety of endogenous and environmental antigens have been suggested to be involved. The deposits in the glomeruli are believed to be predominantly polymeric forms of IgA$_1$, perhaps combined with an environmental or autologous antigen. Several diseases may be associated with similar IgA deposits,

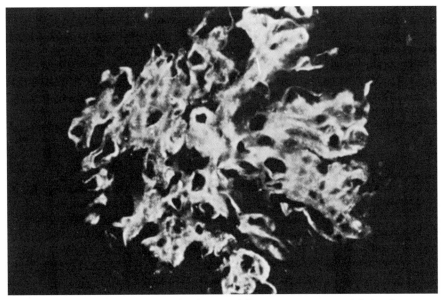

Fig. 15-5. Fluorescent-antibody study, showing diffuse, coarse immunoglobulin deposits located predominantly in the glomerular mesangium. This finding is characteristic of a large group of diseases that often demonstrate focal or diffuse mesangial proliferative glomerulonephritis by light microscopy, including IgA nephropathy.

including Henoch-Schönlein purpura, chronic liver disease, malignancies (especially carcinoma of the lung), seronegative spondyloarthropathies, celiac disease, mycosis fungoides, and psoriasis [1, 75].

Clinically, IgA nephropathy is most commonly associated with recurring episodes of macroscopic hematuria with or without proteinuria [1, 75]. Nephrotic syndrome is seen at presentation in less than 10 percent of patients, and RPGN is rare. Episodes of reversible acute renal insufficiency may be seen in association with upper respiratory infection and bouts of macroscopic hematuria. These events resemble the acute nephritic syndrome. Unlike postinfectious glomerulonephritis, a latent period is not seen, and the onset of hematuria is contemporaneous with the onset of symptoms of the upper respiratory infection.

IgA nephropathy has been encountered throughout the world but is most common in the Asian-Pacific areas [1, 74]. Males appear to be more commonly affected than females. Blacks are uncommonly affected. The disorder is principally seen in adolescents and young adults, with a peak prevalence between the ages of 20 and 30 years of age. The disorder is uncommon in patients over the age of 50. Renal function is typically normal at the time of discovery. Serum complement levels are normal. Blood pressure may be elevated, sometimes to severe levels. IgA-fibronectin complexes may be elevated in 70 to 80 percent [79], IgA rheumatoid factor present in 80 percent [80], and serum IgA levels and IgA containing immune complexes are increased in 50 percent of cases [80]. IgA ANCA may be present [82]. Familial cases have been described. IgA nephropathy has also been associated with thin-basement-membrane nephropathy. Rarely, IgA nephropathy may evolve to full-blown Henoch-Schönlein purpura [1].

The clinical course of IgA nephropathy is prolonged and difficult to predict. Complete remissions are uncommon but do occur [83]. Bouts of gross hematuria following upper respiratory infections or exercise are common; sometimes these may be associated with spontaneously reversible episodes of acute renal failure [1, 13]. Slowly progressive renal failure is seen in about 25 percent of patients. Overall, about 1 percent of patients will develop end-stage renal failure each year of follow-up. A poor prognosis is found in patients with persisting proteinuria (>1.0 g/day), poorly controlled hypertension, impaired renal function at discovery, and chronic tubulointerstitial lesions, advanced glomerulosclerosis, and arteriolar lesions at initial biopsy [1, 84].

The treatment of IgA nephropathy is controversial [1, 85, 86]. Most patients do not require treatment, since they do not have a progressive course. Patients with features indicative of a poor prognosis could be treated with high-dose oral omega-3 fatty acids (12.0 g/day) or with combinations of low-dose warfarin and dipyridamole [87, 88]. Long-term alternate-day glucocorticoids may be helpful, but their value has not been proved by long-term prospective randomized trials [89]. ACE inhibitors are indicated for the control of blood pressure [90]. Alkylating cytotoxic agents or cyclosporine is not indicated due to the chronic and unpredictable nature of the disease and the attendant side effects of these agents. Chronic therapy with azathioprine and glucocorticoids may be useful in some patients with a progressive course [91]. Aggressive treatment with intravenous glucocorticoids, cytotoxic agents, and plasma exchange may be indicated in the treatment of the rare patient with RPGN associated with extensive crescentic involvement of glomeruli [1]. High-dose intravenous immunoglobulins may be helpful in the exceptional patient with severe disease and a progressive course (see also Henoch-Schönlein purpura) [92]. An antigen elimination (hypoallergenic) diet may have some utility; however, this has not been proved in a prospective manner [93].

Thin-Basement-Membrane Nephropathy

Thin-basement-membrane nephropathy is characterized by exceptionally thin and attenuated GBM (<200–250 nM) [1, 94, 95]. The light-microscopic appearance is usually normal, and immunoglobulin and complements are inconsistently found. The pathogenesis is unknown but could be related to a genetically based defect in basement membrane biosynthesis or turnover. Typically, patients present with persisting microscopic hematuria in the absence of significant proteinuria [94, 95]. Renal function is normal and hypertension absent. Familial cases have been described, suggesting autosomal dominant inheritance [95]. Deafness or extrarenal abnormalities are absent, thus distinguishing this disorder from Alport's syndrome. Occasionally, IgA nephropathy may be concomitantly present [96]. The prognosis is excellent, and progressive renal failure is unusual. There is no known therapy.

Other Primary Glomerular Diseases

Fibrillary glomerulonephritis and *immunotactoid glomerulonephritis* are heterogeneous disorders having in common the glomerular accumulation of fibrillary deposits that are Congo red negative (e.g., nonamyloid) [1, 97, 98]. The deposits also frequently contain immunoglobulin. The fibrils are randomly arrayed and are usually 12 to 20 nm in diameter in fibrillary glomerulonephritis, and in the immunotactoid variants the fibrils consist of closely packed microtubules 30 to 50 nm in diameter [97, 100]. Cryoglobulins, collagen, and fibronectin deposits can give rise to similar deposits. Clinically, a broad age range may be affected, but the peak prevalence is between 40 and 60 years of age [100]. Whites are predominantly affected. Hypertension, hematuria, nephrotic syndrome, and progressive renal insufficiency are common. End-stage renal disease develops in about 50 percent of patients by the fifth year of follow-up. Extrarenal manifestations are uncommon but do rarely occur. RPGN with superimposed extensive crescentic involvement may develop [100]. Overall, no therapy has yet been demonstrated to be effective. Immunotactoid glomerulonephritis may be associated with monoclonal paraproteinemia or B-cell neoplasia [100]. Recurrence in renal transplant may develop [100].

Lipoprotein deposition disease is a rare disorder associated with deposition of lipid in the glomeruli (typically apolipoprotein E) [101]. *Collagen deposition disease* (collagenofibrotic glomerulopathy) is a rare disorder associated with the deposition of type III collagen in glomeruli [102]. There are no systemic manifestations of the disease. The pathogenesis of the deposits of these proteins in glomeruli is unknown.

Glomerulopathies Associated with Infectious Diseases

Poststreptococcal Glomerulonephritis

Infection of the throat or skin with certain M protein subtypes of group A β-hemolytic streptococci may evoke acute glomerulonephritis [1, 103]. A latent period of 5 to 14 days or longer is present between the first manifestation of infection and the first sign of nephritis. Shorter latent periods usually signify the exacerbation of underlying chronic renal disease, such as IgA nephropathy, rather than de novo acute glomerulonephritis. The clinical expression of poststreptococcal glomerulonephritis (PSGN) varies widely [1, 103]. Most common manifestations include dysmorphic hematuria (and red blood cell casts), proteinuria, edema, hypertension, circulatory congestion, and reduced GFR [1, 103, 104]. Acute oliguria may develop in a minority of cases. A frank nephrotic syndrome is relatively uncommon, developing in about 20 percent or less of hospitalized patients. The GFR is nearly always decreased. Circulatory congestion may dominate the picture and produce pulmonary edema. Hypertension is usually mild to moderate and not accompanied by severe retinopathy, although encephalopathy with seizures and focal neurologic deficits may be the presenting feature, particularly among children. Less severe cases may be manifested only by changes in the urinary sediment with or without proteinuria and mild sodium retention. In about 5 percent of patients, acute PSGN will evolve into the picture of RPGN with delayed recovery.

The laboratory findings in PSGN are more or less distinctive. An antibody response to one or more of the streptococcal exoenzymes (streptolysin O, DNase, hyaluronidase, and NADase) is frequently found [1, 103]. The antibody response to streptolysin O in pyoderma-associated nephritis is typically weak. Antibody response to exoenzymes may be blunted by early antimicrobial therapy. The serum level of total hemolytic complement (CH_{50}) is reduced regularly during the acute phase but returns to normal within 8 weeks of the development of nephritis [105]. The serum level of C3 parallels the CH_{50} activity, but early-acting complement components C2, C4, and C1q are infrequently decreased, indicating prominent activation of the alternative pathway of complement. A mild hyperchloremic, hyperkalemic (type IV) renal tubular acidosis may be found. Urinary protein excretion is less than 3 g/day in the majority of cases. Anemia is typically normocytic and normochromic and largely dilutional in origin. Serum cholesterol may be transiently increased, and serum albumin is modestly decreased.

Renal biopsies performed early in the course of PSGN (<8 weeks) reveal diffuse endocapillary proliferative glomerulonephritis, often accompanied by infiltration with polymorphonuclear leukocytes and monocytes [1, 103, 106]. A few segmental crescents may also be seen; extensive crescent formation usually signifies a progressive course. Vasculitis is rare. Immunofluorescence reveals prominent granular deposits of C3 and IgG but seldom C1q and C4 [106]. Three patterns of immunoglobulin deposits in gomeruli are found [107]: the *garland* pattern, with granular immunoglobulin deposits in a lobular pattern; the *mesangial* pattern, with granular deposits of immunoglobulin exclusively in a mesangial distribution; and the *starry sky* pattern, with granular deposits of immunoglobulin irregularly scattered throughout the mesangium and peripheral capillary walls. The garland pattern is associated with a poor prognosis and often is associated with persistent proteinuria. Electron microscopy reveals typically discrete subepithelial electron-dense deposits ("humps") [106] (Fig. 15-6) and variable degrees of mesangial and subepithelial deposits. Biopsies performed later in the course (after 8–10 weeks) will reveal resolving mesangial hypercellularity, focal and segmental proliferation, and/or glomerular sclerosis. Mesangial deposits of C3 may persist for several years, but the subepithelial electron-dense deposits usually resolve rapidly.

The pathogenesis of PSGN is unknown [103, 108]. Glomerular deposition of circulating immune complexes may be involved. Prominent activation of the alternative pathway of complement suggests involvement of a polysaccharide antigen. An in situ nonglomerular antigen-antibody complex mechanism is an equally tenable concept on the basis of available data [108]. Certain streptococcal antigens may be "planted" in capillary walls and/or mesangium because of a charge-dependent or lectinlike affinity for glomerular structures.

The short-term prognosis of PSGN is quite favorable, with very few patients dying of electrolyte imbalance, pulmonary edema, uncontrolled hypertension, or uremia [1, 103]. Long-term prognosis remains controversial [1, 103, 109, 110]. The vast majority of cases of children and young adults with PSGN occurring in conjunction with epidemics of nephritogenic streptococci will completely resolve, even

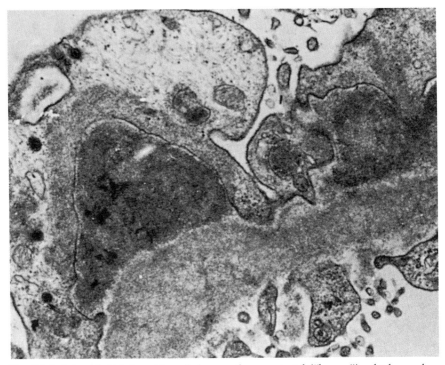

Fig. 15-6. Subepithelial deposition of electron-dense material ("humps"), which may be found in several types of immune complex glomerulopathies and is characteristic of poststreptococcal diffuse endocapillary proliferative glomerulonephritis.

though the urinary sediment may remain abnormal for several years. The prognosis in adults with epidemic PSGN, especially with prolonged azotemia, severe protein-uria, and crescents on renal biopsy specimens, is less certainly favorable. With few exceptions, sporadic PSGN seems unlikely to lead to progressive renal failure in children, although abnormal clinical features may persist for several years after apparent clinical recovery. Sporadic PSGN in adults may evolve into chronic pro-gressive glomerulonephritis in as many as 30 to 40 percent of cases, although this high prevalence of progressive PSGN remains a controversial topic [1, 109]. The descriptions of "progressive" PSGN in the older literature (before 1968) may have inadvertently included patients with exacerbations of IgA nephropathy, thus biasing the analysis toward progressive disease.

The treatment of PSGN is supportive only [1, 109]. Antimicrobial therapy is given primarily to halt the spread of potentially nephritogenic organisms among family members or close contacts. Such therapy does not seem to be very effective in aborting or ameliorating the clinical course of PSGN. Loop diuretics (e.g., furose-mide) should be used for patients with circulatory congestion and hypertension. Peripherally acting vasodilators (e.g., hydralazine) are quite effective in the manage-ment of hypertension not benefited by diuresis alone. Peritoneal dialysis or hemodialysis may be required for oliguric patients presenting with severe circulatory conges-tion or hyperkalemia [1]. Digitalis preparations should not be employed unless abnormal myocardial contractility can be documented by appropriate hemodynamic measurements. Fluid, protein, and electrolyte restriction should be appropriate to fluid balance and azotemia. Bed rest need not be continued beyond the acute phases of the disease. Except in cases of RPGN, steroids, cytotoxic agents, and anticoagu-lants have no proved value and may be harmful.

Nephritis Associated with Other Microbial Organisms

A large number of infectious diseases other than group A β-hemolytic streptococcal infection may also be associated with glomerulonephritis [2, 111]. These include pneumococcal pneumonia, meningococcemia, typhoid fever, infective endocarditis, visceral sepsis, and a variety of viral, protozoal, and fungal diseases. These diseases evoke a variety of clinical syndromes: acute nephritis, RPGN, nephrotic syndrome, asymptomatic hematuria, and non-nephrotic proteinuria. Similarly, a spectrum of morphologic lesions, including mild diffuse mesangial cell proliferation, membra-nous glomerulonephritis, crescentic glomerulonephritis, and focal and segmental proliferative glomerulonephritis, may ensue. Presumably, in each instance, the le-sions are mediated by the glomerular deposits of immune complexes containing microbial antigens and their respective antibodies.

Glomerulonephritis associated with infective endocarditis is mediated by the glo-merular deposition of antigen-antibody complexes [2, 112, 113]. The organisms responsible may vary from the usual *Streptococcus viridans* to *Staphylococcus aureus* and various gram-negative organisms [2]. The major glomerular lesions observed are focal and segmental proliferative glomerulonephritis, diffuse proliferative glo-merulonephritis, and crescentic glomerulonephritis. Clinical manifestations include hematuria and proteinuria of a moderate degree and varying degrees of renal function impairment. The nephrotic syndrome is uncommon. Serum complement compo-nents (C3, C1q, and C4) are generally decreased when the glomerulonephritis is active. Rheumatoid factor tests are positive, and cryoimmunoglobulins are fre-quently detectable. The renal lesion may be reversible if the underlying infection is treated before glomerular scarring has occurred. A similar sequence of events has been seen in children in whom ventriculoatrial shunts (shunt nephritis) have been implanted for the relief of internal hydrocephalus and in whom chronic bloodstream infection has ensued with a cutaneous contaminant, such as *Staphylococcus albus*, *Propionibacterium acnes*, or diphtheroids [114].

The acute nephritic or nephrotic syndromes have also been associated with con-genital and secondary syphilis, in which the proliferative and membranous lesions are associated with granular deposits of immunoglobulin, treponemal antigens, and subepithelial electron-dense deposits [115]. The nephrotic syndrome may also occur in leprosy [116]. Occult visceral sepsis, accompanying undetected or inadequately treated pulmonary or retroperitoneal abscesses, may also be associated with glomeru-lonephritis [117]. Malaria and toxoplasmosis have been associated with glomerulo-nephritis [118, 119]. Quartan malarial infection is the major cause of nephrotic syndrome among schoolchildren in East and West Africa. The disease follows a variable course, depending to some degree on the severity of the glomerular lesions. Corticosteroids and cytotoxic agents have had a beneficial effect on some patients.

Chronic infection with hepatitis B or hepatitis C virus can evoke a lesion similar to membranous or MPGN [120, 121]. Cryoglobulinemia and vasculitis can also be seen with hepatitis B or hepatitis C. Chronic infection with hepatitis C often leads to a syndrome of mixed IgG/IgM cryoglobulinemia, purpura, splenomegaly, cutaneous necrosis, and MPGN (type I). Such patients may temporarily benefit from glucocorticoids and interferon-α. Schistosomiasis and filariasis have also been associated with glomerular lesions, principally membranous glomerulonephritis, MPGN, and the nephrotic syndrome [118, 122].

A new entity presumably caused by chronic infection with HIV has been described. It is called *HIV-associated nephropathy* and is found among asymptomatically infected individuals, those with acquired immune deficiency syndrome (AIDS), and those with AIDS-related complex [123–125]. Morphologically, the glomerular lesion is focal and segmental glomerulosclerosis with extensive tubulointerstitial lesions consisting of infiltration with mononuclear cells, dilated tubules, large casts, and tubuloreticular inclusions in endothelial cells [125]. Clinically, heavy proteinuria, progressively impaired renal function, and large kidneys are found [2, 123, 124]. There is no proven therapy available, but treatment with zidovudine (AZT) protease inhibitors or glucocorticoids may produce temporary benefit. Other lesions found in patients with HIV infection include amyloidosis, proliferative glomerulonephritis, membranous glomerulonephritis (often hepatitis B or hepatitis C related), crescentic glomerulonephritis, and hemolytic-uremic syndrome.

Glomerulopathies Associated with Drugs

Exposure to a variety of environmental chemical agents has been associated with glomerular disease [2, 126]. The principal clinical manifestation has been proteinuria, most often massive and accompanied by other features of the nephrotic syndrome. Microscopic or gross hematuria may also be seen. On occasion, RPGN and/or vasculitis has been observed. The association of organic mercurial compounds with nephrotic syndrome may account for its previous association with congestive heart failure and constrictive pericarditis [2, 127]. Elemental mercury has also been reported to provoke nephrotic syndrome. Inorganic mercury compounds, found in mercurous chloride teething powders and topical ammoniated mercury ointments used in the treatment of various cutaneous disorders, have also been known to produce the nephrotic syndrome. Membranous glomerulopathy is the most common lesion in mercury-related diseases. The use of oral or parenteral organic gold compounds in the treatment of rheumatoid arthritis may be complicated by the development of membranous glomerulopathy in approximately 5 to 10 percent of instances [2, 128]. Microscopic hematuria and dermatitis may be associated findings. Ordinarily, the manifestations of nephrotic syndrome in the glomerular disease will disappear on withdrawal of these agents; however, several years may elapse before complete restitution of normality.

Lithium therapy may occasionally be associated with nephrotic syndrome [129]. The use of D-penicillamine in the treatment of Wilson's disease, cystinuria, and rheumatoid arthritis has been associated with the nephrotic syndrome and/or RPGN [130]. Patients developing renal complications from gold and penicillamine therapy have an increased prevalence of HLA-DR3 antigen.

Captopril therapy of hypertension has on occasion been associated with the development of membranous glomerulopathy and the nephrotic syndrome [131]. Nonsteroidal anti-inflammatory agents may provoke acute renal failure and nephrotic syndrome on a hypersensitivity basis. Minimal change lesions and acute interstitial nephritis are observed [132].

Chronic heroin abuse may be associated with a variety of glomerular lesions, most commonly focal and segmental glomerular sclerosis [2, 133]. This lesion has a tendency to progress rapidly, even if heroin abuse is discontinued. Heroin-associated nephropathy can be distinguished from HIV-associated nephropathy on morphologic grounds. In addition, large kidneys are found in HIV-associated nephropathy, while the kidneys tend to atrophy quickly in heroin-associated nephropathy. Sulfonamides may be associated with a hypersensitivity vasculitis and glomerulonephritis, and intravenous methamphetamine abuse has been noted to be associated with a polyarteritis-like picture. Probenecid and the anticonvulsant drugs mephenytoin, trimethadione, and paramethadione have resulted in the nephrotic syndrome with minimal glomerular changes or membranous glomerulopathy with light microscopy. Antilymphocyte globulin used in the treatment of allograft rejection has been rarely associated with glomerulonephritis due to the presence of contaminating antibodies to human GBM antigens. Acute serum sickness with glomerulonephritis may complicate the treatment of snakebite, tetanus or other clostridial infections, and diphtheria with heterologous antisera. Intravenous radiocontrast agents have rarely been associated with glomerular disease. Rifampicin, allopurinol, and hydralazine have also been associated with RPGN [2].

Glomerulopathies Associated with Pregnancy

Preeclampsia

The glomerular lesion of preeclampsia is characterized by marked endothelial cell swelling and obliteration of capillary lumina [2, 134, 135]. Fibrinogen-fibrin deposits may be found in mesangium. The renal lesion may not be as reversible as once thought, as glomerular changes may persist for 6 months or longer postpartum in up to 33 percent of cases. Patients who have once had preeclampsia may be more likely to have recurrent hypertension with subsequent pregnancies. Fixed hypertension has been commonly observed in these cases. Severe proteinuria may occur in the course of preeclampsia and may from time to time produce the biochemical features of the nephrotic syndrome. Ordinarily, the proteinuria will abate with delivery. In severe cases, associated with cortical necrosis, there may be a microangiopathic hemolytic anemia.

Glomerulopathies Associated with Diseases of Specific Organs

Liver Disease

At autopsy, patients with chronic liver disease (alcoholic, postnecrotic, and biliary) frequently are noted to have a diffuse, glomerular sclerotic lesion often referred to as cirrhotic glomerulosclerosis [2, 136]. This glomerular lesion has seldom been associated with any serious clinical manifestations other than mild proteinuria. Patients with alcoholic cirrhosis have also been demonstrated to have extensive IgA and C3 deposits in the mesangium [2, 137]. The mechanisms underlying this phenomenon are unknown, but it could be due to shunting of enteric antigens or IgA-containing immune complexes into the systemic circulation. Chronic hepatitis B and C viral infection may lead to a variety of glomerular lesions, including membranous glomerulopathy and type I MPGN [138]. α_1-Antitrypsin deficiency may be associated with chronic liver disease and type I MPGN. The prevalence of PSGN may be increased in patients with alcoholic cirrhosis.

Cardiac Disease

Severe congestive heart failure, constrictive pericarditis, and tricuspid insufficiency with markedly raised peripheral venous pressures may be associated with modest proteinuria or may aggravate the quantity of protein excretion when glomerular disease is already present [2]. It is doubtful that raised venous pressure per se can provoke the biochemical features of nephrotic syndrome. It is more likely that mercurial diuretics used in the past for the relief of the cardiac edema led to glomerular disease on an immunologic basis. Cyanotic congenital heart disease may be associated with an increase in glomerular size and mesangial proliferation but seldom evokes any clinical manifestations [139], although focal glomerular sclerosis may be a late sequela. Endocarditis may be associated with glomerular disease (discussed previously). Cardiac and renal amyloidosis frequently coexist in patients with primary amyloidosis.

Pulmonary Disease

A variety of pulmonary infections can evoke acute, chronic, or rapidly progessive glomerulonephritis. These include pneumococcal pneumonia, *Klebsiella pneumoniae*, toxoplasmosis, cytomegalovirus, varicella pneumonia, and chronic bacterial pulmonary abscesses. Legionnaire's disease may provoke acute renal failure and interstitial nephritis but not glomerulonephritis. Bronchiectasis and chronic pulmonary tuberculosis may be associated with renal amyloidosis. α-Antitrypsin deficiency may at times be associated with a proliferative glomerulonephritis and the nephrotic syndrome. Carcinoma of the lung has been associated with the development of membranous nephropathy syndrome, presumably on the basis of tumor-antitumor immune complexes (see following discussion), or it can be associated with IgA nephropathy or crescentic glomerulonephritis.

Glomerulopathies Associated with Malignancy and Paraproteinemia

Carcinoma

The nephrotic syndrome has been associated with several solid tumors, including carcinoma of the colon, bronchus, pleura (mesothelioma), kidney, stomach, breast, cervix, bladder, prostate, and ovary [2, 140–143]. Immunopathologic studies have shown granular deposits of immunoglobulin and usually a membranous glomerulopathy or type I MPGN. On occasion, tumor-associated antigens have been localized in these deposits. Minimal change disease has been associated with carcinoma of the pancreas, mesothelioma, renal cell carcinoma, oncocytoma, and prostatic carcinoma [2]. An important aspect of the association of glomerulopathies and malignancies is that manifestations of the glomerular lesion may *precede* any overt manifestations for the underlying malignancy in about one-third of all cases in which a renal lesion arises in association with neoplasia. Therefore, it is worthwhile to evaluate patients for occult malignancy when they present with glomerular disease that has immunopathologic characteristics suggesting immune complex deposition, principally membranous glomerulopathy. Removal of the tumor has been associated with a remission of the glomerular disease, while it recurs on reappearance of metastatic deposits.

Lymphoma and Leukemia

The nephrotic syndrome has been associated with Hodgkin's disease, non-Hodgkin's lymphoma, Burkitt's lymphoma, and chronic lymphatic leukemia [2, 144–146]. In Hodgkin's disease, the nephrotic syndrome may antedate the expression of the disease by several months, and proteinuria may subside with adequate chemotherapy or irradiation [145]. Although minimal change disease has been the glomerular lesion most commonly seen in patients with Hodgkin's disease with the nephrotic syndrome, an immune complex variety of glomerulonephritis has also been described [2, 146]. Renal amyloidosis may also occasionally complicate the clinical picture in lymphomas.

Paraproteinemias

Multiple Myeloma

Multiple myeloma may be associated with glomerular lesions, most commonly amyloidosis [2, 147]. Approximately 10 percent of patients with multiple myeloma will develop renal amyloidosis and nephrotic syndrome. Amyloidosis in a patient with multiple myeloma has serious prognostic implications, since it usually means progressive renal failure will occur. A histologic picture resembling nodular diabetic glomerulosclerosis has also been described in patients with excessive formation of monoclonal light chains (typically kappa chain). Other disorders associated with excessive production of monoclonal immunoglobulin proteins (such as heavy chain disease) have also been associated with glomerulonephritis. As mentioned previously, immunotactoid glomerulonephritis may rarely be associated with paraproteinemia.

Waldenström's Macroglobulinemia

Waldenström's macroglobulinemia may be associated with the development of glomerular lesions characterized by deposits resembling thrombi on the endothelial aspect of the basement membrane, sometimes so extensive as almost to occlude capillary lumina [2, 148]. Immunofluorescence analysis of these deposits suggests that they contain IgM exclusively. Treatment of the macroglobulinemia with intensive plasma exchange and cytotoxic drugs may be beneficial. Amyloidosis may also develop on occasion.

Cryoimmunoglobulins

Cryoimmunoglobulins consisting of polyclonal IgG and monoclonal IgM have been described in association with the syndrome of purpura, weakness, arthralgia, and RPGN [2, 149]. The renal lesion is a proliferative glomerulonephritis with polymorphonuclear and mononuclear leukocyte infiltration. Immunofluorescence studies show IgG and IgM in a granular pattern along the capillary wall, and electron microscopy shows electron-dense deposits. Elevated rheumatoid factor titers and hypergammaglobulinemia are found, along with lymphadenopathy, splenomegaly, Sjögren's syndrome, and thyroiditis. Most of the cases can be shown to be due to chronic infection with hepatitis C virus (see previous discussion) [2, 121]. The IgM component is approximately 60 percent of the total cryoimmunoglobulin and exhibits anti-IgG (rheumatoid factor) activity. Total serum hemolytic complement is usually reduced, and C4 levels are often, but not invariably, reduced. Favorable short-term responses have been reported to high-dose intravenous methylprednisolone and interferon-α [2, 121]. Intensive plasma exchange is another form of treatment that may be beneficial.

Amyloidosis

Amyloidosis is commonly associated with renal involvement [2, 150, 151]. Kidney involvement occurs in approximately 25 to 50 percent of patients with primary amyloidosis and commonly in patients with amyloidosis secondary to multiple myeloma, osteomyelitis, tuberculosis, leprosy, rheumatoid arthritis, or familial Mediterranean fever. Renal amyloidosis may be associated with nephrogenic diabetes insipidus, renal bicarbonate wasting, and retroperitoneal fibrosis. The nephrotic syndrome, with heavy proteinuria, may develop in up to 50 percent of patients, but hypertension is a relatively infrequent finding [2].

Amyloidosis may be diagnosed unexpectedly on renal biopsy in up to 10 percent of older patients with apparently "idiopathic" nephrotic syndrome. Although the kidneys usually appear large or normal in size, they may also be small, particularly when renal failure is present. Systemic amyloidosis may also be diagnosed by a surgical biopsy of the rectal mucosa or a needle aspiration of the abdominal fatty tissue and staining the specimen with Congo red.

Typical morphologic findings of glomerular involvement in amyloidosis include hypocellular glomeruli infiltrated with Congo red–positive material exhibiting apple-green birefringence by polarized light microscopy [2]. Immunofluorescence reveals amorphous deposits of immunoglobulin, monoclonal light chain, complement, and other plasma proteins. The electron-microscopic findings are characteristic, consisting of a network of fibrils, 8 to 11 nM in diameter, in various orientations that can be readily distinguished from collagen because of their lack of periodicity. The fibrils in fibrillary and immunotactoid glomerulonephritis are larger (12–50 nM) and are Congo red negative.

The amyloid proteins in primary amyloidosis and multiple myeloma are homologous with the variable regions of the light chain of immunoglobulin. The amyloid proteins associated with some forms of secondary amyloidosis (e.g., infection, chronic inflammation) represent a unique protein that has its counterpart in normal plasma (serum amyloid A protein). In primary amyloidosis and that associated with familial Mediterranean fever, progressive renal failure generally occurs. Cardiac involvement confers an ominous prognosis [2, 152, 153]. Successful treatment of a chronic infection (e.g., tuberculosis) may at times be associated with reversal of amyloidosis.

The treatment of primary amyloidosis has been unsatisfactory, although occasionally reversal of amyloid deposits with intensive treatment using steroids and cytotoxic agents (melphalan) has been described [2, 152]. If no contraindications exist, it is probably worthwhile to try intermittent melphalan plus prednisone therapy in patients with primary amyloidosis and renal involvement. The addition of colchicine to the regimen might be beneficial, but this has not yet been proved [153]. Colchicine has also been beneficial in familial Mediterranean fever and in some patients with primary amyloidosis [154].

Glomerulopathies Associated with Multisystem Disease of Poorly Defined Etiology

Lupus Nephritis

Abnormalities of structure and function of the kidney are very common, perhaps universal, among patients with SLE [2, 155–157]. Many theories have been advanced, but the etiology of SLE is still unknown. In fact, it seems likely that several processes underlie the syndrome. Studies of the murine analogues of human SLE have indicated that genetic, viral, and immunologic aberrations interact to result in disease. A genetic influence in human SLE is also supported by family studies and clustering of HLA haplotypes among patients with SLE and SLE-like syndromes, particularly those associated with hereditary C2 deficiency [2].

Patients with SLE produce a variety of autoantibodies to cell constituents. Abnormalities of cell-mediated immunity are also present, primarily defects in T cell–mediated suppression and cytotoxicity. B-cell hyperactivity seems to be a general phenomenon in SLE. Not surprisingly, if sufficient autologous or viral-directed antigen is present in the circulation under such circumstances, circulating immune complexes may be generated, and their deposition in various organs (e.g., glomeruli, lung, skin, joints) may evoke inflammation. Thus, many investigators believe that SLE is a prototypical human example of a circulating immune complex–mediated disease [2]. The principal autologous antigen-antibody systems operative in human SLE appear to be species of DNA, either single-stranded (ss, denatured) or double-stranded (ds, native) DNA, and their respective antibodies.

Recently, several alternative mechanisms to the classic circulating immune complex pathogenesis of lupus nephritis have been proposed. One involves the initial binding of circulating DNA and/or histones with GBM and/or mesangium, followed by formation of immune complexes locally within the glomerulus [2, 158, 159]. This pathogenic mechanism does not require the formation of immune complexes in the circulation for glomerular damage to ensue. Alternatively, autoantibodies arising in SLE could react with native constituents of basement membrane such as collagen, laminin, or proteoglycan [160], or histone proteins could bind to the basement membrane with secondary localization of DNA and anti-DNA antibodies [159]. Finally, congenital deficiencies of complement components (particularly C2 deficiency) are frequently associated with SLE and SLE-like disorders [161]. It is possible that a defect in the normal complement-dependent clearing mechanisms for viral infection may eventuate in an immune complex–type disease process.

In summary, the fundamental etiologic and pathogenetic processes involved in SLE remain elusive. A genetically based susceptibility to autoimmune disease, perhaps involving the immune response genes located in the vicinity of the major histocompatibility complex, aberrant B-cell hyperresponsiveness, and defective T-cell responses all seem to be interrelated in the production of glomerular disease in SLE. The bulk of evidence suggests that the glomeruli are damaged by the deposition or in situ formation of immune complexes composed of a variety of endogenous antigen-antibody systems, principally DNA–anti-DNA.

Despite the uncertainty regarding both the etiology and the fine details of pathogenesis is SLE, certain immunopathologic features are common to all patients with renal involvement in SLE. These include (1) deposition of immunoglobulins (IgG, IgM, IgA, and/or IgE) and complement components (C1q, C4, C3), in a granular pattern at various sites in the glomerular capillary network; (2) electron-dense deposits, sometimes of an organized nature, in various sites within the glomerular capillary network; and (3) the presence of nonglomerular antigens in the immune deposits (chiefly DNA).

Renal Lesions in Systemic Lupus Erythematosus

The immunopathologic alterations that characterize SLE evoke a spectrum of morphologic renal abnormalities [2, 162]. The following is a summary of the morphologic spectrum of renal lesions seen in SLE as modified from the classification of Baldwin and colleagues and the World Health Organization (WHO) [2, 155, 162, 163].

Minimal Change Lupus Nephritis (WHO Class I). Light microscopy reveals little or no alteration of the glomerular capillary or mesangial architecture in minimal change lupus nephritis. However, by immunofluorescence, immunoglobulins (IgG, IgM, IgA) often associated with complement components are found exclusively in the mesangium. Electron-microscopic studies reveal scattered electron-dense deposits in the mesangial matrix, but none is associated with the peripheral capillary walls. The interstitium, tubules, and vessels are normal. This lesion is found in patients with few or no clinical manifestations of renal disease and, in the absence of evolution to other lesions, has a favorable prognosis.

Mesangial Proliferative Lupus Nephritis (WHO Class II). Mesangial proliferative lupus nephritis resembles minimal change lupus nephritis, but by light microscopy an easily discernible increase in the cellularity of the glomeruli is present, mostly confined to the mesangium. The immunoglobulin and electron-dense deposits in the mesangium are more marked than in minimal change lupus nephritis, but the capillary walls are relatively free of deposits. The interstitium, vessels, and tubules are normal or show only a few widely scattered mononuclear cell infiltrates. This lesion is found among patients with few clinical manifestations of renal disease, chiefly abnormal urinary sediment with or without mild proteinuria. Nephrotic syndrome is uncommon. The GFR is usually normal. In the absence of evolution to more severe proliferative nephritis, the prognosis is favorable.

Focal and Segmental Proliferative Lupus Nephritis (WHO Class III). Focal and segmental proliferative lupus nephritis is similar to mesangial proliferative lupus nephritis, except that portions of the capillary tufts of individual glomeruli reveal a pronounced increase in cellularity often associated with capsular adhesions and local epithelial cell proliferation and sometimes with cell necrosis and fibrinoid changes. Not all glomeruli are affected (usually <50%). Immunofluorescence and electron-microscopic findings are similar to those of mesangial proliferative glomerulonephritis; however, occasional peripheral capillary loops may be involved with deposits. This lesion is chiefly found in patients with abnormalities of urinary sediment (especially hematuria) with or without proteinuria. Nephrotic syndrome and decreased GFR are uncommon. The course and prognosis are similar to those of diffuse proliferative lupus nephritis.

Diffuse Proliferative Lupus Nephritis (WHO Class IV). Generalized and diffuse endocapillary proliferation, often associated with fibrinoid necrosis and "wire loops," is characteristic of diffuse proliferative lupus nephritis. The immunoglobulin deposits involve multiple immunoglobulin isotypes (IgG, IgM, IgA) and involve most or all peripheral capillary loops and mesangium, primarily in a subendothelial or intramembranous location. The deposits may be quite large and obstruct the lumina or become organized ("fingerprinting"). *Hematoxylin bodies may be found and are the only pathognomonic lesion for SLE* [2]. Varying degrees of tubulointerstitial and vascular changes may also be found. Immunoglobulin deposits in the tubular basement membrane, Bowman's capsule, and vessels are very common. Crescents may be superimposed. The course and prognosis are poor, but the lesions may respond to therapy.

Membranous Lupus Nephritis (WHO Class V). Membranous lupus nephritis is characterized by diffuse thickening of the glomerular capillary wall due to uniformly distributed subepithelial deposits containing multiple immunoglobulins, C1q, C3, and C4 revealed as electron-dense deposits by electron microscopy. In contrast to idiopathic membranous glomerulopathy, electron-dense deposits and immunoglobulins are also often found in the mesangium. There may be various degrees of interstitial and tubular lesions, and granular tubular basement membrane deposits of immunoglobulin may be pronounced. Tubuloreticular inclusions may be found in endothelial cells [166]. Nephrotic syndrome with well-preserved GFR is common in this category. Several variations exist in which other lesions, including mesangial proliferation, focal and segmental proliferation, or diffuse proliferation, are superimposed on membranous glomerulonephritis. These variants take on the prognostic and therapeutic connotations of the superimposed lesion.

Sclerosing Lupus Nephritis (WHO Class VI). This category is characterized by diffuse or focal sclerosis often superimposed on varying degrees of other proliferative lesions. Immunoglobulin deposits may be scanty, and electron-dense deposits may be confined to the mesangium and scattered in various sites in the peripheral capillary walls. This lesion appears to be a late stage in the evolution of the other lesions just described. It is often associated with a well-developed tubulointerstitial lesion and arteriolonephrosclerosis. Slowly progressive renal failure and hypertension are common in this category.

Necrotizing Lupus Nephritis and Thrombotic Microangiopathy. Necrotizing lupus nephritis and disseminated vasculitis is a rare lesion characterized by severe destructive and necrotizing alteration of the glomerular capillary loops associated with inflammation and fibrinoid necrosis of small vessels and arterioles [2]. Lesions resembling those of malignant hypertension or the hemolytic-uremic syndrome may also be found, as well as segmental renal infarction [164]. Severe hypertension, thrombopenia, hemolysis, and progressive renal failure are common in this category. Some patients will have circulating autoantibody to phospholipids (anticardiolipin, "lupus anticoagulant").

Interstitial Lupus Nephritis. Rarely, tubulointerstitial nephritis may be found with only mild glomerular disease [2, 165]. Extensive peritubular and tubular basement membrane immunoglobulin and electron-dense deposits are seen in interstitial lupusnephritis. Tubuloreticular inclusions resembling myxovirus may be seen in endothelial and tubule cells [166].

These lesions seldom exist as discrete entities among patients with SLE, and forms not readily classified into a particular group are sometimes observed. Transformations from one category to another are not infrequently observed [2, 167]. Mesangial or focal proliferative lupus nephritis may transform into diffuse proliferative lupus nephritis, particularly among patients with heavy proteinuria and/or more extensive subendothelial electron-dense deposits in peripheral glomerular capillaries. Diffuse proliferative lupus nephritis may regress under the influence of therapy. Membranous lupus nephritis may occasionally evolve into diffuse proliferative nephritis and vice versa. On the other hand, a given morphologic lesion may remain stable for years and show no tendency to evolve into other lesions. This seems to be particularly true for membranous lupus nephritis.

It has also been clearly shown that the various lesions described here may exist in the total absence of any clinical manifestations of renal disease (e.g., proteinuria, abnormal urinary sediment, decreased GFR). Notwithstanding these observations, there are some very reasonable correlations between clinical features and extent and severity of underlying renal lesions. For example, among patients with the combination of heavy proteinuria, active urinary sediment, and abnormal GFR, the majority will reveal diffuse proliferative lupus nephritis. Extrarenal signs of SLE correlate poorly or not at all with the nature and extent of renal disease. Florid fever, arthritis, thrombocytopenia, rash, or cerebritis may be present with minimal clinical or histologic evidence of renal disease.

Activity and Chronicity Indices

In addition to the WHO classification of lesions described, the renal lesions of SLE may be classified according to activity and chronicity [2, 168]. Such classifications may be useful in predicting prognosis and may be used as a guide to therapy, but this is not generally agreed on, partly due to poor reproducibility [169]. By assigning a numerical value to these parameters, a semiquantitative index of activity or chronicity can be developed. Table 15-7 outlines the parameters in the scoring systems as utilized by the group at the National Institutes of Health (NIH) [2, 169, 170]. High activity scores with low chronicity scores indicate a high degree of reversibility and a low likelihood of progression [170]. On the other hand, high chronicity scores with low activity scores imply poor reversibility and a high likelihood of progression to end-stage renal failure, at least among the group of patients studied at NIH. Other investigators have not been able to reproduce these findings [169].

The foregoing observations have suggested to some that *all* patients with SLE should undergo an initial renal biopsy for the purpose of staging the nature and extent of renal disease, in hopes of guiding therapy and estimating prognosis more accurately. Unfortunately, no study has as yet demonstrated that such an approach in fact contributes favorably to the survival of patients or decreases the subsequent morbidity in SLE. Obviously, renal biopsy is a static observation of a dynamic

Table 15-7. Lupus nephritis: Activity and chronicity indices

Activity	Chronicity[a]
Proliferation/hypercellularity	Sclerotic glomeruli
Leukocytic infiltration	Fibrous crescents
Necrosis/karyorrhexis[b]	Tubular atrophy
Cellular crescents[b]	Interstitial fibrosis
Hyaline deposits	
Interstitial mononuclear cell infiltration	

[a] Lesions are scored 0 to 3 +.
[b] Lesions are weighted by a factor of 2.
Source: Modified from H. A. Austin, III, L. R. Mueng, K. M. Joyce, et al., Prognostic factors in lupus nephritis: Contribution of renal histologic data. *Am. J. Med.* 75:382, 1983.

process. Serial studies of some more readily available noninvasive factor seem more likely to be valuable. Indeed some workers have concluded from retrospective analyses that renal biopsy in SLE provides generally redundant information and is not much more predictive of prognosis than simple clinical assessment [2, 171, 172]. Renal biopsy may provide evidence of the futility of hazardous treatment or confirm the clinical suspicion of a relatively benign lesion in patients who have manifestations such as proteinuria or abnormal urinary sediment. There is ample justification for performing renal biopsy if a patient has abnormal clinical findings, especially proteinuria, abnormal urinary sediment, or modest decrease in GFR. At the present time, renal biopsy in patients with SLE who have normal renal function, urinalysis, and blood pressure should be regarded as investigational.

Serologic Studies in Systemic Lupus Erythematosus

Much has been written about the value of serologic studies in SLE [2, 173]. Clearly, serologic tests, especially fluorescent antinuclear antibody (FANA) and anti-dsDNA antibodies, are of great value in making a clinical diagnosis; indeed, they have been incorporated into the revised American Rheumatism Association criteria for diagnostic classification of SLE [174]. However, the role of serologic tests in determining the nature and significance of renal lesions, in determining prognosis, and in monitoring the response to therapy is much less well established.

Antinuclear Factors. Approximately 10 percent of patients with SLE and clinically overt nephritis will have *negative* tests for antinuclear antibodies as performed by the FANA technique [175]. In general, the FANA titer shows a poor correlation with the severity of underlying glomerular disease, and monitoring the titer has no value in prognosis or therapy.

Antibodies to dsDNA and ssDNA. Anti-dsDNA antibody levels as determined by the Farr or *Crithidia lucillae* techniques show a rough but inconsistent correlation with the severity of the underlying glomerular disease [2, 176]. Some investigators have shown that the complement-fixing, precipitating antibodies to dsDNA are more likely to be associated with underlying diffuse proliferative lupus nephritis, whereas nonprecipitating, poorly complement-fixing antibodies to dsDNA will coincide with the presence of membranous lupus nephritis. IgM class anti-dsDNA antibody may be associated with milder disease. In individual patients, a rising titer of anti-dsDNA antibody may herald an exacerbation of renal or extrarenal disease, but a persistently high titer of anti-dsDNA antibody may remain even with relatively quiescent clinical disease. Treatment based on rising titers of anti-dsDNA may avoid clinical exacerbations [2]. Overall, only a weak correlation exists between the activity of renal disease and the titer of anti-dsDNA antibodies [2, 177]. Correlations with clinical activity can be improved by examining only complement-fixing, high-affinity anti-dsDNA antibody. Other antibodies to nuclear antigens may also be found in SLE. Anti-Sm antibody is highly specific for SLE but of low sensitivity. Antihistone antibodies are typically associated with drug-induced SLE (e.g., procainamide hydrochloride [Pronestyl] or hydralazine).

Complement Components. Since much of the autoantibody formed in SLE is of the IgG and IgM classes, activation of the *classic* complement cascade with consumption of the early-acting components C1q, C4, and C3 is often found in SLE [2, 178, 179]. Serum C4 and C3 levels are particularly depressed in active SLE, particularly in WHO class IV lupus nephritis. C4 levels fall earlier and to a greater extent than C3 levels in exacerbations of disease [180]. *Alternative* pathway activation of the complement cascade also occurs in SLE. Unfortunately, neither the depressed serum complement component levels nor the total hemolytic activity (CH_{50}) of serum has a good correlation with the presence or severity of glomerular disease [181]. Patients with membranous lupus nephritis most often have normal C3 levels. Among the complement components conveniently assayed, C3 levels are said to have the best correlation with activity of renal disease. Normal C3 and C4 levels with reduced CH_{50} may indicate a coexistent congenital C2, C1r, or C1s deficiency. Some investigators have found that therapy designed to normalize C3 and/or C4 complement values may be associated with an improved prognosis. Severe exacerbations of lupus nephritis may be heralded by a decline in C3 and/or C4 complement components (and a rise in anti-dsDNA antibody), and serial measurements of these proteins may be of value in planning stepwise alterations in the intensity of therapy [181, 182].

Circulating Immune Complexes. Circulating immune complexes are readily found in most patients with active SLE, irrespective of the nature of severity of renal disease [2, 181]. The relationship of these immune complexes to those found in the kidney is unknown. Such circulating immune complexes can be detected and quantified by any of a number of techniques; however, serial measurements have very limited usefulness in management or prognosis. They provide generally redundant information that can be ascertained by other means (complement assay, urinalysis, renal function).

Renal Function in Systemic Lupus Erythematosus Nephritis
Several caveats relating to the measurement of renal function and proteinuria in SLE nephritis are in order. Endogenous creatinine clearance greatly overestimates true GFR in lupus nephritis, and correspondingly serum creatinine values underestimate the severity of depression of renal function [183]. This is due to enhanced but variable tubular secretion of creatinine in lupus nephritis. This abnormality can be corrected by giving an oral dose of cimetidine prior to the measurement of endogenous creatinine clearance to block the tubular secretion of creatinine [184]. Alternatively, GFR can be measured isotopically using radiolabeled iothalamate. The abnormal proteinuria in lupus nephritis is due to an enhancement of the "shunt pathway" (see also Chap. 14), and this involves the excretion of large neutral globular proteins such as IgG. Thus, an unchanged total protein excretion may hide an improvement in the fraction of macromolecules passing through the "shunt pathway." Fractional excretion of IgG is a better measurement of the severity of glomerular disease than is total protein excretion [2, 185].

Treatment of Lupus Nephritis
The treatment of lupus nephritis continues to be surrounded by controversy [2, 155, 186, 187]. Several factors need to be considered: (1) What is the long-term prognosis

of the lesion if *only* the extrarenal manifestations of the disease are symptomatically controlled? (2) What is the extent of reversibility of the lesion? (3) What are the expected side effects of therapy? (4) What parameters are most useful in guiding the response to therapy? (5) Is a renal biopsy needed to assess the type of lesion and its activity and chronicity?

In reaching a decision regarding treatment, one must assess the *risk-benefit ratio* and have the means to determine the effectiveness of treatment and the specific side effect profile of the agents to be used. All patients should regularly undergo a careful examination of urinary sediment and a quantitative measure of protein excretion. Serial measurement of the serologic factors just mentioned may be useful (especially anti-dsDNA antibody, C3, and C4). Careful measurement of renal function, using endogenous creatinine clearance after cimetidine or isotopic methods, and evaluation of fractional IgG excretion may also be of help. Some studies suggest that renal biopsy also contributes significantly to the assessment of prognosis and likelihood of a beneficial response to aggressive therapy with combinations of prednisone and an immunosuppressive agent. Renal biopsies with active inflammatory lesions and mild to moderate lesions of chronicity are associated with a more favorable long-term response to therapy, whereas renal biopsies revealing advanced lesions of chronicity are associated with a poor prognosis regardless of treatment regimens. The following represent tentative recommendations concerning therapy.

Minimal Change and Mesangial Proliferative Lupus Nephritis. Treatment should be primarily directed at the extrarenal manifestations of the disease in minimal change, mesangial proliferative, and some cases of focal proliferative lupus nephritis [2]. The minimum steroid dosage required to maintain the patient relatively symptom free should be employed. If nonsteroidal anti-inflammatory agents are effective, they should be used instead of steroids. One should be aware, however, that these agents may cause a decrease in GFR. Antimalarial agents, such as hydroxychloroquine sulfate (Plaquenil), may be useful, especially for patients with severe skin disease or persistent joint complaints. Serial studies of antibody to dsDNA, C3, and/or C4 concentrations should be undertaken and renal function followed at least at monthly intervals. Persistently low C3 and/or C4 levels, accompanied by rising or persistently elevated antibody to dsDNA, in the absence of active extrarenal disease, should be watched with great care, and any sudden change in serum creatinine or renal function, urinary sediment, or proteinuria may be an indication for renal biopsy or a change in treatment. With such an approach, the 10-year survival from the time of initial observation should be in excess of 85 percent, provided the lesions have not transformed into those of a more severe nature and that life-threatening extrarenal disease (particularly cerebritis) does not supervene.

Focal and Diffuse Proliferative Lupus Nephritis. In the presence of very active extrarenal disease or in the face of rapidly deteriorating renal function or new-onset nephrotic syndrome, large dosages of parenteral glucocorticoids, such as 10 to 30 mg/kg kilogram (maximum single dose, 1000 mg) of methylprednisolone for three to five doses daily, followed by 60 mg of oral prednisone daily for 1 month, followed by gradual tapering of dosage, have been quite effective in some patients [2, 188, 189].

In patients with non–life-threatening extrarenal disease and normal or near-normal renal function with or without the nephrotic syndrome, and in the absence of well-established chronic glomerular or tubulointerstitial lesions (e.g., glomerulosclerosis, tubular atrophy, interstitial fibrosis), therapy could be initiated with oral prednisone (1 mg/kg/day) for 4 to 8 weeks. The addition of an immunosuppressive cytotoxic or cytostatic agent to a regimen of oral prednisone should probably be considered in most patients with diffuse proliferative or severe focal proliferative lupus nephritis, particularly when nephrotic syndrome, progressive renal functional impairment, or a very active urinary sediment is present.

The choice of immunosuppressive agent is not easily established because of the paucity of well-controlled prospective randomized trials. In relatively mild cases, the addition of azathioprine (2 mg/kg/day) may exert a steroid-sparing effect and allow safe tapering of oral corticosteroids to a more acceptable maintenance level of 0.1 to 0.2 mg/kg/day without great risk of exacerbation. In more severe cases, particularly those with nephrotic syndrome, impaired renal function, serologic parameters indicative of systemic activity, and renal biopsy demonstration of a high activity index and a low to moderate chronicity index, it is probably wiser to add oral cyclophosphamide (2 mg/kg/day), a more potent immunosuppressive agent than azathioprine. The choice between continuous daily oral cyclophosphamide and monthly intravenous pulses of cyclophosphamide (0.5–1.0 g/m^2 body surface area) is not easily established [190, 192]. Both are probably equally effective over the short term in controlling the activity of disease and preventing flare-up of disease when corticosteroids are tapered. However, intravenous cyclophosphamide may be safer and associated with fewer side effects (e.g., hemorrhagic cystitis or infection). Both routes of administration may produce profound leukopenia, and careful monitoring of hematologic indices is required during treatment. Both probably share some tendencies toward increased oncogenicity, although the data currently available would suggest that intravenous cyclophosphamide is less oncogenic. Intravenous pulses of cyclophosphamide, when given monthly, must be adjusted to ensure that a modest leukopenia (3500–4000 leukocytes/mm) is produced 7 to 10 days after the infusion [190–192]. Each infusion must be accompanied by adequate oral and/or intravenous hydration, and because nausea is an important complication, the infusion is generally accompanied by infusion of antiemetics. When impaired renal function is present, reduced dosage is indicated. Repeated intravenous courses of cyclophosphamide may be given at monthly intervals for up to 6 months and then every 3 months for up to several years [192]. Oral cyclophosphamide should be given as a single morning dose with adequate hydration. Repeated pulses of intravenous methylprednisolone (500–1000 mg repeated daily for three doses) may be given for acute exacerbations [193]. If a remission of extrarenal and renal manifestations is induced, the patient can often be placed on a long-term maintenance schedule of low-dose, intermittent or daily oral corticosteroids combined with modest doses of azathioprine. Oral cyclophosphamide should probably not be given for periods in excess of 12 months. Intermittent intravenous cyclophosphamide may be administered for longer periods; however, very few data are available regarding the long-term effectiveness of this approach. Severe relapses may occur following rapid discontinuance of cytotoxic drugs. Cyclosporine could be used for therapy-resistant patients [194].

Alkylating agents should be used with great caution in azotemic and elderly patients. These drugs may potentially increase the risk of subsequent neoplastic transformation, especially lymphatic leukemia. The risk of enhancing opportunistic infection, aggravating latent infectious disease (e.g., tuberculosis), and serious bone marrow depression must be taken into account as a real hazard of combined steroid-cytotoxic therapy. Permanent sterility is a risk of prolonged cyclophosphamide therapy.

In patients presenting with potentially reversible lesions, without advanced renal failure and with non–life-threatening extrarenal disease, the 10-year survival (with renal function) should be approximately 70 to 85 percent. When advanced glomerulosclerosis, tubular atrophy, or interstitial fibrosis is present, or crescentic disease has developed (particularly in association with vasculitis and severe hypertension), the mortality is much higher and the response to therapy much lower.

Membranous Lupus Nephritis. In the face of normal renal function and easily controlled manifestations of nephrotic syndrome, treatment with steroids in an amount necessary to control extrarenal disease would seem appropriate on the basis of available date. However, if renal function is declining, or if the severity of the nephrotic syndrome per se is life-threatening, regimens similar to that described for idiopathic membranous glomerulonephritis involving combinations of methylprednisolone, prednisone, and chlorambucil or cyclophosphamide could be used, keeping in mind that the benefit of such an approach has not been proved in a suitably controlled study [195]. Cyclosporine, in dosages of 4 to 5 mg/kg/day combined with low-dose glucocorticoids, may also be beneficial [196]. If renal function is rapidly deteriorating, the patient should undergo rebiopsy to detect conversion to diffuse proliferative nephritis or the development of concomitant interstitial nephritis or crescentic glomerulonephritis. In the absence of developing crescentic disease or serious extrarenal disease such as cerebritis, 10-year survival from the time of diagnosis may be as high as 80 to 90 percent.

Chronic Progressive Renal Failure in SLE. Patients with advanced chronic renal disease (e.g., serum creatinine >4 mg/dl) should not be treated aggressively unless extrarenal disease mandates it. Such patients seem to undergo clinical remission of systemic symptoms as the azotemia progresses, do well with chronic dialysis, and are excellent candidates for renal transplantation [197, 198]. It has been demonstrated that SLE seldom recurs in the renal allograft [197].

Mixed Connective Tissue Disease

Mixed connective tissue disease consists of a mixture of features of scleroderma, polymyositis, and SLE in association with a pronounced autoantibody response to a saline-extractable nuclear RNP antigen [199]. The serum complement component concentrations are typically normal. Patients may present with Raynaud's phenomenon, sclerodactyly, dysphagia, myalgia, weakness, and arthritis. Renal disease is found in about 25 percent or less of cases, chiefly manifested as proteinuria. The underlying renal lesions are usually membranous glomerulonephritis or MPGN. Renal disease is seldom progressive, cerebral involvement rare, and the response to corticosteroid treatment generally favorable [2, 199].

Rheumatoid Arthritis

Renal involvement in rheumatoid arthritis is relatively uncommon [2, 200]. Renal disease is most often a complication of therapy (organic gold or penicillamine) or a manifestation of the development of secondary amyloidosis; however, bona fide cases of glomerular disease in the absence of therapy or complicating amyloidosis have been described. Membranous glomerulonephritis is the most common lesion observed; however, mesangial proliferative and focal proliferative glomerulonephritis may also be observed [201]. Occasional patients with severe and long-standing rheumatoid arthritis develop a disseminated form of vasculitis with fever, necrotizing skin lesions, neuritis, hypertension, circulating immune complexes, and hypocomplementemia [202]. Renal findings in such "malignant rheumatoid disease" with vasculitis include a necrotizing arteriolitis similar to that seen in malignant hypertension.

Henoch-Schönlein Purpura
(Anaphylactoid Purpura)

Henoch-Schönlein purpura is characterized by a nonthrombocytopenic vascular (palpable) purpura, abdominal pain, arthralgias, and renal disease [2, 203]. It is chiefly seen in the pediatric age group, usually between the ages of 2 and 8 years, but is by no means rare in young and older adults. Males are affected more often than females. The syndrome often follows 1 to 3 weeks after a nonspecific upper respiratory infection or drug exposure. No specific etiologic agent has ever been clearly identified. The characteristic cutaneous feature is a symmetric, nonpruritic macular rash beginning over the lower legs and buttocks and gradually progressing to frank palpable purpura. Skin biopsies reveal leukocytoclastic vasculitis of the postcapillary venules [204]. Abdominal pain may be severe, colicky in nature, and mimic an acute "surgical" abdomen. Gastrointestinal bleeding may be present. Joint pain and swelling are most often mild and limited to the knees and ankles. Joint deformities do not occur.

Renal involvement is very common, perhaps universal, as in SLE [2, 203]. A variety of clinical features of renal disease may be present; however, they may be quite evanescent and therefore easily overlooked. Recurrent microscopic or macroscopic hematuria with or without proteinuria is very common. The acute nephritic syndrome and even RPGN may develop. Nephrotic syndrome is relatively uncommon and, if present, is often associated with azotemia [2, 205]. Serum complement component levels are typically normal, although in exceptional cases a slight reduction in C3 may be found. Serum IgA levels are elevated in about 50 percent of cases. Cryoglobulins and circulating immune complexes containing IgA and/or IgG have been found in most cases. IgA rheumatoid factor may be present. IgA fibronectin levels are elevated, and IgA ANCA may be present. The frequency of HLA-Bw35 is increased in some, but not all series. This antistreptolysin O titer may be increased.

Skin biopsies of unaffected or affected skin reveal dermal capillary deposits of IgA, IgG, C3, and fibrin-reactive antigens (FRA) but not C4 or IgA secretory piece. Renal biopsies reveal a spectrum of lesions, but focal and segmental proliferative glomerulonephritis and diffuse proliferative glomerulonephritis with or without crescents may be seen in patients with more severe proteinuria or abnormal GFR [2, 203]. Extensive crescent formation is seen among those with RPGN. Characteristically, immunofluorescence studies reveal IgA and, to a lesser extent, IgG deposits in a diffuse, granular mesangial pattern accompanied by C3, J-chain, and FRA but not C1q, C4, or IgA secretory piece. The IgA deposits are typically polymeric IgA1. The observations are similar, if not identical, to those found in the cutaneous capillaries of the skin and suggest local activation of the alternative pathway of complement by deposition of circulating IgA-containing immune complexes. Electron microscopy reveals electron-dense deposits in the mesangium, occasionally accompanied by fibrin polymers. Based on these findings, the disorder is believed to be a systemic form of IgA nephropathy.

The prognosis is quite variable, although in general favorable [2, 204, 206]. Young children presenting with features of hematuria with or without proteinuria and only transient azotemia can be expected to recover fully [207]. A few such patients may go on to develop chronic renal disease 2 to 5 years later. Adult patients seem to develop more fulminant disease and have a worse prognosis. Patients with persistent azotemia and heavy proteinuria and in whom renal biopsies demonstrate diffuse proliferation, with or without crescents, may be more likely to develop chronic renal disease.

No effective form of treatment is as yet available. Patients with severe crescentic glomerulonephritis have been treated in a fashion similar to that described in idiopathic crescentic glomerulonephrits, with some success. Corticosteroids are said to be useful in controlling some of the severe extrarenal features (such as abdominal pain or recurrent rash), but this has not been proved in a suitable controlled study.

Systemic Necrotizing Angiitis (Polyangiitis)

Polyangiitis encompasses a very heterogeneous group of diseases having in common widespread inflammatory lesions of blood vessels including arteries, arterioles, capillaries, venules, and vein [2, 208]. SLE, Henoch-Schönlein purpura, rheumatoid vasculitis, Takayasu's arteritis, temporal arteritis, and localized cutaneous vasculitis are included in this category but will not be discussed further here.

Microscopic Polyangiitis (Hypersensitivity Angiitis)

Microscopic polyangiitis is characterized pathologically by the predominant involvement of small vessels (<100 μm diameter), frequently including those of the skin, viscera, lung, and kidney [209]. It is often associated with drug exposure of various types and tends to be associated with prominent clinical manifestations of visceral involvement, particularly the lung and kidney. Fever, arthralgia, neuropathy, and skin rash (palpable purpura) may be found. Eosinophilia may be particularly striking among patients with pulmonary involvement. A high percentage (>80%) of patients can be demonstrated to have circulating ANCAs, chiefly, but not exclusively, directed to myeloperoxidase [2, 210, 211]. When the kidney is the sole organ involved, the patients are regarded as having pauci-immune necrotizing and crescentic glomerulonephritis [2, 212]. Serum complement component levels are variable but are often increased. The erythrocyte sedimentation rate is greatly increased (often > 100 mm/hr). Renal involvement may be mild or severe and is frequently progressive. Necrotizing and crescentic glomerulonephritis may produce a clinical picture of RPGN (see Crescentic Glomerulonephritis). Immunofluorescence findings reveal scanty granular deposits of IgG or IgM in vessels or glomerular capillaries.

Untreated, the disease has a grave prognosis [213]. High-dose parenteral corticosteroids seem to be effective, and the addition of cyclophosphamide in all probability improves the prognosis further [2]. Intensive plasma exchange plus cytotoxic drugs and glucocorticoids may be beneficial for those with a rapidly evolving form of renal failure. The overall effectiveness of such an aggressive approach to therapy has not yet been proved by a randomized trial.

Macroscopic Polyangiitis (Polyarteritis Nodosa)

Macroscopic polyangiitis is characterized by a tendency for greater involvement of larger vessels (>100 μm diameter) and a lesser tendency for pulmonary involvement [2, 208]. It is frequently accompanied by hypertension, peripheral neuropathy, and features indicating ischemic infarction of various visceral organs (spleen, gallbladder, appendix, and kidney) [2, 214]. It may be associated with drug abuse or chronic hepatitis B infection. Angiograms of various visceral organs (including the kidney) may reveal aneurysms of the vessels due to inflammatory destruction of the elastic lamina [2, 215]. Circulating ANCAs are sometimes (10–30%) found. This form of polyangiitis is associated with slowly progressive renal failure, often accompanied by severe hypertension. Rapidly progressive renal failure is uncommon. Treatment with steroids and cytotoxic agents may be less effective than that described for microscopic polyangiitis.

Wegener's Granulomatosis

Wegener's granulomatosis is characterized by necrotizing and granulomatous vasculitis in the upper and lower respiratory tract associated with visceral involvement, most often the kidney [2, 216]. Limited forms sparing the kidney have been described. Affected patients, like others in the polyangiitis category, have normal complement component levels. Over 90 percent of patients can be shown to have circulating ANCAs principally directed to a neutral proteinase (proteinase 3) [2, 217]. The level of autoantibody falls quickly with therapy and often rises in advance of a relapse. Focal and segmental proliferative and necrotizing glomerulonephritis associated with hematuria and mild proteinuria is an early feature, but in the absence of treatment it will progress to fulminant renal disease including crescentic glomerulonephritis with rapidly progressive renal failure. Immunofluorescence studies reveal scanty immunoglobulin deposits in a granular pattern.

The overall prognosis is ominous if untreated, but the early administration of alkylating agents, especially cyclophosphamide with corticosteroids, has been dramatically effective for both renal and pulmonary manifestations [2, 216]. Many patients undergoing such treatment have entered into long-term remissions even following discontinuance of therapy. Intensive plasma exchange with cytotoxic drugs and steroids has also been effective in cases when extensive crescentic glomerulonephritis has developed and produced advanced renal failure.

Goodpasture's Disease

Goodpasture's disease, an uncommon disorder, consists of a triad of findings: (1) glomerular disease, (2) pulmonary hemorrhage, and (3) anti-GBM antibody production [2, 218]. Glomerular disease may be mild, consisting only of the immunopathologic finding of linear deposition of IgG (or rarely IgA) along the basement membrane without any light-microscopic changes. Most commonly, however, the lesions are evident and consist of diffuse and extensive extracapillary (crescentic) glomerulonephritis with or without glomerular capillary necrosis. Hematuria, red cell casts, proteinuria, and occasionally the nephrotic syndrome may be the presenting features clinically. Rapid deterioration of renal function is seen among the group with extensive crescentic disease.

The pulmonary aspects of the disease consist of covert or overt hemoptysis [2, 208]. Such intrapulmonary bleeding may lead ultimately to an iron-deficiency anemia out of proportion to renal disease. The hemosiderin sequestered in pulmonary macrophages may appear in the sputum. Fluffy perihilar alveolar densities are found on chest x-ray, and arterial oxygen tension may be diminished during severe episodes of intrapulmonary bleeding. The pulmonary uptake of carbon monoxide increases during bouts of hemoptypsis. Pulmonary bleeding may recur in distinct episodes, and fatal bouts may develop in the absence of clinical manifestations of renal disease. Cigarette smoking or inhalation of volatile hydrocarbons or other pulmonary irritants may also evoke bouts of pulmonary hemorrhage. Lung biopsies reveal intraalveolar hemorrhage without vasculitis. Linear IgG (or rarely IgA) deposits are inconsistently found on the alveolar capillary basement membrane. It must be emphasized that pulmonary hemorrhage with evidence of renal disease may also occur in SLE, Henoch-Schönlein purpura, disseminated polyangiitis, cryoglobulinemia, thrombotic thrombocytopenic purpura, pulmonary edema associated with coagulation disturbances in advanced uremia, pulmonary embolism with renal vein thrombosis, and Legionnaire's disease. Thus, the coexistence of pulmonary hemorrhage and renal disease does not always indicate Goodpasture's disease.

The third and essential element of the triad of Goodpasture's disease is the production of anti-GBM antibody. This aspect may be documented by observing linear IgG (or rarely IgA) deposits along the glomerular capillary or alveolar capillary basement membrane in association with crescentic glomerulonephritis and/or pulmonary hemorrhage [2, 218]. It may also be conveniently defined by the detection of circulating anti-GBM antibody using indirect immunofluorescence or radioimmunoassay techniques [2, 219]. Linear deposits of IgG are accompanied by C3 deposits in about two-thirds of instances. Several patients have been described in which anti-GBM antibody and ANCA coexist. Rarely, IgM ANCA may be associated with severe pulmonary hemorrhage, mimicking Goodpasture's syndrome.

This disorder most commonly affects young males, but individuals of nearly any age, except very young children, have been described with the disease [2]. The onset may be abrupt or insidious. Hypertension is usually absent, and serum complement components are normal. Antistreptolysin O titer is normal, and antinuclear antibodies are absent. Fever and skin rash are usually not found. A flulike illness and/or exposure to hydrocarbon fumes may antedate the onset of the illness. The frequency of HLA-DR2 is greatly increased. Cigarette smoking greatly increases the risk of pulmonary hemorrhage [2, 220].

The prognosis depends on the severity of pulmonary and renal involvement and the stage of renal disease present when the patient is first seen. Severe episodes of pulmonary hemorrhage will often respond to high doses of parenteral corticosteroids but may recur in association with a reduction in dose or the development of intercurrent bacterial infection. Intensive plasma exchange, used in conjunction with cytotoxic agents and oral steroids, is also dramatically effective in terminating life-threatening episodes of pulmonary hemorrhage and is associated with rapid lowering of serum level of anti-GBM antibody. Extensive crescentic glomerulonephritis, when associated with oliguric renal failure, responds poorly to any form of therapy, but current evidence strongly suggests that if therapy is initiated at *early* stages of the disease before oliguria develops, significant improvement in renal function can be expected to occur [2, 218, 221, 222]. At present, intensive plasma exchange associated with cytotoxic drugs and corticosteroids appears to be the most effective form of therapy, especially if initiated *before* serum creatinine has risen above 6 mg/dl. Anti-GBM antibody–mediated glomerulonephritis may recur in the transplanted kidney. There is no contraindication to undertaking renal transplantation so long as the patient does not have detectable levels of circulating anti-GBM antibody [223].

Glomerulonephritis in Renal Allografts and Isografts

The development of glomerular lesions in renal transplants can be explained by several processes: recurrence of the original disease (recurrent glomerulonephritis), de novo glomerulonephritis unrelated to the process of rejection, and glomerular alterations consequent to chronic rejection [2, 224–226]. Recurrent glomerulonephritis can *only* be defined if one knows the characteristics of the original disease, which may be difficult to ascertain in advanced disease. Table 15-8 summarizes the glomerular diseases that have been documented to recur in the grafted kidney [224, 225]. Some of these recur as a morphologic lesion with few clinical manifestations (e.g., type II MPGN, or dense deposit disease), while others recur in a fulminant fashion, sometimes destroying renal function in the graft (e.g., crescentic glomerulo-

Table 15-8. Causes of recurrent glomerulonephritis in the transplanted kidney

Disorder	Relative risk of morphologic* recurrence	Relative risk of clinical recurrence
Focal glomerular sclerosis	30–40%, higher in patients with "malignant" course	30–40%, higher in patients with "malignant" course
Membranous glomerulopathy	Uncommon	Uncommon
MPGN, type I	Low	Low
MPGN, type II (dense deposit disease)	Nearly universal	Common
SLE	Very rare	Very rare
Goodpasture's disease	20–30%	Uncommon
Polyangiitis	Unknown	Unknown
Henoch-Schönlein purpura	Low (?)	Low
IgA nephropathy	50%	Rare
Diabetes mellitus	High	Low (?)
Alport's syndrome	None	None
Amyloidosis	Low	Low
Fibrillary/immunotactoid glomerulonephritis	Moderate	Moderate

MPGN = membranoproliferative glomerulonephritis; SLE = systemic lupus erythematosus.
* Lesion detectable by light, immunofluorescence, or electron microscopy.

nephritis). Some diseases paradoxically have a low prevalence of recurrent disease (e.g., SLE). The clinical features of recurrent glomerulonephritis are similar to those of the original disease, although the prognosis may differ because of the superimposition of immunosuppressive therapy for prevention of rejection. It is noteworthy that recurrent glomerulonephritis is quite common among identical twin transplant recipients. Such patients have customarily not received prophylactic immunosuppressive therapy. De novo glomerular disease related to infection (e.g., endocarditis) may also occur in renal transplants. For unknown reasons, the presence of vesicoureteric reflux seems to predispose to the development of MPGN in the graft, independent of original disease. Membranous glomerulopathy is the most common de novo glomerulopathy developing in allografts [224, 225].

Chronic allograft rejection may lead to ischemic alterations of glomeruli or on occasion to a picture resembling membranous or MPGN. A transplant glomerulopathy consisting of thickening of the capillary wall with relatively electron-lucent subendothelial deposits has been described [226]. This may be the consequence of repeated episodes of rejection-related, intraglomerular coagulation, since FRA deposits are commonly found in the glomerular capillary. There is no known therapy for the transplant rejection-related glomerulopathy, although long-term anticoagulants and antithrombotic agents have been suggested. Nephrotic syndrome is a common manifestation of this progressive lesion.

Glomerulopathies Associated with Heredofamilial, Biochemical, and Metabolic Diseases

Diabetic Nephropathy

After 15 years or more of insulin-dependent diabetes mellitus, over 50 percent of patients show some degree of renal involvement [2, 227]. For poorly understood reasons, 40 to 50 percent of patients *never* develop renal involvement. A similar fraction of patients with non–insulin-dependent diabetes mellitus also develop glomerular lesions. The most common glomerular lesion seen in patients with renal involvement in diabetes is diffuse glomerulosclerosis with thickening of the basement membrane and an increase in the mesangial matrix. Nodular diabetic glomerulosclerosis is very specific for this disease (Fig. 15-7) but is seen in association with the diffuse lesion in only about 10 to 20 percent of patients with diabetic renal disease [2, 228]. The pathogenesis of the diabetic glomerular lesion is unknown. Some believe it is related to a hemodynamic disturbance associated with the abnormal endocrine environment. Increased GFR and renal plasma flow regularly precede the development of albuminuria, and excessive nephron filtration (hyperfiltration) or capillary hypertension may be injurious to the capillary wall or mesangium [229]. Others have suggested that the disease is related to nonenzymatic glycosylation of

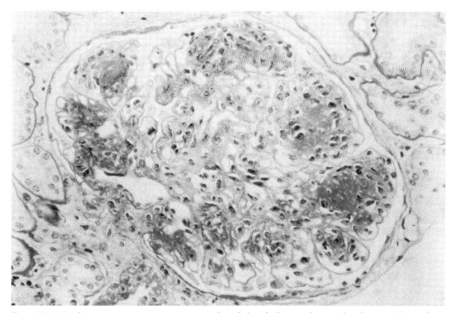

Fig. 15-7. Light-microscopic appearance of nodular diabetic glomerulosclerosis. Note the relatively acellular intercapillary nodule and diffuse increase in mesangial matrix. (Courtesy of Dr. Arthur H. Cohen.)

glomerular proteins with resultant dysfunction of the capillary wall or hyperglycemia-initiated production of cytokines and/or growth factors which promote extracellular matrix accumulation [2].

The principal clinical manifestations of diabetic glomerular disease are initially abnormal proteinuria and later reduced GFR. The first outward manifestation of incipient diabetic nephropathy is an increased excretion rate of albumin (>15 μg/min), often referred to as microalbuminuria [2, 227]. Such microalbuminuria seldom appears before 5 years' duration of insulin-dependent diabetes mellitus, but once established, the rate of albumin excretion slowly rises such that overt proteinuria (>200 μg/min of albumin excretion or >500 mg of total protein excretion/24 hr) is detectable by usual semiquantitative means over the next 5 to 7 years [2, 227, 230]. Nephrotic-range proteinuria commonly supervenes, particularly as azotemia develops. The nephrotic syndrome of diabetic glomerulosclerosis is frequently associated with hypertension. End-stage renal disease with a need for dialysis or transplantation appears within 3 to 5 years of the onset of azotemia in the absence of specific treatment. Papillary necrosis and pyelonephritis, congestive heart failure, and adverse reaction to x-ray contrast media may also complicate a relatively stable course of diabetic nephropathy and may often lead to rapid clinical and renal functional deterioration. In the typical case, diabetic glomerular disease is associated with other signs of diabetic microvascular disease, such as neuropathy and retinopathy. In exceptional cases, however, diabetic glomerular sclerosis, either diffuse or nodular, may arise in patients totally lacking clinical evidence of microvascular disease, even by careful fluorescein retinography. Very rarely, typical diabetic glomerulosclerosis appears in the total absence of carbohydrate intolerance [2, 231].

The development of nephrotic syndrome has been described in children as early as 1 month after the discovery of diabetes mellitus and the initiation of treatment with insulin. In these cases, the nephrotic syndrome responded to corticosteroid therapy and had the morphologic characteristics of minimal change disease. The cause of the early appearance of nephrotic syndrome and its relationship to the diabetic state in those cases are not clear.

Most, if not all patients with diabetic nephropathy reveal a linear pattern of deposition of albumin and IgG along the GBM without concomitant complement deposition or associated circulating anti-GBM antibody. Such a pattern of protein deposition is thought to be the consequence of an alteration in basement membrane biochemistry and not the result of any specific immune reaction.

A similar sequence of events is believed to occur in non–insulin-dependent diabetes mellitus, although precise data are difficult to obtain because of the uncertainty regarding the onset of the diabetic state [2, 227]. Unlike insulin-dependent diabetes mellitus, glomerular hyperfiltration is less common, and microalbuminuria may be observed even in the absence of progressive renal disease. Nevertheless, abnormal excretion rates of albumin in patients with non–insulin-dependent diabetes mellitus are often associated with hypertension and vascular disease in several organs, including the coronary vessels.

While much is unknown regarding the pathogenesis of diabetic nephropathy, the risk of development of this lesion is in part related to the magnitude of hyperglycemia and in part to the severity of raised arterial pressure. Early and vigorous metabolic control reduces the risk of diabetic nephropathy and, in the intensification of insulin therapy in patients with insulin-dependent diabetes mellitus, can reverse microalbuminuria [232]. However, once overt nephropathy manifested by persistent easily detectable proteinuria is present, or once GFR begins to progressively decline, tight glycemic control of diabetes mellitus is of little value in retarding the rate of further progression [2, 233, 234]. Modest elevations of mean arterial pressure commonly occur in concert with the onset of microalbuminuria. Vigorous antihypertensive management, particularly with ACE inhibitors, will reduce microalbuminuria and may eventually retard the rate of progression to overt nephropathy [234]. ACE inhibitor therapy of overt nephropathy when serum creatinine is between 1.5 and 2.5 mg/dl will definitely delay the onset of end-stage renal disease and slow the rate of decline in GFR [233]. Both dialysis and transplantation are satisfactory renal replacement therapies for advanced disease; however, with continued poor metabolic control, diabetic nephropathy may recur in the renal allograft [2, 226]. Simultaneous pancreas and kidney allografting may be the best form of therapy for this disorder. Unfortunately, the mortality of patients with diabetic nephropathy remains increased even with satisfactory control of renal failure due to concomitant coronary, peripheral, and cerebral vascular disease.

Alport's Syndrome

Alport's syndrome or hereditary nephritis with deafness is an autosomal dominant or X-linked disease associated with hematuria, proteinuria, or progressive renal failure [2, 235]. The gene responsible for some of its variants has been identified and is responsible for the synthesis of a portion of the $\alpha 5$ chain of type IV collagen [236, 237]. Progressive renal failure in Alport's syndrome may occur early or late in adult life [2]. Afflicted male subjects have a less favorable prognosis than do female subjects. Some variants have been described in which deafness is absent or mild. Some patients also have prominent eye findings such as anterior lenticonus. By light microscopy, the renal lesions are variable and include focal proliferative glomerulonephritis, focal and segmental glomerulosclerosis, and interstitial nephritis [238, 239]. Immunoglobulin and complement deposits are not present. Lipid-staining foam cells are present in the kidneys of approximately 25 to 50 percent of the patients but are not specific for the disease. A unique laminated and attenuated appearance of the GBM on ultrastructural analysis has been described, but the specificity of the lesion is disputed (Fig. 15-8). Some investigators have also demonstrated that the basement membrane of patients with Alport's syndrome fails to react with antibody to GBM obtained from patients with Goodpasture's disease, indicating a concomitant deficiency of the Goodpasture's epitope on the NC-1 domain of the $\alpha 3$ chain of type IV collagen [2, 240]. Amyloid P component is also absent from the basement membrane.

The most common clinical presentation is that of recurring bouts of macroscopic hematuria sometimes associated with low-grade proteinuria. Hypertension is not a prominent finding until advanced renal failure occurs. Nephrotic syndrome is rare. Serum complement component levels are normal. Megathrombocytopenia and esophageal leiomyomas may develop in some patients [2, 235]. While end-stage

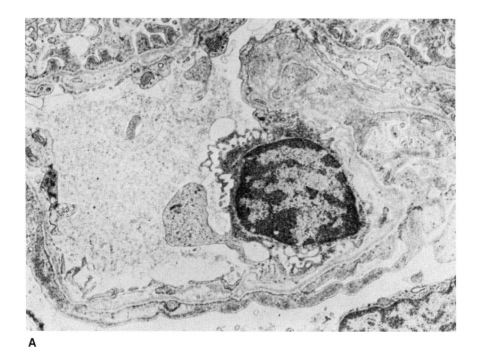

A

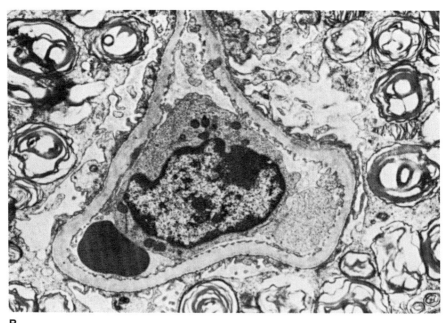

B

Fig. 15-8. (A) Electron-microscopic appearance of the lesion in Alport's syndrome. Note the thin, altered glomerular basement membrane. (B) Electron-microscopic appearance of the lesion in Fabry's disease. Note the whorled "myelin" figures in the epithelial cells. (Courtesy of Dr. Arthur H. Cohen.)

renal failure develops in most male patients between the ages of 20 and 40, female patients may show only persistent microscopic hematuria during the course of a normal life span. No form of therapy is effective in this disorder, and there are no reports of recurrence of the disease in patients who have received renal allografts. Rarely, an anti-GBM antibody–mediated form of crescentic glomerulonephritis may develop de novo in the renal allograft that contains the Goodpasture's antigen lacking in the recipient [226].

Fabry's Disease

Fabry's disease is an X-linked disorder of glycosphingolipid metabolism due to a deficiency of ceramide trihexosidase [2, 241]. Cutaneous angiokeratomas, chiefly about the scrotum, buttocks, and trunk, are characteristic. The accumulation of glycosphingolipids in glomerular epithelial cells results in a characteristic lesion consisting of foamy epithelial cell cytoplasm and shoaled myelin figures by electron microscopy (see Figure 15-8). Proteinuria, microscopic hematuria, and slowly progressive renal failure are the principal clinical manifestations. Other associated findings are acroparesthesias, anhidrosis, and premature coronary artery or cerebrovascular disease due to the infiltration of nerves and vessels with the abnormal lipids. There is no known effective treatment, although enzyme replacement (renal transplantation) may be feasible.

Nail-Patella Syndrome

Nail-patella syndrome is a rare disease with autosomal dominant inheritance, linked to the ABO system, which is characterized by onychodystrophy, absence of the patella, and iliac horns [2, 242, 243]. Characteristic lesions found on renal biopsy consist of intramembranous collagen fibers (type III) by electron microscopy. The principal renal manifestation is mild proteinuria and an occasional nephrotic syndrome progressing to renal failure. There is no known effective therapy.

Sickle Cell Disease

The autosomal recessive conditions of sickle cell disease (SS hemoglobin) and sickle cell trait (SA hemoglobin) may be complicated by a variety of renal abnormalities [2, 244, 245]. Papillary sclerosis and/or necrosis with nephrogenic diabetes insipidus and an incomplete form of renal tubular acidosis are not uncommon. Glomerular lesions are relatively rare and in some instances may be traced to an acquired chronic hepatitis B or C infection due to multiple transfusions. Occasionally, proteinuria, nephrotic syndrome, and progressive azotemia are found in the absence of infection or drug-related causes. The glomerular lesions are those of membranous glomerulonephritis or MPGN with granular IgG deposits. No form of effective therapy is known.

Familial and Congenital Nephrotic Syndrome

The term *familial nephrotic syndrome* is applied to cases in which several children in one family develop nephrotic syndrome [2, 242]. In some instances, the onset is within the first year of life, but the disorder is *not present at birth*. A variety of glomerular lesions have been found to underlie this syndrome. Those with minimal change lesions tend to be responsive to steroids, whereas those with structural glomerular lesions (e.g., focal sclerosis) tend to be steroid unresponsive.

Another form of familial nephrotic syndrome known as *congenital nephrotic syndrome* appears at birth and is associated with a large placenta, polycythemia, and increased alpha-fetoprotein in the amniotic fluid and maternal blood [2, 242, 246]. It is an autosomal recessive trait often found in families of Finnish extraction. The histologic lesion in the Finnish type of congenital nephrotic syndrome consists of microcystic disease of the proximal tubules within immature glomeruli. Immunoglobulin and complement deposits are absent. The principal clinical features of the congenital nephrotic syndrome include corticosteroid resistance, frequent infections, severe bone lesions, and a relentlessly fatal course. Some children can survive long enough to receive renal allografts.

Lecithin-Cholesterol Acyltransferase Deficiency

Lecithin-cholesterol acyltransferase deficiency is an autosomal recessive condition associated with deficiencies of the enzyme lecithin-cholesterol acyltransferase, which is responsible for cholesterol esterification [2, 247]. Affected patients have hematuria, proteinuria, progressive renal failure, increased triglyceride and variably elevated cholesterol levels, corneal opacities, and abnormal forms of high-density and low-density lipoprotein. Hyperuricemia may be observed. Ultrastructural features are quite distinctive, with large lucent zones in the mesangium and in the basement membrane, which contain rounded dense structures. No effective therapy is known; however, plasma or blood transfusions may transiently raise plasma enzyme levels. The disorder may recur in renal transplants.

References

1. Glassock R, Cohen A, Adler S: Primary Glomerular Diseases. In Brenner B (ed): *The Kidney* (5th ed). Philadelphia: Saunders, 1995, pp 1392–1497.
2. Adler S, Cohen A, Glassock R: Secondary Glomerular Diseases. In Brenner B (ed): *The Kidney* (5th ed). Philadelphia: Saunders, 1995, pp 1498–1596.
3. Wilson CB: The Renal Response to Immunologic Glomerular Injury. In Brenner B (ed): *The Kidney* (5th ed). Philadelphia: Saunders, 1995, pp 1253–1391.
4. Glassock R: General Concepts of Immunopathology. In Massry S, Glassock R (eds): *Textbook of Nephrology* (3rd ed). Baltimore, Williams & Wilkins, 1995, pp 623–626.
5. Hellmark T, Johansson C, Wieslander J: Characterization of anti-GBM antibodies involved in Goodpasture's syndrome. *Kidney Int* 46:823–829, 1994.
6. Kelly PT, Haponik EF: Goodpasture's syndrome: Molecular and clinical advances. *Medicine* (Baltimore) 73:171–185, 1994.
7. Couser WG, Salant DJ: In situ immune complex formation and glomerular injury. *Kidney Int* 17:1, 1980.
8. Border WA, Kamil ES, Ward HJ, Cohen AH: Antigenic charge as a determinant of immune complex localization in the rat glomerulus. *Lab Invest* 45:442, 1981.
9. Main IW, Nikolic-Paterson D, Atkins R: T cells and macrophages and their role in renal injury. *Semin Nephrol* 12:395–407, 1992.

10. Hebert L, Cosio F, Birmingham D: Role of complement system in renal injury. *Semin Nephrol* 12:408–427, 1992.
11. Sedor J: Cytokines and growth factors in renal injury. *Semin Nephrol* 12:428–440, 1995.
12. Lianos E: Eicosanoids in immune mediated renal injury. *Semin Nephrol* 12:428–440, 1995.
13. Glassock R: Hematuria and Pigmenturia. In Massry R, Glassock R (eds): *Textbook of Nephrology* (3rd ed). Baltimore, Williams & Wilkins, 1995, pp 557–566.
14. Glassock R: Proteinuria. In Massry R, Glassock R: *Textbook of Nephrology* (3rd ed). Baltimore, Williams & Wilkins, 1995, pp 600–614.
15. Feraille E, Vogt B, Stoerman C, Favre H: New Insights into the Pathogenesis of Nephrotic Edema. In Andreucci V, Fine L (eds): *Internat Yearbook of Nephrology, 1995*. Oxford, Oxford University Press, 1995, pp 16–26.
16. Perico N, Remuzzi G: Renal handling of sodium in the nephrotic syndrome. *Am J Nephrol* 13:413–414, 1993.
17. Nadasdy T, Silva I, Hogg R: Minimal Change Nephrotic Syndrome: Focal Sclerosis Complex (Including IgM Nephropathy and Diffuse Mesangial Cell Hypercellularity). In Tisher CC, Brenner BM (eds): *Renal Pathology* (2nd ed). Philadelphia, Lippincott, 1994, pp 330–389.
18. Savin VJ, Chonko AM, Sharma R, et al: Factor present in serum of patients with minimal change nephrotic syndrome or focal sclerosing glomerulopathy causes an immediate increase in glomerular protein permeability in vitro. *J Am Soc Nephrol* 1:567, 1990.
19. Carrie BJ, Salyer WR, Myers BD: Minimal-change nephropathy: An electrochemical disorder of the glomerular membrane. *Am J Med* 70:262, 1982.
20. Neuhaus T, Barratt M: Minimal Change Disease. In Massry S, Glassock R (eds): *Textbook of Nephrology* (3rd ed). Baltimore, Williams & Wilkins, 1995, pp 710–718.
21. Alfiler CA, Roy LP, Doran T, et al: HLA-DRw7 and steroid-responsive nephrotic syndrome of childhood. *Clin Nephrol* 14:71, 1980.
22. Noss G, Bachmann HJ, Olbing H: Association of minimal change nephrotic syndrome (MCNS) with HLA-B8 and B13. *Clin Nephrol* 15:172, 1981.
23. Korbet SM, Schwartz MM, Lewis EJ: Minimal-change glomerulopathy of adulthood. *Am J Nephrol* 8:29, 1988.
24. Arbeitsgemeinschaft fur Pediatrische Nephrologie: Effect of cytotoxic drugs on frequently relapsing nephrotic syndrome with and without steroid dependence. *N Engl J Med* 306:457, 1982.
25. Arbeitsgemeinschaft fur Pediatrische Nephrologie: Cyclophosphamide treatment of steroid-dependent nephrotic syndrome: Comparison of 8-week with 12-week course. *Arch Dis Child* 62:1101, 1987.
26. Meyrier A, Simon P: Treatment of corticoresistant idiopathic nephrotic syndrome in the adult: Minimal-change disease and focal and segmental glomerulosclerosis. *Adv Nephrol* 17:127, 1988.
27. Ponticelli C, Passerini P: Treatment of the nephrotic syndrome associated with primary glomerulonephritis. *Kidney Int* 46:595–604, 1994.
28. Cade R, Mars D, Privette M, et al: Effect of long-term azathioprine administration in adults with minimal-change glomerulonephritic and nephrotic syndrome resistant to corticosteroids. *Arch Intern Med* 146:737, 1986.
29. British Association for Pediatric Nephrology: Levamisole for corticosteroid-dependent nephrotic syndrome in childhood. *Lancet* 337:1555–1557, 1991.
30. Churg J, Bernstein J, Glassock R (eds): *Renal Disease: Classification and Atlas of Glomerular Disease* (2nd ed). New York, Ingaku-Shoin, 1995, pp 49–66.
31. Meyrier A: Focal Segmental Glomerulosclerosis. In Massry S, Glassock R (eds): *Textbook of Nephrology* (3rd ed). Baltimore, Williams & Wilkins, 1995, pp 719–725.
32. Detwiler RK, Falk RJ, Hogan SL, Jennette JC: Collapsing glomerulopathy: A clinically and pathologically distinct variant of focal segmental glomerulosclerosis. *Kidney Int* 45:1416–1424, 1994.
33. Pei Y, Cattran D, Delmore T, et al: Evidence suggesting undertreatment in adults with idiopathic focal segmental glomerulosclerosis. *Am J Med* 82:938, 1987.
34. Banfi G, Moriggi M, Sabadini E, et al: The impact of prolonged immunosuppression on the

outcome of idiopathic focal-segmental glomerulosclerosis with nephrotic syndrome in adults: A collaborative retrospective study. *Clin Nephrol* 36:53–59, 1991.

35. Korbet S, Schwartz M, Lewis E: Primary focal segmental glomerulosclerosis: Clinical course and response to therapy. *Am J Kidney Dis* 23:773–783, 1994.

36. Dantal J, Bigot E, Bogers W, et al: Effect of plasma protein adsorption on protein excretion in kidney-transplant recipient with recurrent nephrotic syndrome. *N Engl J Med* 330:7–14, 1994.

37. Bhaduri S, Low C, Sharma R, et al: The impact of plasmapheresis on recurrent focal glomerular sclerosis in renal allografts (abstract). *J Am Soc Nephrol* 6:1073, 1995.

38. Cohen A, Adler S: Mesangial Proliferative Glomerulonephritis. In Massry S, Glassock R (eds): *Textbook of Nephrology* (3rd ed). Baltimore, Williams & Wilkins, 1995, pp 739–741.

39. Cohen AH, Border WA, Glassock RJ: Nephrotic syndrome with glomerular mesangial IgM deposits. *Lab Invest* 38:610, 1978.

40. Rosen S, Tonroth T, Bernard D: Membranous Glomerulonephritis. In Tisher C, Brenner B (eds): *Renal Pathology* (2nd ed). Philadelphia, Lippincott, 1994, pp 258–293.

41. Short C, Mallick N: Membranous Glomerulopathy. Massry S, Glassock R (eds), *Textbook of Nephrology* (3rd ed). Baltimore, Williams & Wilkins, 1995, pp 726–733.

42. Couser WG, Schulze M, Pruchno CJ: Role of C_{5b-9} in experimental membranous nephropathy. *Nephrol Dial Transplant* 7:S-25–S-31, 1992.

43. Neale TJ, Ojha PP, Exner M, et al: Proteinuria in passive Heymann nephritis is associated with lipid peroxidation and formation of adducts on type IV collagen. *J Clin Invest* 94:1577–1584, 1994.

44. Cybulsky AV, Rennke HG, Feintzeig ID, Salant DJ: Complement-induced glomerular epithelial cell injury: Role of the membrane attack complex in rat membranous nephropathy. *J Clin Invest* 77:1096, 1986.

45. Donadio JV, Torres VE, Velosa J, et al: Idiopathic membranous nephropathy: The natural history of untreated patients. *Kidney Int* 33:708–716, 1988.

46. Schieppati A, Mosconi L, Perna A, et al: Prognosis of untreated patients with idiopathic membranous nephropathy. *N Engl J Med* 329:85–89, 1993.

47. Remuzzi G, Bertani T, Schieppati A: Idiopathic membranous nephropathy. *Lancet* 342:1277–1280, 1993.

48. Cameron JS: Membranous nephropathy and its treatment. *Nephrol Dial Transplant* 7:S-72–S-79, 1992.

49. Hogan S, Muller K, Jennette C, Falk R: A review of therapeutic studies in idiopathic membranous glomerulopathy. *Am J Kidney Dis* 25:862–875, 1995.

50. Ponticelli C, Zucchelli P, Passerini P, et al: A 10 year follow-up of a randomized study with methylprednisolone and chlorambucil in membranous nephropathy. *Kidney Int* 48:1600–1604, 1995.

51. West ML, Jindal KK, Bear RA, Goldstein MB: A controlled trial of cyclophosphamide in patients with membranous glomerulonephritis. *Kidney Int* 32:579, 1987.

52. Mathieson PW, Turner AN, Maidment CGH, et al: Prednisolone and chlorambucil treatment in idiopathic membranous nephropathy with deteriorating renal function. *Lancet* 2:869, 1988.

53. De Santo N, Capodicasa G, Giordano C: Treatment of idiopathic membranous nephropathy unresponsive to methylprednisolone and chlorambucil with cyclosporin. *Am J Nephrol* 7:742–749, 1987.

54. Williams PS, Bone JM: Immunosuppression can arrest renal failure due to idiopathic membranous glomerulonephritis. *Nephrol Dial Transplant* 4:181–186, 1989.

55. Palla R, Cirami C, Panichi V, et al: Intravenous immunoglobulin therapy of membranous nephropathy: Efficacy and safety. *Clin Nephrol* 35:98–104, 1991.

56. Glassock RJ: Secondary membranous glomerulonephritis. *Nephrol Dial Transplant* 7:S-64–S-71, 1992.

57. Sarasin FP, Schifferli JA: Prophylactic oral anticoagulation in nephrotic patients with idiopathic membranous nephropathy. *Kidney Int* 45:578–585, 1994.

58. Churg J, Bernstein J, Glassock R: *Renal Disease Classification and Atlas of Glomerular Disease* (2nd ed). New York, Igaku-Shoin, 1995, pp 133–135.

59. Jennette C, Falk R: Crescentic Glomerulonephritis. In Massry S, Glassock R (eds), *Textbook of Nephrology* (3rd ed). Baltimore, Williams & Wilkins, 1995, pp 742–745.
60. Couser WG: Idiopathic rapidly progressive glomerulonephritis. *Am J Nephrol* 2:57, 1982.
61. Falk RJ, Hogan S, Carey TS, Jennette JC, and the Glomerular Disease Collaborative Network: Clinical course of anti-neutrophil cytoplasmic autoantibody–associated glomerulonephritis and systemic vasculitis. *Ann Intern Med* 1131:656–663, 1990.
62. Bonsib SM, Goeken JA, Kemp JD, et al: Coexistent anti-neutrophil cytoplasmic antibody and antiglomerular basement membrane antibody associated disease: Report of six cases. *Mod Pathol* 6:526–530, 1993.
63. Angangco R, Thiru S, Esnault VLM, et al: Does truly "idiopathic" crescentic glomerulonephritis exist? *Nephrol Dial Transplant* 9:630–636, 1994.
64. Savage COS, Pusey CD, Bowman C, et al: Anti–glomerular basement membrane antibody–mediated disease in the British Isles 1980–1984. *Br Med J* 292:301, 1986.
65. Glassock RJ: Intensive plasma exchange in crescentic glomerulonephritis: Help or no help? *Am J Kidney Dis* 20:270–275, 1992.
66. Holley K, Donadio JV: Membranoproliferative Glomerulonephritis. In Tisher CC, Brenner BM (eds): *Renal Pathology* (2nd ed). Philadelphia, Lippincott, 1995, pp 294–329.
67. Barbiano di Belgiojoso G, Femario F: Membranoproliferative Glomerulonephritis. In Massry S, Glassock R (eds): *Textbook of Nephrology* (3rd ed). Baltimore, Williams & Wilkins, 1995, pp 734–738.
68. Knoll G, Rabin E, Burus B: Antiglomerular antibody induced nephritis with normal pulmonary and renal function. *Am J Nephrol* 13:494–496, 1993.
69. Cameron JS, Turner DR, Heaton J, et al: Idiopathic mesangiocapillary glomerulonephritis: Comparison of types I and II in children and adults and long-term prognosis. *Am J Med* 74: 175, 1983.
70. McEnery PT, McAdams AJ: Regression of membranoproliferative glomerulonephritis type II (dense deposit disease): Observation in six children. *Am J Kidney Dis* 12:138, 1988.
71. Faedda R, Satta A, Tanda F, et al: Immunosuppressive treatment of membranoproliferative glomerulonephritis. *Nephron* 67:59, 1994.
72. Donadio JV, Anderson CF, Mitchell JC, et al: Membranoproliferative glomerulonephritis: A prospective trial of platelet inhibitor therapy. *N Engl J Med* 310:1421, 1984.
73. Curtis JJ, Wyatt RJ, Bhathena D, et al: Renal transplantation for patients with type I and type II membranoproliferative glomerulonephritis: Serial complement and nephritic factor measurements and the problem of recurrence of disease. *Am J Med* 66:216, 1979.
74. Habib R, Niaudet P, Levy M: Schönlein-Henoch Purpura Nephritis and IgA Nephropathy. In Tisher CC, Brenner BM (eds): *Renal Pathology* (2nd ed). Philadelphia, Lippincott, 1994, pp 472–523.
75. Julian B, ven den Wall Bake AWL: IgA Nephropathy. In Massry S, Glassock R (eds): *Textbook of Nephrology* (3rd ed). Baltimore, Williams & Wilkins, 1995, pp 752–759.
76. D'Amico G: The commonest glomerulonephritis in the world: IgA nephropathy. *Q J Med* 64:709, 1987.
77. Emancipator S, Schena FP (eds): Immunoglobulin A nephropathy. *Semin Nephrol* 7:275, 1987.
78. van Es LA: Pathogenesis of IgA nephropathy. *Kidney Int* 41:1720–1729, 1992.
79. Baldree LA, Wyatt RJ, Julian BA, et al: Immunoglobulin A–fibronectin aggregate levels in children and adults with immunoglobulin A nephropathy. *Am J Kidney Dis* 22:1–4, 1993.
80. Sinico RA, Fornasieri A, Oreni N, et al: Polymeric IgA rheumatoid factor in idiopathic IgA mesangial nephropathy (Berger's disease). *J Immunol* 137:536, 1985.
81. Jones CL, Powell HR, Kincaid-Smith P, Robert DM: Polymeric IgA and immune complex concentrations in IgA-related renal disease. *Kidney Int* 38:323–331, 1990.
82. Savige JA, Gallicchio M: IgA antimyeloperoxidase antibodies associated with crescentic IgA glomerulonephritis. *Nephrol Dial Transplant* 7:952–955, 1992.
83. Costa RS, Droz D, Noel LH: Longstanding spontaneous clinical remission and glomerular involvement in primary IgA nephropathy (Berger's disease). *Am J Nephrol* 7:440, 1987.
84. D'Amico G: Influence of clinical and histological features on actuarial renal survival in adult

patients with idiopathic IgA nephropathy, membranous nephropathy, and membranoproliferative glomerulonephritis: Survey of the recent literature. *Am J Kidney Dis* 20:315–323, 1992.

85. Clarkson AR, Woodroffe AJ, Bannister KM, et al: Therapy in IgA nephropathy. *Contrib Nephrol* 104:189–197, 1993.

86. Clarkson AR, Woodroffe AJ: Therapeutic perspectives in mesangial IgA nephropathy. *Contrib Nephrol* 40:187, 1984.

87. Woo KT, Lee GSL, Lau YK, et al: Effects of triple therapy on the progression of mesangial proliferative glomerulonephritis. *Clin Nephrol* 27:56, 1987.

88. Donadio JV Jr, Bergstrand EJ, Offord KP, et al, for the Mayo Nephrology Collaborative Group: A controlled trial of fish oil in IgA nephropathy. *N Engl J Med* 331:1194–1199, 1994.

89. Julian BA, Barker C: Alternate-day prednisone therapy in IgA nephropathy. *Contrib Nephrol* 104:198–206, 1993.

90. Cattran DC, Greenwood C, Ritchie S: Long-term benefits of angiotensin-converting enzyme inhibitor therapy in patients with severe immunoglobulin A nephropathy: A comparison to patients receiving treatment with other antihypertensive agents and to patients receiving no therapy. *Am J Kidney Dis* 23:247–254, 1994.

91. Goumenos D, Ahuja M, Shortland J, Brown C: Can immunosuppressive drugs slow the progression of IgA nephropathy? *Nephrol Dial Transplant* 10:1173–1181, 1995.

92. Rostoker G, Desvaux-Belghiti D, Pilatte Y, et al: High-dose immunoglobulin therapy for severe IgA nephropathy and Henoch-Schonlein purpura. *Ann Intern Med* 120:476–484, 1994.

93. Ferri C, Puccini R, Longombardo G, et al: Low-antigen-content diet in the treatment of patients with IgA nephropathy. *Nephrol Dial Transplant* 8:1193–1198, 1993.

94. Kincaid-Smith P: Thin Basement Membrane Nephropathy. In Massry S, Glassock R (eds): *Textbook of Nephrology* (3rd ed). Baltimore, Williams & Wilkins, 1995, pp 760–764.

95. van Es LA: Pathogenesis of IgA nephropathy. *Kidney Int* 41:1720–1729, 1992.

96. Cosio FG, Falkenhain ME, Sedmak DD: Association of thin glomerular basement membrane with other glomerulopathies. *Kidney Int* 46:471–474, 1994.

97. Korbet SM, Schwartz M, Rosenberg B, et al: Immunotactoid glomerulopathy. *Medicine* (Baltimore) 64:228–243, 1995.

98. Iskander SS, Falk RJ, Jennette JC: Clinical and pathologic features of fibrillary glomerulonephritis. *Kidney Int* 42:1401–1407, 1992.

99. Fogo A, Qureshi N, Horn RG: Morphologic and clinical features of fibrillary glomerulonephritis versus immunotactoid glomerulopathy. *Am J Kidney Dis* 22:367–377, 1993.

100. Korbet SM, Schwartz MM, Lewis EJ: The fibrillary glomerulopathies. *Am J Kidney Dis* 23:751–765, 1994.

101. Saito T, Sato H, Kudo K, et al: Lipoprotein glomerulopathy: Glomerular lipoprotein thrombi in a patient with hyperlipoproteinuria. *Am J Kidney Dis* 13:148–153, 1989.

102. Ikeda K, Yokoyama H, Tomosugi N, et al: Primary glomerular fibrosis: A new nephropathy caused by diffuse intra-glomerular increase in atypical type III collagen fibers. *Clin Nephrol* 33:155–159, 1990.

103. Rodriguez-Iturbe B: Post-streptococcal Glomerulonephritis. In Massry S, Glassock R (eds): *Textbook of Nephrology* (3rd ed). Baltimore, Williams & Wilkins, 1995, pp 698–702.

104. Tejani A, Ingiulli A: Post-streptococcal glomerulonephritis: Current clinical and pathologic concepts. *Nephron* 55:1–5, 1990.

105. Hebert LA, Cosio FG, Neff JC: Diagnostic significance of hypocomplementemia. *Kidney Int* 39:811–821, 1991.

106. Fish AJ, Herdman RC, Michael AF, et al: Epidemic acute glomerulonephritis associated with type 49 streptococcal pyoderma: II. Correlative study of light, immunofluorescent and electron microscopic findings. *Am J Med* 48:28, 1970.

107. Sorger K, Gessler U, Hubner FK, et al: Subtypes of post-infectious glomerulonephritis: Synopsis of clinical and pathological features. *Clin Nephrol* 17:114, 1982.

108. Lang K, Treser G: Acute poststreptococcal glomerulonephritis: Mechanisms and sequelae—attempts at a unifying concept. *Clin Nephrol* 1:55, 1973.

109. Baldwin DS, Gluck MC, Schacht RG, Gallo G: The long-term prognosis of post-streptococcal glomerulonephritis. *Ann Intern Med* 80:342, 1974.

110. Popovic-Ralovic M, Kostic M, Antic-Pew A, et al: Medium and long-term prognosis of patients with acute post-streptococcal glomerulonephritis. *Nephron* 58:393–399, 1991.
111. Chugh K, Sakhuja V: Glomerulonephritis Due to Other Infections. In Massry S, Glassock R (eds): *Textbook of Nephrology* (3rd ed). Baltimore, Williams & Wilkins, 1995, pp 703–709.
112. Bayer AS, Theophilopoulous AN, Eisenberg R, et al: Circulating immune complexes in infective endocarditis. *N Engl J Med* 295:1500, 1976.
113. Morel-Maroger L, Sraer JD, Herreman G, Godeau P: Kidney in subacute endocarditis: Pathological and immunofluorescent findings. *Arch Pathol* 94:205, 1972.
114. Adler SG, Cohen AH: Glomerulonephritis with Bacterial Endocarditis, Ventriculo-vascular Shunts and Visceral Infections. In Schrier RS, Gottschalk CW (eds), *Diseases of the Kidney* (5th ed). Boston, Little, Brown, 1993, pp 1681–1688.
115. Sanchez-Bayle M, Ecija JL, Estepa R, et al: Incidence of glomerulonephritis in congenital syphilis. *Clin Nephrol* 20:27, 1983.
116. Cologlu AS: Immune complex glomerulonephritis in leprosy. *Lepr Rev* 50:213, 1979.
117. Beaufils M, Morel-Maroger L, Sraer JD, et al: Acute renal failure of glomerular origin during visceral abscesses. *N Engl J Med* 295:185, 1976.
118. Chugh KS, Sakhuja V: Glomerular diseases in the tropics (editorial). *Am J Nephrol* 10:437–450, 1990.
119. Shanin B, Popadopanton ZL, Jenis EH: Cogenital nephrotic syndrome associated with congenital toxoplasmosis. *J Pediatr* 85:366, 1974.
120. Pucello LP, Agnello V: Membranoproliferative glomerulonephritis associated with hepatitis B and C viral infections: From virus-like particles in the cryoprecipitate to viral like particles in para-mesangial deposits, problematic investigations prone to artifacts. *Curr Opin Nephrol Hypertens* 3:465–470, 1994.
121. Johnson R, Gretch D, Couser W, et al: Hepatitis virus glomerulonephritis: Effect of γ-interferon therapy. *Kidney Int* 46:1700–1704, 1994.
122. Barsoum RS: Schistosomal glomerulopathies. *Kidney Int* 44:1, 1993.
123. Rao TK, Filipone EJ, Nicastri AD, et al: Associated focal and segmental glomerulosclerosis in the acquired immunodeficiency syndrome. *N Engl J Med* 310:669, 1984.
124. Seney FD, Burns DK, Silva FG: Acquired immunodeficiency syndrome and the kidney. *Am J Kidney Dis* 16:1–3, 1990.
125. Cohen AH, Nast CC: HIV-associated nephropathy: A unique combined glomerular, tubular and interstitial lesion. *Mod Pathol* 1:87, 1988.
126. Filastre J-P, Druet P, Mery J-P: Proteinuric Nephropathies Associated with Drugs and Substances of Abuse. In Cameron JS, Glassock RJ (eds): *The Nephrotic Syndrome*. New York, Marcel Dekker, 1983, pp 697–744.
127. Becker GG, Becker EL, Maher JF, Schreiner GE: Nephrotic syndrome after contact with mercury: A report of five cases, three after use of ammoniated mercury ointment. *Arch Intern Med* 110:178, 1962.
128. Hall C, Fothergill N, Blackwell M, et al: The natural course of gold nephropathy: A long-term study in 21 patients. *Br Med J* 295:745, 1987.
129. Richman AV, Masco HL, Rifkin SI, Acharya MK: Minimal change disease and the nephrotic syndrome associated with lithium therapy. *Ann Intern Med* 92:70, 1980.
130. Lang K: Nephropathy induced by D-penicillamine. *Clin Nephrol* 10L:63, 1978.
131. Prins EJL, Hoorntje SJ, Weening JJ, Donker AJM: Nephrotic syndrome in patients on captopril. *Lancet* 2:306, 1979.
132. Brezin JH, Katz SM, Schwartz AB, Chinitz JL: Reversible renal failure and nephrotic syndrome associated with non-steroidal anti-inflammatory drugs. *N Engl J Med* 301:1271, 1979.
133. Cunningham EE, Brentjens JR, Zielezny MA, et al: Heroin nephropathy: A clinicopathologic and epidemiologic study. *Am J Med* 68:47, 1980.
134. Katz A, Lindheimer D: Kidney Disease and Hypertension in Pregnancy. In Massry S, Glassock R (eds): *Textbook of Nephrology* (3rd ed). Baltimore, Williams & Wilkins, 1995, pp 1148–1168.
135. Paller M, Ferris T: The Kidney and Hypertension in Pregnancy. In Brenner B (ed): *The Kidney* (5th ed). Philadelphia, Saunders, 1995, pp 1731–1763.
136. Kawaguchi K, Koike M: Glomerular lesions associated with liver cirrhosis: An immunohistochemical and clinicopathologic analysis. *Hum Pathol* 17:1137, 1986.

137. Callard P, Feldmann G, Prandi D, et al: Immune complex type of glomerulonephritis in cirrhosis of the liver. *Am J Pathol* 80:329, 1975.
138. Strife CF, Hug G, Chuck G, et al: Membranoproliferative glomerulonephritis and alpha$_1$-antitrypsin deficiency in children. *Pediatrics* 71:88, 1983.
139. Spear GS: The glomerulus in cyanotic congenital heart disease and primary pulmonary hypertension: A review. *Nephron* 1:238, 1964.
140. Eagen JW, Lewis EJ: Glomerulopathies of neoplasia. *Kidney Int* 11:297, 1977.
141. Cotran RS, Alpers CE: Neoplasia and glomerular injury. *Kidney Int* 30:465, 1986.
142. Dabbs D, Striker LM-M, Mignon F, Striker G: Glomerular lesions in lymphoma and leukemia. *Am J Med* 80:63, 1986.
143. Brueggemeyer CD, Ramirez G: Membranous nephropathy: A concern for malignancy. *Am J Kidney Dis* 9:23, 1987.
144. Rault R, Holley JL, Banner BF, El-Shahawy M: Glomerulonephritis and non-Hodgkin's lymphoma: A report of two cases and review of the literature. *Am J Kidney Dis* 20:84–89, 1992.
145. Delmez JA, Safdar SH, Kissane JM: The successful treatment of recurrent nephrotic syndrome with the MOPP regimen in a patient with a remote history of Hodgkin's disease. *Am J Kidney Dis* 23:743–746, 1994.
146. Korzets Z, Golan E, Manor Y, et al: Spontaneously remitting minimal change nephropathy preceding a relapse of Hodgkin's disease by 19 months. *Clin Nephrol* 38:125–127, 1992.
147. Hill GS, Morel-Maroger L, Mery JP, et al: Renal lesions in multiple myeloma: Their relationship to associated protein abnormalities. *Am J Kidney Dis* 2:423, 1983.
148. Morel-Maroger L, Basch A, Danon F, et al: Pathology of the kidney in Waldenstrom's macroglobulinemia. *N Engl J Med* 283:123, 1970.
149. Cordonnier D, Vialfel P, Renversy J, et al: Renal disease in 18 patients with mixed type II IgM-IgG cryoglobulinemia: Monoclonal lymphoid infiltration (2 cases) and membranoproliferative glomerulonephritis (14 cases). *Adv Nephrol* 12:177, 1983.
150. Gertz AG, Kuyle RA: Primary systemic amyloidosis: A diagnostic primer. *Mayo Clin Proc* 64:1505, 1989.
151. Cohen AS: Amyloidosis (review). *N Engl J Med* 277:522, 574, 628, 1967.
152. Gertz MA, Kyle RA, Greipo PR: Response rates and survival in primary systemic amyloidosis. *Blood* 77:257, 1991.
153. Cohen AS, Rubinow A, Anderson JJ, et al: Survival of patients with primary (AL) amyloidosis: Colchicine-treated cases from 1976 to 1983 compared with cases in previous years (1961 to 1973). *Am J Med* 82:1182, 1987.
154. Zemer D, Pras M, Sohar E, et al: Colchicine in the prevention and treatment of the amyloidosis of familial Mediterranean fever. *N Engl J Med* 314:1011, 1986.
155. Appel G, D'Agati V: Lupus Nephritis. In Massry S, Glassock R (eds): *Textbook of Nephrology* (3rd ed). Baltimore, Williams & Wilkins, 1995, pp 787–796.
156. Cameron JS: Lupus nephritis in children. *Adv Nephrol* 22:59–117, 1993.
157. Balow J: Lupus nephritis (NIH conference). *Ann Intern Med* 106:79, 1987.
158. Raz E, Brezis M, Rosenmann E, et al: Anti-DNA antibodies bind directly to renal antigens and induce kidney dysfunction in the isolated perfused rat kidney. *J Immunol* 142:3076, 1989.
159. Termaat RM, Assmann KJM, Dijkman HBPM, et al: Anti-DNA antibodies can bind to the glomerulus via two distinct mechanisms. *Kidney Int* 43:1363–1371, 1992.
160. D'Cruz DP, Houssiau FA, Ramirez G, et al: Antibodies to endothelial cells in systemic lupus erythematosus: A potential marker for nephritis and vasculitis. *Clin Exp Immunol* 85:254, 1991.
161. Howard PF, Hochberg MC, Bias WB, et al: Relationship between C4 null genes, HLA-D region antigens, and genetic susceptibility to systemic lupus erythematosus in Caucasian and black Americans. *Am J Med* 91:187, 1986.
162. Appel BG, Silva FG, Pirani CL, et al: Renal involvement in systemic lupus erythematosus (SLE): A study of 56 patients emphasizing histologic classification. *Medicine* (Baltimore) 57:371, 1978.
163. Churg J, Bernstein J, Glassock RJ: *Renal Disease: Classification and Atlas of Glomerular Disease* (2nd ed). New York, Igashu-Shoin, 1995, pp 151–155.

164. Banfi G, Bertani T, Boeri V, et al: Renal vascular lesions as a marker of poor prognosis in patients with lupus nephritis. *Am J Kidney Dis* 18:240, 1991.
165. Schwartz MM, Fennell JS, Lewis EJ: Pathologic changes in the renal tubule in systemic lupus erythematosus. *Hum Pathol* 13:534, 1982.
166. Gyorkey F, Min KW, Sincovics JG, et al: Systemic lupus erythematosus and myxovirus. *N Engl J Med* 280:333, 1969.
167. Niaudet P, Berterottiere D, Lacoste M, et al: Evolution des lesions renales du lupus erythemateux dissemine. *Ann Pediatr* (Paris) 38:427, 1991.
168. Austin HA III, Mueng LR, Joyce KM, et al: Prognostic factors in lupus nephritis: Contribution of renal histologic data. *Am J Med* 75:382, 1983.
169. Schwartz MM, Lan S-P, Bernstein J, et al: Irreproducibility of the activity and chronicity indices; their utility in the management of severe lupus glomerulonephritis. *Am J Kid Dis* 21:374–379, 1993.
170. Austin H, Boumpas D, Vaughan E, Balow J: Predicting renal outcomes in severe lupus nephritis contributions of clinical and histologic data. *Kidney Int* 45:544–550, 1994.
171. Esdaile JM, Levinton C, Federgreen W, et al: The clinical and renal biopsy predictors of long-term outcome in lupus nephritis: A study of 87 patients and review of the literature. *Q J Med* 72:779, 1989.
172. Fries JF, Porta J, Liang MH: Marginal benefit of renal biopsy in system lupus erythematosus. *Arch Intern Med* 138:1386, 1978.
173. Reichlin M: Diagnosis, Criteria and Serology. In Schur P (ed): *Clinical Management of Systemic Lupus Erythematosus*. New York, Grune & Stratton, 1983, Chap. 5.
174. Tan EM, Cohen AS, Fries JF, et al: The 1982 revised criteria for the classification of systemic lupus erythematosus. *Arthritis Rheum* 25:1271, 1982.
175. Maddison PJ, Provost TT, Reichlin M: Serological findings in patients with "ANA-negative" systemic lupus erythematosus. *Medicine* (Baltimore) 60:87, 1981.
176. Emlen W, Pisetsky D, Taylor R: Antibodies to DNA: A perspective. *Arthritis Rheum* 29:1417, 1986.
177. Balow JE: Clinicopathologic correlation in lupus nephritis. *Ann Intern Med* 91:587, 1979.
178. Hill GS, Hinglais N, Iron F, Vach JF: Systemic lupus erythematosus: Morphologic correlations and clinical data at the time of biopsy. *Am J Med* 64:61, 1978.
179. Garin EH, Donnelly WH, Shulman ST, et al: The significance of serial measurements of serum complement C3 and C4 components and DNA binding capacity in patients with lupus nephritis. *Clin Nephrol* 12:148, 1979.
180. Williams PG, Peters DK, Fallows J, et al: Studies of serum complement in the hypocomplementemic nephritides. *Clin Exp Immunol* 18:391, 1974.
181. Valentijn R, van Overhagen H, Hazevoet HM, et al: The value of complement and immune complex determinations in monitoring disease activity in patients with systemic lupus erythematosus. *Arthritis Rheum* 28:904, 1985.
182. Laitman RS, Glicklich D, Dablay L, et al: Effect of long-term normalization of serum complement levels on the course of lupus nephritis. *Am J Med* 87:132, 1989.
183. Carrie B, Golbety H, Michaels A, Myers B: Creatinine: An inadequate filtration marker in glomerular disease. *Am J Med* 69:177–183, 1980.
184. Roubenoff D, Draw H, Mayer M, et al: Oral cimetidine improves the accuracy and precision of creatinine clearance in lupus nephritis. *Ann Intern Med* 113:501–504, 1990.
185. Chagnac A, Kiberd B, Farinas C, et al: Outcome of the acute glomerular injury in lupus nephritis. *J Clin Invest* 84:922, 1989.
186. Albert DA, Hadler NM, Ropes MW: Does corticosteroid therapy affect the survival of patients with systemic lupus erythematosus? *Arthritis Rheum* 22:945, 1979.
187. Donadio JV, Glassock RJ: Immunosuppressive drug therapy in lupus nephritis. *Am J Kidney Dis* 21:239, 1993.
188. Cathcart E, Idelson BA, Scheinberg MA, Couser WG: Beneficial effects of methylprednisolone "pulse" therapy in diffuse proliferative lupus nephritis. *Lancet* 1:163, 1976.
189. Kimberly RP, Lockshin MD, Sherman RL, et al: High dose intravenous methylprednisolone pulse therapy in systemic lupus erythematosus. *Am J Med* 70:817, 1981.

190. Donadio JV, Holley KE, Ferguson RH, Ilstrup DM: Treatment of lupus nephritis with prednisone and comined prednisone and cyclophosphamide. *N Engl J Med* 299:1151, 1978.

191. Steinberg AD, Steinberg SC: Long-term preservation of renal function in patients with lupus nephritis receiving treatment that includes cyclophosphamide versus those treated with prednisone only. *Arthritis Rheum* 34:945, 1991.

192. Boumpas DT, Austin HA III, Vaughn EM, et al: Controlled trial of pulse methylprednisolone versus two regimens of pulse cyclophosphamide in severe lupus nephritis. *Lancet* 340:741–745, 1992.

193. Ponticelli C, Zucchelli P, Banfi G, et al: Treatment of diffuse proliferative lupus nephritis by intravenous high dose methylprednisolone. *Q J Med* 201:16, 1982.

194. Miescher PA, Miescher A: Combined Cyclosporine-Steroid Treatment of Systemic Lupus Erythematosus. In Schindler R (ed): *Cyclosporin in Autoimmune Diseases*. Berlin, Springer-Verlag, 1985, p 334.

195. Nanra RS, Kincaid-Smith P: Lupus Nephritis: Clinical Course in Relation to Treatment. In Kincaid-Smith P, Mathew TH, Becker EL (eds): *Glomerulonephritis: Morphology, Natural History, and Treatment*, Part II. New York, Wiley, 1973, p 1193.

196. Radhakrishnan J, Kunis CL, D'Agati V, et al: Cyclosporine treatment of lupus membranous nephropathy. *Clin Nephrol* 42:147, 1994.

197. Coplon NN, Deskin CJ, Petersen J, et al: The long-term clinical course of systemic lupus erythematosus in end-stage renal disease. *N Engl J Med* 308:186, 1983.

198. Cattran DC, Aprile M: Renal transplantation in lupus erythematosus. *Ann Intern Med* 114:991, 1991.

199. Sharp GC, Irvin WG, Tan EM, et al: Mixed connective tissue disease: An apparently distinct rheumatic disease syndrome associated with a specific antibody to an extractable nuclear antigen (ENA). *Am J Med* 52:148, 1972.

200. Bourke BE, Woodrow DF, Scott JT: Proteinuria in rheumatoid arthritis: Drug induced or amyloid? *Ann Rheum Dis* 40:240, 1981.

201. Higuchi A, Suzuki Y, Okada T: Membranous glomerulonephritis in rheumatoid arthritis unassociated with gold or penicillamine treatment. *Ann Rheum Dis* 46:488, 1987.

202. Kuznetsky KA, Schwartz MM, Lohmann LA, Lewis EJ: Necrotizing glomerulonephritis in rheumatoid arthritis. *Clin Nephrol* 26:257, 1986.

203. Haycock GB: Henoch-Schönlein purpura. In Massry S, Glassock R (eds): *Textbook of Nephrology* (3rd ed). Baltimore, Williams & Wilkins, 1995, pp 814–817.

204. Allen DM, Diamond LK, Howell PA: Anaphylactoid purpura in children (Schönlein-Henoch syndrome). *Am J Dis Child* 99:147, 1960.

205. Smila S, Kouvalainen K, Lanning M: Serum immunoglobulin levels in the course of anaphylactoid purpura in children. *Acta Paediatr Scand* 66:537, 1977.

206. Cream JH, Gumpel JM, Peachey RDG: Schönlein-Henoch purpura in the adult: A study of 77 adults with anaphylactoid or Schönlein-Henoch purpura. *Q J Med* 39:461, 1970.

207. Goldstein AR, White RHR, Akuse R, Chantler C: Long-term follow-up of childhood Henoch-Schönlein nephritis. *Lancet* 339:280, 1992.

208. Cameron JS: Vasculitis. In Massry S, Glassock R (eds): *Textbook of Nephrology* (3rd ed). Baltimore, Williams & Wilkins, 1995, pp 802–813.

209. Savage CO, Winearls C, Evans D, et al: Microscopic polyarteritis: Presentation, pathology and prognosis. *Q J Med* 56:467, 1985.

210. Falk RJ, Jennette JC: Anti-neutrophil cytoplasmic autoantibodies with specificity for myeloperoxidase in patients with systemic vasculitis and idiopathic necrotizing and crescentic glomerulonephritis. *N Engl J Med* 318:1651, 1988.

211. Van der Woude FJ, Rasmussen N, Lobatto S: Autoantibodies against neutrophils and monocytes: Tool for diagnosis and marker of disease activity in Wegener's granulomatosis. *Lancet* 1:425, 1985.

212. Droz D, Noel LH, Leibowitch M, Barbanel C: Glomerulonephritis and necrotizing angiitis. *Adv Nephrol* 8:343–363, 1979.

213. Balow JE: Renal vasculitis [clinical conference]. *Kidney Int* 27:954–964, 1985.

214. Davson J, Ball J, Platt R: The kidney in periarteritis nodosa. *Q J Med* 17:175, 1948.

215. Dornfeld I, Lecky JW, Peter JB: Polyarteritis and intrarenal renal artery aneurysms. *JAMA* 215:1950, 1971.
216. Savage COS, Pottinger BE, Gaskin G, et al: Vascular damage in Wegener's granulomatosis and microscopic polyarteritis: Presence of anti-endothelial cell antibodies and their relation to anti-neutrophil cytoplasm antibodies. *Clin Exp Immunol* 85:14, 1991.
217. Bini P, Gabay JE, Teitel A, et al: Antineutrophil cytoplasmic auto-antibodies in Wegener's granulomatosis recognize conformational epitopes on proteinase 3. *J Immunol* 149:1409, 1992.
218. Glassock R: Goodpasture's Disease. In Massry S, Glassock R (eds): *Textbook of Nephrology* (3rd ed). Baltimore, Williams & Wilkins, 1995, pp 818–822.
219. Butkowski RJ, Langewild JPM, Wieslander J, et al: Localization of the Goodpasture syndrome to a novel chain of basement membrane collagen. *J Biol Chem* 262:7874, 1977.
220. Lechleitner P, Defregger M, Lhotta K, et al: Goodpasture's syndrome: Unusual presentation after exposure to hard metal dust. *Chest* 203:956, 1993.
221. Lockwood CM, Boulton-Jones JM, Lowenthal RM, et al: Recovery from Goodpasture's syndrome after immunosuppressive treatment and plasmapheresis. *Br Med J* 2:252–254, 1975.
222. Lockwood CM, Pussell B, Wilson CB, Peters DK: Plasma exchange in nephritis. *Adv Nephrol* 8:383, 1979.
223. Bergrem H, Jervell J, Brodwall EK, et al: Goodpasture's syndrome: A report of seven patients including long-term follow-up of three who received a kidney transplant. *Am J Med* 68:54, 1980.
224. Ramos EL, Tisher CC: Recurrent diseases in the kidney transplant. *Am J Kidney Dis* 24:142–154, 1994.
225. Cameron JS: Recurrent renal disease after renal transplantation. *Curr Sci* 3:602–607, 1994.
226. McKay D, Milford E, Sayegh M: Clinical Aspects of Renal Transplantation. In Brenner B (ed): *The Kidney* (5th ed). Philadelphia, Saunders, 1995, pp 2602–2652.
227. Ritz E, Fliser D, Siebels M. Diabetic Nephropathy. In Massry S, Glassock R (eds): *Textbook of Nephrology* (3rd ed). Baltimore, Williams & Wilkins, 1995, pp 894–911.
228. Watkins PJ, Blamey JD, Brewer DB, et al: The natural history of diabetic renal disease. *Q J Med* 41:437, 1972.
229. Ortola FV, Ballermann BJ, Anderson S, et al: Elevated plasma atrial natriuretic peptide levels in diabetic rats: Potential mechanisms of hyperfiltration. *J Clin Invest* 80:670, 1987.
230. Morgensen CE: Microalbuminuria predicts clinical proteinuria and early mortality in maturity-onset diabetes. *N Engl J Med* 310:356, 1984.
231. Suzuki S, Maruyama Y, Nakamura T, et al: Nodular glomerulosclerosis of unknown origin associated with the nephrotic syndrome. *Nephron* 66:462–469, 1994.
232. The Diabetes Control and Complication Trial Research Group: The effect of intensive treatment of diabetes on the development and progression of long-term complications in insulin-dependent diabetes mellitus. *N Engl J Med* 329:977, 1993.
233. Lewis EJ, Hunsicker LG, Bain RP, et al: The effect of angiotensin converting enzyme inhibition on diabetic nephropathy. *N Engl J Med* 329:1456, 1993.
234. Brichard SM, Santoni JP, Thomas JR, et al: Long-term reduction of microalbuminuria after 2 years of angiotensin converting enzyme inhibition by perindopril in hypertensive insulin-treated diabetic patients. *Diabetes Metab* 16:30, 1989.
235. Kashtan C: Alport Syndrome. In Massry S, Glassock R (eds): *Textbook of Nephrology* (3rd ed). Baltimore, Williams & Wilkins, 1995, pp 869–872.
236. Chugh KS, Sakhuja V, Agarwal, A, et al: Hereditary nephritis (Alport's syndrome): Clinical profile and inheritance in 28 kindreds. *Nephrol Dial Transplant* 8:690–695, 1993.
237. Trygvasson K, Zhou J, Hostikka SL: Shows TB: Molecular genetics of Alport syndrome. *Kidney Int* 43:38, 1993.
238. Grunfeld J-P: The clinical spectrum of hereditary nephritis. *Kidney Int* 27:83, 1985.
239. Zollinger HU, Mihatsch MJ: *Renal Pathology in Biopsy: Light Electron and Immunofluorescent Microscopy and Clinical Aspects.* Berlin, Springer-Verlag, 1978, p 466.
240. McCoy RC, Johnson HK, Stone WJ, Wilson CB: Absence of nephritogenic GBM antigen(s) in some patients with hereditary nephritis. *Kidney Int* 21:642, 1982.
241. Desnick RJ, Astrin KH, Bishop DF: Fabry disease: Molecular genetics of the inherited nephropathy. *Adv Nephrol* 18:113–128, 1989.

242. Barratt TM: Congenital Nephrotic Syndrome. In Cameron S, Davison J, Grunfeld JP, Ritz E (eds): *Oxford Textbook of Clinical Nephrology*. London, Oxford Medical Publishers, 1992, pp 2218–2220.

243. Hoyer JR, Michael AF, Vernier RL, Sisson S: Renal disease in nail patella syndrome: Clinical and morphologic studies. *Kidney Int* 2:231, 1972.

244. Buckalew VM Jr: Sickle Cell Nephropathy. In Robinson RR (ed): *Nephrology*. New York, Springer-Verlag, 1984, p 916.

245. Falk R, Jennette JC: Sickle cell nephropathy. *Adv Nephrol Necker Hosp* 23:133–146, 1994.

246. Mahan JD, Mauer SM, Sibley RK: Cogenital nephrotic syndrome: Evolution of medical management and results of renal transplantation. *J Pediatr* 105:549, 1984.

247. Gjone E: Familial lecithin-cholesterol acyltransferase deficiency: A new metabolic disease with renal involvement. *Adv Nephrol* 10:167, 1981.

Index

Numbers followed by the letter *f* indicate figures; numbers followed by the letter *t* indicate tables.